ENCYCLOPEDIA OF
BIOETHICS

3RD EDITION

EDITORIAL BOARD

ENCYCLOPEDIA OF
BIOETHICS

3RD EDITION

EDITED BY

STEPHEN G. POST

VOLUME

2

D – H

MACMILLAN
REFERENCE
USA™

THOMSON
GALE

New York • Detroit • San Diego • San Francisco • Cleveland • New Haven, Conn. • Waterville, Maine • London • Munich

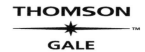

Encyclopedia of Bioethics, 3rd edition

Stephen G. Post
Editor in Chief

While every effort has been made to
ensure the reliability of the information
presented in this publication, The Gale Group,
Inc. does not guarantee the accuracy of
the data contained herein. The Gale Group,
Inc. accepts no payment for listing; and
inclusion in the publication of any
organization, agency, institution, publication,
service, or individual does not imply
endorsement of the editors or publisher.
Errors brought to the attention of the
publisher and verified to the satisfaction of
the publisher will be corrected in future
editions.

Library of Congress Cataloging-in-Publication Data

Encyclopedia of bioethics / Stephen G. Post, editor in chief.— 3rd ed.
   p. cm.
Includes bibliographical references and index.
   ISBN 0-02-865774-8 (set : hardcover : alk. paper) — ISBN
0-02-865775-6 (vol. 1) — ISBN 0-02-865776-4 (vol. 2) — ISBN
0-02-865777-2 (vol. 3) — ISBN 0-02-865778-0 (vol. 4) — ISBN
0-02-865779-9 (vol. 5)
   1. Bioethics—Encyclopedias. 2. Medical ethics—Encyclopedias. I.
Post, Stephen Garrard, 1951-
QH332.E52 2003
174'.957'03—dc22

                                                            2003015694

This title is also available as an e-book.
ISBN 0-02-865916-3 (set)
Contact your Gale sales representative for ordering information.

Printed in the United States of America
10 9 8 7 6 5 4 3 2 1

Front cover photos (from left to right): Custom Medical Stock;
Photo Researchers; Photodisc; Photodisc; AP/Worldwide Photos.

D

DAOISM, BIOETHICS IN

• • •

Daoism is an ancient and multifaceted element of traditional Chinese culture. Its origins and scope are debated by modern scholars, Chinese and Western alike. Most understand "Daoism" in terms of the naturalistic thought seen in ancient texts like those of Lao-tzu (the *Dao te ching*) and Chuang-tzu (see Lau, 1982; Graham, 1981). But to others, "Daoism" denotes primarily a religious tradition that emerged around the second century C.E. and has endured to the present (Seidel, 1990; Robinet, 1991, 1993). Specialists today generally employ a comprehensive approach, interpreting both of those elements as aspects of a broad and inclusive cultural tradition, interwoven both historically and thematically (Schipper).

Daoism may be characterized as a holistic worldview and ethos, including a variety of interrelated moral and religious values and practices. Daoism lacks any coherent conceptual structure, so there have never been any "Daoist positions" regarding ethics or any other issues. Yet, most segments of the tradition share certain assumptions and concerns. One is an assumption that human reality is ultimately grounded in deeper realities; humans are components of a cosmos, a harmonious universe in which all things are subtly but profoundly interrelated (Kirkland, 1993). Daoism is devoted to the pursuit of greater integration with the cosmos, in social as well as individual terms. Daoists vary widely in their understandings of how that integration is best expressed and pursued.

The first section of this entry outlines the elements of classical "Lao-Chuang" Daoism, and the history, teachings, and practices of the much-misunderstood "Daoist religion."

The subsequent exploration of the Daoist moral life focuses upon (1) the ideals of refinement (*lien*) and "fostering life"; (2) the ideals of balance and harmony; and (3) the issue of death. Throughout, one should bear clearly in mind that many issues that are considered central in contemporary bioethical debate are completely alien to the traditional Daoist worldview. Daoists not only lacked the concepts of "good" and "evil," but they were simply never interested in arguments over "right or wrong" on any terms. One should thus beware assuming that contemporary issues could ever be translatable into Daoist terms.

The Daoist Heritage

CLASSICAL THEMES. In the ancient texts *Lao-tzu* and *Chuang-tzu,* integration with the cosmos is generally expressed in terms of returning to the natural rhythm or flow of life—to the Dao, an impersonal reality that constitutes simultaneously the source of the cosmos, the subtle structures of the cosmos in its pristine state, and the salutary natural forces that—in that pristine state—maintain all things in a natural and healthy alignment. In "Lao-Chuang" Daoism, all the world's problems are attributed to humanity's digression from the Dao, particularly to a loss of proper perspective upon the nature of reality. The goal of Lao-Chuang Daoism is to regain that perspective and thereby return to the original integration with the natural world and its constituent forces and processes. The eponymous Lao-Chuang texts are vague about the means to be employed in achieving that end. Later Lao-Chuang writings (e.g., in texts like the *Kuan-tzu* and *Huai-nan-tzu*) present a more detailed analysis of the human constitution, and suggest specific spiritual and physiological practices to reintegrate the individual and realign him or her with the natural forces of the cosmos (Roth). Suffice it to note that all such theory assumes none of the dichotomies of mind/matter or body/spirit that underlie much of Western medicine and moral theory. Moreover, it is a mistake to assume (as do most in twentieth-century Asia and the West) that Daoism was essentially individualistic: the basic Lao-Chuang writings (most notably the *Dao te ching*) often addressed broader problems of human society in both moral and political terms. The later Daoist tradition is generally an extension of the ideals and values seen in these earlier writings.

THE DAOIST RELIGIOUS TRADITION: NEW PERSPECTIVES.
Until recently, virtually all educated people dismissed postclassical Daoism (often misnamed "popular Daoism") as a mass of disreputable superstitions created and perpetuated by the ignorant masses. Such was certainly not the case. The problem is that before the 1970s, few intellectuals, Chinese or Western, had any firsthand knowledge of later Daoism, in terms of either its modern practice or its historical tradition. As scholars began serious analysis of the Daoist texts preserved in the massive collection known as the *Dao-tsang*, and researched the roles that Daoism played in traditional Chinese history and society, they started to develop a far different perspective, though this new perspective has yet to reach the educated public.

Until the 1980s, religious Daoism was often said to have been focused on individual practices intended to confer longevity and/or physical immortality. The pursuit of physical longevity did exist in China from early times, but it is wrong to associate such pursuits with "religious Daoism."

Western scholars generally have placed emphasis on certain practices or crafts that they suppose have been particularly "Daoist," notably the quest for physical immortality, breath control, techniques of sexual union, herbalism, dietetics, and alchemy. In such a view, though, as in the question of doctrine in general, there is some ambiguity between what is specifically Daoist and what is simply Chinese (Strickman, pp. 1044–1045).

Extensive research has generally demonstrated that such practices have little or no intrinsic connection to the traditions of religious Daoism.

THE EVOLUTION OF THE DAOIST RELIGION.
The Daoist religion has been compared to a river formed by the confluence of many streams. Its origins lie in the Han dynasty (206 B.C.E.–221 C.E.). During that period, Chinese intellectuals (like the Confucian theorist Tung Chung-shu) were seeking a comprehensive explanation for worldly events. From such roots, imperial advisers called *fang-shih* produced a series of sacred texts that culminated in the *T'ai-p'ing ching,* which is generally regarded as the first Daoist scripture. According to the *T'ai-p'ing ching,* ancient rulers had maintained an "ambience of Grand Tranquillity" (*t'ai-p'ing*) by observing *wu-wei* (nonaction)—a behavioral ideal of avoiding purposive action and trusting instead to the world's natural order (the Dao). When later rulers meddled with the world, the "Grand Tranquillity" was disrupted. Now, the scripture says, one must return to the Dao by looking within oneself. The text provides specific directions for pursuing union with the Dao, including moral injunctions and instructions for meditation, as well as recommendations for enhancing one's health and longevity through hygienic practices (such as breath control), medicine, acupuncture, and even music therapy. The focus of the *T'ai-p'ing ching* is thus upon providing the people with practical advice for reintegrating with the natural order (Kaltenmark).

In late Han times, the *T'ai-p'ing ching* helped inspire several social movements. One was led by Chang Dao-ling, who claimed to have received a divine mandate to replace the now-effete Han government with a new social order. Claiming the mantle of "Celestial Master," Chang and his heirs oversaw a religious organization in which male and female priests healed the sick by performing expiatory rituals. This organization, generally called "Celestial Master Daoism," was based on the idea that a healthy society depended upon the moral, physical, and spiritual health of all its members.

In the fourth century C.E., northern China was invaded by peoples from the northern steppes, and the leaders of the Celestial Master movement fled south. There they found a rich indigenous religious culture centered upon the pursuit of personal perfection through ritual activity. Unlike the Celestial Master tradition, the religion of southern China took little interest in ideals of a healthy society: its focus was almost exclusively upon the individual. Modern writers, Chinese and Western, have often mistakenly cited certain of its texts (like the *Pao-p'u-tzu* of the maverick Confucian Ko Hung) as representative of religious Daoism. In so doing, they have completely neglected the rich heritage of the *T'ai-p'ing ching* and most of the subsequent Daoist tradition.

The fourth century C.E. was a period of rich interaction among such diverse traditions, and there were two new developments, both of which occurred as the result of revelations from celestial beings. The first, known as the Shang-ch'ing (Supreme Purity) revelation, was received from angelic beings called "Perfected Ones" who dwelt in distant heavens of that name. The Perfected Ones revealed methods by which the diligent practitioner could ascend to their heavens, particularly visualizational meditation (Robinet,

1993). But Shang-ch'ing Daoism also subsumed the older southern pursuit of personal perfection through alchemy, a transformative spiritual process expressed in chemical terms. Alchemy, often misrepresented as a "typical" element of religious Daoism, actually arose quite independently, though it was embraced by certain Shang-ch'ing Daoists as a practice thought to elevate the aspirant's spiritual state for eventual ascent to the heavens (Strickmann). What the alchemical tradition shared with Daoism was a vital concern with self-perfection based on an assumption that the individual's being is a unified whole. For exceptional aspirants, alchemy provided secret knowledge that permitted control of the forces of the cosmos that inhere within the constitution of the individual. Outsiders often misunderstood the whole undertaking as a pursuit of physical longevity. But within Daoism, alchemy was actually a method of moral and spiritual self-refinement: through proper knowledge and action, one could pare away the grosser elements of one's being and eventually ascend to a higher plane of existence. Nonetheless, alchemy was, for most, a purely theoretical interest. The "average" Daoist practiced meditation and morality, and in later ages Daoists discarded the theory of "external alchemy" in favor of "inner alchemy"—a meditative pursuit of reunion with the Dao that employed the language of alchemy metaphorically.

The Shang-ch'ing revelations were immediately followed by a quite different set of revelations, known by the term *Ling-pao* (Numinous Treasure). *Ling-pao* Daoism is distinguished by (1) elements influenced by Mahayana Buddhism, and (2) a renewed concern with the human community. *Ling-pao* scriptures (such as the *Tu-jen ching*, "Scripture for Human Salvation") tell of a great cosmic deity—a personification of the Dao—who is concerned to save humanity. By ritual recitation of the scripture, one may participate in its salvific power. In the fifth century, the *Ling-pao* tradition was refocused by Lu Hsiu-ching, who reconfigured its ritual activities and formulated a new set of liturgies that continue to influence contemporary Daoist practice. A central liturgy is the *chiao,* a lengthy series of rituals that renew the local community by reintegrating it with the heavenly order. Other liturgies, called *chai,* had diverse aims. One was designed to prevent disease by expiating moral transgressions through communal confession. Another labored for the salvation of deceased ancestors. A third was intended to forestall natural disasters and reintegrate the sociopolitical order with the cosmos. Through these liturgies, Daoism incorporated ritual frameworks from all segments of society, from the imperial court to the local village, and unified them through the activity of priests (*Dao-shih*), some of whom were women (Kirkland, 1991a).

"Liturgical Daoism" soon became central to life at all levels of Chinese society. Admiring emperors sought to bolster their legitimacy by associating with Daoist masters, and by having them perform liturgies for the sake of state and society. During the T'ang dynasty (618–906 C.E.), cultural leaders in every field associated with such masters, and were deeply influenced by Daoist religious, artistic, and literary traditions. Prominent Daoists like Ssu-ma Ch'eng-chen not only maintained the liturgical tradition but also refined the meditative practices that had always been central to the Daoist spiritual life (Engelhardt, 1987). In addition, certain Daoists became known for their achievements as physicians. The social prominence of liturgical Daoism changed drastically during the twelfth and thirteenth centuries C.E., when China was again invaded by northern peoples. The foreign rulers often suspected religious organizations of fostering rebellious activities, so Chinese who sought social or political advancement began to dissociate themselves from such organizations. Hence, in late imperial China, liturgical Daoism became divorced from the elite segments of society, and endured primarily among the less affluent and less educated (Kirkland, 1992). The broadly based, ecumenical Daoist tradition of T'ang times dissipated, to be replaced by new, smaller sects. One of the earliest examples was Ch'ing-wei Daoism: founded by a young woman about 900, it introduced "thunder rites," by which a priest internalized the spiritual power of thunder to gain union with the Dao, then healed illnesses. In T'ien-hsin Daoism, founded by a twelfth-century scholar, priests healed mental illness by drawing spiritual power from stars. The most traditional of the new sects was T'ai-i Daoism, which stressed ritual healing and social responsibility, and was popular with some rulers, including the Mongol Khubilai Khan. None of those sects had much lasting influence. One that did endure was Cheng-i (Orthodox Unity) Daoism, which flourished under imperial patronage from the eleventh to eighteenth centuries and is still practiced in Taiwan. It preserves traditional liturgies, adding rituals for exorcism and personal protection. None of the new sects that arose during the "Daoist reformation" was in any way concerned with the pursuit of immortality. Rather, priests of all those sects ministered to the community by healing and performing other ritual services.

Modern Daoism has maintained the pursuit of individual self-perfection through meditation. Earlier Daoist meditation took a variety of forms. But from the eleventh century on, most Daoist meditation was couched in terms of "inner alchemy." Employing terminology from ancient Lao-Chuang texts, "inner alchemy" aims at self-perfection through cultivating "spirit" (*shen*) and "vital force" (*ch'i*) (Robinet, 1989).

These practices were embraced in Ch'üan-chen (Complete Perfection) Daoism, a monastic movement founded in the twelfth century. Ch'üan-chen institutions flourished into the twentieth century, as did some of its teachings on self-perfection through meditation.

The Ethical Dimensions of Daoism

Many accounts of Daoism lead one to question whether there is—or could be—such a thing as a Daoist ethic, suggesting quite incorrectly that Daoist values were intrinsically egocentric. In fact, all segments of the Daoist tradition fostered a personal ethic, and most segments taught a social ethic as well. At times, in fact, it is clear that Daoism assumed a universalistic ethic that extended not only to all humanity but also to the wider domain of all living things (Kirkland, 1986). These values were not borrowings from Confucianism or Buddhism, but a natural extension of fundamental elements of the Daoist worldview, rooted in the ancient heritage of the *Dao te ching* and the *T'ai-p'ing ching*. That worldview was interwoven with an ethos that encouraged individuals and groups to engage in activities intended to promote the healthy integration of the individual, society, nature, and cosmos.

THE MORAL LIFE: IDEALS OF REFINEMENT AND "FOSTERING LIFE." The Daoist view of personal identity and human values contrasts sharply with that of Confucianism. Confucians understand humans to be innately distinct from and superior to all other forms of life, because of humans' social inclinations and moral consciousness. Daoism, by contrast, locates the value of humanity not in what separates it from the rest of the natural world but in what humans share with the rest of the world. A constant if not universal goal of Daoism is to propel the individual's attention to ever higher and broader perspectives, to move as far as possible not only beyond the isolated concerns of the individual but also beyond the socioculturally defined concerns of the unreflective. The Daoist goal is not to ignore socioculturally defined concerns but to transcend them.

For that reason, despite all its insistence upon restoring harmony with the natural order, Daoism is not consistent with the activist tendencies of modern environmentalism. No Daoist of any persuasion ever embraced goal-directed action as a legitimate agency for solving problems. The *Dao te ching* in fact implies that, contrary to appearances, nature is ultimately more powerful than all human endeavor, and that if humans will refrain from taking any action, however well-intentioned, nature itself will inevitably rectify any problems.

Daoists insist that we must focus our concern upon ourselves, seeking (re)integration with the deeper realities of the cosmos through a process of personal refinement (*lien*). In some of Lao-Chuang Daoism, that process at times appears so rarefied that it involves no more than altered perceptions: one learns to reject conventional "truths" in pursuit of a deeper state of awareness. But most later Daoists understand the process of refinement as a more comprehensive undertaking, involving a transformation or sublimation of one's physical reality as well. Such "biospiritual" ideals are often couched in terms of the imperative of "fostering life" (*yang-sheng*). Some writers have identified *yang-sheng* with physiological practices designed to enhance individual health and prolong physical life. But in the Daoist context, at least, the term connotes much more:

> Indeed, the very idea of life or health, including as it does both physical and spiritual dimensions, evokes an archaic aura of religious meaning—that the fullness of life is supranormal by conventional standards—and symbolically is closely linked with a generalized Daoist notion of the mystic and religious, individual and social, salvational goal of reestablishing harmony with the cosmic life principle of the Dao. (Girardot, p. 1631)

Within the Daoist worldview, *yang-sheng* presupposed a personal ethic of moral and spiritual cultivation (Kirkland, 1991b). That ethic, moreover, assumed a dedication not only to the perfection of the individual self but also to reestablishment of a broader, universal harmony.

The term *yang* means "to foster, nourish, or care for." Thus the *Dao te ching* sometimes presents the Dao in imagery that suggests a loving parent who exerts no control, and oft-overlooked passages encourage altruistic attention to the needs and interests of others (Kirkland, 1986). In that context, *yang-sheng* can be interpreted as selfless concern with fostering others' lives as well as one's own.

In fact, rather than being promoted by a Confucian sense of social service, hospitals, orphan care, and community quarantine procedures were linked to the activities of the Daoist and Buddhist monasteries during the Six Dynasties period.... The root of this concern for community healthcare would seem to be most strongly influenced by the Buddhist idea of universal compassion (*karuna*), but in Daoism this idea could be interpreted as an aspect of the selfless kindness and concern for human health extended to all persons in the practice of *wu-wei*. (Girardot, p. 1636)

Medieval Daoist literature abounds in stories of exemplary men and women who earned recognition—and, on occasion, the boon of immortality—by secretly performing compassionate acts, particularly for people and animals disdained by others (Kirkland, 1986; Cahill). Such values have sometimes been attributed to Buddhist influence, but they are actually rooted in elements of the ancient Daoist worldview. The Daoist ethos started with the individual, and redirected his or her attention to a broader life context: from body to spirit, from self to community, from humanity to nature. In addition, it presented the would-be Daoist with a moral responsibility to live for a purpose greater than oneself.

Daoist conceptions of history, humanity, and cosmos also undercut some of the paternalistic tendencies so common in other traditions, including Confucianism. Human lives are to mirror the operation of the Dao, which contrasts markedly with Western images of God as creator, father, ruler, or judge. The Dao is not an external authority, nor a being assumed to possess a moral right to control or intervene in the lives of others. Moreover, the *Dao te ching* commends "feminine" behaviors like yielding, as explicitly opposed to "masculine" behaviors of assertion, intervention, or control. There is thus little temptation for a Daoist to "play God," whether in medicine, government, or law.

THE MORAL LIFE: IDEALS OF BALANCE AND HARMONY. While Daoism did not create the ideals of balance and harmony, it embraced them to an extent unequaled by other traditions. A fundamental Daoist assumption, applicable to any facet of life, was that disorder is a result of imbalance, whether physical or spiritual, individual or social. Physical illness was generally understood as an indicator of what might be called a biospiritual imbalance within the individual. In many presentations of Chinese medicine, disease is explained as a result of a misalignment of *ch'i*, the natural life force (which eludes the distinction of "body" from "spirit"). In the minds of the peasantry, such misalignment was often understood as the result of moral misdeeds, and some Daoists who were anxious to involve the common people incorporated such ideas into their writings and practices. But in a broader theoretical context, the imbalances that result in disease might better be attributed to a kind of natural entropy. Ancient Chinese thought assumed that the present state of the world represents a degeneration from an earlier state of universal peace and harmony. The goal of life for Confucians and Daoists alike was to restore that original harmony. Certain Daoists took a profound interest in the problem of restoring the harmony of individuals through treating physical maladies (Girardot). But disease and healing were never understood in purely materialistic terms, and the goal of medicine was never simply the alleviation of physical suffering. Like healers in many traditional cultures,

Daoists of most periods assumed that all physical symptoms remit when one restores the biospiritual integrity of the individual and reestablishes a state of balance and harmony with the deeper realities of life. Consequently, some Daoists worked to restore health through therapeutic ritual activity (Strickmann).

Restoring harmony, however, was never a purely individual matter, for the Daoist any more than for the Confucian. Just as a physical disorder was understood as resulting from a biospiritual imbalance within the individual, so sociopolitical disorder was generally understood as resulting from a biospiritual imbalance on a larger scale. Daoists and Confucians of classical times and the later imperial period felt a responsibility to rectify that imbalance, to play a managerial role in restoring *T'ai-p'ing,* "Grand Tranquillity." *T'ai-p'ing* connoted a well-ordered society, both in universal terms and in terms of the local community. But it was not merely a political concept:

> It was a state in which all the concentric spheres of the organic Chinese universe, which contained nature as well as society, were perfectly attuned, communicated with each other in a balanced rhythm of timeliness, and brought maximum fulfillment to each living being. (Seidel, 1987a, p. 251)

Daoist priests of all periods assumed a special responsibility to tend to the spiritual dimensions of upholding *T'ai-p'ing,* complementing the real and symbolic activities of the emperor and local magistrate. Until Mongol times, that understanding of the role of the Daoist priest was accepted at all levels of society, and emperors frequently relied upon Daoist priests to provide both advice and ritual support in keeping state and society in harmony with the cosmos.

The Daoist concern with balance and harmony extended to participation in religious activities. While the *Dao te ching* had commended "feminine" behavioral models, the early Daoist religious community offered participation to women, apparently on an equal basis with men. Though it is not clear how often women performed the same priestly functions as men, medieval texts describe women's spirituality in terms that make it only subtly distinguishable from that of men (Cahill; Kirkland, 1991a). The marginalization of liturgical Daoism after the twelfth century coincided with a more general diminution of opportunities for women throughout Chinese life, and from then on, few women appear in the Daoist tradition.

Daoist attitudes toward sexuality were quite vague. Daoists never articulated any specific sexual ethic. Aside from Confucian moralists, few Chinese regarded sexuality as morally problematic, and most regarded it as a valuable component of human life. Some Daoists took an interest in reproductive forces as the most readily accessible manifestation of the natural forces of the cosmos. The imagery of "inner alchemy" was sometimes applied to those forces, resulting in biospiritual practices aimed at total sublimation and concomitant personal perfection. Particularly in later centuries, some men and women focused their efforts at self-transformation upon the physical or metaphorical transformation of sexual forces. But once again, it is questionable whether such activities ought to be called specifically "Daoist," for they have little in common with the activities of any of the liturgical Daoist organizations.

DAOIST ATTITUDES TOWARD DEATH. One of the most intensely debated issues in modern discussions of Daoism is that of its attitude(s) toward death. The controversy stems from some interpreters' insistence that religious Daoists struggled to *avert* death, while the earlier Lao-Chuang Daoists had espoused an *acceptance* of death as a natural conclusion to the cycle of life. There is evidence to support that interpretation, but there are also passages in the *Dao te ching* and other Lao-Chuang texts that suggest the possibility of obviating death and the desirability of attaining a deathless state. A natural conclusion would be that "religious Daoism" focused upon those passages, and set about devising practical methods of attaining such a state. But while none can dispute the commonness of texts describing such methods, it is again questionable whether they can be considered representative of "religious Daoism." It should be noted that the most famous proponent of the pursuit of immortality—the fourth-century Ko Hung—actually repudiated the Daoist tradition. On the other hand, the architects of the Daoist liturgical tradition seldom even alluded to immortality as a desirable goal.

Daoists of all periods would be puzzled by the insistence of modern Western medicine that the prevention of human death transcends all other concerns. To Daoists, the reality of one's life extends far beyond the biological activity of one's body, and extending the latter *for its own sake* would hardly seem even desirable. The Daoist goal is always harmony with the deeper dimensions of life, and in those terms a medical model that defines "life" in strictly biological terms seems perverted.

In reality, Daoist attitudes toward death are hardly reducible to any clear, unequivocal proposition. But one may safely affirm that a pursuit of immortality for its own sake—that is, a search for some trick that would obviate the death event—was never a Daoist goal (Kirkland, 1991b). Rather, Daoists consistently pursued a state of spiritual perfection. Frequently, they expressed that state of perfection as a state that was not subject to death. Chinese literature (by no means specifically Daoist) is replete with stories of *hsien*—wondrous male and female beings who live outside the realm of ordinary life and death. Daoist writers sometimes employed such imagery to suggest the final fruits of spiritual development. Some writings suggest that rare individuals underwent a transformation that merely simulated death (Robinet, 1979). But one must beware mistaking metaphor for reality (Bokenkamp). When read carefully, most Daoist writings actually present a "postmortem immortality"; that is, a deathless state can indeed be achieved, but biological death remains a necessity (Strickmann; Seidel, 1987b). Daoist attitudes toward death thus remain a paradox.

Conclusion

Though some Daoist writings do present moral injunctions, Daoism never developed any real ethical code, for such an idea makes little sense in a Daoist context. For instance, since there was no divine Lawgiver, Daoists never developed an ethic conceived as obedience to divine authority. Daoists of various periods did accept the existence of divinities, and some Daoist writings incorporated popular concepts of a heavenly hierarchy that dispenses posthumous rewards and punishments. But acceptance of such beliefs was never considered mandatory, and most Daoist literature lacks such ideas.

Similarly, Daoists lacked the notion that the individual— or even the human species—is an independent locus of moral value. In fact, Lao-Chuang Daoism can easily be read as a concerted effort to disabuse humans of the absurd notions of self-importance that most people tacitly embrace as natural and normal. Hence, the very concept of "rights"— for individuals or groups, humans or animals—makes no sense in Daoist terms.

Daoism might appear to embody a virtue ethic. Indeed, the term te in the title of the *Dao te ching* is generally translated "virtue." But the Daoist perspective is quite distinct from the virtue ethic developed by Confucians like Mencius. Mencius clearly articulated virtues like *jen* (benevolence), and insisted that proper cultivation of such virtues would result in the perfection of individual, family, society, and state. Much of Daoism seems to suggest a similar model, with the substitution of *te* for *jen*. But though Mencius attributed human moral impulses to a natural inheritance from "Heaven," Lao-Chuang Daoists frequently criticized most Confucians as seeking answers to life's issues in terms that were excessively humanistic. Confucians often seem ambivalent concerning the relevance or even the existence of transhuman realities. And it was upon precisely such realities that Daoism centered itself.

To understand the moral dimensions of Daoism, one must understand the "vague and elusive" concept of the Dao—transcendent yet immanent, divine yet inherent in humanity and all of nature. Most important, since the Dao never acts by design, Lao-Chuang Daoists ridicule the notion that good could result from conscious evaluation of possible courses of action. Such deliberate "ethical reflection," they argue, blinds one to the natural course of action, which is the course that one follows when living spontaneously, without the arrogant and destructive imposition of rationality and intentionality. The ethical dimensions of Daoism are thus real but subtle. Since Daoists never embraced normative expressions of any kind, to perceive the ethical dimensions of Daoism, one must peer deeply and carefully into the entire tradition, extrapolating from a plethora of sources from different segments of a highly diverse tradition. In doing so, one forms the impression that to live a proper Daoist life is to live in such a way that one restores and maintains the world's holistic unity. The Daoist life involves dedication to a process of self-refinement, which is considered one's natural contribution to the health and well-being of both nature and society. In a sense, to be a Daoist is to accept personal responsibility for taking part in a universal healing, doing one's part to restore the health and wholeness of the individual, society, nature, and cosmos.

RUSSELL KIRKLAND (1995)

SEE ALSO: *Buddhism, Bioethics in; Compassionate Love; Confucianism, Bioethics in; Death: Eastern Thought; Medical Ethics, History of South and East Asia: China; Population Ethics: Religious Traditions*

BIBLIOGRAPHY

Bokenkamp, Stephen R. 1989. "Death and Ascent in Ling-pao Taoism." *Taoist Resources* 1(2): 1–20.

Cahill, Suzanne. 1990. "Practice Makes Perfect: Paths to Transcendence for Women in Medieval China." *Taoist Resources* 2(2): 23–42.

Engelhardt, Ute. 1987. *Die klassische Tradition der Qi-Übungen: Eine Darstellung anhand des Tangzeitlichen Textes Fuqi jingyi lun von Sima Chengzhen.* Wiesbaden: Franz Steiner.

Girardot, Norman J. 1978. "Taoism." In vol. 4 of *Encyclopedia of Bioethics*, pp. 1631–1638; ed. Warren T. Reich. New York: Macmillan.

Graham, Angus C. 1981. *Chuang-tzu: The Seven Inner Chapters and Other Writings from the Book Chuang-tzu.* London: Allen and Unwin.

Kaltenmark, Max. 1979. "The Ideology of the *T'ai-p'ing ching.*" In *Facets of Taoism*, pp. 19–45, eds. Holmes Welch and Anna Seidel. New Haven, CT: Yale University Press.

Kirkland, Russell. 1986. "The Roots of Altruism in the Taoist Tradition." *Journal of the American Academy of Religion* 54(11): 59–77.

Kirkland, Russell. 1991a. "Huang Ling-wei: A Taoist Priestess in T'ang China." *Journal of Chinese Religions* 19: 47–73.

Kirkland, Russell. 1991b. "The Making of an Immortal: The Exultation of Ho Chih-Chang." *Numen* 38(2): 214–230.

Kirkland, Russell. 1992. "Person and Culture in the Taoist Tradition." *Journal of Chinese Religions* 20: 77–90.

Kirkland, Russell. 1993. "A World in Balance: Holistic Synthesis in the *T'ai-p'ing kuang-chi.*" *Journal of Sung-Yuan Studies* 23: 43–70.

Kohn, Livia, ed. 1993. *The Taoist Experience: An Anthology.* Albany: State University of New York Press.

Lao-tzu. 1982. *Tao te ching,* tr. D. C. Lau. Hong Kong: Chinese University of Hong Kong Press.

Robinet, Isabelle. 1979. "Metamorphosis and Deliverance from the Corpse in Taoism." *History of Religions* 19(1):37–70.

Robinet, Isabelle 1989. "Original Contributions of *Neidan* to Taoism and Chinese Thought." In *Taoist Meditation and Longevity Techniques,* pp. 297–330, ed. Livia Kohn. Ann Arbor: University of Michigan Center for Chinese Studies.

Robinet, Isabelle. 1991. *Histoire du Taoïsme dès origines au XIVe siècle.* Paris: Editions du Cerf.

Robinet, Isabelle. 1993. *Taoist Meditation: The Mao-shan of Great Purity,* tr. Julian Pas and Norman Girardot. Albany: State University of New York Press.

Roth, Harold D. 1991. "Psychology and Self-Cultivation in Early Taoistic Thought." *Harvard Journal of Asiatic Studies* 51(2): 599–650.

Schipper, Kristofer M. 1993. *The Taoist Body,* tr. Karen C. Duval. Berkeley: University of California Press.

Seidel, Anna. 1980. "Taoism, History of." In *New Encyclopaedia Britannica,* Macropedia, vol. 17, pp. 1044–1050. Chicago: Encyclopaedia Britannica.

Seidel, Anna. 1985. "Therapeutische Rituale und das Problem des Bösen im frühen Taoismus." In *Religion und Philosophie in Ostasien,* pp. 185–200, ed. Gert Naundorf, Karl-Heinz Pohl, and Hans-Hermann Schmidt. Würzburg: Königshausen und Neumann.

Seidel, Anna. 1987a. "T'ai-p'ing." In vol. 14 of *Encyclopedia of Religion,* pp. 251–252. New York: Macmillan.

Seidel, Anna. 1987b. "Post-Mortem Immortality; or, The Taoist Resurrection of the Body." In *GILGUL: Essays on Transformation, Revolution and Permanence in the History of Religions,* pp. 223–237, ed. Shaid Shaked, David Shulman, and Gedaliahu G. Strousma. Leiden: E. J. Brill.

Seidel, Anna. 1990. *Taoismus: Die inoffizielle Hochreligion Chinas.* Tokyo: Deutsche Gesellschaft für Natur- und Völkerkunde Ostasiens.

Strickmann, Michel. 1979. "On the Alchemy of T'ao Hung-ching." In *Facets of Taoism,* pp. 123–192, ed. Holmes Welch and Anna Seidel. New Haven, CT: Yale University Press.

DEATH

• • •

I. CULTURAL PERSPECTIVES

What is death? How do we understand its meaning? Since death cannot be directly apprehended by straightforward scientific means, culture provides the key medium for comprehending the final boundary between our existence as living beings and the eventual end of that existence. Death is a fact of life, but awareness of mortality is a social, not a biological reality. Knowledge about death and its meaning and value is socially constructed. How should we account for profound differences across the world and throughout history? In some societies, elders choose to end their own life via exposure to the elements, to avoid being a burden to the wider community—the perhaps apocryphal Eskimo on an ice floe narrative—which provides a powerful image whether supported by the ethnographic evidence or not. Or mothers may withdraw their love and attention from an infant deemed unlikely to survive in an impoverished environment like the slums of northeastern Brazil.

In contemporary U.S. society, through a combination of technical prowess, institutional arrangements, and bioethics-governed procedures and practices, we elect to maintain the liminal—betwixt and between—existence of patients suffering from persistent coma, maintaining their biological lives in specialized ventilatory-care units. Others may decide to have their brains or bodies "cryopreserved" after the moment of physical, cardiopulmonary death, in response to internet advertisements. The native inhabitants of the Amazon, called the Wari, respect their dead, and assuage their grief, by engaging in ritual mortuary cannibalism. How might the profound range of cultural variability in organizing death inform bioethics debates about the morally right management of death and the end of life?

This entry examines the intersection of death, culture, and bioethics, taking the disciplinary perspective of anthropology, the field most associated with the analysis of culture.

The scope is both broad, examining conceptually the ways in which the experience of death is culturally constructed within particular social and historical moments, and narrow, detailing the growing body of knowledge about the influence of an increasingly globalized biomedicine (and "the ethics" of that medicine, bioethics) on the experience of death and dying in multi-cultural societies (Kaufman; Conklin; Scheper-Hughes).

Intersections of Death, Culture and Bioethics

When *cultural* difference is considered, we generally think of differences among people from varied ethnic backgrounds in a diverse society, or of clashes emerging in the face of immigration or forced migration of populations. In homogenous societies, for example, when healers', patients', and broad social expectations about death are concordant, cultural difference may be transparent and cultural conflicts rare. In diverse societies, ethnic and cultural background influences all aspects of healthcare, nowhere more profoundly than when death is near. Even patients and families who appear well integrated into a diverse society such as the United States may draw heavily on the resources of cultural background (particularly spirituality) when experiencing and responding to death. When cultural gaps between families and healthcare providers are profound, accentuated by language barriers and varied experience shaped by social class, negotiating the difficult transitions on the path from life to death, always a daunting challenge, becomes even more difficult.

We argue that all domains of end-of-life care are shaped by culture, including:

the meaning ascribed to illness;

the actual language used to discuss sickness and death (including whether death may be openly acknowledged);

the symbolic value placed on an individual's life (and death);

the lived experience of pain and suffering;

the appropriate expression of pain;

the styles and background assumptions about family decision making;

the correct role for a healer to assume,

the care of the body after death, and

appropriate expressions of grief.

When the patient's family and healthcare providers do not share fundamental assumptions and goals, the challenges are daunting. Even with excellent and open communication—the foremost goal of culturally, and ethically, appropriate care—barriers remain. Differences in social class and religious background may further accentuate the profound challenge of defining and implementing "good" end-of-life care in healthcare systems serving increasingly diverse societies. The conceptual challenge for bioethics is defining the good in such situations, and making certain that recommendations for respecting cultural difference serve both pragmatic and principled goals (Sprio, McCrea Curnen, and Wandel).

When dealing with concepts as totalizing, but slippery as culture, and as seemingly precise as death, it is useful to begin by considering the definitions and basic concepts used by other disciplines.

Anthropological vs. Philosophical Approaches to Death

It is helpful to consider how taking an anthropological or cultural approach to the study of death differs from the approaches taken within philosophy, where the mystery of death has been a topic of debate and discussion for thousands of years. Philosophy has attempted to account for death conceptually, and more recently in terms of developing criteria for judging when death has occurred. Death is a state following upon the end of life; it is the absence of life. Death is a mystery, but is it more mysterious than other phenomena that we do not understand? Philosophers have tried to ask what death is, and in general have encountered serious definitional difficulties, stemming primarily from the problem of how one defines *life*.

A question of key philosophical interest was posed by the Epicurean philosophers, and most clearly articulated by Lucretius, who asked, "Is death bad for you?" His basic argument, that since the dead person no longer exists, death cannot be "bad" for the individual who dies, has been influential in the subsequent philosophical discourse on death. By contrast, cultural critiques begin with a set of *social* questions that move beyond the individual: How do different societies manage the existential fact that all members will eventually die, and the practical implications of the death of individuals, including the reintegration of survivors of a death? What role do healers and healing systems play, if any. Ethnographers, whether of tribal and hunter-gatherer societies or of a contemporary intensive care units, have a quite different task than the philosopher: describing the range of culturally patterned responses to the existential realities of eventual human frailty and death.

Death and the Birth of Bioethics

Death has been an essential focus of bioethics since the inception of the field nearly four decades ago (Jonsen).

Dealing with the challenges of a dramatically changed biomedical landscape was, in fact, one of the main driving forces in the field's birth. One could argue that bioethics in its current form exists partly in relationship to its encounters with death, to birth pains peculiar to the unique cultural environment of the United States, where the field first crystallized into a new discipline. Following the successes of post-World War II clinical medicine, in particular the development of the mechanical ventilator, and its increasing use outside of its original site—in operating theaters and post-anesthesia recovery—the question arose: When is a patient beyond hope for a meaningful recovery and when is a patient whose heart and lungs are being continued by artificial means actually dead? (Veatch). The first heart transplant in 1968 added the complexity of figuring out when someone was "dead enough" for their organs to be harvested for transplant recipients.

A series of seminal legal cases, many receiving widespread attention, such as the cases of Baby Doe and Karen Ann Quinlan, revealed the fundamental ambiguities of medicine's power to combat death. Recognition of these ambiguities lead to the creation of a series of presidential commissions to debate and reflect on topics such as criteria for establishing brain death, and appropriate procedures for withholding or withdrawing potentially life-sustaining technologies.

Cultural analysis takes account of developments in technology but does not require a determinist position. The argument is *not* that new medical technologies transform cultural understandings of death in a straightforward, linear way. Rather, the meaning of any new medical procedure to forestall death will be developed and gain significance against a specific cultural background. Since understandings of technologies are inevitably culturally shaped, they are never *neutral* but their development is affected by the existing cultural milieu and once in use, cultural context affects how they are used. Thus, most researchers in science studies accept a view that the meanings of new medical technologies are *co-constructed,* rather than determined, they are in a way amalgams of social practices and technical objects; one must understand both in order to have the full picture. A totally implantable defibrillator to save patients from sudden death will not have a specific meaning in an environment where medicine's goal is to intervene in every death. Another society might question the use of certain procedures, such as resuscitation, in the situation of an expected death. The same dynamic affects "low tech" interventions like feeding tubes. Against the background of a long-standing cultural adage that "dying on an empty stomach" is a horrific fate, the surgically-implanted feeding tube will take on one sort of meaning. In another environment, where freedom from tubes and bodily interventions is highly valued, another outcome is likely. As the use of technologies intensifies, indeed, as patients begin to be defined as dying only after they have failed all readily available interventions, we might speak of death occurring in technological time (Muller and Koenig 1988).

Cultural Perspectives on Death

Exact definitions of culture are elusive, like the concept itself. At the most general level, culture is defined as those aspects of human activity that are socially rather than genetically transmitted. Thus culture is patterns of life passed among humans. Definitions are often so broad as to be meaningless, applying to every domain in society: religious beliefs, folk practices, language use, material objects, worldview, artistic expression, etc. According to pioneering anthropologist Robert Lowie, culture "is, indeed, the sole and exclusive subject-matter of ethnology [anthropology], as consciousness is the subject matter of psychology, life of biology, electricity as a branch of physics" (orig. 1917). "In explanatory importance and in generality of application it is comparable to such categories as gravity in physics, disease in medicine, evolution in biology," Alfred Kroeber and Clyde Kluckhohn wrote in 1952 (see Kuper for an overview).

With a category this broad, boundaries are difficult to delineate. Anthropologists have become critical of the application of the culture concept (Kuper). The work of Clifford Geertz moved the field of anthropology in the direction of interpretation, transforming culture from a passive noun to an active verb. "Man is an animal suspended in webs of significance he himself has spun; I take culture to be those webs, and the analysis of it to be, therefore, not an experimental science in search of law, but an interpretive one in search of meaning (p. 5)." In biomedicine the dangers of an essential view of culture are clear. We cannot simply *read* culture in patients facing death or indeed any clinical encounter, discerning their views, desires, and needs with false security based on knowledge that culture *A* holds view *B* about disclosing a terminal prognosis to a patient, and culture *C* holds view *D*.

The origins of the culture concept date back to the work of early post-Enlightenment folklorists, such as Herder, who made use of the concept to avoid the uniform, totalizing theories of human capabilities that were characteristic of the late eighteenth century. The modern concept of culture developed much later, partly in response to racist (and biological determinist) ideologies of the nineteenth century, most incorporating an evolutionary framework based on social Darwinism. The species *homo sapiens* was viewed as divided into separate sub-species or races, each with engrained, essential characteristics, a system that included a hierarchy of moral worth.

Philosophers maintain that a general problem with the culture concept is that it is often linked with a naïve relativism which precludes judgments about the unique cultural practices found around the world. Indeed, in some instances this criticism is warranted; attention to the diversity of cultures and the need to judge each on its own terms is central to the field. However such attention to cultural relativism at the empirical level does not necessarily lead to a stance of ethical relativism. Often practices dealing with death that were unsettling to Europeans, such as head hunting and cannibalism, were the focus of disproportionate attention, supporting efforts to justify and document a radically different "other" (Conklin).

The history of anthropological engagement with mortality dates back to the origins of the discipline, and is bound up with concerns about the origins of religion. Early theorists focused on small scale societies where magic, science, and religion are not separate cultural domains. For example the nineteenth century anthropologist Edward Tyler, who worked from an evolutionary paradigm of explanation, saw the origins of human society and culture in efforts to explain mortality, and in particular, in the recurrence of dreams and other visions about deceased close kin. The "savage philosopher" reflected on everyday experience and developed the notion of the soul. In *Magic, Science and Religion* Malinowski wrote,

> Of all sources of religion, the supreme and final crisis of life—death—is of the greatest importance. Death is the gateway to the other world in more than the most literal sense. According to most theories of early religion, a great deal, if not all, of religious inspiration has been derived from it.... Man has to live his life in the shadow of death, and he who clings to life and enjoys its fullness must dread the menace of its end. Death and its denial—immortality—have always formed, as they form today, the most poignant theme of man's forebodings. [Experience] at life's end condensed into one crisis which provokes a violent and complex outburst of religious manifestations. (p. 47)

Social theorists influential to the development of anthropology, such as Émile Durkheim, and later Robert Hertz, argued that all societies exert institutional controls to protect and preserve the lives of members, including rules governing appropriate and inappropriate killing. Many actions that appear to be individual choices, such as suicide or the expression of emotion during grieving, are actually socially patterned, as studies such as Durkheim's comparative analysis of suicide rates, one of the first uses of statistics in social science, illustrate (1951 [1897]). Hertz used cross cultural comparisons of mourning rituals to suggest that the human expression of grief can also be best understood as a *social fact,* particular to each society (1960 [1907]).

For reasons that have been the subject of extensive internal critique within anthropology (Rosaldo; Behar), until fairly recently the field concerned itself primarily with the rituals following death. This included ceremonies that focus on the disposal of the dead body and occur *after* cardiopulmonary death generally, although not always. This concern with ritual practices and symbolic meaning precluded a full engagement with the profound emotional significance of the process of dying, grief, and loss. Scholars focused on the recurrence throughout the world of death rituals that expressed fertility and rebirth (Bloch and Parry). The emphasis on sexuality, and the connection between sex and death, fit well with interpretations of ritual behavior that emphasized function. Death rituals serve the function of reintegration of society following a death, focusing on reproduction.

In some societies this symbolic link between death and regeneration is expressed explicitly; funerary practices incorporate the abandonment off usual standards of sexual propriety for a confined time period, or allow and encourage sexual relationships between categories of kin where such contact was generally excluded (Barley). These *rites de passage* seemed designed to guide the passage of humans through dangerous, liminal transitions, marking the boundary between life and death. Thus van Gennep (1960 [1909]) saw associations between funerals and other rites of transition, such as initiation ceremonies. In contemporary U.S. hospitals, the practices of bioethics developed in the last decades have become the *new* rituals guiding these transitions between life and death. A number of studies in anthropology (and medical sociology) examine contemporary death practices in biomedical settings, such as Bluebond-Langner's 1978 account of disclosure of a terminal diagnosis to children under treatment for leukemia, or Sudnow's 1967 account of dying in a public hospital. Christakis examines contemporary practices in foretelling death (1999). Other recent ethnographies chronicle the experience of death and extreme old age for specific populations, for example elderly Jewish immigrants (Myerhoff).

Defining the Boundary Between Life and Death

The concept of "social death" has been of considerable utility in describing the varied boundaries between life and

death throughout the world. Nigel Barley, who has written an accessible account of the range of cultural practices surrounding death, describes his alarm and confusion when an African informant tells him casually that his wife "died" that morning, in the midst of a conversation asking him for a cigarette. In reality, she had been, in western terms "unconscious," but the Dowayo make no distinction, either linguistically or conceptually, between death-like states that are reversible (what we might call coma, persistent vegetative state or perhaps suspended animation) and that which continues permanently. This view of death provides a sharp contrast to biomedical definitions that assume irreversibility. (Although it is important to remember that even in the West, belief in resurrection calls the finality of death into question for many, and forms a core of religious belief.)

Studying ideas of death, of course, also reveals views on life and what it means to be human. The idea of social death is intimately tied up with notions of personhood, and who counts as a person within a society. Social death has utility in analyses at both ends of the human lifespan. Anthropologists have observed and documented societies in which full term infants are not considered fully alive, and thus members of the social group, until they have survived the first month of life (perhaps not by chance the period of highest vulnerability for a newborn) and received a name in a formal naming ceremony. Those who die before naming are not considered fully human—we might say that the social group does not recognize the infant' *personhood*—and thus do not warrant ritual attention, such as funerals or elaborate mourning rituals. Such practices are in sharp contrast with contemporary obstetrics practices in the first world, where developing fetuses are named and ultrasound images are exchanged prior to birth. Indeed, the very survival of extremely premature infants in neonatal intensive care units is best understood as an artifact of culture. In other societies specific kinds of birth—such as twins—or certain infants may be judged as incompatible with life, and thus viewed as already dead or infanticide may be allowed. In Bariba society (in Africa), certain infants are understood to be witches, and thus mothers are not allowed to grieve the loss because the infant is defined as not human (Sargent).

Social death is also a useful concept for describing practices near the end of life. In some societies, ritual mourning practices may begin before cardiopulmonary death occurs, since the ill or extremely aged person is viewed as meeting cultural criteria for social death. Or those who are very old may be viewed as almost dead. Many have argued that the warehousing of the elderly in sub-standard U.S. nursing homes constitutes a form of social death. In a series of pioneering ethnographic studies of hospital-based death in the U.S.—in the immediately "pre-bioethics" period—Glaser and Strauss conceive of the isolation of the dying as a form of social death (1965; 1968).

Arguably the most important example of social death in contemporary biomedicine is the notion of "brain death." A body maintained in a modern intensive care unit, pink, with heart beating and lungs inflating and deflating, appears to most observers as a living being. Yet a diagnosis of brain death results in that person's abrupt transition to a socially recognized state of death, and transforms the corpse into a container to house organs awaiting harvesting for another donor. A detailed analysis of the historical development of the concept of brain death, as well as a chronicle of contemporary brain death debates is found in Margaret Lock's 2002 *Twice Dead*. Lock uses a classic anthropological technique called the comparative method to reveal how culture shapes seemingly technical scientific and medical practices. The state of brain death appears to follow the straightforward application of a set of technical criteria about the functioning of the human brain. Lock tells the story of Japanese resistance to organ transplants that require the use of a brain dead patient. By contrasting Japan and the U.S., she reveals how the category of social death can only be understood in cultural context. In Japan, the core site or physical location of personhood is associated with the heart, not the brain. However, Lock makes it clear that the story is not simply about "traditional beliefs," rather many features of contemporary Japanese society—including distrust of the medical profession—play a role in widespread resistance to organ harvesting from brain dead donors.

New Rituals of Dying

For most in the wealthy, developed world the idea that death is an evil to be prevented at all cost, including the use of aggressive therapies like the totally implantable artificial heart, is commonplace. Buoyed by past successes, the arc of medical practice has extended to the moment of death, which increasingly is seen as a process to be stopped whenever possible. As new technologies became available, seeing a patient in cardiac arrest necessitated an action. Resuscitation, in reality attempts at resuscitation, became routinized and normalized at the moment of death (Timmermans). By the late 1960s dying within the sphere of biomedicine became defined as a problem in need of a solution.

The outcome of the many commissions, legal cases, and academic discussions described by Jonsen in the *Birth of Bioethics* (1998) is a set of novel, autonomy-based practices that seek to enhance the self-determination of the dying, and protect patients from the abuses of overzealous physicians

"programmed" by their instrumental training to over treat, prolonging the dying process. These practices incude:

1. formal implementation of advance care planning (and execution of advance directives), institutionalized by law following the passage of the American "Patient Self-Determination Act" in 1991;

2. explicit discussion and decision making about the use of cardiopulmonary resuscitation, or DNR orders;

3. open discussion of diagnosis/prognosis and shared decision making about foregoing or withdrawing curative interventions; and

4. transition to "palliative care" or, in some cases, hospice.

Of course this ideal narrative is rarely followed. All of these practices required a commitment to open and full disclosure of information about death and detailed discussions about how one wishes to die, and assumed that the patient himself—and a gendered pronoun is used purposefully—was in full control of his destiny and fate. The model is gendered male by the focus on individual agency and control, as opposed to the inevitable interdependence of a dying person with her social environment.

What Differences Make a Difference?

Thus far, only broad cultural responses to death have been considered. With increased border crossing and south/north migrations throughout the world, how should we view and define difference in bioethics? Turning to contemporary biomedicine, considerable research documents the relevance of ethnic or cultural and religious differences in the experience of death and dying and in clinical approaches to end-of-life care. However, health researchers and clinicians generally do a poor job of making clear analytic distinctions among the key elements of difference, in answering the question, "What differences make a difference?" When we talk about *cultural* difference, do we mean a patient or family's voluntarily adopted and expressed *ethnic identity*, their nation of origin if recent immigrants, their *race* as assigned by a government enforcing discriminatory laws such as segregation or apartheid, or their adoption of specific health-related practices such as diet or use of medicinal herbs? In healthcare research there is considerable confusion in terminology, particularly with regard to the use of the term "race."

The lack of consistency in the use of terminology for concepts of race, ethnicity, ancestry, and culture is manifest in the wide variance in terms used to describe individual and group identities. Terms such as white, Caucasian, Anglo, and European are routinely used interchangeably to refer to certain groups, whereas black, colored, Negro, and African-American are used to refer to comparison groups. Also, white-black comparisons are straightforward in contrast to the confused use of terms such as Hispanic and Asian. Both of these labels, one based on linguistic criteria and the other on continental origin, lump together many populations of people reflecting enormous variability in factors related to health and medical care. The terms we use gloss over enormous diversity.

Debates in the biomedical literature focus on the appropriate use of terms such as race, ethnicity, and culture. Asking how race is relevant to bioethics, death, and end-of-life care is relevant, but caution is needed whenever the category of race is invoked. Much is "at stake" in how these categories of difference are utilized when conducting research or in designing programs to improve the care of patients, by way of enhancing the *cultural competence* of healthcare providers who must aid patients and families in decision making at the end of life. In particular, approaches to conceptualizing disease etiology or health outcomes may have moral significance if one naïvely assumes that culture predicts behavior in a precise way or that something essential or *inherent* in a certain population leads to poor health outcomes or barriers to healthcare access (Gunaratnam).

In the case of black-white differences in infant mortality or homicide rates, for example, how one thinks about causation, and the relative contribution of genes, environment, and social structure, may determine the type of intervention recommended. Meaningful genetic and biological differences do not always map clearly onto social categories of human difference, whether defined as race, ethnicity, or culture. American patients who self-identify as African American generally seek more aggressive care and are underrepresented in hospice services. If we talk about *racial* differences about preferences for palliative care services, what exactly do we mean? In the United States efforts to tease apart the independent contributions of *race* and socioeconomic status (SES) when analyzing healthcare outcomes may be daunting.

Although the dimensions of difference most relevant to end-of-life care are likely to be social or cultural, biological or genetic variation may also be germane. For example, the field of pharmacogenomics tracks individual and group differences in drug metabolizing enzymes to predict response to medications such as chemotherapy or pain medicines. Although classic understandings of human "races" do not parallel actual genetic variation at the molecular level, there may be frequency differences among socially defined populations relevant to pharmacogenomics. It has been known for decades that there is ethnic or cultural variation in the expression of pain or painful symptoms (Zbrowski;

Garro); the degree of variation in the actual experience of pain—possibly modulated through the action of pain medicines—remains unexplored.

Immigration status is another key category of cultural difference. Recent immigrants provide challenges to the healthcare system, particularly in end-of-life care. In much of the world, the American ideal of open disclosure of information about diagnosis and prognosis is not the norm (Gordon and Paci; Die Trill and Kovalick). In fact, patients and families may experience the directness about diagnosis characteristic of U.S. healthcare as needlessly and aggressively brutal, violating norms espousing "protection" of the ill. Although children may be seen as more in need of protection than adults, much pediatric palliative care literature recommends openness, appropriate to an ill child's age, as preferable to concealment. U.S. bioethics procedures governing end-of-life care may seem unfathomable to those newly in this country, but it is perhaps the assumptions of bioethics that are culturally bound. As Die Trill and Kovalick note, "Those who argue that children always should be told the truth about having cancer must recognize that the truth is susceptible to many interpretations" (p. 203). Whether the dying person is a child or an adult, family members who object to sharing the full differential diagnosis with an ill child may be accused of being "in denial" about the severity of the patient's illness, their concerns "psychologized" rather than understood. Lastly, the experience of those immigrants who are refugees from political violence or war adds another dimension. The effects of multiple losses on family members—including the death of other children and adults in the family, one's country, one's entire history—are difficult to predict but clearly shape a family's response to the serious illness and threatened loss. Responses may appear to be overly stoic or overly emotional.

When considering societies with histories of deep racial divisions, it is especially important to separate analytically the concepts of culture, ethnicity, and race from the effects of social and economic status. Historically underserved populations may have special barriers to end-of-life care that have little to do with difficulties in communication and are not related to their identification with a certain set of ethnic traditions. Culturally specific values and beliefs often exist, but may not be of signal importance. In a ground-breaking study, an American physician documented the lack of availability of narcotic analgesics in minority communities such as Harlem (a low income, historically African American and Hispanic neighborhood in New York City); pharmacies simply did not carry the opiates that are "state-of-the-art" drugs for pain control (Morrison, Wallenstein, and Natale et al.). The American "drug wars," including the recent battles about the abuse of time-release opiates like oxycontin, are often fought in poor neighborhoods with limited access to legitimate employment. Patients from minority backgrounds may not receive adequate pain control if drugs are not prescribed because of fears of theft or abuse. When members of the healthcare team are hesitant to prescribe narcotics it may be a legitimate concern based on factual information about a particular family's drug history, or it may be the exercise of racial stereotyping. The end result is the same: patients may be denied needed pain relief.

The experience of people with sickle cell disease, whose pain is often undertreated because of concerns about drug abuse, is another example of stereotyping. Culture thus contributes to inadequate symptom management, but indirectly, through the actions of healthcare providers, not the essential cultural characteristics of a population. Research in a Los Angeles emergency department documented that Hispanic patients with injuries identical to whites were given less analgesic medication (Todd, Samaroo, and Hoffman). Do patients in such situations have different cultural values about analgesia? Can they exercise full autonomy when faced with decisions about foregoing or withdrawing life prolonging therapies? Surely not, without the assurance of adequate analgesia and palliative care.

Karla Holloway's *Passed On: African American Mourning Stories* (2002) vividly reveals how the unique history of Blacks in the U.S.—including the legacy of slavery, Jim Crow policies, and violent death, such as lynching—shape the experience of death for patients receiving care in hospitals that were segregated two generations ago. Clearly *difference* is relevant to bioethics; assuming that end-of-life procedures and practices have universal applicability is at best naïve and at worst harmful. In addition to the varieties of cultural and social class differences described here, other domains of difference that intersect with culture, such as gender, sexual orientation, disability, and religious background, must also be considered within bioethics (Parens).

Culture Matters: Bioethics, End-of-Life Care and Decision Making

In its report detailing needed changes in care of the dying, the Institute of Medicine has recommended attention to cultural diversity as a national policy objective (Field and Cassel). There is a growing literature based on empirical studies documenting the cultural dimensions of end-of-life care for patients and families. (For reviews see Kagawa-Singer and Blackhall; Koenig and Davies; Crawley, Marshall, and Koenig). Based on this literature, it is possible to identify the key domains of clinical significance in caring for patients from diverse ethnocultural backgrounds who are unlikely to survive.

In general, the cultural challenges of end-of-life care can be divided into two fundamental categories: those that do, and those that do not, violate the healthcare team's foundational cultural values, norms that may also be enforced by legal requirements in some societies. In the first category are cultural values or practices that call into question the biomedical goal of combating disease and extending life at all costs. A family who refused to allow a potentially curative limb amputation for a female child with osteosarcoma because of beliefs about the need to preserve bodily integrity, and a daughter's marriageability, would immediately create consternation for healthcare team members. By contrast, another family who wished to engage a spiritual healer to pray for a successful outcome to the same potentially life-saving surgery would *not* create a cultural crisis, since the family's goals could easily and effortlessly be incorporated into the clinicians' care plan.

Generally, issues such as care of the body after death do not provide a fundamental challenge to biomedical values and beliefs; thus customs prescribing particular approaches to post-death care are relatively easy to implement unless they violate laws governing disposal of the body. However, even in post-death care there may be situations that lead to cultural conflict, such as requests for autopsy or organ donation in situations where the wholeness of the body is highly valued. And the domain of grief counseling and bereavement care may or may not elicit conflict. For medical specialists focused on cure, less is "at stake" once a patient has died and can no longer be saved, but conflicts may still emerge over differing definitions of acceptable grieving practices.

Family Roles and Responsibilities in Shared Decision Making

Within the current conventions of bioethical decision making about end-of-life care for a competent adult patient, the decisions are left up to the individual; theoretically the family or broader community is not critical to the patient's choices. Autonomy is the primary value at play. In the case of children or the severely mentally incapacited, where family members become surrogate decision makers, the situation is much more complex. A growing body of research documents how autonomy-focused bioethics practices may not adequately meet the needs of patients from diverse backgrounds. The value of respect for individual autonomy is not universal. Patients may express confusion and ambivalence when asked to participate in advance care planning about death (Frank, Blackhall, and Michel).

Disagreements about the goals of care, although rare, are emotionally difficult for all. In many cross-cultural situations, the Western view that individual patients will (and should) make decisions about care may be too narrow. In some societies a social unit beyond the nuclear family may also have considerable decision-making authority. Elders in an extended family or clan group may expect to be involved, and patients may desire this. Integrating extended family or kin groups into care in a Western hospital, hospice, or nursing home is hard but may be desirable. Gender may play a role as well. In traditional male-dominated societies, mothers may never have experienced the level of decision-making authority automatically granted to both parents in the United States. This may be a source of tension. Similarly, the evolving practice in pediatrics of requesting "assent" to care by older children, especially girls, may create tensions within the family.

A further dynamic may result from the ideal "shared decision-making" model. Tilden and colleagues have documented stress among family members involved in decisions to withhold treatment. The impact of family involvement in decisions to terminate treatment has not been studied extensively. Inexperienced clinicians or trainees may present decisions about limiting painful or aggressive procedures, sometimes an opening to a transition to palliative or hospice care, in an insensitive way, making it appear that the family decision makers must give "permission" for futile care to be withheld. Although the family's involvment in making decisions on behalf of their loved one is expected, few individuals, regardless of their cultural background, are able to do this easily. In fact, the resistance to giving up hope and explicitly limiting therapies found among families from diverse backgrounds may be appropriate. Models of care that do not require that curative therapies be abandoned in order to obtain excellent palliative services may ultimately lessen this problem. Patients or family members should never be told that care will be withheld; rather the focus should be on meeting the needs of the patient and family.

Varied Understandings of the Role of Health Professionals or Healers

Just as the appropriate role of parents or family members caring for a seriously ill person may vary, the families' expectation of the role played by health professionals may differ. In some societies, healers are expected to make a diagnosis almost magically, perhaps by feeling the pulse without asking any questions. Healers may exert considerable power and authority; they may expect and receive deferential behavior. Patients and families schooled in these traditions may be confused by the shared decision-making ideals of Western practice. They may lose confidence in

physicians who do not appear to know unequivocally the correct course of action but instead ask for the patient's views.

In many societies the roles of healer and religious specialist intersect. "Each religious tradition has its own images and ideals of the doctor, in which the individual engaged in healing is defined as enacting some of the highest ideals of the tradition itself" (Barnes, Plotnikoff, Fox, and Pendleton). The healer's role at the end of life may be particularly meaningful, or it may be proscribed to take on the care of those not expected to survive, as in the Hippocratic tradition.

Families who have been denied access to healthcare providers may also question the trustworthiness of the "establishment" health system, worried that those in power do not have their best interest at heart. The disparities in morbidity and mortality across U.S. populations suggest that often African-American patients receive less intensive care. The irony is that research on end-of-life decision making in adults reveals that minority patients may actually desire more aggressive care near the end of life (Caralis, Davis, Wright, and Marcial; Tulsky, Cassileth, and Bennett).

Communication Barriers: The Need for Translation

Negotiation about the appropriateness of clinical services for patients nearing the end-of-life is a complex task when healthcare professionals, patients, and family members share fundamental goals and assumptions. By no means has a successful "formula" for such communication been established. When cultural barriers exist, particularly those created by language, the goal of open and effective communication is exceptionally difficult. Language translators may be available only intermittently, and are often poorly trained. In 2002, two hospitals in Brooklyn, New York, that routinely serve large numbers of Spanish-speaking patients were sued for failure to provide translation services, examples of a number of such legal actions dating back several decades.

The task of language translation in the arena of ethical decision making and end-of-life care is particularly complex. How does one translate a discussion about a "do not resuscitate" decision to a family with no previous experience of cardiopulmonary resuscitation (CPR), and no prior knowledge of the American bioethics tradition of requiring permission not to offer CPR, even to a patient who is actively dying an "expected" death, or may be frail because of extreme old age? What if the language characters representing resuscitation are interchangeable with those suggesting the religious concept of resurrection? Although it sounds odd from the perspective of Western, scientific understandings of death, who would not elect to have themselves or their dying loved one brought back to life if offered the choice in those words? How might medical interventions at the moment of death be understood among practitioners of Buddhism who believe that rituals spoken during the dying process guide the "soul" through dangerous spiritual territory and ultimately determine where and how a person will be reborn? How do you negotiate with a family about the location of death—home versus hospital—against a cultural background where speaking of an individual's death is thought to bring it about or where certain illnesses cannot be named? The use of family members as interpreters, which may be unavoidable, may make discussions such as these even more problematic. Family members may see their primary role as protecting others in the family from harm and thus "shield" them from information viewed as harmful. Such shielding is counter to bioethics norms of open disclosure.

Furthermore, models of professional translation, such as those employed in courtrooms where relationships are fundamentally adversarial rather than collaborative, assume that language interpreters should function as neutral "machines." Healthcare providers need to be aware that translation services such as those available by phone from AT&T may be based on legal models of interpretation. This stance ignores the interpreter's potential value in providing information about the family's cultural background, as well as providing language interpretation. When interpreters are engaged as full partners in providing care, they may aid in negotiations about difficult end-of-life dilemmas (Kaufert, Putsch, and Lavallee). When included as part of the healthcare team—for example, in programs where native speakers of commonly encountered languages are employed as bilingual medical assistants—interpreters can also serve the useful function of explaining the culture of biomedicine, and the seemingly peculiar assumptions of bioethics, to families.

Integration of Alternative and Complementary Medicine into Palliative Care

Patients and their families may be subject to strong pressures to utilize "ethnomedical" practices and procedures believed to be efficacious. Recent immigrants may utilize products obtained abroad or from Mexico and Central America. Practices vary widely, including acupuncture for pain, cupping or coining, dietary prohibitions based on "hot-cold" belief systems, Chinese herbal products, Ayurvedic patent medicines, and full-blown rituals including chanting and the sacrifice of animals. A skilled practitioner creates an open

environment in which the patient, family, and perhaps a ritual specialist from the community may openly discuss the appropriate blending of biomedically sanctioned medicines and procedures with ethnomedical products. Although some patent medicines and food supplements are known to be harmful and may actually contain potent pharmaceuticals, the healthcare team is unlikely to obtain a full accounting of all treatments used for a particular dying patient unless a nonjudgmental attitude is maintained. This may be a challenge when a healthcare provider must compromise his or her own "ideal" care.

The need to integrate alternative and complementary medicine into palliative care is not limited to patients from particular ethnocultural communities. Research documents that a large percentage of Americans have utilized "alternative" medicine in the recent past (Eisenberg, Davis, Ettner et al.), with prayer being the most widely utilized practice (82 percent of Americans believe in the healing power of personal prayer) (Barnes, Plotnikoff, Fox, and Pendleton).

The Meaning of Pain and Suffering

End-of-life care has as a primary goal the relief of pain and suffering. Cultural difference is relevant to pain management in multiple ways. The effectiveness of symptom management may be lessened by economic barriers to medicines or special treatments. Cross-cultural research with adult patients has documented differences in the way people experience and express pain (Garro). What is considered acceptable way to express painful symptoms? Is stoicism rewarded? Are there gender differences in outward discussion of painful symptoms? Spirituality may have an impact on the meaning of suffering and hence on the management of symptoms. A study of infants and children with a rare genetic disease (recombinant 8 syndrome) in long-time Spanish-speaking residents of the American Southwest revealed the complexity of suffering. The experience of affected children in these devout Catholic families was thought to mirror Christ's suffering, providing meaning to an otherwise unexplainable tragedy (Blake).

Defining the Boundary of Life and Death

Biomedical definitions of death, including the concept of brain death, appear to be clear cut. However, when examined closely considerable ambiguity remains. Even among biomedical professionals one frequently hears confusion in language when speaking, say, about an organ donor who is technically brain dead, but may appear to be as "alive" as adjacent patients in an ICU. Linguistically, these brain-dead bodies experience a second "death" once organs are retrieved for transplantation and ventilatory support is removed (Lock). It is thus not surprising that patients and families can also become quite confused about states resembling death, including brain death, the persistent vegetative state, or coma (Kaufman).

Disputes arise when a patient meets the biomedical criteria for "brain death," but the family refuses to allow withdrawal of "life" support. In a masterful essay, Joseph Fins describes two clinical negotiations about withdrawing life support from children defined as brain dead (1998). In one case, the hospital team engages the family's orthodox rabbi and other religious authorities in a complex series of negotiations, respecting throughout the family's view that the patient is not truly dead and that only God can declare death. A more contentious case involves an African-American family who maintains a stance of mistrust toward the healthcare establishment in spite of every effort on the part of the clinical team. The family's past experience shaped its understanding of the team's intentions in spite of great effort to gain their trust. Disputes such as these are the "hard" cases, revealing cultural clashes that cannot be ameliorated simply by motivated clinicians, sensitivity, or excellent communication skills, although clearly those things may keep conflict to a minimum or may keep small cultural disputes from erupting into major pitched battles.

Work has focused on care of the body after death, particularly the question of autopsy, since in some societies the body is considered inviolable after death; its contents sacred and necessary for the individual's appropriate survival into the afterlife. These cultural practices were most fully-developed in Egyptian dynasties, where funeral practices and preparation for life after death—including mummification and building of elaborate tombs—consumed the society's symbolic attention and material resources. The acceptability of autopsy, or other uses of the body following death, is deeply sensitive to cultural and religious prohibitions. Knowledge about the acceptability of autopsy, or requests for organ donation in the case of acute trauma, cannot usually be guessed by "reading" a family's background.

Furthermore, different ethnocultural groups may have varied understandings of the nature, meaning, and importance of cognitive impairment in a patient. In a society where social relationships are a core value, esteemed more highly than individual achievement, disabilities that affect intellectual functioning but do not interfere with the ill person's role in the family may be more readily "accepted." By contrast, in some societies severely handicapped people may experience a form of social death, isolated from the broader community.

Acceptance of Hospice Philosophy

Utilization of hospice care programs is not identical across racialized U.S. populations. African Americans utilize hospice services at a lower rate than do European Americans. Home death is often considered an ideal within the hospice philosophy. A *good death* is often characterized as one that takes place at home, surrounded by family and/or friends, with pain and symptoms under control, spiritual needs identified and met, and following appropriate good-byes. Traditionally, this ideal good death required giving up curative interventions. At the moment in U.S. history, the 1970s, when hospice care became a viable alternative, aggressive end-of-life interventions were commonplace, and efforts to secure patient participation in decision making were not yet fully realized. Thus, the home became a refuge from the ravages of hospital death. Even though the strict implementation of a six-month prognosis requirement for hospice is changing, it remains difficult to predict the terminal or near-terminal phase of common illnesses, particularly cardiac, pulmonary, and metabolic conditions, in contrast with cancer. Acknowledging that death is near may be particularly difficult. Home death may not be valued in ethnocultural groups where it is considered inappropriate, dangerous, or polluting to be around the dead. Among traditional Navajo, the dying were removed from the Hogan dwelling through a special door to a separate shed-like room to avoid the catastrophe of a death occurring in the Hogan, which would then have to be destroyed. Burial practices were organized to make certain that ghosts could not find their way back to the Hogan, and family members did not touch the dead body. This task was relegated to outsiders. These issues remain salient for those practicing in the Indian Health Service. In some Chinese immigrant communities a death at home may affect the value of a particular property on resale.

Culture, Grief, and Mourning

Bioethics practices generally focus on decision making prior to death. Clinical interventions to aid the bereaved—increasingly seen as a critical component of services provided to patients and families—must take into account cultural differences. It is critical to acknowledge that Western ways of grieving and disposing of the body are not universally accepted as the *right* way. It is also likely that our theories of grief and mourning, including definitions of *normal,* are inappropriately based on Western behavioral norms. For example, a standard way in the West of dealing with grief is to talk-about one's experience, one's relationship with the deceased, one's feelings. But in some cultures, talking may disrupt hard-earned efforts to feel what is appropriate, and to disrupt those efforts may jeopardize one's health. In some cultures, talk is acceptable, but one must never mention the name of the deceased person. In other cultures, talk is acceptable as long as it doesn't focus on oneself. Even in the West, however, not everyone is open to talking. It is important not to label those who do not openly express their emotions as *pathological*. In fact, the concept of pathological grief is primarily a Western construction. A mother in the slums of Cairo, Egypt, locked for seven years in the depths of a deep depression over the death of a child is not behaving pathologically by the standards of her community (Wikan). There is enormous variation in what is considered appropriate behavior following death. The ideal among traditional Navajo is to express no emotion, while in tribal societies a death may be met with wild outpourings of grief, including self-mutilation (Barley). In contrast to clinical notions of pathological grief, in some Mediterranean societies widowhood was considered a permanent state of mourning, and mourning clothes were worn for years, if not decades. In a compelling book titled *Consuming Grief*, Conklin describes how native Amazonians assuage their grief by consuming the body of their dead kin (2001). A number of anthologies provide examples of the range of cross-cultural variation in post-death management (Counts and Counts; Metcalf and Huntington; Irish, Lundquist, and Jenkins Nelsen; Parkes, Laungani, and Pittu; Rosenblatt, Walsh, and Jackson).

The Need for Clinical Compromise: A Challenge for Bioethics

Respecting cultural difference may offer a profound challenge to healthcare practitioners' most fundamental values. In perhaps the best "text" explaining the cultural dynamics underlying the treatment of a critically ill patient, Anne Fadiman, in *The Sprit Catches You and You Fall Down* (1997), offers a detailed account of how the physicians caring for a young Hmong child with life-threatening, difficult-to-control epilepsy ultimately fail her because of their desire to offer her "state-of-the-art" care identical to that offered to any of their other patients. Through her detailed ethnographic account, Fadiman reveals how in this case the physician's quest for the "perfect" treatment was the proverbial "enemy of the good." The parents of the child, Lia Lee, were refugees from the American war in Southeast Asia, illiterate in their own language, with ideas about the cause of epilepsy and its appropriate treatment that were completely at odds with the views of the Western healthcare team. They were not, however, the only participants in the exchange shaped by cultural background and context. Fadiman's work documents the culture of biomedicine,

explaining with great clarity how the physician's uncompromising dedication to perfection kept them from negotiating a treatment regimen acceptable to all.

Often in cross-cultural settings it is imperative to learn to compromise one's own clinical goals in order to meet the patient "halfway." Fadiman's book recounts the profound miscommunication between the pediatricians and family physicians involved in Lia's care, the Lee family, and the broader Hmong community. When her parents are unable to carry out a complex regimen of anti-epilepsy drugs, the child is turned over to the state's child protective services agency, provoking a profound and deepening spiral of tragedies. In the end, the physicians wish they had compromised their goals and prescribed a more simple medication schedule. Ironically, the parents' observation that the medicines were making Lia sick proved true in that one of the antiepileptic drugs contributed to an episode of profound sepsis that resulted in Lia's persistent vegetative state. A number of American medical schools assign this book as a required text in cultural sensitivity training. Its brilliance lies in revealing both sides of a complex equation: a Hmong enclave transported to semi-rural California and a group of elite, Western-trained physicians and healthcare practitioners caught up in a drama they cannot understand, not because the Lee family's cultural practices are so esoteric but because they fail to recognize how their own cultural assumptions and deeply held values limit their ability to help the ill child.

The Culture of Biomedicine and Biomedical Death Reflect Features of U.S. Society

National efforts to improve end-of-life care often include the notion that *cultural change* or promotion of *cultural readiness* is essential for reform efforts to be successful (Moskowitz and Nelson). Yet, what this cultural change would look like and what barriers to such change exist are rarely itemized. National public awareness campaigns such as "Last Acts" have used a variety of strategies to change the *culture of dying* in America, including working with the media. For example, one strategy has been to sponsor scriptwriting conferences to encourage widely viewed television programs, such as "ER," to include realistic stories about patients near the end of life. In fact, one episode focused on end-stage cystic fibrosis. Narratives created for television might convey the idea that a comfortable, pain-free death is possible and should be *demanded* by patients and families as an essential feature of a comprehensive healthcare system. The stories might convey the important lesson that physicians and other caregivers may forgo their most aggressive efforts at cure without abandoning patients.

Unfortunately, these efforts at promoting cultural change ignore a fundamental and problematic social fact—a profound cultural resistance to foregoing high technology interventions and giving up hope for recovery. narratives of hope and recovery compete with stories of patients abandoning efforts at cure after a valiant struggle with disease.

Research by Koenig and her team revealed that patients from minority backgrounds, in particular recent immigrants, seemed to lack a sense of the narrative structure of end-of-life care that English-speaking, middle-class European-American families understood more readily. In particular, the idea that patients and families would make an explicit choice to abandon curative therapy, followed by the "limiting" of aggressive interventions like intensive care and cardiopulmonary resuscitation, did not seem to be a story patients understood. Recent Chinese immigrant patients could not answer questions that presupposed a transition from curative to palliative goals; it was simply beyond their experience (Hern, Koenig, Moore, and Marshall). In their worldview, doctors do not *stop* treating patients. Efforts to change the culture through engagements with the media— encouraging op-ed pieces in newspapers, scriptwriting workshops, and so forth—may educate potential patients about existing approaches in palliative and hospice care.

One cultural barrier is particularly difficult to surmount. Before physicians can recommend palliative care and before patients and families agree to it, in our current system one must first accept the possibility that death is imminent or at least that one's likely survival is seriously limited. Eventually, current reform efforts to introduce palliative care early in a trajectory of disease or illness may decrease the need for patients or families to embrace their own death in order to make a clear transition between curative and palliative modalities of treatment. But it is unlikely that the tension caused by the need to balance conflicting goals will ever dissipate totally.

Even if one embraces the narrative of limiting aggressive treatment and adopting comfort care, including attention to spiritual and interpersonal goals, as a good idea "in principle" for those facing death, there still exists the radically difficult and jarring transition itself, the need to imagine you or your family member as now taking center stage in a particular EOL narrative. It is no longer theoretical but real. The resistance to seeing oneself (or a loved one) in this role is considerable and may prove insurmountable for many. A set of powerful cultural narratives operates to feed this resistance and encourage its perpetuation. Consider, as one example, the heroic narratives of successful research and triumphant cure that are much more often portrayed by the media than stories of failed therapy and excellent end-of-life care (Koenig). The content of public relations materials produced by medical centers and ads published by drug companies conveys powerful cultural metaphors that are directly counter to the mundane realities of palliative care, often focused on managing symptoms such as constipation. Hospital ads suggest that it is vital to "keep shopping" and eventually you will find the program offering the experimental or innovative therapy that will lead to cure. The heroic search for cure is celebrated in media accounts such as the film *Lorenzo's Oil* or news accounts of a family seeking gene therapy to cure their child's severe, life-limiting genetic illness (Canavan disease). A full analysis of the culture of dying in the United States must acknowledge these powerful counter images.

It is important to bear in mind that such stories and advertisements are features of a particular political economy of healthcare. Unlike providing palliative care, which does not generate an economic surplus for hospitals, administering chemotherapy generates profits even when the likelihood of its success is low or nonexistent. One recent study documents that curative chemotherapy is often given very close to the end of life, when its use may be futile (Emanuel et al.). This is not to suggest that individual physicians are primarily motivated by financial gain when they prescribe chemotherapy that they know has little chance of success. The full picture is a much more complex mix of faith in research, trust in therapeutic rituals as opposed to inaction, genuine prognostic uncertainty, and unwillingness to acknowledge the likely poor outcome of patients one knows well. But it is critical to acknowledge that the economic structure of U.S. healthcare for children creates few barriers for the use of advanced life-prolonging therapies such as chemotherapy or days in an intensive care unit, at least for those with insurance or access to government-funded programs. The most intensive services often generate the highest profits. By contrast, hospice and palliative care programs are often supported by philanthropy; providing excellent palliative care is at best revenue neutral and more often a money loser for medical centers. Thus, the political economy of healthcare supports what Daniel Callahan has called "technological brinkmanship," or the aggressive use of technology until the last possible moment, often leading to its overuse. Culture shapes the realities of care at many levels.

Conclusion: Bioethics, Culture, and Globalization

The experiences of death are culturally constructed within particular social and historical moments. An anthropological account of death takes into account the network of human relationships within which behaviors and practices associated with death and mourning are situated. A cultural analysis of the rituals and symbols evoked by death and dying also suggest the powerful role of social and economic conditions that necessarily define and constrain death experiences, including the treatment of bodies, burial practices, and reactions to grief. Viewed from a cultural perspective, death practices provide an important foundation for understanding the meaning of human suffering in response to loss.

Cultural analysis using ethnographic methods provides unique insights into the nature of bioethics practices that have become the new rituals of dying. These insights will be of increasing use in the context of a globalized biomedicine, which moves bioethics practices into multiple settings, often quite different from the social and historical context that shaped their development. When implemented in societies characterized by an increasing degree of cultural diversity, the limitations of these practices, and their cultural roots and sources, are revealed. Cultural analysis—particularly studies that highlight the response of ethnically different others to bioethics practices—is incomplete if not augmented by attention to the political economy of healthcare. Cultural variability does not *determine* ones views about death. Rather, we are all shaped by culture, and in turn contribute to dynamic change.

There is a naïve hope that cultural competency training will lead effortlessly to improved outcomes. It may under some circumstances, but significant cultural difference inevitably brings with it true conflicts that may not be resolved, even with ideal, open communication and mutual respect. In some situations, the distance between families and the healthcare team may be too profound to overcome in spite of considerable efforts by all. Anne Fadiman recounts a physician involved in the care of Lia Lee, who lamented that even if it had been possible to send the Lee family to medical school with an interpreter, the difference in world views separating a refugee Hmong family from mainstream Western pediatrics would remain insurmountable.

How one thinks about culture matters. A serious flaw in current cultural competency training in biomedical settings is a simplistic and unsophisticated account of culture itself. It is almost as if there is a belief that culture codes for—and predicts—behavior in the same way that DNA codes for a certain protein. Reductionist approaches to education in cultural difference will inevitably fail because, at best, they teach a few general clues that must be verified through interaction with a family and, at worst, they model an unsophisticated approach to culture that leads to simple stereotyping, thus doing more harm than good. Educational techniques and programs that emphasize an interpretive approach to understanding cultural difference are more likely to be successful.

If one accepts that analyzing the nature of ethical practice, and ultimately improving end-of-life care, is a fundamental goal of bioethics, then bioethics scholars must take account of culture in their work. Culture must be engaged at many levels, not just through a focus on *the other*. Ethnic and cultural difference in response to bioethics practices—the new end-of-life rituals—must be respected in a sophisticated manner, free of harmful stereotyping. But we must not stop there. Those working in bioethics must engage in a critical analysis of the culture of biomedical science and practice. And finally, they must be active students of the cultural assumptions underlying bioethics itself, interrogating the foundations of the field.

BARBARA A. KOENIG
PATRICIA A. MARSHALL

SEE ALSO: *Aging and the Aged: Old Age; Anthropology and Bioethics; Autonomy; Body: Cultural and Religious Perspectives; Care; Grief and Bereavement; Harm; Holocaust; Human Dignity; Infanticide; Life; Life, Quality of; Life Sustaining Treatment and Euthanasia; Literature and Healthcare; Narrative; Palliative Care and Hospice; Pediatrics, Intensive Care in; Right to Die, Policy and Law; Suicide; and Virtue and Character; Warfare;* and other *Death* subentries

BIBLIOGRAPHY

Barley, Nigel. 1997. *Grave Matters: A Lively History of Death around the World.* New York: Henry Holt.

Bluebond-Langner, Myra. 1978. *The Private Worlds of Dying Children.* Princeton, NJ: Princeton University Press.

Barnes, Linda L.; Plotnikoff, Gregory A.; Fox, Kenneth; and Pendleton, Sara. 2000. "Spirituality, Religion, and Pediatrics: Intersecting Worlds of Healing." *Pediatrics* 104(6): 899–908.

Behar, Ruth. 1996. "Death and Memory: From Santa Maria del Monte to Miami Beach." In *The Vulnerable Observer: Anthropology that Breaks Your Heart,* ed. Ruth Behar. Boston: Beacon Press.

Blake, Deborah. 2000. Unpublished manuscript, Regis University, Denver, CO.

Bloch, Maurice, and Parry, Jonathan. 1982. *Death and the Regeneration of Life.* New York: Cambridge University Press.

Callahan, Daniel. 2000. *The Troubled Dream of Life: In Search of a Peaceful Death.* Washington, D.C.: Georgetown University Press.

Caralis, P. V.; Davis, B.; Wright, K.; and Marcial, E. 1997. "The Influence of Ethnicity and Race on Attitudes toward Advance Directives, Life-Prolonging Treatments, and Euthanasia." *Journal of Clinical Ethics* 4(2):155–165.

Christakis, Nicholas A. 1999. *Death Foretold: Prophecy and Prognosis in Medical Care.* Chicago: University of Chicago Press.

Conklin, Beth A. 2001. *Consuming Grief: Compassionate Cannibalism in an Amazonian Society.* Austin: University of Texas Press.

Counts, David R., and Counts, Dorothy A., eds. 1991. *Coping with the Final Tragedy: Cultural Variation in Dying and Grieving.* Amityville, NY: Baywood.

Crawley, La Vera M.; Marshall, Patricia A.; and Koenig, Barbara A. 2001. "Respecting Cultural Differences at the End of Life." In *Physician's Guide to End-of-Life Care,* ed. T. E. Quill and L. Snyder. Philadelphia: American College of Physicians.

Die Trill, M., and Kovalcik, R. 1997. "The Child with Cancer: Influence of Culture on Truth-Telling and Patient Care." *Annals of New York Academy of Sciences* 809: 197–210.

Durkheim, Émile. 1951 (1897). *Suicide: A Study in Sociology,* trs. John A. Spaulding and George Simpson. Glencoe, IL: Free Press.

Emanuel, Ezekiel J., et al. 2001. "How Much Chemotherapy Are Cancer Patients Receiving at the End of Life?" Abstract Presented at the American Society for Clinical Oncology.

Eisenberg, David M.; Davis, Roger B.; Ettner, Susan L.; et al. 1998. "Trends in Alternative Medicine Use in the United States, 1990–1997: Results of a Follow-Up National Survey." *Journal of the American Medical Association* 280: 1569–1575.

Fadiman, Anne. 1997. *The Spirit Catches You and You Fall Down: A Hmong Child, her American Doctors, and the Collision of Two Cultures.* New York: Farrar, Straus, and Giroux.

Field, Mmarilyn J., and Cassel, Christine K., eds. 1997. *Approaching Death: Improving Care at the End of Life.* Washington, D.C.: National Academy Press.

Fins, Joseph J. 1998. "Approximation and Negotiation: Clinical Pragmatism and Difference." *Cambridge Quarterly of Healthcare Ethics* 7(1): 68–76.

Frank, Geyla; Blackhall, Leslie J.; Michel, Vicki, et al. 1998. "A Discourse of Relationships in Bioethics: Patient Autonomy and End-of-Life Decision Making among Elderly Korean Americans." *Medical Anthropology Quarterly* 12: 403–423.

Garro, Linda C. 1990. "Culture, Pain, and Cancer." *Journal of Palliative Care* 6(3): 34–44.

Glaser, Barney G., and Strauss, Anselm. 1965. *Awareness of Dying.* Chicago: Adine.

Glaser, Barney G., and Strauss, Anselm. 1968. *Time for Dying.* Chicago: Adine.

Gordon, Deborah R., and Paci, Eugenio. 1997. "Disclosure Practices and Cultural Narratives: Understanding Concealment and Silence around Cancer in Tuscany, Italy." *Social Science and Medicine* 4: 1433–1452.

Gunaratnam, Yasmin. 1997. "Culture Is Not Enough: A Critique of Multi-Culturalism in Palliative Care." In *Death, Gender, and Ethnicity,* David Field; Jenny Hockey; and Neil Small, eds. London: Routledge.

Hern, H. Eugene; Koenig, Barbara A.; Moore, Lisa J.; and Marshall, Patricia A. 1998. "The Difference that Culture Can Make in End-of-Life Decision Making." *Cambridge Quarterly of Healthcare Ethics* 7: 27–40.

Hertz, Robert. 1960 (1907). *Death and the Right Hand,* trs. Rodney Needham and Claudia Needham. Glencoe, IL: Free Press.

Holloway, Karla F. C. 2002. *Passed On: African American Mourning Stories.* Durham, NC: Duke University Press.

Huntington, R. and Metcalf, P. 1980. *Celebrations of Death,* 2nd edition. Cambridge, Eng.: Cambridge University Press.

Irish, Donald P.; Lundquist, Kathleen F.; and Jenkins Nelson, Vivian. 1993. *Ethnic Variations in Dying, Death, and Grief: Diversity in Universality.* Washington, D.C.: Taylor and Francis.

Jonsen, Albert R. 1998. "Who Should Live? Who Should Die? The Ethics of Death and Dying." In *The Birth of Bioethics.* New York: Oxford University Press.

Kagawa-Singer, Marjorie, and Blackhall, Leslie J. 2001. "Negotiating Cross-Cultural Issues at the End of Life: 'You Got to Go Where He Lives.'" *Journal of the American Medical Association* 286(23): 2993–3001.

Kaufert, Joseph M.; Putsch, Robert W.; Lavallee, M. 1999. "End-of-Life Decision Making among Aboriginal Canadians: Interpretation, Mediation, and Discord in the Communication of 'Bad News'." *Journal of Palliative Care* 15(1): 31–38.

Kaufman, Sharon R. 2000. "In the Shadow of 'Death with Dignity': Medicine and Cultural Quandaries of the Vegetative State." *American Anthropologist* 102(1): 69–83.

Koenig, Barbara A. 2001. "When the Miracles Run Out: In America, Care for Dying Patients Fails to Measure Up" *San Jose Mercury News.* August 7, 2001.

Koenig, Barbara A., and Davies, Betty. 2003. "Cultural Dimensions of Care at Life's End for Children and Their Families." In *When Children Die: Improving Palliative and End-of-Life Care for Children and their Families,* ed. Marilyn J. Field and Richard E. Behrman. Washington, D.C.: National Academy of Sciences.

Kuper, Adam. 1999. *Culture: The Anthropologists' Account.* Cambridge, MA: Harvard University Press.

Lock, Margaret. 2002. *Twice Dead: Organ Transplants and the Reinvention of Death.* Berkeley: University of California Press.

Lucretius. 1951. *On the Nature of the Universe,* tr. R. E. Latham. London: Penguin.

Malinowski, Bronislaw. 1992 (1916–1926). *Magic, Science and Religion (and other essays).* Prospect Heights, IL: Waveland Press.

Metcalf, Peter, and Huntington, Richard. 1991. *Celebrations of Death: The Anthropology of Mortuary Ritual,* 2nd edition. New York: Cambridge University Press.

Morrison, R. Sean; Wallenstein, Sylvan; Natale, Dana K.; et al. 2000. "'We Don't Carry That'—Failure of Pharmacies in Predominantly Nonwhite Neighborhoods to Stock Opioid Analgesics." *New England Journal of Medicine* 342(14): 1023–1026.

Moskowitz, Ellen H., and Nelson, James L. 1995. "Dying Well in the Hospital: The Lessons of SUPPORT." *Hastings Center Report* 25(Special Supplement), Nov.-Dec.(6).

Muller, Jessica H., and Koenig, Barbara A. 1988. "On the Boundary of Life and Death: The Definition of Dying by Medical Residents." In *Biomedicine Examined,* ed. Margaret Lock and Deborah R. Gordon. Boston: Kluwer.

Myerhoff, Barbara. 1994. *Number Our Days: Culture and Community among Elderly Jews in an American Ghetto.* New York: Meridian.

Parens, Erik, ed. 1998. "What Differences Make a Difference?" In *Cambridge Quarterly of Healthcare Ethics* special issue, 7(1).

Parkes, Colin M.; Laungani, Pittu; and Young, Bill, eds. 1997. *Death and Bereavement across Cultures.* Routledge: London.

Rosaldo, Renato. 1989. *Culture and Truth: The Remaking of Social Analysis.* Boston: Beacon Press.

Rosenblatt, Paul C.; Walsh, R. Patricia; and Jackson, Douglas A. 1976. *Grief and Mourning in Cross Cultural Perspective.* New Haven, CT: HRAF Press.

Sargent, Carolyn F. 1988. "Born to Die: Witchcraft and Infanticide in Bariba Culture." *Ethnology* 27(1): 79–95.

Scheper-Hughes, Nancy. 1992. *Death without Weeping : The Violence of Everyday Life in Brazil.* Berkeley: University of California Press.

Spiro, Howard M.; McCrea Curnen, Mary G.; and Wandell, Lee Palmer. 1996. *Facing Death: Where Culture, Religion, and Medicine Meet.* New Haven, CT: Yale University Press.

Sudnow, David. 1967. *Passing On: The Social Organization of Dying.* Englewood Cliffs, NJ: Prentice-Hall.

Tilden, Virginia P.; Tolle, Susan W.; Nelson, Christine A.; and Fields, Jonathan. "Family Decision-Making to Withdraw Life-Sustaining Treatments from Hospitalized Patients." *Nursing Research* 50(2): 105–115.

Timmermans, Stefan. 1999. *Sudden Death and the Myth of CPR.* Philadelphia: Temple University Press.

Todd, Knox H.; Samaroo, Nigel; Hoffman, Jerome R. 1993. "Ethnicity as a Risk Factor for Inadequate Emergency Department Analgesia." *Journal of the American Medical Association* 269(12): 1537–1539.

Tulsky, James A.; Cassileth, Barrie R.; and Bennett, Charles L. 1997. "The Effect of Ethnicity on ICU Use and DNR Orders in Hospitalized AIDS Patients." *Journal of Clinical Ethics* 8(2): 150–157.

van Gennep, Arnold. 1960. *The Rites of Passage,* tr. Monika B. Vizedom and Gabrielle L. Caffee. Chicago: University of Chicago Press.

Veatch, Robert M. 1976. *Death, Dying, and the Biological Revolution: Our Last Quest for Responsibility.* New Haven: Yale University Press.

Wikan, U. 1988. "Bereavement and Loss in Two Muslim Communities: Egypt and Bali Compared." *Social Science and Medicine* 27: 451–460.

Zborowski, Mark. 1969. *People in Pain.* San Francisco: Jossey-Bass.

INTERNET RESOURCE

Last Acts. 2003. Available from <http://www.lastacts.org>.

II. EASTERN THOUGHT

Unlike other species, humans can reflect on death. One response to the mystery and fear humans associate with death is to create systems of religious meaning that give purpose to life in the face of death. A corollary of the fact that people can reflect on death is their realization that it is possible for them intentionally to end life. Religion constrains this possibility in the interest of human survival; only a few exceptions to the taboo against killing humans are allowed. Animals, by contrast, cannot decide to kill themselves and seldom kill members of their own species.

Concepts of death in Asian religions include two basic types: natural—for example, death by disease and old age; and unnatural—for example, death by an accident, by the intention of another person (homicide), or by one's own intention. The latter, here called self-willed death, may be subdivided into three types: (1) suicide (self-willed death out of depression or passion, an irrational and private act); (2) heroic (self-willed death by warriors, and sometimes their wives, to avoid being killed or captured by an enemy, and therefore shamed; or to follow a leader in death because of loyalty); and (3) religious (self-willed death as a rational and public act sanctioned by a religion; for example, in cases of terminal illness or debilitating old age, or as a means to achieve heaven or enlightenment).

Hinduism

THE CONCEPT OF NATURAL DEATH. In no small measure, Vedic (Brahmanical) religion (1500–600 B.C.E.), its sequel now called Hinduism, and other Indian religions (Jainism and Buddhism) inherited views of death from the Indo-Europeans who came to India, probably from eastern Anatolia. Because life expectancy in the prehistoric world was about thirty years, on account of disease, natural calamities, and warfare, people turned to religion for help, performing rituals for health, physical security, longevity, or immortality.

A proto-Indo-European myth about death involved a primordial sacrifice in which Manu (literally Man), the first priest, sacrificed Yemo, his twin and the first king, to create the cosmos, including the realm of the dead. Located to the south, symbolizing warmth, the realm of the dead was described as a paradise where cold, suffering, labor, injustice, evil, darkness, aging, sickness, and death were unknown (Lincoln). According to one Indian version found in the *Rgveda* (10.13.4)—the earliest and most authoritative Hindu scripture—Manu sacrificed King Yama, who showed the path to where the forebears of old had gone: The *Rgveda* considered this place either the southern world or the highest region—a paradise with light, beauty, and joy. (In later texts, Yama was demoted to preside over a hell; the fetters that once bound him as the sacrificial victim for creation were now used by him to fetter sinners.) In another early Indian version, the Puruṣasūkta (Ṛgveda, 10.90), Man, the sacrificial victim, was bound, killed, and dismembered. His mind became the moon; his eye, the sun; his mouth, the fire; his breath, the wind; his feet, the earth. Henceforth, each sacrifice repeated the cosmogonic one, with animals representing the human victims of earlier Indo-European myths or rituals, to ensure the continued existence of the cosmos. A symbolic reenactment of the cosmogonic sacrifice occurred in the funeral ritual; according to Ṛgveda 10.16, different parts of a dead person went to various parts of the universe.

The Vedas prescribed a life of one hundred years, indicating a desire for longevity and natural death. For those who died a natural death, the funeral ritual (śrāddha) would be performed; this would provide them the status of ancestor, ensuring rebirth as a human or existence as a god (hence creating a double buffer against death as annihilation).

Drawing on their pastoral practice of seasonal migration, the Indo-Europeans referred to the dead as traveling along a pathway. In India, the Vedas also referred to the paths of the dead. The straight and easy one ascended to a luminous paradise where the gods lived; the tortuous and difficult one descended to a dark netherworld. By performing sacrifices and funerals, people gained access to the former (Ṛgveda, 10.2.3). The most common Indo-European image of the dead following a path involved crossing a river or ocean by means of a ferry guided by a ferryman, the personification of old age, to paradise (Lincoln). During their migrations into India, the Indo-Europeans conquered settlements at fords (tīrtha) to cross rivers. A popular Vedic myth alludes to this: The warrior god Indra killed the native serpent demon Vrtra, thus creating a passage from drought to water, barrenness to prosperity, death to survival, danger to security, darkness to light, and chaos to order (Young, 1980). Hence the Vedic notion of figuratively crossing over dangers to arrive happily on the other shore, to make a way through experience or suffering, and to penetrate the real or the true.

Some of these ideas prefigured a new worldview that led to a dramatic transformation of Vedic religion and the birth of two new religions (Jainism and Buddhism) around the sixth century B.C.E. This period witnessed a great increase in life expectancy. Seeing the miseries of frailty and old age, however, led many people to increasing anxiety over the end of life (Tilak). This gave rise to reflections on old age, the meaning and purpose of life, and ways to move beyond death. The path no longer led to another realm *within* the cosmos; it now crossed the cosmos (symbolized as the ocean of *saṃsāra*, characterized by the cycles of time, rebirth, finitude, suffering, and ignorance) to liberation.

One of the Vedic texts that elaborated on the ritual, the Śatapatha Brāhmaṇa, said the Vedic sacrifice was a boat; the priests, oars; and the patron, a passenger who would reach heaven if no error were made in performing the ritual (4.5.10). Sacrifice also became a way of overcoming death by moving beyond *saṃsāra*, the cycles of death and rebirth (2.3.3.7). A personification of death demanded what would happen to him. He was told by the other gods that he had dominion over the body but not over immortality, which would occur without him. In other words, the god of death controlled the process and time of dying, but he could not influence those who attained enlightenment because they were beyond the cycles of death and rebirth (10.4.3.1–9).

In the *Upaniṣads* (philosophical speculations said to reveal the supreme truth of the Vedas but, from a historical perspective, beginning the transformation of Vedic religion to Hinduism), this extracosmic liberation (*mokṣa*) was characterized by the realization of eternal consciousness, called Brahman. This could be achieved during life; at death the body would disappear forever. Or it could be achieved by a postmortem passage to a supreme heaven where there would be eternal life with a supreme God. Some Upaniṣadic texts spoke of sacrifice leading to the path of the forefathers (*pitṛyāna*) and thus to rebirth (indicating a demotion of the status of Vedic rituals), whereas others spoke of self-knowledge leading to the path of the gods (*devayāna*). Still others spoke of a passage to liberation made possible by religious discipline (*sādhana*) and the guidance of a teacher (guru) leading to supreme knowledge. This notion was expressed as a boat guided by a pilot, ferrying the individual across to the other shore. In *Kauṣītaki Upaniṣad* 1.4, for example, the deceased proceeded to the river Vijarā (literally, "apart from old age", shaking off their good and bad deeds. Their good deeds were transferred to relatives for a better rebirth; their bad ones, to other people. Beyond deeds and dualities, the deceased approached the god Brahmá. Although the human body represented bondage, it also provided the only opportunity for liberation (an argument that was probably necessary to inspire humans to pursue a path to liberation in this life, because they might be reborn as plants or animals).

Closely associated with this development was the law of karma, according to which actions (karma) determined destiny. People were reborn higher or lower in the scale of beings (from high-caste people down to plants), depending on the quantity of good (*puṇya*) or bad (*pāpa*) karma they had accumulated. With an excess of good karma, they had a temporary vacation in a paradise; with an excess of bad karma, they descended to a hellish realm. But with an extraordinary religious effort (based on knowledge or devotion), they could negate the law of karma by removing the bondage of action and the perpetual cycles of rebirth. Despite the highly individualistic nature of this karma doctrine (people reap what they sow), some versions allowed the transfer of merit from an extraordinary person, or divine grace from a deity, in order to redirect destiny and ultimately achieve liberation.

After the sixth century B.C.E., the idea of crossing over, signified in the term *tīrtha,* became associated with various bodies of water; these were sacred places where people could cross over to a better rebirth, a vacation in a cosmic paradise (*svarga*), or liberation beyond the cosmos (*mokṣa*). To facilitate crossing over, they followed a religious path characterized by action (*karmayoga*), knowledge (*jñānayoga*), and devotion (*bhaktiyoga*); different schools order the three in different ways.

Even today, most Hindus want to die on the banks of the Ganges—believed to be the river of heaven, the nectar of immortality, a goddess, a mother, or even a physician, since this allows them to cross over to liberation. From all parts of India, the dying come to Banaras to live on its banks. They spend their final days in a hospice where spiritual help but no medicine is provided. Hearing the names of the gods chanted continually, they eat sacred *tulsī* leaves and drink Ganges water, focusing their thoughts exclusively on God. Śiva, Lord of Death, whispers the ferryboat mantra into their ears. After they die, their corpses are taken to the cremation ground, given a final bath in the Ganges, decked with garlands of flowers, and honored as a guest or deity. Then the last sacrifice (*antyeṣṭi*) is performed. The eldest son circumambulates the corpse counterclockwise (reversal symbolizing death) and lights the pyre. Relatives are silent, for wailing is inauspicious or even painful for the dead. Finally, the eldest son turns his back to the pyre, throws water over his shoulders to douse the embers, and leaves the pyre without looking back. For the next eleven days, during the performance of the *śrāddha* rituals, ideally at Banaras or another holy place, rice balls are offered to the dead; on the twelfth day, the departed soul reaches its destination (Eck). It is said that when people die in Banaras, their souls attain liberation—though the idea that transitional souls (*preta*) are transformed into ancestors (*pitr*) is also maintained, as are a host of other ideas about destiny.

If dying by the Ganges is impossible, dying at some other *tīrtha* in India may be a substitute, for the Ganges is said to be there, too, just as all rivers are said to be in the Ganges. And if even that is impossible, simply thinking about the Ganges at the moment of death may influence destiny. Casting the bones that remain after cremation into a *tīrtha* is also effective. Ascetics are buried, however, because

they have given up their ś₍rauta fires (the locus of the Vedic rituals) and their sacrificial implements (Kane). Hindus perform the annual sraddha ceremonies for the dead (offering rice balls to three generations of male ancestors, pitṛs) at the Ganges or any other *tīrtha,* since this will either sustain the ancestors until rebirth as humans or allow them a long vacation as gods (*viśvadeva*) in heaven. In short, the Hindu tradition offers a number of safeguards against annihilation at death: rebirth, a visit to another realm, liberation. Individuals can influence destiny or others can help them by the transfer of merit. Gods, through their grace, also may influence an individual's destiny. There is always hope. The sting is taken out of death, for it is said that even mosquitoes are liberated in Banaras (Eck).

THE CONCEPT OF SELF-WILLED DEATH IN HINDUISM. According to the traditional law books, funeral rituals were not to be performed for those who died in unnatural ways. This may have been used as a deterrent against suicide; the Hindu tradition disapproved of suicide, which was defined as killing oneself because of depression, passion, or uncontrollable circumstance. But unnatural death was not always viewed negatively; death by violence (war, murder, or accident) was viewed as powerful, leading to heaven or deification. The type of unnatural death that has relevance for bioethics is the self-willed death, which is given religious sanction. During the late classical and medieval periods, Hinduism came to accept a rational decision either (1) to kill oneself as a way to destroy bad karma, create good karma, and thus attain heaven or liberation; or (2) if liberated in life, to remove the body. Such self-willed death (*iṣṭamṛtyu*), took many forms. People could walk without food or drink until they dropped dead (*mahāprasthāna*); bury themselves alive and meditate (*samādhimāraṇa*); abstain from food and wait in a seated posture for the approach of death (*prāyopaveśana*); or jump into fire, over a cliff, into sacred water, or under the wheels of a temple cart. The terminally ill and the extremely old who were no longer able to perform their religious duties and rituals sometimes killed themselves by one of these methods. Such self-willed death was religiously permitted. *Sati* (a woman's self-immolation on the funeral pyre of her husband) was a variant of self-willed death that produced a surplus of merit that ensured heaven for both spouses. Despite efforts to prevent abuse, it appears that there was some, for by the tenth century, with the Kalivarjya Prohibitions, all forms of killing oneself—*except sati*—were prohibited (in theory though not in practice).

Some families continued to endorse *sati* because the alternative was lifelong support for widows or, as in Bengal, a share in the inheritance. After additional criticism by both Muslims and Christians in the following centuries, this practice virtually ended. The Indian Penal Code in 1860 made suicide and abetting suicide crimes; judges interpreted suicide as any form of self-willed death and used that interpretation to stop *sati* as well as other practices of self-willed death (Young, 1989). There have been isolated incidents since then, including the widely publicized case of Roop Kanwar in 1987. Almost 160 years after *sati* was declared culpable homicide, Roop Kanwar, an eighteen-year-old Rajasthani woman, performed *sati*. The government alleged that she was forced onto the pyre and pinned down with heavy firewood. This caused the Indian parliament to pass another law in December 1987 to check the practice. According to the new law, the death penalty is imposed for those who help carry out the ritual of *sati*; the woman who tries to perform *sati* may be sentenced to six months in jail; those who glorify *sati* may be given prison sentences up to seven years; and the government is empowered to dismantle memorials and temples related to *sati*. Accordingly, her brother-in-law, who lit the pyre, was charged with murder and twenty-two others received lesser charges.

IMPLICATIONS OF HINDU VIEWS OF DEATH FOR BIOETHICS. According to the *Caraka Saṁhitā* (a classical text on medicine with religious legitimation written about the first century B.C.E.), physicians were not to treat incurable diseases (a policy to establish the benefits of the fledgling science of medicine and to protect the physician's reputation as a healer). This refusal could provide traditional religious legitimation for modern withdrawal of treatment by physicians in cases of terminal disease.

Physicians also were not to reveal the possibility of impending death, unless there was a specific request, so that negative thoughts would not be imposed on the patient that might create bad karma and hasten death. Rather, the process of death should be peaceful and auspicious, because it was the prelude to rebirth or final liberation. The implication of this view for modern medicine is that pain relief provided by a physician might make the dying process peaceful and therefore auspicious in Hindu terms; however, the refusal to inform the patient about terminal illness unless directly asked would be against the modern concept of mandatory truth-telling by the physician and the patient's right to know the prognosis. But another view also existed in traditional Indian religions: a person's last thought influences destiny. In this case, the individual should know of impending death and should not allow anything to cloud the mind. The implication of this view for modern medicine is that pain relief should be given only to the extent that the person remains alert.

Finally, the long tradition of self-willed death, especially fasting to death, in cases of terminal illness or debilitating old age, can be used to give religious legitimation for refusal or withdrawal of treatment in modern India, for it accords with the voluntary and public nature of living wills requesting refusal or withdrawal of treatment and nutrition. Whether it will be used to invoke precedent for active euthanasia depends on the assessment of assistance and whether there had been a slippery slope in the practice of self-willed death. As for the first issue, the Hindu tradition was quite careful to insist on the voluntary nature of self-willed death, though once there was a public declaration and the person could not be discouraged from his or her decision, assistance was allowed, at least in the case of *sati*. For instance, priests were allowed to hold a woman down during her self-immolation if they had been convinced that the decision for *sati* had been her own. As for the second issue, the types of self-willed death and possibly their numbers increased over the centuries; since there was criticism of the practice internal to the religion by the tenth century, there was probably the perception of a slippery slope.

Jainism

THE CONCEPT OF NATURAL DEATH. Jainism is an Indian religion that developed about the sixth century B.C.E. The Jains speak of the twenty-four *tīrthaṅkaras,* such as their founder Mahāvīra, who are the makers of the path or causeway to liberation, enabling people to cross over *saṁsāra.* The Jain view of death is related to its view of liberation: Because karmas (actions) cause bondage in the cycles of existence (reincarnation), they should be eliminated by fasting and meditation leading to the realization of liberation, the radical autonomy of pure consciousness (*kaivalya*).

THE JAIN CONCEPT OF SELF-WILLED DEATH. According to tradition, Mahāvīra fasted to death. Henceforth, the ideal form of death for Jain monastics was a "final fast" to death known by different names—*bhaktapratyākhyāna, inginī, prāyopagamana, samādhi, pañcapada, sallekhanā, ārādhanā*—depending on variants in the practice such as whether there is the assistance of others, whether one dies meditating or chanting, whether the body is to be eliminated by emasculation after initiation, or whether death occurs after the attainment of wisdom (Settar, 1990). Jainism was the first Indian religion to legitimate self-willed death. Initially, the fast to death was to be done only by monastics late in life but before debilitating old age or terminal illness, so that they would be in full control of the meditative and fasting process. Some centuries later, however, the practice was extended to the Jain laity as a legitimate form of death in times of public crisis (natural calamities and military defeat) or personal crisis (debilitating old age and terminal illness).

IMPLICATIONS OF JAIN VIEWS OF DEATH FOR BIOETHICS.

Although self-willed death is illegal in India, Jains are arguing for the decriminalization of suicide so that they can restore the traditional practice of fasting to death. They argue that this practice legitimates refusal or withdrawal of nutrition and life-support systems in modern medical contexts for the terminally ill. They also argue that prolongation of the dying process is immoral, because it increases suffering or depletes the resources of the family or community; thus the fast to death is a way to "permit oneself the honour of dying without undue prolongation of the process" (Bilimoria). But since the fast to death was also practiced traditionally in nonmedical contexts, it was not always a way to avoid the prolongation of dying; on the contrary, it was a way of hastening death by the cultural act of fasting when the body was not about to die of natural causes. Although the fast to death was generally understood to be voluntary and planned (and in a category distinct from both homicide and suicide), there were several exceptions. According to some, severely handicapped newborns were allowed to die (*bālamarana*) when permission was given by parents or a preceptor. In the *Bhāva Pāhuḍa Ṭīku*, *bālamarana* is classified as: "The death of the ignoramus, or a foolish process of meeting death … *Bāla* means childish, undeveloped, or yet-to-be-developed, premature and silly" (Settar, 1990, p. 15). It includes the death of infants and those who have an infantile knowledge—who are ignorant, who do not understand the moral codes, or who have a wrong notion of the faith and kill themselves by fire, smoke, poison, water, rope, suffocation, or jumping. While the original classification indicated simply a subdivision of natural death that would lead to rebirth, it seems that at some point in the tradition or perhaps in the modern period, the classification *bāla-marana* has been reinterpreted. Accordingly, Bilimoria (reporting on statements made by Jain informants) observes that

> in principle there appeared to be no reason why a child afflicted with or suffering from the kinds of conditions described earlier should not be given the terminal fast (*sallekhanā*). Parental permission would be required where there is contact, failing which a preceptor (for instance in an ashram) may be in a position to make a pronouncement. Consent of the recipient is not necessary (hence, a case of *nonvoluntary* terminal fast). One who has fallen in a state of unconsciousness, again, can be given the fast … even if the person had made no requests while she was conscious, though parents or kin would be consulted. It seemed evident that 'consent,' either of the individual or a proxy, or of the parent, does not seem to be a necessary condition for commending [a] final fast. This would seem to constitute a case of *involuntary sallekhanā*.… When … asked whether it would be acceptable to inject lethal poison to bring on the impending death, the response was that under extreme conditions where the pain and suffering is unendurable and not abating.… (p. 347)

It is argued by Jains that the history of fasting to death demonstrates that self-willed death need not lead to other forms of self-willed or other-willed death. While it is true that in the past there were a number of safeguards (permission of the head of the monastery, a formal public vow, established ascetic discipline, evidence of courage and will rather than cowardice) and the history of fasting to death was without any extreme abuse in India, there was still a change in the number of groups involved (from monastics to lay people) indicating extension or popularization of the practice. Moreover, the fact that Jainism was the first Indian religion to legitimate a form of self-willed death means that it set an example, which may have inspired legitimation of self-willed death without such careful safeguards by other Indian religions (Young, 1989). In other words, its indirect contribution to a slippery slope in Indian religions cannot be ruled out despite Jain disclaimers. When the Indian penal code made suicide illegal, fasting to death was included. Despite the fact that any form of self-willed death is still illegal in India, there are between six and ten reported Jain fasts to death annually (Bilimoria).

Buddhism

THE CONCEPT OF NATURAL DEATH.

The imagery of crossing the ocean or river of *saṁsāra* to the other shore of enlightenment is used by Buddhists as well as Hindus. Theravāda (one of the main branches of Buddhism, which purportedly continues the early tradition and is still found in Sri Lanka, Burma, Thailand, Cambodia, and Vietnam) metaphorically considers the Buddha's teaching (*dhamma*) a boat and the individual its pilot. For instance, in Burma, a coin called "ferry fare" is placed in the mouth of a dead person (Spiro).

The Buddha thought often about the nature of death. According to Aśvaghosa's version of his life, the *Buddhacarita,* the future Buddha was surrounded by royal luxury as a youth, sealed off from the real world in a palace. When he finally ventured into the world, he was overwhelmed by his first sight of a sick person, an old person, and a dead person. These shocking revelations about dimensions of human existence beyond anything he had known so troubled him that he left his life of ease to become an ascetic and search for meaning. Later, on the verge of enlightenment, he recalled his own previous lives, meditated on the cycles of rebirth common to all creatures, and came to understand that all beings are propelled into repeated lives by ignorance and desire. The Buddha spent his life teaching others how to blow out (*nibbāna*) the flame of ignorance and desire by realizing that all beings are composite and impermanent (subject to suffering, decay, and death). In the final analysis, there was no "person" who died; there was only the process of dying. As narrated in the *Mahāparinibbāna Sutta,* written down about the first century B.C.E., the Buddha attained final release from his body (*parinibbāna*) at the age of eighty. After falling ill, he chose the time and place of his departure: Telling those present that all composite things must pass away and advising them to strive diligently for liberation, he meditated with complete equanimity and took his last breath.

Despite the Buddha's emphasis on liberation, subsequent generations of monks and nuns took precautions in case they were to be reborn. The *Mulāsarvāstivāda-vinaya* (a text composed at the end of the seventh century) describes the monastic funeral: A gong was sounded; the body was taken to the cremation ground and honored; verses on impermanence were recited; merit from this act was transferred to the deceased, suggesting extra insurance in case the monastic was to be reborn; ownership of property was transferred; and cremation was performed. Finally, Buddhist sacred monuments (*stūpa* or *caitya*) were worshipped by the living, who then took a sacred bath (Schopen). Laypeople tried to attain a better rebirth by practicing morality, accumulating merit, reflecting on the nature of suffering, and disengaging from activities during old age. They were helped by merit transferred to them through the religious activities of families and friends, especially during the dying process, the funeral, and subsequent ancestral rituals.

As in Hinduism, the moment of death was important, because the final thought influenced rebirth. Even today, according to the popular religion of Burma, relatives chant Buddhist texts or have monks chant the *paritta,* canonical verses for protection against danger, to calm those who are dying; good thoughts thus arise and lead them either to a better rebirth or to a heavenly reward (Spiro). In popular forms of Theravāda Buddhism, ideas of the soul often replace the doctrine of no soul (*anatta*). The soul, or ghost, lurks around the house for some days after death and must be ritually fed, placated, and induced to leave the world of the living. Death rituals, ideally involving food and gifts for the monks, not only eliminate the danger posed by a ghost but also allow for the transfer of merit to the dead person, as do rituals performed by relatives on the anniversaries of the death.

Mahāyāna (the other main branch of Buddhism, which originated in India but eventually became popular in Tibet, China, Korea, and Japan) also conceives of the teaching as a boat, but views the pilot as a *bodhisattva,* a salvific figure who refuses enlightenment until all sentient creatures are saved, graciously steering the boat across to the other shore. Nevertheless, Mahayana maintains that ultimately there is no boat, no pilot, and no shore, since all is nothingness (*śunyatā*).

In Tibet, monastics meditated on death and simulated the process of dying to attain enlightenment; they also protected themselves against a bad rebirth by certain funerary rituals. Laypeople focused mainly on rebirth and sought help to ensure a good destiny. A spiritual teacher performed the ritual *gzhan po wa,* by which a disciple went to a paradise. Or the *Tibetan Book of the Dead,* which describes the journey from the moment of death through an intermediate state to rebirth, was read to the deceased over a number of days. Each of the three stages, or *bardos,* offered an experience of past karma along with a vision of both peaceful and wrathful divine figures. These provided more opportunities to attain enlightenment (Buddhahood) or a better rebirth, even though each succeeding one was more difficult than the last. Only by recognizing that the deities were ultimately illusory, for all was emptiness (*śunyatā*), would one attain liberation. These beliefs and practices are still found in Tibetan communities.

In China, Mahayana views of death were reinterpreted in several ways: (1) The notion of heaven was modeled on both Daoist ideas of paradise and its images of Confucian kingdoms complete with palaces, courts, and bureaucracy; the notion of hell was based on Daoist hells and Confucian prisons. (2) Some Chinese argued that the existence of a soul was implied in the theory of reincarnation, in the storehouse of consciousness, or in the Buddhahood of all living creatures. (3) Transferring merit from monastics or relatives became extremely popular. Buddhist monks instituted the annual All Souls festival based on the story of Maudgalyāyana (Mu-lien), who rescued his mother from the lowest hell, as told in the *Ullambana Sūtra* of Central Asian origin (Smith). Food, clothing, and other gifts were offered to rescue seven generations of ancestors from their sufferings in various hells, and the story was reenacted at Chinese funerals (Berling). (4) Pure Land Buddhism, which became particularly popular in China, promoted, in some versions, an otherworldly paradise attained through faith in Amida (a savior whose grace allows people to be reborn in a paradise called the Land of Bliss until they reach *nirvāṇa*) and calling out his name at the moment of death. According to Pure Land philosophers, this paradise was not real, however, but a product of the mind. (5) Ch'an claimed that the Buddha nature was in all sentient beings, truth was near at hand, and Earth was the Lotus Land; enlightenment was the realization that nothing existed beyond the realm of *saṃsāra*. Consequently, death meant reabsorption into nature.

Just as Chinese Buddhism had absorbed Daoist ideas of death and native Confucian ancestor worship, so Japanese Buddhism assimilated, in turn, native Shintō views of death and ancestor worship. According to ancient Shintō, death was a curse; the corpse, polluting; and the spirit of the deceased, frightening. Buddhism contributed rituals to purify the spirits of the dead and transform them into gods: Spirits were deified thirty-three years after death and henceforth worshipped with the Shintō *kami* (entities with a spiritual function that inspire awe). In the seventh century, Empress Saimei ordered that the *Ullambana Sūtra* be taught in all the temples of the capital and that offerings be made on behalf of the spirits of the dead. The Japanese version of the All Souls festival, called Bon, dates from this time. The association of Buddhism with ancestor worship was reinforced in the anti-Christian edicts of the seventeenth century, which insisted on the formal affiliation of every Japanese household with a Buddhist temple and its death rituals (Smith).

Modern Japanese Buddhism has been primarily associated with death: In addition to funerals, there are seventh-day, monthly, hundredth-day, seventh-month, and annual rituals (Smith). Besides these, the collectivity of the spirits of the household dead is given daily offerings and honored at festival times. The Japanese hold conflicting opinions about where the spirits live: (1) Spirits may live peacefully in ancestor tablets on the altar in the home. (2) As depicted in Nō plays, those who suffered tragedy during life or died violently haunt their graves or former homes. (3) Spirits may have a continued existence as buddhas. Curiously, the dead are referred to as buddhas (*hotoke*). The Japanese misunderstood the term *nibbāna,* "to blow out" (in Japanese, *nehan*). Whereas in Indian Buddhism it expressed the metaphorical idea of blowing out the flames of desire in life and thereby achieving enlightenment, in Japanese Buddhism it was understood literally: People attained continued existence as buddhas when life was "blown out," a euphemism for death (Smith); this may have inspired self-willed death. (4) By chanting Amida's mantra (according to Hōnen) or having faith in him (according to Shinran), spirits enter paradise. (5) Spirits go to mountains such as Osore or Morinoyama with its Sōtō Zen and Jōdo-shin shrines. Many of these beliefs and rituals are dying out. The breakdown of the extended family due to mobility and urbanization has contributed to the lessening of interest in ancestor worship.

Now, memory and prayers are for the immediate ancestors; tablets and altars, therefore, are becoming smaller (Smith).

BUDDHIST VIEWS OF SELF-WILLED DEATH. Despite his discussion of the body as the locus of suffering, the Buddha did not endorse self-willed death for everyone. He himself lived out his natural life span. An incident is recorded in the *Pārājika* (a text of the Pāli Canon, the scripture of Theravāda Buddhism) about how, when some monks became depressed in their meditation on the impurity of their bodies, a sham monk encouraged them—up to sixty in one day—to take their lives or be killed by him so that they could cross *saṃsāra* immediately. When he heard about this, the Buddha changed the form of meditation to a breathing exercise and declared that intentionally encouraging or assisting another person to die would lead to expulsion from the monastery. The Buddha also condemned, on the basis of nonviolence (*ahimsā*), any monk who told people to do away with their wretched lives. It is possible that the Buddha, known as the "good physician," allowed one exception to this general principle: From the accounts of the cases of Vakkali, Godhika, Channa, Assaji, Anāthapiṇḍika, and Dīghāvu, it seems that if people were experiencing unbearable pain in dying, they could kill themselves. There is some controversy over such an interpretation, however, for good palliative care had been offered and there were serious attempts to dissuade people from taking their lives. Moreover, neither the Buddha nor the monks gave explicit permission for these monastics and laypeople to take their lives, although the account implies that the act was condoned, perhaps because there were no options aside from physical force to restrain them.

According to an observation of I-Ching, a Chinese pilgrim who traveled to India (671–695), the practice of self-willed death was not popular among the Buddhists in India. Several centuries later, however, its popularity may have grown. In China, some Buddhist monks chose the time, place, and manner of death to bring its uncertainty under their control. It is possible that a story in the *Saddharmapuṇḍarīka* about how the *bodhisattva* Bhaisajyarāja, who was so dissatisfied with his worship that he set himself on fire, may have inspired the Chinese practice. But the fact that Chinese monks fasted to death in a yogic posture in underground pits (as in the Indian *samādhimāraṇa*), and after death their bodies were smoked, wrapped, lacquered, and installed in temples as objects of great veneration (Welch), suggests a different Indian Buddhist influence. This may have been combined with Daoist techniques to achieve immortality. Finally, it has been argued that self-willed death was popularized in China by a misunderstanding of Pure Land Buddhism, which suggested that people should kill themselves to reach the Pure Land more quickly. Shan-Tao's disciple, for example, jumped out of a tree to reach the Pure Land (Kato).

Some sects of Japanese Pure Land continued this idea. Kūya (903–972) and Ippen (1239–1289), both charismatic leaders among the masses, killed themselves by drowning in order to reach the Pure Land. Before his death Ippen instigated Nyudo to drown while meditating on Amida (a story illustrated on many scrolls). Ippen's death prompted six disciples to drown in sympathy. These examples were further popularized by a tradition of drowning to reach the Pure Land; ordinary people who lost their nerve would be hauled ashore by a rope attached around their waist (Becker). Devotees were told to "Delight in dying" and "Hasten your death" (Kato).

These Pure Land practices inspired more secular forms of self-willed death. There are over forty-five terms in Japanese to describe the various forms of self-willed death; for example, the tradition of parents killing first their children and then themselves to avoid further suffering; the tradition of abandoning old women in distant mountains; and the tradition of *joshi* or love-killing, also known as *oshinjuo* or *aitai-shi* (a death pact between two people, such as lovers who want to attain a happier realm) (Kato). Such practices (which also included death by fasting or fire), collectively called *shashinojo*, came under scrutiny by subsequent Pure Land leaders who argued that such acts of self-willed death were a denial of Amida's grace.

Some views held by Zen leaders may have been misinterpreted, inspiring self-willed death; Dogen, for example, says to throw away your "body-mind." Zen inspired the samurai warriors and helped them cultivate a stoicism to face death. In medieval Japan, *harakiri* or *seppuku* was practiced by warriors to expiate crimes, apologize for errors, escape disgrace, redeem friends, or express devotion to their master by following him in death. These forms of warrior self-willed death are similar to the forms of heroic death by warriors in India. Sometimes *seppuku* was assisted by a relative or friend. By the Tokugawa period (1603–1867), it involved an elaborate ceremony and, for the famous, burial in a Buddhist tomb.

The popularity of self-willed death in Japan may have been derived in part from ancient Shintō views of death. The lack of a definitive boundary between life and death led to a feeling of intimacy with death and a desire to take refuge in holistic being, understood as *kami* (nature). This Shintō idea was combined with the concept of the Dao (the transcendent and immanent reality of the universe, represented by vacuity or emptiness because of its being formless and imperceptible) or the concept of the Buddha as nothingness

(*śunyatā*), pure consciousness, or nature. It was also combined with the Buddhist idea of life as suffering and transience, which could be escaped by attaining the Pure Land (Kato).

The Buddhist practice of self-willed death has acquired political significance in the modern period. Known as "falling down like cherry blossoms" or "dying with a smile" (Kato), this way of dying belonging to *bushido,* the way of the warriors, contributed to the psychology of the Japanese kamikaze pilots of World War II. In Vietnam, the monk Thich Quang Duc's selfimmolation in Saigon (1963) focused world attention on the plight of the Vietnamese under Ngo Dinh Diem's oppressive regime.

IMPLICATIONS OF BUDDHIST VIEWS OF DEATH FOR BIOETHICS. Assessments of the importance of Buddhist views of death for bioethics vary considerably, depending on whether Theravāda or Mahāyāna is the focus and what the commentator thinks about issues such as withdrawal of treatment and euthanasia. Pinit Ratanakul (1988) observes, for instance, that in Thailand the Buddhist principle of the sanctity of life is maintained and self-willed death is not condoned as a rule, even in cases of pain and suffering. Two reasons are given: (1) suffering is a way for bad karma to come to fruition rather than be transferred to the next life; and (2) a person who assists suicide or performs euthanasia will be affected by such an act, since it involves repugnance toward suffering and his or her own desire to eliminate that which arouses a disagreeable sensation. But one exception is allowed: self-willed death when incurably ill, in order to attain enlightenment. These comments suggest that Thailand has maintained a reluctance to endorse self-willed death, in line with its Theravāda tradition, but continues to acknowledge the precedent established by the cases of the terminally ill Vakkali, Godhika, Channa, and others reported in the Palī Canon.

Current Japanese views show a greater acceptance of euthanasia, which is to be predicted, given the history of self-willed death in Japanese Buddhism. It is striking that the modern word for euthanasia is *anraku-shi* (literally, "ease—pleasure—death"), also a name for the Pure Land, though now some Japanese prefer the term *songen-shi* (death with dignity). Carl B. Becker, a Western scholar who has discussed this topic with Japanese people, argues that the Buddha accepted or condoned "many" cases of suicide but gives only three examples. He also argues that Buddhists view death as a transition, not an end; therefore, it is the state of mind at the moment of death that is important, not whether the body lives or dies. Those who are not fruitful members of society should be able to die, according to his assessment of Japanese views. Once consciousness (which he takes as brain activity) has permanently dissociated itself from the body, there is no reason to maintain the body, "for the body deprived of its *skandhas* [the constituents of human existence] is not a person" (Becker, p. 554). In short, all that matters is clarity of mind at the moment of death. We must be careful in using Becker's analysis of the data. In point of fact, the Buddha was very reluctant to condone self-willed death if indeed he did so; it was only a few people who possibly killed themselves with the Buddha's blessing, because they were suffering from terminal illness and because they desired enlightenment. The other examples were simply threats. Becker also ignores the fact that the Buddha called the mere encouragement for others to perform self-willed death—or to provide the means—a deplorable act that would lead to expulsion from the monastery. One traditional commentator on the Parajita includes poison in the list of means. Because Buddhist monks were often physicians in ancient India, it is noteworthy that they were told not to perform abortions nor provide the means or even information to facilitate it; moreover, they must not help a family to kill a physically dependent member. This amounts to a strong position against physician-assisted suicide.

Shigeru Kato is much more cautious in his assessment of the Japanese practice of self-willed death and current Japanese interest in self-willed death, but for different reasons. After noting that some prominent Japanese jurists are advocating the legalization of euthanasia, he reflects on Japan's reputation of being "a kingdom of suicides" and relates the fact that it has the largest number of suicides among all Buddhist countries to its tendency to beautify suicide or absolve it of a sense of wrong. Kato argues that "Human beings have no right to manipulate arbitrarily and selfishly their 'own' lives, which are transiently borrowed and must be returned soon to the holistic Being" (p. 71). He opines that "We can never dismiss this religious holism as an outdated superstition; we must keep it as a brake against the drive toward euthanasia" (pp. 78–79). He also looks to the formation of a better hospice organization in Japan in the 1980s as a way of resolving the "euthanasia problem" through the practice of withdrawal of treatment combined with dialogue and religious and aesthetic care. In the final analysis, however, he is willing to entertain active euthanasia as the right to die "with dignity" and to consider the merits of each case.

Confucianism and Daoism

CONCEPTS OF NATURAL DEATH. Confucian concepts of death are closely associated with ancestor worship, which was practiced as early as the first historical dynasty, the Shang (ca. 1500–1045/1046 B.C.E.). Judging from the written record provided by inscriptions of oracles written on bones, the dead were consulted by means of divination, as if they were living. Everything needed for the next life was put in the tombs of the kings and nobles. Originally servants, entertainers, and others were buried with them. Later, pottery figures were substituted. (In modern times, paper effigies of servants are used.) The cult of the ancestors must also have been practiced by commoners, because it was considered an ancient and widespread practice by Confucius in the sixth century B.C.E.

The ancestor cult was based on rituals, or *li*. It assumed the continuity of life after death, communication between the living and the dead, the legitimacy of a social hierarchy, and a virtual deification of the ancestors. In his *Analects,* Confucius upheld the ancient practices, refusing to shorten the period of mourning (XVII.21). Nevertheless, he taught that the spirits should be kept at a distance, so as not to preoccupy the living (VII.20; XI.11). He also thought that mourning rituals should be moderate; they should express grief rather than fear (III.3). Four centuries later, details of the mourning rituals were described in the ritual text *Yi Li.* Now elaborate, they were to last for three years. During the first year, the eldest son (as chief mourner) had to wear sackcloth, live in a hut outside the home, wail periodically, and eat very little food. Over the next two years, the restrictions were gradually lifted. Even after life returned to normal, though, he reported family business to the ancestors. In Confucianism, as in other patrilineal traditions, the performance of funerary and ancestral rites by the eldest son has contributed to a preference for sons. As a result, female infanticide has sometimes been practiced unofficially.

The Chinese developed two other perspectives on death: a return to nature and physical immortality. The Daoist philosopher Chuang Tzu (365–290 B.C.E.) wrote that life and death were two aspects of the same reality, mere differences of form. Death was a natural and welcomed release from life, and was to be neither feared nor desired. Because individuals were reabsorbed into nature, both birth and death were as natural as the progression of the four seasons. Other Daoists were interested in alchemy, macrobiotic diets, exercises, fasting, and meditation. Besides desiring health, youth, and longevity, they wanted immortality. They had several views of the latter: the physical body would rise to heaven; the "real body," not the physical one in the tomb, would rise; the physical body would go to the Isles of the Blessed, said to be off the northeast coast of China; or the self would emerge from the body at death, like the butterfly from its cocoon, to wander freely about the universe or go to the realm of the immortals.

In Taiwan, the Chinese still practice ancestor worship. They believe that people are related to common ancestors and to each other by an elaborate kinship system in which status is symbolized by the length of time spent mourning and authority is passed through the eldest son. They also believe in two souls: the *hun,* living in a tablet at the shrine, and the *p'o,* living in the grave. Both souls may influence the living. Kin meet periodically in the ancestral temple for sacrifices to the *hun*; the latter are offered wine, food, rice, and first fruits in exchange for health, longevity, prosperity, offspring, virtue, and a peaceful death. They are also remembered by preserving extensive genealogical records and documents written by the deceased. Families visit graves to communicate with or pay respect to the *p'o* and thus ensure the *p'o*'s goodwill toward the living.

The Taiwanese euphemistically call death "longevity"; after fifty, a person begins to prepare for death by making "longevity clothes" in the Han style of the second century B.C.E., a coffin, and if possible, a tomb. At the time of death, the eldest son of the deceased person eats "longevity noodles" and puts on the "longevity clothes" inside out. Then he puts these garments on the corpse, whose personal name henceforth may not be spoken. Other family members don sackcloth, leave their hair uncombed, and wail periodically (Thompson). The *hun* is first given a temporary resting place in a paper sword, placed in front of the corpse to receive prayers. After processions to and from the grave, this sword is transferred to a home shrine where the son and relatives offer it food. Finally it is burned, and the spirit is thus transferred to a permanent tablet in the shrine. To keep the *p'o,* the body's orifices are plugged. The body is then rubbed with an elixir, placed in a coffin, and buried. Sometimes it is placed in a strong, watertight tomb to prevent decay. Coffins and graves are positioned according to exact rules for magical protection. If mistreated, the *p'o* causes trouble and threatens to become a ghost (*kuei*). Ritual specialists are then asked to inspect the grave, coffin, or bones to see why the p'o is unhappy (Berling). Daoist and Buddhist priests participate in the rituals of families who can afford them. For instance, priests hold services for seven weeks, during which they chant and pray for the soul to pass quickly through purgatory. Clearly, the Taiwanese try to ensure every advantage for the soul by incorporating practices from many religions.

In Taiwan, death remains associated with the ancestor cult. In the People's Republic of China, by contrast, there have been attempts to reform and even destroy ancestor worship. Communists have argued that traditional funeral rites and customs are remnants of the feudal economy and social structure; those lower in the clan hierarchy are exploited, and women, who cannot attend banquets in the ancestral temple, are excluded. Mourning clothes, moreover, waste cotton; wooden coffins waste timber; graves and tombs waste land; lavish funerals put families into debt; and beliefs in the afterlife instill superstition. Consequently, Communists have recommended the following: simple memorial services for the cadre, factory, village, or cooperative; the replacement of mourning clothes by arm bands; and the introduction of cremation (MacInnis).

CHINESE CONCEPTS OF SELF-WILLED DEATH. Some of these concepts have already been discussed in the section on Buddhism. But it is important to point out that there were practices of self-willed death in the warrior circles of China as well. In fact, it was the obligation, not only the privilege of warriors to practice self-willed death under certain circumstances. This tradition, which had once been found among the elite, became common among the lower classes when warriors began to be recruited from them in the late Chou Dynasty. Later, members of the Mohist school of philosophy, which had links with the lower-class warriors, maintained a tradition of absolute loyalty to their leader. In one incident, eighty-three disciples followed their leader in death (Fung Yu-lan, p. 83).

IMPLICATIONS OF CHINESE VIEWS OF SELF-WILLED DEATH FOR BIOETHICS. According to a report by Shi Da Pu (1991), euthanasia in China, once a taboo topic, has been discussed since the 1980s in the magazine *Medicine and Philosophy*. After the controversial case of the active euthanasia of a patient named Xia in 1986, which led to a court case being filed by her two daughters against their brother, who had authorized it, the topic was hotly debated in the media. It was also debated by the Chinese Dialectical Institute and Beijing Medical Ethics Academy, which concluded that active euthanasia was permissible for patients with no hope of cure. When the widow of former premier Zhou En-lai wrote that euthanasia was a "proper point of dialectical materialism" in need of discussion, there followed even more public debate. Some argued that it represented the height of civilization because it was a pure act of freedom; others, that it was "the result of the infection in the area of medicine from sick Western customs and morality … sharply against our socialist ethical values" (Shi Da Pu, p. 133). In 1988, a survey of 400 people (health professionals and nonprofessionals) showed that 80 percent were in favor of euthanasia. Both withdrawal of treatment and active euthanasia are being quietly practiced; though they are illegal, no one has been charged. Shi Da Pu concludes that most experts in China think that euthanasia should be regarded as part of the agenda of modernization, that the country should develop appropriate legislation to legalize it, and that the press should be enlisted to spread the dialectical materialist teaching about it.

Conclusion

Four major views of natural death emerge when Asian religions are compared: (1) the cosmic, (2) the existential, (3) the familial, and (4) the natural. Hinduism has focused on the cosmic dimension of death, though it has also included the familial in connection with ancestor worship and the existential because of its long interaction with Buddhism. Buddhist views of death are existential in philosophical texts and some monastic circles; cosmic in the popular religion of both Theravāda and Mahāyāna countries; and familial (in countries with traditions of ancestor worship). Chinese religions emphasize the familial aspect of death, though cosmic dimensions are derived from Buddhism and popular Daoism, along with natural ones from philosophical Daoism.

Some of the Asian religions legitimated self-willed death (and sometimes assistance) in certain circumstances—such as a way to attain heaven or enlightenment, or a way to cope with a crisis such as terminal disease or extreme old age—as an exception to natural death. Although there were attempts to distinguish such self-willed death and assistance from suicide and homicide, respectively, some of the religions decided that the practice had created problems over time.

Each religion has a tendency to assimilate many, often contradictory, views, as if these provide extra antidotes against death. When views are too this-worldly—for example, the desire to eliminate suffering or mundane problems—or too otherworldly—for example, promises of easy heaven or liberation by self-willed death—premature death may occur. People, it seems, need to balance respect for the body and transcendence of it in order to live with health and purpose, thereby doing justice to their full humanity.

KATHERINE K. YOUNG (1995)

SEE ALSO: *Anthropology and Bioethics; Autonomy; Body: Cultural and Religious Perspectives; Buddhism, Bioethics in; Care; Compassionate Love; Confucianism, Bioethics in; Daoism, Bioethics in; Grief and Bereavement; Harm; Hinduism, Bioethics in; Holocaust; Human Dignity; Infanticide; Jainism, Bioethics in; Life; Life, Quality of; Life Sustaining Treatment and Euthanasia; Literature and Healthcare; Narrative; Paliative Care and Hospice; Pediatrics, Intensive Care in; Right to Die, Policy and Law; Sikhism, Bioethics in; Suicide; Virtue and Character; Warfare;* and other *Death* subentries

BIBLIOGRAPHY

Becker, Carl B. 1990. "Bioethics and Brain Death: The Recent Discussion in Japan." *Philosophy: East and West* 40(4): 543–556.

Berling, Judith A. 1992. "Death and Afterlife in Chinese Religion." In *Death and Afterlife: Perspectives of World Religions,* pp. 181–192, ed. Hiroshi Obayashi. New York: Greenwood Press.

Bilimoria, Purushottama. 1992. "A Report from India: The Jaina Ethic of Voluntary Death." *Bioethics* 6(4): 331–355.

Blackburn, Stuart H. 1985. "Death and Deification: Folk Cults in Hinduism." *History of Religions* 24(3): 255–274. Chicago: University of Chicago Press.

Caillat, Colette. 1977. "Fasting unto Death According to Ayaranga-Sutta and to Some Paninnayas." In *Mahavira and His Teachings,* pp. 113–117, ed. Adinath N. Upadhye et al. Bombay: Bhagavan Mahavira 2500th Nirvana Mahotsava Samiti.

Eck, Diana L. 1982. *Banaras: City of Light.* Princeton, NJ: Princeton University Press.

Fung Yu-lan. 1953. *History of Chinese Philosophy.* 2 vols. Princeton, NJ: Princeton University Press.

Fusé, Toyomasa. 1980. "Suicide and Culture in Japan: A Study of Seppuku as an Institutionalized Form of Suicide." *Social Psychiatry* 15: 57–63.

Gunaratna, V. F. 1966. *Buddhist Reflections on Death.* Kandy, Ceylon: Buddhist Publication Society.

Holck, Frederick H., ed. 1974. *Death and Eastern Thought: Understanding Death in Eastern Religions and Philosophies.* Nashville, TN: Abingdon Press.

Jaini, Padmanabh S. 1979. *The Jaina Path of Purification.* Berkeley: University of California Press.

Kaltenmark, Max. 1969. *Lao Tzu and Taoism,* tr. Roger Greaves. Stanford, CA: Stanford University Press.

Kane, Pandurang Vaman. 1968. *History of Dharmasastra: Ancient and Mediaeval Religious and Civil Law,* 2nd edition. Poona, India: Bhandkarkar Oriental Research Institute.

Kato, Shigeru. 1990. "Japanese Perspectives on Euthanasia." In *To Die or Not to Die? Cross-Disciplinary, Cultural, and Legal Perspectives on the Right to Choose Death,* pp. 85–102, ed. Arthur S. Berger and Joyce Berger. New York: Praeger.

Keith, Arthur Berriedale. 1961. "Suicide (Hindu)." In vol. 12 of *Encyclopaedia of Religion and Ethics,* pp. 33–35, ed. James Hastings, John A. Selbie, and Louis H. Gray. New York: Charles Scribner's Sons.

Lati, Rinbochay, and Hopkins, Jeffery. 1985. *Death, Intermediate State and Rebirth.* Ithaca, NY: Snow Lion.

Lay, Arthur Hyde. 1974. "A Buddhist Funeral in Traditional Japan." In *Religion in the Japanese Experience: Sources and Interpretations,* pp. 62–64, ed. H. Byron Earhart. Encino, CA: Dickenson.

Lincoln, Bruce. 1991. *Death, War, and Sacrifice: Studies in Ideology and Practice.* Chicago: University of Chicago Press.

Lodru, Lama. 1987. *Bardo Teachings: The Way of Death and Rebirth.* Ithaca, NY: Snow Lion.

MacInnis, Donald E., comp. 1972. *Religious Policy and Practice in Communist China: A Documentary Reader.* New York: Macmillan.

Mullin, Glenn H. 1985. *Death and Dying: The Tibetan Tradition.* London: Arkana.

Obayashi, Hiroshi, ed. 1992. *Death and Afterlife: Perspectives of World Religions.* New York: Greenwood Press.

Poussin, Louis de La Vallée. 1961. "Suicide (Buddhist)." In vol. 12 of *Encyclopaedia of Religion and Ethics,* pp. 24–26, ed. James Hastings, John A. Selbie, and Louis H. Gray. New York: Charles Scribner's Sons.

Pu, Shi Da. 1991. "Euthanasia in China: A Report." *Journal of Medicine and Philosophy* 16(2): 131–138.

Ratanakul, Pinit. 1988. "Bioethics in Thailand: The Struggle for Buddhist Solutions." *Journal of Medicine and Philosophy* 13(3): 301–312.

Reynolds, Frank E., and Waugh, Earle H., eds. 1977. *Religious Encounters with Death: Insights from the History and Anthropology of Religions.* University Park: Pennsylvania State University Press.

Schopen, Gregory. 1992. "On Avoiding Ghosts and Social Censure: Monastic Funerals in the *Mūlasarvāstivada-Vinaya.*" *Journal of Indian Philosophy* 20(1): 1–39.

Settar, Shadakshari. 1989. *Inviting Death: Indian Attitude Towards the Ritual Death.* Leiden: E. J. Brill.

Settar, Shadakshari. 1990. *Pursuing Death: Philosophy and Practice of Voluntary Termination of Life.* Dharward, India: Institute of Indian Art History, Karnatak University.

Sharma, Arvind; Ray, Ajit; Hejib, Alaka; and Young, Katherine K. 1988. *Sati: Historical and Phenomenological Essays.* Delhi: Motilal Banarsidass.

Smith, Robert J. 1974. *Ancestor Worship in Contemporary Japan.* Stanford, CA: Stanford University Press.

Spiro, Melford E. 1970. *Buddhism and Society: A Great Tradition and Its Burmese Vicissitudes.* New York: Harper and Row.

Thakur, Upendra. 1963. *The History of Suicide in India, an Introduction.* Delhi: Munshi-ram Manohar-lal.

Thapar, Romila. 1981. "Death and the Hero." In *Mortality and Immortality: The Anthropology and Archaeology of Death,* pp. 293–315, ed. Sarah C. Humphreys and Helen King. London: Academic Press.

Thompson, Laurence G. 1975. *Chinese Religion: An Introduction,* 2nd edition. Encino, CA: Dickenson.

Tilak, Shrinivas. 1987. *Religion and Aging in the Indian Tradition.* Albany: State University of New York Press.

Tukol, T. K. 1976. *Sallekhanā Is Not Suicide.* Ahmedabad: L. D. Institute of Indology.

Welch, Holmes. 1967. *The Practice of Chinese Buddhism: 1900–1950.* Cambridge, MA: Harvard University Press.

Wiltshire, Martin G. 1983. "The 'Suicide' Problem in the Pali Canon." In *Journal of the International Association of Buddhist Studies* 6(2): 124–140.

Woos, Fleur. 1993. "Pokkuri-Temples and Aging: Rituals for Approaching Death." In *Religion and Society in Modern Japan: Selected Readings;* ed. Mark R. Mullins, Shimazono Susumu, and Paul L. Swanson. Berkeley, CA: Asian Humanities Press.

Young, Katherine K. 1980. "*Tirtha* and the Metaphor of Crossing Over." *Studies in Religion* 9(1): 61–68.

Young, Katherine K. 1989. "Euthanasia: Traditional Hindu Views and the Contemporary Debate." In *Hindu Ethics: Purity, Abortion, and Euthanasia,* pp. 71–130, ed. Harold G. Coward, Julius J. Lipner, and Katherine K. Young. Albany: State University of New York Press.

Young, Katherine K. 1993. "Hindu Bioethics." In *Religious Methods and Resources in Bioethics,* pp. 3–30, ed. Paul F. Camenisch. Dordrecht, Netherlands: Kluwer.

Young, Katherine K. 1994. "A Cross-Cultural Historical Case Against Planned Self-Willed Death and Assisted Suicide." *McGill Law Journal* 39(3, Sept.).

III. WESTERN PHILOSOPHICAL THOUGHT

For both humankind generally and each living person individually, the recognition of the universality and inevitability of death is but the beginning of the problem of death. Indeed, recognizing death as the individual and collective fate of human beings, and of all living creatures, creates the problem of death: Why does it happen? What does it mean? Is death final? Is death a good thing or a bad thing? At least as often these questions emerge for us in their mirror image, still provoked by death: What is the meaning of life, its purpose? Can life be meaningful if it ends in death? What purposes could outlast the inevitability of my death?

Philosophers have struggled with a human fear of death. Recognizing the inevitability of death is very different from supposing death is final. At a very general level, philosophical reflections on death divide those who deny the finality of death and suppose there is ongoing, usually individual, self-consciousness after death, and those who regard bodily death as final, as the destruction of consciousness, but who offer consolation meant to assuage fear of the inevitability of personal extinction. A very few philosophers have found death to be inevitable, final, and horrible. What binds all together in a recognizably *Western* tradition are the analytically and argumentatively philosophical approaches each group takes and the exclusively human-centered character of their views.

Probably the single most persistent theme in Western philosophical reflection on death is the view that death is not the annihilation of the self but its transformation into another form of existence. The conviction that individual human beings survive death, perhaps eternally, has been very differently grounded and elaborated in the history of philosophy, but in some form has persisted and frequently dominated through antiquity, the long era of Christian theologizing, modernity, and into contemporary *postmodern* thinking. Considerably less attended to is the attempt to reconcile human beings to death's finality, to death as the end of individual human experiencing beyond which there exists no consciousness.

The Pre-Socratic Philosophers

The tension in Western philosophy between regarding death as transformation and thinking of death as final appears at the very outset of what is conventionally regarded as the beginning of Western philosophy, in the fragmentary remains of writing that have survived from thinkers in the early Greek colonies of Asia Minor, especially the Ionians. Anaximander (ca. 610–547 B.C.E.) and Heraclitus (ca. 533–475 B.C.E.) in particular were singularly impressed with the transitoriness of all things, as captured in the best-known corruption of a Heraclitean fragment, "One cannot step into the same river twice" (Kirk and Raven, fr. 217). The attempt to reconcile opposites—such as life and death—and to perceive the underlying unity, even harmony, in all of reality was preeminent for the pre-Socratics.

The very earliest surviving pre-Socratic fragment, from a book attributed to Anaximander, contains a passage that allows one to see both of the subsequent views about death—death as final and death as transitory—that have dominated Western thinking:

> And the source of coming-to-be for existing things is that into which destruction, too, happens, "according to necessity; for they pay penalty and retribution to each other for their injustice according to the assessment of Time." (Kirk and Raven, fr.112)

Jacques Choron, to whom all subsequent accounts of death in Western philosophy are indebted, reads this passage as evidence of how impressed Anaximander was with the terrible fact that things perish, but also as expressing the hope "that somewhere and somehow death shall have no dominion" (p. 35). Further, there is the suggestion that despite appearances, death is not annihilation: In the everlasting boundlessness (*aperion*), individual death is not meaningless, perhaps not even final.

In what is now southern Italy, Pythagoras (ca. 572–497 B.C.E.) struggled with these same realities, teaching that the soul suffered from embodiment, longed for release and reunion with the divine, possibly at death experienced transmigration into possibly other life forms, and could be purified in part through the process of rebirth. For the purification needed to overcome death and to be evermore united with the divine, it was most important to live a philosophical life, especially one that paid considerable attention to the contemplation of mathematical truth. This very abstract, highly intellectual element in Pythagoreanism distinguished it from the Orphic cults and Dionysian predecessors that so influenced it, and gave Pythagoreanism considerable appeal for Plato.

Continuity and change, constancy through flux, permanence and impermanence, death, extinction, and recurrence are the enduring concerns of pre-Socratic philosopher/ scientists. If, as mathematician and philosopher Alfred North Whitehead (1861–1947) has suggested, the whole of Western philosophy is but a series of footnotes to Plato, it might equally be said that the history of Western philosophy on death is but a series of footnotes to Plato's predecessors.

Socrates, Plato, and Aristotle

What we know of Socrates's (ca. 470–399 B.C.E.) view of death is largely detached from a theoretical context replete with ontological and metaphysical doctrines. His views seem to be rooted in the immediacy of his experience and circumstances, at a time when he is first anticipating, then under, a death sentence. It is the example Socrates sets, more than the words that Plato (or Xenophon) reports him to have said, that have influenced generations of students.

Early in *Apology* (29Aff.), Socrates is tentative in his assertions about death, saying only that "To be afraid of death is only another form of thinking that one is wise when one is not; it is to think that one knows what one does not know." Later, having been sentenced to death, Socrates ventures that death is either dreamless sleep from which, it seems, we do not awaken (annihilation) or transport to a place where we might ever after commune with those who precede us in death. The first is not fearsome; the second is to be joyfully celebrated (41B–42A). Socrates's deepest and most influential conviction, however, may have been that "Nothing can harm a good man, either in life or after death" (41D).

Socrates's courage and equanimity in the face of a manifestly unjust death sentence is universally admired. But exactly why he was so compliant with injustice at the end of his life is a continuing mystery (Momeyer, 1982).

Less mysterious is how Socrates could go from the cautious and skeptical views on death expressed in *Apology* to the far more metaphysically burdened opinions of *Phaedo*. The accepted explanation here is that in *Phaedo*, written later than *Apology* and *Crito*, Socrates has been transformed into a spokesperson for Plato (ca. 428–348 B.C.E.). As such, *Phaedo* is best read as the most complete case that Plato makes for his views on the immortality of the soul, with only the final death scene bearing any likely resemblance to Socrates's actual words.

Plato's view of death is inseparable from his doctrine of the soul, his identification of the soul with personhood, and ultimately the theory of Forms. Curiously, Plato's arguments are directed more to establishing the immortality of the soul than to the logically prior task of showing that the soul is the person. Whether the soul is identical to the person is a matter of continuing controversy in bioethical debates over the definition of death and criteria for personhood.

In *Phaedo,* Plato reminds readers that knowledge is recollection and shows that the soul must have existed before birth and embodiment in order for us to know most of what we do know during life. While this does not show that the soul survives death, it is suggestive in that it implies the soul's independence from the body. Other arguments attempt to show that the soul is *simple,* that is, not composed of parts and hence not subject to dissolution; that the soul resembles immortal gods in ruling the body; and that since the essence of the soul is life, it cannot admit of its negation or opposite any more than fire can be cold. Similarly, Plato holds that since the soul is capable of apprehending the eternal and immutable Forms or Ideas, it must be of a similar nature, eternal and divine.

It is not clear how seriously Plato intends most of these arguments to be taken, nor how seriously he himself takes them. But at least two central Platonic views are relevant and seriously maintained. The first is the reality of ideas, a domain of pure, unchanging essences the apprehension of which, however imperfect, is as close to real knowledge as living human beings can get. Second, Plato's suspicion of the body—construed by much later followers to be outright disdain—and his longing to be free of its burdens are consistent throughout his work. In Plato's judgment, intellectual pursuits are the most noble, but these are consistently and constantly hindered by bodily appetites and bodily limitations of sensory experience. Hence the true philosopher aspires to death, we are assured in *Phaedo,* and lives to die, in the expectation that only the soul's liberation from embodiment will make possible the fullest attainment of knowledge.

Plato's premier student began his own philosophizing in *Eudemos,* espousing Platonic views on the immortality of the soul and how individual selves survive death. Soon, however, Aristotle (384–322 B.C.E.) departed substantially from his mentor, and in *De anima* sees the soul as almost entirely physical, the entelechy of the body. More than being physically inseparable from the body, Aristotle argues, the soul is logically inseparable, as vision is logically inseparable from the seeing eye. The closest Aristotle will allow us to

come to immortality is in the same fashion other creatures experience it, in successive generations of progeny. (Aristotle, 1941).

Aristotle does allow for the possibility that part of the soul survives death, the part that distinguishes us from other animals: reason, our divine element. But Aristotle's writings on these matters are fraught with ambiguity, and it is not clear that he thinks there is any survival of individual personalities.

In any case, the strongest imperative for Aristotle is to live a life of reason, an important part of which requires one to overcome a natural fear of death through courage and virtue. It seems to be Aristotle's considered judgment that individual selves do not survive death, and no benign deity watches over us; yet life is still meaningful so long as we are awed by the beauty and order of nature, and meet life's misfortunes with courage and perseverance.

Aristotle's death in 322 B.C.E. brought an appropriate close to the Hellenic period of philosophizing and provided some of the central themes in reflections on death for the Hellenistic schools that followed. Chief among these were Epicureanism and Stoicism.

Hellenistic Schools: Epicureanism and Stoicism

Where death had been a distinctly secondary concern for Socratic thinking, it soon became a primary one for Hellenistic philosophers. For Epicurus, Lucretius, and Zeno, then Seneca, Epictetus, and Marcus Aurelius, discovering how to live life and confront death were the central tasks of philosophy.

Although Epicureans and Stoics differed on what they most valued in life, they equally valued attaining equanimity in the face of imminent death. Epicureans in particular saw no reason to fear death, believing that at death the soul, composed of the finest atoms, simply dissipated, so that there was nothing left to have experiences. Epicurus argued that one need not fear an unpleasant afterlife, for there was no afterlife; nor need one fear death as annihilation, for as soon as it occurred, one no longer existed to suffer anything. Epicurus's view is well captured in his memorable letter to Menoecus, in which he asserts:

> Death ... is nothing to us, since so long as we exist, death is not with us; but when death comes, then we do not exist. It does not then concern either the living or the dead, since for the former it is not, and the latter are no more. (Epicurus, 1926, p. 85)

Epicurus may well be on strong ground in urging us to regard death as final and afterlife as nonexistent, for this claim at least is supportable by overwhelming empirical evidence: People die, and they do not return. His second assurance, however—that the living need not fear death because once it occurs, they no longer exist to experience it—is far more problematic.

Epicurus's argument seems to be the following: Only that which is experienced can be evil and fearful. But death is a condition in which nothing is experienced, for the subject of experience no longer exists. Hence, it is unreasonable to fear death.

The problematic assumption here is that only that which is experienced is harmful. Deception, betrayal, and ridicule behind one's back are all capable of doing great harm, though one may never be aware of them, know of the damage they do, or be able to mind the harm. Consequently, it is legitimate to argue, contrary to Epicurus, that death is a harm (even though not experienced) precisely because it is the irrevocable loss of opportunity, of the continued good of life. Death is the deprivation of life, and were one not dead, possibilities for satisfying experiences could be realized (cf. Nagel).

The Stoics pursued a rather different strategy than the Epicureans in attempting to accommodate people to their mortality. Though we have only the most minimal fragments from the early Stoics—Zeno of Citium (ca. 336–264 B.C.E.), Cleanthes of Assos (ca. 331–232 B.C.E.), and Chrysippus of Soli (ca. 280–206 B.C.E.)—it is clear that they were much influenced by Heraclitus and emphasized discoveries in logic and cosmology. In ethics, they were early natural-law theorists, urging the unity of physical and moral universes and the duty to live a life as orderly as the cosmos, always striving for *autarkeia* (autonomy) of the virtuous person. Socrates, especially during his trial and execution, was a model and inspiration for Stoics of all eras.

Most closely identified with Stoicism are the later Stoics of the first two centuries of the Christian era in imperial Rome. The most prominent of these were Seneca (ca. 4 B.C.E.–65 C.E.), Epictetus (ca. 50–130 C.E.), and Marcus Aurelius (121–180 C.E.). What bound these philosophers together was their commitment to virtue, understood as willing behavior in accord with reason (or nature) and unresisting resignation before what was uncontrollable.

The art of mastering the fear of death is not easily learned. Stoics recommend emulating great men [sic], virtuously living the life of a philosopher, and always remembering that living well is by far the most important thing. Reminders of the futility of fearing or resisting death are also prevalent in their writings. For all of its inevitability, death need not be our imposed fate before which impassibility is required. No philosopher more than Seneca recommended

so enthusiastically and vigorously, nor practiced so decisively, taking control of death by choosing it in the form of suicide. In a remarkable letter he says the following:

> For mere living is not a good, but living well. Accordingly, the wise man will live as long as he ought, not as long as he can.… soon as there are many events in his life that give him trouble and disturb his peace of mind, he sets himself free.… It is not a question of dying earlier or later, but of dying well or ill. And dying well means escape from the danger of living ill.… Just as I shall select my ship as I am about to go on a voyage … so shall I choose my death when I am about to depart from life.… Every man ought to make his life acceptable to others besides himself, but his death to himself alone. The best form of death is one we like. (Seneca, 1970, Letter No. 70)

Seneca was not, in practice, so casual about self-killing as some of the above implies. Still, when Nero accused him of conspiring against the state, and ordered him to take his own life, Seneca is reported to have paused only long enough to remind his followers of the philosophical precepts they had striven to live by before slashing his wrists and bleeding to death.

The Long Transition to a Modern View of Death

In tracing our theme through Western philosophy—whether death is final or whether some notion of afterlife is envisioned—there is very little more to say about this between the time of Stoicism's greatest influence and the onset of a secular, scientific modern renaissance. For over 1,200 years Christian religious views held sway, and philosophy, dominated by theology, had little of substance and still less that was novel to say about death. Enormously important philosophical work was done during this long era, but little of it had much new to contribute to Western philosophical thought on death.

Western philosophical thought on death did not take a turn back to the secular until Francis Bacon (1561–1626) promoted an increasingly scientific methodology and worldview, and René Descartes (1596–1650) reordered the philosophical agenda. Both reflect on death with the aim of excising the fear of death (which in the late Middle Ages, overwhelmed by both plague and superstition, reached new heights). Bacon, however, does so by emphasizing the continuity of dying with living, such that once we learn to live fearlessly, we will be assured of dying fearlessly. Descartes chooses to assuage fears of death by the now more traditional route of arguing for the immortality of the soul.

And as is well known, Descartes's argument to this end relies upon a radical division of persons into different substances, body and soul, mysteriously and problematically united, which sets the stage for much subsequent philosophizing.

Most of modern philosophy pursues Cartesian themes, and the variety of responses is considerable. Rationalist philosophers have generally sought to salvage hopes of surviving death. (Benedict Spinoza [1632–1677] is a notable exception.) But the philosophers of the eighteenth century, and the empiricists they often looked to, came to regard doctrines of the immortality of the soul as *priestly lies*. French writer Voltaire (1694–1778), through Candide's misadventures in "The Best of All Possible Worlds," savagely ridicules Gottfried Wilhelm Leibniz's (1646–1716) faith in universal harmony, and other philosophers look back to the Epicureans and Stoics for inspiration on how to face the prospects of death as annihilation.

But it was David Hume (1711–1776) who most systematically and rigorously called into question doctrines of the soul's immortality. His attack is two-pronged: First he argues against the notion of substance, specifically the self as a substance, and second, he directs a series of arguments against the notion that some part of a person survives death. In his essay "On the Immortality of the Soul" (1777), Hume characterizes *substance* as a "wholly confused and imperfect notion," an "aggregate of particular qualities inhering in an unknown something" (p. 591). As for the self as a substance, he states in *A Treatise of Human Nature* (1739):

> There is no impression constant and invariable. Pain and pleasure, grief and joy, passions and sensations, succeed each other, and never all exist at the same time. It cannot therefore be from any of these impressions, or from any other, that the idea of self is derived; and consequently there is no such idea. (1978, bk. I, pt. 4, sec. 6)

Hume claims to be "insensible of *myself*," for the self is "nothing but a bundle or collection of different perceptions which succeed each other with an inconceivable rapidity, and are in a perpetual flux and movement." All that binds perceptions together is memory and constancy, but it is futile to ask what it is that "has" memory or experiences constancy of conjoined perceptions (1978, bk. I, pt. 4, sec. 6).

Hume's more vigorous critique of immortality is reserved for benighted attempts to settle questions of fact by a priori metaphysical speculation, which is what is done by all doctrines of *immaterial substance* and all attempts to identify personhood with an immaterial *soul* substance that is individuated and survives the demise of the body. Placing his faith in the conviction that all natural processes have some point (if not purpose), Hume notes the universal fear of death and remarks that "Nature does nothing in vain, she would never give us a horror against an *impossible* event" (p. 598).

The only admissible arguments on such a question of fact as whether human beings survive death are those from experience, and these, Hume asserts, are "strong for the mortality of the soul." What possible argument could prove a "state of existence which no one ever saw and which in no way resembles any that ever was seen?" Body and mind grow together, age together, ail together, and, from all experience conveys to us, perish together. (p. 598).

Moral arguments that turn on a just Deity's desire to punish the wicked and reward the good fare no better than metaphysical ones when attempting to prove immortality. It would be a "barbarous deceit," "an injustice in nature," Hume asserts, to restrict "all our knowledge to the present life if there be another scene still waiting us of infinitely greater consequence." Still worse, it would be monstrous for a loving God to base a judgment of how each of us will spend eternity upon the all too finite experience of one human lifetime. (p. 593)

Notwithstanding that it was Immanuel Kant's (1724–1804) reading of Hume that woke him up from a comfortable immersion in conventional dogmas. Kant advanced his own version of a moral argument for the immortality of the human soul. Kant agrees with Hume that no argument from nature (i.e., experience) can demonstrate the immortality of a human soul, and he even concedes that *pure reason* is not up to the task. Nonetheless, Kant is firmly convinced that a compelling metaphysical/moral argument will do the job.

Kant apparently never doubted his belief in human immortality, and his argument to show the soul's immortality is both elegant in its simplicity and rich in the number of fundamental Kantian tenets that it incorporates or presupposes. Kant asserts in the *Critique of Practical Reason* (1788) that the most basic requirement of the moral law is the attainment of perfection. Such an achievement is not possible in a finite life, however. But the moral law can command only what it is possible for moral agents to do. Hence the necessity of an immortal soul so that moral agents will have the opportunity to do what they ought to do.

One of the more interesting features of Kant's *proof* is that it breaks with the long tradition that sees afterlife as occurring in paradise. In Kant's moral universe, there must still be pain and suffering in the hereafter, for these are inseparable features of the moral life. Further, doubt, uncertainty, and struggle for constant improvement must accompany our disembodied journey through eternity. The moral law would appear to be nearly as powerful as God.

The soundness of Kant's argument turns on the truth of at least the following Kantian doctrines: Objective reality must conform to the essential structure of the human mind; moral certainty is as sure a route to knowledge as the logical demonstrations of reason; moral perfection is required of all who would live a moral life; human beings exist, simultaneously, in two worlds, one phenomenal, the other noumenal. If any of these dogmas fail—and all have been extensively criticized—Kant's argument for the immortality of the human soul fails as well. Any number of philosophers after Kant, less enamored of metaphysical arguments, have turned his argument around and observed that if perfection is not possible in a human life span, the moral law cannot require perfection of human beings. Far from showing human immortality, Kant's insight into morality shows the limits of what a reasonable morality can demand of mortal creatures.

Toward Postmodernism

Variations on religious, usually Christian, views of death and immortality continued in the writings of eighteenth- and nineteenth-century philosophers, including most notably the idealism of Georg W. F. Hegel (1770–1831) and the atheistic pessimism of Arthur Schopenhauer (1788–1860). Not until a real break with modern thought occurred did genuinely novel views about the significance of death and the possibility of immortality arise. In the thought of Friedrich Nietzsche (1844–1900) many now find both the culmination of ancient and modern approaches to death and the transition to a postmodern worldview. And it is certainly true that in Nietzsche's various writings, one can find many different historically grounded and historically transcendent approaches to the problem of death.

While still a student, Nietzsche read Schopenhauer's *The World as Will and Idea* (1819). Profoundly moved and deeply disturbed, he sought escape from Schopenhauer's pessimism and atheism, and saw the task of philosophy as overcoming the former while taking responsibility for the latter (*Ecce Homo,* 1888). Physical pain and mental suffering were lifelong companions; staring into the abyss of despair and coping with the guilt of killing God, Nietzsche tried a number of different strategies for finding life worth continuing.

Through classical studies and art, Nietzsche supposed, one might escape the profound misery of existence (*The Birth of Tragedy,* 1872). The consolations of *beautiful dreams* soon faded, however, and Nietzsche turned to a detached, critical search for knowledge, and the "*interesting* illusion of science replaces the *beautiful* illusion of art" (Choron, p. 201).

Objective knowledge, or its semblance, proved unsatisfying as well, and Nietzsche then began to develop the idea of the *superman* as the disciplined Dionysian man capable of living a pain-filled life with full creativity. Truth is painful and, to all but the superman, unbearable. Above all, one must love fate (*amor fati*), which becomes possible with the Eternal Recurrence of the Same:

> Everything goes, everything returns; eternally rolls the wheel of existence. Everything dies, everything blossoms forth again; eternally runs the year of existence … All things return eternally and we ourselves have already been numberless times, and all things with us. (*Also Sprach Zarathustra,* 1891 quoted by Choron, p. 202)

At least Heraclitus's voice seems to recur here.

How such a view of the one life we have and the one death we experience, albeit endlessly repeated, solves the problem of death is not clear. Sometimes Nietzsche suggests that recognizing the Eternal Recurrence of the Same should lead us to passionately embrace and affirm life, to live with as much conviction and determination as we can muster, for life might otherwise be all the more miserable for its endless repetition. But Nietzsche, who attempted suicide three times, must have been terrified at the prospect of such recurrence. It is the ultimate test of the superman to love fate while recognizing precisely what fate has in store.

Contemporary Philosophy

The problem of death has not often been seen by contemporary philosophers as a choice between devising consolations for our finitude and demonstrations of our eternalness. For many, perhaps most philosophers early in the twenty-first century, the death of God is more than a century past, the grieving finished more than half a century ago. The problem of death, understood as the struggle to make life meaningful in an increasingly secular age plagued by the temptations of nihilism, continues. The little that philosophers in the present time have had to say about death—outside of chiefly moral concerns centering on choosing death—has tended to suppose death is final, not, in any form, to be survived.

German philosopher Martin Heidegger (1889–1976), once a student of Edmund Husserl (1859–1938), took as his project the application of phenomenological method to the fundamental question of metaphysics, the study of *Being-as-such.* To this philosophically most contentious enterprise in the twentieth century, Heidegger brought a particular concern for death. Since Heidegger is addressing the issue of why there is something rather than nothing, it is not non-existence of Being that concerns him, but rather how individual beings—most particularly, individual self-conscious human beings (*Dasein*)—can possibly come to not exist.

Heidegger uses language in highly idiosyncratic ways, so when he talks about possibility and non-possibility and impossibility it is best to leave our conventional (and philosophical) understandings of these terms behind and attend to Heidegger's peculiar uses.

Understanding our own being at a deep level requires the attainment of wholeness and authenticity, which enables life to be lived with integrity and clear thinking. Nothing is more central to this quest than an appreciation of temporality and possibility, which provides insight into Being in general and Dasein in particular.

Dasein aspires to wholeness, but has future possibilities open to it only so long as it exists and can freely choose. But so long as Dasein exists and can make free choices, it cannot be whole. Death appears to us an end of Dasein and of possibility, but is it the attainment of wholeness? How can non-existence constitute completion?

Heidegger's resolution of these paradoxes involves an analysis of the unique way in which Dasein has possibilities and of how these are limited. Dasein's possibilities are ever limited by *the possibility of the impossibility of existing,* which in Heidegger's discourse is a synonym for death. Yet Heidegger maintains that his view of death leaves open the question of afterlife.

Death creates for Dasein its *ownmost possibility,* one that invites a uniquely free choice in response to mortality from each individual. The certainty of death is the ultimate realization of each Dasein, experienced alone and not shared by another. Attaining authenticity requires *Vorlaufen,* literally a *running forwards,* metaphorically, an ever self-conscious anticipation of death—a *being towards death*—that will free one from life's trivia and focus on using freedom to create an authentic self.

Jean Paul Sartre (1905–1980) in philosophy, and Carl Gustav Jung (1875–1961) in psychoanalytic theory, were both influenced by Heidegger's thinking. Jung developed Heidegger's notion of being towards death as a central focus of his psychoanalytic theory, and Sartre, along with French writers Simone de Beauvoir (1908–1986) and Albert Camus (1913–1960) articulated some of the most distinctive things to say about the problem of death in the twentieth century. Building on Nietzsche's alienation from convention, despair at the death of God, and attraction to nihilism, and struggling with revelations of the distinctly human capacity for genocide revealed during the Holocaust and the era of nuclear weaponry, existentialists have sought ways to affirm against all odds the meaningfulness of individual human existence. A good deal of the spirit of this distinctive approach to death is captured in de Beauvoir's unsettling judgment on the very difficult dying of her mother:

There is no such thing as a natural death: nothing that happens to a man is ever natural, since his presence calls the world into question. All men must die: but for every man his death is an accident and, even if he knows it and consents to it, an unjustifiable violation. (p. 123)

Far from providing assurances of immortality or consolations designed to meet death with equanimity, existentialists recommend a rebellious, often angry response to the *cosmic injustice* that human beings die. Rebellion against or resistance toward death, however, is not recommended as a strategy for overcoming death; no illusions are allowed as to the inevitability and finality of death. Rather, for Camus especially, such resistance is recommended as an affirmation of one's decency, caring about life, and personal integrity. Nowhere is this better illustrated than in Camus's novel *The Plague,* an extended allegory about any number of evils, not the least of which is death itself. Dr. Bernard Rieux and his closest friend, Jean Tarrou, struggle mightily against the ravages of the plague in the seaside town of Oran in Algeria. In time, however, Tarrou succumbs to the plague, and Rieux reflects on what it means:

Tarrou had lost the match, as he put it. But what had he, Rieux, won? No more than the experience of having known plague and remembering it, of having known friendship and remembering it, of knowing affection and being destined one day to remember it. So all a man could win in the conflict between plague and life was knowledge and memories. But Tarrou, perhaps, would have called that winning the match. (Camus, p. 262)

Afterword

Most Western philosophical views on death have been singularly human-centered, driven by the assumption of human uniqueness. Even atheistic existentialists, for whom God is displaced altogether from the universe, seem lost with no center, and substitute human beings and a kind of humanism as their moral center.

We have only just begun to explore the post-Darwinian implications of regarding human beings as a natural kind—as creatures like other creatures known to us, evolved from simpler life forms without conscious direction. The moral implications of such a change in worldview are getting considerable attention from philosophers at present—in reflections on ecology and the moral status of nonhuman animals, in more sympathetic treatments of rational suicide and euthanasia, in greater openness about the difficulties of dying—but the larger ontological and metaphysical consequences are infrequently addressed. If there is to be any substantial breakthrough in our philosophical thinking about death, it might well come only with the displacement of human self-centeredness, with seeing human beings as one among many natural kinds on a solitary planet in an ordinary solar system that is on the fringes of one of many billions of galaxies in an apparently infinitely expanding universe. Such a potentially revitalized naturalism need not imply that life is meaningless for solitary, mortal human beings, nor does it guarantee significant life, but it might suggest that our plight is not unique, not unshared by others, and not, finally, to be resolved (or dissolved) by exclusive self-centered speciesist concerns.

But maybe not. Even such a revitalized naturalism might prove to be but one more variation on one side of the recurrent debate between those who seek a satisfactory means to reconcile each of us to the finality of death, and those who, on the other hand, seek to sustain the hope that life does not end with death and that individual consciousness continues beyond the grave.

RICHARD W. MOMEYER (1995)
REVISED BY AUTHOR

SEE ALSO: *Anthropology and Bioethics; Autonomy; Body: Cultural and Religious Perspectives; Care; Grief and Bereavement; Harm; Holocaust; Human Dignity; Infanticide; Life; Life, Quality of; Life Sustaining Treatment and Euthanasia; Literature and Healthcare; Narrative; Palliative Care and Hospice; Pediatrics, Intensive Care in; Right to Die, Policy and Law; Suicide; Triage; Value and Valuation; Virtue and Character; Warfare;* and other *Death* subentries

BIBLIOGRAPHY

Aristotle. 1941. *The Basic Works of Aristotle,* ed. Richard McKeon. New York: Random House.

Beauvoir, Simone de. 1965. *A Very Easy Death,* tr. Patrick O'Brien. New York: Penguin.

Camus, Albert. 1948. *The Plague,* tr. Stuart Gilbert. New York: Modern Library.

Choron, Jacques. 1963. *Death and Western Thought.* New York: Collier Books.

Epicurus. 1926. *Epicurus, the Extant Remains,* tr. Cyril Bailey. Oxford: Clarendon Press.

Guttmann, James. 1978. "Death: Western Philosophical Thought." In *The Encyclopedia of Bioethics,* ed. Warren T. Reich. New York: Macmillan.

Heidegger, Martin. 1996. *Being and Time,* tr. Joan Stambaugh. Albany: State University of New York Press.

Hume, David. 1978. *A Treatise of Human Nature,* 2nd edition, ed. L. A. Selby-Bigge. Oxford: Clarendon Press.

Hume, David. 1985. *Essays: Moral, Political and Literary,* ed. Eugene F. Miller. Indianapolis, IN: Liberty Classics.

Kant, Immanuel. 1949. *Critique of Practical Reason and Other Writings in Moral Philosophy,* tr. and ed. Lewis White Beck. Chicago: University of Chicago Press.

Kirk, Geoffrey S., and Raven, John E., tr. and eds. 1960. *The Presocratic Philosophers.* Cambridge, Eng.: Cambridge University Press.

Momeyer, Richard W. 1982. "Socrates on Obedience and Disobedience to Law." *Philosophy Research Archives* 8: 21–54.

Momeyer, Richard W. 1988. *Confronting Death.* Bloomington: Indiana University Press.

Nagel, Thomas. 1979. "Death." In *Mortal Questions.* Cambridge, Eng.: Cambridge University Press.

Nietzsche, Friedrich Wilhelm. 1977. *A Nietzsche Reader,* tr. and ed. R. J. Hollingdale. New York: Penguin.

Oates, Whitney Jennings, ed. 1940. *The Stoic and Epicurean Philosophers: The Complete Extant Writings of Epicurus, Epictetus, Lucretius, Marcus Aurelius.* New York: Random House.

Plato. 1961. *The Collected Dialogues of Plato,* ed. Edith Hamilton and Huntington Cairns. Princeton, NJ: Princeton University Press.

Seneca, Lucius Annaeus. 1970. "On the Proper Time to Slip the Cable." In *Ad Lucillum Epistulae Morales,* vol. 2, tr. Richard M. Gummere. Cambridge, MA: Harvard University Press.

Voltaire. 1966. *Candide,* tr. and ed. Robert M. Adams. New York: Norton.

IV. WESTERN RELIGIOUS THOUGHT

Death in Biblical Thought

There is no "biblical view of death" as such. This lack of a single scriptural understanding of death is hardly surprising, given the fact that the Bible is sacred scripture for three world religions and that its contents were written and compiled over a period of a thousand years or more. But the history of literary and religious development embedded within the Bible itself does allow for a kind of "archaeology" of death in biblical thought. Though admittedly vastly oversimplified, the following narrative of the Bible's evolving views on death can be traced backward through their random branchings and read forward toward their studied convergences.

Put in its simplest terms, an ancient desert god named Yahweh came to be regarded not only as the national god of a holy nation, but ultimately as the one and only God of the universe. These momentous shifts in the biblical understanding of God were paralleled by remarkable changes in biblical views of death, beginning with the denial and concluding with the affirmation of individual postmortem existence.

THE HEBREW BIBLE. Hebrew religion emerged out of the tribal polytheisms of ancient Mesopotamia. The protagonists of Yahwism only gradually succeeded in establishing their deity as the national god of the various Semitic tribes that were finally welded together, during the latter half of the second millennium B.C.E., into the people known as the Israelites. A key weapon in their struggle to establish Yahweh's supremacy was the suppression of prevailing beliefs and practices dealing with death. In two very different responses to death, Mesopotamian culture had preserved primitive notions of life after death as a continuation of the life before death. On the one hand, mortuary cults affirmed a significant afterlife for the powerful and privileged who commanded the worship and fealty of the living. On the other hand, postmortem existence was limited to an awful underworld where the departed dead were shrouded in darkness and subsisted on clay. In either case, the realm of the dead was under the control of the gods of the underworld. For that reason, the champions of Yahwism denounced the polytheistic beliefs and practices of both the mortuary cults and the "house of dust."

Against the mortuary cults, the Yahwists presented a view of human nature and destiny that undercut all ancestor worship and necromancy. In the Yahwist creation myth, the protohuman couple was created from the soil and destined to return to the soil (Gen. 3:19). Human beings are material bodies animated by a life force (*nephesh* or *ruach*) residing in the breath or the blood. Death comes when the life force leaves the body and returns to Yahweh. Thus, a common fate awaits all persons upon death—master and slave, rich and poor, good and bad—all descend beneath the earth to the place of the dead called She'ol, where they continue a shadowy existence, but only for a brief period of time. This land of the dead was variously described as an awful pit shrouded in darkness or a walled city covered with dust. Although reminiscent of the Mesopotamian underworld, the Yahwist notion of She'ol excluded any divine ruler of the infernal regions. Neither a god of the underworld nor Yahweh himself was involved with the denizens of She'ol. Yahweh reigned supreme over the community of the living, meting out collective rewards and punishments only in the present life. In other words, mortality was accepted as a fact of life. Premature and violent deaths were feared as great evils and regarded as punishments for sin. As such, the untimely or agonizing death remained under the control of Yahweh (Isa. 45:7). But death at the end of a long and happy life was accepted, if not welcomed (Gen. 25:8; Job 5:26). What mattered were those things which survived the mortal individual: a good reputation (Prov. 10:7), male offspring (Isa. 56:3–5), the promised land (Gen. 48:21), and the God of Israel (Ps. 90).

Precisely this emphasis on present existence contributed to the eventual transformation of Yahwism. The naive assumption that Yahweh rewards the pious with prosperity and a long life while punishing the wicked with misfortune and a brief life was obviously contradicted by communal and individual experience. Especially the disasters that befell Israel between the eighth and the sixth centuries B.C.E. raised radical doubts about Yahweh's justice and omnipotence, because the entire social and religious order of Israel was disrupted and eventually destroyed.

This massive destruction evinced two distinctive responses. On the one hand, most of the great prophets of Israel responded to these dire circumstances by reaffirming collective retribution and promising collective restoration (Isa. 11:10–16; Ezek. 36:16–36). Some prophets moved beyond communal responsibility and punishment (Jer. 21:3), but their new emphasis on the individual only heightened the tension between divine power and justice in the face of innocent suffering (Job 10:2–9). On the other hand, an apocalyptic school of thought slowly emerged that anticipated a miraculous deliverance of the faithful living and dead at the end of time. Envisioned in this apocalyptic outlook was the final defeat of death itself, which had increasingly been personified as a destructive evil force. Thus, by the end of the second century B.C.E., two sharply contrasting views of death dominated the Hebraic worldview. The older notion that death marked the end of life remained the traditional view among those who came to be known as the Sadducees. The newer view that affirmed postmortem divine judgment and human resurrection flourished among such sectarian movements as the Pharisees and the Essenes. For these sectarians, the powers of death would eventually be overcome by the power of God.

THE INTERTESTAMENTAL LITERATURE. This sectarian transformation of the Hebraic view of death during the so-called intertestamental period was immense (ca. 200 B.C.E. to 50 C.E.). A number of disparate ideas were combined into a dramatically new eschatology. The Book of Daniel marked a watershed in Hebrew religious thought by promising Yahweh's final intervention in history to rescue his people from their enemies and to resurrect past generations from the dead to participate in this ultimate restoration. To be sure, this final restoration was limited to the nation of Israel. But, under the impact of speculative thought and foreign influences concerning life after death, the prospect of a final resurrection and judgment for all humankind appeared in the later apocalyptic literature, much of which is contained in the Apocrypha. In this apocalyptic literature, human consciousness and the life force were fused into an entity (*psyche* or *pneuma*) which, unlike the earlier conceptions of *nephesh* or *ruach*, survived the cessation of bodily functions in some spiritual fashion. She'ol was reconceived as a holding place for the dead until their ultimate fate was decided at a final judgment. More significantly, She'ol was divided into compartments reflecting the moral character of the dead, wherein rewards and punishments were already meted out in anticipation of the catastrophic end of the existing world order (Enoch 22:9–14). Thus, death held no terror for the righteous. In fact, death through martyrdom was seen as a seal of divine favor (2 Macc. 6:30–31) and even premature death from serious illness freed the righteous from further suffering (Wisd. of Sol. 4:11). Death was only a threat and curse to the wicked. Reminiscent of the older Yahwist traditions, the apocalyptic emphasis remained largely on the collective aspects of human destiny, for it is the nations that are arraigned for the final judgment (2 Ezd. 7:32–38). The postmortem survival of the individual became an affirmation of faith within certain Jewish circles only following the shattering of the Jewish state in 70 C.E.

THE NEW TESTAMENT. Primitive Christianity emerged out of Jewish apocalyptic expectations of the catastrophic end of the existing world order and the final judgment of the living and the dead. These apocalyptic expectations had been joined in the popular imagination with the older prophetic Messianic traditions in which a divinely appointed and endowed figure would crush the enemies and restore the glories of Israel. So far as the New Testament Gospels allow for historical reconstruction, the message of Jesus centered in the nearness of the Day of the Lord, when the chosen people of Yahweh would be vindicated before the nations of the world. Jesus called his compatriots to prepare themselves for the Coming Judgment through repentance and obedience to the written and oral Law of God. But, unlike the earlier nationalistic preoccupations of Jewish apocalypticism, this newer eschatology emphasized the eternal destiny of individuals in accordance with their moral achievements (Matt. 25:40–46). After his death and resurrection, the followers of Jesus identified him as the promised Messiah who would restore the righteous and judge the wicked. This same "Christianized" apocalyptic tradition informs the Revelation to John, which so profoundly influenced later Christian views of human death and destiny. Here the "end of the world" was described in elaborate detail as a cataclysmic establishment of the millennial reign of Christ and the saints on earth, after which the righteous are rewarded with eternal life and the wicked are punished with eternal death. Thus, the earliest Christian view of life after death was heavily influenced by, but not identical with, Jewish apocalypticism. Jesus was heralded by his early followers as their resurrected Lord who would shortly return in supernatural power and glory to preside over the Final Judgment of the living and the dead.

A somewhat different interpretation of the message and mission of Jesus was offered by Paul in his outreach to a Gentile audience. Paul regarded the death of Christ as a divinely planned event to rescue humankind from enslavement to the demonic powers of evil and death that ruled the world. Although influenced by apocalyptic thought, Paul's interpretation of a divine Savior's death and resurrection involved an eschatology very different from the apocalyptic scheme of things. No longer was obedience to the Twofold Law the basis on which the living and the dead would be judged; instead, faith in the crucified and risen Lord became the crucial factor. The ritual of baptism, which reenacted the death, burial, and resurrection of Christ, initiated believers into immortal life while still living in their material bodies. The baptized Christian, having become a new creation *in Christo,* had already passed from death to life. Thus, the imminent return of Christ and the end of the world held no fear for baptized believers, for their final judgment and destiny had already been settled.

With the Roman overthrow of the Jewish state in 70 C.E., the Mother Church of Jerusalem disappeared and eventually Pauline Christianity became the normative interpretation of Christ. Elements of the earlier apocalyptic eschatology were carried over into this form of faith. Christianity became a salvation religion centered in a Savior God who would shortly return to bring the existing world to a catastrophic end and to judge those who had oppressed the faithful. But the continuing delay of the second coming of Christ forced the Church to rethink its notions of eschatological fulfillment. The Church could no longer think of itself as an eschatological community awaiting the imminent return of their Lord. Rather, the Church developed a hierarchical structure and a sacramental system to shepherd believers through the perils and pitfalls of life from birth to death. Accordingly, Christ was reconceived as the heavenly mediator between God and humankind. Despite these doctrinal and ecclesiological developments, the apocalyptic vision of the catastrophic end of the world was retained, raising anew all sorts of problems about the status of the dead before the final day of resurrection and judgment. Over time, these problems were resolved in ever more vivid and complicated schemes of postmortem paradisal bliss for the saints and purgatorial torment for the sinners until the day of Final Judgment (Luke 16:19–26).

ETHICAL IMPLICATIONS. As noted above, the Bible is a diverse literature containing a variety of religious perspectives on death. Religious affirmation of the triumph of life over death is a common theme running through the whole of scripture, but how, where, and when this victory is won differs dramatically among biblical perspectives. For that reason, the Bible offers no consensus of direct guidelines on death and dying. Nevertheless some application of the biblical tradition to modern "end of life" ethical issues can be ventured.

1. Biblical views of death are greatly influenced by the wider cultural milieu. As human conditions and needs changed, so did prevailing religious beliefs and practices concerning death. Thus, the Bible itself seems to allow for changing definitions and responses to death in the light of new social conditions, scientific knowledge, and religious insights.

2. The biblical tradition's intimate connection between body and spirit is not only a mandate for medical care as treatment of the whole person but also grounds for regarding human life as more than biological functioning. While the Bible does not authoritatively establish when death occurs, it defines death as the separation of the spirit from the body. Thereby, the Bible provides indirect warrants for withholding or withdrawing extraordinary means of life support when the vital bond between body and spirit has been dissolved or destroyed.

3. The biblical tradition never accords absolute power or independent status to death. Death, whether viewed as a natural event or an evil force, is always subordinated to the power and purposes of God. While the Bible speaks of sin as both a cause and a consequence of death, even the death of the sinner remains under divine control and serves the divine will. God's sovereignty over death serves as a caution against simplistic religious warrants for directly or indirectly terminating the lives of the suffering.

4. Biblical support can be found both for death as a natural part of life and death as an evil power opposed to life. Those who regard death as an "enemy" that must be battled at all costs will find more support for their view in the New Testament. Those who see death as a "friend" that can be welcomed at the end of life will feel more kinship with the Hebrew Bible. But both Jewish and Christian scriptures regard untimely and violent deaths as evils to be avoided and enemies to be combatted by all legitimate means that do not compromise religious or moral duties. Of course, death by coercive martyrdom can be affirmed as a seal of great faith, and even premature death from debilitating illness can be welcomed by the believer as a deliverance from great suffering.

5. Taken as a whole, the Bible does not unambiguously affirm individual life after death. But where postmortem existence is affirmed in the Bible, the grounds are theological rather than anthropological. The individual's survival beyond death is a divine possibility rather than a human certainty. Immortal life is a "supernatural" endowment rather than a "natural" attribute. In other words, a belief in life after death is neither a given of human nature nor a constant of human culture. Thus, the idea of life after death cannot become an explicit warrant for public policies or ethical decisions regarding "end of life" issues in a pluralistic society.

Death in Systematic Religious Thought

The classical doctrines and rituals of Judaism and Christianity are no less complicated and diverse than their biblical backgrounds. Neither the Judaic nor the Christian tradition is monolithic. Both faiths have been developed over extended periods of time in response to changing historical circumstances and cultural influences. But these theological complexities can be simplified for purposes of comparing and contrasting their respective views of death. Just as there are elements of continuity and mutuality within the Hebrew Bible and the New Testament, so are there broad similarities between Judaism and Christianity in their traditional beliefs and practices regarding death.

POSTBIBLICAL JEWISH BELIEFS AND PRACTICES. A long and slow transformation took place from the completion of the Hebrew Bible (ca. 200 B.C.E.) to the completion of the Talmud (ca. 500 C.E.), during which time biblical Hebraism emerged as rabbinic Judaism. The Talmud brought together eight hundred years of rabbinic commentary on scripture that was broadly categorized as *halakhah* (law) and *haggadah* (story), the former describing the obligations, the latter explaining the meaning of God's covenant with Israel. This massive compendium of rabbinic thought explicated the scripture's "moralization" of life and death in vast and vivid detail. For example, heaven (*Gan Eden*) and hell (*Gehinnom*) were each divided into five separate chambers, reflecting different levels of eternal rewards for the righteous and punishments for the wicked. Similarly, the rabbis described 903 forms of death. The hardest way of dying is by asthma and the easiest, which is reserved for the righteous, is "like drawing a hair from milk." Death following five days of illness was considered ordinary. Death after four days or less indicated increasing degrees of divine reprimand. Those who died before fifty were "cut off," sixty years was "ripe age," and above seventy was "old age." Despite all this moralizing about death, comparatively few rabbis held that death as such was the wages of sin. Against those who taught that Adam's sin brought death into the world, the majority of rabbis taught that Adam's mortality was given with his creation. Death was an integral part of the good world that God created in the beginning. Thus, sin hastens death but does not cause it in the first place.

In other words, only the timing and manner of death are affected by moral conditions. Acts of benevolence and confessions of sins can delay the hour of death as surely as sins of impurity and injustice can speed it. But there is no avoiding death once the angel of death receives the order from God. Given God's permission to destroy, the angel of death makes no distinction between good and bad, but wields the sword against royalty and commoner, old and young, pious and pagan, animal and human alike. While both the wicked and the righteous must die, their deaths are as different as their lives. The wicked perish to pay for their sins while the righteous die to be freed from their sins. Death is a punishment for the sins of the wicked but an atonement for the sins of the righteous. Put another way, the righteous are still alive even though dead, while the wicked are already dead though still alive.

When death occurs, the soul leaves the body with a silent cry that echoes from one end of the world to the other. The soul's departure from the body is marked by the absence of breathing, heartbeat, and pulse. The slightest sign of movement is an indication that death has not yet occurred. Where the soul goes was a matter of considerable dispute among the rabbis. Some taught that the soul sleeps until the resurrection of the dead and the final judgment. Others believed that the soul passes into an interim state of consciousness and activity. But they all agreed that the body that remains must be treated with dignity and given a proper burial. Desecration of the body, such as mutilation or burial with missing body parts, is forbidden, and burial must be before nightfall if possible. Interment must be in the ground to fulfill the biblical mandate ("Dust you are and to dust you shall return") and to complete the atoning process ("May my death be an atonement for all my sins"). A speedy and simple burial also accorded with widespread popular beliefs that the soul is free to complete its journey to the other world only when the body has decomposed.

These beliefs about death were reflected in a number of customs and rituals surrounding the dying and mourning process. A dying person (*goses*) was given special consideration by loved ones who gave support and comfort during the last hours. The dying person was never to be left alone. Last wishes and spiritual advice were to be faithfully observed. When nearing the end, the dying were encouraged to make a confession such as the following: "I acknowledge unto Thee, O Lord my God, and God of my fathers, that both my cure and my death are in Thy hands. May it be Thy will to send me a perfect healing. Yet if my death be fully determined by Thee, I will in love accept it at Thy hand. O, may my death be an atonement for all my sins, iniquities, and transgressions of which I have been guilty against Thee." This confession was followed with the traditional Jewish affirmation of faith: "Hear, O Israel: The Lord is our God, the Lord is One" (Deut. 6:4).

When death had occurred, the eyes and mouth were closed by the eldest son or nearest relative. The arms were extended alongside the body, which was placed on the floor with the feet toward the door and covered by a sheet. A lighted candle was placed close to the head. Mirrors were turned to the wall or covered. Water in the death room was poured out, reflecting the ancient legend that the angel of death washes its bloody sword in nearby water. The windows of the death chamber were opened to allow the spirits to enter and depart. The dead body was never left alone, whether on weekdays or the Sabbath, until the funeral. Thus, the entire deathbed drama was structured to allow the dying to face the future realistically, yet within a reassuring framework of family and faith.

The theological and literary diversity of the talmudic period yielded two very different developments of the Jewish tradition during the Middle Ages (ca. 1100–1600). A mystical school emerged whose teachings concerning death and the afterlife went far beyond rabbinical Judaism. An emphasis on divine immanence and human transcendence lay at the heart of the *Kabbalah*, the most commonly used term for the esoteric teachings of medieval Judaism. Human life is the journey of the soul from God and back to God. During the interim period of life on earth and in the body, the soul must attain the "knowledge of the mysteries of the faith," which will purify and prepare it for its return to God. Since this esoteric knowledge is seldom learned in a single life, the soul transmigrates from one embodiment to another until all sins are purged and all duties fulfilled. In this mystical scheme of things, death is simply a threshold marking the passage from one life to another in the soul's ascent to God.

By contrast, a scholastic approach emerged, which codified talmudic beliefs and practices concerning death and dying. The greatest halakist of medieval Judaism was Rabbi Joseph Caro. His sixteenth-century work, *Shulhan Arukh,* became the authoritative code of Jewish law by synthesizing and reconciling the three giants of medieval *halakhah*— Isaac Alfasia, Moses Maimonides, and Asher B. Jehiel. Unlike Maimonides, who reinterpreted traditional Jewish teachings in Aristotelian terms, Caro did not subject Jewish law to speculative criticism. Rather, he brought order out of chaos by investigating each stage of development of every single law, finally arriving at a decisive interpretation and application of that law. His work has remained the indispensable guide to the development and interpretation of Jewish laws and customs for two millennia. Included in *Shulhan Arukh* are the detailed halakic rites and duties surrounding death, burial, and mourning observed throughout Orthodox Jewry to this day.

In the modern period, a variety of reform movements have modified many traditional Jewish beliefs and practices concerning death. Orthodox Jews have for the most part remained loyal to rabbinic eschatology, with its emphasis on the final resurrection, but they diverge on whether the resurrection awaits all humankind, the righteous of every age, or only the Jewish people. These otherworldly notions of Messianic redemption and divine judgment have largely faded into the background for Conservative Jewish thinkers. They interpret the Messianic Hope historically in terms of the restoration of the nation of Israel, and spiritually in terms of the immortality of the soul. References to the resurrection of the dead in Jewish rituals of death, burial, and mourning are retained, but the language of resurrection is assimilated to teachings about the immortality of the soul.

Reform Judaism has gone even further in rejecting doctrines of bodily resurrection and the Messianic Age. The "Pittsburgh Platform" of Reformed Judaism (1885) excluded all bodily notions of heaven and hell as abodes for everlasting punishment and reward. Indeed, some liberal Jewish thinkers have rejected the idea of individual immortality entirely, though they affirm the lasting value of each human life within the everlasting life of God. These reformulations of Jewish belief have also produced liberalizations in the areas of Jewish death, burial, and mourning rites. Curiously enough, this turn away from the otherworld and afterlife has fueled a profound concern for the salvation of humankind in the full reality of their historical existence. Thus, many Reformed Jews have returned full cycle to the essentially "humanistic" outlook of the great prophets of ancient Israel.

POSTBIBLICAL CHRISTIAN BELIEFS AND PRACTICES. The traditional Christian understanding of death developed largely in response to two challenges facing the Church at the close of the first century. Internally, the delay of the second coming of Christ forced Christian thinkers to deal with the state of the soul between death and resurrection. For the most part, primitive Christians believed that the dead slept until the Last Day, at which time they would be resurrected from the grave to receive their everlasting rewards or punishments. But, as this period of time lengthened, questions about the interim between individual death and universal judgment became ever more pressing. Externally, the pervasive view of death in Hellenistic religion and philosophy called for some theological response. The Greeks believed that the immortal soul is released from its bodily entrapment by death. This understanding of death was so widespread that some Christian assimilation of the soul's immortality and the body's inferiority was inevitable. Taken together over time, the delay of the return of Christ and the appropriation of Greek ideas of immortality fostered an elaborate system of Christian beliefs and practices concerning the active life of the soul during the period between one's death and the general resurrection at the end of the age. In time, this new eschatology displaced the apocalyptic vision of the Last Days, which vision survived for the most part in millenarian or chiliastic sects, who looked forward to the return of Christ and the establishment of the Kingdom of God on earth.

The church fathers adopted many of the categories of Greek philosophy but retained most of the substance of Pauline Christianity. They affirmed the immortality of the soul but rejected the ultimate separability of soul and body, along with all Hellenistic notions of reincarnation and immediate judgment. The soul is the vivifying principle and as such is incomplete without a body. Indeed, had Adam and Eve not sinned, humankind never would have experienced death. But all must suffer the separation of soul and body in death as punishment for their sins. Their souls, however, cannot perish because they are immortal. Therefore, these souls must eventually be reunited with "the dust of bodies long dead" (Augustine) in order to receive their final inheritance of everlasting salvation or eternal damnation. Surprisingly, there was little speculation among the church fathers about this interim between individual death and general resurrection. Since the soul is immaterial during this period, the dead could experience no sense of place or time, no awareness of comfort or pain, until the resurrection.

Given its finality, death thus became a decisive moment in the soul's destiny. The hour of death sealed the fate of the saved and damned alike. Those who died with their sins forgiven were destined for heaven's bliss. Those who died "while yet in their sins" were condemned to hell's agony. This emphasis on penance in relation to God's mercy and judgment fueled the more elaborate view of heaven, hell, and purgatory that characterized medieval Christianity. The materials for that view were already available in the earlier periods, but an adequate conceptual framework was lacking. The notion of a fire that cleanses the righteous and consumes the wicked at the final resurrection belonged to the earliest biblical traditions. Pushing this purgation of sins back from the final judgment into the interim period after death was encouraged by pietistic and penitential practices. Prayers to the saints and masses for the dead whose sins require expiation implied an active existence for souls following death and suggested a postmortem purgation of sins. But these implications were not fully worked out until the High Middle Ages (1200–1500).

Drawing on Aristotelian philosophy, Thomas Aquinas worked out an eschatology that combined an active spiritual afterlife with the traditional biblical notions of a general resurrection and last judgment. While the soul actualizes the body as its matter, it contains within itself to a degree all the perfections of physical and spiritual existence. Thus, the infliction of punishment or the bestowal of reward on the soul begins immediately after its separation from the body. But neither ultimate happiness nor ultimate misery is possible for a disembodied soul and, therefore, both must await the reunion of soul and body at the resurrection. Moreover, the soul that is ultimately rewarded must be entirely purified, either during or after this life. In other words, the existence of purgatory was a logical correlate of the immortal soul and the sacrament of penance, which requires contrition and satisfaction for all sins committed after baptism.

This thirteenth-century theological synthesis ineluctably shifted the emphasis to the individual's judgment at death rather than the universal judgment of humankind at the final resurrection of the dead. The Church's official view retained the two judgments, but in popular belief and practice they were in effect merged into one. People simply went to heaven, hell, or purgatory at the moment of death. Accordingly, the hour of death became overloaded with urgency. Dying in a state of grace meant eternal salvation, in a state of sin, eternal damnation, while dying with unconfessed sin required purgatorial cleansing. Thus, dying became more important than living. This focus on death was most obvious in the medieval *Ars moriendi* art of dying manuals that gave step-by-step advice to the dying and to the persons attending the dying to ensure a "good death." Of greater significance was the increasing importance of the sacrament of extreme unction, which was administered to the dying for all sins of sight, hearing, smell, speech, touch, and action. For those believers who died ill-prepared, there were masses for the dead and indulgences for the remission of sin for those in purgatory. In other words, a whole arsenal of beliefs and practices were mobilized against the terror of dying outside the state of grace.

What was developed in the thirteenth century as gifts of divine grace became in the fourteenth and fifteenth century marks of human folly. Or so the Protestant reformers claimed. Abuses surrounding the sacraments and indulgences for the dying were rife in the late medieval Church. These abuses were a precipitating cause of the sixteenth-century reform movements that swept both church and society. In point of fact, neither Luther nor Calvin broke with the fundamental worldview of medieval Christianity. Both challenged current beliefs and practices from within the medieval tradition. Thus, with regard to eschatology, the reformers retained the concept of the soul's immortality and eternal destiny. But they both undercut the entire penitential system with a different understanding of divine mercy and justice. The blood of Christ is the sole satisfaction for the sins of believers. Thus, medieval notions of a purgatorial state and a treasury of merits fell to the ground because these practices compromised the sole ground of salvation in Christ through faith. What remained for the reformers was an affirmation of the imperishable soul, which immediately enters its eternal reward or punishment upon separation from the body in death. The older idea of a general resurrection and judgment at the End of the Age was retained, but this last state of the soul only ratifies and perfects the fate of the saved and the damned at death.

In the modern world, mainline Catholic theologians have for the most part remained faithful to the position of Thomas Aquinas. The lurid images and frantic piety surrounding death and the afterlife in the Middle Ages have long since been rejected by educated Catholics. But the devout Catholic can still face the enemy of death armed with the traditional sacramental graces and doctrinal truths of life everlasting. To be sure, some contemporary Catholic theologians interpret these traditional beliefs and practices in symbolic rather than literal terms. For them, the experience of death is viewed as pilgrimage in faith rather than punishment for sin. Death is seen as "the law of human growth," whereby each stage of growth requires a tearing away from previous environments, which have become like so many prisons. In death, one's own body, like the mother's body at birth, is abandoned so that personal growth may continue. Alternatively, death allows the soul to enter into a new all-embracing unity. At death the soul is freed from the limitation of being related to one particular human body and becomes related to the whole universe. The pouring out of the self at death leads to a pan-cosmic level of personal and communal existence. But for the most part, contemporary Roman Catholics simply "look forward to the resurrection of the dead and the life of the world to come," in the words of the Nicene Creed.

Modern Protestant theologians have been even more innovative than their Catholic counterparts. To be sure, mainline Protestants have followed the guidelines laid down by the Reformers. They have combined an emphasis on postmortem rewards and punishments for the soul at death with some notion or another of a Final Consummation of the Age. But a growing freedom from ecclesiastical authority and biblical literalism allowed for a wide range of Protestant theological innovations. These new theologies were usually developed in response to the challenges of modern science and in partnership with one or another modern philosophy.

Beginning in the eighteenth century, the Christian faith was interpreted within such diverse philosophical frameworks as rationalism, romanticism, empiricism, existentialism, and process thought. Not surprisingly, each philosophical theology has dealt with the problem of death and the afterlife in its own distinctive way. These liberal theological experiments share certain convictions about life after death. They reject apocalyptic schemes of history and literalistic views of the afterlife. They empty the afterlife of all ideas of eternal torment, preferring instead to speak of either the total annihilation or eventual salvation of the wicked. But their concrete notions of eternal life run the gamut from the soul's immaterial existence in heaven to the self's authentic existence while on earth. Despite these wide-ranging theological reflections on death, most present-day Protestants hold to the idea of death as the soul's passage to its immortal destiny, either in eternal communion with or eternal separation from God and the people of God.

ETHICAL IMPLICATIONS. The long histories of Judaism and Christianity reveal disagreements within as well as differences between these religious traditions. And yet there are striking parallels between the ways they deal with death over the centuries. Of course, both traditions come out of the same Hebraic background and confront the same broad cultural challenges. But of greater importance is the fact that both traditions are preoccupied with the issue of theodicy. There must be some ultimate justification of the brute fact that the righteous suffer and die along with the wicked. The stubbornly moral character of the Judaic and Christian traditions militates against either indiscriminate immortality or universal annihilation. Thus, for all their differences, Judaism and Christianity are bound together by their efforts to reconcile ethics and eschatology. Not surprisingly, Judaism and Christianity respond in similar ways to a number of "end of life" ethical issues.

1. For the most part, Judaism and Christianity traditionally define death as the moment the spirit leaves the body. The accepted signs of the spirit's departure are the absence of breathing, heartbeat, and pulse. But there is nothing in these theological traditions that directly rules out more precise empirical signs of death, such as a flat brain wave. Most Christian theologians, and many Jewish thinkers, have accepted a brain-oriented definition of death, but some, especially within Orthodox Judaism, oppose such a definition, focusing instead on breathing as the definitive indicator of life. Some contemporary theologians are openly embracing higher-brain oriented definitions of death as modern equivalents of the departure of the spirit from the body.

2. Regardless of the etiology of death, the Jewish and Christian traditions regard death as an evil to be endured rather than a good to be embraced. Though death is inevitable, it is an event to be held at bay by every possible and honorable means that is not excessively burdensome or morally ambiguous. Therefore, most traditional Jews and Christians are categorically opposed to suicide and active euthanasia, or "mercy killing." Since martyrdom is not considered suicide, choosing death over life in service to one's faith or for the sake of others is allowable if it cannot be avoided in an honorable way.

3. Although all must die, not all deaths are the same in the Jewish and Christian traditions. Clearly, there are better and worse ways of dying. The best of deaths is the death of a person at peace with God who is "full of years," relatively free of pain, and surrounded by loved ones. The worst of deaths is to die "before your time," in rebellion against God, and alienated from family and friends. Recognition of these different ways of dying lends at least indirect religious sanctions to modern-day concerns about the "good death." There are no clear-cut religious obligations to prolong the dying process by extraordinarily burdensome means of life support. Indeed, the moral permissibility of withholding or withdrawing heroic means of life support from the terminally ill enjoys wide support among contemporary Jews and Christians alike, even though some Jewish scholars, particularly among the Orthodox, prefer to provide support, whenever possible, until the patient is moribund.

4. For both Jews and Christians, death is a reality that cannot be ignored or wished away. Whether death comes slowly or suddenly, the worst time to deal with death is after it happens. Believers should be prepared to deal with the heartache and havoc it brings before illness or tragedy strikes. We are ready to live only when we are prepared to die. While such preparation need not require the cultivated preoccupation with death of the medieval *Ars moriendi*, it should include a recognition of human mortality and an acceptance of human limits. In principle, such preparation might include the execution of advanced directives regarding terminal care.

5. Although the soul is infinitely more valuable than the body, the bodies of the dead deserve to be treated with care and love. For traditional Jews, such respect for the human body ordinarily excludes mutilation of the body, although sanctions against autopsies and dissection may yield to the superior value of protecting life or punishing crime. Some contemporary Jewish thinkers extend this overriding obligation to preserve life to the justification of organ harvesting for transplantation. Despite centuries of theological opposition, traditional Christians have reconciled themselves to the

legitimacy of anatomical dissection and organ harvesting in the interests of science and medicine, perhaps reflecting the Christian view that the resurrected body is a new creation of God. But more liberal Jews and Christians are untroubled by any of these postmortem procedures, provided they do not disgrace the corpse or disturb the family.

6. Both the Jewish and Christian emphasis on death is, in reality, the obverse of an even greater emphasis on life. At best, death serves as a motive for a creative and responsible life. At worst, death looms as a menace to a courageous and generous life. Either way, death lends an urgency to life that would be utterly lacking without it. Death enhances rather than cheapens the value of life.

7. For both Jews and Christians, there is hope that death does not have the final word in human experience. For many, death is a corridor that leads to a life free of sorrow, suffering, and separation. For others, death is powerless to cut off the faithful from the life of the community and the life of God. On either reckoning, death is incorporated as a meaningful stage in the life cycle. Both the Jewish and Christian traditions, strengthened by centuries of suffering and surviving, provide a variety of ways of affirming life in the face of death.

LONNIE D. KLIEVER (1995)
BIBLIOGRAPHY REVISED

SEE ALSO: *Anthropology and Bioethics; Authority in Religious Traditions; Autonomy; Body: Cultural and Religious Perspectives; Care; Christianity, Bioethics in; Compassionate Love; Grief and Bereavement; Harm; Holocaust; Human Dignity; Infanticide; Islam, Bioethics in; Judaism, Bioethics in; Life; Life, Quality of; Life Sustaining Treatment and Euthanasia; Literature and Healthcare; Narrative; Palliative Care and Hospice; Pediatrics, Intensive Care in; Right to Die, Policy and Law; Suicide; Triage; Value and Valuation; Virtue and Character; Warfare;* and other *Death* subentries

BIBLIOGRAPHY

BIBLICAL THOUGHT

Bailey, Lloyd R., Sr. 1979. *Biblical Perspectives on Death.* Philadelphia: Fortress Press.

Brandon, Samuel George Frederick. 1967. *The Judgment of the Dead: An Historical and Comparative Study of the Idea of a Post-Mortem Judgment in the Major Religions.* London: Weidenfeld and Nicolson.

Brueggeman, Walter. 1976. "Death, Theology of." In *The Interpreter's Dictionary of the Bible: An Illustrated Encyclopedia,*

Supplementary Volume, pp. 219–222, ed. Keith Crim, Lloyd R. Bailey, Sr., Victor P. Furnish, and Emory S. Bucke. Nashville, TN: Abingdon.

Charles, Robert Henry. 1963. *Eschatology: A Doctrine of a Future Life in Israel, Judaism, and Christianity: A Critical History.* New York: Schocken.

Jacob, Edmond. 1962a. "Death." In vol. 1 of *The Interpreter's Dictionary of the Bible: An Illustrated Encyclopedia,* pp. 802–804, ed. George Arthur Buttrick, Thomas S. Kepler, John Knox, Herbert G. May, Samuel Terrien, and Emory S. Bucke. Nashville, TN: Abingdon.

Jacob, Edmond. 1962b. "Immortality." In vol. 2 of *The Interpreter's Dictionary of the Bible: An Illustrated Encyclopedia,* pp. 688–690, ed. George Arthur Buttrick, Thomas S. Kepler, John Knox, Herbert G. May, Samuel Terrien, and Emory S. Bucke. Nashville, TN: Abingdon.

Kaiser, Otto, and Lohse, Eduard. 1981. *Death and Life,* tr. John E. Seely. Nashville, TN: Abingdon.

Keck, Leander E. 1969. "New Testament Views of Death." *Perspectives on Death,* pp. 33–98, ed. Liston O. Mills. Nashville, TN: Abingdon.

Silberman, Lou H. 1969. "Death in the Hebrew Bible and Apocalyptic Literature." *Perspectives on Death,* pp. 13–32, ed. Liston O. Mills. Nashville, TN: Abingdon.

POSTBIBLICAL JUDAISM

Gordon, Audrey. 1975. "The Jewish View of Death: Guidelines for Mourning." *In Death: The Final Stage of Growth,* pp. 44–51, ed. Elisabeth Kübler-Ross. Englewood Cliffs, NJ: Prentice-Hall.

Heller, Zachary I. 1975. "The Jewish View of Death: Guidelines for Dying." *In Death: The Final Stage of Growth,* pp. 38–43, ed. Elisabeth Kübler-Ross. Englewood Cliffs, NJ: Prentice-Hall.

Jakobovits, Immanuel. 1959. *Jewish Medical Ethics: A Comparative and Historical Study of the Jewish Religious Attitude to Medicine and Its Practice.* New York: Bloch.

Kayser, Rudolf. 1972. "Death." In vol. 5 of *Encyclopaedia Judaica,* pp. 1419–1427. New York: Macmillan.

Kohler, Kaufmann. 1964. "Death, Angel of." In vol. 4 of *The Jewish Encyclopedia,* pp. 480–482, ed. Cyrus Adler and Isidore Singer. New York: Ktav.

Kohler, Kaufmann, and Einstein, J. D. 1964. "Death, Views and Customs Concerning." In vol. 4 of *The Jewish Encyclopedia,* pp. 482–486, ed. Cyrus Adler and Isidore Singer. New York: Ktav.

Lamm, Maurice. 1969. *The Jewish Way in Death and Mourning.* New York: J. David.

Mackler, Aaron L. 2001. "Respecting Bodies and Saving Lives: Jewish Perspectives on Organ Donation and Transplantation." *Cambridge Quarterly of Healthcare Ethics* 10(4): 420–429.

Riemer, Jack, ed. 1974. *Jewish Reflections on Death.* New York: Schocken.

Riemer, Jack, and Nuland, Sherwin B., eds. 2002. *Jewish Insights on Death and Mourning* Syracuse, NY: Syracuse University Press.

Scholem, Gershom. 1972. "Kabbalah." In vol. 10 of *Encyclopaedia Judaica*, pp. 490–654. New York: Macmillan.

Weiss, Abner. 1991. *Death and Bereavement: A Halakhic Guide.* Hoboken, NJ: Ktav.

POSTBIBLICAL CHRISTIAN THOUGHT

Badham, Paul. 1987. "The Christian Hope Today." *Death and Immortality in the Religions of the World*, pp. 37–50, ed. Paul Badham and Linda Badham. New York: Paragon House.

Brady, Bernard V. 1998. *The Moral Bond of Community: Justice and Discourse in Christian Morality* Washington, D.C.: Georgetown University Press.

Eber, George. 1997. "End-of-Life Decision Making: An Authentic Christian Death." *Christian Bioethics* 3(3): 183–187.

Engelhardt, H. Tristram Jr. 1998. "Physician-Assisted Suicide Reconsidered: Dying as a Christian in a Post-Christian Age." *Christian Bioethics* 4(2): 143–167.

Engelhardt, H. Tristram Jr. 1998. "Physician-Assisted Death: Doctrinal Development vs. Christian Tradition." *Christian Bioethics* 4(2): 115–121.

Gatch, Milton McCormick. 1969. *Death: Meaning and Mortality in Christian Thought and Contemporary Culture.* New York: Seabury.

Hick, John. 1976. *Death and Eternal Life.* New York: Harper & Row.

Jinkins, Michael. 2002. *The Church Faces Death: Ecclesiology in a Post-Modern Context.* New York: Oxford University Press.

McGown, Thomas. 1987. "Eschatology in Recent Catholic Thought." *Death and Immortality in the Religions of the World*, pp. 51–70, ed. Paul Badham and Linda Badham. New York: Paragon House.

Miller, Arlene B.; Kilner, John F.; and Pellegrino, Edmund D., eds. 1996. *Dignity and Dying: A Christian Appraisal* Grand Rapids, MI: Eerdmans.

Miller-McLemore, Bonnie J. 1988. *Death, Sin and the Moral Life: Contemporary Cultural Interpretations of Death.* Atlanta, GA: Scholars Press.

Stempsey, William E. 1997. "End-of-Life Decisions: Christian Perspectives." *Christian Bioethics* 3(3): 249–261.

Thomasma, David C. 1998. "Assisted Death and Martyrdom." *Christian Bioethics* 4(2): 122–142.

Young, Alexey. 1998. "Natural Death and the Work of Perfection." *Christian Bioethics* 4(2): 168–182.

COMPARATIVE STUDIES

Ariés, Philippe. 1974. *Western Attitudes Toward Death: From the Middle Ages to the Present*, tr. Patricia M. Ranum. Baltimore: Johns Hopkins University Press.

Choron, Jacques. 1963. *Death and Western Thought.* New York: Macmillan.

Eckardt, A. Roy. 1972. "Death in the Judaic and Christian Traditions." *Social Research* 39(3): 489–514.

Hockey, Jennifer Lorna. 1990. *Experiences of Death: An Anthropological Account.* Edinburgh: University Press.

Kabir, Ananya Jahanara. 2001. *Paradise, Death, and Doomsday in Anglo-Saxon Literature (Cambridge Studies in Anglo-Saxon England, Vol. 32).* New York: Cambridge University Press.

Stannard, David E., ed. 1975. *Death in America.* Philadelphia: University of Pennsylvania Press.

Stephenson, John S. 1985. *Death, Grief, and Mourning: Individual and Social Realities.* New York: Free Press.

V. DEATH IN THE WESTERN WORLD

This entry, by the late Talcott Parsons, is reprinted from the first edition. It is followed immediately by a Postscript, prepared by Victor Lidz for the purposes of updating the original entry.

That the death of every known human individual has been one of the central facts of life so long as there has been any human awareness of the human condition does not mean that, being so well known, it is not problematical. On the contrary, like history, it has needed to be redefined and newly analyzed, virtually with every generation. However, as has also been the case with history, with the advancement of knowledge later reinterpretations may have some advantages over earlier ones.

Some conceptualization, beyond common sense, of a human individual or "person" is necessary in order to understand the set of problems presented by death. Therefore, a few comments on this topic are in order before proceeding to a reflection on some of the more salient features of death as it has been understood in the Western world.

The Person and the Problematic of Death

The human individual has often been viewed in the Western world as a synthesized combination of a living organism and a "personality system" (an older terminology made the person a combination of "body" and "mind" or "soul"). It is in fact no more mystical to conceive of a personality analytically distinct from an organism than it is to conceive of a "culture" distinct from the human populations of organisms who are its bearers. The primary criterion of personality, as distinct from organism, is an organization in terms of symbols and their meaningful relations to each other and to persons.

Human individuals, in their organic aspect, come into being through a process of bisexual reproduction. They then go through a more or less well-defined "life course" and eventually die. That human individuals die as organisms is indisputable. If any biological proposition can be regarded as firmly established, it is that the mortality of individual organisms of a sexually reproducing species is completely normal. The death of individuals has a positive survival value for the species.

As Sigmund Freud said, organic death, while a many-faceted thing, is in one principal aspect the "return to the inorganic state." At this level the human organism is "made up" of inorganic materials but is organized in quite special ways. When that organization breaks down—and there is evidence that this is inevitable by reason of the aging process—the constituent elements are no longer part of the living organism but come to be assimilated to the inorganic environment. Still, even within such a perspective on the human individual as an organism, life goes on. The human individual does not stand alone but is part of an intergenerational chain of indefinite durability, the species. The individual organism dies, but if he or she reproduces, the line continues into future generations.

But the problematic of human death arises from the fact that the human individual is not only an organism but also a user of symbols who learns symbolic meanings, communicates with others and with himself or herself through them as media, and regulates his or her behavior, thought, and feelings in symbolic terms. The individual is an "actor" or a "personality." The human actor clearly is not born in the same sense in which an organism is. The personality or actor comes into being through a gradual and complicated process sometimes termed "socialization."

Furthermore, there is a parallel—in my judgment, something more than a mere analogy—between the continuity of the actor and that of the organism. Just as there is an intergenerational continuity on the organic side, so is there an intergenerational continuity on the personality or action side of the human individual. An individual personality is generated in symbiosis with a growing individual organism and, for all we know, dies with that organism. But the individual personality is embedded in transindividual action systems, both social and cultural. Thus the sociocultural matrix in which the individual personality is embedded is in an important sense the counterpart of the population-species matrix in which the individual organism is embedded. The individual personality dies, but the society and cultural system, of which in life he or she was a part, goes on.

But what happens when the personality dies? Is the death of a personality to be simply assimilated to the organic

paradigm? It would seem that the answer is yes, for just as no personality in the human sense can be conceived as such to develop independently of a living organism, so no human personality can be conceived as such to survive the death of the same organism. Nevertheless, the personality or actor certainly influences what happens in the organism—as suicide and all sorts of psychic factors in illnesses and deaths bear witness. Thus, although most positivists and material-ists would affirm that the death of the personality must be viewed strictly according to the organic paradigm, this answer to the problem of human death has not been accepted by the majority in most human societies and cultures. From such primitive peoples as the Australian aborigines to the most sophisticated of the world religions, beliefs in the existence of an individual "soul" have persisted, conceivably with a capacity both to antedate and to survive the individual organism or body. The persistence of that belief and the factors giving rise to it provide the framework for the problematic of death in the Western world.

Christian Orientations toward Death

Because the dominant religious influence in this history of the Western world has been that of Christianity, it is appropriate to outline the main Christian patterns of orientation toward death.

There is no doubt of the predominance of a duality of levels in the Christian paradigm of the human condition, the levels of the spiritual and the material, the eternal and the temporal. On the one hand, there is the material-temporal world, of which one religious symbol is the "dust" to which humankind is said to return at death. On the other hand, there is the spiritual world of "eternal life," which is the location of things divine, not human. The human person stands at the meeting of the two worlds, for he or she is, like the animals, made of "dust," but is also, unlike the animals, made in the image of God. This biblical notion of humanity, when linked to Greek philosophical thought, gave rise to the idea in Catholic Christianity that the divine image was centered in the human soul, which was conceived as in some sense an emanation from the spiritual world of eternal life. Thus arose the notion of the "immortal soul," which could survive the death of the organism, to be rejoined to a resurrected body. The hope of the resurrection, rooted in the Easter faith of the Christian community, was from the beginning a part of the Christian faith and provided another dimension behind the teaching on the immortality of the soul.

The Christian understanding of death as an event in which "life is changed, not taken away," in the words of the traditional requiem hymn, *Dies irae,* can be interpreted in terms of Marcel Mauss's paradigm of the gift and its reciprocation (Parsons, Fox, and Lidz). Seen in this way, the life of the individual is a gift from God, and like other gifts it creates expectations of reciprocation. Living "in the faith" is part of the reciprocation, but, more important to us, dying in the faith completes the cycle. The language of giving also permeates the transcendental level of symbolism in the Christian context. Thus, Mary, like any other woman, *gave* birth to Jesus, God also *gave* his only begotten Son for the redemption of humankind. Finally, Jesus, in the Crucifixion and thus the Eucharist, gave his blood for the same purpose. By the doctrine of reciprocation humankind assumes, it may be said, three principal obligations: to accept the human condition as ordained by the Divine Will, to live in the faith, and to die in the faith (with the hope of resurrection). If these conditions are fulfilled, "salvation," life eternal with God, will come about.

This basically was the paradigm of death in Catholic Christianity. Although the Reformation did collapse some elements in the Catholic paradigm of dualism between the eternal and the temporal, it did not fundamentally alter the meaning of death in societies shaped by the Christian faith. Still, the collapse of the Catholic paradigm did put great pressures on the received doctrine of salvation. The promise of a personal afterlife in heaven, especially if this were conceived to be eternal—which must be taken to mean altogether outside the framework of time—became increasingly difficult to accept. The doctrine of eternal punishment in some kind of hell has proved even more difficult to uphold.

The primary consequence of this collapsing was not, as it has often been interpreted, so much the secularization of the religious component of society as it was the sacralization of secular society, making it the forum for the religious life—notably, though by no means exclusively, through work in a "calling" (as Max Weber held).

Though John Calvin, in his doctrine of predestination, attempted to remove salvation from human control, his doctrine could not survive the cooling of the effervescence of the Reformation. Thus, all later versions of Protestantism accepted some version of the bearing of the individual's moral or attitudinal (faith) merit on salvation. Such control as there was, however, was no longer vested in an ecclesiastical organization but was left to the individual, thus immensely increasing religious and moral responsibility.

The concept of a higher level of reality, a supernatural world in which human persons survived after death, did not give way but became more and more difficult to visualize by simple extrapolation from this-worldly experience; the same problem occurred with the meaning of death as an event in which one gave life back to its Giver and in return was initiated into a new and eternal life. In addition to the changes in conceptualization set in motion by the Reformation, the rise of modern science, which by the eighteenth century had produced a philosophy of scientific materialism, posed an additional challenge to the Christian paradigm of death, manifesting itself primarily in a monism of the physical world. There was at that time little scientific analysis of the world of action, and there was accordingly a tendency to regard the physical universe as unchanging and hence eternal. Death, then, was simply the return to the inorganic state, which implied a complete negation of the conception of eternal life, since the physical, inorganic world was by definition the antithesis of life in any sense.

Contemporary Scientific Orientations

The subsequent development of science has modified, or at least brought into question, the monistic and materialistic paradigm generated by the early enthusiasm for a purely positivistic approach. For one thing, beginning in the nineteenth century and continuing into the twentieth, the sciences of organic life have matured, thanks largely to placing the conception of evolutionary change at the very center of biological thought. This resulted in the view, which has been already noted, that death is biologically normal for individual members of evolving species.

A second and more recent development has been the maturing of the sciences of action. Although these have historical roots in the humanistic tradition, they have only recently been differentiated from the humanistic trunk to become generalizing sciences, integrating within themselves the same conception of evolutionary change that has become the hallmark of the sciences of life.

The development of the action sciences has given rise, as already noted, to a viable conception of the human person as analytically distinct from the organism. At the same time these sciences, by inserting the person into an evolutionary sociocultural matrix analogous to the physico-organic species matrix within which the individual organism is embedded, have been able to create an intellectual framework within which the death of the personality can be understood to be as normal as the death of the organism.

Finally, the concept of evolutionary change has been extended from the life sciences (concerned with the organism) and the action sciences (concerned with the person-actor) to include the whole of empirical reality. And at the same time we have been made aware—principally by the ways in which Einstein's theory of relativity modified the previous assumptions of the absolute empirical "givenness" of physical nature in the Newtonian tradition—of the relative character of our human understanding of the human condition.

Thus there is now a serious questioning of absolutes, both in our search for absolutely universal laws of physical nature and in our quest for metaphysical absolutes in the philosophical wake of Christian theology.

The Kantian Impact and the Limits of Understanding

The developments in a contemporary scientific understanding of the human condition are both congruent with, and in part anticipated and influenced by, Immanuel Kant, whose work during the late eighteenth century was the decisive turning point away from both physical and metaphysical absolutism. Kant basically accepted the reality of the physical universe, as it is humanly known, but at the same time he relativized our knowledge of it to the categories of the understanding, which were not grounded in our direct experience of physical reality but in something transcending this. At the same time Kant equally relativized our conceptions of transcendental reality, whose existence he by no means denied, to something closer to the human condition. Indeed, it may be suggested that Kant substituted procedural conceptions of the absolute, whether physical or metaphysical, for substantive propositions.

While relativizing our knowledge both of the physical world, including the individual human organism, and of the metaphysical world, with its certitude about the immortality of the soul, Kant nonetheless insisted on a transcendental component in human understanding and explicitly included belief in personal immortality in the sense of eternal life.

With respect to the bearing of Kant's thought and its influence through subsequent culture on the problem of the meaning of death, I have already noted that he prepared the way, procedurally, for the development of the action sciences and their ability to account intellectually for the personality or actor experienced as one aspect of the human individual without the need to infer, of necessity, the existence of a spiritual soul existentially and not merely analytically distinct from the living organism. The action sciences, in a very real sense, attempt to provide a coherent account of human subjectivity, much as Kant attempted to do in his *Critique of Judgment,* without collapsing the difference of levels between the physical and what may be called the telic realm.

The framework provided by Kant's thought is indeed congenial to the scientific perspective on the normality of the death of a person, conceived as an actor whose coming into existence is in symbiosis with a growing individual organism and whose individual personality, while continuing into a new generation in the same sociocultural system, can be understood to die in symbiosis with the same organism. Nonetheless, if Kant was right in refusing to collapse the boundaries of the human condition into the one vis-à-vis the physical world, the meaning of human individual death can no more be exhausted by that of the involvement of the human individual in a sociocultural system of more comprehensive temporal duration than can the meaning of our sensory experience of empirical reality be exhausted by the impressions emanating from that external world, or even the theoretical ordering of those impressions.

If Kant's fundamental position is accepted, then his skepticism about absolutes must apply to both sides of the fundamental dichotomy. Modern biology certainly must be classed as knowledge of the empirical world in his sense, and the same is true of our scientific knowledge of human action. In his famous terminology, there is no demonstrable knowledge of the thing in itself in any scientific field.

In empirical terms organic death is completely normal. We have, and according to Kant we presumably can have, no knowledge of the survival of any organic entity after death, except through the processes of organic reproduction that enable the genetic heritage to survive. Kant, however, would equally deny that such survival can be excluded on empirical grounds. This has an obvious bearing on the Christian doctrine of the resurrection of the body. If that is meant in a literal biological sense (though this is by no means universally the way in which Christians understand it), then the inference is clearly that it can never be proved, but it can still be speculated about and can be a matter of faith, even though it cannot be the object of either philosophical or scientific demonstration.

The same seems to hold for the personality-action component of the human individual. Empirically, the action sciences can account for its coming-to-be and its demise without postulating its survival. But they cannot exclude the possibility of such survival. Thus the eternal life of the individual soul, although metaphysically unknowable, can, like resurrected bodies, be speculated about and believed in as a matter of faith.

Thus, included in the victims of Kant's skepticism or relativization is belief in the cognitive necessity of belief in the survival of human individuality after death as well as belief in the cognitive necessity of belief in the nonsurvival of human individuality after death. Kant's relativization of our knowledge, both empirical and metaphysical, both closed and opened doors. It did, of course, undermine the traditional specificities of received beliefs; but at the same time, and for the very same reason, it opened the door, by contrast to scientific materialism, not merely to one alternative to received Christian belief but to a multiplicity of them.

This leaves us with the position that the problem of the meaning of death in the Western tradition has, from a position of relative closure defined by the Christian syndrome, been "opened up" in its recent phase. There is above all a new freedom for individuals and sociocultural movements to try their hands at innovative definitions and conceptions. At the same time, the viability of their innovations is subject to the constraints of the human condition, both empirical and transcendental, noted by Kant.

The grounding of this door-opening process lies in Kant's conception of freedom as the central feature of what he called "practical reason." In essence, the human will, as he called it, can no more be bound by a set of metaphysical dogmas than a person's active intellect can be bound by alleged inherent necessities of the empirical, relevant *Ding an sich.* This doctrine of freedom, among other things, opens the door to Western receptivity to other, notably Oriental, religious traditions. Thus, Buddhist tradition, on the whole by contrast with Christian, stresses not individuality except for this terrestrial life but, rather, the desirability of absorption, after death, into an impersonal, eternal matrix (as opposed to a personal eternal life). The recent vogue of Oriental religion in Western circles suggests that this possibility has become meaningful in the West.

The problem of the meaning of death in the West is now in what must appear to many to be a strangely unsatisfactory state. It seems to come down to the proposition that the meaning of death is that, in the human condition, it cannot have any "apodictically certain" meaning without abridgment of the essential human freedom of thought, experience, and imagination. Within limits, its meaning, as it is thought about, experienced for the case of others, and anticipated for oneself, must be autonomously interpreted. But this is not pure negativism or nihilism, because such openness is not the same as declaring death, and of course with it individual life, to be meaningless.

Conclusion

So far as Western society is concerned, I think the tolerability of this relatively open definition of the situation is associated with the activistic strain in our values, the attitude that human life is a challenging undertaking that in some respects may be treated as an adventure—by contrast with a view that treats human life as a matter of passively enduring an externally imposed fate. Even though Western religion has sometimes stressed humanity's extreme dependency on God, and indeed the sinfulness of asserting independence, on the whole the activistic strain has been dominant. If this is the case, it seems that humans can face their deaths and those of others in the spirit that whatever this unknown future may portend, they can enter upon it with good courage.

Insofar as it is accessible to cognitive understanding at all, the problem of the meaning of death for individual human beings must be approached in the framework of the human condition as a whole. It must include both the relevant scientific understanding and understanding at philosophical levels, and must attempt to synthesize them. Finally it must, as clearly as possible, recognize and take account of the limits of both our scientific and our philosophical understanding.

We have contended that the development of modern science has so changed the picture as to require revision of many of the received features of Christian tradition, both Catholic and Protestant. This emergence of science took place in three great stages marked by the synthesis of physical science in the seventeenth century, that of biological science in the nineteenth, and that of the action sciences in the nineteenth to twentieth.

The most important generalizations seem to be the following. First, the human individual constitutes a unique symbiotic synthesis of two main components, a living organism and a living personality. Second, both components seem to be inherently limited in duration of life, and we have no knowledge that indicates their symbiosis can be in any radical sense dissociated. Third, the individualized entity is embedded in, and derives in some sense from, a transgenerational matrix that, seen in relation to individual mortality, has indefinite but not infinite durability.

From this point of view, death, or the limited temporal duration of the individual life course, must be regarded as one of the facts of life that is as inexorable as the need to eat and breathe in order to live. In this sense, death is completely normal, to the point that its denial must be regarded as pathological. Moreover, this normality includes the consideration that, from an evolutionary point of view, which we have contended is basic to all modern science, death must be regarded as having high survival value, organically at least to the species, actionwise to the future of the sociocultural system. These scientific considerations are not trivial, or conventional, or culture-bound but are fundamental.

There is a parallel set of considerations on the philosophical side. For purposes of elucidating this aspect of the problem complex, I have used Kant's framework as presented in his three critiques. On the one hand, this orientation is critical in that it challenges the contention that absolute knowledge is demonstrable in any of the three aspects of human condition. Thus, any conception like that of the ontological essence of nature, the idea of God, or the notion of the eternal life of the human soul is categorized as *Ding an sich,* which in principle is not demonstrable by rational cognitive procedures.

At the same time, Kant insisted, and I follow him here, on the cognitive necessity of assuming a transcendental component, a set of categories in each of the three realms, that is not reducible to the status of humanly available inputs from either the empirical or the absolute telic references of the human condition. We have interpreted this to mean that human orientation must be relativized to the human condition, not treated as dogmatically fixed in the nature of things.

The consequence of this relativization that we have particularly emphasized is that it creates a new openness for orientations, which humans are free to exploit by speculation and to commit themselves in faith, but with reference to which they cannot claim what Kant called apodictic certainty.

If the account provided in the preceding sections is a correct appraisal of the situation in the Western world today, it is not surprising that there is a great deal of bafflement, anxiety, and downright confusion in contemporary attitudes and opinions in this area. Any consensus about the meaning of death in the Western world today seems far off, although the attitude reflected in this entry would seem to be the one most firmly established at philosophical levels and the level of rather abstract scientific theory.

A very brief discussion of three empirical points may help to mitigate the impression of extreme abstractness. First, though scientific evidence has established the fact of the inevitability of death with increasing clarity, this does not mean that the experience of death by human populations may not change with changing circumstances. Thus, we may distinguish between inevitable death and "adventitious" death, that is, deaths that are premature relative to the full lifespan, and in principle preventable by human action (Parsons and Lidz). Since about 1840, this latter category of deaths has decreased enormously. The proportion of persons in modern populations over sixty-five has thus increased greatly, as has the expectancy of life at birth. This clearly means that a greatly increased proportion of modern humans approximate to living out a full life course, rather than dying prematurely. Individuals living to "a ripe old age" will have experienced an inevitably larger number of deaths of persons who were important to them. These will be in decreasing number the deaths of persons younger than themselves, notably their own children, and increasingly deaths of their parents and whole ranges of persons of an older generation, such as teachers, senior occupational associates, and many public figures. Quite clearly these demographic changes will have a strong effect on the balance of experience and expectations, of the deaths of significant others, and of anticipation of one's own death.

Second, one of the centrally important aspects of a process of change in orientation of the sort described should be the appearance of signs of the differentiation of attitudes and conceptions with regard to the meaning of the life cycle. There has already been such a process of differentiation, apparently not yet completed, with respect to both ends of the life cycle (Parsons, Fox, and Lidz). With respect to the beginning, of course, this centers on the controversy over the legitimacy of abortion and the beginning of life. And concomitant with this controversy has been an attempt at redefinition of death. So far the most important movement has been to draw a line within the organic sector between what has been called brain death, where irreversible changes have taken place, destroying the functioning of the central nervous system, and what has been called metabolic death, where, above all, the functions of heartbeat and respiration have ceased. The problem has been highlighted by the capacity of artificial measures to keep a person alive for long periods after the irreversible cessation of brain function. The main point of interest here is the connection of brain function with the personality level of individuality. An organism that continues to live at only the metabolic level may be said to be dead as an actor or person.

Third, and finally, a few remarks about the significance for our problem of Freud's most mature theoretical statement need to be made. It was printed in the monograph published in English under the title *The Problem of Anxiety.* In this, his last major theoretical work, Freud rather drastically revised his previous views about the nature of anxiety. He focused on the expectation of the loss of an "object." For Freud the relevant meaning of the term "object" was a human individual standing in an emotionally significant relation to the person of reference. To the growing child, of course, the parents became "lost objects" in the nature of the process of growing up, in that their significance for the growing child was inevitably "lost" at later ages. The ultimate loss of a concrete human person as object—of cathexis, Freud said—is the death of that person. To have "grown away" from one's parents is one thing, but to experience their actual deaths is another. Freud's account of the impact on him of the death of his father is a particularly relevant case in point.

Equally clearly, an individual's own death, in anticipation, can be subsumed under the category of object loss, particularly in view of Freud's theory of narcissism, by which he meant the individual's cathexis of his or her own self as a love object. Anxiety, however, is not the actual experience of object loss, nor is it, according to Freud, the fear of it. It is an anticipatory orientation in which the actor's own emotional security is particularly involved. It is a field of rather free play of fantasy as to what might be the consequences of an anticipated or merely possible event.

Given the hypothesis that, in our scientifically oriented civilization, there is widespread acceptance of death—meant as the antithesis of its denial—there is no reason why this should lead to a cessation or even substantial diminution of anxiety about death, both that of others and one's own. Indeed, in certain circumstances the levels of anxiety may be expected to increase rather than the reverse. The frequent assertions that our society is characterized by pervasive denial of death may often be interpreted as calling attention to pervasive anxieties about death, which is not the same thing. There can be no doubt that in most cases death is, in experience and in anticipation, a traumatic event. Fantasies, in such circumstances, are often characterized by strains of unrealism, but the prevalence of such phenomena does not constitute a distortion of the basic cultural framework within which we moderns orient ourselves to the meaning of death.

Indeed, the preceding illustrations serve to enhance the importance of clarification, at the theoretical and philosophical levels, to which the bulk of this entry has been devoted. This is essential if an intelligible approach is to be made to the understanding of such problems as shifts in attitudes toward various age groups in modern society, particularly the older groups, and the relatively sudden eruption of dissatisfaction with the traditional modes of conceptualizing the beginning and the termination of a human life, and with allegations about the pervasive denial of death, which is often interpreted as a kind of failure of "intestinal fortitude." However important the recent movements for increasing expression of emotional interests and the like, ours remains a culture to which its cognitive framework is of paramount significance.

TALCOTT PARSONS (1995)

BIBLIOGRAPHY

Bellah, Robert N. 1964. "Religious Evolution." *American Sociological Review* 29(3): 358–374.

Burke, Kenneth. 1961. *The Rhetoric of Religion: Studies in Logology.* Boston: Beacon.

Chomsky, Noam. 1957. *Syntactic Structures.* The Hague, Netherlands: Mouton.

Durkheim, Émile. 1933. *The Division of Labor in Society,* ed. and tr. George Simpson. Glencoe, IL: Free Press.

Durkheim, Émiffle. 1974. *Sociology and Philosophy,* enl. edition, tr, D. F. Pocock. New York: Free Press.

Durkheim, Émile. 1976. *The Elementary Forms of the Religious Life,* tr. Joseph Ward Swain, 2nd edition. London: Allen and Unwin.

Freud, Sigmund. 1953–1974 (1920). *Beyond the Pleasure Principle.* In *The Standard Edition of the Complete Psychological Works of Sigmund Freud,* vol. 18, ed. James Strachey, Anna Freud, Alix Strachey, and Alan Tyson. London: Hogarth Press.

Freud, Sigmund. 1953–1974 (1923). *The Ego and the Id.* In *The Standard Edition of the Complete Psychological Works of Sigmund Freud,* vol. 19, ed. James Strachey, Anna Freud, Alix Strachey, and Alan Tyson. London: Hogarth Press.

Freud, Sigmund. 1953–1974. (1926). *Inhibitions, Symptoms, and Anxiety.* In *The Standard Edition of the Complete Psychological Works of Sigmund Freud,* vol. 20, ed. James Strachey, Anna Freud, Alix Strachey, and Alan Tyson. London: Hogarth Press.

Freud, Sigmund. 1953–1974 (1927). *The Future of an Illusion.* In *The Standard Edition of the Complete Psychological Works of Sigmund Freud,* vol. 21, ed. James Strachey, Anna Freud, Alix Strachey, and Alan Tyson. London: Hogarth Press.

Freud, Sigmund. 1953–1974. *The Standard Edition of the Complete Psychological Works of Sigmund Freud,* 24 vols., ed. James Strachey, Anna Freud, Alix Strachey, and Alan Tyson. London: Hogarth Press.

Freud, Sigmund. 1954. *The Origins of Psycho-analysis: Letters to Wilhelm Fliess, Drafts and Notes, 1887–1902,* ed. Marie N. Bonaparte, Anna Freud, and Ernst Kris and tr. Eric Mosbacher and James Strachey. New York: Basic.

Henderson, Lawrence Joseph. 1913. *The Fitness of the Environment: An Inquiry into the Biological Significance of the Properties of Matter.* New York: Macmillan.

Henderson, Lawrence Joseph. 1917. *The Order of Nature: An Essay.* Cambridge, MA: Harvard University Press.

Henderson, Lawrence Joseph. 1935. *Pareto's General Sociology: A Physiologist's Interpretation.* Cambridge, MA: Harvard University Press.

Kant, Immanuel. 1929. *Critique of Pure Reason,* tr. Norman Kemp Smith. London: Macmillan.

Kant, Immanuel. 1949. *Critique of Practical Reason and Other Writings in Moral Philosophy,* tr. and ed. Lewis White Beck. Chicago: University of Chicago Press.

Kant, Immanuel. 1952. *Critique of Judgment,* tr. James Creed Meredith. Oxford: Clarendon Press.

Leach, Edmund R. 1969. *Genesis as Myth and Other Essays.* London: Jonathan Cape.

Lévi-Strauss, Claude. 1963–1976. *Structural Anthropology,* 2 vols., tr. Claire Jacobson, Brooke Grundfest Schoepf, and Monique Layton. New York: Basic.

Lovejoy, Arthur Oncken. 1936. *The Great Chain of Being: A Study of the History of an Idea.* Cambridge, MA: Harvard University Press.

Mauss, Marcel. 1954. *The Gift: Forms and Functions of Exchange in Archaic Societies,* tr. Ian Cunnison. Glencoe, IL: Free Press.

Nock, Arthur D. 1933. *Conversion: The Old and the New in Religion from Alexander the Great to Augustine of Hippo.* London: Oxford University Press.

Parsons, Talcott. 1977. *Social Systems and the Evolution of Action Theory.* New York: Free Press.

Parsons, Talcott; Fox, Renée C.; and Lidz, Victor M. 1973. "The 'Gift of Life' and Its Reciprocation." In *Death in American Experience,* ed. Arien Mack. New York: Schocken. First published in *Social Research* 39(3) [1972]: 367–415.

Parsons, Talcott, and Lidz, Victor M. 1967. "Death in American Society." In *Essays in Self-Destruction,* ed. Edwin S. Shneidman. New York: Science House.

Warner, William Lloyd. 1959. *The Living and the Dead: A Study of the Symbolic Life of Americans.* New Haven, CT: Yale University Press.

Weber, Max. 1930. *The Protestant Ethic and the Spirit of Capitalism,* tr. Talcott Parsons. New York: Scribners.

Weber, Max. 1963. *The Sociology of Religion,* tr. Ephraim Fischoff. Boston: Beacon.

POSTSCRIPT

Talcott Parsons's entry "Death in the Western World" addresses the changing and conflicting orientations toward death in contemporary culture. Parsons sought to connect these orientations to broad cultural frameworks that have shaped Western civilization over hundreds of years. His effort was an extension of his previous writings on American orientations toward death and on more general patterns of Western civilization (Parsons and Lidz; Parsons; Parsons, Fox, and Lidz).

In the 1960s and 1970s, a number of authors argued that Americans "deny" death in a defensive manner (Mitford; Becker). They cited particular funeral and mourning customs as evidence, especially the preparing of remains to appear lifelike and peaceful for ritual viewing and the expectation that formal mourning need divert the family of a deceased person from other social obligations for only a brief time. Parsons, however, perceived that if there were a generalized denial of death, it would conflict with the pragmatic realism rooted in American culture since Puritan times.

Instrumental Activism

Parsons drew on German sociologist Max Weber's (1864–1920) characterization of the Puritan religious ethic as an "inner-worldly asceticism" that sought to engage the harsher realities of life to transform them into elements of the "kingdom of God on earth" (Weber, 1930). While agreeing with Weber's analysis, he preferred the term *instrumental activism* to characterize the basic values and worldview

of American society. This term underscored that American civilization had secularized the Puritan emphasis on mastery over the given conditions of life and made it the ethical basis for a wide range of worldly social institutions. Thus, secular variants of the mastery ethic now guide the formation of institutions in science and technology, formally rational law and bureaucracy, the market system and entrepreneurship, and motives of personal self-discipline and improvement (Parsons). Highlighting consistency with this basic cultural theme, Parsons found not "denial" of death but mastery over its disrupting effects on personal and social life.

While death is inevitable, its social impact is meliorable. Parsons explored two respects in which this is true (Parsons and Lidz; Parsons, Fox, and Lidz). First, medical and public health technologies have reduced premature death and now typically enable members of society to use "God-given" talents to advance their vocations in good health over long lives. The demographic changes of the late nineteenth and twentieth centuries, and related efficiencies in the use of human talents, thus flowed from an effort to master death. Second, when individuals die, the resulting experiences of social loss can be controlled. Measures ranging from life insurance to retirement planning in business to estate planning in personal affairs to psychotherapy for grief and loss reduce harms ensuing from death (Zelizer, 1983). Similarly, American mourning customs emphasize austerely supporting the bereaved in overcoming grief and guilt, so they are able to return to their routine social obligations without long delay.

Parsons recognized that, despite sharing the values of "instrumental activism," Americans disagree over many matters related to death. Abortion, capital punishment, licensing of firearms, euthanasia, medical care for the terminally ill, and organ transplantation, for example, were matters of public controversy when Parsons wrote and remain so today. "Death in the Western World" attempts to explain why this particular domain of contemporary culture has been chronically ridden with controversy. Parsons sought an answer in the rationalism of the Enlightenment, focusing on its synthesis in the philosophy of Immanuel Kant (1724–1804).

Secular Rationalism

Kant epitomized the Enlightenment's elevation of Reason as a force of human betterment and a method of transforming culture (Cassirer). Ever since the Enlightenment, Reason has provided a principle for critique of traditional culture, social institutions, and customary practices. Over time, critique of the traditional has gradually given way to the articulation of new principles of legitimacy. Since the eighteenth century, the appeal to Reason has given rise to a secular moral culture as the primary ground of legitimation for the major institutional frameworks of modern society—for the institutional complexes that Weber characterized as having "rational-legal" legitimation (Weber, 1968; Lidz, 1979a, 1979b). Parsons epitomized this long and complex process of cultural change by focusing on Kant's writings and their long-term impact on the creation of new intellectual disciplines and moral-political ideologies.

In Parsons's view, Kant's critique of Newtonian physics became a model for assessing the intellectual legitimacy of new disciplines. It led to the opening of the domain of methodically developed and evaluated knowledge to new forms. Thus, from Kant's time to ours, there has been continuous growth in specialized scientific and scholarly disciplines. Kant's critiques of the human faculties of judgment and practical reason proved no less important, as they legitimated the voice of moral Reason and, as Parsons emphasized, undercut all claims to ultimate moral certainty. Ever since, Western civilization has been engulfed in ever-renewed moral and ideological controversies on almost every topic of social import. As Parsons expected, orientations toward death, given their irreducible significance to humanity, have been caught up in a range of the controversies.

Varying Worldviews

Across the Western world, one observes considerable variation in the adoption of principles of instrumental activism and secular rationalism. Parsons concentrated on a predominant American pattern, but one that many parts of Western civilization, including important groups in American society, have adopted only with qualifications. Catholic societies have generally shown more attachment to tradition, to historical continuity, and to sustaining community structures, and thus less activism in transforming traditional institutions and less individualism. Lutheran societies have given more emphasis to the inner moral cultivation of the individual and less to mastery of the outer world. Fundamentalist Protestantism has been less accepting of secular rationalism and has tended to maintain the emphasis of the Reformation on immediate mastery of morally problematic situations. Anglo-American versions of Enlightenment rationalism have been profoundly individualistic, while French rationalism has been more collectivistic, and German rationalism more focused on transcendental frames of judgment (Mead). In an article published in 2002, Hans Joas criticized Parsons's treatment of the gift of life as a basis of religious ethics in Western Christianity for having overlooked the continuing variation in worldviews. One may add that the variation in outlooks contributes importantly to contemporary controversies, sustaining the disagreements and adding to the anxiety over difficulties in resolving them.

Parsons's emphasis on Enlightenment rationalism as a foundation of modern intellectual disciplines and public moral discourse helps one to understand the nature of contemporary bioethics. Research on the history of bioethics shows that the field has emerged in the mold of an academic specialty that, although interdisciplinary, is dominated by philosophers (Messikomer, Fox, and Swazey). Philosophers trained in the field of ethics have successfully asserted the centrality of their expertise for resolving bioethical issues. Although the relevance of issues of life, death, illness, suffering, incapacity, and worry would seem to create a large role for theologians and religious philosophers in the field of bioethics, they have in fact been marginalized by the prestige of academic philosophy (Messikomer, Fox, and Swazey). Moreover, given the extent to which key innovations in biomedicine have been concentrated in the United States and that the issues created by such innovations have been suffused with the problematics of American moral discourse, the individualism and positivism of Anglo-American philosophy has predominated in bioethics internationally. This process has been further supported by the strategic role that American governmental regulations have assumed in the international structures of biomedical research, in particular regarding clinical trials for new medications and medical devices.

Recent Evolution of Cultural Conflicts

Although Parsons expected death-related matters to remain controversial, he could not foresee the recent evolution of cultural conflicts. The intense social criticism of funeral and mourning customs has subsided, though practices have changed little. How "life" and "living being" should be defined before birth and at the approach of death remain effervescent issues. Public debates over abortion not only have persisted but have grown in intensity, bitterness, and political importance. Issues of end-of-life care and the use of extreme measures to maintain life continue to figure in public discussion, often in connection with legal cases. Procedures once viewed as extreme, such as kidney, liver, and heart transplants, have become routine at many medical centers, but discussion continues around such issues as who should be treated—for example, whether persons with alcohol dependence should receive new livers or smokers new lungs, or whether HIV-positive patients qualify for organ transplants. The public attends with ever greater interest to advances in medicine, with new findings and procedures featured routinely on television and in newspapers. Coverage of heroic lifesaving procedures in particular resonates deeply in American moral culture, dramatizing shared beliefs in the unique value of each life. Themes of self-improvement pervade reports on the health food, antismoking, physical exercise, environmental, and even animal-rights movements.

Despite impressive institutions to master death, contemporary civilization remains acutely insecure over life (Fox and Swazey). The mass media's increasing attention to medicine, and especially to life-threatening conditions, has left the public less secure about health and more readily made anxious over environmental threats and even endemic conditions. The intensity of public fears over apparent "hot spots" of breast cancer in particular communities, over risks of anthrax infection following "terroristic" mailings of a small number of letters containing anthrax spores in the autumn of 2001, and over small risks of West Nile virus in the summer of 2002 are instances. In the context of anxiety over health, matters of personal habit and lifestyle, including diet, exercise, work schedules, and even sexual practices, are adjusted by many whenever new knowledge suggests possible effects on well-being or longevity. Parsons would have viewed such changes in personal habits as efforts to extend mastery over the conditions of life, including death.

In attending patients with highly cultivated medical insecurities, physicians have a limited fund of trust to draw upon, a situation that promotes the practice of "defensive medicine." When the lives of patients are genuinely at risk, pressures build to use the most advanced technologies and extreme measures to show that everything possible is being attempted. This is sometimes the case even when the chances of success are small and when the quality of the lives that may be extended will be quite limited. These tendencies persist while the public also worries over the rising aggregate costs of medical care and health insurance.

In the context of post-Enlightenment secular beliefs about human rights, Western societies have generally established a right of citizens to receive medical care. Different institutions have been established to secure this right, including government single-payer, publicly subsidized private, employer-paid, and combined health insurance systems. The United States stands out among Western nations for not having established universal healthcare or health insurance, although Medicare for the elderly and Medicaid for the poor cover many economically vulnerable citizens.

From the mid-1990s, U.S. national policy has engaged the issue of further democratization of access to medical care. The public has become aware that large sectors of the population lack medical insurance and, hence, access to healthcare independent of personal ability to pay for it. Although the desirability of providing better care to citizens of modest means and the poor is generally accepted, proposals about how to manage the costs while protecting the freedom of doctor–patient relationships are controversial. Proposals that appear to restrict the freedom of relationships between patients and practitioners, whether rights of patients to select their practitioners or the rights of practitioners to treat patients as they believe correct, are widely opposed. Moreover, new plans for cost containment have not directly confronted public sentiments favoring use of "heroic measures" and experimental procedures regardless of cost—sentiments that become especially forceful when physicians and family members face a patient's impending death. Eventual policy remains uncertain, but a system of national health insurance would extend "instrumental activism" in medicine by offering more secure protection from illness, suffering, and death for less affluent citizens.

Shaken Optimism about Modern Medicine

Parsons believed, along with many scientists in the 1960s and 1970s, that modern medicine verged on conquering all major infectious diseases, at least for societies with effective systems of sanitation and public health. The appearance in the 1980s of the human immunodeficiency virus (HIV) and acquired immunodeficiency syndrome (AIDS) has shaken such optimism. It has now become clear that humankind faces a major pandemic that, despite modern science and technology, will take scores of millions of lives globally (WHO). Twenty years of research has failed to produce an effective vaccine. New antiretroviral medications are extending the life and health of many patients with HIV/AIDS, but not all patients are helped, and how long the others will benefit remains unclear (IAPAC). In the meantime, many patients do not receive the new treatments because they have not been diagnosed, are not willing to face the consequences of an HIV/AIDS diagnosis, lack access to care or means of paying for treatment, or do not trust medical institutions to help them (Klitzman).

The costs of the new medications for HIV/AIDS are prohibitively high for most of the populations in non-Western nations, and an active controversy in the early 2000s concerned ways of making them available at reduced cost in African, Asian, and Latin American societies. Until there is an effective vaccine or a less expensive cure, prevention programs must play a prominent role in overall HIV/AIDS policy. In the United States, prevention programming still faces challenges in communicating effectively with sectors of the population most seriously at risk, in part because of political constraints on frank communication with adolescents and young adults regarding sexual practices and condom use and on laws affecting availability of sterile injection paraphernalia.

Western nations have had the public health resources to stabilize rates of HIV infections at low or moderate levels. According to World Health Organization (WHO) data from 2002, Thailand and Uganda had managed to reduce formerly high rates of infection. In a number of nations in sub-Saharan Africa, however, the continued rapid spread of HIV, as of 2003 affecting more than 28.5 million people, in some countries over 30 percent of adults in their reproductive years, is radically changing demographic structures and life-cycle patterns. In Parsons's terms, a major feature of the epidemic is that it afflicts mainly youths, young adults, and people in early middle age. People who become diseased and die are losing their most productive years. Their deaths represent unfulfilled lives, with future achievements, relationships, and experiences all lost. The economic impact on whole regions and nations is becoming immense, as is the burden of caring for children whose parents have died. WHO reported in 2002 that India, China, Burma, Indonesia, and perhaps Russia also had rapidly growing epidemics and were at risk of experiencing similar effects on regional if not national bases.

In Western societies, where HIV infection is concentrated in homosexual men, injection drug users, and, increasingly, women sex partners of injection drug users and of men who have sex with men (CDC), its transmission has often involved stigmatized behavior. HIV, with the ugly image of a wasting, disfiguring, and dementing disease, has added vastly to the burdens of prior stigmas. Many people with HIV disease have experienced intense feelings of guilt, shame, and self-blame as an added dimension of their suffering (Klitzman). Moreover, many have experienced great loss. In social circles where HIV has become common, many individuals still in early adulthood have lost many friends and associates, an otherwise rare experience in modern societies, given the generally thorough control of death before old age. Many are burdened by the "survivors' guilt" typical of people who live through disasters that have claimed the lives of many others (Erikson). They often find that any attempt at a spirited resumption of everyday activities is complicated by feelings that their futures are hopeless or meaningless without the individuals who have been lost. People not infected but aware of being at risk of infection may feel that they will inevitably become diseased—even that they are already "dead," although still walking around. Efforts to change personal conduct in order to avoid exposure to HIV may be complicated by beliefs that it is impossible to stay well or that it would be better to accompany friends in heroic suffering and death (Weitz). In some

Western communities and in African and Asian nations, lassitude engendered by the HIV epidemic, through social loss, fear of death, and guilt, is causing immense social dislocation and will likely cause more in the future.

Conclusion

Parsons's entry highlighted the distinctive pattern of Western institutions relating to death. In comparative perspective, Parsons argued, the modern West has uniquely endeavored to "master" death. Such mastery has involved a range of institutions, including scientific medicine and public health services designed to protect life; insurance, retirement, and estate planning to manage the practical consequences of deaths; and mourning customs that emphasize recovery of survivors' abilities to perform ordinary social roles soon after the death of family members, friends, and associates. Some elements of these institutions remain closely tied to the "instrumental activism" of Western cultural values, while other elements, such as the techniques of scientific medicine or the actuarial tables and formulas of the insurance industry, have transcultural validity now that they have been developed. A matter for future investigation concerns the ways in which these universal elements will be institutionalized in sociocultural settings where they may be disconnected from Western value orientations. Scientific medicine is now practiced almost the world over, but in some non-Western societies it is generally reserved for patients from elite status groups, combined with traditional healing in ways that create different doctor and patient roles, or may be linked to personal relationships of political patronage (Kleinman; Scheper-Hughes). In these settings, the bioethical cultures that emerge in the future may prove to be very different from Western frameworks of the past several decades, not least because they will rest on different value orientations toward life and death. Comparative study of bioethical cultures may become a powerful way of building on, correcting, and refining the analysis developed by Parsons in his writings on Western orientations toward death.

VICTOR LIDZ (1995)
REVISED BY AUTHOR

SEE ALSO: *Autonomy; Body: Cultural and Religious Perspectives; Christianity, Bioethics in; Grief and Bereavement; Harm; Holocaust; Human Dignity; Infanticide; Islam, Bioethics in; Judaism, Bioethics in; Life; Life, Quality of; Life Sustaining Treatment and Euthanasia; Literature and Healthcare; Narrative; Palliative Care and Hospice; Pastoral Care and Healthcare Chaplaincy; Pediatrics, Intensive Care in; Right to Die, Policy and Law; Suicide; Triage;*

Value and Valuation; Virtue and Character; Warfare; and other Death subentries

BIBLIOGRAPHY

Becker, Ernest. 1973. The Denial of Death. New York: Free Press.

Cassirer, Ernst. 1955. The Philosophy of the Enlightenment. Boston: Beacon.

Centers for Disease Control and Prevention (CDC). 2002. HIV/AIDS Surveillance Report 14(1) (June 2002). Atlanta, GA: Author.

Erikson, Kai T. 1976. Everything in Its Path: Destruction of Community in the Buffalo Creek Flood. New York: Simon and Schuster.

Fox, Renée C. 1979. "The Medicalization and Demedicalization of American Society." In Essays in Medical Sociology: Journeys into the Field. New York: Wiley.

Fox, Renée C., and Swazey, Judith P. 1992. Spare Parts: Organ Replacement in American Society. New York: Oxford University Press.

International Association of Physicians in AIDS Care (IAPAC). 2001. "Guidelines for the Use of Antiretroviral Agents in HIV-Infected Adults and Adolescents." IAPAC Monthly 7(1) supplement.

Joas, Hans. 2002. "The Gift of Life: The Sociology of Religion in Talcott Parsons' Late Work." Journal of Classical Sociology 1(1): 127–141.

Kleinman, Arthur. 1980. Patients and Healers in the Context of Culture: An Exploration of the Borderland between Anthropology, Medicine, and Psychiatry. Berkeley: University of California Press.

Klitzman, Robert. 1997. Being Positive: The Lives of Men and Women with HIV. Chicago: Ivan R. Dee.

Lidz, Victor. 1979a. "The Law as Index, Phenomenon, and Element: Conceptual Steps toward a General Sociology of Law." Sociological Inquiry 49(1): 5–25.

Lidz, Victor. 1979b. "Secularization, Ethical Life, and Religion in Modern Societies." In Religious Change and Continuity, ed. Harry M. Johnson. San Francisco: Jossey-Bass.

Mead, George Herbert. 1936. Movements of Thought in the Nineteenth Century. Chicago: University of Chicago Press.

Messikomer, Carla M.; Fox, Renée C.; and Swazey, Judith P. 2001. "The Presence and Influence of Religion in American Bioethics." Perspectives in Biology and Medicine 44(4): 485–508.

Mitford, Jessica. 1963. The American Way of Death. New York: Simon and Schuster.

Parsons, Talcott. 1971. The System of Modern Societies. Englewood Cliffs, NJ: Prentice-Hall.

Parsons, Talcott; Fox, Renée C.; and Lidz, Victor M. 1973. "The 'Gift of Life' and Its Reciprocation." In Death in American Experience, ed. Arien Mack. New York: Schocken. First published in Social Research 39(3) [1972]: 367–415.

Parsons, Talcott, and Lidz, Victor M. 1967. "Death in American Society." In Essays in Self-Destruction, ed. Edwin S. Shneidman. New York: Science House.

Scheper-Hughes, Nancy. 1992. Death without Weeping: The Violence of Everyday Life in Brazil. Berkeley: University of California Press.

Weber, Max. 1930. The Protestant Ethic and the Spirit of Capitalism, tr. Talcott Parsons. New York: Scribners.

Weber, Max. 1968. Economy and Society, 3 vols., ed. Guenther Roth and Claus Wittich. New York: Bedminster Press.

Weitz, Rose. 1991. Life with AIDS. New Brunswick, NJ: Rutgers University Press.

World Health Organization (WHO). 2002. Report on the Global HIV/AIDS Epidemic, 2002. New York: United Nations.

Zelizer, Viviana. 1983. Morals and Markets: The Development of Life Insurance in the United States. New Brunswick, NJ: Transaction Books.

VI. PROFESSIONAL EDUCATION

Palliative care represents a new health professional discipline in the United States focused on the care of seriously ill and dying patients, although not necessarily just for patients at the end of their lives. There is widespread agreement that all facets of the end-of-life experience have been neglected in health professional education, including, but not limited to, pain and symptom management, communication skills, ethics, personal awareness and hospice care. Educational initiatives have emerged, especially within medicine and nursing, to address these deficiencies. This discussion will focus primarily on physician education within palliative care, although the discussion is directly applicable to other health professions.

Requirements for End-of-Life Physician Education in the United States

Until recently, few medical schools offered comprehensive training in end-of-life care. The training that existed was largely elective, in lecture format, and with limited patient contact. Although some U.S. medical schools developed dedicated palliative care courses or comprehensive curricula, this was the exception until very recently. The Liaison Committee on Medical Education (LCME), the accrediting authority for United States medical schools, mandated in 2000 that all medical schools provide instruction in end of life care, which may improve the situation.

Graduate physician education requirements for end-of-life training are also highly variable. Since 1997 the oversight educational committees for Geriatrics, Family Medicine, Internal Medicine, Neurology, General Surgery and Hematology/Oncology have added requirements for end-of-life training. In the realm of testing, the National Board of Medical Examiners started work in 1999 to review, re-write and expand end-of-life content on test questions administered to all medical students and interns.

Although there is no national requirement for physicians already in practice to attend continuing education courses in end-of-life care, the American Medical Association (AMA) has encouraged all its member physicians to participate in *Education for Physicians on End-of-life Care* (EPEC), a comprehensive training program. In addition, starting in 2000, the state of California began requiring that all applicants for a medical license successfully complete a medical curriculum that provides instruction in pain management and end-of-life care. As with the LCME requirement for medical schools, the exact criteria to determine what constitutes end of life instruction have not been defined.

Curriculum Guides for End-of-Life Physician Education

Several groups have worked to define the components of a comprehensive end-of-life and palliative care curriculum. Curriculum guidelines have been developed for Canadian medical schools and separate guidelines exist for medical student training in Great Britain and Ireland. Palliative care teaching objectives for U.S. physicians were first published in 1994. In 1997, a national consensus conference on U.S. undergraduate and graduate education was held, outlining curriculum features and opportunities for education across different educational venues (e.g. ambulatory care, inpatient care). Although each venue presented somewhat different aspects of end-of-life care education, there is broad similarity on the major educational domains (see Table 1). Finally, a consensus document was developed by participants from eleven U.S. medical schools working on an end of life curriculum project. This document outlines goals and objectives for medical student education along with a discussion of potential student assessment measures and curriculum implementation strategies.

The American Academy of Hospice and Palliative Medicine (AAHPM) developed a curriculum designed for medical educators and practicing physicians. This curriculum includes twenty-two modules, each containing a listing of learning objectives and core content for key domains in symptom control, communication, hospice care, and ethics. The AAHPM curriculum was originally designed for physicians working as hospice medical directors, but can easily be adapted for other levels of physician education. The EPEC project, designed for physicians in practice, contains a comprehensive palliative care curriculum including pain

TABLE 1

Domains and Locations for Palliative Care Physician Education

Educational Domains

- Pain assessment and treatment
- Non-pain symptom assessment and treatment
- Ethical principles and legal aspects of end-of-life care
- Communication skills; Personal reflection
- Psychosocial Aspects of Death and Dying:
    Death as a life-cycle event
    Psychological aspects of care for patient/family
    Cultural and spiritual aspects of end-of-life care
    Suffering/Hope
    Patient/family counseling skills
- Working as part of an interdisciplinary team

Care Locations

- Hospital
- Hospice/ Palliative Care Consultation Service or Inpatient Unit
- Outpatient Clinic
- Home
- Residential Hospice
- Long-term care facility

SOURCE: Author.

and symptom control, communication skills, ethics, and legal aspects of care. The most recent curriculum for medical oncologists and oncology trainees, developed in 2001 by the American Society of Clinical Oncology, includes twenty-nine modules covering symptom control, communication skills, and related aspects of palliative care. Curriculum standards for palliative care fellowships have been proposed by the American Board of Hospice and Palliative Medicine and the AAHPM. An extensive listing of peer-reviewed educational tools, curriculum guides, reference articles, and palliative care links are available at the End-of-Life Education Resource Center.

In parallel to physician education, the nursing profession has been working to develop curriculum guidelines and materials for nursing education. Palliative care education content has been reviewed in nursing textbooks and two educational products have been developed for nursing education, *ELNEC* (end-of-life nursing education consortium) and *TNEEL* (the toolkit for nursing excellence at end-of-life transitions) (Ferrell et al.). In addition, a national consortium of nursing groups has come together to plan for institutional changes in nursing education and practice surrounding palliative care (Palliative Care).

Planning an End of Life Education Program

The first step in the design of any educational intervention is to conduct a needs assessment, to understand the gap between what is being taught and evaluated and the ideal. A variety of multidimensional palliative care needs assessments have been reported for different populations of learners.

Once the needs assessment has defined important domains for focused education, specific learning objectives can be developed. Objectives communicate to the learner what is expected of the educational encounter and form the basis for evaluating the impact of training. Learning objectives are broadly defined as those directed at attitudes, knowledge or skills. Given the pervasive and often negative attitudes, which shape caring for the dying, it is advisable to include a mixture of attitude, knowledge, and skill objectives in all training experiences. Thus, it is also desirable to include a mixture of teaching methods in each educational exercise. Addressing attitudes tends to be the most challenging feature of end-of-life education. It is a truism of medical education that attitudes can not be taught. Rather, a shift in attitudes requires the learner to feel safe and respected enough to give up one attitude (e.g. I am afraid to use opioids for fear of causing addiction) for another (e.g. opioids rarely lead to addiction, they are safe and improve quality of life). Providing information to address knowledge objectives can be done via lectures, self-study guides, journal articles, videotapes and audiotapes. Teaching directed at skill objectives requires the learner to practice and demonstrate a defined skill such as patient counseling, calculating equianalgesic doses or pronouncing death.

As with teaching methods, different assessment methods work best when appropriately matched to the learning objective. Attitudes are best assessed through personal interactions, directed questioning and surveys. Knowledge can be assessed via oral or written examinations and skills through direct observation, feedback from patients, or written problem solving (e.g. calculating opioid equianalgesic doses).

Awareness of adult learning principles is essential when developing an end-of-life educational encounter. These include keeping the experience *learner-centered,* with relevant information keyed to the learners *need to know,* and understanding that adult learners make choices about their participation (e.g. they leave the room if the information is not relevant to their needs).

Educational Issues for Specific End-of-Life Domains

PAIN EDUCATION. Pain must be controlled before physicians can assist patients with the myriad of physical, psychological, and spiritual problems at end-of-life. Yet, physicians frequently fail to apply accepted standards of care for acute or chronic pain management. Moreover, it is clear that despite a multitude of clinical guidelines, position papers,

workshops, lectures, grand rounds, journal articles, and book chapters written about pain management, clinical practice is still far from ideal.

The primary reason that conventional education formats fail to translate into a change in clinical practice is that physicians harbor a host of attitudes about pain and pain management that inhibit the appropriate application of knowledge and skills. These attitudes fall into two broad categories. First are physician attitudes about pain that reflect societal views about the meaning of pain and pain treatment. Second are the fears and myths about opioid analgesics. These include fears of addiction, respiratory depression, and regulatory scrutiny, along with the secondary consequences of these fears—malpractice claims, professional sanctions, loss of practice privileges, and personal guilt about potential culpability for causing death.

In addition to attitudes, deficits in pain knowledge and skills are widespread. These include how to conduct a pain assessment, clinical pharmacology of analgesic medications, use of non-drug treatments, and skills in patient education and counseling. Educational techniques and results from various pain education programs have been reported; key findings from these include the following principles: pain education must include attention to attitudinal issues along with knowledge and skills; pain education must be longitudinal across all years of medical training; and pain education must be coupled to other elements of institutional change, such as quality monitoring, team building with non-physicians, development of routine assessment, and documentation and analgesic standards development.

ETHICS, LAW AND COMMUNICATION SKILLS EDUCATION. There is considerable content overlap between ethics and communication skills. For example, to effectively care for patients, trainees need to understand both the ethical and legal framework of advance directives *and* the communication skills necessary to discuss these with patients. Similarly, trainees need to understand the ethical and legal background to make decisions about treatment withdrawal *and* to acquire the skills to discuss these issues with patients and families.

There is a rich literature on educational methods and outcomes in ethics and communication skills education. Although ethics is generally considered a preclinical course in medical school, it is advisable that training in ethics be incorporated throughout medical school, residency, and fellowship training. As the level of professional responsibility increases with each year of training, such responsibility imposes demands on the trainee to make increasingly complex and ethically challenging decisions. Such decisions often strain the trainee's personal understanding of professionalism and altruism and thus merit dedicated time for self-reflection and mentoring. Although both ethics and communication skill training require attention to attitudes and knowledge deficits, communication skill training requires special and dedicated attention to the acquisition and demonstration of specific skills. Notably, trainees must be able to demonstrate their ability to give bad news and discuss treatment goals, treatment withdrawal, and issues surrounding hospice and palliative care empathetically and professionally.

CLINICAL TRAINING EXPERIENCES. Hospital-based palliative care teams are a valuable venue for clinical education in end-of-life care. Trainees, both physicians and nurses, can learn how to work within a multidisciplinary group and experience a collaborative process with the educational focus enlarged to include the physical, psychological, social, and spiritual dimensions of care. Since 1992 many medical schools and residency programs have established successful clinical experiences in hospice and palliative care at acute care hospitals, hospice residence facilities, and at home.

PERSONAL AWARENESS TRAINING. Very few health professionals have had formal training in how to deal with the emotions that arise when caring for patients with progressive fatal illness. Undergraduate course, residency, and fellowship directors have a number of options that can help trainees gain the needed personal awareness including support groups, family of origin group discussions, meaningful experiences discussion, personal awareness groups, literature in medicine discussion groups, and psychosocial morbidity and mortality conferences.

Future Directions

One important avenue to improve of end of life care is through health professional education. Much progress has been made since the early 1990s in defining curriculum content and establishing standards for education for medical students and primary care residencies. The most recent development in end of life education is the focus on training existing academic faculty and fellows in palliative care. Faculty development is needed if the established goals and standards in undergraduate and graduate palliative care education are to be met. Several courses have been developed in the United States, with the explicit goal of training academic faculty to become role models for end-of-life education. Fellowship training in palliative care is needed to prepare medical trainees for community or academic careers focused on care of the seriously ill and dying. In 2003 there are approximately twenty-five fellowship programs in the United States.

DAVID E. WEISSMAN

SEE ALSO: *Care; Compassionate Love; Emotions; Life Sustaining Treatment and Euthanasia; Literature and Healthcare; Medical Education; Nursing, Theories and Philosophy of; Nursing Ethics; Palliative Care and Hospice; Suicide;* and other *Death* subentries

BIBLIOGRAPHY

Billings, J. Andrew, and Block, Susan D. 1997. "Palliative Care in Undergraduate Medical Education." *Journal of the American Medical Association* 278: 733–743.

Billings, J. Andrew; Block, Susan D.; Finn, John W.; et al. 2002. "Initial Voluntary Program Standards for Fellowship Training in Palliative Medicine." *Journal of Palliative Medicine* 5: 23–33.

Branch, William; Lawrence, Robert S.; and Arky, Ronald. 1993. "Becoming a Doctor: Critical Incident Reports from Third-Year Medical Students." *New England Journal of Medicine* 329: 1130–1132.

Ferrell, B.; Virani, R.; Grant, M.; and Juarez, G. 2000. "Analysis of Palliative Care Content in Nursing Textbooks." *Journal of Palliative Care* 16(1): 39–47.

Lo, Bernard; Quill, Timothy; and Tulsky, James. 1999. "Discussing Palliative Care with Patients." *Annals of Internal Medicine* 130: 744–749.

Novak, Dennis H.; Suchman, Anthony L.; Clark, William; et al. 1997. "Calibrating the Physician: Personal Awareness and Effective Patient Care." *Journal of the American Medical Association* 278: 502–509.

Ross, Douglas D.; Fraser, Heather C.; and Kutner, Jean S. 2001. "Institutionalization of a Palliative and End-of-Life Care Educational Program in a Medical School Curriculum." *Journal of Palliative Medicine* 4: 512–518.

Schonwetter, Ronald S., ed. 1999. *Hospice and Palliative Medicine: Core Curriculum and Review Syllabus,* American Academy of Hospice and Palliative Medicine. Dubuque, IA: Kendall/l/Hunt.

Simpson, Deborah E. 2000. "National Consensus Conference on Medical Education for Care Near the End-of-Life: Executive Summary." *Journal of Palliative Medicine* 3: 87–91.

Simpson, Deborah E.; Rehm, Judy; Biernat, Kathy; et al. 1999. "Advancing Educational Scholarship Through the End of Life Physician Education Resource Center." *Journal of Palliative Medicine* 2: 421–424.

von Gunten, Charles F.; Ferris, Frank D.; and Emanuel, Linda. 2000. "Ensuring Competency in End of Life Care Communication and Relational Skills." *Journal of the American Medical Association* 284: 3051–3057.

Weissman, David E. 2000. "Cancer Pain as a Model for the Training of Physicians in Palliative Care." In *Topics in Palliative Care*, ed. Russell K. Portenoy and Eduardo Bruera. New York: Oxford University Press.

Weissman, David E., and Abrahm, Janet. 2002. "Education and Training in Palliative Care." In *Principles and Practice of Palliative are and Supportive Oncology*, 2nd edition, ed. Ann M. Berger, Russell K. Portenoy, and David E. Weissman. Philadelphia: Lippincott Williams and Wilkins.

INTERNET RESOURCES

Emanuel, Linda L.; von Gunten, Charles F.; and Ferris, Frank D., eds. 1999. *The EPEC Curriculum: Education for Physicians on End-of-life Care.* Available from <www.EPEC.net>.

End-of-Life/Palliative Education Resource Center. Available from <www.eperc.mcw.edu>.

Palliative Care web site. 2003. Available from <www.palliative carenursing.net>.

DEATH, DEFINITION AND DETERMINATION OF

• • •

I. CRITERIA FOR DEATH

Before the middle of the twentieth century there was no major dispute about the criteria for death. In the nineteenth century several isolated cases of premature burial from around the world raised some alarm, and safeguards (e.g., coffins equipped with alarms) were established to minimize the possibility of that practice. However, concern about the accuracy of diagnosing death largely abated by the turn of the twentieth century.

Beginning with the advent of more effective artificial respirators in the 1940s, major technological breakthroughs in modern medicine raised serious questions about the traditional ways of diagnosing death. Before the widespread use of respirators, defibrillators, intensive-care units, and cardiopulmonary resuscitation failures of cardiac, respiratory, and neurological functions were closely linked. When one system failed, the other two inevitably failed as well. However, respirators and other advanced life-support systems can sustain cardiac, respiratory, and other autonomic functions for prolonged periods even after neurological functions have ceased.

Terminology

With the advent of those new technologies neurological specialists became aware of certain new neurological syndromes, to which an array of confusing and inconsistent terms were applied.

Several landmark medical events stand out in the early days of the new neurologic syndromes. In 1959 the French first described the syndrome of brain death (*coma dépassé*) (Mollaret and Coulon), in 1968 a special committee of the Harvard Medical School formulated specific neurological criteria to diagnose brain death ("Definition of Irreversible Coma"), and in 1972 Bryan Jennett of Scotland and Fred Plum of the United States first used the term *persistent vegetative state*, or PVS (Jennett and Plum).

A variety of terms have been used to describe the medical syndrome of brain death: *cerebral death, coma dépassé,* and *irreversible coma.* Terms used as imprecise equivalents for the persistent vegetative state have included *apallic state, neocortical death, irreversible coma,* and *permanent unconsciousness* It also became necessary to distinguish the new neurological syndromes from common and well-accepted neurological conditions such as coma and dementia. Many newer terms, for example, *persistent vegetative state,* were used solely to describe the clinical condition. Others, such as the *apallic state* and *neocortical death,* were used in an attempt to correlate the loss of neurological functions with the underlying pathological changes in the brain.

As of 1994 there were two different legal/philosophical positions about what it means to be dead in terms of brain functions. Proponents of the whole-brain-oriented position consider a person dead if there is an irreversible loss of all the functions of the entire brain (brain death). Under the other position, which is not law in any jurisdiction in 2003, a person will be pronounced dead when there is an irreversible loss of higher brain functions (permanent unconsciousness).

Dilemmas surrounding these new syndromes, such as when it is appropriate to stop treatment and when death has occurred, have raised fundamental questions about the meaning of medical concepts such as consciousness, awareness, self-awareness, voluntary interactions with the environment, purposeful movement, pain, and psychological and physical suffering.

Neurological specialists are achieving a much greater understanding of these syndromes and their similarities and differences and are reaching a degree of consensus on terminology. However, they have not reached universal agreement on several major issues related primarily to the persistent vegetative state. A historical example illustrates how difficult it can be to reach consensus on terminology. The Harvard Committee ("Definition of Irreversible Coma,") equated irreversible coma with brain death, as did many neurological specialists in the 1970s. Others, equally knowledgeable and experienced, equated irreversible coma with the persistent vegetative state. Still others used the term in a much broader fashion to denote any form of permanent unconsciousness. Because this term has gathered so many different and contradictory meanings, the only reasonable alternative for neurological specialists was to drop it entirely.

Traditional Criteria

With all the controversy surrounding neurological criteria for death, the traditional criteria related to heartbeat and breathing have remained largely unchanged and undisputed except in the University of Pittsburgh Medical Center's program in which organs are taken from certain patients as soon as possible after expected cardiopulmonary death (Lynn). No major legal or ethical concerns have been raised about the traditional criteria for death. Medical organizations around the world have not felt it necessary to establish specific clinical criteria for the diagnosis of death that are based on the irreversible loss of cardiac and respiratory functions. The medical consultants to the President's Commission for the Study of Ethical Problems in Medicine and Biomedical and Behavioral Research recommended that the clinical examination disclose at least the absence of consciousness, heartbeat, and respiratory effort and that irreversibility be established by persistent loss of these functions for an appropriate period of observation and trial of therapy ("Guidelines for the Determination of Death"). However, these consultants recommended no specific length of time for this period of observation.

Brain Death

The neurological syndrome of brain death has been accepted by the medical profession as a distinct clinical entity that experienced clinicians can diagnose with an extremely high degree of certainty and usually can distinguish easily from other neurological syndromes. Brain death is defined as the irreversible cessation of all the functions of the entire brain, including the brainstem. If the brain can be viewed simplistically as consisting of two parts—the cerebral hemispheres (higher centers) and the brainstem (lower centers)—brain death is defined as the destruction of the entire brain, both the cerebral hemispheres and the brainstem. In contrast, in the permanent vegetative state the cerebral hemispheres are damaged extensively and permanently but the brainstem is relatively intact (Cranford, 1988).

An understanding of the pathological sequence of events that leads to brain death is essential if one is to appreciate fully why brain death is a unique syndrome and why it can be differentiated readily from other neurological syndromes with a high degree of certainty. Although a variety of insults can cause the brain to die, head trauma, cardiorespiratory failure, and intracerebral hemorrhage are the most common causes. Regardless of the underlying cause, the pathological sequence is essentially the same in almost all cases. The acute massive insult to the brain causes brain swelling (cerebral edema). Because the brain is contained in an enclosed cavity, brain swelling gives rise to a massive increase in intracranial pressure. In brain death the increased intracranial pressure becomes so great that it exceeds the systolic blood pressure, thus causing a loss of blood flow to both the cerebral hemispheres and the brainstem. Whatever the primary cause of brain death, this end result of loss of blood flow results in the destruction of the entire brain. This sequence of events usually occurs within a matter of hours after the primary event, and so brain death can be diagnosed within a short period of time with an extraordinarily high degree of certainty.

The loss of both cerebral hemisphere and brainstem functions is usually clearly evident to an experienced clinician from the clinical bedside examination. The patient is in a coma, the deepest possible coma, a sleeplike state associated with a loss of all brainstem functions, such as pupillary reaction to light; gag, swallowing, and cough reflexes; eye movements in response to passive head turning (the oculocephalic response) and in response to cold caloric stimulation (oculovestibular response); and spontaneous respiratory efforts.

However, whereas respirations are completely dependent on the functioning of the brainstem, cardiac function can continue independent of brain destruction because the heart has an independent mechanism for spontaneously firing (semiautonomous functioning). With modern life-support systems continued cardiac and blood pressure functions can persist for hours, days, or even longer. Extremely rare cases of continued cardiovascular functions for over a year in the presence of the loss of all brain functions have been reported. The first cases of prolonged somatic survival in brain death usually occurred in the context of brain-dead pregnant women who were maintained on life-support systems for several months so that a viable fetus could be delivered (Wijdicks). However, the most extraordinary case of prolonged somatic survival of a patient with well-documented brain death involved a young adult age twenty-two who for eighteen years has been without any brain functions (Shewmon, 1998; Cranford, 1998; Shewmon, 2000).

In the 1970s and 1980s numerous medical organizations in the United States and around the world developed specific medical criteria for the diagnosis of brain death (Bernat). In the United States major criteria were published by Harvard University, the University of Minnesota, the National Institutes of Health, Cornell University, and the President's Commission. Major international criteria emerged from Sweden, Japan, the United Kingdom, and Canada. All those standards essentially agreed on three clinical findings: coma, apnea (loss of spontaneous respirations), and absence of brainstem reflexes.

The critical issue distinguishing these international criteria was not the clinical findings but how best to establish irreversibility. The United Kingdom, deemphasizing the use of laboratory studies such as electroencephalography, focused on the basic diagnosis as clinical and asserted that the best way to establish irreversibility was to preclude any reversible processes before making a final determination of brain death (Conference of Royal Colleges). Reversible processes that could mimic brain death include a variety of sedative medications and hypothermia (low body temperature, below 32.2° Centigrade). The British also recommended a period of observation of at least twelve hours. In contrast, the Swedish criteria focused less on the period of observation and more on the need for definitive laboratory studies to document a loss of blood flow to the brain, such as intracranial angiography.

In the United States the earlier standards emphasized the use of electroencephalography to establish electrocerebral silence (a loss of all electrical activity of the brain); more recent standards focused on establishing a loss of intracranial circulation by means of radioisotope angiography. The 1981 report of the medical consultants to the President's Commission, which became the definitive medical standard in the United States, recommended a period of observation of at least six hours combined with a confirmatory study, such as tests measuring intracranial circulation ("Guidelines for the Determination of Death"). If no confirmatory laboratory studies were performed, an observation period of at least twelve hours was suggested, assuming that all reversible causes of loss of brain functions had been excluded. In cases of damage to the brain caused by the lack of blood or oxygen (hypoxic-ischemic encephalopathy) the consultants recommended an observation period of at least twenty-four hours if confirmatory studies were not performed.

The diagnosis of brain death in newborns, infants, and children is often more difficult than is the diagnosis in adults. A major reason for this difficulty is that the usual pathological sequence of events in adults that leads to increased intracranial pressure and loss of all blood flow to the brain does not apply to newborns and infants because the cranial cavity in those patients has not yet closed completely. Thus, the mechanism for brain death in newborns and infants may be different from what it is in older children and adults.

To address this question a task force for the determination of brain death in children representing several neurological and pediatric specialty organizations in the United States developed specific diagnostic criteria for the younger age groups (Task Force for the Determination of Brain Death in Children). That task force stated that it would be extremely difficult to establish brain death in newborns less than seven days old. It recommended that in infants seven days to two months of age there should be two separate clinical examinations and two electroencephalograms separated by at least forty-eight hours; for infants two months to one year of age, two clinical examinations and two electroencephalograms separated by at least twenty-four hours; and for children over one year of age, criteria similar to those established for adults.

Beginning in the early 1990s, the University of Pittsburgh and a few other large transplants centers developed protocols for removing organs from patients whose hearts had stopped beating but who were not brain-dead (non-heartbeating organ donors, or NHBOD) (DeVita et al.). In cases of brain death and organ donation the patient is first pronounced dead after the medical diagnosis of brain death has been established, including a period of time to establish irreversibility. The patient then is transferred to the operating room for organ removal while life-support systems are continued. After the transplantable organs are removed, life-support systems are discontinued, but the cessation of heartbeat at this time has no clinical or legal significance. In cases of non-heartbeating organ donors, patients who are terminally ill or have sustained severe irreversible brain damage and are ventilator-dependent are transferred to the operating room, where the respirator is removed, with the resultant loss of heartbeat, usually within minutes. After two minutes of pulselessness, apnea, and unresponsiveness the patient is pronounced dead on the basis of cardiorespiratory criteria. Organ removal then occurs as expeditiously as possible before the organs incur ischemic damage from lack of perfusion. The entire process is carried out in the most humane and caring way possible, including full disclosure to the appropriate surrogate decision makers and the obtaining of their consent (Ethics Committee, American College of Critical Care Medicine). The success and limitations of this controversial procedure have been reported by some of the pioneering transplant centers.

Permanent Unconsciousness

The syndromes of permanent unconsciousness include two major types. The first is a permanent coma: an eyes-closed, sleeplike form of unarousable unconsciousness. The second is the permanent vegetative state: an eyes-open, wakeful form of unconsciousness (U.S. President's Commission for the Study of Ethical Problems). This entry takes no position on the ethical and legal issues involved in choosing between the whole-brain and higher-brain formulations of death but describes the neurological syndromes of permanent unconsciousness that would be considered the medical basis for the higher-brain formulation of death.

A permanent coma is an uncommon neurological syndrome because most patients with damage sufficient to cause brainstem impairment resulting in permanent coma die soon either naturally or because a decision is made to discontinue treatment as a result of the poor prognosis. Cases of prolonged (more than a few weeks) permanent coma do occur but are extremely uncommon.

The vegetative state has three major classes, depending on the temporal profile of the onset and the progression of the brain damage. The first form is the acute vegetative state. This occurs when the onset of brain damage is sudden and severe, such as with head trauma (traumatic vegetative state) or loss of blood flow to the brain caused by sudden cardiorespiratory insufficiencies (hypoxic-ischemic vegetative state). The second form is the degenerative, or metabolic, vegetative state, in which the brain damage begins gradually and progresses slowly over a period of months to years. In adults the most common form of the degenerative vegetative state is the final stage of Alzheimer's disease, whereas in children it is the final stage of a variety of degenerative and metabolic diseases of childhood. The third form is the congenital vegetative state secondary to a variety of severe congenital malformations of the brain that are present at birth, such as anencephaly.

The vegetative state is considered persistent when it is present longer than one month in the acute form and permanent when the condition becomes irreversible. The exact prevalence is unknown, but it is estimated that in the United States there are approximately 10,000 to 25,000 adults and 4,000 to 10,000 children in a vegetative state (Multi-Society Task Force on PVS). When it becomes permanent, this syndrome is the major neurological condition that is the prototype for the higher-brain formulation of death.

Vegetative State

The vegetative state is characterized by the loss of all higher brain functions, with relative sparing of brainstem functions. Because brainstem functions are still present, the arousal mechanisms contained in the brainstem are relatively intact and the patient therefore is not in a coma. The patient has sleep/wake cycles but at no time manifests any signs of consciousness, awareness, voluntary interaction with the environment, or purposeful movements. Thus, the patient can be awake but is always unaware: a mindless wakefulness.

Unlike brain death, in which the pathology and sequence of changes are relatively uniform regardless of the primary cause of the brain damage, the pathological changes in the vegetative state vary substantially with the cause of the unconsciousness. Although there are a variety of causes, the two most common causes of the acute form are head trauma and hypoxic-ischemic encephalopathy. In head trauma the major damage is due to shearing injuries to the subcortical white matter (the fiber tracts that connect the cell bodies of the cerebral cortex with the rest of the brain) of the cerebral hemispheres. With hypoxic-ischemic encephalopathy the primary damage is to the neurons in the cerebral cortex. These different patterns of brain damage are important for several reasons, among them the fact that the chances for recovery of neurological functions and the time necessary to establish irreversibility vary with the underlying cause.

For patients, both adults and children, in a hypoxic-ischemic vegetative state that lasts longer than three months the prognosis for recovery is uniformly dismal. The vast majority who recover and do well after a hypoxic-ischemic insult to the brain are those who have regained consciousness in the first three months. Among adults in a traumatic vegetative state the majority who do well usually will have regained consciousness within six months of the injury. The prognosis for the recovery of children in a traumatic vegetative state is slightly more favorable than that for adults (Council on Scientific Affairs and Council on Ethical and Judicial Affairs). However, in both children and adults a period of observation of at least twelve months may be appropriate before permanency is established (Multi-Society Task Force on PVS).

Although specific medical criteria for brain death have been established by numerous organizations around the world, no comparable criteria have been established for the diagnosis of the vegetative state. It is unlikely that any criteria as specific as those for brain death will be formulated in the near future because the diagnosis of the vegetative state is not nearly as precise and definitive. The determination of irreversibility in brain death usually takes hours and does not vary according to etiology, whereas it may take months to establish irreversibility in patients who are in the permanent vegetative state, and the time necessary to establish this irreversibility varies substantially with cause and age (Institute of Medical Ethics Working Party on the Ethics of Prolonging Life and Assisting Death).

Because all vegetative state patients are unconscious, they are unable to experience suffering of any kind, psychological or physical. These patients normally manifest periods of eyes opening and closing with accompanying sleep/wake cycles. They also may demonstrate a variety of facial expressions and eye movements that originate from the lower centers of the brain and do not indicate consciousness. They may appear at times to smile and grimace, but observation over prolonged periods reveals no evidence either of voluntary interaction with the environment or of self-awareness (Executive Board, American Academy of Neurology). Neuroimaging studies such as computerized axial tomography (CAT) and magnetic resonance imaging (MRI) may be helpful in establishing the severity and irreversibility of the brain damage. After several months in a vegetative state the brain begins to show progressive shrinkage (atrophy), primarily of the cerebral hemispheres. The loss of consciousness and the inability to experience suffering, which are established on the basis of clinical observations, have been supported by measuring the metabolism of glucose and oxygen at the level of the cerebral cortex by means of positron emission tomography (PET) scanning. These studies have shown a 50 to 60 percent decrease in cerebral cortical metabolism, a level consistent with unconsciousness and deep anesthesia (Levy et al.).

Long-term survival of vegetative state patients at all ages is reduced drastically compared with the normal population. Life expectancy in adult patients is generally about two to five years; the vast majority do not live longer than ten years. In elderly patients the prognosis for survival is even worse; many do not survive for more than a few months. Infants and children may survive longer than adults do, but probably not significantly longer. Some studies have shown the average life expectancy to be four years for infants up to two months of age and about seven years for children seven to eighteen years old (Ashwal et al.).

Cases of prolonged survival—longer than twenty years—have been reported but are rare. One patient, Elaine Esposito from Tarpon Springs, Florida, lived for 37 years and 111 days without regaining consciousness, from age six to age forty-three. Another patient, Rita Greene, a surgical nurse from Wheeling, West Virginia, who survived for 47 years, 100 days from age twenty-four to age seventy-one, is probably the longest survivor in a permanent vegetative state ("Woman Lived Since '51 in Comalike State"). Considering

the total estimated number of patients in a persistent vegetative state and the small number of well-documented cases of survival beyond fifteen years, the probability of an individual patient having such a prolonged survival is extremely low, probably less than 1 in 15,000 to 1 in 75,000 (Multi-Society Task Force on PVS).

It is more difficult to make the diagnosis of the vegetative state in newborns and infants. Generally, the diagnosis cannot be made below the age of three months except in the case of the condition of anencephaly. Anencephaly is the congenital malformation form of the permanent vegetative state (Stumpf et al.). This extensive and severe congenital malformation of the brain can be diagnosed with an extraordinarily high degree of certainty. At birth it is readily apparent by visual observation alone that the child has only rudimentary cerebral hemispheres and no skull except in the rear of the head. These children have variable degrees of brainstem functions but usually not enough functions to sustain life for any length of time. The vast majority are dead within two months, and most die within a few weeks.

The Locked-In Syndrome and the Minimally Conscious State

Brain death and the vegetative state should be contrasted with two other contemporary neurological syndromes of severe brain damage: the locked-in syndrome and the minimally conscious state. The locked-in syndrome, first named by Fred Plum and Jerome Posner in 1966, is characterized by a severe paralysis of the entire body, including the extremities and facial muscles, but with normal or nearly normal consciousness. This often results from a severe stroke to the brainstem that spares the cerebral hemispheres (in one sense the reverse of the vegetative state), and these patients often appear to be unconscious; however, a careful history and neurological examination uncover a high degree of cognitive functioning. Some physicians use this term to denote patients with any degree (e.g., mild to moderate) of disparity between paralysis and cognitive functioning. However, this term, when used properly, means a profound disparity between paralysis (severe) and consciousness (normal or nearly normal).

Unlike brain death, the vegetative state, and the locked-in syndrome, all of which are fairly well characterized and accepted by the medical profession, the term *minimally conscious state* is of relatively recent vintage, and its acceptance and potential usefulness as a distinct neurological syndrome are far from settled. Formally called the minimally responsive state, the minimally conscious state is defined as a condition of "severely altered consciousness in which minimal but definite behavioral evidence of self or environmental awareness is demonstrated," in other words, a condition of severely to profoundly impaired cognitive functioning (Giacino et al.). This diagnosis is made by the demonstration on a reproducible or sustained basis of one or more of the following behaviors: following simple commands, gestural or verbal yes/no responses, intelligible verbalization, and purposeful behavior such as appropriate smiling or crying, pursuit eye movement, and sustained visual fixation. Even though the difference between being vegetative and thus completely unconscious and being "minimally" conscious may seem to be a subtle distinction and even though some have argued that being minimally conscious is a medical fate worse than being vegetative, the courts in recent landmark decisions and many healthcare professionals have treated these syndromes radically differently from a medical, ethical, and legal standpoint (Rich).

Conclusion

The criteria for diagnosing cardiorespiratory death and brain death have been well established and accepted by the medical profession. Even though there are differences in how physicians may apply these criteria in individual cases and even though the standards may vary somewhat in different countries, there are no major disputes about the medical diagnosis itself.

The syndromes of permanent unconsciousness, in contrast, are much more variable than are those of brain death. The three major forms of the vegetative state—acute, degenerative, and congenital—are substantially different in terms of causes, type of brain damage, and length of time necessary to establish irreversibility. Thus, the criteria for a higher-brain formulation of death are far more complex and uncertain than are those for the whole-brain formulation of death.

RONALD E. CRANFORD (1995)
REVISED BY AUTHOR

SEE ALSO: *Body: Cultural and Religious Perspectives; Conscience, Rights of; Consensus, Role and Authority of; Judaism, Bioethics in; Life; Metaphor and Analogy; Organ and Tissue Procurement; Public Policy and Bioethics;* and other *Death, Definition and Determination of* subentries

BIBLIOGRAPHY

Ashwal, Stephen; Bale, Jr., James F.; Coulter, David L.; et al. 1992. "The Persistent Vegetative State in Children: Report of the Child Neurology Society Ethics Committee." *Annals of Neurology* 32(4): 570–576.

Bernat, James L. 1991. "Ethical Issues in Neurology." In *Clinical Neurology,* ed. Robert J. Joynt. Philadelphia: Lippincott.

Conference of Royal Colleges and Faculties of the United Kingdom. 1976. "Diagnosis of Brain Death." *Lancet* 2: 1069–1070.

Council on Scientific Affairs and Council on Ethical and Judicial Affairs, American Medical Association. 1990. "Persistent Vegetative State and the Decision to Withdraw or Withhold Life-Support." *Journal of the American Medical Association* 263(3): 426–430.

Cranford, Ronald E. 1988. "The Persistent Vegetative State: Getting the Facts Straight (The Medical Reality)." *Hastings Center Report* 18: 27–32.

Cranford, Ronald E. 1998. "Even the Dead Are Not Terminally Ill Anymore." *Neurology* 51(6): 1530–1531.

DeVita, Michael A.; Snyder, James V.; Arnold, Robert M.; et al. 2000. "Observations of Withdrawal of Life-Sustaining Treatment from Patients Who Became Non-Heart-Beating Organ Donors." *Critical Care Medicine* 28(6): 1709–1712.

Ethics Committee, American College of Critical Care Medicine. 2001. "Recommendations for Non-Heart-Beating Organ Donation: A Position Paper by the Ethics Committee, American College of Critical Care Medicine, the Society of Critical Care Medicine." *Critical Care Medicine* 29(9): 1826–1831.

Executive Board, American Academy of Neurology. 1989. "Position of the American Academy of Neurology on Certain Aspects of the Care and Management of the Persistent Vegetative State Patient." *Neurology* 39(1): 125–126.

Giacino, Joseph T.; Ashwal, Stephen; Childs, Nancy; et al. 2002. "The Minimally Conscious State: Definition and Diagnostic Criteria." *Neurology* 58: 349–353.

"Guidelines for the Determination of Death: Report of the Medical Consultants on the Diagnosis of Death to the U.S. President's Commission for the Study of Ethical Problems in Medicine and Biomedical and Behavioral Research." 1981. *Journal of the American Medical Association* 246(19): 2184–2186.

Institute of Medical Ethics Working Party on the Ethics of Prolonging Life and Assisting Death. 1991. "Withdrawal of Life-Support from Patients in a Persistent Vegetative State." *Lancet* 337(8733): 96–98.

Jennett, Bryan, and Plum, Fred. 1972. "Persistent Vegetative State after Brain Damage: A Syndrome in Search of a Name." *Lancet* 1(7753): 734–737.

Levy, David E.; Sidtis, John J.; Rottenberg, David A.; et al. 1987. "Differences in Cerebral Blood Flow and Glucose Utilization in Vegetative versus Locked-in Patients." *Annals of Neurology* 22(6): 673–682.

Lynn, Joanne. 1993. "Are the Patients Who Become Organ Donors under the Pittsburgh Protocol for `Non-Heart Beating Donors' Really Dead?" *Kennedy Institute of Ethics Journal* 3(2): 167–178.

Mollaret, Pierre, and Coulon, M. 1959. "Le Coma Dépassé." *Revue Neurologique (Paris)* 101: 5–15.

"The Definition of Irreversible Coma: Report of the Ad Hoc Committee of the Harvard Medical School to Examine the

Definition of Brain Death." 1968. *Journal of the American Medical Association* 205(6): 337–340.

The Multi-Society Task Force on PVS (American Academy of Neurology, Child Neurology Society, American Neurological Association, American Association of Neurological Surgeons, American Academy of Pediatrics). 1994. "Medical Aspects of the Persistent Vegetative State." *New England Journal of Medicine* 330(2): 1499–1508, 1572–1579.

Plum, Fred, and Posner, Jerome E. 1980. *The Diagnosis of Stupor and Coma,* 3rd edition. Philadelphia: F.A. Davis.

Rich, Ben A. 2002. "The Tyranny of Judicial Formalism: Oral Directives and the Clear and Convincing Evidence Standard." *Cambridge Quarterly of Healthcare Ethics* 11: 292–302.

Shewmon, D. Alan. 1998. "Chronic 'Brain Death' Meta-Analysis and Conceptual Consequences." *Neurology* 51(6): 1538–1545.

Shewmon, D. Alan. 2000. "Seeing Is Believing: Videos of Life 13 Years after 'Brain Death.'" *Third International Symposium on Coma and Brain Death.* Havana, Cuba, February 22–25.

Stumpf, David A.; Cranford, Ronald E.; Elias, Sherman; et al. 1990. "The Infant with Anencephaly." *New England Journal of Medicine* 322(10): 669–674.

Task Force for the Determination of Brain Death in Children (American Academy of Neurology, American Academy of Pediatrics, American Neurological Association, Child Neurology Society). 1987. "Guidelines for the Determination of Brain Death in Children." *Neurology* 37(6): 1077–1078.

U.S. President's Commission for the Study of Ethical Problems in Medicine and Biomedical and Behavioral Research. 1983. *Deciding to Forego Life-Sustaining Treatment: Ethical, Medical, and Legal Issues in Treatment Decisions.* Washington, D.C.: U.S. Government Printing Office.

Wijdicks, Eelco F. M. 2001. *Brain Death.* Philadelphia: Lippincott Williams & Wilkins.

"Woman Lived Since '51 in Comalike State." 1999. *The Intelligencer,* Wheeling, WV, February 2, pp. 1, 3.

II. LEGAL ISSUES IN PRONOUNCING DEATH

The following is a revision and update of the first-edition entry "Death, Definition and Determination of, II. Legal Aspects of Pronouncing Death" by the same author.

The capability of biomedicine to sustain vital human functions artificially has created problems not only for medical practitioners but for the public and its legal institutions as well. In some cases, determining that people have died is no longer the relatively simple matter of ascertaining that their heart and lungs have stopped functioning. Mechanical respirators, electronic pacemakers, and drugs that stimulate functioning and affect blood pressure can create the appearance of circulation and respiration in what is otherwise a corpse. The general public first recognized the need to update public policy concerning when and how death could

be declared when Christiaan Barnard performed the first human-to-human heart transplant in Cape Town, South Africa, on December 3, 1967. Beyond amazement at the technical feat, many people were astonished that a heart taken from a woman who had been declared dead conferred life on a man whose own heart had been removed.

Cardiac transplantation provides the most dramatic illustration of the need for clear standards to classify the outcomes of intensive medical support (e.g., respirators). But only a handful of the moribund, unconscious patients maintained through intensive support long after they formerly would have ceased living become organ donors (U.S. President's Commission). Sometimes such medical intervention is ended because it has succeeded in enabling the patient to recover; more often, it is terminated because the patient's bodily systems have collapsed so totally that circulation and respiration cannot be maintained. But for a significant number of patients, artificial support can be continued indefinitely with no prospect that consciousness will ever return. For some of this latter group of patients—especially those who can eventually be weaned from the respirator and require only nutrition and hydration by tube—the question arises whether to withdraw treatment and allow death to occur. But for others who have suffered great brain damage, the need arises to recognize that death has occurred and that further attempts to keep the patient alive are therefore no longer appropriate even before the point (usually within several weeks) when physiological processes in the body can usually no longer be maintained.

Beginning in the 1960s, the response of the medical profession was to develop new criteria, such as those articulated in 1968 by an ad hoc committee at Harvard Medical School. Experts in the United States tend to rely on certain clinical signs of the absence of any activity in the entire brain (Ad Hoc Committee); British neurologists focus on the loss of functioning in the brain stem, while doctors in certain European countries search for conditions for brain function, such as intracranial blood circulation (Van Till). Despite differences in technique, the medical profession arrived at a consensus that the total and irreversible absence of brain function is equivalent to the traditional cardiorespiratory indicators of death (Medical Consultants).

The story of the law's response to these new medical criteria can be divided into three parts. The first, largely played out in the late 1960s and the 1970s, concerned an issue of process—how ought society respond to the divergence between new medical precepts and practices, on the one hand, and the common understanding of the lay public of rules embodied in custom and law, on the other? (Anglo-American common law, for example, had traditionally defined death as the total cessation of all vital functions.) The second phase, from the 1970s through the 1980s, centered on the specific changes being made in the law. In the third period, which is still continuing, commentators (principally philosophers and a few physicians) have raised questions about the appropriateness of the legal standards that have been adopted and called for various changes in those standards.

Phase One: Framing Definitions

A MEDICAL MATTER? A number of routes were advanced for arriving at what was often termed a new definition of death that would encompass the neurological understanding of the phenomenon of death that emerged in the 1960s and has since been further refined. (The common shorthand phrase "definition of death" is misleading since "definition" suggests an explanation of a fact whereas the task at hand is specifying the significance of particular facts for the process of determining whether, and when, a person has died.) Early commentators proposed that the task should be left to physicians, because the subject is technical and because the law might set the definition prematurely, leading to conflicts with developments that will inevitably occur in medical techniques (Kennedy). Yet the belief that defining death is wholly a medical matter misapprehends the undertaking. At issue is not a biological understanding of the inherent nature of cells or organ systems but a social formulation of humanhood. It is largely through its declaration of the points at which life begins and ends that a society determines who is a full human being, with the resulting rights and responsibilities.

Since physicians have no special competence on the philosophical issue of the nature of human beings and no special authority to arrogate the choice among definitions to themselves, their role is properly one of elucidating the significance of various vital signs. By the 1970s, it became apparent that a new definition should be forthcoming, not simply to accommodate biomedical practitioners' wishes but as a result of perceived social need and of evidence that tests for brain function were as reliable as the traditional heart-lung tests.

JUDICIAL DECISIONS? If not physicians, then who should frame the definition? One answer was, "Let the courts decide." In the United States and other common-law countries, law is to be found not only on the statute books but in the rules enunciated by judges as they resolve disputes in individual civil and criminal cases. Facing a factual situation that does not fit comfortably within the existing legal rules, a court may choose to formulate a new rule in order to more accurately reflect current scientific understanding and social viewpoints.

Nonetheless, problems of principle and practicality emerged in placing primary reliance on the courts for a redefinition of death. Like the medical profession, the judiciary may be too narrowly based for the task. While the judiciary is an organ of the state with recognized authority in public matters, it still has no means for actively involving the public in its decision-making processes. Judge-made law has been most successful in factual settings embedded in well-defined social and economic practices, with the guidance of past decisions and commentary. Courts operate within a limited compass—the facts and contentions of a particular case—and with limited expertise; they have neither the staff nor the authority to investigate or to conduct hearings in order to explore such issues as public opinion or the scientific merits of competing "definitions." Consequently, a judge's decision may be merely a rubber-stamping of the opinions expressed by the medical experts who appeared in court. Moreover, testimony in an adversary proceeding is usually restricted to the "two sides" of a particular issue and may not fairly represent the spectrum of opinion held by authorities in the field.

Furthermore, in the U.S. cases in which parties first argued for a redefinition, the courts were unwilling to disturb the existing legal definition. Such deference to precedent is understandable, because people need to be able to rely on predictable legal rules in managing their affairs. As late as 1968, a California appellate tribunal, in a case involving an inheritorship issue, declined to redefine death in terms of brain functioning despite the admittedly anachronistic nature of an exclusively heart-lung definition (Cate and Capron).

The unfortunate consequences for physicians and patients of the unsettled state of the common-law definition of death in the 1970s is illustrated by several cases. In the first, *Tucker v. Lower,* which came to trial in Virginia in 1972, the brother of a man whose heart was taken in an early transplant operation sued the physicians, alleging that the operation was begun before the donor had died. The evidence showed that the donor's pulse, blood pressure, respiration, and other vital signs were normal but that he had been declared dead when the physicians decided these signs resulted solely from medical efforts and not from his own functioning, since his brain functions had ceased. At the start of the trial, the judge indicated that he would adhere to the traditional definition of death, but when charging the jury, he permitted them to find that death had occurred when the brain ceased functioning irreversibly. Although a verdict was returned for the defendants, the law was not clarified since the court did not explain its action.

The other two cases arose in California in 1974, when two transplant operations were performed using hearts removed from the victims of alleged crimes. The defendant in each case, charged with homicide, attempted to interpose the action of the surgeons in removing the victim's still-beating heart as a complete defense to the charge. One trial judge accepted this argument as being compelled by the existing definition of death, but his ruling was reversed on appeal, and both defendants were eventually convicted. This graphic illustration of legal confusion and uncertainty led California to join several other jurisdictions in the United States, Canada, and Australia that, beginning in 1970, followed a third route to redefining death, the adoption of a statutory definition.

STATUTORY STANDARDS? The legislative process allows a wider range of information to enter into the framing of standards for determining death, as well as offering an avenue for participation of the public. That is important because basic and perhaps controversial choices among alternative definitions must be made. Because they provide prospective guidance, statutory standards have the additional advantage of dispelling public and professional doubt, thereby reducing both the fear and the likelihood of cases against physicians for malpractice or homicide.

Not all countries have adopted legislation. In Great Britain, for example, the standards for determining death reside not in a statute but in medically promulgated codes of practice, which have been indirectly accepted in several judicial decisions (Kennedy and Grubb). Yet in the United States and among most commentators internationally, the first period in policymaking on a new definition of death produced wide agreement that an official response was necessary in light of the changes wrought by medical science, and that this response ought to be statutory.

Phase Two: The Contours of a Statute

By 1979 four model statutes had been proposed in the United States; in addition to those from the American Bar Association (ABA), the American Medical Association (AMA), and the National Conference of Commissioners of Uniform State Laws (NCCUSL), the most widely adopted was the Capron-Kass proposal, which grew out of the work of a research group at the Hastings Center (U.S. President's Commission, 1981). Ironically, the major barrier to legislation became the very multiplicity of proposals; though they were consistent in their aims, their sponsors tended to lobby for their own bills, which in turn produced apprehension among legislators over the possible importance of the bills' verbal differences. Accordingly, the President's Commission worked with the three major sponsors—the ABA, the AMA,

and the NCCUSL—to draft a single model bill that could be proposed for adoption in all jurisdictions. The resulting statute—the Uniform Determination of Death Act (UDDA)—was proposed in 1981 and is law in more than half of U.S. jurisdictions, while virtually all the rest have some other, essentially similar statute. In four states the law derives from a decision by the highest court recognizing cessation of all functions of the brain as one means of determining death (Cate and Capron).

The UDDA provides that an individual who has sustained either (1) irreversible cessation of circulatory and respiratory functions, or (2) irreversible cessation of all functions of the entire brain, including the brain stem, is dead. A determination of death must be made in accordance with accepted medical standards. This statute is guided by several principles. First, the phenomenon of interest to physicians, legislators, and the public alike is a human being's death, not the "death" of his or her cells, tissues, or organs. Indeed, one problem with the term "brain death" is that it wrongly suggests that an organ can die; organisms die, but organs cease functioning. Second, a statute on death will resolve the problem of whether to continue artificial support in only some of the cases of comatose patients. Additional guidance has been developed by courts and legislatures as well as by professional bodies concerning the cessation of treatment in patients who are alive by brain or heart-lung criteria, but for whom further treatment is considered (by the patients or by others) to be pointless or degrading. This question of "when to allow to die?" is distinct from "when to declare dead?"

Third, the merits of a legislative definition are judged by whether its purposes are properly defined and how well the legislation meets those purposes. In addition to its cultural and religious importance, a definition of death is needed to resolve a number of legal issues (besides deciding whether to terminate medical care or transplant organs) such as homicide, damages for the wrongful death of a person, property and wealth transmission, insurance, taxes, and marital status. While some commentators have argued that a single definition is inappropriate because different policy objectives might exist in different contexts, it has been generally agreed that a single definition of death is capable of being applied in a wide variety of contexts, as indeed was the traditional heart-lung definition. Having a single definition to be used for many purposes does not preclude relying on other events besides death as a trigger for some decisions. Most jurisdictions make provision, for example, for the distribution of property and the termination of marriage after a person has been absent without explanation for a period of years, even though a person "presumed dead" under such a law could not be treated as a corpse were he or she actually still alive (Capron).

Fourth, although dying is a process (since not all parts of the body cease functioning equally and synchronously), a line can and must be drawn between those who are alive and those who are dead (Kass). The ability of modern biomedicine to extend the functioning of various organ systems may have made knowing which side of the line a patient is on more problematic, but it has not erased the line. The line drawn by the UDDA is an arbitrary one in the sense that it results from human choice among a number of possibilities, but not in the sense of having no acceptable, articulated rationale.

Fifth, legislated standards must be uniform for all persons. It is, to say the least, unseemly for a person's wealth or potential social utility as an organ donor to affect the way in which the moment of his or her death is determined. One jurisdiction, in an attempt to accommodate religious and cultural diversity, has departed from the general objective of uniformity in the standards for determining death. In 1991, New Jersey adopted a statute that allows people whose religious beliefs would be violated by the use of whole-brain criteria to have their deaths declared solely on the traditional cardiorespiratory basis (New Jersey Commission).

Sixth, the UDDA was framed on the premise that it is often beneficial for the law to move incrementally, particularly when matters of basic cultural and ethical values are implicated. Thus, the statute provides a modern restatement of the traditional understanding of death that ties together the accepted cardiopulmonary standard with a new brain-based standard that measures the same phenomenon.

Finally, in making law in a highly technological area, care is needed that the definition be at once sufficiently precise to determine behavior in the manner desired by the public and yet not so specific that it is tied to the details of contemporary technology. The UDDA achieves this flexible precision by confining itself to the general standards by which death is to be determined. It leaves to the developing judgment of biomedical practitioners the establishment and application of appropriate criteria and specific tests for determining that the standards have been met. To provide a contemporary statement of "accepted medical standards," the U.S. President's Commission assembled a group of leading neurologists, neurosurgeons, pediatricians, anesthesiologists, and other authorities on determination of death (Medical Consultants). Their guidelines, which provide the basis for the clinical methodology used in most American institutions, have since been supplemented by special guidance regarding children (Task Force).

Phase Three: The Continuing Points of Debate

As a practical matter, the law nearly everywhere (most recently including Japan) (Akabayashi) recognizes that death may be diagnosed based upon the determination that the brain as a whole has ceased functioning. In the United States, this consensus is embodied in the UDDA, which has therefore become the focus of criticism from certain people—principally some philosophers, but also physicians and lawyers—who are not comfortable with this consensus. Their objections can be summarized in three challenges to the UDDA.

WHOLE-BRAIN VERSUS HIGHER-BRAIN DEATH. The strongest position against the UDDA is mounted by those who would substitute for its "whole brain" standard a "higher brain" standard. Many philosophers have argued that certain features of consciousness (or at least the potential for consciousness) are essential to being a person as distinct from merely a human being (Veatch; Zaner). The absence of consciousness and cognition—as occurs, for example, in patients in the permanent vegetative state (PVS)—thus results in the loss of personhood. A related argument rests on the ontological proposition that the meaning of being a person—that is, a particular individual—is to have a personal identity, which depends on continuity of personal history as well as on self-awareness. The permanent loss of consciousness destroys such identity and hence means the death of that person, even if the body persists.

Consideration of the implications of these theories for determination of death takes several forms. On a conceptual level, the specific characteristics deemed by philosophers to be essential for personhood have varied widely from John Locke's focus on self-awareness to Immanuel Kant's requirement of a capacity for rational moral agency (Lizza). Thus, while certain definitions would exclude only those who lack any capacity for self-knowledge, such as PVS (persistent vegetative state) patients, other conceptions would encompass senile or severely retarded patients who cannot synthesize experience or act on moral principles.

On a practical level, trying to base a definition of death on cessation of higher-brain functions creates at least two problems. The first is the absence of agreed-upon clinical tests for cessation of these functions. Although certain clinical conditions such as PVS that involve the loss of neocortical functioning when brainstem functions persist can be determined sufficiently reliably for prognostic purposes (such as when deciding that further treatment is no longer in the best interests of a dying patient), the greater complexity and uncertainty that remain prevent testing with the same degree of accuracy as with the whole-brain standards. The practical problems increase enormously if the higher-brain definition is grounded on loss of personhood or personal identity, because loss of such a characteristic is not associated with particular neurologic structures.

More fundamentally, patients who are found to have lost (or never to have had) personhood because they lack higher-brain functions, or because they no longer have the same personal identity, will still be breathing spontaneously if they do not also meet whole-brain standards such as those of the UDDA. While such entities may no longer be "persons," they are still living bodies as "living" is generally understood and commonly used. "Death can be applied directly only to biological organisms and not to persons" (Culver and Gert, p. 183). To regard a human being who lacks only cerebral functions as dead would lead either to burying spontaneously respiring bodies or to having first to take affirmative steps, such as those used in active euthanasia, to end breathing, circulation, and the like. Neither of these would comport with the practices or beliefs of most people despite widespread agreement that such bodies, especially those that have permanently lost consciousness, lack distinctive human characteristics and need not be sustained through further medical interventions. Perhaps for this reason, in proposing a statute that would base death on cessation of cerebral functions, Robert Veatch condones allowing persons, while still competent, or their next of kin to opt out of having their death determined on the higher-brain standard. No state has adopted a "conscience clause" of this type, and the New Jersey statute mentioned above does not endorse the higher-brain standard (Olick).

The major legal evaluation of the higher-brain standard has arisen in the context of infant organ transplantation because of several highly publicized attempts in the 1980s to transplant organs from anencephalic infants (babies born without a neocortex and with the tops of their skulls open, exposing the underlying tissue). In 1987–1988, Loma Linda Medical Center in California mounted a protocol (a formal plan for conducting research) to obtain more organs, particularly hearts, from this source. The protocol took two forms. At first, the anencephalic infants were placed on respirators shortly after birth; but such infants did not lose functions and die within the two-week period the physicians had set, based on historical experience that virtually all anencephalics expire within two weeks of birth. In the second phase of the protocol, the physicians delayed the use of life support until the infants had begun experiencing apnea (cessation of breathing). Yet by the time death could be diagnosed neurologically in these infants, the damage to other organs besides the brain was so great as to render the organs useless. No organs were transplanted under the Loma Linda protocol.

Proposals to modify either the determination of death or the organ-transplant statutes to permit the use of organs from anencephalic infants before they meet the general criteria for death have not been approved by any legislature, nor was the Florida Supreme Court persuaded to change the law in the only appellate case regarding anencephalic organ donation. In that case, the parents of a child prenatally diagnosed with anencephaly requested that she be regarded as dead from the moment of birth so that her organs could be donated without waiting for breathing and heartbeat to cease. The Florida statute limits brain-based determinations of death to patients on artificial support. Turning to the common law, the court held that it established the cardiopulmonary standard, and the court then declined to create a judicial standard of death for anencephalics in the absence of a "public necessity" for doing so or any medical consensus that such a step would be good public policy (T.A.C.P.).

Although the Loma Linda protocol for using anencephalic infants as organ sources attempted to comply with the general consensus on death determination, it also proved that the "slippery slope" is not merely a hypothetical possibility. While the program was ongoing and receiving a great deal of media attention, the neonatologist who ran the pediatric intensive-care unit where potential donors were cared for reported receiving offers from well-meaning physicians of infants with hydrocephalus, intraventricular hemorrhage, and severe congenital anomalies. These physicians found it difficult to accept Loma Linda's rejection of such infants, whom the referring physicians saw as comparable on relevant grounds to the anencephalic infants who had been accepted. Beyond the risk of error in diagnosing anencephaly, it is hard to draw a line at this one condition, since the salient criteria—absence of higher-brain function and limited life expectancy—apply to other persons as well. The criterion that really moves many people—namely, the gross physical deformity of anencephalic infants' skulls—is without moral significance. Thus, a decision to accept anencephaly as a basis for declaring death would imply acceptance of some perhaps undefined higher-brain standard for diagnosing any and all patients.

CHANGING CLINICAL CRITERIA. Some medical commentators have suggested that society should rethink brain death because studies of bodies determined to be dead on neurological grounds have shown results that fail to accord with the standard of "irreversible loss of all functions of the entire brain" (Truog and Fackler). Specifically, some of these patients still have hypothalamic-endocrine function, cerebral electrical activity, or responsiveness to the environment.

Although the technical aspects of these various findings differ, similar reasoning can be applied to assessing their meaning for the concept of brain death. For each, one must ask first, are such findings observed among patients diagnosed through cardiopulmonary as well as neurological means of diagnosing death? Second, are such findings inconsistent with the irreversible loss of integrative functioning of the organism? Finally, do such findings relate to functions that when lost do not return and are not replaceable?

If some patients diagnosed dead on heart-lung grounds also have hypothalamic-endocrine function, cerebral electrical activity, or environmental responses, then the presence of these findings in neurologically diagnosed patients would not be cause for concern that the clinical criteria for the latter groups are inaccurate, and no redefinition would be needed.

Plainly, in many dead bodies some activity (as opposed to full functions) remains temporarily within parts of the brain. The question then becomes whether the secretion of a particular hormone (such as arginine vasopressin, which stimulates the contraction of capillaries and arterioles) is so physiologically integrative that it must be irreversibly absent for death to be declared. Depending upon the answer, it might be appropriate to add to the tests performed in diagnosing death measurements of arginine vasopressin or other tests and procedures that have meaning and significance consistent with existing criteria.

Such a modest updating of the clinical criteria is all that is required by Truog and Fackler's data and is preferable to the alternative they favor, modifying the conceptual standards to permanent loss of the capacity for consciousness while leaving the existing criteria for the time being. Not only does this change fail to respond to their data that testing can evoke electrical activity in the brain stem, despite the absence of such activity in the neocortex (called electrocerebral silence); it also has all the problems of lack of general acceptability that attach to any standard that would result in declaring patients with spontaneous breathing and heartbeat dead because they are comatose (i.e., deeply unconscious).

THE MEANING OF IRREVERSIBILITY. The final challenge to the UDDA is less an attempt to refute its theory than it is a contradiction of the standards established by the statute and accompanying medical guidelines. Under a protocol developed at the University of Pittsburgh in 1992, patients who are dependent on life-support technology for continued vital functions and who desire to be organ donors are wheeled into the operating room and the life support disconnected,

leading to cardiac arrest. After two minutes of asystole (lack of heartbeat), death is declared based upon the "irreversible cessation of circulatory and respiratory functions," at which point blood flow is artificially restored to the organs which are to be removed for transplantation (Youngner et al., 1993). Yet the failure to attempt to restore circulatory and respiratory functions in these patients shows that death had not occurred according to the existing criteria. The requirement of "irreversible cessation" must mean more than simply the physician "chose not to reverse." If no attempt is made to restore circulation and respiration before organs are removed it is not appropriate to make a diagnosis of death—merely a prognosis that death will occur if available means of resuscitation continue not to be used.

The reason for alternative standards for determining death is not because there are two kinds of death. On the contrary, there is one phenomenon that can be viewed through two windows, and the requirement of irreversibility ensures that what is seen is virtually the same thing through both. To replace "irreversible cessation of circulatory and respiratory functions" with "choose not to reverse" contradicts the underlying premise, because in the absence of the irreversibility there is no reason to suppose that brain functions have also permanently ceased.

A different, and more potent, challenge to the irreversibility requirement is posed by the prospect inherent in current research on human stem cells that some time in the future it may be possible to restore brain functions whose loss is at present beyond repair. Should such treatments become a clinical reality, the present standards for determining death will need to be reconsidered because the occurrence of death will in all cases turn on the decision whether or not to attempt repair.

Conclusion

The movement toward a modern legal formulation of the bases for pronouncing death has not been completed, and it is not clear that a complete consensus is possible (Younger, Arnold, and Shapiro, 1999). In some societies, that task may be left to the medical profession, since the problems faced in medical practice provide the impetus for change. Tradition as well as sound policy suggests, however, that the ground rules for decisions about individual patients should be established by public authorities. Whether the new legal definition of death emerges from the resolution of court cases or from the legislative process, it will be greatly influenced by opinion from the medical community. Recognition that the standards for determining death are matters of social and not merely professional concern only serves to underline the education of the public on this subject as an important ethical obligation of the profession.

ALEXANDER MORGAN CAPRON (1995)
REVISED BY AUTHOR

SEE ALSO: *Body: Cultural and Religious Perspectives; Consensus, Role and Authority of; Judaism, Bioethics in; Law and Bioethics; Law and Morality; Life; Metaphor and Analogy; Organ and Tissue Procurement; Public Policy and Bioethics;* and other *Death, Definition and Determination of* subentries

BIBLIOGRAPHY

Ad Hoc Committee of the Harvard Medical School to Examine the Definition of Brain Death. 1968. "A Definition of Irreversible Coma." *Journal of the American Medical Association* 205(6): 337–340. The original guidance on the means for determining an irreversible loss of total brain functioning, unfortunately mislabeled "irreversible coma."

Akabayashi, Akira. 1997. "Japan's Parliament Passes Brain-death Law." *The Lancet* 349: 1895. The law adopted by Japan in 1997 recognizes brain death but accommodates traditional religious beliefs by allowing the patient's family to veto this diagnosis.

Capron, Alexander Morgan. 1973. "The Purpose of Death: A Reply to Professor Dworkin." *Indiana Law Journal* 48(4): 640–646. Argues for developing a definition that comports with social reality and that can be employed in as many legal settings as it suits.

Capron, Alexander Morgan, and Kass, Leon R. 1972. "A Statutory Definition of the Standards for Determining Human Death: An Appraisal and a Proposal." *University of Pennsylvania Law Review* 121: 87–118. Discusses the procedures and objectives for lawmaking and provides a model that was widely adopted.

Cate, Fred H., and Capron, Alexander Morgan. 2003. "Death and Organ Transplantation." In *Treatise on Health Care Law*, pp. 45–60, ed. Michael G. Macdonald, Robert M. Kaufman, Alexander M. Capron, and Irwin M. Birnbaum. New York: Matthew Bender.

Culver, Charles M., and Gert, Bernard. 1982. *Philosophy in Medicine: Conceptual and Ethical Issues in Medicine and Psychiatry.* New York: Oxford University Press.

Kass, Leon R. 1971. "Death as an Event: A Commentary on Robert Morison." *Science* 173(998): 698–702. Refutes Morison's thesis that death does not occur at an identifiable time and explores the social rules that follow from this view.

Kennedy, Ian McColl. 1971. "The Kansas Statute on Death: An Appraisal." *New England Journal of Medicine* 285(17): 946–949. Criticizes the first American statute and urges that defining death be left in medical hands.

Kennedy, Ian McColl, and Grubb, Andrew. 1989. *Medical Law: Text and Materials.* London: Butterworths.

Lizza, John P. 1993. "Persons and Death: What's Metaphysically Wrong with our Current Statutory Definition of Death?" *Journal of Medicine and Philosophy* 18(4): 351–374.

Medical Consultants on the Diagnosis of Death to the President's Commission for the Study of Ethical Problems in Medicine and Biomedical and Behavioral Research. 1981. "Guidelines for the Determination of Death." *Journal of the American Medical Association* 246(19): 2184–2187. This statement, signed by nearly all the leading American authorities on the subject, became the prevailing standard for pronouncing death.

New Jersey Commission on Legal and Ethical Problems in the Delivery of Health Care. 1991. The New Jersey Advance Directives for Health Care and Declaration of Death Acts: Statutes, Commentaries and Analysis. Trenton, NJ: Author. Proposes and defends state's unique statute on determination of death.

Olick, Robert S. 1991. "Brain Death, Religious Freedom, and Public Policy: New Jersey's Landmark Legislative Initiative." *Kennedy Institute of Ethics Journal* 1(4): 275–288. Discusses New Jersey's religious exemption and offers a defense of the conscience clause in law and policy.

T.A.C.P., In re. 609 So.2d 588–95 (Fla. Sup. Ct. 1992).

Task Force for the Determination of Brain Death in Children. 1987. "Guidelines for the Determination of Brain Death in Children." *Annals of Neurology* 21(6): 616–621. Provides special standards for pediatric death determination.

Truog, Robert D., and Fackler, James C. 1992. "Rethinking Brain Death." *Critical Care Medicine* 20(12): 1705–1713.

U.S. President's Commission for the Study of Ethical Problems in Medicine and Biomedical and Behavioral Research. 1981. *Defining Death: Medical, Legal, and Ethical Issues in the Determination of Death.* Washington, D.C.: U.S. Government Printing Office. Explanation of concepts and rationale for Uniform Determination of Death Act by federal bioethics commission, which operated from 1980 to 1983.

Van Till-d'Aulnis de Bourouill, Adrienne. 1975. "How Dead Can You Be?" *Medicine, Science and the Law* 15(2): 133–147. Compares American diagnostic criteria with those used in France, Austria, and Germany; also differentiates ceasing artificial maintenance from murder or active euthanasia.

Veatch, Robert M. 1976. *Death, Dying, and the Biological Revolution: Our Last Quest for Responsibility.* New Haven, CT: Yale University Press. Argues for regarding death as the loss of cerebral functions and provides a statute to achieve this end.

Youngner, Stuart; Arnold, Robert M.; and Shapiro, Renie. 1999. *The Definition of Death.* Baltimore, MD: Johns Hopkins University Press. Identifies problems with defining death, including ethical, historical, cultural, and international arguments.

Youngner, Stuart, and Arnold, Robert M., for the Working Group on Ethical, Psychosocial, and Public Policy Implications of Procuring Organs from Non-Heart-Beating Cadaver Donors. 1993. "Ethical, Psychosocial, and Public Policy Implications of Procuring Organs from Non-Heart-Beating Cadaver Donors." *Journal of the American Medical Association* 269(21): 2769–2774. Reviews issues that are raised by using as organ donors patients whose hearts stop beating when life-sustaining treatment is discontinued.

Zaner, Richard M., ed. 1988. Death: Beyond Whole-Brain Criteria. Dordrecht, Netherlands: Kluwer Academic Publishers. A symposium on the debate between whole- and higher-brain standards, with essays favoring the latter by such leading figures as Edward T. Bartlett and Stuart J. Youngner, H. Tristram Engelhardt, Robert M. Veatch, and Richard M. Zaner.

III. PHILOSOPHICAL AND THEOLOGICAL PERSPECTIVES

The bioethics debate concerning the definition and criteria of human death emerged during the rise of organ transplantation in the 1960s, prompted by the advent of functional mechanical replacements for the heart, lungs, and brain stem, and by the ability to diagnose the pervasive brain destruction that is termed *brain death.* Previously, there had been no need to explore the conceptual or definitional basis of the established practice of declaring death or to consider additional criteria for determining death, since the irreversible cessation of either heart or lung function quickly led to the permanent loss of any other functioning considered a sign of life. New technologies and advances in resuscitation changed all this by permitting the dissociated functioning of the heart, lungs, and brain. In particular, society experienced the phenomenon of a mechanically sustained patient whose whole brain was said to be in a state of irreversible coma. And there were an increasing number of *vegetative* patients sustained by feeding tubes, whose bodies had been resuscitated to the status of spontaneously functioning organisms, but whose higher brains had permanently lost the capacity for consciousness. Such phenomena as these pressed a decision as to whether the irreversible loss of whole or higher-brain functioning should be considered the death of the individual, despite the continuation of respiration and heartbeat. With mounting pressure to increase the number of viable organs for transplant within the unquestioned constraint of the Dead Donor Rule which requires that the organ donor be dead before organ removal, the debate concerning whole-brain death arose.

The Beginnings of the Debate

The debate opened in 1968, when the Ad Hoc Committee of the Harvard Medical School to Examine the Definition of Brain Death (Harvard Committee) recommended an *updating* of the criteria for determining that a patient has died. The Harvard Committee put forth a set of clinical tests it claimed was sufficient to determine the death of the entire brain. It then recommended that whole-brain death be considered direct and sufficient evidence of the death of the patient. Thus arose the suggestion, which has become entrenched practice in the United States, that a binary standard be used for determining death: that in addition to the traditional heart and lung criteria still applicable in the vast majority of cases, a whole-brain death criterion be used to determine death for respirator-dependent, permanently unconscious patients.

This was the modest beginning of the so-called *definition-of-death* debate. Rather than having resolved over the last thirty-five years, this debate has evolved and intensified due to fascinating and complex constellations of philosophical, clinical, and policy disagreements. To best appreciate these disagreements, one must understand the definitional debate as one that has three logically distinct, yet interdependent levels: (1) the conceptual or definitional level; (2) the criteriological level; and (3) the medical diagnostic level. Let us look at each of the three levels in turn.

THE THREE LEVELS OF THE DEBATE. *Level One: The conceptual or definitional level.* At level one, the question is, What is human death? While some people think basic definitions such as this one are somehow written on the face of reality for our discernment, defining death is in fact a normative activity that draws on deeply held philosophical, religious, or cultural beliefs and values. The definition or concept of death reflects a human choice to count a particular loss as death. The level two and level three activities of deciding which physiological functions underlie that loss (i.e., choosing a criterion for determining death), and of specifying the medical tests for determining that the criterion is fulfilled, are medical/scientific activities. The conceptual question can be answered in a general, yet uninformative way by saying that human death is the irreversible loss of that which is essentially significant to the nature of the human being. No one will take issue with this definition, but it does not go far enough. There is still a need to decide what is essentially significant to the nature of the human being.

People differ radically in their views on the distinctive nature of the human being and its essentially significant characteristic(s). Because their fundamentally different perspectives on human nature flow from deeply rooted beliefs and values, the difficult policy question arises concerning the extent to which a principle of toleration should guide medical practice to honor the alternative definitions of human death that exist.

The discussion later in this section will show that the human being can be thought of as a wholly material or physical entity, as a physical/mental amalgam, or as an essentially spiritual (though temporarily embodied) being. The way the human is thought of will influence the view of what is essentially significant to the nature of the human being, and ground one's view about the functional loss that should be counted as human death. A metaphysical decision concerning the kind of being the human is, is the ultimate grounding for the normative choice of criteria for determining that an individual human being has died. There could be no more interesting or important a philosophical problem, then, than the problem of deciding: What is human death? Why? And, there could be no more interesting an ethical/policy problem than that of deciding whether and how to tolerate and enable a diversity of answers to these questions.

Level Two: The criteriological level. Based on the resolution of the ontological and normative questions at the conceptual level, a criterion for determining that an individual has died, reflecting the physiological function(s) considered necessary for life and sufficient for death, is specified. That is, the essentially significant human characteristic(s) delineated at the conceptual level is (are) located in (a) functional system(s) of the human organism. The traditional criteria center on heart and lung function, suggesting that the essentially significant characteristics are respiration and circulation. The whole-brain-death criterion is said by its proponents to focus on the integrated functioning of the organism as a whole. The higher-brain-death criterion centers on the irreversible absence of a capacity for consciousness.

Level Three: The diagnostic level. At this level are the medical diagnostic tests to determine that the functional failure identified as the criterion of death has in fact occurred. These tests are used by medical professionals to determine whether the criterion is met, and thus that death should be declared. As technological development proceeds, diagnostic sophistication increases. The Harvard Committee believed that the death of the entire brain could be clinically diagnosed using the tests it identified in its report, and recommended that the whole-brain-death criterion be used to determine death in cases of respirator dependency. However, it provided no conceptual argument (i.e., no answer to the level one question, What is human death?) to support the criterion and practice it recommended.

These three levels—conceptual, criteriological, and diagnostic—provide a crucial intellectual grid for following the complex definition-of-death debate since 1968. The debate encompasses all three levels. In any reading and reflection associated with this complex debate, it is essential to remember what level of the debate one is on, and what sort of expertise is required on the part of those party to the debate at that level. Further, any analysis and critical assessment of suggested criteria for determining death require that one attend to the important interconnections among tests, criteria, and concepts. Criteria without tests are useless in practice; criteria without concepts lack justification. It is the

philosophical task of constructing an adequate concept or definition of human death that becomes central to a justified medical practice of declaring death. As Scot philosopher and historian David Hume (1711–1776) said centuries ago, "Concepts without percepts are blind." At the beginning of the twenty-first century, a criterion for determining death without a philosophical analysis of what constitutes death is equally blind. All in all, there ought to be coherence among concept, criterion, and clinical tests. At least this is the way one would normally wish to operate. Among other things, the definition-of-death debate can be expressed as a debate among alternative formulations of death: the traditional cardio-pulmonary, whole-brain and higher-brain formulations.

The Traditional Cardio-Pulmonary Formulation

Initially, many objected to the whole-brain formulation because they saw it to be a change in our fundamental understanding of the human being, and a dramatic change from the essentially cardiac-centered concept and criterion for determining death (the traditional cardio-pulmonary criteria, which required the final stoppage of the heart). Several have called for a return to the use of the traditional criteria, consistent with an understanding of death as the irreversible loss of the integrative functioning of the organism as a whole. The claim has been that whether mechanically or spontaneously sustained, a beating heart signifies the ongoing integrated functioning of the organism as a whole, whether or not the patient is *brain-dead.* On this view, death has not occurred until the heart and lungs have irreversibly ceased to function. Some religious traditions adhere steadfastly to this concept of death, and consider the brain-death criterion an unacceptable basis on which to declare death.

The Whole-Brain-Death Formulation: Concept and Criterion

When the Harvard Committee recommended that a whole-brain-death criterion be used to determine death in respirator-dependent patients, thus creating an exception to the use of the traditional cardio-pulmonary criteria for a specific category of patients, controversy arose over whether the adoption of this criterion constituted a departure from the concept of death implicit in the use of the traditional cardio-pulmonary criteria for the determination of death.

Some saw the use of the brain-death criterion to be a blatantly utilitarian maneuver to increase the availability of transplantable organs. Some opposed it because it was inconsistent with their view of the human self and/or failed to protect and respect dying patients. While others agreed that the neurological focus represented an alternative understanding of the self, they saw the move to be eminently logical: What argument could one have with the notion that someone whose whole brain is dead, is dead? Others continued to affirm that life was essentially a heart-centered reality rather than a brain-centered reality: They saw the shift to a neurological focus on the human to be a discounting of the relevance of the spontaneous beating of the heart and the mechanically sustained functioning of the lungs. So, representatives of some cultures and faith traditions opposed the shift to the brain-death criterion, suggesting that it was a radically unacceptable way of understanding and determining the death of a human being.

The Harvard Committee report was a clinical recommendation, not a philosophical argument. It made recommendations at levels two and three (the criteriological and the diagnostic), and prompted but did not answer a number of level one definitional questions. What is death, such that either the traditional criteria or the whole-brain-death criterion may be used to determine its occurrence? Do the traditional criteria and the brain-death criterion presuppose the same definition of death? If not, should human death be *redefined* in response to technological change? It gave rise to a philosophical debate that is ongoing on the question, What is so essentially significant to the nature of a human being that its irreversible loss should be considered human death?

The literature has been replete with answers to this question, including the irreversible loss of the flow of vital fluids, the irreversible departure of the soul from the body, the irreversible loss of the capacity for bodily integration, the irreversible cessation of integrative unity (i.e., of the antientropic mutual interaction of all of the body's cells and tissues), the irreversible loss of the integrated functioning of the organism as a whole, and the irreversible loss of the capacity for consciousness or social interaction. Without such an account of what is essentially significant, the criterion used as a basis for determining death lacks an explicit foundation. However, the plurality of thoughtful answers to this fundamental conceptual question raises the issues of whether a consensus view can be fashioned, whether to tolerate diverse understandings of human death, and of how to assure societal stability concerning the determination of death.

While the Harvard Committee provided no philosophical defense of its position, adherents of the whole-brain formulation have continued to argue over the years that the traditional criteria and the whole-brain-death criterion share a common concept of death—the irreversible loss of the capacity for integrated functioning of the organism as a whole. Not everyone has agreed with this position, however. Some resist the adoption of the brain-death criterion for this reason, considering the shift to a new understanding of human death to be philosophically unjustifiable. However, others have welcomed the change: Reflecting on the contingency of the definition of death under circumstances of technological change, some have argued in favor of redefining death even further. In their view, the philosophical concept of death said to underlie the whole-brain-death criterion inadequately reflects the essentially significant characteristic of human existence: existence as an embodied consciousness. A more adequate concept of human death, they contend, would center on the permanent cessation of consciousness (requiring a higher-brain-death criterion), not on the permanent cessation of the integrated functioning of the organism. Advocates of the higher-brain formulation of death oppose the whole-brain formulation on the ground that the latter unjustifiably defers to the characteristics biological organisms have in common and ignores the relevance of the distinctively human characteristics associated with life as a person.

If the whole-brain formulation is essentially an organismically-based concept, and the higher-brain formulation is essentially a person-based concept, the controversy between whole- and higher-brain formulations suggests that in order to answer the question, What is human death? another layer of philosophical reflection is required. The central normative question concerning what is essentially significant to the nature of the human being requires a prior account of the nature of the human being. In philosophical terms, such an account of the nature of a being is referred to as an ontological account. One's view of the nature of the human being is informed by philosophical, theological and/or cultural perspectives on the nature of human existence, its essentially significant characteristics, and the nature of its boundary events. In the case of the human, there appear to be two logically distinct choices concerning the nature of the human being: one either sees it as one organism among others, for which meanings-in-common of life and death should be sought; or one sees the human being as distinctive among organisms for the purpose of characterizing its life and death, in ways we signify by the term *person*. In short we need to make and defend a decision concerning the way we look at the human—as organism or as person—for the purpose of determining what constitutes human death.

The Whole-Brain Formulation: Public Policy

In 1981 the whole-brain-death formulation originally advanced by the Harvard Committee was articulated in a major U.S. policy document. The President's Commission for the Study of Ethical Problems in Medicine and Biomedical and Behavioral Research published its report, *Defining Death: A Report on the Medical, Legal, and Ethical Issues in the Determination of Death*. In this document, it provided a model law called the Uniform Determination of Death Act, to encourage the uniform adoption in each of the United States of the traditional criteria and the brain-death criterion as alternative approaches to declaring death. The supporting framework they offered for this recommendation was this: The concept of human death is the irreversible cessation of the integrated functioning of the organism as a whole. This, they claimed, is a function of the activity of the entire brain, not just a portion of the brain, and its occurrence can be measured, depending on the patient's circumstances, either by the traditional criteria or the brain-death criterion.

Questioning the Whole-Brain Formulation

The whole-brain formulation has been attacked at the conceptual level, and on the ground that the answers at each level collectively provide an incoherent account of concept, criterion and clinical tests for determining death. The President's Commission's concept or definition of death has been objected to by those who favor one centered on the essential features of a personal life, as well as by those who favor a circulatory concept and consider that only the irreversible cessation of circulation adequately signals death.

In addition, since 1981, clinical findings have confirmed that what has come to be called whole-brain death is not in fact synonymous with the death of the brain in all of its parts. There are instances of isolated continued functioning in the brain-dead brain. Those wishing to support the established consensus around the use of the brain-death criterion argue that such *residual functioning* in the brain-dead brain is insignificant to the determination of death. Specifically, then, they refuse to allow that these kinds of residual brain functioning have significance: (i) persistent cortical functioning as evidenced by electroencephalograph (EEG) activity, and in rare cases a sleep/wake pattern; (ii) ongoing brainstem functioning as evidenced by auditory or visual evoked potential recording; and (iii) preserved antidiuretic neurohormonal functioning. Such instances of residual functioning suggest that brain death, as customarily diagnosed, does not include the hypothalamus and the posterior pituitary. Most importantly, the third instance of residual functioning just cited actually plays an *integrative* role in the life of the organism as a whole. Hence, one of the residual functions fulfills the concept of life implicit in the definition of death underlying the whole-brain formulation.

So, the clinical tests used to establish the death of the entire brain have been shown to reflect a pervasive but nonetheless *partial* death of the brain only, opening wide the question, If brain death is to remain a reasonable basis upon which to declare death, which brain functions are so essentially significant that their irreversible loss should be counted as brain death? Why?

Both philosophically and clinically speaking, then, many feel that a rethinking of the U.S. societal adherence to the brain-death criterion is warranted. It rests on a contested understanding of what human death is, raising the issue of whether the brain-death criterion should be used to declare someone dead who holds philosophical/theological/cultural objections to it. It lacks coherence among its levels because (1) the brain-death criterion does not correlate with the irreversible loss of the integrated functioning of the organism as a whole; and (2) because the clinical tests for brain death fail to reflect the death of the entire brain. No important societally established practice can be imagined to be so highly problematic as this one.

The supporters of the whole-brain formulation have nonetheless stood their ground, claiming that the instances of residual cellular and subcellular activities occurring in the brain are irrelevant to the determination of the life/death status of the patient. In their view, the brain-death criterion should continue to be used, despite that it really reflects a pervasive albeit partial brain death.

The basic challenge to the whole-brain formulation has been that its defenders need to provide criteria for distinguishing between brain activity that is relevant and irrelevant for the purpose of determining death. Some have argued that the only bright line that could be drawn in this regard is between the brain functions essential for consciousness and those that are not; others have argued that the brain should be abandoned entirely as a locus for establishing that a human being has died. In point of fact then, advocates of the whole-brain formulation have embraced a partial-brain-death criterion but have failed to provide a non-question-begging, principled basis for it.

Another aspect of the whole-brain formulation that has been challenged concerns its reliance on the non-spontaneous function of the lungs to support the claim that the irreversible cessation of the integrated functioning of the organism as a whole has occurred. They claim that the integrated functioning continues, and that the manner of its support is irrelevant. Their point is that as long as the respirator is functioning, it seems something of a word game to say that the organism is not functioning as an integrated whole.

While in brain death the brain stem is no longer playing its linking role in the triangle of function along with lungs and heart, the respirator is standing in for the brain stem, just as it might if there were partial brain destruction in the area of the brain stem. If the patient were conscious, but just as dependent on the respirator in order to continue functioning as an organism, there would be no inclination to pronounce the patient dead. Hence, it would seem that even the brain-dead patient is exhibiting integrated organismic functioning until the respirator is turned off, the lungs stop, and the heart eventually stops beating. The phenomenon of a mechanically-sustained brain-dead pregnant woman producing a healthy newborn certainly seems to bear out their insight: Whatever the sort of organismic disintegration possessed in such a case, it seems most unfitting to call it death. Integrated organismic functioning is present in brain death, so if brain death *should be* considered the death of the human being, it is not because brain death signals the irreversible loss of the integrated functioning of the organism as a whole.

As this last point makes clear, the real reason so many people are inclined to agree that the brain-dead patient is dead has much more to do with the fact that the brain-dead patient is permanently unconscious than with the facts of brain stem destruction and respirator dependency. It is this loss of the self, the loss of consciousness and thus of embodiment as a self, that is for many of us a good reason to consider the brain-dead patient dead. This suggests that the concept of human death underlying people's willingness to adopt the brain-death criterion may have more to do with the loss of the capacity for embodied consciousness than with the loss of the capacity for integrated organismic functioning.

The Higher-Brain Formulation

Consistent with this insight, some contributors to the definition-of-death debate propose a higher-brain-death criterion for the determination of death, contending that this criterion presupposes a different and preferable view of what is essentially significant to the nature of the human being. They hold that consciousness, sometimes characterized as a capacity for social interaction, is the *sine qua non* of human existence, and that the criterion used to determine death should reflect this loss. In their view, requiring that the brain-death criterion be used when the patient is permanently unconscious is biologically reductionistic. That is, the brain-death criterion attaches primary significance to the functional connection of the brainstem, lungs and heart, and not the conscious capacity that that functioning supports. Unless the concept of human death reflects what is essentially significant to the nature of the human being as a person—conscious awareness—it fails to provide a community with an effective moral divide between the living and the dead.

Questioning the Higher-Brain Formulation

Critics of the higher-brain formulation object that the emphasis on consciousness and person-centered functions of the human being places us on a *slippery slope* that will eventually lead to a broadening of the definition of death to include those who are severely demented or only marginally or intermittently conscious. They argue further that the adoption of a higher-brain basis for determining death would require us to bury spontaneously respiring (and heart beating) *cadavers*.

These arguments have little to recommend them. First there is a bright and empirically demonstrable line between those who are in a permanent vegetative state (recall the cases of Karen Quinlan, Paul Brophy, Nancy Cruzan, and others) and those who retain the capacity for higher-brain functioning. The slippery slope worry that we would begin to declare conscious patients dead is unfounded. By contrast the slippery slope objection is telling in relation to the whole-brain-death criterion, which does not in fact measure the death of the brain in its entirety. Whole-brain-death adherents have failed to provide criteria for identifying some brain functions as residual and insignificant, so the opportunity for the unprincipled enlargement of the residual functioning category is ever present.

Finally, for aesthetic reasons as well as reasons of respect, society does not permit certain forms of treatment of the dead. There is no reason to think that a consciousness-based concept of death would lead to the abandonment of long-held understandings of the dignified and appropriate treatment of the body of the deceased person. One would not bury a spontaneously breathing body any more than one would bury a brain-dead body still attached to a respirator. A higher-brain advocate might argue that stopping residual heart and lung function would be as morally appropriate in the case of a permanently unconscious patient as the discontinuation of the ventilator is in the case of a brain-dead patient.

Questioning the Irreversibility of Death

Still laboring under the power of the Dead Donor Rule and a concern to increase the supply of transplantable organs, a 1990s effort to update the clinical tests associated with the cardiac-centered traditional criteria occurred. Several transplant centers began the practice, in the case of a dying patient who had consented in advance to be an organ donor and to forego both life-sustaining treatment and resuscitative efforts, of declaring death two minutes after the patient's last heartbeat, as the measure of the patient's irreversible loss of cardiopulmonary function. This approach to assessing the irreversible loss of cardiopulmonary function challenged people to accept a particular and unprecedented definition of *irreversibility* in relation to declaring patients dead. Both common understanding and the Uniform Determination of Death Act were understood to require irreversibility of functional loss in the stronger sense that the functional loss could in no way be recovered or restored.

If death is declared two minutes after the loss of cardiopulmonary function, when, conceivably, the heart could resume functioning on its own (auto-resuscitation) or resuscitation could successfully restart the heart, in what sense is the loss of function irreversible? It appears that irreversibility is only a function of a morally valid decision on the part of a patient or perhaps a surrogate to forego resuscitation. Is this change in the association of death with the irreversible loss of function ethically acceptable?

The interest in declaring death as close to the cessation of cardiopulmonary function as possible arises from the need to remove organs before warm ischemia destroys their viability for transplantation. But what sense of the concept of irreversibility should be required to assess a loss of critical function sufficient to ground a declaration of death? In the weak moral sense indicated above, two minutes after the last heartbeat when resuscitation has been refused? In the relatively stronger sense that auto-resuscitation of the heart has become physiologically impossible? Or in the strongest sense, that the heart cannot be restarted by any means?

While many hold the religious belief that the self survives the death of the body, the commonly held view is that the death of the body is a finished, non-reversible condition. The Uniform Determination of Death Act requires that the cessation of brain function be irreversible in the sense that all function throughout the entire brain is permanently absent, or it requires that cardiopulmonary function has ceased in the sense that the patient can never again exhibit respiration or heartbeat. Clearly, then, because it entails a novel understanding of the conceptual connections between death and irreversibility, the variation in the application of the cardiopulmonary criterion adopted by many transplant centers after 1992 requires philosophical justification.

In addition this new strategy for determining death raises interesting issues about the overall consistency of alternative approaches to determining death. It has always been the case that a patient declared brain-dead could not be declared dead using the traditional criteria, since the respirator was maintaining lung and heart functions. Those functions were effectively ruled out as signs of life. Yet after only two minutes of cardiac cessation, the patient is arguably not yet brain-dead, raising a question: Is the non-heart beating donor (NHBD) whose heart has stopped for two minutes but whose brain retains some functional capacity *really* dead? In order to be declared dead, should a patient be required to fulfill at least one but not necessarily all extant criteria and their associated clinical tests for the determination of death? Which way of being determined dead is more morally appropriate when surgery to procure organs is to be undertaken?

In sum, the definition-of-death debate goes on. The deep and disturbing irony in this debate surrounds the disagreement among ethicists as to whether the public should be informed about the degree of dissension on the conceptual, clinical, and policy issues central to the debate. Despite the rather stable practice in the United States of using the brain-death criterion to determine death, the definition-of-death debate is at loggerheads. The situation is such that, some have argued, parties to the debate should share none of this dissension with the public lest they disturb the acceptance of the brain-death criterion and the improved access to transplantable organs it allows over the traditional criteria for determining death. Others argue that every question in this debate, including the question of the kind of irreversibility that should ground the determination of deaths, is still an open question, and that the public should be informed and polled for its views. Yet others have suggested that one of the prime movers in the definitional debate, the Dead Donor Rule, should be rethought, and the practices of declaring death, discontinuing life-sustaining treatment, and removing organs for transplantation should be decided independently of one another.

Public Policy for a Diverse Society

The public policy issue in the definition-of-death debate arises because there are diverse, deeply held understandings concerning the nature of the human and human death. Because these views derive from fundamental philosophical, religious, or cultural perspectives, should people have any say in the concept and criteria for determining death that might be applied to them? If, for example, a person is aware that being declared dead under the brain-death criterion contradicts his or her religiously-based understanding of death, should that person be allowed to conscientiously object to the use of this criterion? Some argue that toleration in such matters is imperative because of the extraordinary damage done to persons by ignoring and disrespecting their foundational understandings. They claim that individuals should be allowed to use a conscience clause to express their wishes. Others claim that diversity on such a fundamental matter as the determination of when someone has died can only lead to social and legal instability. The next section explores the diverse philosophical perspectives that might be taken on human death. On this basis, the reader must decide on the importance and practicality of a conscience clause for those who disagree with the concept and criteria for determining death that have become established U.S. policy.

Philosophical and Theological Perspectives: Preliminaries

Human groups engage in different behaviors upon the death of one of their members. They do so because they have different understandings of the nature of the individual self and, consequently, of the death of the self. Yet every human society needs a way of determining when one of its members has died, when the quantum change in the self that both requires and justifies *death behaviors* has occurred, when the preparation of the bodily remainder of the individual for removal from the sphere of communal interaction both may and must begin.

This need for a line of demarcation between life and death suggests that for societal purposes, the death of an individual must be a determinable event. There has been debate, however, about whether death is an event or a process. Those engaged in this debate have appealed to the biological phenomena associated with the shutting down of a living organism. Some of them have argued that death is a discrete biological event; others, that it is a biological process. In fact, neither biological claim settles the philosophical question of whether death is an event or a process. Different communities decide whether to view the biological phenomena associated with death as an event or a process. For societal/cultural reasons, it is essential that some terminus be recognized.

Death is a biological process that poses a decisional dilemma because, arguably, the biological shutdown of the organism is not *complete* until putrefaction has occurred. Human communities have a need to decide when, in the course of the process of biological shutdown, the individual should be declared dead; they must decide which functions are so essentially significant to human life that their permanent cessation is death. For a variety of reasons, death has come to be associated with the permanent cessation of functions considered to be vital to the organism rather than with the end of all biological functioning in the organism. These vital functions play a pervasive and obvious role in the functioning of the organism as a whole, and so their use as lines of demarcation is reasonable. With their cessation, the most valued features of human life cease forever, and it is reasonable to regard that as the event of a person's death. Advances in medical technology, permitting the mechanical maintenance of cardiac and respiratory functions in the absence of consciousness, force us to evaluate the functions

we have always associated with life, and to choose which of them are essentially significant to human life or so valuable to us that their permanent loss constitutes death. The ancient and (until the late-twentieth century) reasonable assumption has been that death is an irreversible condition, so it should not be declared until the essentially significant functions have irreversibly ceased.

In pretechnological cultures, humans undoubtedly drew on the functional commonalities between other animal species and themselves to decide that the flow of blood and breathing were essentially significant functions. When either of these functions stopped, no other *important* functions continued, and predictable changes to the body ensued. Since it was beyond human power to alter this course of events, the permanent cessation of heart and lung functioning became the criterion used to determine that someone had died.

This choice has clearly stood the test of time. Often referred to as the traditional cardio-pulmonary criteria, there is certainly no reason to impugn this choice for a society lacking the technological life-support interventions characteristic of modern medicine. But it is important to see that even in a pretechnological culture, the choice of the traditional cardiopulmonary criteria was a choice, an imposition of values on biological data. It was a choice based on a decision concerning significant function, that is, a decision concerning what is so essentially significant to the nature of the human being that its irreversible cessation constitutes human death. Such a decision is informed by fundamental beliefs and values that are philosophical/theological/cultural in nature.

If a technologically advanced culture is to update its criteria for declaring death, it must reach to the level that informs such a decision. Deciding the normative issue concerning the essentially significant characteristic of a human being is impossible without an ontological account of the nature of the human being. The assumptions and beliefs we hold on these matters form the combined philosophical/theological/cultural basis upon which we dissect the biological data and eventually bisect them into *life* and *death*.

Such assumptions and beliefs constitute the most fundamental understandings and function as the often unseen frame through which people view, assess, and manipulate reality. As a rule, this frame is inculcated through the broad range of processes that a social group uses to shape its members. The frame itself consists of assumptions and beliefs that are used to organize and interpret experience. They are deeply yet pragmatically held beliefs that may be adjusted, adapted, discarded, or transformed when they cause individual or social confusion, cease to be useful, or no longer make sense. Arguably, changes in the capacity to resuscitate and support the human body in the absence of consciousness have brought that society to such a point of non-sense. To respond fully to this crisis, people must consider the various philosophical and theological perspectives in their culture that inform thinking about human nature and death.

Representative Philosophical and Theological Perspectives

Death is the word we use to signify the end of life as we know it. As stated above, individuals and groups hold different understandings of the existence and the death of the self. These understandings are the background for the *nuts and bolts* medical decision that a person has died, when death should be declared, and what ought/ought not be done to and with the physical remains of the person who has died.

As individuals and as cultural groups, humans differ in their most basic assumptions and beliefs about human death. For some the death of the body marks the absolute end of the self; for others it is a transition to another form of existence for the continuously existing self. This transition may be to continued life in either a material or an immaterial form. Despite these differences, every human community needs a way of determining when one of its members has died, a necessary and sufficient condition for considering the body as the remainder of the individual that can now be treated in ways that would have been inappropriate or immoral before, and for preparing the body for removal from the communal setting. Different philosophical and theological perspectives on the nature of death, the individual self, and the death of the self will yield different choices of criteria for the determination of death, just as these differing perspectives yield very different death practices or death behaviors. To see why this is the case, various philosophical and theological views of death and the self must be reviewed.

In the Hebrew tradition of the Old Testament, death is considered a punishment for the sin of disobedience. It is an absolute punishment. This tradition does not hold a concept of an afterlife following the punishment of death. But it would be misleading to say that this tradition has no conception of immortality, since the communal setting of the individual's experience and life remains the arena of that person's identity and impact, even after the death of the body. Although the conscious life of the person ceases, the person lives on in the collective life, unless he or she lived badly. Thus, immortality is the community's conscious and unconscious memory of the person.

Another view, originating in Platonic philosophy and found in Christian and Orthodox Judaic thought, and in Islam and Hinduism, holds that death is not the cessation of conscious life. The conscious self, often referred to as the soul, survives in a new form, possibly in a new realm. The experience of the self after the death of the body depends on the moral quality of the person's life. The body is the soul's temporary housing, and the soul's journey is toward the good, or God, or existence as pure rational spirit without bodily distractions. Thus, death is the disconnection of the spiritual element of the self (mind, soul, spirit) from the physical or bodily aspect of the self.

Traditions believing in eternal life differ in their view of the soul and its relationship to the body. This has implications for the criteria that might be used to determine death, as well as for the appropriate treatment of the body after death. The soul is viewed by some as separate and capable of migrating or moving into different bodies as it journeys toward eternal life. The Christian tradition, by contrast, posits the self as an eternally existing entity created by God. The death of the body is just that—the person continues, with body transformed, either punished in hell for living badly or rewarded in heaven for having faith and living righteously. These diverse views have a common belief: Everyone survives death in some way. This may influence the understanding of what constitutes the death of the body as well as of what ought/ought not to be done to the body of the person who has died. For some traditions, certain bodily functions are indicative of life, whether or not those functions are mechanically supported, and damage to the body is damage to the self.

In contrast to these theological conceptions of death and the self, three philosophical perspectives, secular in that they hold materialist views of the self, figure in Western thought: the Epicurean, the Stoic, and the existential. A materialist view of the self considers the human to be an entirely physical or material entity, with no soul or immaterial aspect. The Epicurean view of the self holds that humans are fully material beings without souls. The goal of life is to live it well as it is and not to fear death since death is the end of experience, not something one experiences. Therefore, there is no eternal life for souls; the body dies and disintegrates back into the material nature from which it sprang. The death of the body marks the end of consciousness, and thus the death of the self. A materialist holding a view such as this could conclude that the cessation of consciousness itself should be considered death, whether or not the body continues to function in an integrated manner.

The Stoic view acknowledges death as the absolute end of the conscious self but directs persons to have courage about its inevitability and to resign to it creatively. This creative resignation is achieved by focusing on the inevitability of death in such a way that one treats every moment of life as a creative opportunity. The necessity of death becomes the active inspiration for the way one lives. Like the Epicurean view, the Stoic conception ties the self to the body; the end of the self to the death of the body. But it is the consciousness supported by the body that is the creative self.

In contrast existential thought believes that the absoluteness of death renders human life absurd and meaningless. The other materialist views of the self saw death as the occasion for meaning in life, not the denial that life has meaning. Rather than infusing meaning into life and inspiring a commitment to striving, existentialism holds that death demonstrates the absurdity of human striving. While individuals may pursue subjective goals and try to realize subjective values during their lives, there are no objective values in relation to which to orient one's striving, and so all striving is ultimately absurd. Since death is the end of the self, there is nothing to prepare for beyond the terms of physical existence and the consciousness it supports.

Without critiquing these theological and philosophical perspectives on death and the self, an inquiry into their diversity is relevant to a discussion of the debate in bioethics about the criteria for determining that a human being has died. The earlier demonstration that the criteria rest on a decision of functional significance, and that a decision of functional significance is philosophically/theologically informed, coupled with this demonstration of philosophical/theological diversity on the fundamental concepts of self and the death of the self, together show that criteria are acceptable only if they are seen to be consistent with an accepted philosophical/theological frame, and that what is acceptable in one frame may be unacceptable in another.

Further, while it might be the case that virtually every tradition has agreed on the appropriateness of the traditional heart and lung criteria for declaring death, they may do so for vastly different reasons deriving from their specific understanding of death and the self. There may be ways of reconciling virtually every ontological view to the use of the traditional criteria but not to the use of consciousness-centered criteria like the higher brain-death criterion, or even the brain-death criterion (which appears, to a tradition like Orthodox Judaism, to deny that the still-functioning body is indicative of life, even when the entire brain is dead).

Philosophical and theological commitments relate centrally to society's death practices, including conclusions concerning the acceptability of traditional, and whole-brain, and higher-brain formulations of death. How philosophically and theologically sophisticated has the bioethics debate on the definition of death been, over the years?

The Persistence of the Debate

Why do arguments concerning the definition and criteria of death persist? The debate has been intractable since 1968. One important reason is that the concepts of self and death that inform the various positions in the debate are based on fundamental beliefs and values that suggest that they will remain irreconcilably different. While it is true that persons holding different philosophical/theological/cultural premises may assent to the use of the same criteria for determining death, they may well do so for very different reasons. Because of this, it is reasonable to seek and adopt a broadly acceptable societal standard for the determination of death.

For example, the several materialist views of the self that were examined earlier suggest a consciousness-centered concept of self and death that further recommends a higher-brain formulation of death. But equally, the prevailing Judeo-Christian understandings of the self and death—that of death as the dissociation of consciousness from the body, the end of embodied consciousness—are also compatible with a higher-brain formulation of death.

Some traditions, like Orthodox Judaism, and certain Japanese and Native American perspectives, resist the use of the brain-death criterion because they understand death to be a complete stoppage of the vital functions of the body. The self is not departed until such stoppage has occurred. Such groups will be uncomfortable with the use of the brain-death criterion because it permits the determination of death while vital functions continue. This kind of philosophical/theological difference in perspective on the human self, intimately linked to a person's religious and cultural identity, raises serious questions about how a pluralistic culture should deal with deeply held differences in designing a policy for the determination of death.

Given that there are a finite number of possible perspectives on the human person and on human death, and given the rootedness of these perspectives in conscientiously held philosophical and religious views and cultural identities, public policy on the determination of death in a complex and diverse culture could well manage to service conscience through the addition of a conscience clause in a determination-of-death statute. Similar to and perhaps in conjunction with a living will, a person could execute a conscience-clause exclusion to the statute's implicit concept of death. For instance, an Orthodox Jew could direct that death be determined using the traditional criteria alone, and also indicate personal preferences concerning the use of life-sustaining treatment such as ventilator support in the situation of brain death.

The fact that a conscience clause would permit some to reject the use of the brain-death criterion need not hinder the law from specifying punishable harms against others on the basis of considerations additional to whether death was caused. The exotic life-sustaining technologies now available have already generated arguments concerning whether the person who causes someone to be brain-dead or the person who turns off the ventilator on that brain-dead patient causes the patient's death.

Life-sustaining technologies as well as the alternative concepts of death underscore the need for more precise legal classifications of punishable harms to persons. Such a classification should recognize permanent loss of consciousness as a harm punishable to the same extent as permanent stoppage of the heart and lungs.

The self can be thought of in a variety of ways: as an entirely material entity, as an essentially mental entity, and as a combined physical/mental duality. In contemporary language, the human being may be thought of as a physical organism, as an embodied consciousness (which we often call person), or as an amalgam of the two. As one examines the definition-of-death debate, one sees that fundamentally different ontological perspectives on the human have been taken.

Once such an ontological perspective on the human being has been chosen, a further decision as to what is essentially significant to the nature of the human being can be made. When a conclusion is reached as to which function is essentially significant to the human being, the potential exists for settling on the criterion (or criteria) for determining death. To the extent that these two steps of philosophical analysis support attention to the brain as the locus of the relevant human functions, views may divide on whether a whole-brain or a higher-brain formulation of death is adopted.

A complex entity that manifests its aliveness in a variety of ways has the potential to engender dispute about the ontological perspective that should be taken toward it, as well as about what is essentially significant to it. Hence, there may be no agreement on the definition of death that should be applied. Instead, the greatest achievement may be to articulate a policy on the determination of death that honors a plurality of philosophical/theological perspectives.

KAREN G. GERVAIS

SEE ALSO: *African Religions; Bioethics, African-American Perspectives; Buddhism, Bioethics in; Christianity, Bioethics in; Eastern Orthodox Christianity, Bioethics in; Embryo and Fetus: Religious Perspectives; Hinduism, Bioethics in; Infanticide; Islam, Bioethics in; Life Sustaining Treatment and Euthanasia; Moral Status; Right to Die, Policy and Law; Utilitarianism and Bioethics;* and other *Death, Definition and Determination of* subentries

BIBLIOGRAPHY

Ad Hoc Committee of the Harvard Medical School to Examine the Definition of Brain Death. 1968. "A Definition of Irreversible Coma: A Report of the Ad Hoc Committee." *Journal of the American Medical Association* 205(6): 337–340.

Becker, Lawrence C. 1975. "Human Being: The Boundaries of the Concept." *Philosophy and Public Affairs* 4(4): 335–359.

De Vita, Michael A., and Snyder, James V. 1993. "Development of the University of Pittsburgh Medical Center Policy for the Care of Terminally Ill Patients Who May Become Organ Donors After Death Following the Removal of Life Support." *Kennedy Institute of Ethics Journal* 3(2): 131–143.

Gervais, Karen G. 1986. *Redefining Death.* New Haven, CT: Yale University Press.

Gervais, Karen G. 1989. "Advancing the Definition of Death: A Philosophical Essay." *Medical Humanities Review* 3(2): 7–19.

Green, Michael, and Wikler, Daniel. 1980. "Brain Death and Personal Identity." *Philosophy and Public Affairs* 9(2): 105–133.

Halevy, Amir. 2001 "Beyond Brain Death?" *Journal of Medicine and Philosophy* 26(5): 493–501.

Hoffman, John C. 1979. "Clarifying the Debate on Death." *Soundings* 62(4): 430–447.

Lamb, David. 1985. *Death, Brain Death and Ethics.* Albany: State University of New York Press.

Lock, Margaret. 1996. "Death in Technological Terms: Locating the End of a Meaningful Life." *Medical Anthropology Quarterly* 10(4): 575–600.

New Jersey. 1994. *Declaration of Death. New Jersey Statutes Annotated,* Title 26, chapter 6A. St. Paul, MN: West.

Potts, Michael. 2001. "A Requiem for Whole Brain Death: A Response to D. Alan Shewmon's *The Brain and Somatic Integration.*" *Journal of Medicine and Philosophy* 26(5): 479–491.

Truog, Robert D., and Fackler, James C. 1992. "Rethinking Brain Death." *Critical Care Medicine* 20(12): 1705–1713.

U.S. President's Commission for the Study of Ethical Problems in Medicine and Biomedical and Behavioral Research. 1981. *Defining Death: A Report on the Medical, Legal, and Ethical Issues in the Determination of Death.* Washington, D.C.: Author.

Veatch, Robert M. 1989. *Death, Dying, and the Biological Revolution: Our Last Quest for Responsibility,* rev. edition. New Haven, CT: Yale University Press.

Veatch, Robert M. 1992. "Brain Death and Slippery Slopes." *Journal of Clinical Ethics* 3(3): 181–187.

Shewmon, D. Alan. 2001. "The Brain and Somatic Integration: Insights into the Standard Biological Rationale for Equating *Brain Death* with Death." *Journal of Medicine and Philosophy* 26(5): 457–478.

Youngner, Stuart J. 1992. "Defining Death: A Superficial and Fragile Consensus." *Archives of Neurology* 49(5): 570–572.

Youngner, Stuart J.; Arnold, Robert M.; and Shapiro, Renie, eds. 1999. *The Definition of Death: Contemporary Controversies.* Baltimore, MD: Johns Hopkins Press.

Zaner, Richard M., ed. 1988. *Death: Beyond Whole-Brain Criteria.* Dordrecht, Netherlands: Kluwer.

DEATH PENALTY

• • •

Fewer and fewer crimes are punishable by death even in countries where execution is legal, and crimes that are widely considered to be extremely serious, such as murder, often lead to prison sentences rather than capital punishment. In 1991, offenses under the laws of over ninety countries carried a penalty of death. In eighty-five, execution was illegal or had ceased to be imposed. These included virtually all of the nations of western Europe, as well as Canada, Australia, Hungary, and Czechoslovakia. In the United States, in addition to military and federal jurisdictions, thirty-six states impose the death penalty. Not all of these states do so regularly, however; and in those where capital punishment has become routine, it is sometimes a relatively new development. From 1967 to 1977 there were no executions in the United States; between 1977 and 1992, there were 190, and over 2,500 people in 34 states were on death row. In a few countries in which the death penalty was still used in the 1980s—Brazil, Argentina, and Nepal—it had been reintroduced (in Brazil and Argentina by military governments) after a long period of abolition.

The reintroduction of capital punishment after centuries of decline has once again raised the question of the morality of execution. No code of law now prescribes death for the theft of fruit or salad, as Draco's code did in ancient Athens; and boiling to death is no longer a recognized punishment for murder by poisoning, as it was in England under the Tudors and Stuarts. Can a principle that explains why these developments are good also explain why it is good that some codes of law no longer prescribe death as punishment for murder? Or can a principle that condemns the death penalty for some crimes also support its imposition for others? These are live questions, for one of the arguments commonly presented against the death penalty turns on the suggestion that retaining it or reintroducing it is a case of being morally behind the times. According to this argument, standards of humane punishment have now risen to a point where killing a human being—even one who is guilty of a terrible crime—can only be understood as cruel, and therefore immoral. Such an argument is sometimes used to counter another that is perhaps even more familiar: that the death penalty is justified because of its power to deter people from violent crime. The argument from deterrence will be examined later.

The Argument from Cruelty

The language of this argument is sometimes taken from the Eighth Amendment of the U.S. Constitution ("Excessive bail shall not be required, nor excessive fines imposed, nor cruel and unusual punishments inflicted"); or from human-rights declarations that outlaw "cruel, inhuman or degrading" treatment or punishment. Thus, a brochure titled *When the State Kills,* issued by the British Section of Amnesty International (1990), contains the following passage under the heading "Cruel, Inhuman and Degrading": "International law states that torture or cruel, inhuman or degrading punishments can never be justified. The cruelty of the death penalty is self-evident."

Certain methods of execution are quite plausibly said to be so painful that any application of them must be cruel. Amnesty International cites the case of a Nigerian military governor who in July 1986 ordered successive volleys of bullets to be fired at convicted armed robbers. The shots would first be aimed at the ankles, to produce painful wounds, and only gradually would the firing squad shoot to kill. Other methods, believed by some authorities to be painless, can undoubtedly cause suffering when clumsily applied. According to eyewitness reports, the first death sentence carried out by use of the electric chair in the United States; in August 1890, was very painful. But these ill effects may not be typical. Certainly the electric chair was not introduced because it was thought to be painful; on the contrary, along with other methods of execution, such as the guillotine, it was thought to spare the convicted person suffering.

Execution by lethal injection is the latest in a series of supposedly humane methods of execution to be introduced. It is now being used in a number of states in the United States. Is this technique cruel? Perhaps not, if severe pain is the test of cruelty. Deliberate poisoning is normally cruel, and Amnesty International classifies the use of lethal injection as deliberate poisoning. But is it clear that poisoning in the form of lethal injection is always cruel? What if the injection is self-administered in a suicide or given at the request of someone who is dying in intense pain? If poisoning is always cruel, then it must be so in these cases. On the other hand, if it is not cruel in these cases, then it is not necessarily cruel in the case of execution. It is true that execution is usually not in line with the wishes of the convicted person, as it is when poison is administered to someone at his or her request. But that by itself cannot make execution cruel, unless virtually all punishment is cruel: Virtually all punishment is inflicted on people against their wishes. If it is not pain and not the unwillingness of the criminal to undergo it that makes lethal injection cruel, then what does? If nothing does—if lethal injection is sometimes painless and not cruel in other respects—then there may be principles that consistently explain why it is good for murderers, for example, to be punished with death (severe crimes deserve severe punishments); why it was bad for murderers to be put to death in the past by boiling (torture is wrong); and why it is not necessarily bad for murderers to be put to death today by lethal injection.

Arguments from Finality and Arbitrariness

Arguments against the death penalty sometimes emphasize its finality. There are several versions of the argument from finality, some religious, some secular. One religious version has to do with the way the death penalty removes all possibility of repentance or a saving change of heart on the part of the offender (Carpenter). Capital punishment writes off the offender in a way that, for example, imprisonment combined with education or religious instruction does not. It arguably refuses the offender the sort of love that Christianity enjoins, and it presumes to judge once and for all—a prerogative that may belong to God alone.

Secular arguments from finality are almost always combined with considerations about the fallibility of judicial institutions and doubt whether people who are accused of crimes are fully responsible agents. In some views, society contributes to the wrongdoing of criminals (Carpenter), so that they are not fully responsible and should not be punished. This argument shows sympathy for those who are accused of wrongdoing, but because it does not take wrong-doers as full-fledged agents it may not show them as much respect as apparently harsher arguments do. As for fallible judicial institutions, certain factors—such as prejudice against some accused people, and poor legal representation—can produce wrong or arbitrary verdicts and sentences; even conscientious judges and juries can be mistaken. When errors occur and the punishment is not death, something can be done to compensate the victims of miscarriages of justice. The compensation may never make up entirely for what is lost, but at least a partial restitution is possible; but where what is lost is the accused person's life, on the other hand, the possibility of compensation is ruled out. This argument is particularly forceful where evidence exists that certain groups (black males in the United States, Tibetans in China) are disproportionately represented among those receiving harsh sentences, including the death sentence (Amnesty International, 1991; Wolfgang and Reidel). In these cases, the possibility of an error with disastrous consequences starts to grow into something like a probability. What is more, the evidence of certain groups being disproportionately represented suggests that the law is not being applied justly. This adds to the argument that the death penalty should not be applied, for it suggests that people are fallible, the background conditions for the existence of justice are not being met, and consequently that some miscarriages of justice result from factors other than honest error.

Arguments from Side Effects

EFFECTS ON PROFESSIONALS. Executions are carried out by officials who are not always hardened to their task, and at times they rely on the services of medical people, who have sworn to preserve life. The burdens of those who officiate and serve in these ways; the suffering of those who are close to the convicted person; and the ill effects on society at large of public hangings, gassings, or electrocutions are sometimes thought to constitute an argument against capital punishment over and above the argument from cruelty to the offender.

The side effects on medical personnel have recently been brought into prominence in the United States by the use of lethal injection. The method involves intravenous injection of a lethal dose of barbiturate as well as a second drug, such as tubocurarine or succinylcholine, that produces paralysis and prevents breathing, leading to death by asphyxiation. Doctors have sometimes had to check that the veins of the convicted person were suitable for the needle used and, where death took longer than expected, to attend and give direction during the process of execution. In Oklahoma, which was the first state to adopt lethal injection as a method of execution, the medical director of the Department of Corrections is required to order the drugs to be injected; the physician in attendance during the execution itself has to inspect the intravenous line to the prisoner's arm and also pronounce him dead.

Of course, doctors have been in attendance at executions carried out by other methods, and some of the moral objections to their involvement are applicable no matter which method is used. What is different about intravenous injection, in the opinion of some writers (e.g., Curran and Cassells), is that it involves the direct application of biomedical knowledge for the taking of life. This practice is often said to be in violation of the Hippocratic Oath (Committee on Bioethical Issues of the Medical Society of the State of

New York); and many national and international medical associations oppose the involvement of doctors in the death penalty. The fear that nurses might assist at executions led the American Nurses Association in 1983 to declare it a "breach of the nursing code of ethical conduct to participate either directly or indirectly in legally authorized execution."

The conflict between providing medical services to further an execution and abiding by the Hippocratic Oath makes the moral problem facing doctors particularly sharp, but other professionals may face difficulties as well. Judges and lawyers may be caught up unwillingly or reluctantly in prosecutions that will lead to the imposition of the death sentence. They, too, have a reason for withdrawing their services if they are sincerely opposed to capital punishment; but if all the professionals with qualms acted upon them, the legal process, and the protections it extends to those accused of capital crimes, might be compromised as well (Bonnie). This argument probably understates the differences between legal and medical professionals: the latter recognize a duty of healing and of relieving pain; the former are committed to upholding the law and seeing that justice is done, which does not necessarily conflict with participation in a regime of execution.

EFFECTS ON PERSONS CLOSE TO THE CONDEMNED AND ON SOCIETY. In addition to the effects of the death penalty on involved professionals, the effects on persons close to condemned prisoners are sometimes cited in utilitarian arguments against the death penalty (Glover). These effects are undoubtedly unpleasant, but it is unclear whether they are to be traced to the existence of capital punishment or to the commission of the crimes classified as capital. As for the effects on society at large, they are harder to assess. Samuel Romilly, who campaigned successfully for a reduction in the very large number of capital offenses recognized in English law at the beginning of the 1800s, maintained that "cruel punishments have an inevitable tendency to produce cruelty in people." In fact, Romilly's success in law reform owed something to the benevolence of juries, who had consistently, and often against evidence, found accused people innocent of capital offenses as minor as shoplifting. Whoever was made cruel by the existence of cruel punishments, it was not ordinary English jurors. Judges avoided imposing the death penalty for minor crimes by transporting criminals to the colonies.

Deterrence

The death penalty has often been introduced to act as a strong deterrent against serious crime, and the deterrence argument is commonly used to justify reintroduction. In a British parliamentary debate on the reintroduction of capital punishment in May 1982, one legislator said, "The death penalty will act as a deterrent. A would-be murderer will think twice before taking a life if he knows that he may well forfeit his own in so doing" (Sorell, pp. 32–33). He went on to argue that the absence of the death penalty had been associated with a rise in the number of ordinary murders, and an increase in the rate of murder of police officers. But the evidence for its having the power to discourage, or for its having a greater such power than imprisonment, is inconclusive (Hood). Indeed, deterrence generally seems to depend on potential offenders expecting to be caught rather than on their judging the punishment for an offense to be severe (Walker). In the case of murder, the deterrent effect is particularly doubtful: Murder is often committed in a moment of high passion or by those who are mentally disturbed (Sorell). Either way, the serious consequences of the act are unlikely to register so as to make the agent hesitate. An American review of statistical studies concludes that the deterrent effect of capital punishment is definitely not a settled matter, and that the statistical methods necessary for reaching firm conclusions have yet to be devised (Klein et al.).

Incapacitation

A purpose of punishment that is more convincingly served by the death penalty is the incapacitation of offenders. The death penalty undoubtedly does incapacitate, but this is just another aspect of its finality, which has already been seen to be morally objectionable from some points of view. Again, for incapacitation to be a compelling general ground for the imposition of the death penalty—that is, a ground that justifies the imposition of the penalty in more than the occasional case—there has to be strong evidence that people who have the opportunity to repeat capital crimes frequently do so. Although killers sometimes kill again, it is not clear that they are *likely* to reoffend. Finally, life imprisonment without parole may be sufficiently incapacitating to make the death penalty unnecessary.

Retribution

Another argument in favor of the death penalty is based on the value of retribution. Here the idea is that the evil of a crime can be counterbalanced or canceled out by an appropriate punishment, and that in the case of the most serious crime, death can be the appropriate punishment because it is deserved. Appropriateness should be understood against the background of the thought that penal justice requires what Immanuel Kant called an "equality of crime and punishment." His examples show that he meant an act of punishment not identical to the crime but proportionate to its severity; Kant held that death was uniquely appropriate to the crime of murder. John Stuart Mill, in a famous speech in favor of capital punishment delivered in the British House of Commons in 1868, argued that only those guilty of aggravated murder—defined as brutal murder in the absence of all excusing conditions—deserved to be executed. Mill called the punishment "appropriate" to the crime and argued that it had a deterrent effect. He meant "appropriate" in view of the severity of the crime.

Retribution should not be confused with revenge. It is generally considered revenge, not retribution, when there is love or sympathy for the one who has suffered an injury; retribution requires a response even to injuries of people no one cares about. Its impersonality makes the injuries of the friendless have as much weight as the injuries of the popular. Again, revenge is still revenge when the retaliation is utterly out of proportion to the original injury, but the retributivist *lex talionis*—an eye for an eye—limits what can be done in return.

One question raised by the retributivist defense of capital punishment is how a punishment can counterbalance or cancel out an evil act. Retributivists sometimes refer in this connection to the ideal case in which the offender willingly undergoes a punishment as a sign of remorse and of wishing to be restored to a community from which he or she has been excluded due to a criminal act (Duff). In that case the punishment is supposed to counterbalance the crime. But it is unnecessary for retributivism to be committed to the idea that a punishment cancels out an offense. One can appeal instead, as Kant did, to a punishment's fitting an offense—being proportional in quality to the quality of the offense—and one can justify the imposition of punishment by reference to the following three considerations: (1) laws have to promise punishment if people who are not wholly rational and who are subject to strong impulses and temptations are to obey the laws, and promises must be kept; (2) offenders who are convicted of breaking laws in a just society can be understood to have been party to a social contract designed to protect people's freedom; and (3) threats of punishment in a just society are intended to prevent encroachments on freedom.

This is not a justification of capital punishment, until one specifies a crime that capital punishment uncontroversially fits. Murder is not always the right choice, since such factors as provocation, the numbers of people who die, and the quality of the intention can make some murders much more serious than others; while crimes other than murder—crimes in which, despite the criminal's best efforts, the victim survives—can be as bad as or worse than those in which death occurs. Aggravated murder is, as Mill maintained, a more plausible candidate for capital crime than is plain murder. But execution even for aggravated murder has something to be said against it: the danger of executing the innocent in error, and the suspicion—which goes to the heart of retributivism—that it is bad for pain or unpleasantness to be visited even on wrongdoers.

TOM SORELL (1995)
BIBLIOGRAPHY REVISED

SEE ALSO: *Conscience, Rights of; Human Rights; Justice; Medicine, Profession of; Nursing, Profession of; Prisoners, Healthcare Issues of; Prisoners as Research Subjects; Profession and Professional Ethics; Race and Racism; Warfare: Medicine and War; Women as Health Professionals*

BIBLIOGRAPHY

Amnesty International. 1989. *When the State Kills: The Death Penalty v. Human Rights.* London: Author.

Amnesty International. 1991. *Death Penalty: Facts and Figures.* London: Author.

Baird, Robert M., and Rosenbaum, Stuart E., eds. 1995. *Punishment and the Death Penalty: The Current Debate.* Buffalo, NY: Prometheus.

Banner, Stuart. 2002. *The Death Penalty: An American History.* Cambridge, MA: Harvard University Press.

Bedau, Hugo A. 1987. *Death Is Different: Studies in the Morality, Law, and Politics of Capital Punishment.* Boston: Northeastern University Press.

Bedau, Hugo A., ed. 1982. *The Death Penalty in America,* 3rd edition. New York: Oxford University Press.

Bonnie, Richard I. 1990. "Medical Ethics and the Death Penalty." *Hastings Center Report* 20(3):12–18.

Carpenter, Canon E. F. 1969. "The Christian Context." In *The Hanging Question: Essays on the Death Penalty,* pp. 29–38, ed. Louis J. Blom-Cooper. London: Duckworth.

Committee on Bioethical Issues of the Medical Society of the State of New York. 1991. "Physician Involvement in Capital Punishment." *New York State Journal of Medicine* 91(1): 15–18.

Curran, William J., and Cassells, Ward. 1980. "The Ethics of Medical Participation in Capital Punishment by Intravenous Drug Injection." *New England Journal of Medicine* 302(4): 226–230.

Duff, R. Antony. 1986. *Trials and Punishments.* Cambridge, Eng.: Cambridge University Press.

Glover, Jonathan. 1977. *Causing Death and Saving Lives: A World-Wide Perspective.* Harmondsworth, Eng.: Penguin.

Hodgkinson, Peter, and Schabas, William A, eds. 2004. *Capital Punishment: Strategies for Abolition.* New York: Cambridge University Press.

Hood, Roger G. 1989. *The Death Penalty.* Oxford: Clarendon Press.

Kant, Immanuel. 1965. *The Metaphysical Elements of Justice: Part 1 of The Metaphysics of Morals,* tr. John Ladd. Indianapolis, IN: Bobbs-Merrill.

King, Rachel. 2003. *Don't Kill in Our Names: Families of Murder Victims Speak Out Against the Death Penalty.* Piscataway, NJ: Rutgers University Press.

Klein, Lawrence; Forst, Brian; and Filatov, Victor. 1978. "The Deterrent Effect of Capital Punishment: An Assessment of the Estimates." In *Deterrence and Incapacitation: Estimating the Effects of Criminal Sanctions on Crime Rates,* pp. 336–361, ed. Alfred Blumestein, Jacqueline Cohen, and Daniel Nagin. Washington, D.C.: National Academy of Sciences.

Leiser, Burton M. 2001. "Capital Punishment and Retributive Justice: A Reasoned Response to Crime." *Free Inquiry* 21(3): 40–42.

Martinez, J. Michael; Richardson, William D.; and Hornsby, D. Brandon, eds. 2002. *The Leviathan's Choice: Capital Punishment in the Twenty-First Century.* Lanham: Totowa, NJ: Rowman and Littlefield.

McDermott, Daniel A. 2001. "Retributivist Argument against Capital Punishment." *Journal of Social Philosophy* 32(3): 317–333.

Mill, John Stuart. 1868. *Hansard's Parliamentary Debates,* 3rd series. London: Hansard.

Nathanson, Stephen. 1987. *An Eye for an Eye? The Morality of Punishing by Death.* Totowa, NJ: Rowman and Littlefield.

Pojman, Louis P., and Reiman, Jeffrey. 1998. *The Death Penalty: "For and Against."* Totowa, NJ: Rowman and Littlefield.

Sarat, Austin. 2002. *When the State Kills: Capital Punishment and the American Condition.* Princeton, NJ: Princeton University Press.

Simon, Rita James, and Blaskovich, Dagny A. 2002. *A Comparative Analysis of Capital Punishment: Statutes, Policies, Frequencies and Public Attitudes the World Over.* Lanham, MD: Lexington Books.

Sorell, Tom. 1987. *Moral Theory and Capital Punishment.* Oxford: Basil Blackwell.

Van den Haag, Ernest. 1991. *Punishing Criminals: Concerning a Very Old and Painful Question.* New York: University Press of America.

Walker, Nigel. 1991. *Why Punish?* Oxford: Oxford University Press.

Wolfgang, Marvin E., and Reidel, M. 1982. "Racial Discrimination, Rape and the Death Penalty." In *The Death Penalty in America,* 3rd edition, ed. Hugo Bedau. New York: Oxford University Press.

Wolpin, Kenneth I. 1978. "An Economic Analysis of Crime and Punishment in England and Wales, 1894–1967." *Journal of Political Economy* 86(5): 815–840.

Zimring, Franklin E. 2003. *The End of Capital Punishment in America.* New York: Oxford University Press.

DEEP BRAIN STIMULATION

• • •

Electrical stimulation of the brain is an important therapy for refractory neurological disorders such as drug resistant Parkinson's disease and severe tremor and has become an area of active clinical research in both neurology and psychiatry. Using a technique called *deep brain stimulation* (DBS), small electrical leads are placed into the brain using stereotactic localization. A special head frame is attached to the skull under local anesthesia, and electrodes are implanted using internal brain targets located with reference to anatomical landmarks determined by brain imaging techniques such as computed tomography (CT) or magnetic resonance imaging (MRI). This technique allows for the precise targeting of specific brain sites or nuclei. Insertion of electrodes can be done without damage to adjacent tissue. These electrodes are connected by a wire to a pacemaker implanted in the chest that generates electrical stimulation. Stimulation parameters can be modified by manipulation of the pacemaker.

Unlike ablative surgery that results in irreversible damage of brain tissue from the intentional destruction of targeted areas, the effects of DBS are reversible. The stimulator can be turned off, and the electrodes can generally be removed without any significant aftereffects. DBS differs from other methods that employ electrical stimulation of the central nervous system. Electroconvulsive therapy (ECT), primarily used to treat severe depression, stimulates the brain using electrodes placed on the scalp. Transcranial magnetic stimulation induces electrical currents in the brain using external magnetic coils. Electrical stimulation in the neck of the vagus nerve has been demonstrated to reduce epileptic seizures. Cortical stimulation of the brain is also employed as a treatment for chronic pain disorders (Greenberg).

Electrical stimulation of the brain is also used as a diagnostic tool in the treatment of epilepsy and as a means to localize specific brain areas in order to avoid injury during surgical procedures. Electrical stimulation has also been applied within the peripheral nervous system for neuroprosthethic applications such as reconstituting motor function in a paralyzed limb.

Historical Considerations

The modern history of electrical stimulation of the brain dates to the nineteenth century During this period the French surgeon and anthropologist Paul Broca (1824–1880) correlated speech with an area in the left hemisphere that is known as Broca's area, and the English neurologist John Hughlings Jackson hypothesized that electrical activity in the cortex could result in seizures. In tandem with these efforts to correlate cerebral structure and function, early neurophysiologists engaged in animal experimentation using electrical stimulation In 1870 the German neurologists Eduard Hitzig and Gustav Fritsch demonstrated motor activity in a dog following stimulation (Thomas and Young). In 1873 the Scottish neurologist David Ferrier induced contralateral seizures in a dog after unilateral hemispheric stimulation.

The first known electrical stimulation of the human brain was conducted by the American neurosurgeon Roberts Bartholow in Cincinnati, Ohio, in 1874 on a terminally ill woman with locally invasive basal cell carcinoma that had eroded her skull and left her brain exposed. Bartholow demonstrated that the dura mater covering the brain was insensate, that motor activity on one side of the body could be induced by stimulation of the opposite hemisphere, and that electrical stimulation of the brain could induce localized seizures and transient loss of consciousness when the amount of current was increased. The patient subsequently died from recurrent seizure activity. Contemporaries harshly criticized Bartholow on ethical grounds because of the fatal complications of the intervention, the uncertain nature of the patient's "consent," and the suffering that she experienced (Morgan).

Early electrical stimulation of the brain was used as a method of mapping cerebral cortical function, matching the site of stimulation of the brain's surface with the patient's response during operations under local anesthesia. Pioneering work was done by two American neurosurgeons: Harvey Cushing in the early twentieth century and Wilder Penfield, who later in the century used electrical stimulation in his study of epilepsy and the mapping of cognitive function. An important advance was the development in 1947 of stereotactic surgery, which enabled brain targets to be precisely located in three dimensions. With this technique, electrodes could now be inserted in the brain without the completion of a full craniotomy in which the entire skull needs to be opened (Gildenberg, 1990).

Robert G. Heath first described electrical stimulation for the control of chronic pain in his 1954 book, *Studies in Schizophrenia*. In the 1960s and 70s investigators demonstrated that deep stimulation of selected targets within the brain was demonstrated to relieve pain In 1985, the Swiss neurosurgeon, Jean Siegfried noted that stimulation of the thalamus for pain control could improve tremor in a patient with Parkinson's disease (Gildenberg, 1998).

The Psychosurgery Debate

Research involving electrical stimulation of the brain was closely linked to the broader debate over psychosurgery in the 1960s and 1970s (Fins, 2003). Commentators from that era worried about the use of electrical stimulation of the brain as a means of behavior control to address social problems such as crime and civic unrest. These concerns were prompted, in part, by the work of José M. R. Delgado who advanced the idea of "psychocivilizing society" using a brain implant that could be operated by remote control. Delgado came to international attention in 1965 when he stopped a charging bull in a bullring using a "stimoceiver" he had developed. Speculation was enhanced by popular novels such as Michael Crichton's *The Terminal Man* whose main character underwent electrical stimulation of the brain to treat violent behavior.

The National Commission for the Protection of Human Subjects of Biomedical and Behavioral Research, authorized by the National Research Act of 1974, was specifically ordered by the U.S. Congress to issue a report on psychosurgery (*National Research Act of 1974. U.S. Statutes at Large*). The National Commission, which issued its report in 1977, included electrical stimulation of the brain under its definition of psychosurgery, noting that "psychosurgery includes the implantation of electrodes, destruction or direct stimulation of the brain by any means" when its primary purpose was to "control, change, or affect any behavioral or emotional disturbance" (National Commission for the Protection of Human Subjects of Biomedical and Behavioral Research). The National Commission's definition of psychosurgery excluded brain surgery for the treatment of somatic disorders such as Parkinson's disease or epilepsy or for pain management.

Of the National Commission, the Behavioral Control Research Group of the Hastings Institute (Blatte), and the American Psychiatric Association's Task Force on Psychosurgery (Donnelly), none found reliable evidence that psychosurgery had been used for social control, for political purposes, or as an instrument for racist repression as had been alleged. Contrary to expectations of the day, the National Commission did not recommend that psychosurgical procedures be banned. Instead, it found sufficient evidence of efficacy of some psychosurgical procedures to endorse continued experimentation as long as strict regulatory guidelines and limitations were in place.

Although allegations of mind control were never substantiated, contemporary media reports about modern deep brain stimulation often allude to these earlier fears This misuse of historical analogy has the potential to distort current policy regarding the regulation of this novel technology (Fins, 2002).

Clinical Applications in Neuromodulation

The modern era of neuromodulation began in 1987 when the French neurosurgeon Alim Benabid noted improvements of parkinsonian tremor following stimulation of the thalamus (Speelman and Bosch). While engaged in mapping with electrodes prior to ablative surgery for Parkinson's disease, Benabid discovered that electrical stimulation of specific targets could modulate motor symptoms and tremor—a technique that came to be known as neuromodulation. These observations inspired him to develop the modern deep brain stimulator in use today (Fins and Schachter).

Deep brain stimulation is viewed as the standard of care for the treatment of refractory Parkinson's disease and is no longer investigational. In 1997 the U.S. Food and Drug Administration (FDA) approved use of the deep brain stimulator for refractory Parkinson's disease and essential tremor (Blank). DBS has been found effective in prospective, double-blind studies in patients with advanced Parkinson's disease (Deep-Brain Stimulation, 2001; Kumar et al.).

Complications can be related to the procedure, device, or stimulation, and they include hemorrhage, infection, seizures, and hardware-related complications. Such complications can necessitate revision or removal of the device at a rate per electrode year of 8.4 percent (Oh et al.). In one large series of patients, there were no fatalities or permanent severe neurological complications, although 6 percent of patients had some persistent neurological complication (Beric et al.).

In addition to being used to treat Parkinson's disease, neuromodulation using DBS has been used to treat chronic pain and manage epilepsy (Kopell and Rezai). Cortical mapping continues, with more electronic sophistication. Such mapping is being used to guide neurosurgical procedures; to prevent injuries to critical areas, such as those associated with speech or movement, during operations on the brain; and to precisely locate areas of the brain involved with epilepsy, occasionally by provoking seizures through stimulation (Feindel).

Investigational Applications

Research in deep brain stimulation is blurring the disciplinary boundaries between neurology and psychiatry. French investigators have discovered that DBS caused transient acute depression in a patient with Parkinson's disease whose motor function had improved markedly through DBS intervention (Bejjani et al.). Investigators are conducting clinical trials for the use of DBS for severe psychiatric illnesses such as obsessive–compulsive disorder using techniques pioneered in the treatment of movement disorders (Roth et al.; Rapoport and Inoff-Germain). Nicholas D. Schiff and colleagues have proposed the use of DBS for the modulation of consciousness after severe traumatic brain injury (Schiff, Plum, and Rezai).

Ethical Considerations

Deep brain stimulation raises special concerns because neuromodulation techniques deal with the direct stimulation of the brain. No other organ is so closely involved with concepts of mind or self, self-determination and consent.

POTENTIAL ALTERATION OF THE SELF. Interventions involving brain structure or function may result in alterations in cognition, memory, or emotions that may have a bearing on personhood. The potential of DBS to alter brain function may lead some to argue categorically against these interventions. This position would fail to appreciate that psychoactive drugs and cognitive rehabilitation alter brain states and that DBS can be used to restore brain functions that had themselves been altered by injury or disease.

The use of DBS as a potential agent of cognitive rehabilitation raises the question of whether helping a patient regain self-awareness is always an ethical good (Fins, 2000). Partial recovery of cognitive function could theoretically lead to greater awareness of impairment and increased suffering. These perceptions, which may also accompany improvement from more conventional rehabilitation, might be reversed with cessation of stimulation or be treated with antidepressant therapy.

THERAPEUTIC VERSUS INVESTIGATIONAL USE. Given the rapid development of this field, it is important to determine whether the application of deep brain stimulation to a particular disease is therapeutic or investigational. Historically, a treatment has moved from investigational use to therapeutic use when it is shown to relieve the symptoms it is intended to relieve with an acceptable degree of risk and when a significant proportion of physicians, especially those working in the field, are convinced that the intended outcome will appear without adverse long- or short-term effects that outweigh the benefits. This delineation between research and therapy has implications for the informed-consent process and the ability of surrogates to provide consent for DBS when a patient or subject lacks decision-making capacity. In the early twenty-first century DBS is recognized as therapeutic for the management of chronic pain, Parkinson's disease, and other movement disorders. It remains investigational for other indications.

Today, the use of a device such as the deep brain stimulator goes through several investigational stages before it is accepted as therapeutic. Formal mechanisms are in place to codify this transition. The FDA uses the investigational device exemption process to regulate devices that pose significant risk, such as the deep brain stimulator (Pritchard, Abel, and Karanian). FDA procedures, which supplement institutional review board (IRB) oversight of clinical trials, are designed to establish the safety and efficacy of devices and are required by law.

Once a device has been approved for use in humans, a clinical trial can proceed to assess the safety and efficacy of the device for a particular indication. Use of a device is deemed therapeutic when its safety and efficacy have been demonstrated in prospective trials, the most rigorous being ones that are double-blinded and randomized (a double-blinded study is one in which during the course of the study neither the subjects nor the conductors of the study know which subjects are in the active therapy or placebo group). Blinded studies can be conducted in the evaluation of DBS. Once the electrodes have been implanted, patients can be blinded to whether they are receiving stimulation, and their responses can be evaluated. Such methodological rigor is essential in the assessment of DBS because of the potential for a powerful placebo effect. The placebo effect has been shown to improve motor performance of patients with Parkinson's disease who were led to believe that they were being stimulated (Pollo et al.).

Demarcating the therapeutic use of DBS from the investigational may be difficult. For example, the use of an approved device does not, in itself, mean that an intervention is therapeutic. In these cases, the intent of the physician or clinical investigator may be important. Many would assert that if the physician's *intent* is to produce effects generally beneficial to the patient that have previously been demonstrated in similar cases, the intervention can be considered therapeutic. But when the investigator intends to use an approved device to increase knowledge of safety or efficacy for an approved indication or use the device at a new anatomical site or for a new indication, such interventions should be considered to be investigational and undergo review by an IRB.

Because investigational uses of DBS require more regulatory oversight, clinicians might be biased to classify borderline uses of DBS as therapeutic When it is unclear whether the use of DBS is therapeutic or investigational, clinicians should seek the guidance of their local IRB to mitigate this potential conflict of interest.

INFORMED CONSENT. The delineation of DBS as either therapeutic or investigational is also critical given ethical norms that govern informed consent. Given the ongoing investigational nature of many DBS procedures, potential candidates for stimulation need to be informed of whether the proposed procedure is therapeutic or experimental. Physicians who obtain consent from patients for therapeutic procedures should explain the risks, benefits, and alternatives so that the patient, or a surrogate authorized to consent for medical treatment, can provide consent.

Clinicians should seek to maintain the patient's voluntariness and ability to make an informed and reasonable decision about treatment with DBS. Those obtaining consent should appreciate that the chronic nature of the illness and desperation may lead a patient to consent to any treatment that promises symptomatic relief.

When individuals are approached for enrollment in an IRB-approved clinical trial, it is especially important to state the investigational nature of the intervention. Investigators should be careful to avoid the suggestion of a "therapeutic misconception" that falsely equates a clinical trial with safe and effective therapy (Applebaum et al.).

DBS RESEARCH IN THE DECISIONALLY INCAPACITATED. Individuals with severe psychiatric illness or head trauma, who may become candidates for enrollment in DBS clinical trials, may lack decision-making capacity. When these individuals are unable to engage in the informed-consent process, they are considered a vulnerable population and in need of special protections. While surrogates are generally allowed to consent to therapeutic procedures, their authority is more constrained when permission is sought for enrollment in a clinical trial unless they have been authorized through an advance directive for prospective research.

The National Bioethics Advisory Commission (NBAC), in its 1998 report, *Research Involving Persons with Mental*

Disorders That May Affect Decisionmaking Capacity, proposed guidelines to regulate the conduct of research on individuals who are unable to provide consent. While the NBAC recommendations were never enacted into law, they do point to the ethical complexity of neuromodulation research in several cases: when subjects lack decision-making capacity, when the research has yet to demonstrate the prospect of direct medical benefit, and when the research poses more than minimal risk.

BALANCING THE PROTECTION OF HUMAN SUBJECTS WITH ACCESS TO RESEARCH. When considering the balance between the protection of human subjects and access to neuromodulation research, it is important to ask whether current ethical norms deprive decisionally incapacitated individuals of interventions that have the potential to promote self-determination by restoring cognitive function (Fins, 2000). While the ethical principles of respect for persons, beneficence, and justice require that decisionally incapacitated subjects are protected from harm, these principles can also be invoked to affirm a fiduciary obligation to promote well-designed and potentially valuable research for this historically underserved population (Fins and Miller; Fins and Schiff). This justice claim becomes especially compelling as developments in neuromodulation demonstrate growing clinical potential (Fins, 2003).

JOSEPH J. FINS

SEE ALSO: *Behaviorism; Behavior Modification Therapies; Electroconvulsive Therapy; Emotions; Freedom and Free Will; Informed Consent: Issues of Consent in Mental Healthcare; Neuroethics; Psychosurgery, Ethical Aspects of; Psychosurgery, Medical and Historical Aspects of; Research Policy: Risk and Vulnerable Groups; Technology*

BIBLIOGRAPHY

Applebaum, Paul S.; Roth, Loren H.; Lidz, Charles W.; et al. 1987. "False Hopes and Best Data: Consent to Research and the Therapeutic Misconception." *Hastings Center Report* 17(2): 20–24.

Bejjani, B.-P.; Damier, P.; Arnulf, I.; et al. 1999. "Transient Acute Depression Induced by High-Frequency Deep-Brain Stimulation." *New England Journal of Medicine* 340(19): 1476–1480.

Beric, A.; Kelly, P. J.; Rezai, A.; et al. 2001. "Complications of Deep Brain Stimulation." *Stereotactic Functional Neurosurgery* 77(1–4): 73–78.

Blank, Robert H. 1999. *Brain Policy: How the New Neuroscience Will Change Our Lives and Our Politics.* Washington, D.C.: Georgetown University Press.

Blatte, H. 1974. "State Prisons and the Use of Behavior Control." *Hastings Center Report* 4(4): 11.

Cushing, Harvey. 1909. "A Note upon the Faradic Stimulation of the Postcentral Gyrus in Conscious Patients." *Brain* 32: 44–53.

Deep-Brain Stimulation for Parkinson's Disease Study Group. 2001. "Deep-Brain Stimulation of the Subthalamic Nucleus or the Pars Interna of the Globus Pallidus in Parkinson's Disease." *New England Journal of Medicine* 345(13): 956–963.

Delgado, José M. R. 1969. *Physical Control of the Mind: Toward a Psychocivilized Society,* ed. Ruth N. Anshen. New York: Harper and Row.

Donnelly, J. 1978. "The Incidence of Psychosurgery in the United States, 1971–1973." *American Journal of Psychiatry* 135(12): 1476–1480.

Feindel, William. 1982. "The Contributions of Wilder Penfield to the Functional Anatomy of the Human Brain." *Human Neurobiology* 1(4): 231–234.

Fins, Joseph J. 2000. "A Proposed Ethical Framework for Interventional Cognitive Neuroscience: A Consideration of Deep Brain Stimulation in Impaired Consciousness." *Neurological Research* 22(3): 273–278.

Fins, Joseph J. 2002. "The Ethical Limits of Neuroscience." *Lancet Neurology* 1(4): 213.

Fins, Joseph J. 2003. "From Psychosurgery to Neuromodulation and Palliation: History's Lessons for the Ethical Conduct and Regulation of Neuropsychiatric Research." *Neurosurgery Clinics of North America* 14(2): 303–319.

Fins, Joseph J., and Miller, Franklin G. 2000. "Enrolling Decisionally Incapacitated Subjects in Neuropsychiatric Research." *CNS Spectrums* 5(10): 32–42.

Fins, Joseph J., and Schiff, Nicholas D. 2000. "Diagnosis and Treatment of Traumatic Brain Injury." *Journal of the American Medical Association* 283(18): 2392.

Gaylin, Willard M.; Meister, Joel S.; and Neville, Robert C., eds. 1975. *Operating on the Mind: The Psychosurgery Conflict.* New York: Basic.

Gildenberg, Philip L. 1990. "The History of Stereotactic Surgery." *Neurosurgery Clinics of North America* 1(4): 765–780.

Gildenberg, Philip L. 1998. "The History of Surgery for Movement Disorders." *Neurosurgery Clinics of North America* 9(2): 283–293.

Greenberg, Benjamin D. 2002. "Update on Deep Brain Stimulation." *Journal of ECT* 18(4): 193–196.

Kopell, Brian Harris, and Rezai, Ali R. 2000. "The Continuing Evolution of Psychiatric Neurosurgery." *CNS Spectrums* 5(10): 20–31.

Kumar, R.; Lozano, A. M.; Kim, Y. J.; et al. 1998. "Double-Blind Evaluation of Subthalamic Nucleus Deep Brain Stimulation in Advanced Parkinson's Disease." *Neurology* 51(3): 850–855.

Morgan, James P. 1982. "The First Reported Case of Electrical Stimulation of the Human Brain." *Journal of the History of Medicine* 37(1): 51–64.

National Bioethics Advisory Commission. 1998. *Research Involving Persons with Mental Disorders That May Affect Decisionmaking Capacity.* Rockville, MD: National Bioethics Advisory Commission.

National Commission for the Protection of Human Subjects of Biomedical and Behavioral Research. 1977. "Use of Psychosurgery in Practice and Research: Report and Recommendations of National Commission for the Protection of Human Subjects of Biomedical and Behavioral Research." *Federal Register* 42(99): 26318–26332.

National Research Act of 1974. U.S. Statutes at Large 88: 342.

Oh, Michael Y.; Abosch, Aviva; Kim, Seong H.; et al. 2002. "Long-Term Hardware Related Complications of Deep Brain Stimulation." *Neurosurgery* 50(6): 1268–1274.

Penfield, Wilder. 1977. *No Man Alone: A Neurosurgeon's Life.* Boston: Little, Brown.

Pollo, Antonella; Torre, Elena; Lopiano, Leonardo; et al. 2002. "Expectation Modulates the Response to Subthalamic Nucleus Stimulation in Parkinsonian Patients." *NeuroReport* 13(11): 1383–1386.

Pritchard, W. F.; Abel, D. B.; and Karanian, J. W. 1999. "The U.S. Food and Drug Administration Investigational Device Exemptions and Clinical Investigation of Cardiovascular Devices: Information for the Investigator." *Journal of Vascular and Interventional Radiology* 10(2): 115–122.

Rapoport, J. L., and Inoff-Germain, G. 1997. "Medical and Surgical Treatment of Obsessive–Compulsive Disorder." *Neurologic Clinics* 15(2): 421–428.

Roth, Robert M.; Flashman, Laura A.; Saykin, Andrew J.; and Roberts, David W. 2001. "Deep Brain Stimulation in Neuropsychiatric Disorders." *Current Psychiatric Reports* 3: 366–372.

Schiff, Nicholas D.; Plum, F.; and Rezai, A. R. 2002. "Developing Prosthetics to Treat Cognitive Disabilities Resulting from Acquired Brain Injuries." *Neurological Research* 24(2): 116–124.

Speelman, J. D., and Bosch, D. A. 1998. "Resurgence of Functional Neurosurgery for Parkinson's Disease: A Historical Perspective." *Movement Disorders* 13(3): 582–588.

Thomas, R. K., and Young, C. D. 1993. "A Note on the Early History of Electrical Stimulation of the Human Brain." *Journal of General Psychology* 120(1): 73–81.

DEMENTIA

• • •

The syndrome of dementia is an irreversible decline in cognitive abilities that causes significant dysfunction. Like most syndromes, dementia can be caused by a number of diseases. In the nineteenth century, for example, a main cause of dementia was syphilis. As a result of dramatic increases in average human life expectancy, dementia is caused primarily by a number of neurological diseases associated with old age. Dementia is distinguished from *pseudo-dementia* because the latter is reversible—for example, depression, extreme stress, and infection can cause dementia but with treatment a return to a former cognitive state is likely (Oizilbash et al.). Dementia is also distinguished from *normal age-related memory loss,* which effects most people by about age seventy in the form of some slowing of cognitive skills and a deterioration in various aspects of memory. But *senior moments* of forgetfulness do not constitute dementia, which is a precipitous and disease-related decline resulting in remarkable disability. Since 1997, a degree of cognitive impairment that is greater than normal age-related decline but not yet diagnosable as dementia has been labeled *mild cognitive impairment* (MCI), with about one-third of those in this category *converting* to dementia each year. These cognitive conditions from normal age-related forgetfulness to dementia form a continuum. Specialized clinics that were once called Alzheimer's Centers are increasingly changing their name to Memory Disorders Centers in order to begin to treat patients at various points along the continuum prior to the onset of dementia.

Although dementia can have many causes, the primary cause of dementia in our aging societies is Alzheimer disease (AD). Approximately 60 percent of dementia in the American elderly and worldwide in industrialized nations is secondary to AD (U.S. General Accounting Office). This discussion will focus on so-called *Alzheimer's dementia* in order to illustrate ethical issues that pertain to all progressive dementias. One epidemiological study in the United States estimated that 47 percent of persons eighty-five years and older (the *old-old*) had probable AD, although this is a widely considered inflated (Evans et al). Epidemiologists differ in their estimates of late-life AD prevalence, but most studies agree roughly on the following: about 1 percent to 2 percent of older adults at age sixty have probable AD, and this percentage doubles every five years so that 3 percent are affected at age sixty-five, 6 percent at age seventy, 12 percent at age seventy-five, and 24 percent by age eighty. While some argue that those who live into their nineties without being affected by AD will usually never be affected by it, this is still speculative. According to a Swiss study, 10 percent of non-demented persons between the ages of eighty-five and eighty-eight become demented each year (Aevarsson). There are very few people in their late forties and early fifties who are diagnosed with AD. Without delaying or preventive interventions, the number of people with AD, in the United States alone, will increase to 14.3 million by 2050 (Evans et al). These numbers represent a new problem of major proportions and immense financial consequences for medicine, families, and society (Binstock et al).

There is a second very rare form of AD which is early onset that is clearly familial. About 3 percent of AD cases are caused by rare autosomal dominant (or causative) single gene mutations, of which three are clearly defined. In these cases of *familial* AD, symptoms usually occur in the early forties or mid- to late-thirties, and death occurs within five years of diagnosis, in contrast to the more typical seven to eight years for ordinary late-onset disease (Post and Whitehouse).

Various stage theories of disease progression have been developed. However, in clinical practice, professionals speak roughly of three stages. In *mild stage dementia,* the newly diagnosed patient has significant cognitive losses resulting in disorientation and dysfunction, and often displays affective flatness and possibly depression. In *moderate stage dementia,* the patient forgets that he or she forgets, thereby gaining relief from insight into losses. Some patients will at this point adjust well emotionally to a life lived largely in the pure present, although some long-term memories are still in place. The recognition of loved ones is usually still possible. However, as many as one-third of patients in the moderate stage will struggle with emotional and behavior problems, including agitation, combativeness, paranoia, hallucinations, wandering, and depression. A small percentage becomes sexually disinhibited. The *advanced stage of dementia* includes a loss of all or nearly all ability to communicate by speech, inability to recognize loved ones in most cases, loss of ambulation without assistance, incontinence of bowel and/or bladder, and some weight loss due to swallowing difficulties. The advanced stage is generally considered terminal, with death occurring on average within two years. AD, however, is heterogeneous in its manifestations, and defies simplistic staging. For example, while most people with advanced AD will have no obvious ability to recognize loved ones, this is not always the case. In late December 2000, for example, the daughter of a man recently deceased sent an e-mail note to the AD networks around the world:

> Hello Dear Friends: As many of you know, my father has been suffering from Alzheimer's disease for the past 4.5. years. It has been a long and often very hard road for him, for my mom, and for me too. However, as of 7 p.m. last night, my father no longer has to struggle with the disease that robbed him of every part of his being, except one. He never once stopped recognizing my mom and never, ever stopped reaching out to her and wanting to give her a kiss. No matter how many parts of his

personality were lost, no matter how many hospital visits full of needles and catheters, no matter how many diapers, he always retained his kind, gentle sweetness and his European manners as a gentleman. In the end, things went very quickly for him. He simply closed his eyes and closed his mouth, indicating no more food or water.

The gentleman described above was in the advanced and therefore terminal stage of AD. Yet he retained the ability to recognize loved ones.

The Fundamental Moral Question: Do People with Dementia *Count*?

Despite the seriousness of dementia and the responsibilities it creates for caregivers, it is ethically important that the person with dementia not be judged by *hypercognitive* values (Post, 1995, 2000a). The self is not cognition alone, but is rather a complex entity with emotional and relational aspects that should be deemed morally significant and worthy of affirmation (Sabat). A bias against the deeply forgetful is especially pronounced in *personhood* theories of moral status in which persons are defined by the presence of a set of cognitive abilities (Kitwood). After discussion of the disparities in bioethical thinking about what constitutes a person, Stanley Rudman concludes, "It is clear that the emphasis on rationality easily leads to diminished concern for certain human beings such as infants, ... and the senile, groups of people who have, under the influence of both Christian and humanistic considerations, been given special considerations" (Rudman, p. 47). Often, the personhood theorists couple their exclusionary rationalistic views with utilitarian ethical theories that are deeply incoherent with regard to life and death. As Rudman summarizes the concern, rationality is too severe a ground for moral standing, "allowing if not requiring the deaths of many individuals who may, in fact, continue to enjoy simple pleasures despite their lack of rationality ..." (Rudman, p. 57). Of course, in the real world of families, love, and care, personhood theories have no practical significance.

The philosophical tendency to diminish the moral status or considerability of people with dementia is also related to a radical differentiation between the formerly intact or *then* self and the currently demented or *now* self. The reality is that until the very advanced and even terminal stage of AD, the person with dementia will usually have sporadically articulated memories of deeply meaningful events and relationships ensconced in long-term memory. It is wrong to bifurcate the self into then and now, as if continuities are not at least occasionally striking (Kitwood, Sabat). This is why it is essential that professional caregivers be aware of the person's life story, making up for losses by providing cues toward continuity in self-identity. Even in the advanced stage of dementia, as in the case presented at the outset of this entry, one finds varying degrees of emotional and relational expression, remnants of personality, and even meaningful nonverbal communication as in the reaching out for a hug.

The fitting moral response to people with dementia, according to western ethical thought as informed by Judaism and Christianity, is to enlarge our sense of human worth to counter an exclusionary emphasis on rationality, efficient use of time and energy, ability to control distracting impulses, thrift, economic success, self-reliance, self-control, *language advantage,* and the like. As Alasdair MacIntyre argues, too much has been made of the significance of language, for instance, obscuring the moral significance of species who lack linguistic abilities, or human beings who have lost such abilities (MacIntyre). It is possible to distinguish two fundamental views of persons with dementia. Those in the tradition of Stoic and Enlightenment rationalism have achieved much for universal human moral standing by emphasizing the spark of reason (*logos*) in us all; yet when this rationality dissipates, so does moral status. Those who take an alternative position see the Stoic heritage as an arrogant view in the sense that it makes the worth of a human being entirely dependent on rationality, and then gives too much power to the reasonable. This alternative view is generally associated with most Jewish and Christian thought, as well as that of other religious traditions in which the individual retains equal value regardless of cognitive decline. As the Protestant ethicist Reinhold Niebuhr wrote, "In Stoicism life beyond the narrow bonds of class, community, and race is affirmed because all life reveals a unifying divine principle. Since the principle is reason, the logic of Stoicism tends to include only the intelligent in the divine community. An aristocratic condescension, therefore, corrupts Stoic universalism." (p. 53). This rationalistic inclusivity lacks the deep universalism of other-regarding or unlimited love (Post, 2000a).

The perils of forgetfulness are especially evident in our culture of independence and economic productivity that so values intellect, memory, and self-control. AD is a quantifiable neurological atrophy that objectively assaults normal human functioning; on the other hand, as medical anthropologists's highlight, AD is also viewed within the context of socially constructed images of the human self and its fulfillment. A longitudinal study carried out in urban China, for example, by Charlotte Ikels, which was published in 1998, indicates that dementia does not evoke the same level of dread there as it does among Americans. Thus, the stigma associated with the mental incapacitation of dementia varies according to

culture. Peter Singer, for example, is part of a *preference utilitarian* philosophical culture that happens to believe that those who do not project preferences into the future and implement them are not persons. According to Singer, those with memory impairment must then ultimately be devalued. While this devaluation is plausible for those human beings in the persistent vegetative state where the essentially human capacities—cognitive, emotional, relational, or aesthetic—no longer survive, people with dementia can experience many forms of gratification. The challenge is to work with remaining capacities. The first principle of care for persons with dementia is to reveal to them their value by providing attention and tenderness in love (Kitwood).

Enhancing Quality of Life

Emotional, relational, aesthetic, and symbolic well-being are possible to varying degrees in people with progressive dementia (Kitwood). Quality of life can be much enhanced by working with these aspects of the person. The aesthetic well-being available to people with AD is obvious to anyone who has watched art or music therapy sessions. In some cases, a person with advanced AD may still draw the same valued symbol, as though through art a sense of self is retained (Firlik).

A sense of purpose or meaning on the part of caregivers can enhance quality of life for the person with dementia. In an important study by Peter V. Rabinsand his colleagues, thirty-two family caregivers of persons with AD and thirty caregivers of persons with cancer were compared cross-sectionally to determine whether the type of illness cared for affected the emotional state of the caregiver and to identity correlates of both undesirable and desirable emotional outcomes. While no prominent differences in negative or positive states were found between the two groups, correlates of negative and positive emotional status were identified. These include caregiver personality variables, number of social supports, and the feeling that one is supported by one's religious faith. Specifically, "emotional distress was predicted by self-reported low or absent religious faith" (Rabins et al., p. 335). Moreover, spirituality predicted positive emotional states in caregiving. Interestingly, the study suggests that it was "belief, rather than social contact, that was important" (Rabins et al., p. 332) Spirituality and religion are especially important to the quality of life of African-American caregivers, for whom it is shown to protect against depression (Picot et al.). Spirituality is also a means of coping with the diagnosis of AD for many affected individuals (Elliot).

In general, quality of life is a self-fulfilling prophesy. If those around the person with dementia see the glass as half empty and make no efforts to relate to the person in ways that enhance his or her experience, then quality of life is minimal. Steven R. Sabat, who has produced the definitive observer study of the experience of dementia, underscores the extent to which the dignity and value of the person with dementia can be maintained through affirmation and an existential perspective.

Specific Clinical Ethical Issues

Nearly every major issue in clinical ethics pertains to AD (Post, 2000b). The Alzheimer's Disease and Related Disorders Association issued an authoritative 2001 publication on ethics issues that covers truth in diagnosis, therapeutic goals, genetic testing, research ethics, respect for autonomy, driving and dementia, end-of-life care, assisted oral feeding and tube feeding, and suicide and assisted suicide. This work borrowed considerably from focus group work that led to the Fairhill Guidelines on Ethics of the Care of People with Alzheimer's Disease (Post and Whitehouse). The Fairhill Guidelines were also the acknowledged baseline for the Alzheimer Canada's national ethics guidelines entitled "Tough Issues" (Cohen et al). The most relevant work on ethics and AD emerges in a grounded way from the affected individuals, their families, and those who serve them in loyal care.

The Association recommends truthtelling in diagnosis because this allows the affected individual, while still competent, to make plans for the future with regard to finances, healthcare, and activities. Most clinicians in the United States and Canada do disclose the probable diagnosis of AD, even though it is only about 90 percent accurate and must be verified upon autopsy. This transition has been encouraged by the emergence of new treatments (Alzheimer's Disease Association).

Genetic testing is frowned on by the Association, except in the early-onset familial cases where a single gene mutation causes the disease. AD is the object of intense genetic analysis. It is a genetically heterogeneous disorder—to date, it is associated with three determinative or causal gene mutations (i.e., someone who has the mutation will definitely get the disease) and one susceptibility or risk gene. The three causal AD genes mutations (located on chromosomes 21, 14, and 1) were discovered in the 1990s. These are autosomal-dominant genes and pertain to early-onset familial forms of AD (usually manifesting between the early 40s and mid-50s) which, according to one estimate, account for possibly fewer than 3 percent of all cases. These families are usually well aware of their unique histories. Only in these relatively few unfortunate families is genetic prediction actually possible, for those who carry the mutation clearly know that the disease is an eventuality. Many people in these families do not wish to know their genetic status, although some do get tested. Currently, there is no clearly predictive test for ordinary late-onset AD that is associated with old age. There is one well-defined susceptibility gene, an apolipoprotein E $\in 4$ allele on chromosome 19 (apoE=protein; APOE=gene), which was discovered in 1993 and found to be associated with susceptibility to late-onset AD (after fifty-five years). A single $\in 4$ gene (found in about one-third of the general population) is not predictive of AD in asymptomatic individuals—it does not come close to foretelling disease, and many people with the gene will never have AD. Among those 2 percent of people with two of the $\in 4$ genes, AD does not necessary occur either (Post et al). Such susceptibility testing can be condoned in a research setting, but is not encouraged in clinical practice because it provides no reliable predictive information upon which to base decisions, it has no medical use, and it may result in discrimination in obtaining disability or long-term care insurance (Post et al., Alzheimer's Disease Association).

The Association's 2001 statement includes the important argument that disclosing the diagnosis early in the disease process allows the person to "be involved in communicating and planning for end-of-life decisions." Diagnostic truthtelling is the necessary beginning point for an ethics of *precedent autonomy* for those who wish to implement control over their futures through advance directives such as durable power of attorney for healthcare, which allows a trusted loved one to make any and all treatment decisions once the person with dementia becomes incompetent. This can effectively be coupled with a living will or some other specific indication of the agent's material wishes with regard to end-of-life care. Unless the person knows the probable diagnosis in a timely way while still competent to file such legal instruments, the risk of burdensome medical technologies is increased. Even in the absence of such legal forms, however, many technologically advanced countries will allow next of kin to decide against efforts to extend life in severe dysfunction. This is important because many patients suffer incapacitating cognitive decline long before having a diagnostic work up; those who are diagnosed early enough to exercise their autonomy can become quickly incapacitated.

The Association does not support mandatory reporting of a probable diagnosis of AD to the Department of Motor Vehicles. There are a number of reasons for this caution, one of which is patient confidentiality. Reporting requirements might discourage some persons from coming into the clinic for early diagnosis at a time early in the course of disease when drug treatments are most clearly indicated. Eventually all people with AD must stop driving when they are a serious risk to self or others. Family members must know that if a loved one drives too long and injures others, they may even be held financially liable and insurers may not be obliged to cover this liability. Ideally, a privilege is never limited without offering the person ways to fill in the gaps and diminish any sense of loss. An *all or nothing* approach can and should be avoided. Compromise and adjustments can be successfully implemented by those who are informed and caring, especially when the person with AD has insight into diminishing mental abilities and loss of competence. The affected person should retain a sense of freedom and self-control if possible (Alzheimer's Disease Association).

AD is on the leading edge of the debate over physician-assisted suicide (PAS) and euthanasia. The policies that emerge from this debate will have monumental significance for people with dementia, and for social attitudes toward the task of providing care when preemptive death is cheaper and easier. The Association affirms the right to dignity and life for every Alzheimer patient, and cannot condone suicide (Alzheimer's Disease Association).

The Association asserts that the refusal or withdrawal of any and all medical treatment is a moral and legal right for all competent Americans of age, and this right can be asserted by a family surrogate acting on the basis of either *substituted judgement* (what would the patient when competent have wanted) or *best interests* (what seems the most humane and least burdensome option in the present).

The Association concludes that AD *in its advanced stage should be defined as a terminal disease,* as roughly delineated by such features as the inability to recognize loves ones, to communicate by speech, to ambulate, or to maintain bowel and/or bladder control. When AD progresses to this stage, weight loss and swallowing difficulties will inevitably emerge. Death can be expected for most patients within a year or two, or even sooner, regardless of medical efforts. One useful consequence of viewing the advanced stage of AD as terminal is that family members will better appreciate the importance of palliative (pain medication) care as an alternative to medical treatments intended to extend the dying process. All efforts at life extension in this advanced stage create burdens and avoidable suffering for patients who could otherwise live out the remainder of their lives in greater comfort and peace. Cardiopulmonary resuscitation, dialysis, tube-feeding, and all other invasive technologies should be avoided. The use of antibiotics usually does not prolong survival, and comfort can be maintained without antibiotic use in patients experiencing infections. Physicians and other healthcare professionals should recommend this less burdensome and therefore more appropriate approach to family members, and to persons with dementia who are competent, ideally soon after initial diagnosis. Early discussions of a peaceful dying should occur between persons with dementia and their families, guided by information from healthcare professionals on the relative benefits of a palliative care approach (Alzheimer's Disease Association).

Avoiding hospitalization will also decrease the number of persons with advanced AD who receive tube-feeding, since many long-term care facilities send residents to hospitals for tube placement, after which they return to the facility. It should be remembered that the practice of long-term tube-feeding in persons with advanced dementia began only in the mid-1980s after the development of a new technique called percutaneous endoscopic gastrostomy (PEG). Before then, such persons were cared for through assisted oral feeding. In comparison with assisted oral feeding, however, long-term tube-feeding has no advantages, and a number of disadvantages (Alzheimer's Disease Association).

In closing this entry, attention will be directed in greater depth to three representative areas of special concern to family and professional caregivers: cognitive enhancing compounds, research risk, and tube feeding.

COGNITIVE ENHANCING COMPOUNDS. Persons with AD and their families greet the emergence of new compounds to mitigate the symptoms of dementia with great hope. These compounds, known as cholinesterase inhibitors, slightly elevate the amount of acetylcholine in the brain, slightly boosting communication between brain cells. In the earlier stages of the disease, while enough brain cells are still functional, these drugs can improve word finding, attentiveness to tasks, and recognition of others for a brief period in the range of six months to two years. Thus, some symptoms can be mitigated for a while, but these drugs have no impact on the underlying course of the disease, and neither reverse nor cure dementia. Some affected individuals, after taking any new compound whether artificial or natural, may exude a burst of renewed self-confidence in their cognitive capacities. But how much of this is due to the compound itself remains unclear. Presumably each person with AD is a part of some relational network that inevitably plays a role in the self-perception of cognitive improvement—indeed, self-perception is dependent on the perceptions of others and their need for a glimmer of hope as caregivers. Realistically, a medication may bring the self-perception of a renewed sense of mental clarity, as though *a fog has lifted,* yet none of the available cognitive enhancing compounds slow the progression of disease.

It is hard for professionals to know how to respond to the passion for the possible. Should unrealistic hopes be indulged for emotional reasons (Post, 1998, 2000b)? Should the money expended for new compounds of relatively marginal efficacy be spent on environmental and relational opportunities? Many clinicians caution both persons with AD and their family caregivers against thinking that the new compound is a miracle cure. Many still remain somewhat skeptical of studies of cognitive testing indicating significant but always minor benefit; no such studies take into account confounding factors such as the quality of relationships, environment, and emotional well-being. Nevertheless, reports of a *fog lifting* are interesting anecdotally. Are statements of future expectations so excessive among some desperate caregivers that hope is easily exploited by pharmaceutical profiteers? Medication needs to be placed within a full program of dementia care (including emotional, relational, and environmental interventions) so as not to be excessively relied on; family members should be respected when they desire to stop medication; even when medication is desired, families need to appreciate the limits of current compounds.

It is possible as well, that the anti-dementia compounds can, in those cases where they may have some capacity to give what is always at best a modest and fleeting cognitive boost,—fleeting because the underlying cognitive decline is intractable—be double-edged swords. While some slight cognitive improvements may occur, these may come at the cost of renewed insight into the disease process on the part of the affected individual, and of relational difficulties in the context of affected individuals and their caregivers. If the kindest point in the progression of AD is when the person with dementia forgets that he or she forgets, and is therefore able to get free of *insight* and related anxiety, then a little cognitive enhancement is not obviously a good thing for quality of life and quality of lives. Is it possible, then, to speak of *detrimental benefits?*

Decisions about these compounds are ethically and financially complex because their efficacy is quite limited, the affected individual remains on the inevitable downward trajectory of irreversible progressive dementia, and there may be nonchemical interventions focusing on emotional, relational, and spiritual well-being that are both cheaper and more effective. This is not to suggest that we should all be pharmacological Calvinists rather than pharmacological hedonists, but does anyone doubt that the pharmaceuticals wield a great deal of power across the spectrum of AD support groups? In the future, as compounds emerge that can actually alter the underlying progression of AD, affected individuals and caregivers will be faced with difficult trade-offs between length of life and quality of life (Post, 1997, 2001a).

Research Risks

The *crucial* unanswered question in AD research is this: What should be the maximal or upper limit for permissible potential risks in any AD research, regardless of whether the

research is characterized as potentially therapeutic for the subject or not? A secondary unanswered question is this: Should proxy consent be permitted in higher risk research, even when there is no potential therapeutic benefit for the participant, just as it is permitted when the research is considered potentially therapeutic? Without agreement on these fundamental questions, the upcoming treatments, promising both greater benefit and greater risk, will not expeditiously reach those in most need.

The Association's 2001 statement is as follows:

(A) For minimal risk research all individuals should be allowed to enroll, even if there is no potential benefit to the individual. In the absence of an advance directive, proxy consent is acceptable.

(B) For greater than minimal risk research *and* if there is a reasonable potential for benefit to the individual, the enrollment of all individuals with Alzheimer disease is allowable based on proxy consent. The proxy's consent can be based on either a research specific advance directive *or* the proxy's judgment of the individual's best interests.

(C) For greater than minimal risk research *and* if there is *no* reasonable potential for benefit to the individual only those individuals who (1) are capable of giving their own informed consent, or (2) have executed a research specific advance directive are allowed to participate. In either case, a proxy must be available to monitor the individual's involvement in the research. (*Note*: this provision means that individuals who are not capable of making their own decisions about research participation and have not executed an advance directive or do not have a proxy to monitor their participation, cannot participate in this category of research.)

The Association's statement is laudable because of its endorsement of surrogate consent in all research of potential benefit to the subject, even if there is potentially a greater than minimal risk. Surrogate consent should always be based on accurate facts about the risks and potential benefits of the clinical research or trial, rather than on understatement of risks or burdens and exaggerated claims of benefit. Participants in all research should be protected from significant pain or discomfort. It is the responsibility of all investigators and surrogates to monitor the well-being of participants.

The Association indicates that surrogates must not allow their hopes for effective therapies to overtake their critical assessment of the facts, or to diminish the significance of participant expressions of dissent. Subject dissent or other expressions of agitation should be respected, although a surrogate can attempt reasonable levels of persuasion or assistance. People with dementia, for example, may initially refuse to have blood drawn or to take medication; once a family member helps calm the situation and explains things, they may change their minds. This kind of assistance is acceptable. Continued dissent, however, requires withdrawal of the participant from the study, even though surrogates would prefer to see the research participation continue.

At this point in time, the most important unresolved issue in dementia research is how much potential risk to those affected by AD should society allow? Research in AD is becoming increasingly physically invasive and biologically complex. Is there any maximal threshold of potential risk beyond which research should be disallowed? Furthermore, how can actual discomforts in research be properly monitored, and what degree of discomfort requires that research be halted? In general, research ethics has not addressed these issues, focusing instead on matters of subject and proxy consent.

END OF LIFE AND PEG TUBES. Gastrostomy tube feeding became common in the context of advanced dementia and in elderly patients more generally after 1981, secondary to the development of the PEG procedure. The PEG procedure was developed by Dr. Michael Gauderer and his colleagues at Rainbow Babies and Children's Hospital in Cleveland from 1979 to 1980 for use in young children with swallowing difficulties. The procedure required only local anesthesia, thus eliminating the significant surgical risk associated with general anesthesia and infection (Gauderer and Ponsky). Gauderer wrote two decades later that while PEG use has benefited countless patients, "in part because of its simplicity and low complication rate, this minimally invasive procedure also lends itself to over-utilization" (p. 879). Expressing moral concerns about the proliferation of the procedure, Gauderer indicates that as the third decade of PEG use begins to unfold, "much of our effort in the future needs to be directed toward ethical aspects …" (p. 882). PEG is being used more frequently even in those patients for whom these procedures were deemed too risky in the past.

For over a decade, researchers have underscored the burdens and risks of PEG tube-feeding in persons with advanced dementia. The mounting literature was well summarized by Finucane and his research colleagues, who found no published evidence that tube-feeding prevents aspiration pneumonia, prolongs survival, reduces risks of pressure sores or infections, improves function, or provides palliation in this population (Finucane, et al.; Gillick; Post, 2001b).

Families often perceive tube-feeding as preventing pneumonia or skin breakdown, and many assume that it extends survival. These perceptions are erroneous. The main benefit of PEG is that it makes life easier for the informal family caregiver who, for reason of competing duties or perhaps physical limitation, cannot find the time or energy to engage in assisted oral feedings. Yet PEG use is not really *easy*, because it has its technological complexities, and the recipient will usually have diarrhea. In some cases, physical restraints are used to keep a person from pulling on the several inches of tube that extend out of the abdomen. One wonders if assisted oral feeding is not easier after all. Regardless, purported technical ease and efficiency do not mean that these technologies should be applied. Should persons with advanced progressive dementia ever be provided with PEGs? In the general, assisted oral feeding and hospice are the better alternative to tube-feeding, although in practice there will be some cases in which the limited capacities of an informal family caregiver do justify tube-feeding as the ethically imperative alternative to starvation when the ability to swallow has begun to diminish. Ideally home health aides would make assisted oral feeding possible even in these cases, but this is not a priority in the healthcare system. Institutions, however, should uniformly provide assisted oral feeding as the desired alternative to tube-feeding, a measure that would profoundly obviate the overuse of this technology.

There will be many family caregivers who have no interest in PEG use and who feel that they are being loyal to their loved one's prior wishes. A physician should expect this response. A study included in-person interviews of eighty-four cognitively normal men and women aged sixty-five years and older from a variety of urban and suburban settings (including private homes, assisted-living apartments, transitional care facilities, and nursing homes). Three-fourths of the subjects would not want cardiopulmonary resuscitation, use of a respirator, or parenteral or enteral tube nutrition with the milder forms of dementia; 95 percent or more would not want any of these procedures with severe dementia (Gjerdingen et al.). These subjects were adequately informed of the burdens and benefits of such interventions.

Physicians and other healthcare professionals should recommend this less burdensome and therefore more appropriate approach to family members, and to persons with dementia who are competent, ideally soon after initial diagnosis. Early discussions of a peaceful dying should occur between persons with dementia and their families, guided by information from healthcare professionals on the relative benefits of a palliative care approach (Volicer and Hurley).

STEPHEN G. POST

SEE ALSO: *Abuse, Interpersonal: Elder Abuse; Advance Directives and Advance Care Planning; Aging and the Aged;*

Artificial Nutrition and Hydration; Autonomy; Beneficence; Care; Christianity, Bioethics in; Compassionate Love; Competence; Confidentiality; Genetic Testing and Screening; Grief and Bereavement; Human Dignity; Informed Consent; Judaism, Bioethics in; Life, Quality of; Life, Sanctity of; Long-Term Care; Medicaid; Medicare; Moral Status; Neuroethics; Palliative Care and Suffering; Research, Unethical; Right to Die, Policy and Law

BIBLIOGRAPHY

Aevarsson, O Skoog I. 1996. "A Population-Based Study on the Incidence of Dementia Disorders Between 85 and 88 Years of Age." *Journal of the American Geriatrics Society* 44: 1455–1460.

Alzheimer Canada. 1997. *Tough Issues: Ethical Guidelines of the Alzheimer Society of Canada.* Toronto: Alzheimer Canada.

Alzheimer's Disease Association. 2001. *Ethical Issues in Alzheimer's Disease.* Chicago: Alzheimer Disease Association.

Binstock, Robert H.; Post, Stephen G.; and Whitehouse, Peter J.; eds. 1992. *Dementia and Aging: Ethics, Values and Policy Choices.* Baltimore, MD: The Johns Hopkins University Press.

Cohen, Carol A.; Whitehouse, Peter J.; Post, Stephen G.; et al. 1999. "Ethical Issues in Alzheimer Disease: The Experience of a National Alzheimer Society Task Force." *Alzheimer Disease and Associated Disorders* 13(2): 66–70.

Elliot, Hazel. 1997. "Religion, Spirituality and Dementia: Pastoring to Sufferers of Alzheimer's Disease and Other Associated Forms of Dementia." *Disability and Rehabilitation* 19(10): 435–441.

Evans, D. A.; Funkenstein, H. H.; Albert, M. S.; et al. 1989. "Prevalence of Alzheimer's Disease in a Community Population of Older Persons: Higher than Previously Reported." *Journal of the American Medical Association* 262: 2551–2556.

Finucane, Thomas E.; Christmas, Colleen; and Travis, Kathy. 1999. "Tube Feeding in Patients with Advanced Dementia: A Review of the Evidence." *Journal of the American Medical Association* 282: 1365–1370.

Firlik, Andrew D. 1991. "Margo's Logo." *Journal of the American Medical Association* 265: 201

Gauderer, Michael. 1999. "Twenty Years of Percutaneous Endoscopic Gastrostomy: Origin and Evolution of a Concept and its Expanded Applications." *Gastrointestinal Endoscopy* 50: 879–882.

Gauderer, Michael, and Ponsly, Jeffrey L. 1981. "A Simplified Technique for Constructing a Tube Feeding Gastrostomy." *Surgery in Gyncology and Obstetrics* 152: 83–85.

Gillick, Muriel R. 2000. "Rethinking the Role of Tube Feeding in Patients with Advanced Dementia." *New England Journal of Medicine* 342(3): 206–210.

Gjerdingen, Dwenda K.; Neff, Jennifer A.; Wang, Marie; et al. 1999. "Older Persons' Opinions About Life-Sustaining Procedures in the Face of Dementia." *Archives of Family Medicine* 8: 421–425.

Ikels, Charlotte. 1998. "The Experience of Dementia in China." *Culture, Medicine and Psychiatry* 3: 257–283.

Kitwood, Tom. 1997. *Dementia Reconsidered: The Person Comes First.* Buckingham, Eng.: Open University Press.

Kitwood, Tom, and Bredin, Kathleen. 1992. "Towards a Theory of Dementia Care: Personhood and Well-being." *Ageing and Society* 12: 269–297.

MacIntyre, Alasdair. 1999. *Dependent Rational Animals: Why Human Beings Need the Virtues.* Chicago: Open Court.

Niebuhr, Reinhold. 1956. *An Interpretation of Christian Ethics.* New York: Meridian Books.

Oizilbash, Nawab; Schneider, Lon S.; Tariot, Pierre; et al., eds. 2002. *Evidence-Based Dementia Practice.* Oxford: Blackwell Press.

Picot, Sandra J.; Debanne, Sara M.; Namazi, Kevin; et al. 1997. "Religiosity and Perceived Rewards of Black and White Caregivers." *Gerontologist* 37(1): 89–101.

Post, Stephen G. 1997. "Slowing the Progression of Dementia: Ethical Issues." *Alzheimer Disease and Associated Disorders* 11(supplement 5): 34–36.

Post, Stephen G. 1998. "The Fear of Forgetfulness: A Grassroots Approach to Alzheimer Disease Ethics." *Journal of Clinical Ethics* 9(1): 71–80.

Post, Stephen G. 2000a. *The Moral Challenge of Alzheimer Disease: Ethical Issues from Diagnosis to Dying,* 2nd edition. Baltimore, MD: The Johns Hopkins University Press.

Post, Stephen G. 2000b. "Key Issues in the Ethics of Dementia Care." *Neurological Clinics* 18(4): 1011–1022.

Post, Stephen G. 2001a. "Anti-Dementia Compounds, Hope, and Quality of Lives." *Alzheimer's Care Quarterly* 2(3): 75–77.

Post, Stephen G. 2001b. "Tube-Feeding and Advanced Progressive Dementia." *The Hastings Center Report* 31(1): 36–42.

Post, Stephen G., and Whitehouse, Peter J. 1995. "Fairhill Guidelines on Ethics of the Care of People with Alzheimer Disease: A Clinician's Summary." *Journal of the American Geriatrics Society* 43(12): 1423–1429.

Post, Stephen G., and Whitehouse, Peter J., eds. 1998. *Genetic Testing for Alzheimer Disease: Ethical and Clinical Issues.* Baltimore, MD: The Johns Hopkins University Press.

Post, Stephen G.; Whitehouse, Peter J.; Binstock, Robert H.; et al. 1997. "The Clinical Introduction of Genetic Testing for Alzheimer Disease: An Ethical Perspective." *Journal of the American Medical Association* 277(10): 832–836.

Rabins, Peter V.; Fitting, Melinda D.; Eastham, James; et al. 1990. "The Emotional Impact of Caring for the Chronically Ill." *Psychosomatics* 31(3): 331–336.

Rudman, Stanley. 1997. *Concepts of Persons and Christian Ethics.* Cambridge, Eng.: Cambridge University Press.

Sabat, Steven R. 2002. *The Experience of Alzheimer's Disease: Life Through a Tangled Veil.* Oxford: Blackwell Publishers.

Singer, Peter. 1993. *Practical Ethics.* Cambridge, Eng.: Cambridge University Press.

U.S. General Accounting Office. 1998. *Alzheimer's Disease: Estimates of Prevalence in the U.S.,* Pub. No. HEHS–98–16. Washington, D.C.: Author.

Volicer, Ladislav, and Hurley, Ann, eds. 1998. *Hospice Care for Patients with Advanced Progressive Dementia.* New York: Springer Publishing.

DENTISTRY

• • •

Most dentists in the United States practice as independent entrepreneurs either individually or in small groups. Nevertheless, dental care generally is not viewed as an ordinary commodity in the marketplace. Instead, the vast majority of dentists and most people in the larger community think of dentistry as a profession. That is, they consider dental care to be a component of healthcare and consider dentists to be experts in the relevant knowledge and skills, committed individually and collectively as professionals to giving priority to their patients' well-being as they practice their expertise. Consequently, when a person becomes a dentist, he or she makes a commitment to the larger community and accepts the obligations and ethical standards of the dental profession. Those obligations and standards are the subject matter of the subdiscipline called dental ethics.

Ethical Dilemmas

Because dentists rarely make life-or-death decisions, some people are unaware that the professional obligations of dentists require careful study. Important human values are at stake in dental care: relieving and preventing intense pain as well as less intense pain and discomfort; preserving and restoring patients' oral function, on which both nutrition and speech depend; preserving and restoring patients' physical appearance; and preserving and restoring patients' control over their bodies. These matters are important, and as a result dentists who are committed to responding to them in accordance with ethical standards often face complex questions.

Ethical dilemmas such as the following are faced regularly by almost every dentist:

1. When examining a new patient, a dentist finds evidence of poor earlier dental work. What should the dentist say to the patient? Should the dentist contact the previous dentist to discuss the matter? Should the dentist contact the local dental society?

2. May a dentist ethically advertise that his or her practice will produce "happy smiles" as well as quality dental care, or is such advertising false or significantly misleading?

3. May a dentist tell a patient that the patient's teeth are unattractive with a view to recommending aesthetic treatment when the patient has not asked for an opinion and has indicated no displeasure with his or her appearance?

4. May a dentist ethically decline to treat a patient with a highly infectious disease? What obligations does the dentist have regarding the information that this patient is a carrier of infection?

5. How should a dentist deal with an adult patient who cannot participate fully in making decisions about about care? Do treatment considerations depend on the reason for that inability? What should a dentist do when the guardian of a minor or an incompetent adult patient refuses to approve the best kind of therapy?

6. What may a dentist do to obtain cooperative behavior from a young or developmentally disabled patient who needs dental care but is uncontrollable in the chair?

7. What obligations does a dentist have and to whom when that dentist learns that another dentist is substance-dependent in a manner that probably affects the care he or she is providing?

Issues and Themes in Dental Ethics

The specific requirements of a dentist's ethical commitments in any aspect of professional practice depend on the specific facts and circumstances of the situation. However, the principal categories of dentists' professional obligations can be surveyed under nine headings:

1. Who are dentistry's chief clients?

2. What is the ideal relationship between a dentist and a patient?

3. What are the central values of dental practice?

4. What are the norms of competence for dental practice?

5. What sacrifices is a dentist professionally committed to, and in what respects do obligations to the patient take priority over other morally relevant considerations?

6. What is the ideal relationship between dentists and coprofessionals?

7. What is the ideal relationship between dentists, both individually and collectively, and the larger community?

8. What should members of the dental profession do to make access to the profession's services available to all those who need them?

9. What are members of the dental profession obligated to do to preserve the integrity of their commitment to its professional values and educate others about them?

THE CHIEF CLIENT. For every profession there is a person or set of persons whose well-being the profession and its members are committed to serving. The patient in the dental chair is the most obvious chief client of a dentist, but dentists also have professional obligations to the patients in the waiting room and all their patients of record, to patients who present with emergency needs, and arguably to the entire larger community, especially in matters of public health. The relative weight of a dentist's obligations to each of these entities when those obligations come into conflict ordinarily is considered to favor the patient in the chair over the others, but comparative judgments of the respective degrees of need also must be made.

THE IDEAL RELATIONSHIP BETWEEN PROFESSIONAL AND PATIENT. What is the proper relationship between the dentist and the patient in the chair as they make judgments and choices about the patient's care? There are a number of different ways of conceiving this ideal relationship when it involves the dentist and a fully competent adult: with the dentist alone making the judgment that determines action, with the judgment resting with the patient alone, and with the judgment shared by both parties.

Since the late 1960s the accepted norm of dental practice in the United States has shifted toward the third type of relationship: shared judgment and shared choice regarding treatment. The legal doctrine of informed consent identifies a minimum standard of shared decision making for dentists and their patients, but it is important to ask whether informed consent fully expresses the ideal relationship between a dentist and a fully capable patient (Segal and Warner; Ozar, 1985; Hirsch and Gert; Ozar and Sokol, 2002).

What is the appropriate relationship between the dentist and a patient who cannot participate fully in treatment decisions? What is the dentist's proper role in this relationship? What is the role of the patient up to the limit of the patient's capacity to participate? What is the proper role of other parties?

In practice most dentists depend on choices made by the parents and guardians of such patients when they are available and when these choices do not involve significant harm to the patients' oral or general health. However, there is no clear consensus about how dentistry should proceed when these conditions are absent. The dental ethics literature has begun a careful discussion of the dentist's relationship with patients of diminished capacity or no capacity for decision making (Bogert and Creedon; Ozar and Sokol, 2002).

A HIERARCHY OF CENTRAL VALUES. Regardless of many professions' rhetoric on the subject, no profession can be expert in fostering the complete well-being of those it serves. There is instead a certain set of values that are the appropriate focus of each profession's particular expertise. These values can be called the central values of that profession. They determine and/or establish parameters for most aspects of a professional's judgments in practice. They are the criteria by which a person is judged to need professional assistance in the first place and by which that need is judged to have been met properly through the professional's intervention.

What, then, are the central values of dental practice, and if there is more than one, how are those central values ranked? One proposal is that the central values of the dental profession are, in the following order:

1. the patient's life and general health;
2. the patient's oral health, which is understood as appropriate and pain-free oral functioning;
3. the patient's autonomy—to the extent that the patient is capable of exercising it—over what happens to his or her body (including the patient's ranking of health, comfort, cost, aesthetic considerations, and other values);
4. preferred patterns of practice on the part of the dentist (including differing philosophies of dental practice);
5. aesthetic considerations from the point of view of skilled dental practice and from the point of view of patients' aesthetic values; and
6. considerations of efficiency, which may include considerations of cost, from the dentist's point of view. (Ozar and Sokol, 2002)

A particular dental intervention may achieve each of these values to a greater or lesser degree, and each value is more or less urgent for a particular patient. The ethical dentist takes the details of each situation into account and attempt to maximize dentistry's central values in accordance with their ranked priority in every encounter with every patient.

COMPETENCE. Every professional is obligated to acquire and maintain the expertise required to undertake his or her professional tasks. Every professional also is obligated to undertake only the tasks that are within his or her competence. Consequently, dentists must be constantly attentive to whether they have sufficient competence to make each specific diagnosis and perform each particular procedure for each patient in light of the clinical circumstances, especially when this involves something nonroutine.

Of necessity the dental community, not the community at large, determines the details of standards of competence because doing this requires dental expertise. However, the larger community is justified in demanding an explanation of the reasoning involved, especially regarding the trade-offs between quality of care and access to care that the setting of such standards inevitably involves.

SACRIFICE AND THE RELATIVE PRIORITY OF THE PATIENT'S WELL-BEING. Most sociologists who study professions and most of the literature of professions speak of "commitment to service" or "commitment to the public" as one of the characteristic features of a profession. Dentistry's self-descriptions are similar in this respect, but these expressions allow many different interpretations with different implications for practice. What sorts of sacrifices, for example, are dentists professionally committed to make for the sake of their patients? What sorts of risks to life and health, financial well-being, and reputation may a dentist be obligated to face?

The related question of the proper relationship between entrepreneurship and commitment to the patient, along with the sacrifice of self-interest this can involve, has been discussed in every age of the dental profession. The consensus is that especially in emergency situations, the patient's oral health and general health require significant sacrifices of personal convenience and financial interest on the part of a dentist. Since the arrival of HIV and AIDS, even more urgent implications of the obligation to give priority to the patient, including accepting an increased risk of infection, also have become part of this discussion.

RELATIONS WITH COPROFESSIONALS. Each profession has norms, usually largely implicit and unstated, concerning the proper relationship between the members of a profession. Should a dentist relate to other dentists as competitors in the marketplace, as cobeneficiaries in the monopoly their exclusive expertise gives them in the marketplace, or in some other way? What is the ideal relationship between dentists, and how is it connected with the fact that they are members of a profession, not only entrepreneurs in the same marketplace?

How should a dentist deal with another dentist's inferior work when its consequences are discovered in the mouth of a new or emergency patient or a patient referred for specialty care? The discovering dentist could inform the patient that bad work has been done or could hide that judgment from the patient. The discovering dentist could contact the dentist whose work had a bad outcome or possibly the local dental society. What is the proper balance between obligations to patients and obligations to one's fellow dentist? As in other professions obligations to the patient ordinarily take priority in dentistry, but this principle does not supply simple or automatic answers to the complexities of such situations.

There are also situations in which members of different professions are caring for the same patients. Many dentists, for example, work very closely with dental hygienists, whose professional skills and central professional values are closely related to but significantly distinct from those of dentists. In the best relationships those differences complement each other to the benefit of the patient, but in other situations the skills of the dental hygienist may be demeaned or the dental hygienist's status as a professional may be challenged. The ethical commitments of these professions imply an obligation to develop a working relationship that is conducive to mutual respect and focused on the well-being of the patient.

RELATIONS BETWEEN DENTISTS AND THE LARGER COMMUNITY. Every profession is involved in numerous relationships with the larger community and with important subgroups in it. Both the dental profession and individual dentists must monitor the quality of dental work and practice and report and address instances of inferior work and unethical practice. They also relate to the community as dental-health educators both through direct educational efforts and by monitoring the dependability and effectiveness of dental-care products offered to the public. Dentistry's relationships with the larger community also include developing proper standards for professional advertising. Dentists play an important role in public-health efforts, preserving public oral health, and addressing serious epidemic diseases such as HIV.

ACCESS TO THE PROFESSION'S SERVICES. Individual dentists and the dental profession as a whole have responsibilities in regard to access to dental care for people with unmet dental needs. Dentists also may be obligated to be educationally and politically active when policies are being made to determine how society will distribute its healthcare resources. Also, organized dentistry has an obligation to monitor access issues and use its resources to promote access for those whose dental needs are not being met.

INTEGRITY AND EDUCATION. A dentist who made no effort to influence patients to incorporate the central values of dental practice into their lives and educate them about how to do that would be falling short as a professional committed to these values. However, dentists influence and educate patients not only through their words and professional interventions at chairside but also by the way they live and act. Thus, there is a ninth category of questions to ask about dentists' professional obligations. What are dentists required to do and what might they be required to avoid to preserve the integrity of the values to which dentistry is committed and to educate others by living in a manner consonant with those values?

Organized Dentistry and Ethics

Ultimately, the content of a profession's obligations is the product of a dialogue between the profession and the larger community that entrusts the profession and its members with a high degree of autonomy in practice, including the power of self-regulation. In the case of dentistry this dialogue is often subtle and informal. Codes of ethics formulated by professional organizations such as the American Dental Association's *Principles of Ethics and Code of Professional Conduct* (American Dental Association, 2002) play an important role in articulating the most fundamental principles of dentistry's professional ethics within American society. However, such codes, like state dental-practice acts, can never articulate more than a small part of the content of a practicing profession's ethics. It therefore is incumbent on both individual dentists and organized groups of dentists to monitor this ongoing dialogue continuously and offer representative statements of its content as they are needed.

If the larger community had no part in this ongoing dialogue, its trust of the dental profession would make no sense. Nevertheless, the community exercises its role in the dialogue more often through passive tolerance than through active articulation. Therefore, the initiative ordinarily falls first to the members of the profession to articulate in word and action the current understanding of the profession's ethical commitments.

Although the dental profession includes every dentist who practices competently and ethically, those who speak for the profession most articulately and are heard the most widely are dentistry's professional organizations. Therefore, those organizations have a special responsibility to foster reflection on and contribute to discussion of dental ethics (Ozar and Sokol, 2002).

Some dental organizations, such as the American Dental Association (ADA), the American College of Dentists (ACD), and some specialty organizations, have contributed actively to the articulation of dentistry's professional standards. Particular issues have temporarily focused the profession's attention on dentistry's ethical commitments. This

occurred when the ADA's Council on Dental Therapeutics first awarded its Seal of Approval to a commercial dentifrice (Dummett and Dummett) and when the ADA first issued a policy statement regarding dentists' obligation to treat HIV-positive patients (American Dental Association, 1991; Ozar, 1993).

Until the late 1970s most dental organizations fulfilled this responsibility chiefly through editorials and other hortatory articles in their journals and sometimes through a published code of conduct. Detailed, carefully reasoned discussions of ethical issues in which assumptions were explicit and alternative points of view were accounted for or that articulated the profession's ethics in more than broad generalities were few and far between. Even the published codes of conduct, significant as they have been as representative articulations of dentistry's professional commitments, have not exhausted the contents of dental ethics, much less effectively addressed new and specific issues as they have arisen.

Since the late 1970s, however, the level of interest in and sophisticated discussion of ethical issues within organized dentistry have increased steadily. Responding to newly significant ethical issues in a rapidly changing social climate, the ADA's Council on Ethics, Bylaws, and Judicial Affairs has regularly prepared, after considerable debate in print and other forums, a number of revisions and amendments of the ADA's *Principles of Ethics and Code of Professional Conduct* (2002). The ADA and its council also have sponsored national workshops and other educational programs on specific ethical issues facing the dental community.

The ACD sponsored several national workshops and a national grassroots educational program to train dentists in more sophisticated forms of reflection on ethical issues as well as national conferences, Ethics Summits I and II, in which representatives from every part of the oral healthcare community worked to develop common understandings of the ethical issues they face and respectful collaboration in dealing with them (American College of Dentists, 1998, 2000). Many other dental organizations have incorporated programs on dental ethics into their meetings and published scholarly and popular articles on those topics in their journals. A number of them also have made major revisions of their codes of ethics.

An organization specifically focused on dental ethics and its teaching, the Professional Ethics in Dentistry Network (PEDNET), was founded in 1982 by a group of dental school faculty members and has grown into a national organization with additional members in full-time practice as well as representatives from organized dentistry, dental hygiene, and the larger healthcare ethics community. The International Dental Ethics and Law Society (IDEALS) was established in 1999 to facilitate dialogue on dental ethics and law around the world.

The literature of dental ethics has grown significantly. In 1988 the *Journal of the American Dental Association* initiated a regular feature on dental ethics, "Ethics at Chairside," which moved in 1991 to *General Dentistry,* the journal of the American Academy of General Dentistry, and a similar series of ethics cases and commentary has appeared in the *Texas Dental Association Journal.* A peer-reviewed series, "Issues in Dental Ethics," supervised by the editorial board of PEDNET began publication in 2000, appearing as a special feature in each quarterly issue of the *Journal of the American College of Dentists.* Also since 2000, the dental journal *Quintessence* has published a series on ethical heroes in dentistry.

Dental Education

The changing climate of dental practice from the late 1970s into the 1980s and a heightened awareness of ethical issues throughout the dental profession in that period also brought about changes in dental schools. Until that time few dental schools had formal programs in dental ethics. Inspirational lectures by respected senior faculty members or local or national heroes were the standard fare (Odom). However, with prompting from the American Dental Education Association (ADEA), then called the American Association of Dental Schools, as well as the ACD, and the ADA, many dental schools began offering formal programs in dental ethics. They identified faculty members with an interest in dental ethics who began to develop curricular materials and network with the faculty in other institutions. For example, the University of Minnesota pioneered an innovative four-year curriculum in dental ethics in the early 1980s. With the founding of PEDNET, dental-ethics educators acquired a major resource for their teaching and a locus for scholarly discussions of issues in dental ethics at the national level both at annual meetings and at biennial workshops on teaching dental ethics.

During the 1990s, several new textbooks were published (Rule and Veatch; Weinstein; Ozar and Sokol, 1994, 2002) and additional educational programs and materials were developed for use in the classroom, in the clinic, and in continuing education programs. By the beginning of the new millennium, most dental schools had multiyear curricula in dental ethics in place (Zarkowski and Graham) and significant efforts were under way to integrate dental ethics education into the innovative patient-centered and problem-based-learning curricula that are the hallmark of contemporary dental school education.

Dentistry in the Twenty-First Century

As dentistry moves into the twenty-first century the focus on ethics will have to be even greater. Two of dentistry's greatest success stories of the twentieth century will yield two of its most important ethical challenges in the twenty-first.

Dentists deeply committed to preventive healthcare for the whole community lobbied successfully during the twentieth century for the fluoridation of water supplies. As a consequence most twenty-first-century dentists' patients will need much less restorative work to remedy the effects of caries than their predecessors' patients did. In these circumstances how will dentists maintain their practices fiscally and still remain true to their fundamental ethical commitments? For many patients and dentists the answer has been an increasing interest in aesthetic dentistry. However, there is a risk here. Too strong a shift in the focus of dental care in this direction could bring about a significant change in the community's view of dentistry, seeing it much more as a taste-driven commercial enterprise and much less as an expertise-grounded, value-based health profession.

The second success story concerns the tremendous advances made in dental research in recent decades. For example, the ways in which laser technology can be used in dental practice have multiplied at least tenfold since the early 1990s. However, these new technologies frequently require extensive training as well as new forms of theoretical understanding so that dentists can employ them safely and skillfully. Because so many patients are fascinated with new technologies, dentists, often fascinated themselves, feel strong pressure to purchase and employ them. The ethical standard of employing only those therapeutic techniques in which one is expert and that truly produce a marginal benefit for the patient compared with older technologies often is strained in these circumstances, and commercial pressures on dentists, both direct fiscal issues within their practices and the pressure of skillful marketing by manufacturers, enhance the challenge for twenty-first-century dentists to choose new technologies wisely and with their patients' best oral healthcare as the goal.

Further complicating both of these issues is the extent to which managed care has had an increased impact on oral healthcare since the early 1990s. More and more frequently dentists must negotiate with patients about treatments in circumstances in which a patient's insurance will pay only for the cheapest acceptable intervention and in which the patient has been poorly informed. The dentist or dental office staff frequently is the bearer of this bad news. Dealing with such situations in a way that preserves an appropriate dentist-patient relationship is often very challenging (Ozar, 2001).

Dentistry as a profession has always taken its professional ethics seriously. However, as a field of study and as a subdiscipline within the study of moral theory and professional ethics dental ethics is still a young field. Nevertheless, as reflection on ethical issues is taken more seriously and participated in more widely by practicing dentists and dental hygienists, dental school and dental hygiene faculty and students, and the leaders of organized dentistry, the dental profession's ethical standards and their implications for daily practice will be understood more clearly and creative dialogue about the ethical practice of dentistry will be more widespread and sophisticated.

DAVID T. OZAR (1995)
REVISED BY AUTHOR

SEE ALSO: *Conflict of Interest; Healthcare Resources; Informed Consent; Profession and Professional Ethics; Professional-Patient Relationship; Public Health; Trust*

BIBLIOGRAPHY

American Association of Dental Schools. 1989. "Curriculum Guidelines on Ethics and Professionalism in Dentistry." *Journal of Dental Education* 53(2):144–148.

American College of Dentists. 1998. "Ethics Summit I." *Journal of the American College of Dentists* 65(3): 5–26.

American College of Dentists. 2000. "Ethics Summit II." *Journal of the American College of Dentists* 67(2): 4–22.

American Dental Association. 1991. *AIDS Policy Statement.* Also incorporated into the ADA Principles of Ethics and Code of Professional Conduct at 4A1.

American Dental Association. 2002. *ADA Principles of Ethics and Code of Professional Conduct, with Official Advisory Opinions.* Chicago: American Dental Association.

Bebeau, Muriel J. 1991. "Ethics for the Practicing Dentist: Can Ethics Be Taught?" *Journal of the American College of Dentists* 58(1): 5, 10–15.

Bebeau, Muriel J.; Spidel, Thomas M.; and Yamoor, Catherine M. 1982. *A Professional Responsibility Curriculum for Dental Education.* Minneapolis: University of Minnesota Press.

Bogert, John, and Creedon, Robert, eds. 1989. *Behavior Management for the Pediatric Dental Patient.* Chicago: American Academy of Pediatric Dentistry.

Burns, Chester R. 1974. "The Evolution of Professional Ethics in American Dentistry." *Bulletin of the History of Dentistry* 22(2): 59–70.

Chiodo, Gary T., and Tolle, Susan W. 1992. "Diminished Autonomy: Can a Person with Dementia Consent to Dental Treatment?" *General Dentistry* 40(5): 372–373.

Dummett, Clifton O., and Dummett, Lois Doyle. 1986. *The Hillenbrand Era: Organized Dentistry's "Glanzperiode."* Bethesda, MD: American College of Dentists.

Hirsch, Allan C., and Gert, Barnard. 1986. "Ethics in Dental Practice." *Journal of the American Dental Association* 113(4): 599–603.

Horowitz, Herschell S. 1978. "Overview of Ethical Issues in Clinical Studies." *Journal of Public Health Dentistry* 38(1): 35–43.

Jong, Anthony, and Heine, Carole Sue. 1982. "The Teaching of Ethics in the Dental Hygiene Curriculum." *Journal of Dental Education* 46(12): 699–702.

McCullough, Laurence B. 1993. "Ethical Issues in Dentistry." In *Clark's Clinical Dentistry,* rev. edition, vol. 1, ed. James W. Clark and Jefferson F. Hardin. Philadelphia: Lippincott.

Odom, John G. 1982. "Formal Ethics Instruction in Dental Education." *Journal of Dental Education* 46(9): 553–557.

Ozar, David T. 1985. "Three Models of Professionalism and Professional Obligation in Dentistry." *Journal of the American Dental Association* 110(2): 173–177.

Ozar, David T. 1993. "AIDS, Ethics, and Dental Care." In *Clark's Clinical Dentistry,* rev. edition, vol. 3, ed. James W. Clark and Jefferson Hardin. Philadelphia: Lippincott.

Ozar, David T. 2001. "A Position Paper: Six Lessons about Managed Care in Dentistry." *Journal of the American College of Dentists,* special section, "Issues in Dental Ethics" 68(1): 33–37.

Ozar, David T., and Sokol, David J. 1994. *Dental Ethics at Chairside: Professional Principles and Practical Applications.* St. Louis: Mosby-Yearbook.

Ozar, David T., and Sokol, David J. 2002. *Dental Ethics at Chairside: Professional Principles and Practical Applications,* 2nd edition. Washington, D.C.: Georgetown University Press.

Professional Ethics in Dentistry Network. 1993. *The PEDNET Bibliography, 1993.* Chicago: Professional Ethics in Dentistry Network.

Rule, James T., and Veatch, Robert M. 1993. *Ethical Questions in Dentistry.* Chicago: Quintessence.

Segal, Herman, and Warner, Richard. 1979. "Informed Consent in Dentistry." *Journal of the American Dental Association* 99(6): 957–958.

Weinstein, Bruce D., ed. 1993. *Dental Ethics.* Philadelphia: Lea & Febiger.

Zarkowski, Pamela, and Graham, Bruce. 2001. "A Four-Year Curriculum in Professional Ethics and Law for Dental Students." *Journal of the American College of Dentists,* special section, "Issues in Dental Ethics" 68(2): 22–26.

INTERNET RESOURCE

American Dental Association. 2002. *ADA Principles of Ethics and Code of Professional Conduct, with Official Advisory Opinions.* Available from <www.ada.org/prof/prac/law/code/index.html>.

DIALYSIS, KIDNEY

• • •

Two principal therapies exist for patients who develop irreversible kidney failure and require renal replacement therapy to survive: kidney dialysis and kidney transplantation. The topic of kidney transplantation is addressed elsewhere in the Encyclopedia. This entry discusses kidney dialysis.

The two main techniques for kidney dialysis are hemodialysis and peritoneal dialysis. In hemodialysis, blood is pumped from a patient's body by a dialysis machine to a dialyzer—a filter composed of thousands of thin plastic membranes that uses diffusion to remove waste products—and then returned to the body. The time a hemodialysis treatment takes varies with the patient's size and remaining kidney function; most patients are treated for three and one-half to four and one-half hours three times a week in a dialysis unit staffed by nurses and technicians. In peritoneal dialysis, a fluid containing dextrose and electrolytes is infused into the abdominal cavity; this fluid, working by osmosis and diffusion, draws waste products from the blood into the abdominal cavity and then is drained from the abdominal cavity and discarded. Most patients on peritoneal dialysis perform four procedures at home daily about six hours apart to drain out the fluid with the accumulated wastes and instill two to two and one-half liters of fresh fluid. This technique is called continuous ambulatory peritoneal dialysis (CAPD). An automated form of peritoneal dialysis at home, called continuous cycling peritoneal dialysis (CCPD), is also available.

Both hemodialysis and peritoneal dialysis require a means to enter the body, called an access. In hemodialysis, access to the blood is obtained by removing blood through needles inserted into surgically created conduits, called fistulas or synthetic grafts, from arteries to veins. In peritoneal dialysis, access to the abdominal cavity is obtained with a plastic catheter, which is surgically implanted into the abdominal wall with the tip of the catheter positioned in the abdominal cavity.

Dialysis is a benefit to patients with severe kidney failure because it removes metabolic waste products and excess fluid, electrolytes, and minerals that build up in the blood when the kidneys are not functioning normally. Without the removal of these substances, patients become very weak, short of breath, and lethargic and eventually die.

While dialysis is lifesaving for these patients and some can return to their prior level of functioning, most do not, because they do not feel well. Despite dialysis and medications, patients may experience anemia, bone pain and weakness, hypertension, heart disease, strokes, infections or clotting of the dialysis access, and bleeding. In addition to these medical problems, dialysis may impose other burdens on dialysis patients and their families, including extra costs for medications and for transportation to the dialysis center, loss of time spent in the treatments and travel to the dialysis center, and loss of control over the patient and family schedule to accommodate dialysis treatments. For these reasons, renal transplantation is considered to be the preferable form of treatment for severe kidney-failure patients who are able to undergo this major surgical procedure.

Kidney dialysis predates other life-sustaining therapies. In 1945 in the Netherlands, Willem Kolff first used hemodialysis to save the life of a woman with acute renal failure. In subsequent years, Kolff and others improved hemodialysis, but it could not be provided to patients with chronic, irreversible renal failure, or what has been called end-stage renal disease (ESRD), until 1960, when Dr. Belding Scribner of Seattle, Washington, used plastic tubes to form a shunt that could be left in an artery and vein for repeated dialysis access.

By most standards, kidney dialysis can be considered a very successful life-sustaining treatment. In the United States alone, since the inception of the Medicare-funded ESRD program in 1973, well over 1 million patients have had their lives sustained by dialysis, and at least some of them have survived for longer than twenty-five years. This program has been costly, however; in 1999, for example, the cost of keeping ESRD patients alive in the United States exceeded 17 billion dollars. Because dialysis preceded many other modern life-sustaining medical technologies, and because initially there was a scarcity of resources to pay for it, many of the ethical concerns subsequently discussed for other modern medical technologies were initially debated regarding dialysis: patient-selection criteria, rationing, access to care, the just allocation of scarce resources, the right to die (by having dialysis withheld or withdrawn), end-of-life care, and conflicts of interest (in dialysis unit ownership). This entry examines a number of these concerns in the United States ESRD program and compares them with those in other countries.

Patient-Selection Criteria and Overt Rationing

The first ethical concern to arise for physicians was how to select patients for dialysis. In the early 1960s in the United

States, 10,000 people were estimated to be dying of renal failure every year, but there were not enough dialysis machines or trained physicians and nurses to treat these patients. Furthermore, the cost of treatment for one patient for one year, $15,000, was prohibitively expensive for most patients. Dialysis centers like the Seattle Artificial Kidney Center, founded in 1962, were able to treat only a small number of patients. It was therefore necessary to restrict the number of patients selected for dialysis; in other words, criteria had to be developed for the rationing of dialysis.

The problem of selecting patients had major ramifications because the patients denied access would die. The solution of the physicians of the Seattle dialysis center was to ask the county medical society to appoint a committee of seven laypersons to make the selection decisions for them from among persons they had identified as being medically appropriate. The doctors recognized that the selection decision went beyond medicine and would entail value judgments about who should have access to dialysis and be granted the privilege of continued life. Historian David Rothman says that their decision to have laypersons engaged in life-and-death decision making was the historic event that signaled the entrance of bioethics into medicine. Bioethics scholar Albert Jonsen believes that the field of bioethics emerged in response to these events in Seattle because they caused a nationwide controversy that stimulated the reflection of scholars regarding a radically new problem at the time, the allocation of scarce lifesaving resources.

The doctors regarded children and patients over the age of forty-five as medically unsuitable, but they gave the committee members no other guidelines with which to work. At first the committee members considered choosing patients by lottery, but they rejected this idea because they believed that difficult ethical decisions *could* be made about who should live and who should die. In the first few meetings, the committee members agreed on factors they would weigh in making their decisions: age and sex of the patient, marital status and number of dependents, income, net worth, emotional stability, educational background, occupation, and future potential. They also decided to limit potential candidates to residents of the state of Washington.

As the selection process evolved, a pattern emerged of the values the committee was using to reach its decisions. They weighed very heavily a person's character and contribution to society (Alexander).

Once public, the Seattle dialysis patient-selection process was subjected to harsh criticism. The committee was castigated for using middle-class American values and social-worth criteria to make decisions (Fox and Swazey). The selection process was felt to have been unfair and to have undermined American society's view of equality and the value of human life.

In 1972, lobbying efforts by nephrologists, patients, their families, and friends culminated in the passage by the U.S. Congress of Public Law 92–603 with Section 2991. This legislation classified patients with a diagnosis of ESRD as disabled, authorized Medicare entitlement for them, and provided the financial resources to pay for their dialysis. The only requirement for this entitlement was that the patients or their spouses or (if dependent children) parents were insured or entitled to monthly benefits under Social Security. The effect of this legislation was to virtually eliminate the need to ration dialysis.

When Congress passed this legislation, its members believed that money should not be an obstacle to providing lifesaving therapy (Rettig, 1976, 1991). Although the legislation stated that patients should be screened for *appropriateness* for dialysis and transplantation, the primary concern was to make dialysis available to those who needed it. Neither Congress nor physicians thought it necessary or proper for the government to determine patient-selection criteria.

By 1978, many U.S. physicians believed that it was morally unjustified to deny dialysis treatment to any patient with ESRD (Fox and Swazey). As a consequence, patients who would not previously have been accepted as dialysis candidates were started on treatment. A decade later, the first report of the U.S. Renal Data System documented the progressively greater acceptance rate of patients onto dialysis (U.S. Renal Data System), and subsequent reports have shown that the sharp rise in the number of dialysis patients could be explained in part by the inclusion of patients who had poor prognoses, especially the elderly and those with diabetic nephropathy (Hull and Parker). By 2000, of the new patients starting dialysis 48 percent were sixty-five years of age or older and 45 percent had diabetes as the cause of their ESRD.

Observers have raised concerns about the appropriateness of treating patients with a limited life expectancy and limited quality of life (Fox; Levinsky and Rettig). Specifically, questions have been raised about the appropriateness of providing dialysis to two groups of patients: those with a limited life expectancy despite the use of dialysis and those with severe neurological disease. The first group includes patients with kidney failure and other life-threatening illnesses, such as atherosclerotic cardiovascular disease, cancer, chronic pulmonary disease, and AIDS. The second group includes patients whose neurological disease renders them unable to relate to others, such as those in a persistent vegetative state or with severe dementia or cerebrovascular disease (Rettig and Levinsky).

The Institute of Medicine Committee for the Study of the Medicare End-Stage Renal Disease Program, which issued its report in 1991, acknowledged that the existence of the public entitlement for treatment of ESRD does not obligate physicians to treat all patients who have kidney failure with dialysis or transplantation (Levinsky and Rettig). For some kidney-failure patients, the burdens of dialysis may substantially outweigh the benefits; the provision of dialysis to these patients would violate the medical maxim: Be of benefit and do no harm. This committee recommended that guidelines be developed for identifying such patients and that the guidelines allow physicians discretion in assessing individual patients. Such guidelines might help nephrologists make decisions more uniformly, with greater ease, and in a way that promotes patient benefit and the appropriate use of dialysis resources. Subsequent studies have demonstrated that nephrologists differ on how they make decisions to start or stop dialysis for patients (Moss et al., 1993; Singer).

Access to Dialysis and the Just Allocation of Scarce Resources

The numbers of dialysis patients steadily grew each year, resulting in an ever increasing cost of the Medicare ESRD program. In the 1980s the United States experienced record-breaking budget deficits, and questions began to be raised about continued federal funding for the ESRD program. Observers wondered if the money was well spent or if more good could be done with the same resources for other patients (Moskop).

Critics of the ESRD program observed that it satisfied neither of the first principles of distributive justice: equality and utility. On neither a macro- nor a microallocation level did the ESRD program provide equality of access. On the macroallocation level, observers asked, as a matter of fairness and equality, why the federal government should provide almost total support for one group of patients with end-stage disease—those with ESRD—and deny such support to those whose failing organs happened to be hearts, lungs, or livers (Moskop; Rettig, 1991). On a microallocation level, only 93 percent of patients with ESRD have been eligible for Medicare ESRD benefits. The poor and ethnic minorities are thought to constitute most of the ineligible. The Institute of Medicine Committee for the Study of the Medicare End-Stage Renal Disease Program recommended that the U.S. Congress extend Medicare entitlement to all citizens and resident aliens with ESRD (Rettig and Levinsky).

From a utilitarian perspective, the ESRD program could not be argued to be maximizing the good for the greatest number. In the 1980s, more than 5 percent of the total Medicare budget was being spent on dialysis and transplant patients, who represented less than 0.2 percent of the active Medicare patient population. A similar disproportionate expense has continued into the twenty-first century. Furthermore, while in 2000 more than 40 million Americans were without basic health insurance, the cost to treat one ESRD patient on dialysis—of whom there were over 300,000—exceeded $50,000 per year. Despite the high cost, ESRD patient unadjusted one-year mortality approached 25 percent; for many, as Anita Dottes noted, life on dialysis was synonymous with physical incapacitation, dependency, chronic depression, and disrupted family functioning (Dottes).

Withholding and Withdrawing Dialysis

After cardiovascular diseases and infections, withdrawal from dialysis is the third most common cause of dialysis-patient death. In one large study, dialysis withdrawal accounted for 22 percent of deaths (Neu and Kjellstrand). Older patients and those with diabetes have been found to be most likely to stop dialysis. Over time, as the percentage of diabetic and older patients (those sixty-five or over) on dialysis increased, withdrawal from dialysis became more common. According to surveys of dialysis units performed in the 1990s, most dialysis units had withdrawn one or more patients from dialysis in the preceding year with the mean being three. (Moss et al., 1993).

Because of the increased frequency of decisions to withhold and withdraw dialysis in the 1980s and 1990s, the clinical practices of nephrologists in reaching these decisions with patients and families generated heightened interest. Discussions of the ethics and process of withholding or withdrawing dialysis became more frequent (Hastings Center, U.S. President's Commission). Two ethical justifications were given for withholding or withdrawing dialysis: the patient's right to refuse dialysis, which was based on the right of self-determination, and an unfavorable balance of benefits to burdens to the patient that continued life with dialysis would entail. Nephrologists and ethicists recommended that decisions to start or stop dialysis be made on a case-by-case basis, because individual patients evaluate benefits and burdens differently. They noted that such decisions should result from a process of shared decision making between the nephrologist and the patient with decision-making capacity. If the patient lacked decision-making capacity, the decisions should be made on the basis of the patient's expressed wishes (given either verbally or in a written advance directive) or, if these were unknown, the patient's best interests. They also advised that in such cases a surrogate be selected to participate with the physician in making decisions for the patient.

Questions were identified to help nephrologists evaluate a patient's request to stop dialysis. For example, why does the patient want to stop? Does the patient mean what he or she says and say what he or she means? Does the patient have decision-making capacity, or is his or her capacity altered by depression, encephalopathy, or another disorder? Are there any changes that can be made that might improve life on dialysis for the patient? How do the patient's family and close friends view his or her request? Would the patient be willing to continue on dialysis while factors responsible for the patient's request to stop are addressed?

If, after patient evaluation based on these questions, the patient still requested discontinuation of dialysis, nephrologists were counseled to honor the competent patient's request. In several studies, nine out of ten nephrologists indicated that they would stop dialysis at the request of a patient with decision-making capacity (Moss et al., 1993; Singer).

In half or more of the cases in which decisions have been made to withdraw dialysis, patients have lacked decision-making capacity. Nephrologists have expressed a willingness to stop dialysis of *irreversibly incompetent* patients who had clearly said they would not want dialysis in such a condition, but they have disagreed about stopping dialysis in patients without clear advance directives (Singer). In general, there has been a presumption in favor of continued dialysis for patients who cannot or have not expressed their wishes. The patient's right to forgo dialysis in certain situations has therefore usually been difficult to exercise.

The Patient Self-Determination Act, which applied to institutions participating in Medicare and Medicaid and which became effective December 1, 1991, was intended to educate healthcare professionals and patients about advance directives and to encourage patients to complete them. Although the ESRD program is almost entirely funded by Medicare, dialysis units were inadvertently left out of the act. Nonetheless, the completion of advance directives by dialysis patients has been specifically recommended for three reasons: (1) the elderly, who constitute roughly half of the dialysis population, are those who are most likely to withdraw or be withdrawn from dialysis; (2) dialysis patients have a significantly shortened life expectancy compared to non-renal patients; and (3) unless an advance directive to withhold cardiopulmonary resuscitation (CPR) is given, it will automatically be provided, and CPR rarely leads to extended survival in dialysis patients (Moss et al., 1992).

When patients lack decision-making capacity and have not completed advance directives, ethically complex issues may arise in the decision whether to start or stop dialysis. Many nephrologists have indicated that they would consult an ethics committee, if available, for assistance in making

decisions in different cases (Moss et al., 1993). Ethics consultations are most frequently requested for decisions regarding the withholding or withdrawing of life-sustaining therapy such as dialysis.

By the end of the twentieth century, nephrologists recognized the need for a guideline on starting and stopping dialysis. Such a guideline, which would address appropriateness of patients for dialysis (patient-selection criteria), had been recommended by the Institute of Medicine Committee for the Study of the Medicare ESRD Program almost a decade earlier. In a 1997 survey of the American Society of Nephrology (ASN) and the Renal Physicians Association (RPA) leadership, the respondents gave the highest priority among twenty-four choices to the development of an evidence-based clinical practice guideline on starting and stopping dialysis. In the context of a changing patient population, the RPA and ASN leaderships believed that an evidence-based clinical practice guideline would assist patients, families, and the nephrology team in making difficult decisions about initiating, continuing, and stopping dialysis. The resultant clinical practice guideline, *Shared Decision-Making in the Appropriate Initiation of and Withdrawal from Dialysis,* was developed by a working group of physicians, nurses, social workers, patients, dialysis administrators, a bioethicist, and a health policy expert (RPA and ASN, 2000). The objectives for the guideline were to:

- Synthesize available research evidence on patients with acute renal failure and ESRD as a basis for making recommendations about withholding and withdrawing dialysis;

- Enhance understanding of the principles and processes useful for and involved in making decisions to withhold or withdraw dialysis;

- Promote ethically as well as medically sound decision-making in individual cases;

- Recommend tools that can be used to promote shared decision-making in the care of patients with acute renal failure or ESRD;

- Offer a publicly understandable and acceptable ethical framework for shared decision-making among healthcare providers, patients, and their families.

The guideline makes nine recommendations. These recommendations encourage the process of shared decision-making, the obtaining of informed consent or refusal for dialysis, estimating prognosis as part of informed dialysis decision-making, systematic approaches to conflict resolution, the use and honoring of advance directives, withholding or withdrawing dialysis for patients under certain circumstances, the use of time-limited trials to assist in reaching decisions about continuing or stopping dialysis, and the use of palliative care for ESRD patients who decide to forgo dialysis. By defining the appropriate use of dialysis and the process to be used in making dialysis decisions, this guideline should also prove to be very useful to ethics consultants when they are called to help resolve conflicts over starting or stopping dialysis (Moss).

End-of-Life Care

In the wake of public dissatisfaction with end-of-life care and efforts to legalize physician-assisted suicide in several states, physician groups, including the RPA and ASN, recognized their ethical responsibility to improve end-of-life care for their patients. In 1997 in a joint position statement on *Quality Care at the End of Life,* the RPA and the ASN urged nephrologists and others involved in the care of ESRD patients to obtain education and skills in palliative care. They noted that palliative care knowledge and skills were especially important for nephrologists because they treat ESRD patients who die from complications despite the continuation of dialysis or after withholding or withdrawing dialysis. For example, in 1999, 48,000 patients died from complications while continuing dialysis and 12,000 died after a decision to stop dialysis.

One issue unresolved in the 1997 position statement was whether cardiopulmonary resuscitation ought always to be provided if cardiac arrest were to occur while patients are receiving dialysis, even if individual dialysis patients preferred not to undergo it. Data suggested that as many as one-third of dialysis units performed cardiopulmonary resuscitation on all patients who arrested while on dialysis, including those who refused the procedure. The concerns driving the uniform resuscitation of dialysis patients were two: The cardiac arrest might be iatrogenic, i.e., due to a complication of the dialysis procedure; and other patients might be troubled if the dialysis team made no attempt at cardiopulmonary resuscitation.

In 1999 the Robert Wood Johnson Foundation convened a series of workgroups to evaluate how end-of-life care could be improved for special populations of patients. The Robert Wood Johnson Foundation included the ESRD population because they perceived a readiness to address end-of-life care issues among the healthcare professionals treating ESRD patients.

In its report the ESRD workgroup noted that

most patients with end-stage renal disease, especially those who are not candidates for renal transplantation, have a significantly shortened life expectancy. In the United States, dialysis patients live about one-third as long as non-dialysis patients of the same age and gender. The unadjusted five-year probability of survival for all incident ESRD patients is only 39 percent; and for the 48 percent of incident ESRD patients who are 65 years of age or older, it is only 18 percent. Life expectancy is also shortened by comorbid conditions. 45 percent of new ESRD patients have diabetes, and many have other comorbid conditions including hypertension, congestive heart failure, ischemic heart disease, and peripheral vascular disease.... It is clear from the foregoing information that the care of ESRD patients requires expertise not only in the medical and technical aspects of maintaining patients on dialysis, but also in palliative care—encompassing pain and symptom management, advance care planning, and attention to ethical, psychosocial, and spiritual issues related to starting, continuing, withholding, and stopping dialysis. (p. 5)

The ESRD workgroup noted the following with regard to the unresolved issue of cardiopulmonary resuscitation in the dialysis unit: (1) research studies of cardiopulmonary resuscitation have indicated that the outcomes for ESRD patients are poor; (2) most dialysis patients express a preference for undergoing cardiopulmonary resuscitation, but over 90 percent believe that a dialysis patient's wish not to undergo cardiopulmonary resuscitation should be respected by dialysis unit personnel (Moss et al., 2001); and (3) it is necessary for nephrologists and other members of the renal team to educate dialysis patients about the likely outcome of cardiopulmonary resuscitation based on patients' particular medical conditions. They recommended that "dialysis units should adopt policies regarding cardiopulmonary resuscitation in the dialysis unit that respect patients' rights of self-determination, including the right to refuse cardiopulmonary resuscitation and to have a do-not-resuscitate order issued and honored" (Robert Wood Johnson Foundation, p. 10). The RPA and the ASN accepted this recommendation and revised their position statement on *Quality Care at the End of Life* in 2002 to include this and other recommendations of the ESRD workgroup.

The Effect of Reimbursement

Reimbursement has affected both dialysis techniques and quality of care provided to dialysis patients. In the 1980s cost was the federal policymakers' primary concern about the ESRD program, and federal reimbursement rates for dialysis were reduced twice. By 1989, the average reimbursement rate—adjusted for inflation—for freestanding dialysis units was 61 percent lower than it had been when the program began (Rettig and Levinsky).

When the U.S. Congress established the Medicare ESRD program, the highest estimate for cost of the program by 1977 was $250 million; the actual cost was approximately $1 billion (Fox and Swazey). At least two major reasons were held to be responsible for the higher cost: the increasing number of patients being started on dialysis, some of whom would have been *unthinkable* dialysis candidates ten years earlier, and the growth of in-center dialysis while the use of less costly home dialysis declined.

Despite inflation and increases in the costs of salaries, equipment, and supplies, there were only two modest increases in the Medicare reimbursement to dialysis providers in the 1990s. By the end of the twentieth century, the rate of reimbursement for dialysis by Medicare adjusted for inflation was only one-third of the amount in 1973. A longstanding historian of the ESRD program, Richard Rettig, observed, "No other part of Medicare has been subjected to this severe, even punitive, economic discipline" (2001, p. 16). Meanwhile, the incidence of ESRD in the United States had tripled compared to twenty years earlier. Almost 100,000 new patients were starting dialysis each year.

Conflicts of Interest

A conflict of interest occurs when there is a clash between a physician's personal financial gain and the welfare of his or her patients. While a conflict of interest generally exists for all physicians who practice fee-for-service medicine, there is a potentially greater conflict of interest for physicians who share in the ownership of for-profit dialysis units in which they treat patients. Physicians who receive a share of the profits are financially rewarded for reducing costs. Although measures to reduce costs may simply lead to greater efficiency, they may also compromise patient welfare if they entail decreasing dialysis time; purchasing cheaper, possibly less effective dialyzers and dialysis machines; and hiring fewer registered nurses, social workers, and dietitians. In the past, for-profit dialysis companies were quite open about their policy of giving physicians a financial stake in their companies. Such companies flourished under the ESRD program (Kolata).

Physicians and dialysis units are paid on a per-patient and per-treatment basis, respectively, under the ESRD program, and the acceptance rate of patients to dialysis in the United States is higher than anywhere else in the world (Hull and Parker). This higher rate has been at least partly attributed to the acceptance on dialysis in the United States of a much greater number of patients with poor prognoses. Some have argued that this high acceptance rate was a sign that nephrologists and dialysis units were seeking to maximize their incomes, while others have commented that

many physicians believed they were obligated to dialyze all patients with ESRD who wanted it (Fox).

In the 1990s, the concerns about conflicts of interest heightened. Two-thirds of ESRD patients were being dialyzed in for-profit units. Short dialysis times were found disproportionately in for-profit units and associated with increased mortality. Patients treated in for-profit dialysis units were noted to have a 20 percent higher mortality rate and a referral rate for renal transplantation 26 percent lower than that for not-for-profit units (Levinsky). The nephrologist who owned all or a share of a for-profit unit was confronted with a clear conflict of interest. In responding to financial pressures created by a dialysis reimbursement rate that failed to keep up with inflation and in instituting cost-cutting measures, he or she was believed to be treading a very fine line between maintaining adequate profit to keep the dialysis unit open and compromising patient care.

A decade earlier, nephrologist and *New England Journal of Medicine* editor Arnold Relman had anticipated the predicament nephrologist owners of dialysis units would face. He had warned that the private enterprise system—the so-called new medical-industrial complex—had a particularly striking effect on the practice of dialysis, and he urged physicians to separate themselves totally from any financial participation so as to maintain their integrity as professionals (Relman). Education of nephrologists about these issues, both in training and in continuing education courses, was advocated to help them to identify present and potential conflicts of interest and resolve them in a way that places patients' interests first.

To hold dialysis units, both for-profit and non-profit, accountable for the quality of care they provide, the Medicare ESRD program through the eighteen ESRD Networks established quality indicators to measure the performance of individual dialysis units and all the dialysis units within a region. These measures monitor adequacy of dialysis, anemia management, vascular access placement, and standardized mortality ratios as well as other indicators.

Racial Disparities

Racial differences in access to effective medical procedures are known to be a problem in the United States. Black patients are less likely than white patients to undergo renal transplantation, coronary artery bypass surgery, and many other procedures. Despite the tendency to undertreatment in other areas, black patients are significantly overrepresented in the dialysis population, comprising 32 percent of all ESRD patients but only 13 percent of the United States population. There is also an overrepresentation of other racial and ethnic minority groups in the ESRD population. The increased susceptibility of nonwhite populations to ESRD has not been fully explained and probably represents a complex interaction of genetic, cultural, and environmental influences. Disparities in treatment for racial minority ESRD patients have been noted, including the following: (1) they are less likely to be referred for home dialysis and renal transplantation; (2) they are more likely to be underdialyzed; and (3) they are more likely to have less desirable synthetic grafts (shorter patency and more complications) rather than fistulas as permanent dialysis access. Nonetheless, blacks have better survival and quality of life compared to whites, and they are also less likely to withdraw from dialysis. The better outcomes despite less than optimal treatment present an opportunity to study and further improve ESRD care for minority patients.

International Perspective

Economics plays the leading role in determining the availability of dialysis in countries throughout the world. The countries with the largest numbers of patients on dialysis are among the richest: the United States, Japan, and Germany. The number of patients per million population treated with dialysis correlates highly with the gross national product per capita. Countries with a per capita gross national product of less than $3,000 per year treat a negligible number of patients with dialysis and transplantation. Approximately three-quarters of the world's population live in these poorer countries.

In parts of the world where dialysis technology and money for healthcare are limited, dialysis is severely rationed. Two sets of criteria have been used to select patients for dialysis. In India, China, Egypt, Libya, Tunisia, Algeria, Morocco, Kenya, and South Africa, money and political influence play an important role in deciding which patients will have access to dialysis and transplantation. In Eastern Europe, ESRD patients with primary renal disease who have a lower mortality and who are more likely to be rehabilitated tend to be selected (Kjellstrand and Dossetor).

Conclusion

Dialysis was one of the earliest life-sustaining treatments. Since its inception, dialysis has raised many ethical issues to be analyzed and resolved. In the 1960s the attempt to make difficult yet socially acceptable ethical decisions about patient-selection criteria and the rationing of dialysis failed because of the use of social worth criteria. The dialysis community and others learned from this experience. In the 1990s, prompted by the dramatic expansion of the ESRD program

and a belief by many that not all patients on dialysis were appropriate for it, the renal professional societies succeeded in developing patient-selection criteria—based on likelihood of benefit and shared decision making—that have been widely endorsed. Other examples of analyzed and resolved ethical issues in dialysis that are broadly applicable are the ethical justifications for allowing patients to forgo dialysis, a life-sustaining treatment, and the development of an approach to hold providers accountable when there is a major and continuing conflict of interest.

Kidney dialysis has succeeded beyond all expectations in its ability to sustain life for hundreds of thousands of patients worldwide. Refinements in the technology have allowed patients who were previously considered not to be candidates for dialysis to experience several or more years of extended life. Its success brings with it three major challenges: how to finance the expensive treatments for a larger and larger number of patients; how to maintain the quality of dialysis care in the United States with the provision of dialysis increasingly being provided by for-profit dialysis corporations who have an inherent conflict of interest; and how to humanely care for an increasingly older, frail population with multiple medical problems and a significantly shortened life expectancy.

Because of the continuing challenges it poses, dialysis will likely continue to break new ground with regard to ethical analyses that will subsequently be helpful to other modern medical technologies.

ALVIN H. MOSS (1995)
REVISED BY AUTHOR

SEE ALSO: *Artificial Hearts and Cardiac Assist Devices; Biomedical Engineering; Body; Cybernetics; Healthcare Resources; Life, Quality of; Lifestyles and Public Health; Life Sustaining Treatment and Euthanasia; Medicaid; Organ and Tissue Procurement; Organ Transplants; Technology; Xenotransplantation*

BIBLIOGRAPHY

Alexander, Shana. 1962. "They Decide Who Lives, Who Dies." *Life* November 9, 1962.

Dottes, Anita L. 1991. "Should All Individuals with End-Stage Renal Disease Be Dialyzed?" *Contemporary Dialysis and Nephrology* 12: 19–30.

Fox, Renée C. 1981. "Exclusion from Dialysis: A Sociologic and Legal Perspective." *Kidney International* 19(5): 739–751.

Fox, Renée C., and Swazey, Judith P. 1978. *The Courage to Fail: A Social View of Organ Transplants and Dialysis,* 2nd edition rev. Chicago: University of Chicago Press.

Hastings Center. 1987. *Guidelines on the Termination of Life-Sustaining Treatment and the Care of the Dying.* Bloomington: Indiana University Press.

Hull, Alan R., and Parker, Tom F., III. 1990. "Proceedings from the Morbidity, Mortality and Prescription of Dialysis Symposium, Dallas TX, September 15 to 17, 1989." *American Journal of Kidney Diseases* 15(5): 375–383.

Jonsen, Albert R. 1990. *The New Medicine and the Old Ethics.* Cambridge, MA: Harvard University Press.

Kjellstrand, Carl M., and Dossetor, John B., eds. 1992. *Ethical Problems in Dialysis and Transplantation.* Dordrecht, Netherlands: Kluwer.

Kolata, Gina Bari. 1980. "NMC Thrives Selling Dialysis." *Science* 208(4442): 379–382.

Levinsky, Norman G. 1999. "Quality and Equity in Dialysis and Renal Transplantation." *New England Journal of Medicine* 341(22): 1691–1693.

Levinsky, Norman G., and Rettig, Richard A. 1991. "The Medicare End-Stage Renal Disease Program: A Report from the Institute of Medicine." *New England Journal of Medicine* 324(16): 1143–1148.

Moskop, John C. 1987. "The Moral Limits to Federal Funding for Kidney Disease." *Hastings Center Report* 17(2): 11–15.

Moss, Alvin H. 2001. "Shared Decision Making in Dialysis: A New Clinical Practice Guideline to Assist with Dialysis-Related Ethics Consultations." *Journal of Clinical Ethics* 12(4): 406–414.

Moss, Alvin H.; Holley, Jean L.; and Upton, Matthew B. 1992. "Outcomes of Cardiopulmonary Resuscitation in Dialysis Patients." *Journal of the American Society of Nephrology* 3(6): 1238–1243.

Moss, Alvin H.; Hozayen, Ossama; King, Karren; et al. 2001. "Attitudes of Patients toward Cardiopulmonary Resuscitation in the Dialysis Unit." *American Journal of Kidney Diseases* 38(4): 847–852.

Moss, Alvin H.; Stocking, Carol B.; Sachs, Greg A.; et al. 1993. "Variation in the Attitudes of Dialysis Unit Medical Directors toward Reported Decisions to Withhold and Withdraw Dialysis." *Journal of the American Society of Nephrology* 4(2): 229–234.

Neu, Steven, and Kjellstrand, Carl M. 1986. "Stopping Long-Term Dialysis: An Empirical Study of Withdrawal of Life-Supporting Treatment." *New England Journal of Medicine* 314(1): 14–20.

Relman, Arnold S. 1980. "The New Medical-Industrial Complex." *New England Journal of Medicine* 303(17): 963–970.

Renal Physicians Association, and The American Society of Nephrology. 1997. *Quality Care at the End of Life.* Washington, D.C.: Renal Physicians Association.

Renal Physicians Association, and The American Society of Nephrology. 2000. *Shared Decision-Making in the Appropriate Initiation of and Withdrawal from Dialysis.* Washington, D.C.: Renal Physicians Association.

Rettig, Richard A. 1976. "The Policy Debate on Patient Care Financing for Victims of End-Stage Renal Disease." *Law and Contemporary Problems* 40(4): 196–230.

Rettig, Richard A. 1991. "Origins of the Medicare Kidney Disease Entitlement: The Social Security Amendments of 1972." In *Biomedical Politics,* ed. Kathi E. Hanna. Washington, D.C.: National Academy Press.

Rettig, Richard A. 2001. "Historical Perspective." In *Ethics and the Kidney,* ed. Norman G. Levinsky. New York: Oxford University Press.

Rettig, Richard A., and Levinsky, Norman G. 1991. *Kidney Failure and the Federal Government.* Washington, D.C.: National Academy Press.

Robert Wood Johnson Foundation Promoting Excellence in End-of-Life Care Program. 2002. *End-Stage Renal Disease Workgroup Recommendations to the Field.* Princeton, NJ: Author.

Rothman, David J. 1991. *Strangers at the Bedside: A History of How Law and Bioethics Transformed Medical Decision Making.* New York: Basic Books.

Singer, Peter A. 1992. "Nephrologists' Experience with and Attitudes Towards Decisions to Forego Dialysis: The End-Stage Renal Disease Network of New England." *Journal of the American Society of Nephrology* 2(7): 1235–1240.

U.S. President's Commission for the Study of Ethical Problems in Medicine and Biomedical and Behavioral Research. 1983. *Deciding to Forego Life-Sustaining Treatment: A Report on the Ethical, Medical, and Legal Issues in Treatment Decisions.* Washington, D.C.: U.S. Government Printing Office.

U.S. Renal Data System. 1989. *Annual Data Report, 1989.* Bethesda, MD: National Institutes of Health, National Institute of Diabetes and Digestive and Kidney Diseases, Division of Kidney, Urologic, and Hematologic Diseases.

DISABILITY

• • •

I. ETHICAL AND SOCIETAL PERSPECTIVES

People who are physically or mentally disabled have many disadvantages. They may have an impairment, such as paralysis, blindness, or a psychiatric disorder, that reduces their ability to do things that nondisabled people do and may interfere with their fulfillment of socially valued roles. Also, disabled people often are subjected to various degrees of exclusion from the social and economic life of their communities. Political movements by disabled people to remove barriers and overcome discrimination, and protective legislation in several countries, have focused attention on the controversial concept of disability and on what constitutes just and compassionate behavior toward the disabled by individuals and institutions, including private employers, providers of public services, and schools. These ethical issues are pressing for all people because everyone can be disabled by trauma and because in societies in which life expectancy is long everyone may expect some impairments in old age.

This entry analyzes the concept of disability and its links to certain other concepts (impairment, handicap, health, and disease), explains the two competing explanatory models of disability, and surveys some of the ethical controversies that pertain to the nature of disability and the relationship between a disabled person and the rest of society.

Defining Disability: Conceptual Issues

The idea of disability and these related concepts are tricky to define. The conditions that often are referred to as disabilities are varied, including sensory losses, learning difficulties, chronic systemic illnesses and their effects (such as constant fatigue and pulmonary insufficiency), mental illnesses, lack of limbs, and lack of mobility. Do all these conditions have a common feature? Does every biological abnormality qualify as a disability? Does the availability of technological aids play a role in determining whether a bodily state is a disability? To what extent does being disabled depend on the environment in which a person lives? The very definition of disability is controversial; there is no single accepted definition.

The World Health Organization (WHO) of the United Nations offered the following definitions, which have been highly influential:

Impairment: Any loss or abnormality of psychological, physiological, or anatomical structure or function.

Disability: Any restriction or lack (resulting from an impairment) of ability to perform an activity in the manner or within the range considered normal for a human being.

Handicap: A disadvantage for a given individual, resulting from an impairment or disability, that limits or prevents the fulfillment of a role that is normal, depending on age, sex, social and cultural factors for that individual. (United Nations, 1983, quoted in Wendell)

Those definitions provide a good starting point but require fine-tuning. The distinction between impairments and disabilities is useful even though in some cases the distinction may be strained. The term *impairment* best captures a loss of or a defect in psychological, physiological,

or anatomic features. Thus, paralysis of an arm muscle is an impairment, and inability to throw something is a disability brought about by that impairment, because it is a lack of the ability to perform an activity (throwing). Inability to throw a baseball is not an impairment or a disability; instead, in a person who would be expected to be able to throw a baseball it may be a handicap: a disadvantageous inability to perform a socially defined activity that is caused by an impairment and a disability.

Thus, not every impairment is disabling. An abnormal shape of the eyeball that prevents light from focusing properly on the lens is an impairment, but if the afflicted person can see perfectly well with glasses or contact lenses and carry out the same activities that other people can, that impairment is not disabling. One also can ask whether a disability is a handicap. Franklin Delano Roosevelt had a disability (he could not walk) that no doubt prevented him from fulfilling some social roles, but it did not prevent him from fulfilling the role of president of the United States, and so in that respect it was not a handicap.

Difficulties with the WHO Definitions

There are two main deficiencies in the definitions given above that should be remedied. First, they contain no account of what is normal or abnormal for human beings either in structure and function (as in the definition of impairment) or in the manner and range of performing an activity (as in the definition of disability). Second, only the definition of a handicap makes reference to disadvantage, yet intuitively, disadvantage, or at least inconvenience, is part of the concept of disability. Below are suggested improvements, although significant imperfections remain.

THE HUMANLY NORMAL AND ABNORMAL. An account of the type of abnormality necessary for the notion of impairment to be applicable is needed. What is normal human physiology, psychology, anatomic structure, and function? The topic is vast and controversial, and it is easy to go wrong.

A statistical account of normal structure and function would be misconceived. Even if all human beings were damaged in a nuclear accident, it would not be humanly normal to suffer from radiation sickness and sterility.

It is also not possible to define normal structure and function simply by listing all the body parts human beings are observed to have, what those parts are observed to do, and how they do it. This is not only because knowledge in this area is incomplete. If one simply observes human organisms, the list will include things frequently observed that never would count as normal. One would observe both sound and decayed teeth, both painful childbirth and painful urination, and both the beating of the heart and myocardial infarction (another thing the heart is seen to do), yet the second item in each pair is abnormal. The concept of a human organ and its function is inseparable from the concept of what is normal for human beings (an evaluative, teleological concept), and any definition of normality that refers to the functions of organs assumes the concept of the normal in the attempt to define it. (The biologist's concept of the function of an organ need not depend on cultural assumptions, however. It only presupposes the distinction between normal and abnormal.)

A partial account of the normal functions and abnormalities of body parts can be derived from an understanding of their role in the survival of the species. As Norman Daniels puts it (p. 28), the biomedical sciences, including evolutionary biology, provide an account of "the design of the organism" and "its fitness to meeting biological goals" relative to which a scientist can specify some normal and abnormal phenomena. However, the usual biological goal assumed in evolutionary theory—transmission of an organism's genes to the next generation—does not entail the abnormality of many intuitively abnormal conditions, such as the diseases of extreme old age.

Rather than abandon hope of a definition, though, it is possible to adopt the following crude and incomplete standard, which suffices for the issues surrounding impairment and disability and leaves the thorniest controversies aside. A state of a human being is an abnormality of the type that can make it an impairment only if the state is such that if all human beings had had it from the beginning of human prehistory and otherwise were as they in fact are now, the human species would have been significantly less likely to survive.

This is a necessary but not a sufficient condition of a state's being abnormal. That is, all abnormal traits are ones that probably would have precluded species survival, but not all states that would have precluded species survival are abnormal. States that are abnormal fulfill certain other conditions. There is no complete list of these conditions, but here are two of them.

The first requires a subsidiary definition. Some traits assist survival when they are present in some members of a population as long as other individuals have a different trait; however, if all individuals had the trait, the population could not survive. These can be called diversity-requiring traits. An obvious one is being male or female. Having some males has been indispensable to the species's survival over time, but if all individuals were male (from prehistory), the species would have died out long ago.

The other condition excludes from the definition characteristics that are universal in but are limited to human beings of a certain developmental stage. It is normal for newborn infants to be unable to walk, for example, even though if all human beings of all ages had always been unable to walk, the species would not have survived.

The definition of abnormality can be supplemented in light of this characterization. Thus, a state of a human being is an abnormality of the type relevant to impairment only if the state is such that if all human beings had had it from the beginning of human prehistory and otherwise were as they in fact are today, the human species would have been unlikely to survive. If the state (1) is of that kind, (2) is not a diversity-requiring trait, and (3) is not a trait that is characteristic of and limited to certain stages of human development, it is abnormal.

With this understanding of abnormality, one can say, with the WHO, that an impairment is any abnormal loss or other abnormality of psychological, physiological, or anatomic structure or function. This standard ensures that the abnormalities that qualify as impairments are ones that characteristically make a difference in living a human life, the typical life of the species, whether or not they cause a great loss for any specific individual in any particular set of circumstances. Thus, extreme myopia (nearsightedness or shortsightedness) is an impairment by this definition because if all human beings had had this characteristic since prehistory and otherwise had been the same as they are today, the human species would have been unlikely to survive. A hunter-gatherer society composed entirely of severely myopic people would be doomed. Yet severe myopia may not cause serious inconvenience to a person in a modern technological society.

IMPAIRMENT AND DISABILITY. The WHO definition of disability says nothing about disadvantage, whereas intuitively that seems to be part of the concept. People would not count it as a disability if someone were unable to perform an activity in the manner normal for human beings if it were an activity that that person, or perhaps everyone, had no interest in performing in that way. It is no disability to someone who has taken a vow of celibacy or has undergone voluntary surgical sterilization that that person is biologically infertile because it does not disadvantage that person even though it is an impairment.

Instead, one can define a disability as any impairment-caused disadvantageous restriction or lack of ability to perform an activity in the manner or within the range that is normal for a human being. The relevant notion of normality is the same one identified above: that manner and range of activity without which the human species as a whole would have been unlikely to survive. Thus, extreme myopia, although it is an impairment, is not a disability for someone who suffers no consequent disadvantage because she or he has glasses or contact lenses that enable her or him to see perfectly.

Some people argue that a disability need not be disadvantageous. Anita Silvers (1994) gives the example of the great violinist Izhak Perlman, who walks with great difficulty yet has had a life of magnificent artistic accomplishment. However, it is surely to Perlman's disadvantage to have difficulty walking, as Bonnie Steinbock (2000) notes. A particular condition may be disadvantageous even for someone who is fortunate overall.

In light of these definitions impairments may disable a person to different degrees or in different ways in different societies, depending not only on the technology available (as with severe myopia) but more generally on the modes of living prevalent in the person's society, for example, whether the society is literate, whether it is agrarian or industrial, and the forms of transportation available in it. People with impairments also may confront varied cultural obstacles. In a society in which those born with bodily defects are regarded as cursed by the gods, for example, people with congenital impairments may be shunned, barred from most vocations, and reduced to begging. For a less extreme example, in a society in which attendant care is available only to those who live in institutions people who need the help of an aide to dress or bathe must be institutionalized. Someone with the same impairment might live in his or her own home in a different society. Consequently, some have argued that disability is purely a social construct. The degree of disability may indeed vary greatly as a result of cultural factors, however, as defined here, the impairment that causes disability is not fundamentally social in nature.

Handicap

The difference between a handicap as defined by the WHO and a disability as it has been defined here is that handicap employs a different concept of normality. A handicap results from impairment or disability, but it is a disadvantage that results from the consequent inability to fulfill roles that are normal, where what is normal is determined by social and cultural factors. Some activities, such as walking and seeing, are normal for human beings regardless of cultural expectations. If one cannot perform them, one is disabled in that respect. Other activities are normal for people in a particular type of society but are not expected or needed in others. If a person cannot perform them, that person will be handicapped in one society but not in another. Reading and using a telephone are normal activities in some societies but not in

others, and so the inability to perform them, for example, because one is dyslexic or deaf, is not culturally abnormal and thus is not a handicap.

However, humanly normal activities may not always be clearly distinguishable from culturally normal activities. Often people perform their normal human activities by carrying out certain social roles that are dictated by their cultural and physical environment. Susan Wendell (1996) points out that a woman with impaired vigor might be able to obtain drinking water in the way that is normal in western Canada (turning on a tap) but unable to obtain it in the way that is normal in rural Kenya (walking a long distance to a well twice daily). Consequently, the distinction between a disability and a handicap is not always sharp.

Disadvantages Resulting from Prejudice

People with disabilities tend to be looked down on, ignored, discriminated against, and otherwise badly treated. Sometimes they are denied education or medical care or excluded from employment. Sometimes they are institutionalized or sterilized against their will. Sometimes they are subjected to violence or other forms of abuse. Often, especially but not only in poor countries, their needs for food and shelter are not met. Many nondisabled individuals are uncomfortable in the presence of the disabled and therefore exclude them from social life. Thus, at times the attitudes of their fellow citizens bar disabled people from carrying out the social roles of students, employees, spouses, and parents, causing their handicaps.

Impairment, Disability, Disease, and Health

The concept of impairment is closely related to the concepts of disease and health. Health commonly is defined as the absence of disease. Chistopher Boorse (1977) defines disease as an impairment of or limitation on functional ability, identifying disease with impairment. (However, he gives a statistically based account of functional ability, which was rejected here.) Norman Daniels (1985) defines disease as a deviation from the natural functional organization of a typical member of the species. He says that in characterizing "natural functional organization," the biomedical sciences draw on evolutionary notions and "claims about the design of the species" (p. 28), yielding an account of what is humanly normal that is close to the account given here. Thus, disease and impairment are nearly equivalent. Impairment is a slightly wider category because it includes the absence of a structure, and this usually is not called a disease. An amputee may be healthy (free of disease), yet that person is impaired.

Disability has been defined as an impairment-caused disadvantageous restriction on the ability to perform normal human activities or to perform them within the normal range. Because diseases are a subset of impairments, many diseases are causes of disability provided that they impose a disadvantage on the persons who have them. Thus, an infection is both a disease and an impairment, and it may cause disability (temporary or permanent) by disadvantageously reducing the ability of an afflicted person to perform humanly normal activities. Nondisease impairments such as the absence of a limb also may cause disability.

Two Models of Disability

There are two opposing, dominant ways of conceiving of disability: the medical model and the minority group model; the latter sometimes is called the disability rights model. These are explanatory models for understanding how and why disabled people are disadvantaged and theories of the appropriate means to ameliorate those disadvantages. These two ways of representing disability influence their advocates' positions on several ethical issues.

THE MEDICAL MODEL. According to the medical model, a disabled person's lack of ability to perform normal human activities can be traced entirely to that person's impairment: the abnormalities in his or her psyche, physiology, or anatomy. A paraplegic cannot get from place to place because her legs are paralyzed; a blind person cannot read because he cannot see. Disability is a result of the state of a disabled person's body. Consequently, the best way to remove the disadvantage is to correct the impairment medically, by means of surgery, drugs, physical therapy, prosthetics, and the like. Proponents of the medical model advocate vigorous treatment to eliminate impairments, extensive research to find cures for impairments for which no treatment is available, and prevention of future impairments. Prevention should be achieved by increasing the use of existing safety devices (e.g., in automobiles), developing new ways to avoid disabling accidents and illnesses, and identifying and encouraging healthful behavior in pregnant women (such as good nutrition and not smoking) to prevent the birth of children with disabilities. Some people also support preventing the birth of affected infants by using prenatal screening and abortion of abnormal fetuses or using genetic engineering when possible.

Many corrective medical interventions are performed successfully to prevent or eliminate disability, but many impairments cannot be corrected. When medicine cannot restore normal structure or function, the extent of the incapacity may be reduced. However, in many cases this cannot be done, and the person remains impaired and disabled. The disadvantages that person experiences may be substantial. At this point the medical model has little to offer to enable a disabled person to overcome her or his disadvantage. Because the disadvantage is understood to arise from the impairment, if nothing can be done to remove the impairment, it follows that nothing can be done to overcome the disadvantage.

THE MINORITY GROUP MODEL. According to the minority group model, although disabled people have physical, sensory, or psychological impairments, the principal source of their disadvantage is not the impairments but the impact on those people of the socially created environment. Because people with impairments are few in number and lack power and influence, they make up a minority group that is not taken into account in the physical and organizational design of facilities and institutions. Consequently, they are excluded from many mainstream activities. Thus, disability and handicap are only to a small degree the result of impairments; the disadvantages they involve, which can range from inability to attend a nightclub to unemployment and poverty, are largely the result of a lack of social inclusion.

Whereas the medical model explains a paraplegic's disadvantage solely in terms of the fact that that person cannot walk, the minority group model explains it by reference to the fact that buildings and streets are built in such a way that a paraplegic cannot maneuver a wheelchair into them or through them and therefore cannot go where he or she needs to go to conduct business, acquire an education, perform a job, or engage in recreation. A paraplegic is disadvantaged because she or he cannot do those things. Anita Silvers (1995) points out that streets and buildings would be made wheelchair-accessible if the majority of people in the society moved about by means of wheelchairs. Silvers makes this statement to show that it is their minority status, not their impairment, that causes the disabled to be excluded from so much of ordinary social life.

In contrast to the medical model, the minority group model claims that a great deal can be done to overcome the disadvantage component of disability for those whose impairments are not medically correctable. Society should be altered to make it much more inclusive. To continue with the example of a person who cannot walk, buildings can be fitted with ramps and elevators, cities can provide buses and taxis with wheelchair lifts, and doorways can be widened, enabling a wheelchair user to lead an independent life that is fully integrated into the community. Thus, a wheelchair user would experience vastly less disadvantage as a result of changes in society rather than by means of medical intervention.

According to the minority group model, in nearly all societies there is rampant discrimination against the disabled. This is the case because the built environment, the chief means of information gathering, and many forms of activity are suitable only for nondisabled people. As an analogy one can imagine that unknown to the builders, a widely used building material gave off radiation that had no effect on most people but gave intolerable shocks to one small ethnic group. Members of that ethnic group thus could not enter many buildings, including places they urgently needed to go to do their banking, pay taxes, and so on. This clearly would be unfair, if unintentional, discrimination.

According to the minority group model, this is exactly the way things are. Barriers to the participation of the disabled are present both in the built environment and in cultural institutions. For example, proceedings in classrooms, courts, and legislatures are impenetrable to people with sensory impairments. According to the minority group view this state of affairs is unjust. It imposes terrible disadvantages on disabled people that could be alleviated, and because it is society that unfairly excludes the disabled, society should remediate the situation.

The tension between the more widely held medical model of disability and the minority group model helps shape some of the crucial ethical debates over the moral treatment of the disabled.

Ethical Issues

Two main categories of ethical issues pertain to disability: issues concerning the value of the lives of disabled people and issues that concern the rights disabled people have and the grounds on which they claim those rights.

THE VALUE OF THE LIVES OF DISABLED PEOPLE. The ethical issues in this category are those related to the withholding of life-prolonging medical treatment, euthanasia, physician-assisted suicide, prenatal screening and abortion of fetuses with likely birth defects, and genetic engineering to prevent impairments in future offspring. Of course, these are areas of great general ethical controversy that raise many other issues.

When nondisabled people hear descriptions of a person's impairments, especially ones that result from sudden trauma to a previously unimpaired individual, they often react by thinking, "I would not want to live like that." That is sometimes the reaction of a disabled individual to his or her own losses. Robert B. White (1975) reports that at one point after his disabling accident Dax Cowart summarized his attitude by saying, "I do not want to go on as a blind and

crippled person." That type of reaction helps explain why many regard the lives of people with disabilities as not worth living. However, those who have had time to adjust to their disabilities or have always lived with them are usually very glad to be alive. Although some disabilities may deprive a person's life of value, this cannot be assumed, and such an assumption, which may be unconscious, could lead to grave wrongdoing by caregivers and the legal system.

Euthanasia, withholding of life-prolonging treatment, and physician-assisted suicide. The question whether an individual should be kept alive by medical means (for example, cardiopulmonary resuscitation) or allowed to die as the result of a disease or injury and the question whether a person's death should be brought about by his or her own agency or that of others often arise when a person is terminally ill. However, they also may arise when a person has an incurable disease or another medical condition but can be expected to live for a considerable amount of time if given fairly standard medical treatments and food and water. Justifications for withholding a standard form of life-prolonging treatment from such a person or for taking steps to bring about that person's death usually appeal to the fact that as a result of the person's wretched medical condition, life is not a good to him or her. This may be the case if the person is mentally competent and requests death (usually because the medical condition causes unbearable suffering) or if the person is in a persistent vegetative state and is unable to have experiences of any kind or is an infant too young to make decisions who faces a very bleak future.

The appeal to autonomy. The refusal of life-prolonging treatment by a mentally competent patient is justified by an appeal to individual autonomy. A patient has a moral right to refuse treatment; this is an aspect of the fundamental moral right to autonomy, including decision-making control over what happens to one's body. Some people doubt whether it is ever morally permissible for a person to exercise the right to refuse treatment for the sole purpose of hastening his or her own death. However, there is wide agreement that if a patient does refuse treatment for any reason, provided that that person is mentally competent and well informed about her or his condition and prospects, it is wrong for anyone else to force the treatment on that person against her or his will. To do so would be an act of assault.

It is far more controversial whether the right to autonomy includes the right to commit suicide (rather than only to refuse treatment), and whether once a competent patient has decided to end his or her life a physician or another person may rightly assist him or her in doing that or may deliberately end that person's life at his or her request. Some defend the legitimacy of suicide as a rational and autonomous act, at least in the face of great and irremediable suffering that deprives life of its value. Others object to it even in such cases on the grounds that suicide is incompatible with respect for life. Physicians sometimes are asked to provide help in dying, for example, by giving lethal doses of drugs. Some argue that in cases in which the patient's life is not a good to the patient assistance with suicide is legitimate and indeed is a compassionate act. Others condemn this practice either because they condemn all suicide and judge it wrong to assist in a wrongful act or because they deem assisting with suicide incompatible with the role of a physician. Finally, some regard active euthanasia as incompatible with respect for life, indeed as murder, even when the killing is requested by the person who is to be killed. Others argue that euthanasia is morally justified when it is fully voluntary and the person's life is not worth living.

The incurable conditions that sometimes cause people to refuse life-prolonging treatment or seek physician-assisted suicide (PAS) or euthanasia (or because of which treatment is refused or euthanasia is sought on people's behalf) are often impairments and/or disabilities or are, like pain and nausea, the causes of impairments and/or disabilities. Among them are such conditions as the extensive brain damage suffered by Nancy Cruzan and diseases (and impairments) such as bone cancer, which causes disability by producing such overwhelming pain that the person cannot engage in normal activities. Thinking of a person who wishes to die as being disabled, as nearly always is the case, may change one's thinking about the ethical issues involved.

For those who oppose all euthanasia and PAS no moral conundrum arises with respect to disabilities in these areas: All such acts are wrong. For proponents of euthanasia and PAS, however, disabilities introduce some special dilemmas.

Many advocates of euthanasia and PAS tend to think of the matter as follows: Disabling conditions such as cerebral palsy, paralysis, and the type of permanent respiratory insufficiency that requires daily use of a respirator are incurable and can deprive life of its value for the afflicted person. If that person is mentally competent and refuses a life-prolonging treatment, saying that he or she prefers to die, these conditions are sufficient reason for that person to do so, and of course the request should be honored because it represents an exercise of individual autonomy. Even the opponents of euthanasia and PAS agree that treatment should not be forced on a person who is competent. If a person requests PAS or euthanasia, these are also sufficient reasons for it to be administered by willing parties according to this view. People with disabilities who seek death by starvation or the removal of a respirator have been hailed as champions of individual autonomy who attempt to exercise their rights against the resistance of officious healthcare institutions.

TWO ARGUMENTS AGAINST THE AUTONOMY-BASED APPROACH. There are two important counterarguments to this way of looking at requests to die made by people with disabilities.

The first is Carol Gill's (1992) suicide-prevention argument. Gill notes that when a nondisabled person undergoes a life crisis and subsequently shows certain behavioral signs and expresses a wish to die, that person is diagnosed with depression and is given counseling. He or she is regarded as less than fully competent because of depression and suicidal ideation. Gill observes a widespread assumption among nondisabled people, including healthcare professionals, that life with a disability is not worth living. Because of this, she argues, when someone with a disability expresses a suicidal wish, it is not classified as a symptom of curable, temporary emotional pathology. Instead, healthcare professionals regard the wish to die as rational because of their revulsion at the thought of living with a disability. They overlook standard clinical signs of depression and may disregard the presence of life crises or disappointments that are not related to the disability, such as loss of employment and divorce. Consequently, instead of providing suicide-prevention services, they encourage withdrawal of life-prolonging treatment, euthanasia, or PAS. If suicide-prevention services were provided, the disabled person might see adequate reason to live regardless of the disability, for once the depression was treated, the person would find life worthwhile. Thus, to advocate a right to die for the disabled is, at least in some cases, not to promote individual autonomy in decisions about life and death but instead to deprive the disabled of the suicide-prevention services routinely offered to nondisabled persons, a form of invidious discrimination.

The second, and related, counterargument arises more directly from the minority group model of disability. There is evidence that in some cases disabled persons seek death not because they find their impairments unendurable but because they are trapped in a dehumanizing social setting. Larry McAfee, for example, became so frustrated with his confinement to a nursing facility that he obtained a legal ruling that his ventilator be disconnected. Disabilities activists helped McAfee obtain job training and arrange to live outside the nursing home; he then decided to continue to live. According to this argument, what makes life unbearable to such people is not their impairments but the social world that subjects them to physical confinement and denies them decision-making power over their lives. Many people who are fairly severely disabled can, with assistance, do what McAfee did. However, government aid programs often refuse to provide the needed services outside an institution or the person is stymied by an unresponsive bureaucracy or excluded from jobs or housing by physical barriers or human prejudices. Thus, the disabled person's misery is caused by the choices and policies of other people. The person may seek death as the only alternative to living without basic dignity. In this view the ethical solution is not to allow or assist in the person's death but to free the members of this minority group from the oppressive conditions under which they are forced to live by implementing policies that promote independent living.

EUTHANASIA OF NEWBORNS WITH IMPAIRMENTS. Because newborn infants cannot make informed decisions about whether to end their lives, those who grant that some euthanasia is legitimate usually argue that such decisions should be made for newborns on the basis of whether a child's life will be of value to the child. The witholding of life-prolonging treatment is treated in the same way because there is no possibility in this case of informed refusal of treatment by the patient. According to the minority group model, infants born with incurable impairments may be wrongly killed because caregivers and parents assume that their lives would be entirely unrewarding even though many people with similar disabilities lead satisfying lives.

PUBLIC POLICY. Even if euthanasia or PAS for some disabled individuals were morally justified and not a result of depression or exclusion from independent living, some authors predict that if those options were made legal and routinely available, many morally unacceptable acts would result. They cite the difficulties of judging the mental competence of suffering patients who request death. In busy or understaffed hospitals people could be put to death who did not really want to die or were not really able to make a decision about it. Those authors mention the further danger that death may be sought not for the benefit of the person who dies but for the benefit of family members overwhelmed by the responsibility of caring for or paying for the care of an incurable individual or for the benefit of insurance companies and publicly funded healthcare programs.

This position creates a conundrum: Is it acceptable to adopt a policy that denies euthanasia and PAS to some people who are morally entitled to it, resulting in their prolonged suffering, to prevent the wrongful killing of others from carelessness, poor administration, or evasion of the law? Some argue that disabled people would be particularly vulnerable to being put to death wrongly under a policy of legal euthanasia or PAS because of the tendency of nondisabled people to expect a life with disabilities to be much worse for a disabled person than it actually is, the corresponding tendency of healthcare professionals and others to overlook the needs for treatment and other services, and the costs of providing for the disabled person's

needs. Any such policy must include rigorous safeguards to prevent abuses and errors, but no safeguards are foolproof.

ABNORMAL FETUSES, PRENATAL SCREENING, AND ABORTION. Testing during pregnancy for a variety of genetic and other congenital abnormalities is available in many places. Familiar examples are the test for Down's syndrome performed by means of amniocentesis or chorionic villus sampling and the blood test for the alpha-fetoprotein level to gauge the likelihood of neural tube defects. Most prospective parents seek prenatal tests with the intention of aborting the fetus or embryo if it is found to have an abnormality. The tests that exist or will exist in the near future are for types of impairments that can be fairly severe, although some exhibit a great range of severity, and tests cannot show how severely or mildly affected a child would be.

Those who regard abortion as wrong in every case or defensible only in very limited cases (e.g., to save the life of a pregnant woman) must regard abortions of impaired fetuses as immoral. Antiabortion arguments usually are based on the thesis that an unborn human being, no matter how primitive its stage of development, has a right not to be killed (and indeed to be kept alive) because it is human. If a human fetus has a right to life from conception onward by virtue of its human genome and if abortion is therefore wrong, abortion is just as wrong when a fetus is affected by spina bifida or another abnormality as it is when a fetus is normal. According to this view these fetuses are surely human, just as are adult disabled people. The most common antiabortion position holds that human fetuses are already full-fledged persons with moral rights. Thus, impaired fetuses are also persons with moral rights.

Those who argue that abortion is wrong because of a being's potential to become a person rather than as a result of its actual personhood may have some flexibility to justify exceptions for fetal abnormality. However, many abnormal fetuses have the potential to fulfill the fundamental criteria of personhood and thus could not rightly be aborted even according to the potentiality theory.

Therefore, an antiabortion position opposes nearly all abortions of impaired fetuses. Some general opponents of abortion try to defend an exception for fetal abnormalities, but it is difficult to make that position logically consistent.

Those who regard abortion as often permissible (those with a "prochoice" position) may hold a range of different views that are based on various ethical principles and countenance abortions at different stages of fetal development or for different purposes. Some regard only early abortion as acceptable, for example, before sentience; others think abortion is acceptable later in pregnancy. Some regard abortion for frivolous reasons as unacceptable, whereas others regard it as legitimate for almost any reason as long as other criteria are fulfilled. However, most defenses of abortion attribute to an embryo or early fetus a moral status below that of persons and for that reason see nothing wrong with an early abortion chosen because the prospective parents would find it burdensome to raise a child in their circumstances. The presence of an impairment in an embryo or young fetus would count as such circumstances for many couples or pregnant women. Therefore, on the whole, according to the prochoice position, early abortion of an abnormal fetus is morally acceptable.

Furthermore, if a prochoice stance is assumed, there are positive reasons for aborting an impaired embryo or fetus. If the child were born, it might experience significant suffering, and raising a disabled child can be a great strain on parents and siblings. Indeed, a good prospective parent tries to produce a normal child rather than a disabled child and to give it advantages whenever possible. Bonnie Steinbock (2000) argues that given the prochoice assumption, selective abortion is a method of disability prevention that is comparable to a pregnant woman's taking folic acid to prevent neural tube defects. It also may be argued that the birth of disabled children is best avoided on the grounds that it drains resources from the healthcare system because those children may require multiple surgeries and other costly interventions.

THE DISABILITY RIGHTS CRITIQUE OF SELECTIVE ABORTION.

Some authors who adopt a generally prochoice stance, however, argue specifically that abortion in response to fetal impairments is wrong. This has been called the disability rights critique of selective abortion. It consists of several distinct arguments, two of which are given below.

The expressive argument. The expressive argument is used both to show that the choice to abort an impaired fetus is wrong and at times that the government should not sponsor prenatal screening services. In this view aborting a fetus solely because it would develop into a disabled child expresses rejection of the disabled and perhaps exhibits the attitude that such children are undesirable or should not be born or the belief that the lives of all disabled people are miserable and lack value.

To express such an attitude is morally wrong for several reasons. For one thing the attitude is both erroneous and unfair. Many disabled people have good lives, and respect for the equal human worth of all individuals is one of the bases of morality. Also, aborting impaired fetuses, it is claimed, perpetuates bias against the disabled, just as selective abortion of female fetuses in certain societies perpetuates bias against women. Also, communicating a message of contempt to disabled people demoralizes them. Public funding of prenatal screening programs that people will use for abortion decisions does particular emotional harm because it shows public contempt and announces that society cares more about eliminating disabled people from the population than about helping those who are already born.

The main counterargument to the expressive position is that people who choose to abort impaired fetuses do not have the feelings or beliefs they are accused of expressing. Instead, their decision may be motivated by perfectly legitimate attitudes. Parents undergo special hardships in raising a disabled child that may include providing arduous or costly care well into the child's adult years. The desire to avoid those hardships is not tantamount to distaste or contempt for disabled people and does not stem from a belief that those people are all wretched. In light of the prochoice assumption, in aborting an early-term fetus with an impairment prospective parents choose not to produce a child who probably will suffer more and have more limited opportunities than a normal child does. The attempt to avoid those outcomes is part of the legitimate effort to do well for their families.

It should be noted that regardless of the actual attitudes of the agent, an action can convey an unintended but hurtful symbolic message, particularly if it is done in a context of widespread discrimination. However, this must be balanced against the central interests of adults in exercising reproductive freedom and making choices that determine the nature of their family life.

The cultural differences/social construction arguments. The arguments in this category focus on society's contribution to the phenomenon of disability. According to the minority group model, mainstream society causes much of the disadvantage inherent in disability by excluding disabled people from its central activities. Disability is socially constructed in this view. The way to eliminate the disadvantages of the disabled, then, is not to eliminate impaired people from the population through prenatal screening and abortion but to restructure society so that the impaired are included in it.

In addition, it is claimed that certain groups of disabled people form a distinct culture that should be respected. Defect-based abortion threatens to destroy that culture. This sometimes is claimed with respect to the Deaf (deaf people who identify with Deaf Culture, with a language such as American Sign as its central component). If too few congenitally deaf children are born, they will not be able to perpetuate their community.

Counterarguments to these claims turn on the shared assumption that appropriately early abortion is generally legitimate because the fetus is not yet a person with rights. Selective abortion does not kill off members of a society or participants in a culture; it simply makes it the case that there will be fewer people eligible to join the culture in the next generation. That harm to the culture must be weighed against the disadvantages impaired children would suffer if they were born. Even if society were made more inclusive, significant disadvantages would remain.

Disability and Genetic Intervention

Developments in human genetics offer the prospect of correcting or preventing impairments by means of genetic intervention. Of course, this would eliminate only impairments that are genetically based; it is irrelevant to impairments with other causes.

One use of genetics—testing for genetic abnormalities followed by the abortion of affected fetuses—was addressed above. There are also other uses. One may screen prospective parents for deleterious genes, and the carriers may choose not to reproduce or to have children by using donor gametes or transplanted embryos. In the future one may be able to modify the somatic genome of an existing person to eliminate impairment or modify a person's germ-cell DNA (the genome of a person's eggs or sperm) to prevent disabling impairments in future generations.

Because no life is terminated in these procedures (not even that of an embryo), there is no ethical objection to them from the perspective of the right to life even among those opposed to abortion in general. The ethical concerns that arise for selective abortion against a prochoice background, however, also apply to genetic techniques that prevent the conception of impaired fetuses, although with less force. For example, choosing not to have children or to use someone else's gametes to avoid producing a disabled child might express an attitude that devalues the disabled, although merely using contraception would do that less forcefully than abortion does. Programs of gamete donation and embryo transfer and techniques for altering genes *in utero* also would reduce the size of the disabled population and the number of participants in subcultures composed of people with particular disabilities, just as abortion does.

However, techniques that "switch off" or replace deleterious genes in living people or in gametes or fetuses that will be allowed to develop have a special defense against such criticisms. First, it is hard to see what could be wrong with treating a gamete, fetus, or already-born individual to correct or prevent a disabling impairment. This would be like treating a child with antibiotics to keep an infection from causing blindness, which is surely legitimate; it is a form of healthcare. Second, individuals who were denied available interventions and went on to develop disabling impairments would have moral grounds for complaint. The claims of disabled people not to be incrementally marginalized by decreases in their numbers and not to be given a discouraging message must be weighed against the claims of other individuals to receive an intervention that spares them from grave disadvantages. To deny them this would be to make them bear a disproportionately steep cost to protect the sensibilities of others.

On the basis of either a liberal or a strictly egalitarian theory of distributive justice, Norman Daniels and others argue that citizens of an affluent industrialized society that spends heavily on healthcare have a right to a broad package of efficacious healthcare services (Daniels; Buchanan et al.). If genetic intervention in living individuals becomes a reliable form of healthcare (once it is beyond the experimental stage), it will become the type of treatment to which such citizens have a right, according to these theories (Buchanan et al.), and failure to provide it will be not only a failure of compassion but an injustice.

There are significant risks in altering the somatic-cell genes of a single individual because the biological processes involved are so complex and the environment may interact with the changed genome in unexpected ways. However, for the most part it is only the individual who is at risk. There is further risk in changing a person's germ-cell DNA so that the change is transmitted to all that person's descendants. The new genome may give rise to new impairments when it is combined with the genes of others during reproduction or in response to shifting environmental influences. Because the technology for those procedures does not exist yet, one can say only that the ethical legitimacy of germ-line intervention to prevent disability will depend on the range of risks involved in each particular procedure. Great caution here is morally obligatory.

EQUAL HUMAN RIGHTS. Western philosophers argue that all human beings, in spite of their many obvious differences in strength, intelligence, and so forth, have equal fundamental human rights. Equal human rights always are thought to include noninterference rights such as the right to autonomy or self-determination and the right to freedom. They often are thought to include rights to goods or services as well, such as the right to a minimum amount to eat or a basic education. Philosophers offer different grounds for these moral rights.

For Immanuel Kant (1996 [1797]) human beings have such rights because they possess reason, including the capacity for rational choice in regard to action. Many recent authors follow Kant in proposing as the basis for the possession of equal rights criteria that depend on the psychological properties of the rights holder: the being's conceptual capacities, its control of its behavior, its emotions, or its capacities for reciprocal social interaction.

Social contract theories such as that of John Rawls (1971) offer a different basis for equal rights for all human beings. Jeffrie Murphy, following Rawls, says that "an individual should be understood as having a right to x if and only if a law guaranteeing x to the individual would be chosen by rational agents in the original position" (p. 8). The original position is a hypothetical situation in which a group of rational agents comes together to agree unanimously to principles and practices to govern their community. Each participant is self-interested, may care deeply about some (but not all) of the others, and knows in general what can happen in human lives but is "behind the veil of ignorance"—does not know his or her future or what his or her role in society will be. Those to whom the items in question are guaranteed need not be rational.

RIGHTS OF THE MENTALLY DISABLED. According to theories that base rights on psychological features of the prospective right holder, mentally competent people with physical disabilities have the same fundamental human rights as other competent adults because they fulfill all the criteria that have been propounded as the bases of human rights. Inability to walk or see does not deprive people of rationality, the capacity for informed choice, or the ability to interact reciprocally with others. According to contractarians, those people also have rights equal to those of the nondisabled because people in the original position know that they themselves might become physically disabled and thus would agree to protect the disabled in their possession of many goods.

In the psychologically based theories, however, a problem arises for people with severe cognitive or emotional disabilities. As Lois Weinberg (1981) points out, these people will not develop the capacities frequently cited as the grounds for equal human rights, such as the capacity for rational choice (in the severely retarded) and the capacity to interact reciprocally with others (in the sociopath). According to these philosophical theories, such individuals do not have any fundamental human rights; but that is implausible. At the very least those with mental or psychological disabilities have the basic human right not to be physically abused, and some argue that they have human rights to minimal care and an appropriate education. Giving them those things is not merely an act of compassion but also one of justice, it is argued, and hence a matter of rights.

The contractarian approach fares better. Murphy (1984) argues that rational agents behind the veil of ignorance would agree to guarantee a certain level of security and training for the mentally disabled because they know that they might become mentally disabled or might have a much-loved mentally disabled child. They would not guarantee autonomy protections to the mentally disabled but would guarantee them rights to basic food, shelter, and freedom from abuse.

AUTONOMY/NONINTERFERENCE RIGHTS AND RIGHTS TO AID. Noninterference or autonomy rights are the rights of rational persons who are capable of deciding their destinies to be left alone to do that: rights not to have others deprive them of life, liberty, or legitimately owned property (Locke, 1975 [1699]). Even for contractarians the full range of these rights belongs only to rational decision-making creatures because of their capacity to guide their behavior through their choices.

Mentally normal people with other types of disabilities are rational choosers, and so there are no grounds to deny that they have noninterference/autonomy rights. It is unjust to coerce them in the making of important life decisions, for example, to subject them to forcible sterilization. Mentally disabled people, depending on the severity of their impairments, may not live up to the standard of rational decision making needed to qualify for noninterference/autonomy rights. Some ethicists think that therefore people whose mental disabilities are significant do not have the moral right to make their own decisions about medical treatment, life-skills training, and finances. Those decisions are rightly made for them and should be made in ways that serve their interests. Others defend some autonomy rights for the mentally disabled.

Apart from noninterference rights, various authors claim that the disabled have the right to have a great assortment of goods and services provided to them by the rest of society. This may include life aids (ventilators and wheelchairs), attendant care, special education or training, the rebuilding of public structures, and income support (for food and shelter and also for healthcare in countries where healthcare is not subsidized for all). It is controversial which, if any, of these things are owed to disabled people by right and on what conceptual basis.

RIGHTS TO THE MEANS OF INCLUSION. For Anita Silvers (1994) all persons, or perhaps all who are mentally competent, have equal rights to participate fully in society on the basis of their individual dignity and self-respect. If any are excluded, justice requires that the barriers to their participation be dismantled or bridged. Thus, equality rights are the grounds on which the disabled have a right to be provided with the means of inclusion. Barriers to full participation are conceived broadly: The lack of a teacher for the visually impaired might qualify as a barrier to a visually disabled child's full participation in her or his school. Thus, the removal of barriers consists not only in the alteration of physical structures but also in the creation of new structures or devices and the provision of trained personnel. The disabled have a right to these things solely because of their right to equal participation, which in this view is a right that everyone has. This equality right to devices and services that remove barriers does not include the right to income support, however, because people do not all equally have that right solely on the basis of their equal dignity and self-respect. Silvers (1995) argues that once disabled people are granted equal access, they will earn their own living. If a few severely disabled people have a right to subsistence support, that has a different and nonuniversal basis.

However, a contractarian view treats the right to the removal of barriers and the right to income support as being on a par. In a contractarian view both are based on the protections rational agents would agree to for their society when choosing behind the veil of ignorance.

Thus, Gregory Kavka (1992) argues on the basis of both Hobbesian and Rawlsian social-contract theory that in advanced societies people with significant disabilities have a right against society that it provide, where feasible, the accommodation, equipment, and training needed to permit the disabled to engage in the productive processes of their society and thus earn an income. The Rawlsian version of the argument says that people in the original position would agree to improve the lot of society's least-advantaged members and that the disabled are among the least advantaged because of the disadvantage inherent in their disabilities and the barriers and prejudices they face in society. The most effective way to better their lot is to give them access to self-respect, which in modern societies depends greatly on work and career identification. Income support will not provide the same basis of self-respect, and so it is not the best means to achieve this end. Thus, although Kavka argues for the subsidized removal of barriers to employment, if the provision of food and shelter were the most effective way to better the condition of the least well off, that is what he would defend. Murphy's argument, similarly appealing to the original position, defends the provision of food and shelter to the mentally disabled.

Vigorous counterarguments are made against these arguments that society should provide the disabled with the means of inclusion. Philosophers who reject Rawls's theory of distributive justice attack the relevant premises. A different sort of counterargument claims that it is too expensive to provide all the goods and services needed by the disabled.

Although giving disabled people access to full social participation would enable many of them to earn a living and not depend on welfare payments, it is an economically inefficient solution, they say, because it would be cheaper to provide income support for all disabled people. Society could use the savings for other important purposes. This need not be a selfish argument; the savings could be used to provide free healthcare to the poor or to build better schools.

Various replies are offered to the efficiency objection. The basic structure of the argument is utilitarian, and it may be criticized on those grounds. The cheaper policy may increase the well-being of some elements in society, such as taxpayers and the nondisabled poor, but may yield a far lower level of well-being for the disabled than would inclusion, and no evidence is provided that the net well-being of all the persons affected will be higher with the less expensive policy. Alternatively, the argument may be rejected on grounds of justice: It may be less expensive to provide nothing but income support, but it is unjust to deny disabled people the bases of self-respect that come from inclusion in society.

Conclusion

This entry has investigated the concepts of disability, impairment, and handicap; defended partial definitions of those concepts; and related them to the concepts of disease and health. It has explained the two prevailing models for understanding disability: the medical model and the minority group model. Those conceptual analyses provided tools for surveying two groups of ethical issues pertaining to disability: issues regarding the value of the lives of the disabled and issues regarding the moral rights of disabled people. In the first category the entry examined permitting the disabled to choose death, abortion of impaired fetuses, and genetic intervention to prevent disabilities. In the second category the entry considered issues of whether the disabled have a right to various kinds of liberties and government assistance, and if so, on what grounds.

RACHEL COHON

SEE ALSO: *Adoption; Anthropology and Bioethics; Autonomy; Care; Christianity, Bioethics in; Chronic Illness and Chronic Care; Dementia; Eugenics; Genetic Testing and Screening: Reproductive Genetic Testing; Human Dignity; Human Rights; Infanticide; Infants, Ethical Issues with; Judaism, Bioethics in; Life, Quality of; Long-Term Care; Mental Illness; Metaphor and Analogy; Moral Status; Pediatrics, Intensive Care in; Rehabilitation Medicine; Value and Valuation; Virtue and Character;* and other *Disability* subentries

BIBLIOGRAPHY

Amundson, Ron. 1992. "Disability, Handicap, and the Environment." *Journal of Social Philosophy* 23(1): 105–119.

Arneson, Richard E. 1990. "Liberalism, Distributive Subjectivism, and Equal Opportunity for Welfare." *Philosophy and Public Affairs* 19(2): 158–194.

Asch, Adrienne. 2000. "Why I Haven't Changed My Mind about Prenatal Diagnosis: Reflections and Refinements." In *Prenatal Testing and Disability Rights,* ed. Erik Parens and Adrienne Asch. Washington, D.C.: Georgetown University Press.

Asch, Adrienne. 2001. "Prenatal Diagnosis and Selective Abortion: A Challenge to Practice and Policy." *GeneWatch: A Bulletin of the Council for Responsible Genetics* 14(2): 5–7, 14.

Benn, Stanley I. 1967/reprinted 1971. "Egalitarianism and the Equal Consideration of Interests." In *Nomos IX: Equality,* ed. J. Roland Pennock and John W. Chapman. New York: Atherton Press. Reprinted in *Justice and Equality,* ed. Hugo A Bedau. Englewood Cliffs, NJ: Prentice-Hall.

Boorse, Christopher. 1977. "Health as a Theoretical Concept." *Philosophy of Science* 44: 542–573.

Bouvia v. Superior Court California Court of Appeals, Second District. 225 Cal.Rptr. 297 (Cal. App. 2 Dist. 1986).

Buchanan, Allen; Brock, Dan W.; Daniels, Norman; and Wikler, Daniel. 2000. *From Chance to Choice: Genetics and Justice.* Cambridge, Eng.: Cambridge University Press.

Cohen, Gerald A. 1993. "Equality of What?: On Welfare Goods and Capabilities." In *The Quality of Life,* ed. Martha Nussbaum. Oxford: Clarendon Press.

Cruzan v. Director, Missouri Department of Health. United States Supreme Court. *United States [Supreme Court] Reports* 497: 261–357 (1990).

Daniels, Norman. 1985. *Just Health Care.* Cambridge, Eng.: Cambridge University Press.

Dworkin, Ronald M. 1985. "Why Should Liberals Care about Equality?" In *A Matter of Principle.* Cambridge, MA: Harvard University Press.

Foot, Philippa. 1977. "Euthanasia." *Philosophy and Public Affairs* 6(2): 85–112.

Gill, Carol. 1992. "Suicide Intervention for People with Disabilities: A Lesson in Inequality." *Issues in Law and Medicine* 8(1): 37–53.

Herr, Stanley S.; Bostrom, Barry A.; and Barton, Rebecca S. 1992. "No Place to Go: Refusal of Life-Sustaining Treatment by Competent Persons with Physical Disabilities." *Issues in Law and Medicine* 8(1): 3–36.

Kant, Immanuel. 1996 (1797). *The Metaphysics of Morals,* tr. and ed. Mary Gregor. Cambridge, Eng.: Cambridge University Press.

Kavka, Gregory S. 1992. "Disability and the Right to Work." *Social Philosophy and Policy* 9(1): 262–290.

Locke, John. 1975 (1699). *Two Treatises of Government.* London: Dent.

Longmore, Paul K. 1987. "Elizabeth Bouvia, Assisted Suicide and Social Prejudice." *Issues in Law and Medicine* 3: 141–153.

Melden, Abraham I. 1977. *Rights and Persons.* Berkeley: University of California Press.

Melden, Abraham I., ed. 1970. *Human Rights.* Belmont, CA: Wadsworth.

Murphy, Jeffrie. 1984. "Rights and Borderline Cases." In *Ethics and Mental Retardation,* ed. Loretta Kopelman and John C. Moskop. Dordrecht, Netherlands: Reidel.

Nelson, James Lindemann. 2000. "The Meaning of the Act: Reflections on the Expressive Force of Reproductive Decision Making and Policies." In *Prenatal Testing and Disability Rights,* ed. Erik Parens and Adrienne Asch. Washington, D.C.: Georgetown University Press.

Parens, Erik, and Asch, Adrienne. 2000a. "The Disability Rights Critque of Prenatal Genetic Testing: Reflections and Recommendations." In *Prenatal Testing and Disability Rights,* ed. Erik Parens and Adrienne Asch. Washington, D.C.: Georgetown University Press.

Parens, Erik, and Asch, Adrienne, eds. 2000b. *Prenatal Testing and Disability Rights,* Washington, D.C.: Georgetown University Press.

Rawls, John. 1971. *A Theory of Justice.* Cambridge, MA: Harvard University Press.

Roemer, John. 1989. "Equality and Responsibility." *Boston Review* 20(2): 3–7.

Silvers, Anita. 1994. "'Defective' Agents: Equality, Difference, and the Tyranny of the Normal." *Journal of Social Philosophy,* 25th Anniversary Special Issue, pp. 154–175.

Silvers, Anita. 1995. "Reconciling Equality to Difference: Caring (f)or Justice for People with Disabilities." *Hypatia* 10(1): 30–55.

Spicker, Paul. 1990. "Mental Handicap and Citizenship." *Journal of Applied Philosophy* 7(2): 139–151.

Steinbock, Bonnie. 2000. "Disability, Prenatal Testing, and Selective Abortion." In *Prenatal Testing and Disability Rights,* ed. Erik Parens and Adrienne Asch. Washington, D.C.: Georgetown University Press.

Thompson, Michael. 1995. "The Representation of Life." In *Virtues and Reasons: Philippa Foot and Moral Theory,* ed. Rosalind Hursthouse, Gavin Lawrence, and Warren Quinn. Oxford: Oxford University Press.

Tremain, Shelley. 1996. "Dworkin on Disablement and Resources." *Canadian Journal of Law and Jurisprudence* 9(2): 343–359.

United Nations. 1983. *International Classification of Impairments, Disabilities, and Handicaps.* Geneva: World Health Organization.

United Nations. 1999. *International Classification of Functioning and Disability, Beta-2.* Geneva: World Health Organization.

Weinberg, Lois. 1981. "The Problem of Defending Equal Rights for the Handicapped." *Educational Theory* 31(2): 177–187.

Wendell, Susan. 1996. *The Rejected Body.* New York: Routledge.

White, Robert B. 1975. "A Demand to Die." *Hastings Center Report* 5: 3.

Williams, Bernard A. O. 1962 (reprinted 1971). *Philosophy, Politics, and Society,* ed. Peter Laslett and Walter G. Runciman. Cambridge, Eng.: Basil Blackwell. Reprinted in Justice and Equality, ed. Hugo A Bedau. Englewood Cliffs, NJ: Prentice-Hall.

INTERNET RESOURCES

Longmore, Paul K. 1997. "Paul Longmore Talks about Terminal Illness and How Society Misses the Real Issues." *The Electric Edge* (Web edition of *The Ragged Edge*). Available from <www.ragged-edge-mag.com/archive/p13story.htm>.

II. LEGAL ISSUES

Persons with disabilities daily face challenges beyond their individual disabilities. Social prejudice and physical barriers often pose far greater hindrances. Prejudice takes the form of the myths, stereotypes, and irrational fears that many people in society associate with impaired functioning. Barriers are those environmental factors, both physical and social, that limit the meaningful involvement of persons with disabilities in normal life activities (Herr, Gostin, and Koh). While a corpus of law has been developed in the United States to protect persons with disabilities, the passage of the Americans with Disabilities Act (ADA) of 1990 (42 U.S.C. 112101–12213 [Supp. II 1990]) marks the most important federal antidiscrimination legislation since the Civil Rights Act of 1964.

The Social Situation of Persons with Disabilities

The ADA was enacted in response to profound inequities and injustice for persons with disabilities (National Council on Disability). Americans with disabilities typically are poorer, less educated, less likely to be employed, and less likely to participate in social events than other groups in society. Social attitudes toward persons with disabilities add to their burdens. Persons with disabilities may be ignored, treated with pity or fear, adulated as *inspirations* for their efforts to overcome their disabilities, or expected to be as *normal* as possible. Moreover, Americans with disabilities have historically lacked a subculture from which to derive a collective strength, primarily due to the disparity of their disabilities and backgrounds. Disability interest groups, offshoots of civil rights groups, have filled this void in the last several decades (West).

Such prejudice and barriers raise a number of legal issues, most notably discrimination. In employment, in education, and in mobility, society often fails in its efforts to effectively accommodate persons with disabilities.

Legal Responses to Disability

Legal responses to disability range from application of constitutional theory to statutory initiatives. It would be comforting to believe that the U.S. Constitution provides meaningful protection to persons with disabilities. Sadly, the Constitution has little to offer persons with disabilities except in egregious cases. The Bill of Rights is applicable principally to government (*DeShaney v. Winnebago County Department of Social Services,* 1989). Since most forms of discrimination take place in the private sector, the Constitution is of limited applicability.

Even where state action can be demonstrated, the Supreme Court has not enunciated a coherent and compelling constitutional doctrine to protect persons with disabilities against discrimination. The Court, for example, has never found disability to be a *suspect classification,* and most government activities do not deprive persons with disabilities of a "fundamental freedom such as liberty" (*City of Cleburne, Texas v. Cleburne Living Center, Inc.,* 1985). Accordingly, the Court might be expected to uphold a state discriminatory action, provided the government could show a reasonable basis for its policy.

The Supreme Court, in one of its few constitutional decisions concerning discrimination against persons with disabilities, did suggest that it would not tolerate clear instances of prejudice or animus in government policies. In *City of Cleburne, Texas v. Cleburne Living Center,* the Court struck down a city zoning ordinance that excluded group homes for persons with mental retardation. The Court, in a particularly thorough search of the record, found no rational basis to believe that mentally retarded people would pose a special threat to the city's legitimate interest (Gostin, 1987).

A convincing constitutional argument could be made that persons with disabilities should have a high level of constitutional protection as is the case with racial minorities and women. Persons with disabilities have a similar history of exclusion and alienation by the wider society. They are often subject to discrimination on the basis of their status without regard to their abilities.

Much of the legal protection afforded to persons with disabilities is under federal and state law. Statutory initiatives in disability law fall into three general categories: (1) programs and services; (2) income maintenance; and (3) civil rights. Such statutes incrementally have sought the legislative goals of full participation and independence for persons with disabilities. While state laws vary in scope and effect, at the federal level three main acts shaped the corpus of disability law prior to enactment of the ADA.

The federal Rehabilitation Act (29 U.S.C. 791–794 [1988 and Supp. I 1989]), enacted in 1973, covers federally funded entities (and continues to cover all federal employees). Section 504 of this act (broadened by amendments in 1987) prohibits discrimination against otherwise qualified disabled persons in any federally funded program, executive agency, or the Postal Service. Sections 501 and 503 require affirmative action hiring plans in the federal government and certain large federal contractors.

The Individuals with Disabilities Education Act (IDEA) (42 U.S.C. 6000–6081 [1975]; 20 U.S.C. 1400 *et seq.* [1991]), enacted in 1975 and amended in 1990, mandates a free and appropriate education for all children with disabilities, encouraging integration (*mainstreaming*) whenever possible.

The Fair Housing Amendments Act of 1988 (42 U.S.C. 3601–3619 [1988]) ensures that persons with disabilities are a protected class in housing discrimination cases, and mandates access requirements for new housing and adaptation requirements for existing housing to ensure that the housing needs of disabled persons are met. This act continues to cover housing discrimination in place of specific provisions in the ADA.

The Americans with Disabilities Act of 1990

While these initiatives were a start, they failed to address cohesively the needs and rights of persons with disabilities. The ADA is a strong response to the needs and rights of persons with disabilities, needs and rights articulated by the growing voice of disability interest groups in America. It offers a potentially important vehicle for safeguarding the rights of persons with disabilities, but the judiciary has been whittling away its protections over recent years (Gostin, 2002).

More specifically, as an outgrowth of civil rights law, the ADA serves as a legal tool because of its broad scope and unique ability to adopt the visions of both equality and special treatment. The ADA recognizes that a person's disabilities often have little to do with his or her inabilities. Often it is society's reactions to the person with disabilities or society's structural barriers that disable the person. The mandate of civil rights law is to destroy those negative reactions and dismantle those barriers in order to restore equal opportunity and full participation in daily life activities with dignity, not charity. The ADA strives to achieve this objective.

The act prohibits discrimination against qualified persons with disabilities in employment, public services, public accommodations, and telecommunications. The principal change in federal law is that the ADA applies to all covered entities, whether or not they receive federal funding. The impact of the ADA on public health departments and communicable-disease law (Gostin, 1991b) and on the healthcare system (Gostin and Beyer) is significant. It will also have a significant impact on other important areas of bioethics, including the duty to treat, the right to health-benefit coverage, and medical testing and examinations by employers (Parmet).

Although the specific titles of the ADA have slightly different provisions, a finding of discrimination is based on adverse treatment of a person (1) with a *disability* who is (2) *qualified* or who (3) would be qualified if *reasonable accommodations* or modifications were made available.

Disability is defined broadly to mean "a physical or mental impairment that substantially limits one or more of the major life activities," a record of such impairment, or being regarded as having such impairment (section 3). The definition of disability theoretically covers a wide range of medical conditions. The courts had construed the Rehabilitation Act to include a wide-range of disabilities that are both genetic (e.g., Down syndrome [*Bowen v. American Hospital Association*], muscular dystrophy [S. Rep. no. 116]); or cystic fibrosis [*Gerben v. Holsclaw*] and multifactorial (e.g., heart disease, schizophrenia, or arthritis [S. Rep. no. 116]). Disability was also construed to include diseases that are communicable (e.g., tuberculosis [*School Board of Nassau County, Florida v. Arline*], hepatitis [*New York State Association of Retarded Children v. Carey*], or syphilis); as well as those that are not (e.g., cerebral palsy [*Alexander v. Choate*], or diabetes [S. Rep. no. 116]). However, a person who is currently using illegal drugs is not considered disabled, but is covered once he or she has been successfully rehabilitated and is no longer using drugs (section 510). Similarly, a range of socially disapproved behavior disorders are excluded from protection, such as most gender-identity disorders, pedophilia, exhibitionism, voyeurism, compulsive gambling, kleptomania, pyromania, and psychoactive drug-use disorders (section 511).

Moreover, a person is disabled if he or she has a *record* of, or is *regarded* as, being disabled, even if there is no actual disability (*Southeastern Community College v. Davis*). A record indicates that a person has, for example, a history of disability, thus protecting persons who have recovered from a disability or disease, such as cancer survivors.

The term regarded includes individuals who do not have disabilities but are treated as if they did. This concept protects people who are discriminated against in the false belief that they are disabled. It would be inequitable for a defendant who intended to discriminate on the basis of disability to successfully raise the defense that the person claiming discrimination was not, in fact, disabled. This provision is particularly important for individuals who are perceived to have stigmatizing or disfiguring conditions such as HIV, leprosy, or severe burns (S. Rep. no. 116).

Although the ADA theoretically covers a wide range of persons with disabilities, the Supreme Court has been significantly narrowing its scope. The first Supreme Court opinion on the ADA was quite hopeful. In its decision in *Bragdon v. Abbott* (1998), the Court held that a person with purely asymptomatic HIV infection was *disabled* within the meaning of the Act.

The *Bragdon* decision makes it more likely that, in the future, the courts will find persons with asymptomatic HIV infection protected under the ADA. The question remains, however, whether other health conditions will satisfy the ADA's definition of disability. As explained above, courts deciding cases under the Rehabilitation Act did not view the definition of disability as a strict obstacle for plaintiffs. The issues did not turn on whether an individual *had* a disability, but rather on whether the disability was the *cause* of the adverse action, or on whether the action was *justified* because a person's disability rendered her unqualified for a job or ineligible for a service. The judicial approach in disability cases was similar to the approach when individuals claim discrimination based on their race or gender. When making decisions regarding race or gender discrimination, courts do not engage in searching inquiries into whether the individual is *really a woman,* or *really an African-American.* Rather, these cases are often lost because individuals are unable to prove they have been discriminated against *because* of their race or gender (Feldblum, 1996).

Nothing during passage of the ADA suggested that courts would adopt a narrow definition of disability. But the legal landscape has changed dramatically (D'Agostino). Courts deciding ADA cases have arrived at a restricted definition of disability through two principal methods. First, many courts analyze whether a plaintiff is substantially limited in the major life activity of working. Courts often conclude that the impairment is not sufficiently limiting because there is a range of jobs that the individual can still perform. This narrow view makes little sense because the ADA was designed to prohibit discrimination against people with disabilities who *can* work, but who are nonetheless discriminated against.

Even if an individual's claim that her impairment limits a major life activity *other* than working is accepted, there is a second method by which courts have restricted coverage under the ADA. Courts scrutinize whether the individual's impairment *substantially* limits a *major* life activity. In *Toyota Motor Manufacturing Kentucky v. Williams* (2002), the Supreme Court adopted a narrow construction of "major life activity." The Court found that a medical diagnosis of carpal tunnel syndrome was not sufficient to qualify a person as disabled; nor is evidence that the person cannot perform "isolated, unimportant, or particularly difficult manual tasks."

Courts have also restricted coverage under the ADA by asking whether the impairment of a major life activity is "substantial." The Supreme Court requires that the impairment be "considerable." For example, in *Albertsons v. Kirkinburg* (1999) the Supreme Court held that a person with monocular vision is not disabled because the condition is not serious enough to substantially restrict his life activities.

The Supreme Court not only requires a substantial limitation in a major life activity, but it also requires that corrective and mitigating measures be considered in determining whether an individual is disabled. In *Sutton v. United Airlines, Inc.* (1999) the Court held that severely myopic job applicants for airline pilot positions are not disabled because eyeglasses or contact lenses mitigate their impairment. Similarly, in *Murphy v. United Parcel Service, Inc.* (1999) the Court held that a driver with high blood pressure is not disabled because his condition could be mitigated with medication. The Court did not claim that individuals with myopia or high blood pressure are not qualified to be pilots or drivers. Rather, the Court held that since the plaintiffs were not disabled, their qualifications for the job were not even relevant considerations under the ADA. Thus, in an ironic twist, although the ADA's goal is to provide anti-discrimination protection to individuals who (perhaps because they are taking medication) are qualified for jobs and eligible for services, such individuals are denied protection precisely because their medical conditions are under control.

The third prong of the definition of disability—which protects individuals who are *regarded as* having a substantially limiting impairment—has been applied quite restrictively by courts. Indeed, the Supreme Court in *Sutton* suggested that the employer or service provider must actually believe the person is substantially limited in a major life activity before receiving protection against discrimination. Thus, a person fired due to irrational fear or prejudice will not receive protection under the ADA provided the employer does not think the individual has a substantial physical or mental limitation.

A person is *qualified* if he or she is capable of meeting the essential performance or eligibility criteria for the particular position, service, or benefit. Thus, a person with a disability is not protected unless he or she is otherwise qualified to hold the job or to receive the service or benefit.

Qualification standards can include a requirement that the person with a disability does "not pose a direct threat to the health or safety of others" (sections 103[b], 302 [b][3]). The *direct threat* standard means that persons can be excluded from jobs, public accommodations, or public services if necessary to prevent a *significant risk* to others (*School Board of Nassau County, Florida v. Arline,* 1987). The significant risk standard originally applied only to persons with infectious disease. However, it was extended by the House Judiciary Committee to all persons with disabilities (H.R. Conference Report no. 101–596).

In order to determine, for example, that a person with mental illness poses a significant risk to others, evidence of specific dangerous behavior must be presented. In the context of infectious diseases such as tuberculosis, the Supreme Court laid down four criteria to determine significant risk:

1. the mode of transmission;
2. the duration of infectiousness;
3. the probability of the risk;
4. the severity of the harm (*School Board of Nassau County, Florida v. Arline*).

The Supreme Court in *Chevron U.S.A. Inc. v. Echazabal* (2002), held that a person with a disability is not "qualified" if she poses a direct threat to herself. This is a form of paternalism that is not in the language of the ADA, but had been supported by the Equal Employment Opportunities Commission. Allowing an employer to balance the benefits and risks for an individual, rather than allotting that power to the individual, opens the door to unfair treatment whenever an employer has reason to believe that workplace conditions or activities may be harmful.

The ADA requires reasonable accommodations or modifications for otherwise qualified individuals (sections 102[b][5], 302[b][2][A][ii]). This requires adaptation of facilities to make them accessible, modification of equipment to make it usable, and job restructuring to provide more flexible schedules for persons who need medical treatment (section 101[9]). To accommodate otherwise qualified persons with infectious conditions, an entity might have to reduce or eliminate the risk of transmission. Employers, for example, might be required to provide infection control and training to reduce nosocomial (disease or condition acquired in the hospital) or blood-borne infections. An employer, however, is not forced to endure an undue hardship that would alter the fundamental nature of the business or would be disproportionately costly. The Eighth Circuit Court of Appeals, for example, held that a school for persons with mental retardation was not obliged to vaccinate employees in order reasonably to accommodate a student who was an active carrier of hepatitis B virus (*Kohl v. Woodhaven Learning Center,* 1989).

Conceptual Foundations of Disability Law

Conceptually, disability law follows two distinct traditions—equal treatment (based on civil rights law) and special treatment (based on social welfare law). The equal treatment perspective means that persons with disabilities should be treated as if their disabilities do not matter. Accordingly, the law mandates businesses, public accommodations, public services, transportation, and communications authorities not to discriminate. This concept of equal treatment is powerfully articulated in the law. At the same time disability law also requires special treatment. The law requires the aforementioned entities to adopt a concept of affirmative action that focuses on the person's disabilities, as well as on societal barriers to equal treatment (Feldblum, 1993). The ADA requires reasonable accommodations or modifications designed to enable or empower the person with disabilities to take his or her rightful place in society. The law, therefore, insists on special treatment when that is necessary to allow a person to perform a job, enter a public building, or receive public service. As the Supreme Court observed over two decades ago, "Sometimes the greatest discrimination can lie in treating things that are different as though they were exactly alike" (*Jenness, et al. v. Fortson*, p. 442).

Disability law, however, does not take either the equal treatment or the special treatment principle to its logical extension. With respect to equal treatment, the Supreme Court has dismantled the statute to such an extent that the ADA does not provide an effective remedy for many individuals with a disability. With respect to special treatment, the ADA does not allocate tax dollars to enable the person to participate equally in society, beyond use of government funds for *reasonable accommodations* in such areas as public transportation. Nor does it require covered entities to spend unlimited amounts to provide equal access and opportunities for persons with disabilities.

Conclusion: A New Vision

The ADA promised to revolutionize the way we view the law's protection and empowerment of persons with disabilities. No longer were we supposed to see persons with disabilities through the lens of charity, sympathy, or benign discretion. Now we were supposed to see persons with disabilities through the lens of civil rights law. Under civil rights law persons with disabilities should not have to not ask for societal favors. They should be able to demand an equal place in a society that has long been structured—physically and sociologically—by and for the able-bodied.

This promise and vision, however, have been sharply curtailed by the Supreme Court. It is no longer realistic to believe that persons with disabilities will receive the same kind of civil rights protection as, say, African Americans and women. For that to happen, Congress will have to amend the ADA to express the vision of true inclusion and protection against discrimination for all Americans with a disability.

LAWRENCE O. GOSTIN (1995)
REVISED BY AUTHOR

SEE ALSO: *Access to Healthcare; Genetic Discrimination; Human Rights; Informed Consent; Law and Bioethics; Medicaid; Patients' Rights; Right to Die; Utilitarianism and Bioethics;* and other *Disability* subentries

BIBLIOGRAPHY

Albertsons v. Kirkinburg. 527 U.S. 555 (1999).

Alexander v. Choate. 469 U.S. 287 (1985).

Americans with Disabilities Act of 1990. 42 U.S.C. 12101–12213 (Supp. II 1990).

Bowen v. American Hospital Association. 476 U.S. 610 (1986).

Bragdon v. Abbott. 524 U.S. 624 (1998).

Chevron U.S.A. Inc. v. Echazabal. 122 S. CT. 2045 (2002).

City of Cleburne, Texas v. Cleburne Living Center, Inc. 473 U.S. 432 (1985).

Civil Rights Act of 1964, codified as amended in scattered sections of 42 U.S.C. (1988).

D'Agostino, Thomas. 1997. "Defining 'Disability' Under the ADA: 1997 Update." *National Disability Law Reporter* Special Report No. 3.

DeShaney v. Winnebago County Department of Social Services. 489 U.S. 189 (1989).

Education for All Handicapped Children Act of 1975. 20 U.S.C. 1400 et seq. (1975).

Fair Housing Amendments Act of 1988. 42 U.S.C. 3601–3619 (1988).

Feldblum, Chai R. 1991. "The Americans with Disabilities Act: Definition of Disability." *Labor Lawyer* 7(1): 11–26.

Feldblum, Chai R. 1993. "Anti-Discrimination Requirements of the ADA." In *Implementing the Americans with Disabilities Act: Rights and Responsibilities of All Americans,* ed. Lawrence O. Gostin and Henry Beyer. Baltimore, MD: Paul H. Brooks.

Feldblum, Chai R. 1996. "The (R)evolution of Physical Disability Anti-discrimination Law: 1976–1996." *Mental and Physical Disability Law Reporter* September–October: 613–625.

Gerben v. Holsclaw. 692 F.Supp. 557 (E.D.Pa. 1988).

Gostin, Lawrence O. 1987. "The Future of Public Health Law." *American Journal of Law and Medicine* 3–4: 461–490.

Gostin, Lawrence O. 1991a. "Genetic Discrimination: The Use of Genetically Based Diganostic and Prognostic Tests by Employers and Insurers." *American Journal of Law and Medicine* 17(1–2): 109–144.

Gostin, Lawrence O. 1991b. "Public Health Powers: The Imminence of Radical Change." *Milbank Memorial Fund Quarterly* 69(Supp. 1–2): 268–290.

Gostin, Lawrence O. 1993. "Impact of the ADA on the Health Care System: Genetic Discrimination in Employment and Insurance." In *Implementing the Americans with Disabilities Act: Rights and Responsibilities of All Americans,* ed. Lawrence O. Gostin and Henry Beyer. Baltimore, MD: Paul H. Brooks.

Gostin, Lawrence O. 2002. "The Judicial Dismantling of the Americans with Disabilities Act." *Hastings Center Report.* November-December 20–22.

Gostin, Lawrence O., and Beyer, Henry, eds. 1993. *Implementing the Americans with Disabilities Act: Rights and Responsibilities of All Americans.* Baltimore, MD: Paul H. Brooks.

Herr, Stanley S.; Gostin, Lawrence O.; Koh, Harold H., eds. 2003. *Different but Equal: The Rights of Persons with Intellectual Disabilities.* Oxford: Oxford University Press.

H.R. Conference Report no. 101–596. 102nd Cong., 1st Sess. (1990).

Individuals with Disabilities Education Act of 1992. 20 U.S.C. 1400 et seq. (1991).

Jenness, et al. v. Fortson. 403 U.S. 431 (1971).

Kohl v. Woodhaven Learning Center. 865 F.2d 930 (8th Cir. 1989).

New York State Association of Retarded Children v. Carey. 612 F.2d 644 (2d Cir. 1979).

National Council on Disability. 1997. *Equality of Opportunity: The Making of the Americans with Disabilities Act.* Washington, D.C.: National Council on Disability.

Parmet, Wendy E. 1990. "Discrimination and Disability: The Challenges of the ADA." *Law, Medicine and Health Care* 18(4): 331–344.

Rehabilitation Act of 1973. 29 U.S.C. 791–794. (1988 and Supp. I 1989).

School Board of Nassau County, Florida v. Arline. 480 U.S. 273 (1987).

Southeastern Community College v. Davis. 442 U.S. 397 (1979).

S. Rep. no. 116. 101st Cong., 1st Sess. (1989).

Sutton v. United Airlines, Inc. 527 U.S. 471 (1999).

Toyota Motor Manufacturing Kentucky Inc. v. Williams. 534 U.S. 184 (2002).

West, Jane. 1993. "The Evolution of Disability Rights." In *Implementing the Americans with Disabilities Act: Rights and Responsibilities of All Americans,* ed. Lawrence O. Gostin and Henry Beyer. Baltimore, MD: Paul H. Brooks.

DIVIDED LOYALTIES IN MENTAL HEALTHCARE

• • •

Physicians have traditionally understood their primarily loyalty as being to the patients they serve. This tradition goes back to at least to the time healers left behind their shamanistic roots, some twenty-five centuries ago. So important is this sacred commitment that it is enshrined in Hippocratic Oath, with which physicians and the public often identify the medical profession. The relationship between physician and patient is understood as a fiduciary relationship, meaning it is based on trust. Other healthcare professions—and indeed other professions—have modeled their self-understanding on this sort of promise to benefit those served.

Situations do arise in which physicians and other professionals experience divided loyalties—divided between allegiance to the patient and allegiance to some other interest. This has traditionally been spoken of as "the dual-agent (or double-agent) problem." A physician or therapist is a dual agent, for example, if he or she owes an allegiance to an employer as well as the patient. In situations of divided loyalties the integrity of a physician's judgment or action may be compromised. Classic examples of this occur when a physician (especially a psychiatrist) works for the military or for a state or federal institution, where confidences cannot be guaranteed. Increasingly, physicians and other providers find themselves asked to serve the broader interests of society; that is, the interests of populations rather than individuals. This is especially true for those working for large organizations, such as health maintenance organizations (HMOs), managed-care organizations, or nationalized health services. In these situations, the physician must recognize an obligation to society, making it more difficult to buffer the unique concern for each individual patient.

From the moral point of view, most dual-agent situations are best seen as cases of conflicting loyalties or clashing duties. The doctor must choose one duty over another (Macklin, 1982). Perhaps most problematic are situations in which the patient assumes (because of the weight of the professions' patient-centered ethic) that the doctor is working for the patients' best interest. A psychiatrist in a pre-arraignment examination might be able to elicit more information then a police interrogation simply by presenting a trusting demeanor. But if the message is not "I am here to help you," then the purpose of the examination should be directly stated. An administrative evaluation in a student health service should clearly state, "You are being evaluated at the request of the dean, who will receive a report of my findings." A health professional should not give the impression that everything a person says is confidential if that is not the case.

While cases in psychiatry and mental health have received the most attention, this attention has increased awareness of the problem of divided loyalties in virtually all areas of healthcare. A quick literature search for "divided loyalties" on the Internet returns results from the following specialties: nursing (Winslow; Dinc and Ulusoy; Chao; Tabik, 1996), ophthalmology (Addison), sports medicine (Sim), occupational medicine (Walsh), physical therapy (Lurie; Bruckner), military medicine (Howe; Camp; Pearn; Hines), transplant medicine (Bennett; Tabik, 1994), clinical researchers (Miller), aviation medicine (McCrary), infectious diseases, obstetrics (Plambeck), student health and those doing administrative evaluations and disability evaluations (Lomas and Berman), and house physicians and residents (Morris; La Puma), as well as psychiatrists, forensic psychiatrists and physicians, and child psychiatrists and pediatricians. Issues of privacy, especially the privacy of medical records, cut across all disciplines in the information age, as do issues of cost containment, reimbursement, and healthcare funding. While all these disciplines face situations of divided loyalties, perhaps nowhere is the conflict more dramatic than it is in nursing, where loyalties have undergone a transformation from loyalty to the individual physician for whom and with whom a nurse works, to the healthcare institution that employs the nurse, to patients more generally, and finally to the principles of medical ethics that inform the values of all professions.

Background and History

Divided-loyalty dilemmas have been most blatant in efforts at social control. Since mental healthcare often deals with deviance in behavior, its conceptions run parallel to society's conceptions of social behavior, personal worth, and morality. Thus, in certain situations, there may be great pressure for mental-health professionals to label patients on the basis of social, ethical, or legal norms, and not on clearly established clinical or laboratory evidence of psychopathology.

Doctors are influenced in their activity and judgment by sociocultural context, by the ideology implicit in their professional training, and by the economic and organizational constraints of the setting in which they practice. Their practice involves multiple and, at times, competing professional roles with different social and ethical requirements, but often with no clear definition of boundaries (Mechanic). The practitioner must always ask the crucial question: Whom do I represent and whom do I serve? History is replete with cases showing that the patient is not always the primary one represented.

Extreme cases put the more mundane cases into perspective. Psychiatrists in the former Soviet Union (as well as in other Eastern European countries and in the People's Republic of China) have come under scrutiny for hospitalizing political dissidents and labeling them psychiatrically impaired (Bloch and Reddaway). Physicians in the military governments of Latin American have (perhaps under coercion themselves) cooperated with the torture of political prisoners, a situation that also occurred in South Africa during the period of apartheid. Nazi physicians conducted experiments in concentration camps that would have previously been unimaginable, giving rise to the safeguards of informed consent now required (Drob; Lifton, 1976, 1986). Nazi doctors acted completely contrary to their own moral and professional commitments, serving the ideology of the state and not their patients. These historic lessons make the need to examine divided loyalties all the more urgent.

The use of psychiatry as an instrument of social control had a long history in the former Soviet Union. Soviet authorities chose to have dissenters from official governmental policy labeled with mental illness designations such as schizophrenia, "sluggish schizophrenia," or paranoid development of the personality. The labeling of persons as mentally ill is an effective way to discredit their beliefs and actions, and to maintain control over those persons of whom a government disapproves.

Although the situation in the former Soviet Union was extreme, there have been examples in other societies in which psychiatry has been used (or abused) to stifle nonconformity, serving the interest of someone other than the patient. Notorious examples include the poet Ezra Pound and the actress Frances Farmer, both of whom where involuntarily hospitalized for political extremism (Arnold).

In cases of controversial religious movements, distressed families have sought help from mental health professionals to "rescue" and "deprogram" their children from such groups or cults. The mental health professional may be caught in a divided-loyalty dilemma between family values and religious liberties, possibly medicalizing religious conversions and then treating them as illnesses (Post). On the other hand, vulnerable young people may be particularly susceptible to coercive group pressure, and mental health professionals have traditionally acted in the "best interest of the child" for autonomous growth and development.

The question of divided loyalty can readily arise in matters of confidentiality. Mental health professionals cherish confidentiality as a prerequisite for psychotherapeutic work, but what is an appropriate limit to confidentiality when a patient reveals plans that might endanger others? This question came dramatically to public attention in 1974, when Tatiana Tarasoff, a college student, was murdered. Lawsuits were subsequently brought by the student's parents against the university, the campus police, and the psychotherapist who had failed to warn Tarasoff of threats made against her life by a fellow student (and patient of the therapist) who had fallen in love with her and whose love was unrequited. The therapist had alerted campus police to the danger his patient posed, but they arrested him, found him harmless, and released him.

The military is an organization whose needs and interests may compete with those of the patient. In the military, mental-health professionals are committed to serving society by supporting their commanders in carrying out military operations (Howe). The psychiatrist who returns a soldier to mental health may be returning him to a battlefield where he could be killed. Robert Jay Lifton highlights this ethical conflict by showing that the soldier's very sanity in seeking escape from the environment via a psychiatric judgment of instability renders him eligible for the continuing madness of killing and dying (a perfect example of Joseph Heller's "Catch-22"). Even in military situations, mental health professionals retain obligations to their profession. Further, their clinical effectiveness requires that they give high priority to the needs and interests of the military personnel they treat. In most cases, the mental health professional's ambiguous position in military medicine as a dual agent allows the person to believe that he or she is participating in both the care of patients and the public interest (Howe).

The prison system has also been the setting for a variety of divided-loyalty dilemmas. The professional may be called upon to evaluate an accused person's competency to stand trial. If treated, the person may become competent to stand trial, but left untreated the psychosis may prevent the person from participating in his or her own defense. In capital cases this can be a matter of life or death. How does a physician understand this obligation to the patient when providing treatment, particularly antipsychotic medication that may ultimately lead to conviction and death?

Conflicting obligations can easily arise in situations where doctors ask their own patients to participate in clinical research. While most doctors comply with their primary obligation to deliver the best possible care to their patients, the demands of adhering to a strict research design can create obligations that compete with those of giving good medical care. The research-oriented physician must maintain special ethical vigilance to assure that the patients' interest comes first, a vigilance that is reinforced by external review of research consent procedures.

Ethical Analysis and Resolution

A first step in resolving divided loyalties is to think of loyalty as an attachment or allegiance to a person or cause, and to see it as expressing a coherent meaning that unifies one's personal and professional conduct (Dwyer). Loyalties develop with the assumption of roles and relationships both inside and outside of professional practice. The professional's identity is connected with the primary role of restoring the patient to health. In approaching a divided-loyalty dilemma, it is necessary to articulate and reflect on the meaning of one's commitments in order to determine how these commitments ought to be ordered or reconciled in a particular case.

A basic principle of medical practice is that health professionals should be loyal to their patients and be advocates for them. This commitment does not always avoid conflict. For example, even when health professionals devote themselves exclusively to the good of the patient and show no allegiance to other persons or causes, conflicts may still arise between what the professional sees as good treatment and what the patient wants and sees as good treatment.

The roots of the confidentiality concept are essentially ethical and not legal, and from the earliest days of medical practice, respect for the patient's confidences has been considered an important part of the obligation owed by the physician to the patient. Communications told in secret and in trust have been guarded and respected. In a situation such as the Tarasoff case, however, while acknowledging the desirability of maintaining patients' confidences, one sees a strong competing ethical obligation. When a patient intends harm to another person, or when information is required for the adjudication of a dispute in court, physicians are faced with the claim that societal interests should take precedence. While absolute confidentiality is no longer the expectation, arguments for protecting and extending confidentiality, even in the face of competing demands, remain strong. The arguments usually rest on both ethical and utilitarian grounds and center on the moral good reflected in protecting private utterances. The arguments relate to the belief that confidentiality promotes desirable goals, such as encouraging potential patients to seek medical care and allowing patients to unburden themselves and provide all the information essential for the doctor to help them. In a healthcare system such as that in the United States, the practitioner's relationship to

the patient is fiduciary—that is, he or she acts for the benefit of the patient. Can modifications be made that do not compromise the fiduciary relationship? Can the doctor–patient relationship be extended to support affirmative duties not only to the patient but also for the benefit of third parties? Ralph Slovenko, an attorney-psychologist, answers this question in the affirmative, stating that a psychiatrist's loyalty to the patient and responsibility for treating the professional relationship with respect and honor do not negate responsibilities to third parties, to the rest of the profession, to science, or to society. Slovenko goes on to say, however, that how these other duties are accepted, how the patient is kept informed, and how the patient is cared for when other duties are carried out can either introduce or help to avoid a divided-loyalty dilemma.

Joan Rinas and Sheila Clyne-Jackson recommend a forthright stance in preventing dual-agent dilemmas. They argue that the mental health professional has obligations to all parties with whom he or she has a relationship. These duties include notifying all parties of their rights, the professional's specific obligations to each party, potential and realistic conflicts that may arise, and limitations in knowledge and service. If, on exchange of this information, the mental health professional concludes that he or she is not the appropriate one to provide the requested service, the patient or the third party should be referred to a professional appropriate and qualified to perform the desired function. Participants in a Hastings Center symposium on double agentry made a similar set of recommendations for addressing divided-loyalty dilemmas (Steinfels and Levine).

The answer to what appears to be a divided-loyalty dilemma in court cases may rest on a particular type of disclosure. Where the psychiatrist is functioning as a friend of the court, the primary loyalty is not to the patient but to society as embodied in the judicial system. In such settings, the doctor–patient relationship does not exist in the traditional sense. Both doctor and patient must understand this from the outset. Divided-loyalty dilemmas are prevented when the psychiatrist advises all parties involved that the relevant materials they provide will be used in the court proceedings and that he or she is functioning as a consultant to the court (Goldzband).

Financial Considerations

Divided loyalties are becoming more prevalent due to efforts at cost containment and the rationing of health services. Society is demanding that healthcare costs be controlled. In response, careful protocols are being developed as to what services can be given, and for how long they can be given.

These cost-containment methods may interfere with what patients realistically need to remedy their health problems, and can therefore compromise the ethical principle of doctor as patient advocate. Ruth Macklin emphasizes that whether doctors cut costs voluntarily in treating their patients or are required to adhere to policies instituted by others, their ability to advocate vigorously for their patients' medical needs is weakened. When rationing becomes a factor in physicians' treatment decisions, such as which patients will be admitted to the hospital and for how long, physicians are forced into a divided-loyalty conflict. Further, the care obligation embraced by medical ethics cannot be accomplished without permitting a physician to strive for "a robust patient–physician relationship, patient well-being, and avoidance of harm" (Wolf, p. 38).

Conclusion

Conflicting responsibilities, contradictory goals, hidden scenarios, and unsigned contracts existing in the changing world of both the patient and the professional serve as reminders that ideal resolutions may be unattainable in many divided-loyalty dilemmas. Professionals must be very sensitive to the possibility that they may become double agents in the routines of their everyday practice with its many ambiguities and subtleties.

Further, review and examination of dual-agent issues should be a continuing obligation of mental health professionals, for that is one way to prevent these issues from disrupting the doctor-patient relationship. These are issues that often come before professional ethics committees, which keep them alive through education, codes, and professional discipline.

In cases of divided loyalties, physicians and other health professionals should give the patient their primary loyalty, and other allegiances should be subordinated to that of the patient. Where this is not possible, any conflicting allegiance should be explicitly disclosed. The goal of maintaining trust is essential for the therapeutic relationship, and anything that erodes that goal diminishes not only the therapy or the treatment, but also the therapist and the profession he or she represents.

JAMES ALLEN KNIGHT (1995)
REVISED BY ALLEN R. DYER
LAURA WEISS ROBERTS

SEE ALSO: *Conflict of Interest; Profession and Professional Ethics; Professional-Patient Relationship; Psychiatry, Abuses of; Research, Unethical*

BIBLIOGRAPHY

Addison, D. J., et al. 1988. "Divided Loyalties?" *Canadian Journal of Ophthalmology* 23(7): 297–298.

Arnold, Williams. 1978. *Shadowland.* New York: McGraw-Hill.

American Psychiatric Association. 2001. *The Principles of Medical Ethics With Annotations Applicable to Psychiatry.* Washington, D.C.: Author.

Arnstein, Robert L. 1986. "Divided Loyalties in Adolescent Psychiatry: Late Adolescence." *Social Science and Medicine* 23(8): 797–802.

Baer, E. D. 1989. "Nursing's Divided Loyalties: A Historical Case Study." *Nursing Research* 38(3): 166–171.

Bennett W. M. 2001. "Divided Loyalties: Relationships between Nephrologists and Industry." *American Journal of Kidney Diseases* 37(1): 210–221.

Block, S., and Reddaway, P. 1977. "Russia's Political Hospitals: The Abuse of Psychiatry in the Soviet Union." London: Gollancz (published in the U.S. as *Psychiatric Terror: How Society Psychiatry Is Used to Suppress Dissent.* New York: Basic Books).

Bruckner, J., et al. 1987. "Physical Therapists As Double Agents. Ethical Dilemmas of Divided Loyalties." *Physical Therapy* 67(3): 383–387.

Camp, N. M., et al. 1993. "The Vietnam War and the Ethics of Combat Psychiatry." *American Journal of Psychiatry* 150(7): 1000–1010.

Chao, T. M. 1995. "Nursing's Values from a Confucian Perspective." *Internation Nursing Review* 42(5): 147–149.

Clouser, K. Danner. "What is Medical Ethics?" *Annals of Internal Medicine* 80: 657–660.

Dinc, L., and Ulusoy, M. F. 1998. "How Nurses Approach Ethical Problems in Turkey." *International Nursing Review* 45(5): 137–139.

Dougherty, Charles J. 1988. "Mind, Money, and Morality: Ethical Dimensions of Economic Change in American Psychiatry." *Hastings Center Report* 18(3): 15–20.

Drob, Sanford L. 1992. "The Lessons from History: Physicians' Dual Loyalty in the Nazi Death Camps." *Review of Clinical Psychiatry and the Law* 3: 167–171.

Dwyer, James. 1992. "Conflicting Loyalties in the Practice of Psychiatry: Some Philosophical Reflections." *Review of Clinical Psychiatry and the Law* 3: 157–166.

Dyer, Allen R. 1988. *Ethics and Psychiatry: Toward Professional Definition.* Washington, D.C.: American Psychiatric Press.

Gellman, R. M., et al. 1986. "Divided Loyalties: A Physician's Responsibilities in an Information Age." *Social Science and Medicine* 23(8): 817–826.

Goldzband, Melvin G. 1992. "Dual Loyalties in Custody Cases and Elsewhere in Child and Adolescent Psychiatry." *Review of Clinical Psychiatry and the Law* 3: 201–207.

Hines, A. H.; Ader, D. N.; Chang, A. S.; and Rundell, J. R. 1998. "Dual Agency, Dual Relationships, Boundary Crosssings, and Associated Boundary Violations: A Survery of Military and Civilian Psychiatrists." *Military Medicine* 163(12): 826–833.

Howe, Edmund G. 1986. "Ethical Issues Regarding Mixed Agency of Military Physicians." *Social Science and Medicine* 23(8): 803–815.

Lifton, Robert Jay. 1976. "Advocacy and Corruption in the Healing Professions." *International Review of Psychoanalysis* 3(4): 385–398.

Lifton, Robert Jay. 1986. *The Nazi Doctors: Medical Killing and the Psychology of Genocide.* New York: Basic Books.

La Puma, J. 1996. "House Physicians: Accountabilities and Possibilities." *Archives of Internal Medicine* 156(22): 2529–2533.

Lomas, H. D., and Burman, J. D. 1983. "Diagnosing for Administrative Purposes." *Social Science and Medicine* 17(4): 241–244.

Lurie, S. G. 1994. "Ethical Dilemmas and Profession Roles in Occupations Medicine." *Social Science and Medicine* 38(10): 1367–1374.

Macklin, Ruth. 1982. *Man, Mind, and Morality: The Ethics of Behavior Control.* Englewood Cliffs, NJ: Prentice Hall.

Macklin, Ruth. 1987. *Mortal Choices: Bioethics in Today's World.* New York: Pantheon.

McCrary, B. F. 1992. "Ethical Concerns in the Practice of Military Aviation Medicine." *Aviation and Space Environmental Medicine* 63(12): 1109–1111.

Mechanic, David. 1981. "The Social Dimension." In *Psychiatric Ethics,* ed. Sidney Bloch and Paul Chodoff. New York: Oxford University Press.

Miller, F. G.; Rosenstein, D. L.; and De Renzo, E. G. 1998. "Professional Integrity in Clinical Research" *Journal of the American Medical Association* 280(16): 1449–1454.

Morreim, Haavi E. 1988. "Cost Containment: Challenging Fidelity and Justice." *Hastings Center Report* 18(6): 20–25.

Morris, M., et al. 1992. "When Loyalties Are Divided between Teachers and Patients." *Journal of Medical Ethics* 18(3): 153–155.

Murray, Thomas H. 1986. "Divided Loyalties for Physicians: Social Context and Moral Problems." *Social Science and Medicine* 23(8): 827–832.

Pearn, J., et al. 2000. "Medical Ethics Surveillance in the Armed Forces." *Military Medicine* 165(5): 351–354.

Pellegrino, E. D. 1993. "Societal Duty and Moral Complicity: The Physician's Dilemma of Divided Loyalty." *International Journal of Law and Psychiatry* 16(3–4): 371–391.

Pellegrino, E. D. 1994. "Ethics." *Journal of the American Medical Association* 272(21): 1668–1670.

Plambeck, Cheryl M. 2002. "Divided Loyalties: Legal and Bioethical Considerations of Physician–Pregnant Patient Confidentiality and Prenatal Drug Abuse." *Journal of Legal Medicine* 23(1): 1–35.

Post, Stephen P. 1993. "Psychiatry and Ethics: The Problematics of Respect for Religious Meanings." *Culture, Medicine, and Psychiatry* 17(3): 363–383.

Rinas, Joan, and Clyne-Jackson, Sheila. 1988. *Professional Conduct and Legal Concerns in Mental Health Practice.* Norwalk, CT: Appleton and Lange.

Roberts, Laura Weiss, and Dyer, Allen R. 2003. *Concise Guide to Mental Health Ethics.* Arlington, VA: American Psychiatric Publishing.

Rodwin, M. A. 1995. "Strains in the Fiduciatry Metaphor: Divided Physician Loyalties and Obligations in a Changing Health Care System." *American Journal of Law and Medicine* 21(2–3): 241–257.

Sim, J. 1993. "Sports Medicine: Some Ethical Issues." *British Journal of Sports Medicine* 27(2): 95–100.

Slovenko, Ralph. 1975. "Psychotherapy and Confidentiality." *Cleveland State Law Review* 24: 375–396.

Steinfels, Margaret O'Brien, and Levine, Carol, eds. 1978. "In the Service of the State: The Psychiatrist as Double Agent." *Hastings Center Report,* spec. supp. 8(2): 1–24.

Szasz, Thomas S. 1970. *Ideology and Insanity: Essays on the Psychiatric Dehumanization of Man.* New York: Anchor.

Tabik N. 1994. "Divided Loyalties and Conflicting Interests: Ethical Dilemmas in Organ Transplantation." *Professional Nursing* 9(9): 592–599.

Tabik, N. 1996. "Informed Consent: The Nurses' Dilemma." *Medical Law* 15(1): 7–16.

Walsh, D. C., et al. 1986. "Divided Loyalties in Medicine: The Ambivalence of Occupational Medical Practice." *Social Science and Medicine* 23(8): 789–796.

Winslow, G. R. 1984. "From Loyalty to Advocacy: A New Metaphor for Nursing." *Hastings Center Report* 14(3): 42–40.

Wolf, Susan M. 1994. "Health Care Reform and the Future of Physician Ethics." *Hastings Center Report* 24(2): 28–41.

DNA IDENTIFICATION

• • •

In 1985, Alex J. Jeffries and his colleagues demonstrated that patterns of molecular markers in human DNA, or *DNA fingerprints,* could serve as uniquely identifying personal traits. This discovery was quickly applied by the criminal justice system, as way of definitively connecting suspects with blood, tissue, or semen from crime scenes. Shortly thereafter, governments at the state and national levels began authorizing the collection of DNA samples from individuals convicted of violent crimes who were considered at high risk for recidivism. By 1998, all fifty states in the United States had enacted such laws, and the U.S. Federal Bureau of Investigation (FBI) was able to launch a national electronic database of DNA profiles from convicted criminals for use in future cases (Hoyle). In the interim, the collection of DNA for personal identification purposes has already become mandatory within the military and has become a mainstay of civilian efforts to clarify the identities of children and kidnap victims, to investigate family lineages, and even to authenticate religious relics. On the horizon, lies the question that civil libertarians anticipate with dread: Why not store personally identifying genetic information on everyone as a matter of course, for the advances in public safety and personal security that can be gained thereby?

Photographs and traditional fingerprints have, of course, also been taken, collected, and used for all these same purposes in the past. But unlike photography and manual fingerprinting, collecting individually identifying DNA patterns (iDNAfication) does involve taking bits of people's bodies from them: nucleated cells and their complements of DNA molecules. For those concerned about the ethical and legal status of body tissues and an individual's ability to control what happens to him or her through use of that tissue, this corporeal side of iDNAfication raises an interesting challenge. Clearly, questions of personal privacy are involved. But unlike most other disputes over body tissues, the issues here are not primarily matters of personal sovereignty.

For example, unlike involuntary sterilization or forced surgeries, the central concern with mandatory iDNAfication does not seem to be the violation of a person's bodily integrity. Compared with the other infringements of personal freedom that legitimately accompany legal arrest, providing a saliva or cheek swab sample seems negligibly invasive (Schultz). Moreover, unlike the creation of marketable human cell lines or the commercialization of organ procurement, it is not the exploitation or misappropriation of the person's body for others's gain that is centrally troubling either. Manual fingerprints and photographs also exploit suspects's bodies in order to incriminate them, without raising special privacy concerns. Moreover, consider the fact that it does not matter to an identical twin whether a DNA sample under scrutiny actually comes from him or his sibling: To the extent that the genetic information it contains describes both their bodies, the privacy of each is endangered.

In fact, the major moral concern about iDNAfication has little to do with whether the DNA analyzed is a piece of the person being identified, the property of the person being identified, or even is forcibly extracted from the person being identified. In most iDNAfication contexts, these physical, proprietary, and decisional privacy considerations are beside the point. Rather, the important feature of iDNAfication is what the DNA analyzed can *disclose about* the person being identified. It is, in other words, individuals's informational privacy that is at stake in the prospect of widespread iDNAfication, and it is in those terms that the policy challenge of iDNAfication should be framed. What

should society be allowed to learn about its citizens in the course of attempting to identify them?

Taking up this challenge means taking seriously the precedents set by society's use of photography and manual fingerprinting, since their primary impact on personal privacy also lies in the identifying information they record rather than the nature of their acquisition. If the collection of mandatory *mug shots* and fingerprint impressions are taken as benchmarks of social acceptance for at least some identification purposes, any iDNAfication methods that conveyed no more personal information than those techniques should also be socially acceptable, for at least the same range of purposes. Thus, where fingerprints of arrestees, inmates, employees and recruits are now taken legitimately, performing iDNAfication should also be justified, if its informational privacy risks were equivalent. Similarly, if society accepts the personal disclosures involved in using photographs on drivers's licenses and identification cards, it should be willing, in theory, to expose an equivalent range of genetic information in any legitimate forms of iDNAfication. One approach to the general challenge of iDNAfication, then, would be to ask the following question: If the ways in which photographs and manual fingerprints are used for legitimate identification purposes are accepted, under what circumstances, if any, might forms of iDNAfication meet the standard those practices set for the disclosure of personal information?

Personal Privacy Considerations

A number of personal privacy risks of iDNAfication have been described and anticipated in the design of some iDNAfication programs. Thus, for example, many have pointed out that if the DNA sequences used as the components of an iDNAfication profile are taken from the regions of the human genome that code for proteins, important biological information about their sources could be revealed, including information about their paternity, current health status, and potential health risks (U.S. Congress Office of Technology Assessment (OTA), National Academy of Sciences). Any risk of disclosing sensitive personal information of these sorts would clearly increase the intrusiveness of iDNAfication beyond that of traditional fingerprinting and photography. In addition, it could expose the person being described to the possibility of discrimination on the basis of a disclosed genotype (Bereano; DeGorgey; Scheck; Sankar) Fortunately, this is a privacy risk that can be almost entirely eliminated by two simple precautions: One need only avoid analyzing biologically informative DNA, and destroy the DNA samples upon analysis.

The first precaution can be accomplished by restricting the sections of DNA that are amplified, analyzed and utilized in the iDNAfication profile to the non-coding regions of DNA between our functional genes. By definition, markers selected from these regions will not disclose any biologically significant information. Rather, like fingerprints, they could merely provide a unique pattern to match in seeking to identify an unknown person. Even photographs are useful mainly as patterns to match, rather than for what they can independently tell us about the person pictured in them. Serendipitously, individual variation is also vastly more pronounced in this so called junk DNA (since mutations can accumulate in these sections without having any adverse effect on genomic function), making it more attractive for iDNAfication purposes on scientific grounds as well.

Thus, the FBI, in establishing standardized forensic iDNAfication markers for use by state laboratories contributing DNA profiles to the latter's National DNA Index System (NDIS), has focused on a set of thirteen loci from non-coding regions that contain series of repeated nucleotide sequences whose length is highly variable between individuals (Hoyle). The exclusive use of these markers in any iDNAfication program would forestall most genetic privacy concerns linked to the biological information content of the DNA profile itself.

The second important step to insuring the genetic privacy of iDNAfication is to destroy the physical samples of DNA once DNA profiles have been generated from them. As long as the DNA samples themselves are retained, the risk remains that they could be retested for their biological informational content. Thus, in its report on forensic DNA analysis, the National Academy of Sciences in 1990 recommended that even samples taken from convicted offenders be destroyed promptly upon analysis, and the FBI has designed its national iDNAfication collection as a databank, not a DNA bank, including only the electronic profiles of non-coding DNA markers (Murch and Budowle).

This second precaution has not been adopted by forensic laboratories at the state level, or by the military at the federal level. Most of these laboratories plan to bank their actual DNA samples indefinitely, on the grounds that the samples may need to be retested as new markers or testing technologies become standard (McEwen). The Department of Defense is storing dried blood samples from its recruits, for genotyping only in the event that the recruits later turn up missing in combat. This effectively undercuts the privacy protections afforded by using non-coding markers in the iDNAfication profile itself, and immediately elevates the privacy risk of any iDNAfication program well beyond that of ordinary fingerprinting. Even if, *contra* the National

Academy of Sciences, this increased risk were tolerable for convicted offenders, it should not be for military recruits, government employees, or arrestees, since the potential intrusion goes well beyond what is required for identification.

Social Policy Considerations

Despite the initial hopes of early enthusiasts like English scientist Francis Galton (1822–1911), large collections of ordinary fingerprints have never been useful for much else besides individual identification. (Rabinow) The informational potential of the human genome, however, does require the designers of iDNAfication systems to consider in advance the range of uses they should accommodate. Even when a DNA profile collection is committed exclusively to use for personal identification purposes, several policy choices present themselves: (1) Should the system be designed to support any type of research involving the stored information? (2) Should the system be designed to aid in the identification of the sources of new DNA samples without clear matches in the database?, and (3) Should the system be designed to support electronic *dragnet* screening of the population in search of particular individuals? In the context of the expanding uses of iDNAfication, these choices raise some important social policy issues that go well beyond issues of personal privacy.

RESEARCH USES. Among the legislatively authorized uses of the existing iDNAfication databanks is their use for various kinds of research. For example, many state statutes, following the FBI's legislative guidelines, provide for the use of convicted offender iDNAfication data in research by state forensic scientists designed to improve iDNAfication techniques and protocols. Although the state statutes vary widely in the security procedures they mandate for containing this research within the crime laboratories and protecting the identities of the sample sources, if they were to implement the protections recommended by the FBI (Murch and Budowle) using such samples would raise few direct privacy issues. However, it is worth noting that to the extent that this research requires access to physical DNA samples, it provides the main impetus for retaining samples in state crime labs after the database profiles have been generated. This opens the door for other research uses of the collection. For example, Alabama allows the use of anonymous DNA samples from its convicted offender collection "to provide data relative to the causation, detection and prevention of disease or disability" and "to assist in other humanitarian endeavors including but not limited to educational research or medical research or development." (Alabama Laws [1994] 1st Spec Sess Act 94–100).

Alabama's generosity towards researchers is presumably premised on the view that the *anonymity* of the samples provides adequate protection of the sources's privacy, and frees the state from having to worry about the usual elements of biomedical research, like informed consent. But on the contrary, from the perspective of research ethics, these samples are not anonymous, nor even *anonymized,* since the iDNAfication database is itself the key to identifying the source of any given sample. Since that existing linkage makes it technically possible to benefit and harm the sample donors with the results of such research, all the usual biomedical research protections should apply (Clayton et. al.). In addition to these personal privacy issues, moreover, open-ended research on iDNAfication samples also poses broader questions of research justice. Collections of DNA samples from criminals or soldiers, for example, are likely to be perceived as particularly rich research resources by those interested in studying genetic factors involved in antisocial or aggressive behavior. Unfortunately, our social experience with such research has not been good (Marsh and Katz). Repeatedly, such studies have succumbed to ascertainment biases that ultimately mischaracterize—and stigmatize—groups of people that are disproportionately represented in the systems under study for social reasons. Two forms of injustice tend to flow from these results. First, genetic claims about individual research subjects, like those concerning XYY syndrome in the 1970s, become generalized to an entire class, simultaneously pathologizing behavior and stigmatizing bearers of the genetic trait. This has the effect of both undercutting personal responsibility and legitimizing draconian medical responses to the targeted behavior, like eugenic sterilization. Second, genetic studies tend to misdirect attention from the overwhelming social causes of the behaviors they purport to explain, by encouraging a determinism that suggests that efforts at social reform are ultimately futile. Where this misdirection reinforces existing social policy inequities, it is likely to have an even more pronounced effect (Wasserman).

PROFILING USES. The third kind of databank that is part of a comprehensive iDNAfication system (in addition to the identified DNA profile collection and the aggregate population polymorphism frequencies database) is an open case file: a collection of DNA profiles taken from crime scenes or battlefields or plane crash sites that come from as yet unidentified sources. Obviously, this collection needs to be comparable to the identified reference collection, which means the same markers should be used to compose the profiles in both. With these collections, however, investigators will be especially tempted to glean as much information as they can from their genetic analyses in their efforts to compose a profile of their missing sample source. One of the areas of highest interest has been in non-coding

polymorphisms that would allow investigators to estimate the *ethnic affiliation* of a sample source (Shriver, et al.). These investigators call their markers *population specific alleles* (PSAs), and the ethnic populations they mark are, once again, just our traditional races: European-Americans, African-Americans, native Americans, and Asian Americans. Should these PSAs be included in or excluded from the panel of markers established for our universal, humanitarian iDNAfication system? Including them would allow the system to support an open case file that could take advantage of the additional information to narrow the search for sample sources. It would also, presumably, take the guesswork out of deciding which racial reference group to assess a particular sample against.

Of course, including PSAs in iDNAfication profiles would elevate the informational content of the profile beyond that of a traditional fingerprint, constituting more of an intrusion on privacy. Moreover, it would do so by reporting a particularly socially sensitive feature of the arrestee: their probable race. But photographs also can reveal race, and we sanction collecting them for identification purposes. How would this be different?

Photography is an illuminating analogy here. Photographs show only the superficial distinctions that we use socially to categorize a person's ethnic affiliation. They leave that categorization itself up to the observer, and make no claims about its merits. Thanks to our large-scale hybridization, in other words, *passing* for one race or another is still possible in mug shots. PSAs, on the other hand, are defined in terms of our society's racial categories, and purport to be able to *appropriately classify* even interethnic individuals into their true (ancestral) categories.

This has several implications. First, it means that genuine secrets might be revealed through PSA screening: for example, shifts in the social (racial) status of the arrestee or her ancestors that have nothing to do with their arrest, but which, if interpreted as normative, could cause psychological and social harm to the individuals and their families by upsetting their social identities. In that sense, PSAs are more threatening to privacy than photographs. Second, as the scientists's own hopes for appropriately classifying hybrids shows, it is hard not make the logical mistake of moving from the use of social categories to define the PSAs to then using PSAs to define our social categories. This mistake raises two important issues about the use of PSAs in iDNAfication schemes.

First, it risks exacerbating racism by reinventing in statistical and molecular terms the arbitrary social apparatus of the *blood quantum* and *the One Drop Rule*: Under PSA screening, one's proportional racial endowment could be quantified, and carrying the defining polymorphisms for any given race would warrant (statistically) *affiliating* one with it for official identification purposes, regardless of one's superficial social identity. In the wake of a program of iDNAfication in which thousands of American's would have their PSAs determined, this could have powerful social consequences. In fact, our bad experiences with other forms of *low tech* racial profiling in law enforcement has already led to court decisions prohibiting the practice as unconstitutional under the Equal Protection clause (Johnson).

The second danger in estimating ethnic affiliation through PSAs is the way it facilitates the reification of (fundamentally unjust) social categories as biological realities. If PSAs are not *genes for race,* they are at least differentially associated with the people we classify in particular races. Genetic association, however, in the public and scientific mind, often comes to imply causation that implies in turn the objective reality of the effect. In other words, if PSAs correlate with racially defined populations, they must be linked somehow with the defining genes of those populations, and if the racial populations have defining genes, races must be real and separable biological entities, not just social constructions. Our society has had recurrent experience with this kind of *hardening of the categories,* all of which has been detrimental to the least well off (Duster) because it fosters a particular form of social harm: the erosion of our sense of solidarity as a community and our empathy for members of other groups, leading to what one scholar has called social policies moral abandonment (Wasserman). Any widespread iDNAfication program that involved PSA-based ethnic affiliation estimations would run the real risk of exacerbating that harm, by fostering the public perception that PSA-based profiles revealed real racial assignments.

DRAGNET USES. Finally, there is a third set of choices about the range of use to which any arrestee iDNAfication system should be put. Given our commitment to the presumption of innocence, should such a system accommodate *sweep searches* of its stored profiles in the pursuit of a criminal suspect? Obviously, in addition to the precise identification of sample sources, the principal purpose of the existing convicted offender iDNAfication databanks in law enforcement is to aid in the identification of suspects by matching unidentified DNA samples from a crime scene with an identified profile in the collection. If in fact we kept the informational content of arrestee iDNAfication under the *pattern matching* standard of manual fingerprinting, could we really complain about police searches of arrestee iDNAfication databases for the same purpose?

On one hand, it is clear that some dragnet uses of iDNAfication would not be acceptable in the United States.

Critics of current forensic iDNAfication programs often point to the 1987 British case in which every male resident in three Leicestershire villages was asked to voluntarily provide a DNA sample to the police in an (ultimately successful) effort to identify a murderer, as an cautionary sign of things to come (Wambaugh). However, given the coercive nature of such a request (police made house calls on those failing to appear for sampling), its effect of shifting the presumption of innocence to one of guilt, its lack of adequate probable cause, and the U.S. Supreme Court's rejection of similar uses of manual fingerprinting, it seems implausible that such a sampling practice would be constitutionally sanctioned in the United States.

However, what if the dragnet were only a matter of searching a database of DNA profiles previously collected by the state for the identification of arrestees? In supporting the existing convicted offender iDNAfication databases, the courts have argued that the public interest in prosecuting crime outweighs any presumption of innocence that criminals may have in future cases, thus justifying the reuse of their DNA fingerprints for forensic matching (*Jones v. Murray,* 1991). Moreover, we already store and reuse arrest photographs and manual fingerprints, even from those arrestees subsequently cleared of their charges, in attempting to identify suspects in future cases. Why should arrestee DNA fingerprints be handled differently?

Here is where the uniquely biological side of iDNAfication reenters the analysis, with its increased claims of physical privacy. U.S. courts have ruled that systematic analyses of tissue samples and body products (as opposed to photos and fingerprints) of suspects (as opposed to convicted criminals) are the sorts of searches that are protected by the Fourth Amendment, even when the samples are already in the state's hands. This suggests that, although one's arrest presumes enough probable cause to justify sampling for *identification* purposes, arrestees have not forfeited as much of their presumption of innocence and the physical privacy that attends it as convicted offenders have, whose samples can be searched at will by the state. If these decisions are accepted as precedents for iDNAfication, efforts to screen forensic DNA against a database of arrestee profiles from citizens who have no convictions would also have to pass the Fourth Amendment's tests, and show probable cause for each attempted match.

Moreover, if anything, the bar to dragnet searches of arrestee iDNAfication collections should be set higher than the bar to searching other tissue samples and body products, because DNA profile matching actually poses a greater risk to privacy than other forms of tissue typing. This is because, unlike both fingerprint and urinalysis screening, the process of matching a forensic sample against an iDNAfication database can reveal familial relationships as well as identities. Unlike fingerprints and photographs, in which the environmental vagaries of human development usually work to obscure any convincing evidence of kinship, DNA profiles can demonstrate those relationships in clear genetic terms.

Thus, when non-coding nuclear DNA markers are used to profile a forensic specimen, the siblings, parents, and children of the specimen source will all show partial matches with the specimen. Their appearance in an arrestee iDNAfication database will not make them direct suspects, because of the mismatching elements of the profile. But their matching elements can reveal that they are related to the suspect, and so will flag their family for further investigation by the police. Moreover, when mitochondrial DNA is used for genotyping, the resulting profiles will almost always be completely shared by the DNA source's mother and siblings, and by her mother and all her siblings as well: They are all essentially mitochondrial clones. In these cases, the appearance of family members in an arrestee database might even make them immediate suspects for investigation. In any case, the disclosure of the identities of a suspect's relatives is not something that fingerprint searches accomplish, which means that iDNAfication puts more personal information at risk. It therefore poses a greater threat to the privacy of both the arrestees and their kin. Moreover, experience from clinical DNA testing within families demonstrates that even in a supportive context, the disclosure of familial relationships can have tremendous psychosocial impact on family members (Juengst). To have those relationships disclosed publicly in the context of a criminal investigation only amplifies the risk that the impact will be negative on both the sample sources and their kin.

It is interesting to note in this regard that some states's convicted offender iDNAfication databanking statutes already include provisions mandating the expungement of a person's DNA profile, and the destruction of their samples, if their convictions are overturned or dismissed on appeal (McEwen and Reilly). The only circumstance in which that this happens with traditional fingerprints is in case of juvenile acquittals, where expungement is justified in terms of the burden of an early criminal record on the life prospects of the acquitted. This suggests that having one's DNA on file with the state is also recognized, at least in some states, to carry privacy risks to the individual that are unfair to impose on citizens cleared of criminal guilt, in the same way it is unfair to impose a criminal record on a reformed youth. But if that is true of those whose convictions are overturned, it should be equally true for those who are never convicted in the first place (Nelkin and Andrews).

ERIC T. JUENGST

SEE ALSO: *Autonomy; Bioterrorism; Confidentiality; Conflict of Interest; Conscience, Rights of; Genetic Discrimination; Genetic Testing and Screening; Human Rights; Public Health; Warfare*

BIBLIOGRAPHY

Bereano, Philip. 1990. "DNA Identification Systems: Social Policy and Civil Liberties Concerns." *International Journal of Bioethics* 1: 146–155.

Chakraborty, Rajit, and Kidd, Kenneth. 1991. "The Utility of DNA Typing in Forensic Work." *Science* 254: 1735.

Clayton, Ellen Wright, et al. 1995. "Informed Consent for Genetic Research on Stored Tissue Samples." *Journal of the American Medical Association* 274: 1786–1792.

DeGorgey, Andrea. 1990. "The Advent of DNA Databanks: Implications for Information Privacy" *American Journal of Law and Medicine* 16: 381–398.

Duster, Troy. 1992. "Genetics, Race and Crime: Recurring Seduction to a False Precision." In *DNA On Trial: Genetic Identification and Criminal Justice,* ed. Paul Billings. Cold Spring Harbor, NY: Cold Spring Harbor Laboratory Press.

Hoyle, Russ. 1998. "The FBI's National DNA Database." *Nature Biotechnology* 16(November): 987.

Jeffries, Alex J.; Wilson, V.; and Thein, S. L. 1985. "Individual-Specific *Fingerprints* of Human DNA." *Nature* 316: 76.

Johnson, Erica. 1995. "A Menace to Society: The Use of Criminal Profiles and Its Effects on Black Males." *Howard Law Journal* 38: 629–664.

Jones v. Murray, 763 F. Supp 842 (W.D. Va 1991).

Juengst, Eric. 1999. "Genetic Testing and Moral Dynamics of Family Life." *Public Understanding of Science* 8(3): 193–207.

McEwen, Jean. 1995. "Forensic DNA Data Banking by State Crime Laboratories." *American Journal of Human Genetics* 56: 1487–1492.

McEwen, Jean, and Reilly, Philip. 1994. "A Review of State Legislation on DNA Forensic Data Banking." *American Journal of Human Genetics* 54: 941–958.

Marsh, Frank, and Katz, Janet, eds.1985. *Biology, Crime and Ethics: A Study of Biological Explanations for Criminal Behavior.* Cincinnati, OH: Anderson Publishing Company.

Murch, Randall, and Budowle, Bruce. 1997. "Are Developoments in Forensic Applications of DNA Technology Consistent with Privacy Protections?" In *Genetic Secrets: Protecting Privacy and Confidentiality in the Genetic Era,* ed. Mark Rothstein. New York: Oxford University Press.

National Academy of Sciences. 1992. *DNA Technology in Forensic Science.* Washington, D.C.: National Academy Press.

Nelkin, Dorothy, and Andrews, Lori. 1999. "DNA Identification and Surveillance Creep." *Sociology of Illness and Health* 21: 689–699.

Rabinow, Paul. 1992. "Galton's Regret: Of Types and Individuals." In *DNA On Trial: Genetic Identification and Criminal*

Justice, ed. Paul Billings. Cold Spring Harbor, NY: Cold Spring Harbor Laboratory Press.

Sankar, Pamela. 1997. "The Proliferation and Risks of Government DNA Databases." *American Journal of Public Health* 87(3): 336–337.

Scheck, Barry. 1994. "DNA Data Banking: A Cautionary Tale." *American Journal of Human Genetics* 54: 931–933.

Schulz, Marjorie. 1992. "Reasons for Doubt: Legal Issues in the Use of DNA Identification Techniques." In *DNA on Trial: Genetic Identification and Criminal Justice,* ed. Paul Billings. Cold Spring Harbor, NY: Cold Spring Harbor Press.

Shriver, Mark, et al. 1997. "Ethnic Affiliation Estimation by Use of Population Specific DNA Markers." *American Journal of Human Genetics* 60: 962–963.

U.S. Congress Office of Technology Assessment. 1990. *Genetic Witness: Forensic Uses of DNA Tests,* OTA-BA-438. Washington, D.C: U.S. Government Printing Office.

Wambaugh, Joseph. 1989. *The Blooding.* New York: William Morrow.

Wasserman, David. 1995. "Science and Social Harm: Genetic Research into Crime and Violence." *Philosophy and Public Policy* 15(Winter): 14–19.

DNR (DO NOT RESUSCITATE)

• • •

In its most simple form, "DNR" is a physician's order directing a clinician to withhold any efforts to resuscitate a patient in the event of a respiratory or cardiac arrest. The literal form, *do not resuscitate,* is more precisely worded as *do not attempt resuscitation.* While originally intended for hospitalized patients, the concept of withholding resuscitative efforts has since been extended to include patients in nursing homes, children with incurable genetic or progressive neurologic diseases, and terminally ill patients in the home or hospice setting.

More broadly, the DNR order has become a part of the ritual of death in American society. For the patient, a DNR order (or the absence of a DNR order) establishes how death will likely ensue. The introduction of DNR orders also marked a pivotal change in the practice of medicine, for it was the first order to direct the withholding of treatment. DNR orders are so commonplace and widely accepted in everyday practice that nearly all physicians and nurses have had some experience in determining whether to invoke or adhere to the order when it is written.

History

Although commonplace and widely accepted today, the development of the do-not-resuscitate order was, and remains, controversial on several fundamental issues at the intersection of medicine and ethics. As with artificial (mechanical) ventilation and artificial nutrition and hydration, the development of advanced cardiopulmonary resuscitation (CPR) techniques created decision points regarding treatment alternatives for both dying patients and their caretakers that had not previously been confronted.

Prior to 1960 there was little that physicians could do for a patient in the event of sudden cardiac arrest. In that year, surgeons at Johns Hopkins Medical Center reported a technique for closed-chest massage combined with "artificial respiration" and designed specifically for patients suffering anesthesia-induced cardiac arrest. This condition was especially conducive to closed-chest massage because it often occurred in otherwise healthy patients who needed only short-term circulatory support while the adverse effects of anesthesia were resolved. In the context for which it was designed—transient and easily reversible conditions in otherwise healthy individuals—the technique at first appeared miraculous for its effectiveness and simplicity. A 1960 article in the *Journal of the American Medical Association* stated: "Anyone, anywhere, can now initiate cardiac resuscitative procedures. All that is needed are two hands" (Kouwenhoven, Jude, and Knickerbocker, pp. 1064–1067).

Partly because of its simplicity, and partly because of uncertainty over who might benefit from the performance of CPR, it soon became the rule and not the exception that any hospitalized patient experiencing cardiac arrest underwent a trial of resuscitative efforts. These attempts often transiently restored physiologic stability, but too often also resulted in prolonged patient suffering. By the late 1960s, articles began appearing in the medical literature describing the agony that many terminally ill patients experienced from repeated resuscitations that only prolonged the dying process (see Symmers).

Soon a covert decision-making process evolved among clinicians regarding the resuscitation decision. When physicians and nurses responded to situations in which they believed that CPR would not be beneficial, they either refused to call a *code blue* or performed a less than full resuscitation attempt. New terms, such as *slow code* and *Hollywood code,* entered the vocabulary of the hospital culture as these partial or half-hearted resuscitation efforts became more pervasive.

Lacking an established mechanism for advanced decision making about resuscitation, some hospitals developed their own peculiar means of communicating who would not receive a full resuscitation attempt in the event of cardiopulmonary arrest. Decisions were concealed as purple dots on the medical record, written as cryptic initials in the patient's chart, or in some cases simply communicated as verbal orders passed on from shift to shift.

The absence of an open decision-making framework about resuscitation decisions was increasingly recognized as a significant problem in need of a solution. Unilateral decision making by clinicians in this context effectively circumvented the autonomy of the patient and prevented the full consideration of legitimate options by the involved parties prior to a crisis. From the patient's perspective, this covert decision making resulted in errors in both directions: some patients received a resuscitation attempt in circumstances where they did not desire it, while others did not receive a resuscitation attempt in circumstances where they would have desired it.

In 1976 the first hospital policies on orders not to resuscitate were published in the medical literature (see Rabkin). These policies mandated a formal process of advance planning with the patient or patient's surrogate on the decision of whether to attempt resuscitation, and also stipulated formal documentation of the rationale for this decision in the medical record. In 1974 the American Heart Association (AHA) became the first professional organization to propose that decisions not to resuscitate be formally documented in progress notes and communicated to the clinical staff. Moreover, the AHA position on DNR stated that "CPR is not indicated in certain situations, such as in cases of terminal irreversible illness where death is not unexpected" (American Heart Association).

Ethical Perspective

Parallel to the development of the DNR order in the medical community was the emergence of a broad societal consensus on patient's rights. The conceptual foundation of this consensus was the recognition that the wishes and values of the patient should have priority over those of medical professionals in most healthcare decisions.

An influential President's Commission further advocated that patients in cardiac arrest are presumed to have given consent to CPR (that is, a resuscitation attempt is favored in nearly all instances). By extension the commission argued that the context in which the presumption favoring CPR may be overridden must be explicit, and must be justified by being in accord with a patient's competent choice or by serving the incompetent patient's well-being

(President's Commission for the Study of Ethical Problems in Medicine and Biomedical and Behavioral Research). Since that time nearly all states have adopted specific statues on the DNR order. The bioethics community, however, has not embraced this view without dissent.

The assumption that CPR is generally beneficial and should be withheld only by exception has been seriously challenged. CPR, the argument goes, is often not beneficial and was never intended to be the standard of care for all situations of cardiac arrest (four of the five patients in the original Johns Hopkins report experienced an unanticipated cardiac arrest in the setting of anesthesia). From this perspective, CPR, like any treatment, should only be offered to those patients for whom it is medically indicated—physicians are not ethically bound to seek consent to refrain from a procedure that is not medically indicated.

Few issues have been more contentious than whether a physician may determine, without patient or surrogate consent, that CPR is not indicated. Some hospitals have adopted a "don't ask, don't tell" approach to this question by allowing *unilateral* or *futility-based* DNR orders without asking or informing the patient of the decision. Still other policies employ a "don't ask, do tell" approach, where unilateral DNR orders can be written at the discretion of the attending physician, who then informs the patient or patient's family of the decision.

Attempts have been made within the medical profession to define *futile, nonbeneficial, inappropriate,* or *not indicated* in specific terms, such as lack of physiological effect or low likelihood of survival. The assumption underlying this approach is that physicians are best qualified to determine whether and when a medical therapy is indicated. Others advocate procedural resolution pathways, in the belief that it is not possible to achieve consensus on an accepted definition of what constitutes futile medical treatment. This approach assumes that end-of-life decisions inherently involve value-laden choices that people will not always agree on.

Who ultimately decides when a treatment is indicated? The original foundation of the consent process in medicine is the principle that permission is needed "to touch," even when the intent of the person who seeks "to touch" is solely to promote health and treat illness. Because the DNR order is an order not to touch—when that touch may be both highly invasive and life-preserving—only a properly informed patient can decide whether touching is wanted or not. This determination is ultimately a value judgment made by the patient, utilizing information as to efficacy (or futility) provided by the physician.

Conclusion

The introduction of the DNR order brought an open decision-making framework to the resuscitation decision, and also did much to put appropriate restraints on the universal application of cardiopulmonary resuscitation for the dying patient. Yet, DNR orders focus upon what will not be done for the patient, as opposed to what should be done for the patient. These deficiencies are being addressed through the palliative care movement, which recognizes that good care at the end of life depends much more on what therapies are provide than upon those that are not.

JEFFREY P. BURNS

SEE ALSO: *Advance Directives and Advance Care Planning; Aging and the Aged: Healthcare and Research Issues; Autonomy; Clinical Ethics: Clinical Ethics Consultation; Conscience, Rights of; Dementia; Human Dignity; Informed Consent; Pain and Suffering; Palliative Care and Hospice; Right to Die, Policy and Law; Surrogate Decision-Making; Technology: History of Medical Technology*

BIBLIOGRAPHY

Alpers, Ann, and Lo, Bernard. 1995. "When Is CPR Futile?" *Journal of the American Medical Association* 273(2): 156–158.

American Heart Association. 1974. "Standards and Guidelines for Cardiopulmonary Resuscitation (CPR) and Emergency Cardiac Care (ECC), V. Mediolegal Considerations and Recommendations." *Journal of the American Medical Association* 227: S864–S866.

Baker, Robert. 1995. "The Legitimation and Regulation of DNR Orders." In *Legislating Medical Ethics: A Study of the New York State Do-Not-Resuscitate Law,* ed. Robert Baker and Martin Strosberg. Boston: Kluwer Academic.

Blackhall Leslie J. 1987. "Must We Always Use CPR?" *New England Journal Medicine* 317(20): 1281–1285.

Helft Paul R; Siegler, Mark; and Lantos, John. 2000. "The Rise and Fall of the Futility Movement." *New England Journal Medicine* 343: 293–296.

Kouwenhoven W. B.; Jude, James R.; and Knickerbocker, G. Guy. 1960. "Closed-Chest Cardiac Massage." *Journal of the American Medical Association* 173: 1064–1067.

President's Commission for the Study of Ethical Problems in Medicine and Biomedical and Behavioral Research. 1983. *Deciding to Forego Life-Sustaining Treatment: A Report on the Ethical, Medical, and Legal Issues in Treatment Decisions.* Washington, D.C.: U.S. Government Printing Office.

Rabkin, Mitchell T.; Gillerman, Gerald; and Rice, Nancy R. 1976. "Orders Not to Resuscitate." *New England Journal of Medicine* 295: 364–366.

Symmers William S. 1968. "Not Allowed to Die." *British Medical Journal* 1: 442.

Tomlinson, Tom, and Brody, Howard. 1990. "Futility and the Ethics of Resuscitation." *Journal of the American Medical Association* 264(10): 1276–1280.

Youngner Stuart J. 1987. "Do-Not-Resuscitate Orders: No Longer Secret, but Still a Problem." *Hastings Center Report* 17(1): 24–33.

Youngner Stuart J. 1988. "Who Defines Futility?" *Journal of the American Medical Association* 260(14): 2094–2095.

DOUBLE EFFECT, PRINCIPLE OR DOCTRINE OF

• • •

Originating in Roman Catholic scholastic moral philosophy, the Principle of Double Effect (hereafter referred to as the PDE or Double Effect) is still widely discussed in the bioethics literature on euthanasia, palliative care, physician assisted suicide, suicide and abortion (Barry; Quill, Lo et al.; Manfredi, Morrison et al.; Stempsey; Kamm, 1999; McIntosh; Shaw). It has also been applied to a range of other issues, including organ donation and transplantation (DuBois). Due in large part to these bioethics discussions, the PDE has been the subject of a resurgence of interest in moral and political philosophy generally. Double Effect has been debated in the philosophy of law as germane to discussions of, among other things, murder, self-defense, capital punishment, and suicide (Frey; Hart; Finnis, 1991, 1995; Aulisio, 1996). In social and political philosophy, it has been put forth as an important principle for rights theory (Quinn, 1989; Bole), and as a partial justification for affirmative action (Cooney). A traditional military ethics application of Double Effect, to distinguish between strategic and terror bombing, remains a subject of debate today as well (Bratman; Kamm, 2000). In addition, the PDE's central distinction, intention/foresight, has been the subject of rigorous analysis in the philosophy of action (Robins; Bratman; Aulisio, 1995; Brand; Harman).

Double Effect is typically applied to conflict situations in which any action (or course of actions) will result in numerous effects, good and bad. Traditionally a four-part principle, contemporary versions of the PDE are usually formulated as two-part principles, along the following lines: An action with multiple effects, good and bad, is permissible if and only if (1) one is not committed to intending evil (bad effects) either as end or means, and (2) there is proportionate reason for bringing about the evil (bad effects). The first condition, a non-consequentialist intention condition, is lexically prior to the second. Most proponents of the PDE consider the second condition, the proportionate reason condition, to be consequentialist in nature while allowing for other considerations as well.

Paradigm Applications

In the Roman Catholic bioethics literature, the PDE has long been invoked to deal with cases of maternal-fetal conflict to distinguish between permissible interventions that may result in the death of the fetus and abortion, which is absolutely forbidden (Barry). Consider the following set of maternal-fetal conflict paradigm cases.

Paradigm 1: Therapeutic Hysterectomy. A thirty-three year old pregnant woman is diagnosed with a highly aggressive form of uterine cancer ten weeks into her pregnancy. The woman is a devout Roman Catholic, strongly opposed to abortion, and is under care at a Catholic hospital. If the woman were not pregnant, her doctors would recommend a therapeutic hysterectomy to prevent the spread of cancer.

Paradigm 2: Hypertensive Pregnancy. A thirty-nine year old woman is diagnosed with dangerously life threatening high blood pressure seventeen weeks into her pregnancy. The woman is a devout Roman Catholic, strongly opposed to abortion, and is under care at a Catholic hospital. An abortion would alleviate the hypertension and remove the threat to the woman's life.

Though it may come as a surprise to some, those familiar with the Roman Catholic double effect literature will know that the therapeutic hysterectomy proposed in the first case above has long been considered permissible by orthodox Roman Catholic moralists. Indeed, this is viewed as a paradigm instance of a *permissible* action under the PDE (Healy; Kelly; O'Donnell). On the traditional view, the physician's intended *end* would be *saving the life of the mother* by stopping the spread of cancer through her intended *means* of removing the cancerous uterus. Fetal death, on the traditional view, would properly be described as a foreseen but unintended (bad) side effect of the (good) act of saving the mother's life.

In contrast, the case of the hypertensive pregnancy has long been considered a paradigm instance of an action that fails the PDE. In particular, the abortion has traditionally been interpreted as the intended means to the good end of saving the life of the mother, thus failing the PDE's lexically prior intention condition (Healy; Kelly; O'Donnell).

The following scenarios illustrate another set of paradigm applications of the PDE, that is, to distinguish between palliative care and euthanasia:

Paradigm 3: Morphine Drip. David, a forty-nine year old HIV patient, is terminally ill and in constant pain. After much discussion with his partner, family, friends and care team, David has decided that he wants only comfort care. He is adamant that he be kept comfortable. David is placed on a morphine drip, which is then periodically adjusted to alleviate David's discomfort. David's physician knows that continued titration to alleviate David's discomfort runs the risk of hastening or even causing death given David's weakened state. David's physician continues to adjust the morphine drip to keep David comfortable.

Paradigm 4: Lethal Overdose. David, a forty-nine year old HIV patient, is terminally ill and in constant pain. After much discussion with his partner, family, friends and care team, David has decided that he no longer wants to go on living. After saying his good-byes to his partner, family, and friends, David asks his physician to give him a lethal injection of morphine. David's physician gives him a lethal overdose of morphine.

Traditionally, Paradigm 3, the Morphine Drip, has been considered permissible under the PDE, while Paradigm 4, the Lethal Overdose, has been considered impermissible. Why? In Paradigm 3, on the traditional view, David's physician's intended end is to alleviate David's pain. The intended means to this end is the administration of a palliative medication, morphine. Given David's excruciating pain and terminal illness, David's physician has proportionate reason to titrate to pain even though he knows this may hasten or even cause death. On the traditional view, should David die, his death is taken to be a foreseen, but unintended, side effect of the doctor's action (Healy; Kelly; O'Donnell).

In Paradigm 4, David's physician has the same end (i.e., to alleviate David's pain). His means, however, is to give David a lethal injection (i.e., to kill him). On the traditional view, Paradigm 4 is taken to fail the intention condition of the PDE because David's death, the bad effect, is intended by his physician as the means to alleviating David's pain. Paradigm 4 is, on the traditional view, a classic instance of mercy killing (Healy; Kelly; O'Donnell).

The application of the PDE to these, and other, types of cases has been challenged. These challenges generally fall into one of three categories: conceptual tenability, practical applicability, and moral significance. Since challenges to the conceptual tenability and practical applicability of the PDE are largely matters for the philosophy of action, they extend well beyond the scope of this entry. In the bioethics literature, challenges to the PDE have focused on its moral significance outside of the absolutist moral framework within which it emerged. In order to understand this type of challenge, however, it is important to consider the historical origins of the PDE.

Historical Origins

In its traditional form, the PDE has four conditions:

1. The act to be done must be good in itself or at least indifferent.
2. The good intended must not be obtained by means of the evil effect.
3. The evil effect must not be intended for itself, but only permitted.
4. There must be proportionately grave reason for permitting the evil effect. (Fagothey)

Most trace the origins of this traditional four-part PDE and its two-part contemporary successor to St. Thomas Aquinas's (1224–1274) discussion of killing in self-defense (Aquinas; Mangan). Aquinas notes that the Christian tradition had, until his time, almost universally forbidden killing in self-defense. This prohibition probably stemmed from a teaching of St. Augustine (354–430) in *De Libero* that Christians should not kill others to save themselves because bodily life is that which "they ought to despise" (I, 5 PL 32, 1228). In his justification of killing in self-defense, Aquinas invoked what later became the essential conditions of the PDE. He argued that:

> A single act may have two effects, of which only one is intended, while the other is incidental to that intention. *But the way in which a moral act is to be classified depends on what is intended,* not what goes beyond such an intention. Therefore, from the act of a person defending himself a twofold effect can follow: one, the saving of one's own life; the other the killing of the aggressor. (IIaIIae, q.64, a.7)

Implicit here is the crucial distinction upon which the PDE depends, namely intention/foresight. An act of self-defense is classified as such provided that it is the saving of oneself and not the killing of the aggressor that is intended. If the killing was intended (*intendere*), and not merely foreseen (*praeter intentionem*), then, for Aquinas, the act would properly be classified as homicide.

It would seem that both conditions one and three of the traditional PDE might be elicited from this passage. Condition three forbids the intending of an evil effect *for itself* (as an end). Yet if acts are to be classified according to what is intended, then a violation of condition three (intending the evil as an end) will also be a violation of condition one (the act will be classified as bad in itself). Furthermore, condition two, that the good intended not be obtained by means of the

evil, though not explicitly stated, can be understood as a plausible explication of conditions one and three as one who intends an end may also be taken as intending the means to his or her end.

Not to have intended evil is a necessary, but not sufficient, condition of justified self-defense for Aquinas. In the same section he offers a second condition:

> An act that is properly motivated may, nevertheless, become vitiated if it is not *proportionate* to the end intended. And this is why somebody who uses more violence than is necessary to defend himself will be doing something wrong. (IIaIIae, q.64, a.7)

What became the fourth condition of the traditional PDE, the proportionality principle, can be elicited from this passage. Though it is not obvious from this passage, nor from the broader context of Aquinas's work, that proportionate is meant to refer to the measure of good and bad effects, later moralists interpreted the condition in this way.

Double Effect and Contemporary Bioethics

As noted at the outset, the contemporary bioethics literature generally treats Double Effect as a two-part principle. Interestingly, the two-part contemporary PDE, as the preceding discussion suggests, is closer to its Thomistic origins. Though its traditional applications to abortion, euthanasia, self-defense and suicide (particularly physician assisted suicide) continue to be discussed, the PDE has been applied to some novel contemporary bioethics cases, such as the separation of conjoined twins and the use of embryos in research, as well (Coughlan and Anscombe). The strong resurgence of interest in Double Effect in bioethics, however, is directly attributable to the rise of the palliative care movement (Cantor and Thomas; Cavanaugh; Quill, Lo et al.; Manfredi, Morrison et al.; Patterson and Hodges; Preston; Shorr; Gilbert and Kirkham; Sulmasy and Pellegrino; Hawryluck and Harvey; Nuccetelli and Seay; Sulmasy; Bernat; Luce and Alpers; Thorns). Indeed, the vast majority of contemporary bioethics discussion of Double Effect has centered its application to *terminal sedation* which, though controversial in some quarters, is usually little more than a logical extension of the morphine drip case considered above (Paradigm 3) (Krakauer, Penson et al.; Wein). A somewhat novel application of Double Effect in terminal sedation is illustrated by the following case.

Terminal Sedation: Agonal Breathing. Mrs. Jones, an eighty-two year old white female, is a vent dependent terminally ill cancer patient. She is conscious and deemed to have decision capacity upon psychiatric evaluation. Though her pain is well controlled, she requests to be removed from the ventilator. She also requests to first be sedated so that she will not have the experience of not being able to breathe once ventilator support is withdrawn.

The use of palliative medicine in the case of Mrs. Jones can plausibly be construed as satisfying the PDE. Here the use of palliative medicine is intended to alleviate the discomfort of agonal breathing and the attendant suffering of Mrs. Jones should she have to experience this. Critics have argued that invoking Double Effect in these types of cases is a thinly veiled attempt to avoid the charge of intentional killing (Quill, Dresser et al.; Kuhse). Such critics argue that, rather than invoking Double Effect as a rationalization for palliative care, it should be acknowledged that there are times when the intentional mercy killing (euthanasia) is appropriate, thus rendering Double Effect concerns irrelevant.

Double Effect and Moral Relevance: Curious Artifact or Bulwark?

Many critics of Double Effect and even some of its proponents have focused on its Roman Catholic origins, questioning its moral relevance outside of absolutist Roman Catholicism (Boyle 1991a, 1991b; Quill, Dresser et al.). Indeed, this is the most common challenge articulated in the bioethics literature. What, then, can be said of the moral relevance of the PDE outside of absolutist Roman Catholicism? Should bioethicists outside of Roman Catholic moral tradition view the PDE as little more than the curious invention of sectarian casuistry?

To understand this challenge, it is important to highlight the fact that the Roman Catholic moral tradition, in which the PDE emerged, absolutely prohibits certain types or classes of action, including active euthanasia, abortion, murder, and suicide (Boyle, 1991b). In such a tradition, the question of appropriate act description and classification is of paramount importance. The intention condition of the PDE helps to delimit what counts as falling into a given class of action (recall Aquinas's claim, cited above, that the way an act is to be classified depends on intention). Provided an act does not fall into one of the absolutely forbidden classes of action, one may then apply the proportionate reason condition to help determine the permissibility of bringing about the evil effect. Thus, the moral relevance of the PDE and, in particular, of the intention/foresight distinction, is easy to establish in the context of Roman Catholicism with its absolute prohibitions on certain types of acts.

The claim that Double Effect is morally relevant only within the context of absolutist Roman Catholicism is highly problematic. As discussed above, the most fundamental element of the PDE is a conceptual distinction between intention and foresight. Arguably, the normative significance of *any* conceptual distinction will depend on the normative framework within which the distinction is operative (Aulisio, 1996, 1997). The central distinction of PDE, intention/foresight, is embedded in ordinary language and common morality, and is arguably important for certain areas of Anglo-American law despite its emphasis on individual autonomy (e.g., law of attempts, distinction between murder one and manslaughter; etc.) (Aulisio, 1996). More importantly, any moral framework, absolutist or not, that incorporates deontic constraints, formulated in terms of intention, on consequentialist considerations may have use of the intention/foresight distinction (and, therefore, the PDE) (Nagel; Kagan; Quinn, 1993; Beauchamp; Kamm, 2001).

If the preceding discussion is on target, given the wide variety of moral frameworks that incorporate deontic constraints formulated in terms of intention, it seems likely that the PDE will continue to be relevant to a range of bioethics issues. This does not mean that proponents of the PDE can rest easily, however. Serious challenges to the PDE remain. Chief among these are challenges to the conceptual tenability and practical applicability of the intention/foresight distinction, and the need for an adequate theory of intention to address these challenges. Though interesting and important in their own right, it seems unlikely that these matters will inhibit continued vigorous bioethics debate concerning the application of the PDE to vexing cases.

MARK P. AULISIO

SEE ALSO: *Abortion, Religious Traditions: Roman Catholic Perspectives; Beneficence; Ethics: Religion and Morality; Life Sustaining Treatment and Euthanasia: Ethical Aspects of; Medical Ethics, History of Europe: Contemporary Period; Palliative Care and Hospice; Right to Die, Policy and Law; Triage*

BIBLIOGRAPHY

Aulisio, Mark P. 1995. "The Intention/Foresight Distinction." *American Philosophical Quarterly* 32(4): 341–354.

Aulisio, Mark P. 1996. "On the Importance of the Intention/Foresight Distinction." *American Catholic Philosophical Quarterly* LXX(2): 189–205.

Aulisio, Mark P. 1997. "One Person's Modus Ponens: Boyle, Absolutist Catholicism, and the Doctrine of Double Effect." *Christian Bioethics* 3(2): 142–157.

Barry, Robert. 1997. "The Roman Catholic Position on Abortion." *Advances in Bioethics* 2: 151–82.

Beauchamp, Thomas L., ed. 1996. *Intending Death: The Ethics of Assisted Suicide and Euthanasia.* Upper Saddle River, NJ: Prentice Hall.

Bernat, James L. 2001. "Ethical and Legal Issues in Palliative Care." *Neurologic Clinics* 19: 969–987.

Bole, Thomas J. 1991. "The Theoretical Tenability of the Doctrine of Double Effect." *Journal of Medicine and Philosophy* 16: 467–473.

Boyle, James. 1991a. "Further Thoughts on Double Effect: Some Preliminary Responses." *Journal of Medicine and Philosophy* 16: 565–570.

Boyle, James. 1991b. "Who Is Entitled to Double Effect?" *Journal of Medicine and Philosophy* 16(October): 475–494.

Brand, Myles. 1984. *Intending and Acting: Toward a Naturalized Action Theory.* Cambridge, MA: MIT Press.

Bratman, Michael E. 1987. *Intention, Plans, and Practical Reason.* Cambridge, MA: Harvard University Press.

Cantor, Norman L., and Thomas, George C. 1996. "Pain Relief, Acceleration of Death, and Criminal Law." *Kennedy Institute of Ethics Journal* 6(June): 107–127.

Cavanaugh, Thomas A. 1996. "The Ethics of Death-Hastening or Death-Causing Palliative Analgesic Administration to the Terminally Ill." *Journal of Pain and Symptom Management* 12: 248–254.

Cooney, William. 1989. "Affirmative Action and the Doctrine of Double Effect." *Journal of Applied Philosophy* 6: 201–204.

Coughlan, Michael J., and Anscombe, Elizabeth. 1990. "Using People." *Bioethics* 4: 55–65.

DuBois, James M. 2002. "Is Organ Procurement Causing the Death of Patients?" *Issues in Law and Medicine* 18: 21–41.

Fagothey, Austin. 1959. *Right and Reason.* St. Louis, MO: C.V. Mosby Co.

Finnis, John. 1991. "Intention and Side-Effects," In *Liability and Responsibility: Essays in Law and Morals,* ed. R.G. Frey and Christopher W. Morris. New York: Cambridge University Press.

Finnis, J. 1995. "Intention in Tort Law," In *Philosophical Foundations of Tort Law,* ed. David G. Owen. New York: Clarendon Press.

Frey, Raymond G. 1975. "Some Aspects to the Doctrine of Double Effect." *Canadian Journal of Philosophy* 5: 259–283.

Gilbert, James, and Kirkham, Stephen. 1999. "Double Effect, Double Bind or Double Speak?" *Palliative Medicine* 13: 365–366.

Harman, Gilbert. 1986. *Change in View: Principles of Reasoning.* Cambridge, MA: MIT Press.

Hart, Herbert L. A. 1982. *Punishment and Responsibility.* New York: Clarendon Press.

Hawryluck, Laura A., and Harvey, William R. 2000. "Analgesia, Virtue, and the Principle of Double Effect." *Journal of Palliative Care* 16(Supplement): S24–S30.

Healy, Edwin F. 1956. *Medical Ethics.* Chicago: Loyola University Press.

Kagan, Shelly. 1989. *The Limits of Morality.* New York: Oxford University Press.

Kamm, Frances M. 1999. "Physician-Assisted Suicide, the Doctrine of Double Effect, and the Ground of Value." *Ethics* 109: 586–605.

Kamm, Frances M. 2000. "Justifications for Killing Noncombatants in War." In *Life and Death: Metaphysics and Ethics,* ed. Peter A. French and Howard K. Wettstein. Boston: Blackwell Publishers.

Kamm, Frances M. 2001. "Toward the Essence of Nonconsequentialism." In *Fact and Value: Essays on Ethics and Metaphysics for Judith Jarvis Thomson,* ed. Judith Jarvis Thomson, Alex Byrne, Robert Stalnaker, et al. Cambridge, MA: MIT Press.

Kelly, Gerald A. 1958. *Medico-Moral Problems.* St. Louis, MO: Catholic Hospital Association of the United States and Canada.

Krakauer, Eric L.; Penson, Richard T.; et al. 2000. "Sedation for Intractable Distress of a Dying Patient: Acute Palliative Care and the Principle of Double Effect." *Oncologist* 5: 53–62.

Kuhse, Helga. 2002. "Response to Ronald M Perkin and David B Resnik: The Agony of Trying to Match Sanctity of Life and Patient-Centered Medical Care." *Journal of Medical Ethics* 28: 270–272.

Luce, John M., and Alpers, Ann. 2001. "End-of-Life Care: What Do the American Courts Say?" *Critical Care Medicine* 29: N40–N45.

Manfredi, Paolo L.; Morrison, R. Sean; et al. 1998. "The Rule of Double Effect." *New England Journal of Medicine* 338: 1390.

Mangan, Joseph. 1949. "An Historical Analysis of the Principle of Double Effect." *Theological Studies* 10: 41–61.

McIntosh, Neil. 2001. "Withdrawing Life Sustaining Treatment and Euthanasia Debate. Double Effect Is Different from Euthanasia." *British Medical Journal (Clinical Research Edition)* 323: 1248–1249.

Nagel, Thomas. 1986. *The View from Nowhere.* New York: Oxford University Press.

Nuccetelli, Susana, and Seay, Gary. 2000. "Relieving Pain and Foreseeing Death: A Paradox about Accountability and Blame." *Journal of Medicine and Ethics* 28: 19–25.

O'Donnell, Thomas J. 1996. *Medicine and Christian Morality.* Staten Island, NY: Alba House.

Patterson, James R., and Hodges, Marian O. 1998. "The Rule of Double Effect." *New England Journal of Medicine* 338: 1389.

Preston, Thomas A. 1998. "The Rule of Double Effect." *New England Journal of Medicine* 338: 1389.

Quill, Timothy E.; Dresser, Rebecca; et al. 1997. "The Rule of Double Effect—A Critique of Its Role in End-of-Life Decision Making." *New England Journal of Medicine* 337: 1768–1771.

Quill, Timothy E.; Lo, Bernard; et al. 1997. "Palliative Options of Last Resort: A Comparison of Voluntarily Stopping Eating and Drinking, Terminal Sedation, Physician-Assisted Suicide, and Voluntary Active Euthanasia." *Journal of the American Medical Association* 278: 2099–2104.

Quinn, Warren. 1993. *Morality and Action.* Cambridge, Eng.: Cambridge University Press.

Quinn, Warren S. 1989. "Actions, Intentions, and Consequences: The Doctrine of Double Effect." *Philosophy and Public Affairs* 18: 334–351.

Robins, Michael H. 1984. *Promising, Intending, and Moral Autonomy.* New York: Cambridge University Press.

Shorr, Andrew F. 1998. "The Rule of Double Effect." *New England Journal of Medicine* 338: 1389–1390.

Stempsey, William E. 1998. "Laying Down One's Life for Oneself." *Christian Bioethics* 4: 202–224.

Sulmasy, Daniel P. 2000. "Commentary: Double Effect—Intention Is the Solution, Not the Problem." *Journal of Law, Medicine and Ethics* 28: 26–29.

Sulmasy, Daniel P., and Pellegrino, Edmund D. 1999. "The Rule of Double Effect: Clearing Up the Double Talk." *Archives of Internal Medicine* 159: 545–550.

Thorns, Andrew. 2002. "Sedation, The Doctrine of Double Effect and the End of Life." *International Journal of Palliative Nursing* 8: 341–343.

E

EASTERN ORTHODOX CHRISTIANITY, BIOETHICS IN

• • •

The Eastern Orthodox church considers itself identical with the Church established by Jesus Christ and believes itself to be guided by the Holy Spirit, continuing that ecclesial reality into the present age as an organic historical, theological, liturgical continuity and unity with the apostolic Church of the first century. Historically, it sees itself as identical with the "One, Holy, Catholic, and Apostolic Church" that suffered the "Great Schism" in 1054 that led to the division of Christendom into Eastern and Western Christianity.

The Orthodox church is organized hierarchically, with an ordained clergy and bishops. A number of national and ethnic Orthodox churches, under the leadership of patriarchs, are united by tradition, doctrine, and spirit rather than by authority, although the Ecumenical Patriarch of Constantinople is accorded a primacy of honor. The church's identity is rooted in the experience of the Holy Spirit in all aspects of its life and in a doctrinal perspective that serves as a matrix for its ethical teachings (Ware; Pelikan). In the sphere of bioethics, this theological matrix forms a coherent source of values for bioethical decision making. At its center is the view that life is a gift of God that should be protected, transmitted, cultivated, cared for, fulfilled in God, and considered a sacred reality. Consequently, there is a high regard for the concerns usually identified with the field of bioethics.

Doctrine and Ethics

In Orthodox belief, the teaching of the church is found in the Old and New Testaments, the writings of the church fathers, and all aspects of the synodical, canonical, liturgical, and spiritual tradition of faith as lived, experienced, and reflected upon in the consciousness of the church, for which the general name "holy tradition" is used.

The Eastern Orthodox church understands ultimate reality to be the Holy Trinity, or God who is a triune unity of persons: the Father, source of the other two fully divine persons; the Son, forever born of the Father; and the Holy Spirit, forever proceeding from the Father. Thus, ultimate uncreated and uncontingent reality is a community of divine persons living in perpetual love and unity.

This divine reality created all else that exists, visible and invisible, as contingent reality. Human beings are created as a composite of body and spirit, as well as in the "image and likeness" of the Holy Trinity. "Image" refers to those characteristics that distinguish humanity from the rest of the created world: intelligence, creativity, the ability to love, self-determination, and moral perceptivity. "Likeness" refers to the potential open to such a creature to become "God-like." This potential for deification, or *theosis,* has been lost through the choice of human beings to separate themselves from communion with God and their fellow human beings; that is to say, sin is a part of the human condition. Though weakened and distorted, the "image" remains and differentiates human existence from the rest of creation.

The work of redemption and salvation is accomplished by God through the Son, the second person of the Holy Trinity who took on human nature (except for sin) in the person of Jesus Christ. He taught, healed, gave direction, and offered himself upon the cross for the sins of humanity, and conquered the powers of death, sin, and evil through his resurrection from the dead. This saving work, accomplished for all humanity and all creation, is appropriated by each human person through faith and baptism, and manifested in continuous acts of self-determination in communion with the Holy Spirit. This cooperation between the human and divine in the process of growth toward the fulfillment of God-likeness is referred to as synergy.

The locus for this appropriation is the Church—specifically, its sacramental and spiritual life. The sacraments, or "mysteries," use both material and spiritual elements, as does the life of spiritual discipline known as "struggle" and "asceticism" (*agona* and *askesis*). Both foster a communion of love between the Holy Trinity and the human being, among human beings, and between humans and the nonhuman creation, making possible continuous growth toward God-likeness, which is full human existence.

Though in this earthly life growth toward Godlikeness can be continuous, it is never completed. In the Eastern Orthodox worldview, the eternal Kingdom of God provides a transcendent referent for everything. The Kingdom is not only yet to come in the "last days," but is now a present reality through Christ's resurrection and the presence of the Holy Spirit. Within this spiritual reality, the goal of human life is understood to be an ongoing process of increasing communion with God, other persons, and creation. This forms the matrix for Orthodox Christian ethics and provides it with the materials and perspectives for articulating the "ought" dimensions of the church's teaching (Mantzaridis).

Among the more important aspects of these teachings for bioethics are (1) the supreme value of love for God and neighbor; (2) an understanding that sees nature fallen but also capable of providing basic norms for living through a foundational and elementary natural moral law; (3) the close relationship of material and spiritual dimensions of human existence and their appropriate relationship and integration; (4) the capacity for self-determination by human beings to make moral decisions and act on them; and (5) the criterion of movement toward God-likeness—all within a framework that is both this and other-world focused.

In practice, ethical norms are arrived at in holy tradition and by contemporary Orthodox ethicists by defining moral questions within this context of faith in a search for ethical guidelines that embody the good, the right, and the fitting (Harakas, 1983).

Bodily Health

Concern for the health of the body, though not central, has a significant place in Eastern Orthodox ethics (Harakas, 1986a). Orthodox Christian ethics calls for "a healthy mind and a healthy spirit with a healthy body." The body is neither merely an instrument nor simply a dwelling place of the spirit. It is a constituent part of human existence, and requires attention for the sake of the whole human being. Thus, in its sinful condition, the body can also be a source of destructive tendencies that need to be controlled and channeled. This is one of the works of asceticism, which seeks to place the body under control of the mind and the spirit. But asceticism is never understood as a dualistic condemnation of the body. As a good creation, under the direction of the proper values, the body is seen as worthy of nurturing care. Thus, everything that contributes to the well-being of the body should be practiced in proper measure, and whatever is harmful to the health of the body ought to be avoided. The Eastern Christian patristic tradition is consistent in this concern (Constantelos; Darling).

Practices that contribute to bodily health and well-being are ethically required. Adequate nourishment, proper exercise, and other good health habits are fitting and appropriate, while practices that harm the body are considered not simply unhealthful, but also immoral. Abuse of the body is morally inappropriate. Both body and mind are abused through overindulgence of alcohol and the use of narcotics for nontherapeutic purposes. Orthodox teaching holds that persons who might be attracted to these passions need to exercise their ethical powers in a form of ascetic practice to overcome their dependence upon them as part of their growth toward God-likeness.

Healing Illness

When illness occurs, Orthodox Christianity affirms an ethical duty to struggle against sickness, which if unaddressed can lead to death. The moral requirement to care for the health of the body indicates it is appropriate to use healing methods that will enhance health and maintain life. Two means are used concurrently: spiritual healing and different forms of medicine. The first is embodied in nearly all services of the church, in particular, the sacrament of healing, or holy unction. There is also a continuing tradition of multiple forms of prayer and saintly intercessions for the healing of body and soul.

The church does not see spiritual healing as exclusive nor as competitive with scientific medicine. In the fourth century, Saint John Chrysostom, one of the great church fathers, frequently referred to his need for medical attention and medications. In his letters to Olympias, he not only speaks of his own use of medications but advises others to use them as well. Saint Basil, another great fourth-century church father, underwent various forms of therapy for his illnesses. In fact, both of these church fathers had studied medicine. Basil offers a classic Christian appreciation of the physician and the medical profession:

> Truly, humanity is the concern of all of you who follow the profession of medicine. And it seems to me that he who would prefer your profession to all other life pursuits would make a proper choice, not straying from the right, if really the most precious of all things, life, is painful and undesirable unless it can be possessed with health. And your profession is the supply vein of health. (Epistle 189, To Eustathius, the Court Physician fourth century, p. 228)

Recent studies have highlighted the Eastern Orthodox church's concern with healing, both in its medical and spiritual dimensions. Orthodox monks established the hospital as a place of healing, a tradition maintained by Orthodox monasticism for almost a thousand years, until it was taken over by the medical establishment (Miller; Scarborough; Harakas, 1990).

Bioethical Concerns and Methods

Bioethics as a distinct discipline is only a few decades old, but some topics included in the discipline, such as abortion, have been addressed by the Christian tradition over the centuries. Many bioethical issues are new, however, and the Orthodox church's views concerning them have yet to be officially stated. The method contemporary Orthodox ethicists use to determine Eastern Orthodox perspectives on bioethical questions is the same as the general method used to make ethical decisions. The general doctrinal stance and ethos of the church form the larger context, delineating basic perspectives. The church requires further study, however, to assess the moral dimensions of newly created bioethical questions.

The ethicist concerned with bioethical questions then consults the tradition, which embodies the mind of the church: Scripture, patristic writings, decisions of the ecumenical councils and other synods, the received doctrinal teachings of the church, canon law, ascetical writings, monastic *typika* (constitutions of monastic establishments), liturgical texts and traditions, *exomologetaria* (penitential books), the exercises of *economia* (a process of judgment that allows for consideration of circumstances in a particular case, but without setting precedents for future normative decision making), and theological studies, for specific references that exhibit the mind of the church in concrete ethical situations. The "mind of the church" is understood as the consciousness of the people of God, together with the formulation of theological opinion, in conjunction with the decisions of the

church in local, regional, and ecumenical synods, conceived and experienced as arising from the guidance of the Holy Spirit. It is a mindset, rather than a set of rules or propositions. The purpose of examining these sources is to determine whether these sources speak either directly, or indirectly, or by analogy, to new questions of bioethics. The historical contexts of these specific sources are kept in mind, and will serve to condition contemporary judgments.

Both general and specific applications can then be made and expressed as theological opinion on topics in bioethics. These views, however, are tentative, until the mind of the church specifically decides. Wherever this has already occurred, it will be noted below. Otherwise, what follows should be understood as thoughtfully considered theological opinion, subject to correction by the mind of the church (Harakas, 1980, 1986b).

The Protection of Life

Orthodox thought holds that life is a gift from God, given to creation and to human beings as a trust to be preserved and protected. Just as the care for one's health is a moral duty for the individual, society's concern for public health is also a moral imperative. The first large division of concern is that existing life be protected. This can be expressed in a number of ethical positions characteristic of an Orthodox perspective.

The protection of life has been a value pursued throughout history by the church. During the early days of the rise and spread of Christianity, abortion was widely practiced in the Roman Empire. The Church, based on its respect for life, condemned this practice in its canon law as a form of murder. The Church considered abortion particularly heinous because of the defenseless and innocent condition of the victim (Kowalczyk). Of course, no moral stance is absolute. In Orthodox traditional teaching, however, abortion is nearly always judged to be wrong. There can be unusual circumstances, such as an ectopic pregnancy that threatens the life of the mother, that might be judged prudentially as calling for an abortion, but such situations are rare.

Historically related to the rejection of abortion was a condemnation of the exposure of infants, that is, their abandonment, a practice that caused their death or led to their exploitation by unscrupulous persons who profited from forcing children into prostitution or begging. These are severe examples of child abuse that unfortunately have continued into the modern age. Every such case, historic or contemporary, violates the moral requirement that adults care for children in a loving and supportive manner.

Modern Medical Technology and Ethics

The development of medical science and technology has raised many new issues, however. Studying these issues from within the mind of the church has produced a body of positions that are expressive of the church's commitment to the protection of life. Some of these follow.

ALLOCATION OF MEDICAL RESOURCES. A bioethical question that finds a response in the concern for the protection of life is the issue of the allocation of scarce medical resources. A healthcare system that fosters the widest possible distribution of healthcare opportunities is the most morally responsible, since it reflects the common human situation before God.

PROFESSIONAL-PATIENT RELATIONSHIPS. In the area of the relationships of providers and recipients of healthcare, the church affirms the existence of patients' rights and requires that the medical profession honor them. The full human dignity of every person under treatment should be among the controlling values of healthcare providers, manifested in their concern to maintain the patient's privacy, obtain informed consent for medical procedures, develop wholesome personal contacts between the patient and the medical team members, and treat the patient as a total human being rather than an object of medical procedures.

HUMAN EXPERIMENTATION. Because of the role it plays in the development of medical therapies and the possible cure of individual persons, human experimentation must be conducted and is morally justified by an appeal to the value of the protection of life. Wherever possible, however, such experimentation should fulfill the following minimal conditions: The patient should be informed of the risks involved and should accept participation in the experiment freely and without coercion, and the experiment should have potential benefit for the patient. Increased knowledge should be secondary to the welfare of the patient.

ORGAN TRANSPLANTATION. Protection of life finds intense application in the area of organ transplantation. This topic may serve as a somewhat more extensive example of Orthodox bioethical reflection. Organ transplantation was unknown in the ancient world. Some Orthodox Christians consider it wrong, a violation of the integrity of the body. Significant as this consideration is, it does not outweigh the value of concern for the welfare of the neighbor, especially since organs for transplants are generally donated by persons who are philanthropically motivated for the protection of life. The sale of organs is seen as commercializing human body parts and therefore unworthy, and is prohibited by a concern for the protection of life and its dignity.

There are two categories of potential donors: the living and the dead. Usually, the potential living donor of a duplicated organ is a relative. In such cases, concern for the well-being of the patient may place undue pressure upon the potential donor. No one has an absolute moral duty to give an organ. Healthcare professionals must respect the integrity of the potential donor as well as the potential recipient. Yet it is certainly an expression of God-likeness for a person to give an organ when motivated by caring concern and love for the potential recipient. Ethical consideration must be given to the physical and emotional consequences upon both donor and recipient and weighed in conjunction with all other factors. When these are generally positive, the option for organ donation by a living person has much to commend it.

In the case of donation of organs from the dead, some of the same considerations hold, while several new issues arise. Organs can be donated in anticipation of death. Some states, for example, encourage people to declare their donation of particular organs (liver, kidney, cornea) in conjunction with the issuance of auto licenses. There do not appear to be serious objections to this practice; many Orthodox consider it praiseworthy. When no expressed wish is known, permission of donation should be sought from relatives. Their refusal should be respected.

Persons may donate organs through bequests associated with their wills. This choice should be made known to responsible survivors before death. In 1989, for example, the Greek Orthodox Archbishop of Athens announced in the press that he had made provision for the donation of his eyes after his death.

BODY DONATION TO SCIENCE. Similarly connected with the protection of life is the issue of donating one's body to science. Much of the answer from an Orthodox Christian perspective has to do with what the representatives of science will do with it. Giving one's body to science means, in nearly all cases, that it will be used for the education of medical students. There has been a bias against this practice in many countries because at the same time that the personal identity of the body is destroyed, the body itself is treated without respect. The alternative to using donated bodies for medical education, however, is that medical students and young physicians will learn surgical skills on living patients. The concern for the protection of life could not, thus, totally disapprove of the practice of body donation. In principle, then, giving one's body for medical education cannot be ethically prohibited. But medical schools should strive to create an atmosphere of reverence and respect for the bodily remains of persons given for this purpose. In some medical schools, this already takes place; in most, it has not. Potential donors of their bodies should inquire about procedures and refuse to donate their bodies to schools that do not show adequate respect for the body. Usually this means making arrangements for ecclesial burial of the remains after their educational use.

THE AGED. The protection of life covers the whole life span. The Orthodox church has always had a special respect and appreciation for the aged. Industrial society, with its smaller, nuclear families, has tended to isolate the aged from the rest of society. The aging themselves ought not to accept such marginalization passively. They should continue to live active and fulfilling lives, with as much independence of movement and self-directed activity as possible. Spiritually, growth in the life of Christ continues to be important. Repentance, prayer, communion with God, service to others, and loving care for others are important in this and every age bracket.

Children and relatives should do everything possible to enhance the quality of life for their aging parents and relatives. But in cases of debilitating conditions and illnesses, it may be necessary to institutionalize them. Many Orthodox Christians feel that this is an abandonment of their moral responsibilities to their parents. If institutionalization is a way of abdicating one's responsibilities to parents for the sake of convenience, then it is wrong. However, it is often the best solution. Even when it is morally indicated, the important values remain; in a nursing home or outside of it, children still have the obligation to express love, care, and respect for their parents.

DEATH. Concern for the protection of life is also present at the end of life. Death should come of itself, without human intervention. God gives us life; God should be allowed to take it away. Proponents of so-called euthanasia hold that persons should be allowed and may even be obliged to end their earthly lives when "life is not worth living." In the church's judgment, this is a form of suicide, which the church condemns. If one does this to another person, it is a case of murder. Orthodox Christian ethics rejects euthanasia as morally wrong.

Modern medical practice has raised some related issues, however. The possibility that vital signs can be maintained artificially, even after death has occurred, raises the complex question of turning off "life-sustaining" machines after brain death is diagnosed. The tradition has never supported heroic intervention in situations where death is imminent and no further therapies exist. It has been Eastern Orthodox practice not only to allow a person to die but also to actively pray for it when, according to the best medical judgment available, a person is struggling to die. If a person is clinically dead but his or her vital organs are kept functioning by mechanical means, turning off the machines is not considered euthanasia. Until the determination of clinical death, both physician and family should seek to maintain the comfort of the patient. Spiritually, all should provide the dying person opportunities for repentance and reconciliation with God and with his or her fellows (Breck, 1989).

SUFFERING. In all serious medical situations, suffering should be relieved as much as possible; this is especially true for the Orthodox patient who has participated in the sacraments of Holy Confession and Holy Communion. Pain that cannot be relieved should be accepted in as redemptive a way as possible. For the church, a "good death" (in Greek, *euthanasia*) is one in which the human being accepts death with hope and confidence in God, in communion with him, as a member of his kingdom, and with a conscience that is at peace. Genuine humanity is achievable even on the deathbed.

The Transmission of Life

The Eastern Orthodox approach to marriage provides the context for discussing procreative and sexual issues. The church sees marriage as a sacramental dimension of human life, with ecclesial and interpersonal dimensions and purposes (Guroian). The Orthodox church sees both men and women as equal before God as human beings and as persons called to grow toward God-likeness. Both men and women are persons in their own right before God and may be endowed with many potentialities that ought to be developed as part of their human growth. Yet the special sacramental relationship of marriage, procreation, and child rearing gives to women, in the mind of the church, a special role. Accompanying it is the role of husband and father in constituting a marriage and creating a family. Most of the bioethical issues regarding the transmission of life arise out of this marital and familial perspective in Orthodox thought.

REPRODUCTIVE TECHNOLOGIES. Artificial insemination assists spouses to procreate when they cannot conceive through normal sexual intercourse. In such cases, the sperm of the husband is artificially introduced into the wife's childbearing organs. There are differences of opinion in the Orthodox church regarding this procedure. A major objection is that this is a totally unnatural practice. But since other "unnatural practices" such as cooking food, wearing clothes, using technical devices such as eye-glasses and hearing aids, and performing or undergoing surgery are considered morally acceptable, this argument loses much of its force.

More cogent is the argument that artificial insemination separates "baby-making" from "love-making," which is a way of emphasizing the unity of the spiritual and bodily dimensions of marriage. In the case of artificial insemination by husband (AIH), the personal, social, and spiritual context seems to indicate that AIH is morally acceptable. The opposite holds true when the semen of a donor is used (AID). The intrusion of a third party in providing the semen violates the psychosomatic unity of the marital couple.

The same pattern of ethical reflection applies to other procedures, such as artificial inovulation and in vitro fertilization. If the sperm and ovum come from the spouses themselves, and the wife bears the child to term, ethical objections to these procedures are lessened. Often, however, fertilized ova are discarded in the procedures. The majority of Orthodox consider this a form of abortion. Others hold that for abortion to take place, implantation in the womb must have previously occurred. Nevertheless, surrogate mothers, egg donation, and sperm donation from parties outside the marriage find no place in an ethical approach that places heavy emphasis on the wholeness and unity of the bodily and spiritual aspects of human life, and of the marital relationship in particular.

STERILIZATION. Where sterilization is intended to encourage promiscuous sexual living, Orthodox Christianity disapproves. A strong ethical case can be made for it when there are medical indications that a pregnancy would be life-threatening to the wife. An as yet unexplored ethical area is the case of almost all older, yet still fertile, married couples, for whom there is a significant likelihood that the children of their mature love would be bearers of serious genetic diseases.

GENETICS. Genetic counseling seeks to provide information to a couple before they conceive children so that potentially serious conditions in newborns can be foreknown. Genetic counseling is also related to genetic screening of population groups that might be carriers of particular genetic illnesses. Genetic screening refines and makes more accurate the earlier practices of the church and of society that sought to reduce the incidence of deformed and deficient children, through the restriction of marriages between persons closely related genetically.

As a procedure that would reduce the number of persons entering into marriages with dangerously high chances for the transmission of genetic illnesses, these procedures ought to be strongly encouraged. Premarital genetic screening of young people with Mediterranean backgrounds, where there is a relatively high incidence of thalessemia B and Tay-Sachs disease, might guide them in the selection of spouses. Once a child is conceived and growing in the womb, however, the church could not consider the termination of the pregnancy as anything other than abortion. An impaired child is still the image of God with a right to life (Harakas, 1982). Since the church strenuously opposes abortion, prenatal diagnostic information indicating the prospective birth of a genetically deformed child cannot justify ending the life of the baby in the womb. Instead, this information serves to prepare the parents to receive their child with the love, acceptance, and courage required to care for such an exceptional baby.

GENETIC ENGINEERING. Concern with genetic engineering as an aspect of the transmission of life provokes a conflicting reaction among Orthodox Christian ethicists. Some Orthodox ethicists value the potential therapeutic possibilities of genetic engineering. In this case, the treatment of the genome to correct deficiencies is looked at positively, as a form of medical therapy. Nevertheless, there is concern when these same techniques are thought of as means for eugenic goals. The potential for misuse and abuse make Orthodox Christian reactions very cautious (Breck, 1991).

Conclusion

The common denominator in all these issues is the high regard and concern of the church for human life as a gift of God. Eastern Orthodox Christianity takes a conservative approach to these issues, seeing in them a dimension of the holy and relating them to transcendent values and concerns. Only an intense respect for human life can curb the modern tendencies to destroy human life both before birth and as it approaches its end. The human person, from the very moment of conception and implantation in the womb, is dependent upon others for life and sustenance. It is in the community of the living—especially as it relates to the source of life, God in Trinity—that life is conceived, nurtured, developed, and fulfilled in communion with God. The trust that each person has in others for the continued well-being of his or her own life forms a basis for generalization. Eastern Orthodox ethics, consequently, functions with a pro-life bias that honors and respects the life of each person as a divine gift that requires protection, transmission, development, and enhancement.

STANLEY S. HARAKAS (1995)

SEE ALSO: *African Religions; Buddhism, Bioethics in; Christianity, Bioethics in; Daoism, Bioethics in; Eugenics and*

Religious Law; Islam, Bioethics in; Jainism, Bioethics in; Judaism, Bioethics in; Medical Ethics, History of: Europe; Mormonism, Bioethics in; Native American Religions, Bioethics in; Reproductive Technologies; Sikhism, Bioethics in; Transhumanism and Posthumanism

BIBLIOGRAPHY

Basil, Saint. 1968. "Epistle 189." *Letters. A Select Library of Nicene and Post-Nicene Fathers of the Christian Church,* ed. Philip Schaff and H. Wace. Grand Rapids, MI: Eerdmans.

Breck, John. 1989. "Selective Nontreatment of the Terminally Ill: An Orthodox Moral Perspective." *St. Vladimir's Theological Quarterly* 33(3): 261–273.

Breck, John. 1991. "Genetic Engineering: Setting the Limits." In *Health and Faith: Medical, Psychological and Religious Dimensions,* pp. 51–56, ed. John Chirban. Lanham, MD: University Press of America.

Constantelos, Demetrios J. 1991. *Byzantine Philanthropy and Social Welfare,* 2nd rev. edition. New Rochelle, NY: A. D. Caratzas.

Darling, Frank C. 1990. *Christian Healing in the Middle Ages and Beyond.* Boulder, CO: Vista Publications.

Guroian, Vigen. 1988. *Incarnate Love: Essays in Orthodox Ethics.* Notre Dame, IN: University of Notre Dame Press.

Harakas, Stanley S. 1980. *For the Health of Body and Soul: An Eastern Orthodox Introduction to Bioethics.* Brookline, MA: Holy Cross Orthodox Press.

Harakas, Stanley S. 1983. *Toward Transfigured Life: The Theoria of Eastern Orthodox Ethics.* Minneapolis, MN: Light and Life.

Harakas, Stanley S. 1986a. "The Eastern Orthodox Church." In *Caring and Curing: Health and Medicine in the Western Religious Traditions,* pp. 146–172, ed. Ronald L. Numbers and Darel W. Amundsen. New York: Macmillan.

Harakas, Stanley S. 1986b. "Orthodox Christianity and Bioethics." *Greek Orthodox Theological Review* 31: 181–194.

Harakas, Stanley S. 1990. *Health and Medicine in the Eastern Orthodox Tradition: Faith, Liturgy and Wholeness.* New York: Crossroad.

Kowalczyk, John. 1977. *An Orthodox View of Abortion.* Minneapolis, MN: Light and Life.

Mantzaridis, Georgios. 1993. "How We Arrive at Moral Judgements: An Orthodox Perspective." *Phronema* 3: 11–20.

Miller, Timothy S. 1985. *The Birth of the Hospital in the Byzantine Empire.* Baltimore: Johns Hopkins University Press.

Pelikan, Jaroslav. 1974. *The Spirit of Eastern Christendom (600–1700). The Christian Tradition: A History of the Development of Doctrine,* vol. 2. Chicago: University of Chicago Press.

Scarborough, John, ed. 1985. *Symposium on Byzantine Medicine: Dumbarton Oaks Papers, Number 38.* Washington, D.C.: Dumbarton Oaks Research Library and Collection.

Ware, Kallistos. 1964. *The Orthodox Church.* Baltimore: Penguin.

ECONOMIC CONCEPTS IN HEALTHCARE

• • •

Healthcare has always been an economic activity; people invest time and other resources in it, and they trade for it with each other. It is thus amenable to economic analysis—understanding the demand for it, its supply, its price, and their interrelationship. Economic analysis, of course, does not merely discern what the supply, demand, and price for healthcare in private or public markets are. It also attempts to understand why they are what they are: What behavior on the part of suppliers affects the demand for healthcare? How does a particular insurance framework affect supply and demand? And so on. Moreover, economic analysis is indispensable in the larger attempt to improve healthcare—to make it more efficient, for example, so that people can accomplish more with their investment in healthcare, or more in life generally with their resources.

The economics of healthcare, in fact, has grown into an established specialty within professional economics. Though virtually every good is in some sense an *economic good,* economists have been quick to notice some differences with healthcare. Final demand seems to be more supplier-created in the case of healthcare than it is with most goods; both the shape of health services and their price are very directly influenced by providers. Other forms of what economists call *market failure* occur in healthcare—for example, when people with a considerable demand for healthcare do not receive services because their high risk to insurers drives prices for even the most basic insurance to unaffordable levels.

As people have become increasingly concerned about rising cost, economic concepts have gained greater general currency in society's consideration of healthcare. Price is seldom *no object,* and the search for efficiency is vigorous. This entry on economic concepts in healthcare will:

1. Clarify the differences between two important forms of efficiency analysis in healthcare;

2. Articulate some of the difficulties in devising and using a common unit of health benefit;

3. Examine the monetary evaluation of one health benefit, life extension;

4. Focus on some of the fundamental moral difficulties that the demand for efficiency poses for clinical practice; and

5. Briefly explore the notions of *externality* and *public good* and their role in health policy.

Many other economic concepts apply to healthcare, but these are some that obviously raise ethical issues and are therefore most appropriate to include in this volume. Throughout, however, it will be important to keep in mind that economists, qua economists, usually think of their primary task as describing the world, not saying what it ought to be.

One should also note that although many economic concepts may appear to be more at home in capitalist than in centralized, collectivist, or socialist economies, they virtually always have a role to play in those other economies, too. For example, cost-effectiveness and cost-benefit analysis are used at least as much in socialist as in more capitalist healthcare systems. While the economic concepts developed here may not be ideology-free, they are hardly confined to free-market frameworks.

Cost-Effectiveness, Cost-Benefit, and Risk-Benefit Analysis

Efficiency involves the basic economic concept of *opportunity cost*: the value sacrificed by not pursuing alternatives that might have been pursued with the same resources. When the value of any alternative use is less than the value of the current service, the current one is efficient; when the value of some alternative is greater, the current service is inefficient. In thinking of the possible alternative uses, our sights can be set either narrowly or broadly. If we focus just on other options in healthcare, wondering whether we can get *more benefit* for our given healthcare dollars, or whether we can get the *same health benefit more cheaply*, we are engaged in cost-effectiveness analysis (CEA). If, on the other hand, we are comparing an investment in healthcare with *all the other things* we might have done with the same time, effort, and money, we are engaged in cost-benefit analysis (CBA). CEA asks whether the money spent on a particular program or course of treatment could produce healthier or longer lives if it were spent on other forms of care. CBA involves an even more difficult query: whether the money we spend on a particular portion of healthcare is *matched* by the benefit. We determine that by asking in turn whether, spent elsewhere, it could produce greater value of another sort, not just healthier or longer lives.

Both kinds of analysis are important. We want to get the most health and life for our investment in healthcare (CEA), but we also want neither to be so occupied with other investments that we ignore improvements in health that would be worth more to us, nor to pass up other things in life because we are investing too much in relatively unproductive healthcare (CBA). CEA is the less ambitious enterprise: We compare different healthcare services, detecting either final differences in expense to achieve the same health benefit or differences in some health benefit (for example, added years of life, and reductions in morbidity). That itself is a tall order, but it is less daunting than CBA. CBA is difficult, of course, because the advantages gained from such other investments often seem incommensurable with health and longevity. Improvements *within* healthcare, though, often seem terribly incommensurable, too: How do we really compare the values of non-life-extending hip replacement, for instance, and life-extending dialysis or transplants?

Formal, economic CBA puts into common *monetary* terms the various benefits of the endeavors in life that are being compared—a life saved with healthcare is seen to have a value, let us say, of $1 million. With the benefits thus monetarized, the conceptual package of resource trading is tied together; we are able to compare the benefits of healthcare and those of other endeavors with each other in the same terms (i.e., monetary ones). If benefits are assigned a monetary value, then, since costs have been stated from the beginning in monetary terms, we can ascertain straightforwardly whether the benefits are worth the costs. If, for example, it will likely take three $500,000 liver transplants to get one lifesaving success, and if a life saved has a monetary value of $1 million, then the transplants cost more than the life they save is worth. Whether we are achieving actual *value for money*—efficiency—now gets an explicit answer (though critics will doubt that we can ever sustain the judgment that a life saved has a monetary value of *only* $1 million).

Another, less formalized kind of analysis is *risk-benefit analysis*: One compares the probabilities of harm presented by a certain course of action with its likely benefits. If another procedure is likely to produce similar benefits with less risk, the latter is obviously preferable. It is not always clear, however, when one risk is *less* than another; the two may be risks of different things—one, say, of paralysis and the other of chronic pain. Moreover, one procedure may harbor lower risk but also promise fewer health benefits; again we are left with non-comparables. Unlike CEA, the beneficial effects in risk-benefit analysis are not all measured on a common scale, and unlike CBA, the benefits are not put in the same terms as the costs or risks.

We use the economic tools of CEA and CBA to discern potential improvements in efficiency. The existence of a potential efficiency improvement, however, does not by itself tell us that we should pursue it. Efficiency is only one goal; we might also need to consider the fairness of distributing goods and resources in the most efficient way. Economists, though, will be quick to note efficiency's especially great moral force in two sorts of circumstance: where the new, more efficient distribution is *Pareto superior* (someone gains, and no one loses), or where the gain to some is sufficient to allow them to compensate the *losers* back to their reference point and still retain some net benefit for themselves. If, for example, so many people gain from water fluoridation that they are better enough off even after being taxed to provide a really ample compensation fund for those who suffer some side effect, then all, even the *losers,* gain by fluoridation.

Health Benefit Units: Well-Years or Quality-Adjusted Life Years (QALYs)

CEA, unlike CBA, does not venture answers to the question of how much money to spend for a given health benefit. It does, however, attempt ambitious as well as modest comparisons within healthcare. What it needs to be able to do this is a common unit of health benefit. In some contexts this will quite naturally be present; suppose we are comparing the respective prolongations of life provided by bypass grafts and coronary *medical management* (drug therapy). The more difficult task for CEA comes in translating widely different health benefits into a common conceptual currency. The notion developed for this purpose goes by various labels: a *well-year,* a *quality-adjusted life year* (QALY, pronounced to rhyme with *holly*), or *health-state utility.* The essential idea is a unit that combines mortality with quality of life considerations—*a year of healthy life,* as one defender of QALYs puts it. We can then compare not only life-prolonging measures with each other but also measures that enhance quality with those that prolong life—hip replacements with kidney dialysis, for example. And then we can also track the health of a population, calculating changes in per capita *years of healthy life.*

Having available a unit that combines mortality and morbidity will be immensely useful if we are trying to maximize the *health benefit* of a given amount of resources invested in healthcare. Suppose dialysis patients' self-stated quality of life is 0.8 (where 0 is death and 1.0 is normal healthy life). They would gain 8.0 QALYs from ten years on $40,000-a-year dialysis, a cost-benefit ratio of $50,000 per QALY. Suppose hip replacements improve fifteen years of life from 0.9 quality ranking to 0.99. That will be a 1.35 QALY gain for the $10,000 operation, a cost of less than

$7,500 per QALY. To achieve greater efficiency, we apparently should expand the use of hip replacements and look toward reducing dialysis.

A sizable literature of CEA has developed, not only studies of particular procedures but also discussions about the construction of common units of health benefit. Take the QALY. Questions abound. Whom does one ask to discern quality-of-life rankings for different sorts of health states—patients with the problems, or other citizens and subscribers who are less dominated by their desire to escape their immediate health need? What questions do we ask them? Those building the QALY and well-year frameworks have used *time trade-off* (how much shorter a life in good health would you still find preferable to a longer lifetime with the disability or distress you are ranking?), *standard gamble* (what risk of death would you accept in return for being assured that if you did survive, you would be entirely cured?), and several others. Whatever question people are asked, it should convey as accurately as possible what might be called the *QALY bargain*: their exposure to a greater risk of being allowed to die should they have an incurable, low-ranking condition, in return for a better chance of being helped to significant recovery or saved for prospectively normal health.

The moral argument for using some such common health benefit unit is more than just some narrow focus on aggregate economic efficiency per se. The major moral argument by many health economists for using both quality adjustment and longevity extension in a serious attempt to maximize the benefit that a plan or an entire healthcare system produces is that it is people themselves who implicitly quality-rank their own lives and thus consent to the allocation priorities that QALYs or well-years generate. Critics charge, however, that maximizing years of healthy life in our lifesaving policies systematically fails to respect the individual with an admittedly lower quality of life. To what interpersonal trade-offs have people consented, even when it might involve themselves? Suppose you yourself now prefer, as you did previously, a shorter, healthier life to a longer, less healthy one. You are now an accident victim who could survive, though paraplegic, while someone else could be saved for more complete recovery. Admittedly, you yourself prefer a life with recovery to one with paraplegia, and you would be willing to take a significant risk of dying from a therapy that promised significant recovery if it succeeded. You do not admit, though (and you never have admitted), that when life itself is on the line, a life with paraplegia is any less valuable to the person whose life it is than life without that disability. *Compared with death,* your paraplegic life could still be as valuable *to you* as anyone else's *better* life is *to them*—that is, you want to go on living as fervently as the nondisabled person does.

Some analysts, in attempting to incorporate points such as this and other ethical criticisms of QALYs, have emphasized a standard distinction in economics, that between individual utility and societal (or *social*) value. Individual utilities convey information about the welfare of an individual, while social values constitute preferences or evaluative claims about communities or relationships between persons. People hold social values, just as they also have preferences about their own lives. For example, they typically believe that those who are more severely ill should get a given healthcare service first before another who is not as severely ill, even if in either case the care produces equivalent improvement in those two persons' individual utilities. They also typically believe that even if the individual utility of a given number of years of life extension is arguably greater for someone in full health than it is for someone with a significant chronic illness, the value of saving either of their lives is equal. Using the *person trade-off* technique for eliciting such social values, some economists and policy analysts (Nord; Menzel et al) have argued for extending empirical value measurement to so-called *cost-value analysis* (CVA). Whether a model for health resource allocation developed along such lines will prove to be ethically superior to standard health economic analysis that focuses on individual utility units such as QALYs will undoubtedly be vigorously debated in the coming decade.

Common health benefit units will undoubtedly continue to be developed and used. Their contested character only indicates that the process of economic analysis into which they fit, systemwide CEA, is itself a morally contested vision for healthcare.

The Monetary Value of Life

CBA, in contrast to CEA, demands the assignment of monetary value to the benefits of a program or procedure. The health benefit whose monetarization has received the most explicit attention in the literature of CBA is life itself. Economic evaluation of life itself, as superficial and distorting as it may sound, is in one sense now an ordinary phenomenon. Now that a great number of effective but often costly means of preserving life are available, we inevitably and repeatedly pass up potential lifesaving measures for other good things, and money mediates those trade-offs. In CBA, however, one goes further and assigns a *particular* monetary value, or range of monetary values, to life. Is that value $200,000 or $2,000,000? Other questions abound. Is the monetary value of a relatively short remaining segment of life (a year, say) simply an arithmetic proportion of the

whole life's value? If we assume that the length of different people's lives that remains to be saved or preserved is equal, is the economic value of their lives the same, or does it vary—for example, with income level, wealth, or future earning power? And if it does vary, should we still use those varying values or instead some common average in doing CBA of healthcare?

Independent of the debates on those questions, economists have developed two main models for translating empirical data into an economic value of life: discounted future earnings (DFE), also known as *human capital,* and willingness to pay (WTP). DFE looks at the future earnings forgone when a person dies. In the economy, those earnings are what is lost when a person dies, so that from the perspective of the *whole economy* (if we can speak of any such thing), it would be self-defeating not to save a life for $200,000 if the value of the person's earnings (after discounting the future figures back to present value) was more than that. While such DFE calculations continue to be used in some CBAs in healthcare, DFE has been largely surpassed in economists' work by WTP. In WTP the value of life is taken to be a direct function of people's willingness to use resources to increase their chances of survival. Suppose one annually demands an extra $500, and only $500 extra, to work in an occupation that runs an additional 1 in 1,000 risk of dying. Then according to WTP, $500,000 (1,000 × $500) is the monetary value one puts on one's life. Within the context of CBA, this would mean it would be inefficient to devote more than $500,000 per statistical life saved to healthcare that eliminates prospective risks of death.

In economic theory, WTP is generally regarded as the superior model; it captures the range of life's subjective, intangible values that DFE seems to ignore. Generally people spend money for reasons of subjective preference satisfaction quite independent of monetary return. That is, economic value incorporates consumption values, not just investment. Despite that firm basis in underlying economic theory, WTP has raised a host of objections. For one thing, questions arise similar to those that afflict DFE. Just as there are in DFEs, there are wide variations in willingness to pay—largely based on people's wealth and income. May those variations in value legitimately affect what is spent on lifesaving measures? If their effect is legitimate, is that only for services privately purchased, or also for those funded publicly? Defenders of WTP have articulated many responses to handle these and other critical questions, but the model may still seem suspicious. Any statement to the effect that "it was efficient not to save his life (now lost)—it was worth only $500,000" is not easily accepted. Consequently, despite its professional popularity, WTP has hardly gained widespread moral acceptance for actual use in health-policy.

The basic problem is simply that in the end the world is such a different place for a loser than it is for a winner. Suppose one refuses to pay more than $500 (when one could) for a CAT scan or magnetic resonance image (MRI) that one knows is likely to eliminate a 1-in-1,000 portion of the risk of dying from one's malady, and that then one later dies because of that decision. Of course one has in some sense consented to what happened, but one never thought anything remotely like "$500,000—no more—is the value of my life," the life that after the fact is irretrievably lost. The move that economists make in WTP to get from an initial trade-off between money and risk to the value of a real, irreplaceable life is puzzling. One critic has claimed that in principle only valuations of life made directly in the face of death are correct reflections of the actual economic value of life (Broome). And as another contributor to this discussion has noted, we do not know of anyone "who would honestly agree to accept any sum of money to enter a gamble in which, if at the first toss of a coin it came down heads, he would be summarily executed" (Mishan, p. 159–160). Some conclude from this that CBA can set no rational limit on what to spend to save a life because no particular finite amount of money is adequate to represent the real value of life.

Even if this point about the actual value of a life is correct, however, it may not render WTP estimates of the value of life irrelevant for use in health policy. In the context of setting policy about whether to include a certain service in our package of insurance, we cannot just assume that the later perspective of an individual immediately in the face of death is the correct one from which to make decisions. Such a perspective may be proper for the legal system to adopt in awarding compensation for wrongful death, for there we are trying to compensate people for losses actually incurred. But perhaps healthcare decisions ought to be made from an earlier perspective. In modern medical economies, after all, most people either subscribe to private insurance plans or are covered by public ones. Once insured, whether in private or public arrangements, subscribers and patients as well as providers find themselves with strong incentive to overuse care and underestimate opportunity costs. Why should we not address the problem of controlling the use of care in the face of these value-distorting incentives at the point in the decision process, *insuring,* where the major cost-expansion pressure starts? In the context of CBA for health policy, while it may not be necessary to claim that willingness to risk life shows us the *value of life,* willingness to risk may still be appropriate to use in any case. Perhaps what is important in decisions to invest resources in healthcare is only that what gets referred to as *the monetary value of the benefits* should be derived from people's decisions to bind themselves in advance to certain restrictions on the provision of care. The

problem with WTP may then be narrower: Many of the *values of life* generated by WTP are not sufficiently close to the actual decisions of people to take risk by limiting their own investment in lifesaving. That would render any resulting CBAs that used them crude and ungrounded, but would not necessarily seal the fate generally of WTP-using CBA.

It is possible that as a formal method of analysis, CBA will never have great influence. Even if that is true, however, the larger enterprise of less formal CBA will remain an active and crucial dimension of the broader attempt to find the proper place of healthcare in our lives overall.

The Difficulties That Economic Concepts Pose for Clinical Practice

Suppose that economic efficiency analysis, whether of the CEA, CBA, or other less formalized sort, lays the groundwork for recommendations about the kind and amount of healthcare to use—fewer diagnostic MRIs in certain low-yield situations and very cautious introduction of new, expensive drugs, for example, and more hip replacements and much more assertive and widely diffused prenatal care. The former, service-reducing steps would not constitute the elimination of merely wasteful procedures that generate no net health benefit. They would constitute something much harder: *genuine rationing,* in which some patients did not get what for them would be optimal care. How does such rationing for efficiency relate to the ethical obligations of healthcare providers? The traditional (at least traditionally professed) ethic of physicians is one of loyalty to individual patients. Generally, in turn, that loyalty is interpreted to mean beneficence: doing whatever benefits a patient the most, within the limits of what the competent patient willingly accepts. If healthcare is to be rationed in order to control the resources it consumes, however, will the basic clinical ethic have to change? This potential clash between traditional ethical obligations and the economic and social demands of the *new medicine* in an age of scarcity is one of the central foci of ethical controversies in medicine as we enter the twenty-first century.

One can divide the potential views here into *incompatibilist* and *reconciliationist* camps: those who think that the demands of societywide (or at least large-group) efficiency cannot be reconciled with the ethical obligations of practitioners, and those who think they can be. The incompatibilists will end up in two different positions: (1) the "well, then, to hell with morality" view in which one is willing to pursue economic efficiency anyhow; and (2) the anti-efficiency stance that opposes rationing in the name of a morality of strict beneficence toward individual patients. Reconciliationist views will also come in distinctly different sorts. (1) Parties more distant from the patient than clinicians should make all rationing decisions, and clinicians should then ration only within pre-determined practice guidelines—the separation-of-roles position. (2) As a provider, one's proper loyalty to a patient, though not dominated by efficiency, is to the patient as a member of a just society; this then enables the clinician to ration with a clean conscience if based on considerations of fairness and justice (Brennan). (3) Patients are larger, autonomous persons; rationing can then be grounded in the consent of the pre-patient subscriber to restrictions on his or her later care (Menzel, 1990). (Why would the patient consent?—to reserve resources for other, more value-producing activities in life.)

The strength of the incompatibilist views may seem to be that they call a spade a spade, but their abiding weakness is that they just dam up the conflict and create later, greater tensions. The reconciliationist views, on the other hand, deal constructively with the conflict and allow conscientious clinical medicine to find roots in a more cost-controlled, socially acceptable aggregate of healthcare. Their weakness may be the great difficulties they face in actual use. The separate-roles view requires extremely clear formulation of detailed care-rationing practice guidelines in abstraction from the medically relevant particulars of individual patients; by contrast, *bedside rationing* in which clinicians make substantive rationing decisions may be preferable and necessary (Ubel). The patient-in-a-just-society model requires a great degree of agreement on what constitutes a just society. And the prior-consent-of-patients solution requires not only accurate readings of what restrictions people are actually willing to bind themselves to beforehand but also a willingness of subscribers and citizens to think seriously about resource trade-offs beforehand and then abide honestly by the results even when that places them on the short end of rationing's stick.

Undoubtedly this discussion is not about to reach immediate resolution soon in societies that are enamored of ever-expanding healthcare technologies, pride themselves on respecting individual patients, and are determined to steward their resources wisely.

Externalities and Public Goods

Externalities and public goods play a prominent role in economics-informed discussions of public policy. Externalities are costs or benefits of a behavior not borne by or accruing to the actor, but by or to others. They pose a distinct problem for the achievement of efficiency in market economies. If I am making and selling an item whose production involves harms or burdens to others for which I do not have to pay, I

will be able to price the product under its true cost and sell it more easily. The solution is to correct incentives by imposing a tax on the item equivalent to its external cost (or a subsidy equivalent to its external benefit). Even better, one could give the proceeds of that tax to the parties harmed by the item's use or production. Externalities, then, immediately propel us into public-policy decisions about taxes and subsidies.

Public goods also directly raise questions of public regulation and taxation. A *public good* in the economist's sense is one whose benefits accrue even to those who do not buy it. If you clean up your yard, I benefit from a somewhat better appearance on the block regardless of whether I clean up my own or help you clean up yours. Or if a large number of people contribute to an educational system in the community, I get some of the benefits of the more civilized culture and productive economy that result even if I never contribute anything. The benefit is thus public and nonexclusive: Once a certain mass of contributors is in place, it is difficult if not impossible to exclude from the benefits an individual who chooses not to contribute. Standard examples of public goods include many of the basic functions of the modern state (public safety, national defense, education, public health, and the reduction of pollution). Thus, public goods constitute a primary justification of the state's coercive power. If I contribute not a penny to a police force, for example, I will still receive most of its benefits; if not taxed, I can thus *free-ride* on others' willingness to fund public safety. The obvious solution is for the collective to tax me my fair share.

The use of both public goods and externalities is undoubtedly on the rise in discussions of healthcare. Note just two examples of the interesting contexts in which these concepts come up.

An example of externalities is the taxing of health-complicating products such as tobacco and alcohol. Smoking and excessive drinking undoubtedly increase certain costs to others—healthcare expenditures for smoking- and drinking-related diseases; lost work time; displeasure, sadness, and pain in dealing with others' destruction of their social and biological lives; and even direct loss of life (from passive smoking, drunk driving, etc.). These externalities provide part of the momentum behind the movement to increase taxes on tobacco and alcohol. Note, however, that the empirical picture can be much more complicated, and in the case of tobacco it certainly is. First-impression, informal cost analysis of smoking (and many published academic studies as well) leads us to think that smokers cost nonsmokers a great deal of money. That conclusion ignores, however, two hidden *savings* of smoking that accrue to others: Because smokers die earlier, and generally near the end of their earning years or shortly thereafter, they save others the pension payouts and the unrelated healthcare expenditures they would have incurred had they lived longer, without losing that saving through significantly reduced earnings. One leading study, in fact, concludes that all the costs that smokers impose on others, including losses from fires and the costs of the U.S. tobacco subsidies justify only a cigarette tax of $.37 per pack (Manning et al.). The typically higher taxes that actually obtain in most states cannot then be justified by any empirically well-grounded externalities argument, nor can the state governments' claims to settlements of hundreds of billions of dollars from tobacco companies (Viscusi). This is not the last word on the net external costs of smoking, but it illustrates the subtleties and hidden costs that increasingly sophisticated economic analysis reveals. Economic analysis may turn up equally surprising results in the future as we turn increasingly to prevention in the hope of controlling healthcare costs; prevention that saves healthcare expense in one respect may lose those gains as its longer-living beneficiaries draw more pension payouts and end up incurring higher aggregate costs of illness in their longer lives.

An example of public goods is sharing in the costs of a healthcare system that provides access to those who otherwise cannot pay. Suppose most people think a good society provides basic care to those who cannot afford it, and that they believe that the financial burdens of the medical misfortunes that people cannot have been expected to control by their own choices ought to be shared equally by well and ill. It is then possible to analyze the situation in the traditional and conservative terms of public goods and the prevention of free-riding. If a considerable amount of charity care is societally provided and access is thus improved, I gain both the security of knowing that I will be helped if I become poor or sick, and the satisfaction of knowing that I live in a society that does not neglect its poor and ill. If I do not contribute financially to make this more secure and arguably better society possible, I free-ride on the largess of others. This free-riding situation generates an essentially conservative justification for requiring people to pay into an insurance pool even when they think they are safe.

Many other interesting and controversial instances of the use of these and other economic concepts in the analysis of healthcare could be cited. Without being targeted accurately on identifiable pockets of market failure, tax breaks for health-insurance premiums would seem to create incentives for inefficient overinvestment in healthcare. If physicians significantly create demand for their own services, their incomes will need to be regulated either by the government or by market forces at work among health plans using salary or capitation payments (as distinct from fee for service) to compensate physicians. And so on and so forth. More generally, how to discern what constitutes efficiency in the investment of resources in healthcare, how to arrange incentives to stimulate efficient use of care, and how the achievement of efficiency is to be compared with the realization of other values central to the whole healthcare enterprise constitute the challenge that economic concepts bring to healthcare in the twenty-first century.

PAUL T. MENZEL (1995)
REVISED BY AUTHOR

SEE ALSO: *Healthcare Allocation; Healthcare Resources; Healthcare Systems; Health Insurance; International Health; Justice; Just Wages and Salaries; Managed Care; Medicaid; Medicare; Pharmaceutical Industry; Profit and Commercialism; Value and Valuation*

BIBLIOGRAPHY

Brennan, Troyen A. 1991. *Just Doctoring: Medical Ethics in the Liberal State.* Berkeley: University of California Press.

Broome, John. 1982. "Uncertainty in Welfare Economics and the Value of Life." In *The Value of Life and Safety: Proceedings of a Conference Held by the "Geneva Association,"* ed. Michael W. Jones-Lee. Amsterdam: North-Holland.

Daniels, Norman. 1986. "Why Saying No to Patients in the United States Is So Hard." *New England Journal of Medicine* 314(21): 1381–1383.

Drummond, Michael F.; O'Brien, Bernie; Stoddart, Greg L.; et al. 1997. *Methods for the Economic Evaluation of Health Care Programmes,* 2nd edition. Oxford and New York: Oxford University Press.

Feldstein, Paul J. 1998. *Health Care Economics,* 5th edition. New York: Delmar Learning.

Feldstein, Paul J. 1999. *Health Policy Issues: An Economic Perspective on Health Reform.* Chicago: Health Administration Press.

Fuchs, Victor R. 1986. "Health Care and the United States Economic System." In Victor Fuchs *The Health Economy* Cambridge, MA: Harvard University Press.

Harris, John. 1987. "QALYfying the Value of Life." *Journal of Medical Ethics* 13(3): 117–123.

Jennett, Bryan. 1986. *High Technology Medicine: Benefits and Burdens.* Oxford: Oxford University Press.

Manning, Willard G.; Keeler, Emmett B.; Newhouse, Joseph P.; et al. 1991. *The Costs of Poor Health Habits.* Cambridge, MA: Harvard University Press.

Menzel, Paul T. 1990. *Strong Medicine: The Ethical Rationing of Health Care.* New York: Oxford University Press.

Menzel, Paul T. 2002. "Justice and the Basic Structure of Health-Care Systems." In *Medicine and Social Justice,* ed. Rosamond Rhodes, Margaret Battin, and Anita Silvers. New York: Oxford University Press.

Menzel, Paul T.; Gold, Marthe; Nord, Erik; et al. 1999. "Toward a Broader View of Cost-Effectiveness Analysis of Health Care." *Hastings Center Report* 29(1): 7–15.

Mishan, Ezra J. 1985. "Consistency in the Valuation of Life: A Wild Goose Chase?" In *Ethics and Economics,* ed. Ellen Frankel Paul, Jeffrey Paul, and Fred D. Miller, Jr. Oxford: Basil Blackwell.

Morreim, E. Haavi. 1991. *Balancing Act: The New Medical Ethics of Medicine's New Economics.* Dordrecht, Netherlands: Kluwer.

Nord, Erik. 1999. *Cost-Value Analysis in Health Care: Making Sense Out of QALYs.* Cambridge, Eng.: Cambridge University Press.

Pellegrino, Edmund D., and Thomasma, David C. 1988. *For the Patient's Good: The Restoration of Beneficence in Health Care.* New York: Oxford University Press.

Phelps, Charles E. 1997. *Health Economics,* 2nd edition. Reading, MA: Addison-Wesley.

Rhoads, Steven E., ed. 1980. *Valuing Life: Public Policy Dilemmas.* Boulder, CO: Westview.

Rice, Thomas. 1998. *Economics of Health Reconsidered.* Chicago: Health Administration Press.

Robinson, James C. 1986. "Philosophical Origins of the Economic Valuation of Life." *Milbank Quarterly* 64(1): 133–155.

Russell, Louise B. 1986. *Is Prevention Better Than Cure?* Washington, D.C.: Brookings Institution.

Sloan, Frank A., ed. 1996. *Valuing Health Care: Costs, Benefits, and Effectiveness of Pharmaceuticals and Other Medical Technologies.* Cambridge, Eng.: Cambridge University Press.

Torrance, George W. 1986. "Measurement of Health State Utilities for Economic Appraisal: A Review." *Journal of Health Economics* 5: 1–30.

Ubel, Peter A. 2000. *Pricing Life: Why It's Time for Health Care Rationing.* Cambridge, MA: The MIT Press.

Viscusi, W. Kip. 2002. *Smoke-Filled Rooms: A Postmostem on the Tobacco Deal.* Chicago: University of Chicago Press.

Walker, Rebecca L., and Siegel, Andrew W. 2002. "Morality and the Limits of Societal Values in Health Care Allocation." *Health Economics* 11: 265–273.

Williams, Alan. 1985. "Economics of Coronary Artery Bypass Grafting." *British Medical Journal* 291(6491): 326–329.

ELECTROCONVULSIVE THERAPY

• • •

Electroconvulsive therapy (ECT) is a highly efficacious treatment in psychiatry (Crowe, Abrams), and yet there is ethical controversy about its use. Some have claimed that ECT should be outlawed because it seriously impairs memory; others, that ECT is best viewed as a crude form of behavior control that psychiatrists frequently coerce patients to accept. Still others claim that, even if coercion is not employed, depressed patients are rarely, if ever, competent to give valid consent to the treatment (Breggin). The complaint is also sometimes voiced that ECT is given more frequently to women patients than to men. There is also ample evidence that, in earlier years, ECT was given in ways that are not used today: higher amounts of electrical current, and sometimes daily or several-times-daily treatments. Undoubtedly, this harmed some patients (Breggin). Probably because of concerns like these, one state, California, has passed legislation making it difficult for psychiatrists to employ ECT without satisfying many administrative regulations (California Welfare and Institutions Code). There also exist several activist groups that are opposed to all ECT and have even tried to criminalize the administration of ECT. Daniel Smith provides an excellent summary of these groups's arguments and activities in his 2001 article "Shock and Disbelief."

The nature of the treatment itself understandably frightens some persons, and there have been gruesome depictions of it in popular films and novels (Kesey). The notion of passing an electrical current through the brain, stimulating a cerebral seizure and causing unconsciousness, may seem forbidding, particularly in view of the fact that ECT's therapeutic mechanism of action remains largely unknown. There are, however, many effective treatments in medicine whose mechanisms are unknown, and there are probably many surgical treatments that would seem equally forbidding if they were observed by a layperson. In appraising the ethical legitimacy of ECT as a treatment, it is important to ask the same questions about ECT that are asked about any treatment: Of what does it consist, what is the likelihood that it will help, what kinds of harm can it cause; and how does its spectrum of benefits and harms compare with those of alternative plausible treatments?

ECT Treatment

There are several excellent reviews of the history, clinical indications, and likely harms and benefits of ECT (Abrams; American Psychiatric Association Task Force on Electroconvulsive Therapy (APA Task Force); Crowe; Ottosson). The essential feature of the treatment is the induction of a cerebral seizure (which is easily measured via concomitant electroencephalography) by means of electrodes attached to the scalp. Current is applied through the electrodes for a fraction of a second. The two electrodes may be attached to the right and left temples (bilateral ECT), inducing a seizure in both hemispheres of the brain, or to anterior and posterior placements on only one side (unilateral ECT), limiting the seizure to that side. Patients are premedicated with a muscle relaxant and anesthetized with a short-acting barbiturate general anesthetic. Patients remain unconscious after the treatment for about five minutes and are usually mildly confused for an hour or so after they awaken. They have no memory of the treatment itself. Treatments are usually given two or three times weekly for two to four weeks.

ECT was used originally as a treatment for schizophrenia on the basis of the now-discredited belief that epilepsy, which ECT was thought to mimic, and schizophrenia did not occur in the same persons. It is used chiefly with patients suffering from severe depression; most psychiatrists suggest its use to patients only when drug treatment and/or psychotherapy have not helped. ECT is also used occasionally with bipolar patients suffering from a life-threatening degree of manic excitement, or to schizophrenic patients suffering from a catatonic stupor, when these conditions do not improve with drug therapy.

Efficacy and Side Effects

The effectiveness of ECT in reversing severe depression seems beyond dispute (Abrams; Crowe; APA Task Force): Many large studies show a significant recovery from depression in 80 to 90 percent of patients who receive ECT, as compared with 50 to 60 percent of depressed patients who respond to antidepressant medication. Patients who do not respond to drugs show a high response rate to ECT: about 50 to 60 percent recover. No study comparing the differential effects of drugs and ECT has ever found that drugs have a greater therapeutic effect. ECT also works more quickly than drugs: Patients who improve typically begin to do so after about one week; drugs, if they work, typically take three to four weeks, sometimes longer, to have a significant effect. Many studies have shown that unilateral and bilateral ECT are equally effective treatments, although a minority have found unilateral ECT to be on average less effective. However unilateral ECT also causes, on average, less cognitive confusion during treatment and less residual memory impairment afterward.

Although ECT can cause death, it does so infrequently that it is difficult to reliably estimate a mortality rate. The largest modern report (Heshe and Roeder) studied 3,438 courses of treatment (22,210 ECTs), and only one death occurred. The APA Task Force estimates a death rate of 1 in 10,000 patients and 1 in 80,000 treatments. When ECT does cause death, it is usually cardiovascular in origin and is related to the use of a general barbiturate anesthesia.

The principal adverse effect of ECT on some patients is to cause one or another kind of memory impairment. Two of these kinds of memory impairment are limited. During the two to three weeks that treatments are given, memory and other cognitive functions are usually mildly to moderately impaired because of the ongoing seizures. Moreover in later years patients are often unable to recall many events that took place shortly before, during, and shortly after the two- to three-week course of treatment. Neither of these effects bothers most patients, as long as they understand ahead of time that they will occur.

The more important and controversial question is how often ECT causes an ongoing, permanent deficit in memory function (an anterograde amnesia). If and when it does, it is possible that the treatment has damaged parts of the brain underlying memory function. This has proven to be an elusive research problem, despite dozens of studies, many quite sophisticated, that have been carried out (Taylor et al., Abrams). Among the many methodological problems involved in doing this research (Strayhorn) is the fact that depression itself often causes cognitive impairment, including memory dysfunction. In fact studies of the effect of ECT on memory have repeatedly shown that the majority of patients actually report improved memory function after ECT, probably due to the diminution of their depression (APA Task Force).

A small minority of patients—the exact percentage seems unknown—do report mild, ongoing, permanent memory problems after ECT; nearly all of them rate the memory problem as annoying but not serious. However, when patients treated with ECT are compared with appropriate control groups, no deterioration in performance on objective tests of memory ability has ever been found. Nonetheless a very small number of patients, perhaps 1 to 2 percent, complain of serious ongoing memory problems. Memory complaints occur more frequently after bilateral than unilateral ECT, which has led many commentators to recommend that unilateral treatment generally be given, and that bilateral treatment be used only in serious conditions and after unilateral ECT has failed.

Ethical Issues

Is ECT so harmful that it should be outlawed? Very few persons maintain this position. ECT has an extremely small risk of causing death. It probably also has a small risk of causing chronic mild memory impairment, and a very small risk of causing chronic serious memory impairment. It is frequently used, however, in clinical settings where other treatments have failed and where the patient is suffering intensely and may be at risk of dying. Severe depression is a miserable and a serious illness: The three-year death rate in untreated or undertreated patients is about 10 percent, while in treated patients, it is about 2 percent (Avery and Winokur). Even if the risks of ECT were substantially greater than they are, it would still be rational in the clinical setting of severe depression for patients to consent to receiving ECT.

As with all other treatments in medicine, the possible harms and benefits of ECT should be explained to the patient during the consent process. The risk of death and of chronic memory dysfunction should be mentioned specifically. The APA Task Force also stipulates that a discussion should be included, during the consent process, "of the relative merits and risks of the different stimulus electrode placements and the specific choice that has been made for the patient. The patient's understanding of the data presented should be appraised, questions should be encouraged, and ample time for decision making should be allowed. Patients should be free to change their minds about receiving ECT, either before the treatments start or once they are under way" (pp. 5–6).

ECT is often suggested to patients only after other treatments have failed. However, although it has slight risks, ECT has several advantages over other treatments: It works more quickly, in a higher percentage of cases, and it does not have the annoying and, for some cardiac patients, possibly dangerous side effects of many antidepressant drugs. Following the general notion that part of an adequate valid consent process is to inform patients of any available rational treatment options (Gert et al.), a strong argument can be made that, from the outset of treatment, seriously depressed patients should be offered ECT as one therapeutic option (Culver et al.). The APA Task Force states: "As a major treatment in psychiatry with well-defined indications, ECT should not be reserved for use only as a *last resort.*"

Do psychiatrists often coerce patients into receiving ECT? This seems doubtful, but there are no data addressing this question. In the overwhelming majority of cases, psychiatrists should not force any treatment on a patient. Nonetheless there are very rare clinical situations in which it is ethically justified to give ECT to patients who refuse it (Group for the Advancement of Psychiatry): for example, patients in danger of dying from a severe depression that has not been responsive to other forms of treatment (Merskey). But this is a special instance of the general ethical issue of justified paternalistic treatment, and no special rules should apply to psychiatric patients or to ECT (Gert et al.).

There seems no reason to believe that the consent or the refusal depressed patients give to undergo ECT is not in most cases valid. If a patient is given adequate information about the treatment, if he or she understands and appreciates this information, and if the patient's choice is not forced, then the decision is valid and, in almost all cases, should be respected. Most psychiatrists would assert that the great majority of depressed patients are like the great majority of all patients: They feel bad, they would like to feel better, and if presented with information about available treatment options, they try to make a rational choice.

Is ECT disproportionally and unjustly given to women patients? There are no data that address this question, and it would be useful to obtain them. However, given the fact that women suffer from clinically significant depression two to three times more frequently than men (Willner), the critical question is not whether more women in total receive ECT, as would be expected, but whether ECT is given at a higher rate to women than to equally depressed men.

CHARLES M. CULVER (1995)
REVISED BY AUTHOR

SEE ALSO: *Behaviorism; Behavior Modification Therapies; Electrical Stimulation of the Brain; Emotions; Freedom and Free Will; Human Dignity; Informed Consent: Issues of Consent in Mental Healthcare; Mental Health Therapies; Mental Illness: Issues in Diagnosis; Neuroethics; Psychiatry, Abuses of; Psychosurgery, Ethical Aspects of; Psychosurgery, Medical and Historical Aspects of; Research Policy: Risk and Vulnerable Groups; Technology*

BIBLIOGRAPHY

Abrams, Richard. 2002. *Electroconvulsive Therapy*, 4th edition. New York: Oxford.

American Psychiatric Association. Task Force on Electroconvulsive Therapy. 2001. *The Practice of Electroconvulsive Therapy: Recommendations for Treatment, Training, and Privileging,* 2nd edition. Washington, D.C.: Author.

Avery, David, and Winokur, George. 1976. "Mortality in Depressed Patients Treated with Electroconvulsive Therapy and Antidepressants." *Archives of General Psychiatry* 33(9): 1029–1037.

Breggin, Peter Roger. 1979. *Electroshock: Its Brain-Disabling Effects.* New York: Springer.

California Welfare and Institutions Code. 1979. §§5325.1, 5326.7, 5326.8, 5434.2.

Crowe, Raymond R. 1984. "Electroconvulsive Therapy—A Current Perspective." *New England Journal of Medicine* 311(3): 163–167.

Culver, Charles M.; Ferrell, Richard B.; and Green, Ronald M. 1980. "ECT and Special Problems of Informed Consent." *American Journal of Psychiatry* 137: 586–591.

Gert, Bernard; Culver, Charles M.; and Clouser, K. Danner. 1997. *Bioethics: A Return to Fundamentals.* New York: Oxford.

Group for the Advancement of Psychiatry. Committee on Medical Education. 1990. *A Casebook in Psychiatric Ethics.* New York: Brunner/Mazel.

Heshe, Joergen, and Roeder, Erick. 1976. "Electroconvulsive Therapy in Denmark." *British Journal of Psychiatry* 128: 241–245.

Kesey, Ken. 1962. *One Flew over the Cuckoo's Nest.* New York: New American Library.

Merskey, Harold. 1991. "Ethical Aspects of the Physical Manipulation of the Brain." In *Psychiatric Ethics,* 3rd edition, ed. Sidney Bloch and Paul Chodoff. Oxford: Oxford University Press.

Ottosson, Jan-Otto. 1985. "Use and Misuse of Electroconvulsive Treatment." *Biological Psychiatry* 20(9): 933–946.

Smith, Daniel. 2001. "Shock and Disbelief." *Atlantic* 287(2): 79–90.

Strayhorn, Joseph M., Jr. 1982. *Foundations of Clinical Psychiatry.* Chicago: Year Book Medical Publishers.

Taylor, John R.; Tompkins, Rachel; Demers, Renée; and Anderson, Dale. 1982. "Electroconvulsive Therapy and Memory Dysfunction: Is There Evidence for Prolonged Defects?" *Biological Psychiatry* 17(10): 1169–1193.

Willner, Paul. 1985. *Depression: A Psychobiological Synthesis.* New York: Wiley.

EMBRYO AND FETUS

• • •

I. DEVELOPMENT FROM FERTILIZATION TO BIRTH

The ethical relevance of studying human development appears when one asks which stages of the human life cycle embody significant ethical concerns. Between birth and death, the human organism is a person, equipped with the full measure of basic human rights. This much is not really controversial, and the debate primarily concerns the prenatal phase of development. Do human rights accrue to the unborn all at once, for instance at fertilization? Do they instead arise in a gradual manner, based on the various progressive steps through which the prenatal human organism acquires significant person–like properties? Besides personal rights, are there other ethically–significant values and properties that would justify a respectful treatment of embryos and fetuses? An understanding of prenatal development is a necessary, albeit in no way sufficient, condition for addressing these issues successfully.

To understand the basic biology of any sexually reproducing organism, one needs to grasp the primary concept of the life cycle. The life cycle of humans includes fertilization, cleavage, gastrulation, organogenesis, fetal development, birth, child development and puberty, gametogenesis and again fertilization. It is through the germ–line that the life cycle persists from generation to generation. On the other hand, the somatic cells (which comprise all the cells of the fetus, child, and adult that are not directly involved in reproduction) belong to an inherently mortal entity, the human organism, whose fate is senescence and death. One turn of the life cycle defines one generation. Fertilization and birth define the beginning and end of the prenatal phase of development, which is comprised of two stages: embryonic and fetal.

The embryonic phase initiates with fertilization, the meeting of the male (sperm) and female (oocyte) gametes, giving rise to the zygote. At fertilization, a new, diploid genome arises from the combination of the two haploid genomes included in the gametes. The zygote divides several times (cleavage stage) to form a blastocyst. The cells of the blastocyst, called blastomeres, are separated into two parts: an outer layer, called the *trophoblast,* that eventually contributes to the placenta; and an inner cell mass that contributes to the future embryo. About six days after fertilization, the blastocyst attaches to the endometrium (the epithelial lining of the uterus). This marks the beginning of pregnancy and further development depends on intricate biochemical exchanges with the woman's body. While the trophoblast invades the uterine wall, the inner cell mass undergoes further stepwise differentiation processes that lead to the formation of the embryonic epiblast (the precursor of the actual human individual) and several extraembryonic structures (Figure 1). The embryo then undergoes gastrulation, the process that starts with the formation of the *primitive streak.* This is the crucial developmental step, common to all animals but the most primitive invertebrates, by which the three basic germ layers of the embryo are formed. These are called ectoderm, mesoderm, and endoderm.

From the third to the eighth week, the process of organogenesis involves the differentiation of the three germ—layers into specific tissues and primordial organs. The earliest stage in organogenesis is called neurulation and starts when a specific area of ectoderm turns into the primordium of the nervous system. During organogenesis, many genes that are crucial to development are activated, and complex cell–to–cell signals insure the proper differentiation of various cell types, as well as the movement and migration of cells to their proper places in the developing embryo. For some cell types, this involves long–range navigation. For instance, the gamete precursors must travel from their initial position near the yolk sac to the primordial gonads.

At the end of the embryonic phase, many important organ systems are in place, at least in rudimentary form. The fetal phase is characterized by further differentiation and maturation of tissues and organs, as well as considerable growth, especially towards the end of pregnancy. In the late fetal phase, the nervous system undergoes an acceleration of synapse formation and maturation of the brain, which is increasingly sensitive to outside cues. This process continues well after birth.

Specific Developmental Stages in Detail

Especially in early development, specific developmental processes seem more meaningful than others in the ethical debate about the moral status of human prenatal life. These are described in more detail.

GAMETOGENESIS AND FERTILIZATION. The embryo is usually defined as coming into existence at fertilization and becoming a fetus when organogenesis is completed (eight weeks after fertilization). These borders are not sharply defined. The definition of an embryo thus cannot avoid being operational and context–dependent. The term *conceptus* is useful to denote any entity resulting from fertilization, when no reference to a more specific stage is intended. An additional complication results from the significant overlap between the final stages of female gametogenesis, fertilization, and initial cleavage.

Gametogenesis involves a special type of cell division called meiosis. When primordial germ cells (which are diploid—i.e., they have two complete sets of chromosomes) enter meiosis, their DNA is duplicated so that there are now four copies of each type of chromosome (a condition called

tetraploidy). In the first meiotic division, there are genetic exchanges within each group of homologous chromosomes, which then separate into diploid daughter cells. In the second meiotic division, there is no further round of DNA duplication. Each chromosome in a pair is allotted to a separate daughter cell, now haploid. Each primordial germ cell thus gives rise to four daughter haploid cells.

In the male, all four cells resulting from meiosis ultimately become functional spermatozoa. In contrast, in the female, only one of the daughter cells becomes an oocyte, the other three cells are discarded as polar bodies. In addition, female meiosis is not completed until after fertilization has occurred. During each ovarian cycle of the sexually mature female, one oocyte progresses partially through meiosis but is arrested in the middle of the second meiotic division at the time it is discharged from the mature ovarian follicle into the oviduct. If the oocyte is fertilized, meiosis is completed. Within the newly fertilized egg, the male and female pronuclei undergo a protracted migration towards each other, while DNA is duplicated within both. Thereafter, both nuclear envelopes disappear and the chromosomes derived from the male and female gamete are involved in the first cleavage division. Thus the first genuine diploid nucleus is observed at the two–cell stage only (30 hours after initial contact of sperm and oocyte). While fertilization usually occurs close to the ovary, the conceptus is gently nudged towards the uterus, a voyage lasting about five days.

Both through recombination of gene segments during the first meiotic division, and through random assortment of homologous chromosomes in gametes, genetic novelty is generated. In other words, gametes are genetically distinctive in relation to their diploid progenitors and do not simply reflect the genetic structure of their parent organism. In a sense, gametes are distinctive "individuals" in relation to the organism that produces them. Fertilization creates genetic novelty of a different sort, by combining two independent paternal genomes. The zygote is genetically distinctive because it represents the meeting of two independent parental lineages. Thus genetic novelty appears twice per turn of the human life cycle.

CLEAVAGE, PLURIPOTENTIALITY, AND TWINNING. During cleavage, the zygote divides into smaller embryonic cells. At the 16–cell stage, the embryo is called a morula and a first differentiation into two cell types is initiated. The trophoblast is the cell layer that will soon connect with the uterine wall, whereas the inner cell mass includes the cells of the later stage embryo. At the blastocyst stage, a central cavity (blastocoel) is formed. If a blastomere is removed from the inner cell

FIGURE 1

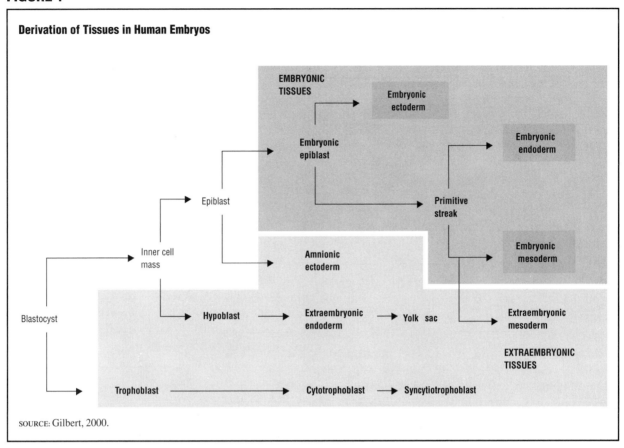

Derivation of Tissues in Human Embryos

SOURCE: Gilbert, 2000.

mass of a blastocyst (as, for instance, in preimplantation diagnosis), the blastocyst is still able to produce a complete late embryo and fetus. This illustrates a fundamental principle called regulation, or regulative development. Within the early embryo, cell fates are not definitely fixed but largely depend on interactions with neighboring cells, so that development adjusts to the presence or absence of specific environmental cues. The molecular basis and the genes responsible for these cues are increasingly well known.

At the blastocyst stage, the inner mass cells are pluripotent (i.e., they have developmental plasticity) and are able to participate in the formation of most cell types of the adult organism, as shown for instance by experiments with cultured immortalized blastomeres, called embryonic stem cells. Recent research does suggest that individual blastomeres acquire some degree of molecular specificity quite early. However, this inherent "bias" that tends to drive every blastomere towards a specific cellular fate can easily be overridden at this stage.

Around day 6, the blastocyst has hatched from the surrounding zona pellucida (the outer envelope of the ovum) and is ready for implantation. As it attaches to the

endometrium, two distinctive layers appear in the inner cell mass. The ventral layer (hypoblast) contributes to the primitive yolk sac. The dorsal layer soon differentiates between the embryonic epiblast that will contribute to the embryo–to–be, and the amniotic ectoderm lining the newly appearing amniotic cavity (day 7–8). This two–layered structure is called the embryonic disk. All this happens as the blastocyst burrows deeper into the uterus wall and the trophoblast comes into close contact with maternal blood vessels. The trophoblast also produces human chorionic gonadotropin (hCG), which is the substance detected in pregnancy tests and is essential to the maintenance of pregnancy. Abnormal conceptuses are very common until that stage and are eliminated, usually without detectable signs of pregnancy. Inversely, fertilization occasionally results in a hydatidiform mole. This structure consists of trophoblastic tissue and therefore mimics the early events of pregnancy (hCG is produced), without their being any actual embryonic tissue present.

The term *pre–embryo* was often used to mark the embryonic stages described so far. This term is sometimes shunned in contemporary discourse, as it has been suspected to be a semantic trick to downgrade the standing of the very early embryo. Yet even writers like Richard A. McCormick belonging to the Catholic tradition, sets great store by the moral standing of the earliest forms of prenatal development, have expressed doubts about the validity of this suspicion (1991). More importantly, doing away with the term "pre–embryo" does not solve the two underlying conceptual problems that this term addresses. The first ensues from the cellular genealogy linking the zygote to the later stage embryo and fetus. Only a small part of the very early embryo is an actual precursor to the late embryo, fetus, and born child. Whatever terminology one wishes to use, no account of early development can avoid sentences such as this, written by Thomas W. Sadler in 2000, "[t]he inner cell mass gives rise to tissues of the *embryo proper*," or terms such as the *embryo–to–be*. This is an inescapable consequence of the fact that the late embryo includes only a small subset of all the cells that originate with the zygote and blastocyst (Figure 1 shows the complex genealogy of embryonic and extraembryonic tissues in human development). The second problem arises from the fact that the early embryo has a degree of freedom as regards its final numerical identity. Until about 12 days after fertilization, twinning can occur. In other words, until that stage, a single embryo still has the potential to divide in two embryos, ultimately developing into two separate persons. Therefore there is no intrinsic one–to–one relationship between the zygote and the late embryo, as there is between the late embryo, the fetus, and the born human.

GASTRULATION. Gastrulation begins with a wave of cellular movements that start at the tail end of the embryo and extend progressively forward. Future endoderm and mesoderm cells slip inside the embryonic disk through a groove called the primitive streak (day 14). The anterior end of the streak is called the node. Of the cells that migrate inside the streak, some form the endoderm and others will lie atop the endoderm and form the mesoderm. Finally, those cells that remain in their initial position on the surface of the embryonic disk become the ectoderm. Gastrulation sets the overall organization of the embryo in a definitive way. The main axes (anterior–posterior, left–right) are defined under the control of two central signaling centers: the node (which is the equivalent of the organizer discovered by embryologists working on frog and chick embryos) and the anterior visceral endoderm.

Recent data from molecular genetics have partially uncovered the molecular basis of axis determination. The determination of the anterior–posterior axis involves the HOX genes, a set of four gene complexes. Since HOX genes located at the "front end" of a HOX complex are expressed

at the "front end" of the embryo, the arrangement of the various genes within each complex remarkably reflects the place at which they are expressed in the embryo along the anterior–posterior axis. The four HOX complexes thus provide four "genetic images" of the lengthwise arrangement of embryonic structures. The left–right asymmetry of the embryo (and thus of the future body plan) is thought to originate with specific cells in the node. In a way that is not fully understood, these cells induce a cascade of protein signals that is different on the left and right side of the embryo. This results in the synthesis of controlling factors that are laterally restricted. It is supposed that these controlling factors and other factors direct the development of asymmetric organs accordingly.

Through gastrulation, the embryo arises as a defined entity endowed with a much higher level of organic unity than at any stage before. The laying down of the head–to–tail axis and other defined spatial features, as well as the loss of pluripotentiality in many cell lineages, mark the beginning of a single individual human organism and thus provide one of the first important dimensions of the ontological continuity typical of the born human.

LATER DEVELOPMENTAL STEPS. In the initial step in organogenesis, the midline axial section of mesoderm—the notochord—instructs the overlying ectoderm to turn into the neural plaque. This structure soon wraps around to form the primitive neural tube, out of which the central nervous system will eventually grow. By the beginning of the fetal period (eighth week), the rudiments of the heart, blood and blood vessels, the major segments of the skeleton and associated muscle groups, the limbs, and many other structures are in place. It is noteworthy that although the primordial nervous system is one of the earliest organ systems to emerge in development, it takes the longest time to mature. Synaptogenesis (the formation of –contacts between nerve cells) starts on a grand scale only late in pregnancy and continues well after birth. This is important to keep in mind when interpreting early movements of the fetus, visualized more and more accurately by ultrasonography. These movements reflect the maturation of local neuromuscular structures and are not due to significant brain function, since there is no "brain" in the sense of the later, much more developed anatomic and functional structure called by that name. This is different later in pregnancy, when fetal movement is more reactive to the environment and when it becomes arguably legitimate to interpret it as "behavior," insofar as it reflects the increased functional capabilities of the central nervous system. Finally, the concept of *viability* basically reflects the ability of fetal lungs and kidneys to support extrauterine life, which is impossible before the twenty-second week.

As mentioned before, the differentiation and migration of early gametes also occurs during the embryonic phase. This separation of the germ cell lineage from all other cell lineages marks a bifurcation in the life cycle. Unlike somatic cells, gamete precursors have a chance of becoming gametes and participating in fertilization, thus contributing to the next generation. In a way, the germ cell lineage is eternal through successive turns of the life cycle, whereas the rest of the embryo, the sum total of somatic cells, is inherently mortal.

Extracorporeal Embryos

Science fiction fantasies about the artificial uterus notwithstanding, only the very first stages of human development can occur outside the female body. Since 1978, in vitro fertilization followed by embryo transfer has been a common treatment of fertility problems. The growth of ovarian follicles is stimulated by the administration of gonadotropins. Oocytes are then collected by laparoscopy and placed in an appropriate culture medium. Sperm is added and cleavage occurs in culture until the blastocyst is transferred in the uterus.

With in vitro fertilization, the early embryo became much more accessible to human intervention, and this has raised ethically perplexing possibilities. Interventional research on early embryos has become possible, raising the question of whether it is ethical to produce human embryos for research purposes, or whether research should be done, if at all, only on "spare" embryos. These occur when some embryos are no longer needed for fertility treatment, even though they resulted from in vitro fertilization performed with therapeutic intent. Additionally, progress in genetic testing techniques using very small amounts of DNA has made preimplantation diagnosis of genetic abnormalities possible. Single blastomeres are removed from in vitro blastocysts, their DNA amplified by polymerase chain reaction (PCR), and subjected to genetic tests with appropriate DNA probes. (Thanks to regulative development, the missing blastomere is soon compensated for.) In this way, embryos can be screened for certain genetic defects and only those free of defects chosen for embryo transfer. This procedure is sometimes suspected of being eugenic, and the controversy around it has led to it being outlawed in certain countries including Germany and Switzerland.

Developmental Steps and Moral Status

The biological processes around fertilization and early embryonic development are often accorded considerable relevance in ethical debates, making a detailed description of these processes necessary. This descriptive effort, however, is not based on the belief that "the facts speak for themselves." They emphatically do not. In fact, many ethical controversies about the ethics of in vitro fertilization, embryo research, therapeutic cloning, abortion and the like, are less about ethics in the strict sense as they are about expressing divergent interpretations of biology. The marshalling of biological fact to support apodictic statements of moral status involves many, usually unspoken, "bridge principles." These principles involve highly complex notions, such as unity, individuality, potentiality, and continuity. It is a common misconception that these theoretical concepts constitute stable, common–sense notions that are merely applied to biological entities and processes. In actuality, these concepts are themselves given new meanings and qualifications in the very process of using them to make sense of biological facts. Between the realm of ontological categories and the empirical domain of biology, there is a two–way street.

It is often said that "human life begins at fertilization." Strictly speaking, this statement is meaningless. Human life does not begin at any point of the human life cycle; it persists through successive generations. The ethically relevant question to ask is at what stage a human individual is first endowed with important ethical value and correlative rights against harm. The difficulty is that no particular step stands forth as a self–evident developmental marker, both because developmental events that appear as sharp discontinuities turn out to be protracted processes upon closer scrutiny (for instance, fertilization is a process, not an instantaneous event), and because the highlighting of one developmental process over another necessarily involves more or less plausible philosophical assumptions.

Three different concepts of individuality appear to be relevant:

- genomic individuality as established trough fertilization;
- numerical identity, defined once twinning is no longer possible;
- identity of the self, as sustained by a functional central nervous system.

Fertilization is important because it newly connects two parental lineages that were independent until then. The meeting of sperm and oocyte gives rise to a uniquely novel diploid genome that is not subject to further change. It will be the genome of the future person or persons arising from this particular fertilization. This fact is often misinterpreted according to a hylomorphic interpretation of the genome, where the latter becomes the formal cause of the future human being (Mauron). (Hylomorphism is the aristotelian and scholastic teaching that concrete objects, especially living things, result from a combination of form [morphê] and substance [hylê].) This interpretation suggests the notion that fertilization is the single crucial step, since the new genome appears at that point. This interpretation fails, not only because of the inherent conceptual problems of the hylomorphic view, but also because there exist biological facts such as twinning and genetic mosaicism that show that there is little connection between genomic individuality as such and personal identity. Monozygotic or identical twins are separate persons, even though they share "the same" genome, that originated from "the same" fertilization. This shows that genomic individuality does not provide any basis for the most essential property of personal identity, namely numerical identity through time. To be one and same person through changes in one's biography is an essential ingredient of any workable concept of the person, and the biological basis for this property does not originate before gastrulation. In fact, much of the organic singularity and coordinated functioning as one organism (rather than several potential organisms) is established only at that stage.

However, one may want a richer interpretation of this basic criterion of personal identity. Having a biography of one's own is not just being the same individual through time, but also experiencing a continuity of mental states, which is linked to an at least minimally-functioning central nervous system. In fact, nothing is more central to the modern conception of the self than the functional persistence of a central nervous system that provides the material substrate of an individual subjective biography. For this biographical, or subjective, identity, it is difficult to quote a definitive starting point. It is plausible to place it in late pregnancy, when the earliest possibility of a continuing self seems to be given, but there is no absolute certainty in this claim.

Conclusion

Ethical reasoning on this topic often shows a common pattern: one takes moral concepts that belong to uncontroversial persons (such as grown humans) and tries to apply them backwards to the fetus and embryo. However, importing intuitions pertaining to the ethics of personal rights and interests onto various forms of prenatal life is increasingly fraught with conceptual difficulties as one moves towards earlier stages. Indeed, the most perplexing problem in bridging human developmental biology and statements of moral standing is perhaps that traditional moral categories tend to be "all-or-none" concepts (either one is a person or not, and if so, one is equal in basic rights to all persons), whereas developmental biology shows mostly gradual change and tends to resolve what appear to be discrete borders into

continuities. One obvious and popular answer to this quandary is to make ethical standing a gradually increasing property of the developing human organism. On the other hand, one may query the underlying assumption that there is a one-dimensional measure of ethical concern. Further reflection may benefit from a recognition that ethical concerns about human prenatal life are multidimensional, and sometimes qualitatively, not just quantitatively, different from the person-centered systems of ethical values and duties.

ALEXANDRE MAURON

SEE ALSO: *Abortion: Medical Perspectives; Alcoholism and Other Drugs in a Public Health Context; Cloning; Death, Definition and Determination of: Criteria for Death; Feminism; Infants; Infanticide; Maternal-Fetal Relationship; Moral Status; Reproductive Technologies: Ethical Issues;* and other *Embryo and Fetus* subentries

BIBLIOGRAPHY

Ford, Norman M. 1988. *When Did I Begin? Conception of the Human Individual in History, Philosophy and Science.* Cambridge, Eng.: Cambridge University Press.

Gilbert, Scott F. 2000. *Developmental Biology,* 6th edition. Sunderland, MA: Sinauer Associates.

Green, Ronald M. 2001. *The Human Embryo Research Debates: Bioethics in the Vortex of Controversy.* Oxford: Oxford University Press.

Mauron, Alex. 2001. "Is the Genome the Secular Equivalent of the Soul?" *Science* 291: 831–832.

McCormick, Richard A. 1991. "Who or What Is the Preembryo?" *Kennedy Institute of Ethics Journal* 1: 1–15.

Robertson, John A. 1991. "What We May Do with the Preembryos: A Response to Richard A. McCormick." *Kennedy Institute of Ethics Journal* 1: 293–302.

Sadler, Thomas W. 2000. *Langman's Embryology,* 8th edition. Baltimore, MD: Lippincott Williams & Wilkins.

INTERNET RESOURCES

Gilbert, Scott F. 2000. "When Does Human Life Begin?" Website to accompany *Developmental Biology,* 6th edition. Available from <www.devbio.com/chap02/link0202a.shtml>.

II. EMBRYO RESEARCH

In previous editions of this encyclopedia, the topic of embryo research was included within the entry on fetal research. However, during the latter part of the twentieth century the issues arising from research involving in vitro fertilized embryos became sharply distinguished from issues in research with already-implanted fetuses. Moreover, new technologies such as the development of embryonic stem cells and the possibility of human cloning raised new ethical concerns in relation to research involving human embryos.

This entry will address the history of human embryo research, public policy on embryo research in the United States and internationally, moral considerations, particularly the debate on the moral status of the human embryo, and the relevance of ethical distinctions that have been proposed, such as the distinction between research use of surplus embryos versus embryos created specifically for research.

The Research Subject

Scientifically the product of conception is called an *embryo* until eight weeks of gestational age, when the name changes to *fetus*. However, contemporary discussions of embryo research customarily restrict the term embryo to the earliest stages of human development before implantation in the uterus occurs. This terminology is supported by the U.S. federal regulations on fetal research, which define the fetus as "the product of conception from implantation until delivery," thus excluding non-implanted embryos from the regulations (45 CFR 46.202).

In practical terms the embryo as subject of research is the embryo in the laboratory, generally the result of in vitro fertilization (IVF), but possibly developed by other means, for example, through flushing naturally-fertilized eggs from the fallopian tube, or through somatic cell nuclear transfer (SCNT) of a body cell into an enucleated egg, a type of cloning procedure.

A variety of terms has been proposed for the embryo as subject of research:

> the *preembryo,*
> the *preimplantation embryo,*
> the *embryo ex utero,*
> the *early embryo.*

In this entry the simple term *embryo* will be used, with the understanding that it refers to the embryo in the laboratory that has not undergone transfer to a woman. Some commentators maintain that only embryos resulting from fertilization of eggs by sperm are properly called embryos. This question will be addressed in later sections when it is relevant.

Early History of Embryo Research

Until the 1990s most research involving human embryos was directed toward improving the chances for pregnancy in laboratory-assisted conception. These investigations, in turn, were based on many years of research with animal models, where virtually all research in the United States has been supported with federal funding. It was hoped that procedures developed in animal studies could later be applied to human reproduction and embryology, especially to the understanding and alleviation of human infertility.

Attempts at laboratory fertilization of human oocytes (precursor eggs) showed some promise as early as 1944 in the work of American obstetrician-gynecologist John Rock and scientist Miriam Menkin. From that time until the birth of the first child conceived through IVF in 1978, various approaches were tried in order to achieve a pregnancy and live birth. The work of Robert Edwards, British reproductive endocrinologist, culminated in the birth of Louise Brown after he collaborated with Patrick Steptoe, an obstetrician who utilized laporoscopy for viewing and recovering a mature ovarian follicle containing an oocyte capable of fertilization.

According to embryologist Jonathan Van Blerkom, most current methods used in laboratory-based treatment of infertility have evolved from those used by Edwards and Steptoe and their predecessors. According to Van Blerkom, this work "established the basic science foundation of clinical IVF" (p. 9). Without these four decades of research on fertilizing oocytes, accompanied by study of the early cleavage and development of fertilized eggs or zygotes, the clinical practice of IVF, which is an almost universally accepted primary treatment for infertility, would not exist.

U.S. Funding and Regulation of Embryo Research

In 1975 the U.S. National Commission for the Protection of Human Subjects recommended guidelines for federal funding of research involving human fetuses, but stipulated that these guidelines did not cover research on IVF or on embryos resulting from IVF. It proposed that an Ethical Advisory Board be appointed to review such protocols, and this recommendation was incorporated into federal regulations. In 1978 an Ethics Advisory Board (EAB) was appointed to recommend a policy on federal funding for research involving IVF.

In its 1979 report the EAB concluded that research on IVF was ethically acceptable for federal funding under these conditions: that all federally funded research is directed toward establishing the safety and efficacy of IVF; all gametes used to develop embryos in research protocols are provided by married couples; and no embryos are preserved in the laboratory beyond fourteen days of development. The EAB's rationale was based on two main points. First, it would be irresponsible to offer clinical IVF without doing the studies necessary to insure its safety and efficacy. Second, given the high rate of embryo loss in natural procreation, a similar rate of loss could be tolerated for the goal of eventually achieving pregnancies and births.

The EAB did not distinguish between embryos created for research purposes and embryos remaining from infertility treatment. In fact, the board implied that at times it might be necessary to create embryos with no intent to transfer them to a woman. For the sake of safety, the results of new types of procedures would have to be studied in the laboratory before the procedures were offered clinically. It would be unethical to transfer to a woman the embryos resulting from unvalidated novel procedures.

The EAB report elicited an outpouring of letters opposing embryo research, and its recommendations were never implemented. When the EAB charter expired in 1980, a subsequent board was not appointed, thus leaving no body to review proposals for federal funding of IVF and embryo research. This situation effectively created a moratorium on federal funding in the United States, though it did not affect research that was privately funded.

Public Policy in Other Countries

It is not possible to review all legislation and policy recommendations throughout the world, but two early initiatives are of particular interest. They come from countries that share a common law tradition with the United States, Australia (Victoria), and the United Kingdom.

AUSTRALIA (VICTORIA). The earliest comprehensive legislation on reproductive technologies was enacted in the State of Victoria, Australia in 1984. The Infertility (Medical Procedures) Act addressed embryo research by prohibiting research that might damage the embryo or make it unfit for implantation. This prohibition appeared to outlaw any IVF or embryo research that was not directed toward benefiting each individual embryo.

In 1986 the review committee established by the act received a proposal for research on the microinjection of a single sperm into an egg. In their application the investigators suggested a novel approach for circumventing the prohibition on embryo research. They proposed to examine the egg after the sperm had penetrated it, but before the genetic contributions of the sperm and egg had fused at the stage known as syngamy. Arguing that fertilization was not completed until syngamy had occurred, researchers claimed that the law did not apply until the time of syngamy, thus giving them approximately twenty-two hours after sperm penetration for conducting their studies.

Since the review committee was uncertain as to whether the 1984 act allowed this interpretation, it recommended that the act be amended to clarify that research was permissible if it ended by the time of syngamy, even if the research destroyed the embryo's potential for implantation. The act was amended according to this recommendation in 1987.

UNITED KINGDOM. The issue of the regulation of reproductive technologies and embryo research was particularly pressing in the United Kingdom because of the publicity given to the birth of Louise Brown in England in 1978. The Warnock Committee was appointed to study the matter, and its 1984 report recommended national regulation of assisted reproduction. It also recommended that research on embryos resulting from IVF be permitted up to the fourteenth day after fertilization, under the jurisdiction of a licensing body.

Based on the Warnock Report, the Human Fertilisation and Embryology Act (HFE Act) of 1990 commissioned a standing body, the Human Fertilisation and Embryology Authority (HFEA), to develop standards for licensing clinical facilities and research protocols, and mechanisms for auditing and oversight. Initially research protocols were restricted to the study of infertility, the causes of congenital diseases, and the detection of gene or chromosome abnormalities in embryos.

Since its establishment in 1991 the HFEA has addressed new types of procedures and research through public consultation processes as well as the advice of experts. If a matter was beyond the scope of authority of the HFEA, it was referred to Parliament. In January 2001 Parliament extended the HFE Act to permit embryo research directed at increasing knowledge about treatments for serious diseases. This provision would allow the HFEA to issue licenses for research on embryonic stem cells, including stem cells derived from blastocysts resulting from somatic cell nuclear replacement (SCNR). However, the Pro-Life Alliance brought a challenge to this provision, arguing that the HFE Act applied only to embryos resulting from the fertilization of eggs by sperm. Despite a Court of Appeal ruling against the Pro-Life Alliance, in June 2002 the House of Lords agreed to hear a final appeal of the case. In March 2003 the House of Lords ruled that the HFE Act applied to all types of embryos, and hence the HFEA had authority over research with embryos created by nuclear transfer as well as embryos resulting from fertilization by sperm.

The U.S. Human Embryo Research Panel

After nearly twenty years of moratorium on federal funding of research involving IVF, the U.S. Congress in 1993 revoked the requirement of EAB review. Through the

National Institutes of Health (NIH) Revitalization Act of 1993, Congress explicitly permitted the NIH to fund research on assisted reproductive technologies with the goal of improving the understanding and treatment of infertility.

Since research on IVF includes the study of IVF-fertilized embryos, the research authorized by Congress included research involving human embryos. Recognizing the controversial issues raised by this research, NIH decided to conduct an examination of ethical issues before funding any research proposals. Consequently, the Director of NIH appointed the Human Embryo Research Panel (HERP) to provide advice and recommendations.

In developing its position and recommendations, the panel focused on two distinct sources of guidance: viewpoints on the moral status of the early human embryo, and ethical standards governing research involving human subjects. It considered a wide range of possible views on the moral status of the embryo, from the position that full human personhood is attained at fertilization, to the argument that personhood requires self-consciousness and is not attained until after birth. In the end, all nineteen members of the panel agreed to the following statement:

> Although the preimplantation embryo warrants serious moral consideration as a developing form of human life, it does not have the same moral status as an infant or child. (Human Embryo Research Panel, p. x)

This conclusion implied that the preimplantation embryo is not a full human subject and thus is not a fully protectable human being. As a result, some research that might be destructive to the embryo could be acceptable for federal funding. But the panel also asserted that the human embryo "warrants serious moral consideration," requiring that it be treated differently from mere human cells or animal embryos. The panel proposed restrictions on embryo research that would express such moral consideration, for example, that human embryos be used in research only as a last resort, that the number of embryos used be carefully limited, and that embryos not be allowed to develop longer than required by a specific research protocol, and in no case longer than fourteen days of development.

In applying the ethical standards governing research involving human subjects, panel members invoked the criteria used by Institutional Review Boards (IRBs) in approving research protocols. Donors of eggs, sperm, or embryos were to be informed of the specific goals, procedures, and risks of research projects. Risks to donors, particularly egg donors, were to be minimized. Eggs for research could be donated only by women who were undergoing diagnostic or therapeutic procedures where egg retrieval would present little additional risk.

The most controversial issue facing the panel was the question of whether human oocytes could be fertilized solely for research purposes. The panel decided to allow such fertilization only under very special circumstances, most particularly, if certain research by its very nature could not otherwise be conducted. For example, research on the laboratory maturation of human oocytes, which could eliminate the need for egg donors as well as infertile women to be subjected to high levels of hormonal stimulation, requires study as to whether such oocytes can be successfully fertilized.

The panel's limited acceptance of the fertilization of oocytes for research purposes aroused strong criticism, and President Bill Clinton immediately announced his opposition.

The Aftermath in the United States and Beyond

Despite President Clinton's directive that NIH not fund research involving the creation of embryos, most types of research on IVF and human embryos were still eligible for federal funding. However, in its next appropriations bill Congress reversed its previous stance and prohibited NIH from funding any research that might involve damaging or destroying human embryos. In 2003 this prohibition was still in effect.

During the 1990s scientific advances raised new questions regarding research with human embryos. In 1998 the first embryonic stem cell lines were developed from the inner cell mass of human blastocysts, and at the same time, similar stem cell lines were produced from the germ cell tissue of aborted fetuses. Deriving stem cells from blastocysts was clearly prohibited for federal funding. However, the derivation of stem cells from the tissue of aborted fetuses was eligible for federal funding under previous legislation (U.S. Public Law 103–43, Manier).

Another discovery was the successful cloning of a variety of nonhuman animals from adult cells, beginning with the cloning of the sheep Dolly in 1997. Research on human cloning arguably involves research on human embryos. These embryos are produced by transfer of somatic cell nuclei into enucleated oocytes, rather than through fertilization of eggs by sperm, yet their development and potential appear to be similar to those of fertilized eggs. Thus cloning research raises similar ethical questions.

The day after the announcement of the cloning of Dolly, President Clinton instructed the National Bioethics Advisory Commission (NBAC) to undertake a thorough review of the technology and to report within ninety days.

Given this short deadline, it is understandable that NBAC had to focus on issues specific to the cloning process. In particular, NBAC decided to "not revisit … the issues surrounding embryo research," since the topic had "recently received careful attention by a National Institutes of Health panel, the Administration, and Congress" (Shapiro).

In contrast, when the President's Council on Bioethics appointed by President George W. Bush issued its report on cloning in 2002, it called for a broader debate on the entire topic of human embryo research. The ten-member majority of the council wanted cloning discussed "in the proper context of embryo research in general and not just that of cloning" (p. 133). Both the majority and minority reports call attention to the fact that human embryo research of all types remains essentially unregulated in the private sector, with the minority noting that "it seems inappropriate to halt promising embryo research in one arena (cloned embryos) while it proceeds essentially unregulated in others" (p. 143).

In the United States, public policy at the national level is focused on what types of research are eligible for public funding. There is essentially no regulation of research in the private sector. This situation contrasts sharply with that of most other countries, where laws apply to all research, regardless of the funding source.

As of April 2003, Germany, Austria, and Ireland prohibit embryo research unless intended to benefit the individual embryo subject. Germany does allow some importation of established stem cell lines for research. France prohibits any embryo research that would harm the embryo. However, in January 2002 the French assembly passed a bill that, if enacted, would permit research using surplus embryos originally created for reproductive purposes. Sweden allows research on surplus embryos up to day fourteen, including research on deriving stem cell lines. Creating IVF embryos solely for research is prohibited, but creating embryos through nuclear transfer is not mentioned in Swedish law and thus has an uncertain legal status. The United Kingdom arguably has the most permissive policies on embryo research within the European Union. It explicitly sanctions the granting of licenses to create embryos, including cloned embryos, for specific research projects.

Because of the diverse views and policies of its member states, the European Union has taken an intermediate position, providing support for research on surplus embryos in countries where that is permitted, but discouraging the creation of embryos for research. In April 2003 the European parliament voted for a ban on cloning or otherwise creating embryos for stem cell research. However, this decision becomes law only if approved by all fifteen member states of the European Union.

In May 2002 the Assisted Human Reproduction Act was introduced into the Canadian Parliament. The act prohibits the creation of a human clone for any purpose. It also prohibits the creation of an IVF embryo for research purposes with the exception of "improving or providing instruction in assisted reproduction procedures." In April 2003 the bill was in its third reading in the House of Commons.

In some non-Western countries, embryo research is proceeding with few restrictions. Chinese laboratories are forging ahead with cloning research to develop stem cells. Though Chinese scientists have been slow to publish their work, they may well be ahead of their Western counterparts (Leggett and Regalado). India has developed a number of internationally recognized stem cell lines, and scientists are developing additional lines. Dr. Firuza Parikh, Director of Reliance Life Sciences in Bombay, links their success to the absence of cultural and political opposition to embryo research (Lakshmi).

The Moral Status of the Early Embryo

In contrast to China and India, most Western countries are deeply divided over ethical issues related to embryo research. Does the embryo merit full protectability from the moment of fertilization, or does it gradually attain full protectability as it moves through a series of developmental stages? If fertilization is not the point of greatest moral significance, is there some later developmental marker beyond which embryo research ought not be conducted?

FERTILIZATION. Fertilization of egg by sperm marks the initiation of a new and unique genotype, that of a human being distinct from either of its progenitors. The zygote or fertilized egg not only contains the plan or blueprint for a new human being, but it has the potential within itself to develop into that human being.

Based on these facts, many would argue that the zygote is a full human being from the moment it comes into existence. This view would preclude any research that might be harmful or destructive to an embryo, unless intended to be therapeutic for that embryo or to improve its chances for implantation. This position has received able defense in contemporary terms by opponents of embryo research (McCarthy and Moraczewski).

It is possible to hold this position while acknowledging that fertilization is a process rather than an instantaneous event, and hence that the new human life begins only when the process of fertilization is completed. At least two possible candidates marking the completion of fertilization have been suggested. The first is the time of syngamy, when the chromosomes from the male and female gametes unite to form the genotype of the embryo. Since syngamy is not completed until about twenty-four hours after the sperm penetrates the egg, this view would allow some study of the early development of the embryo.

A second proposal maintains that the embryo does not begin its life as a new human being until the regulation of its development switches from oocyte genes to embryonic genes. In 1988 Peter Braude and colleagues showed that this occurs at the six- to eight-cell stage, approximately two days after penetration of egg by sperm. Arguably the embryo begins its own life distinct from that of the oocyte at the time that its own internal regulatory mechanism begins to function. This interpretation would allow investigation of questions such as why a large proportion of embryos are arrested in their development during the earliest cell divisions (Van Blerkom).

Such variant views of the process of fertilization do not counter the claim that the human being begins its life at fertilization. Rather, they provide differing interpretations as to what constitutes fertilization, under the assumption that the formation or activation of the unique genotype of the new organism is the crucial event.

IMPLANTATION. Implantation is the process by which the embryo imbeds itself in the uterine wall and begins to take nourishment from the woman, thus marking the beginning of pregnancy. It is at this time that the U.S. federal regulations define the product of conception as a fetus, and the research regulations begin to apply (45 CFR 46.201–207).

From a moral point of view, some have argued that the IVF embryo lacks the potential to develop into a human being as long as it is simply maintained in culture in the laboratory. Only those embryos that are transferred to women and that implant successfully acquire the potential for development. This type of argument has been utilized by politicians like U.S. Senator Orrin Hatch, who support some forms of embryo research while they take pro-life positions in relation to abortion. In his testimony to a Congressional subcommittee in July 2001, Hatch stated, "I believe that a human's life begins in the womb, not in a petri dish or refrigerator."

This view can be linked to a philosophic distinction between *possible* persons, entities that could possibly develop into persons if certain actions were taken with respect to them, and *potential* persons, entities that will develop into persons in the normal course of events unless something happens or is done to interrupt that development. The embryo in the laboratory or freezer is a possible person that might develop into a person if action were taken to transfer it

to a uterus. The already-implanted embryo or fetus is a potential person that, under normal circumstances, will continue to develop into a person. Proponents of this distinction argue that while we may have a moral obligation not to interfere with the development of a potential person, we do not have a similar obligation to bring every possible person into existence (Singer and Dawson; Tauer 1997a).

PRIMITIVE STREAK. In the late twentieth century, scholars were faced with biological data about early embryonic development that led to new perspectives on the ontological and moral status of the early embryo. Particularly within the Catholic tradition, writers such as Norman Ford, John Mahoney, Richard McCormick, and Karl Rahner developed arguments questioning whether the zygote or early embryo is a full human being or human person. Their arguments appealed to the following points:

1. Twinning of the embryo is possible until implantation, and at least through the morula stage, several embryos may aggregate (recombine) to form one embryo. Thus the embryo lacks developmental individuation at this early stage. Philosophic arguments that rely on the continuity of personal identity and religious arguments based on ensoulment must deal with the phenomena of twinning and recombination, which occur naturally and can also be induced scientifically.

2. Until the blastocyst stage at approximately five days after fertilization, the cells of the embryo are totipotent or completely undifferentiated. Each cell has the capacity to differentiate into any of the cell or tissue types of the fetus, or more likely, not to become part of the fetus at all but rather to form placental and other extra-embryonic tissues. The early embryo is a collection of undifferentiated cells rather than an organized individual.

3. At approximately fourteen days after fertilization, the primitive streak appears, the groove along the midline of the embryonic disk that establishes in the embryo its cranio-caudal (head-to-tail) and left-right axes. The primitive streak marks the beginning of the differentiation of cells into the various tissues and organs of the human body, and thus initiates the development of the embryo proper (the cells that will become the fetus) as an organized, unified entity. The primitive streak is also the precursor of the neural system.

4. In normal procreation, during the period between fertilization and the completion of implantation a large proportion of embryos (generally estimated at over 50%) are discarded naturally. Karl Rahner argues that it is implausible that such a large number of human beings could come into existence

and disappear without anyone's knowing about it. Others have argued that given nature's prodigality with human embryos, it ought to be morally acceptable to allow similar types of embryonic losses in research as part of the effort to achieve healthy pregnancies.

These sorts of arguments have been utilized in public policy debates since 1978, and the appearance of the primitive streak has come to be accepted internationally as a marker carrying moral significance. The prohibition of embryo research after fourteen days of development is almost universally accepted.

Opponents of embryo research have responded to claims that the early embryo is not yet a full human being. These commentators find arguments based on twinning and recombination, totipotency of cells, and embryo loss to be unpersuasive (Ashley; Ashley and Moraczewski; Mirkes). In its 2002 report on cloning, the majority members of the U.S. President's Council on Bioethics questioned the significance of the primitive streak as a moral marker, stating:

> Because the embryo's human and individual genetic identity is present from the start, nothing that happens later … —at fourteen days or any other time—is responsible for suddenly conferring a novel human individuality or identity. (p. 97)

GASTRULATION AND NEURULATION. Some persons regard the initiation of the neural system or the presence of brain activity to be the most significant marker for the beginning of the life of a human being. This view is based on the belief that the brain is the essential organ underlying our specifically human capacities. It also represents an effort to identify a criterion at the beginning of human life that is analogous to the criterion of whole-brain death marking the end of life. For those who regard the presence of sentience as a necessary condition for personhood, the neural system is significant since sentience is impossible in the absence of any neural structures.

While there is debate as to the stage at which brain activity first occurs, it is certain that there is no brain activity before fourteen days of gestational age. The emergence of the primitive streak marks the very beginning of the development of the nervous system. If the presence of neural structures is the significant criterion for the beginning of a human life, then it might be permissible to extend embryo research slightly beyond fourteen days of development.

Several possible cut-off points have been suggested. By the completion of *gastrulation* at about seventeen days, the three germ layers of the embryo are in place, with cells of each layer committed to forming tissues and organs of one of three types. Subsequent neural development leads to the beginning of *closure of the neural tube* around twenty-one days, with the primitive nervous system in place by the completion of *neurulation* around twenty-eight days.

However, given the widespread consensus that fourteen days of gestational age is a morally defensible boundary for embryo research, there has been limited discussion of extending research to a later embryonic stage.

Other Moral Considerations

Those who believe that the human embryo is a fully protectable human being have no choice but to oppose embryo research that could not ethically be performed on infants or children. But those who maintain that the early embryo is not yet a full human being, still have to determine how that embryo ought to be treated.

Some have proposed severely restrictive criteria for embryo research. Norman Ford, after providing painstaking arguments to support the conclusion that the embryo cannot be a human individual until fourteen days after fertilization, acknowledges that he could be wrong. In his view, the Catholic Church is right to insist on the principle that "human embryos should be treated as persons," even if they may not be (2001, p. 160). In other words, as long as there is any degree of uncertainty regarding the moral status of the embryo, it must be absolutely inviolate.

A more commonly held view is that the human embryo has an intermediate sort of moral status. While it is not a fully protectable human being, it is not merely cells or tissue. Proponents of this view are generally willing to permit some embryo research with restrictions that acknowledge that the embryo is nascent human life or a developing form of human life. Our ethical obligation toward the embryo is often characterized as *respect* or *profound respect*.

Proponents as well as opponents of embryo research have questioned the concept of respect as a guide for human embryo research. John Robertson, an advocate of scientific freedom with respect to embryo research, believes the notion of respect carries mainly symbolic significance. Hence its practical ramifications are vague, potentially allowing a wide range of types of research. Daniel Callahan, in an essay opposing most embryo research, wonders how one shows respect for a living being while intending to end its life and future potential, even if done for a good purpose such as research on infertility or disease.

In an effort to express respect for the special status of the human embryo, public policy bodies have stipulated conditions for embryo research that are considerably more restrictive than policies on research with human cells or animal embryos. For example, research must have important scientific or medical goals and may involve human embryos only when the research cannot be conducted in any other way. Research projects should be restricted to the smallest number of embryos that is feasible, and for the shortest possible time period. Careful records and security must be utilized to ensure that no embryos are diverted for unapproved purposes and that none are sold.

Bringing Embryos into Existence for Research

One of the most contentious issues in embryo ethics is the question of whether it is ever justifiable to bring human embryos into existence specifically for research purposes. Many would argue that research use of surplus embryos remaining after the completion of infertility treatment is ethically acceptable, since these embryos are destined to be destroyed in any case. At the same time, they may hold that the development of embryos for research purposes, so-called research embryos, is not morally justified.

The development of embryos for research purposes has been characterized as a novel practice that requires particular justification. Referring to embryos created through nuclear cell transfer, the President's Council on Bioethics in 2002 claimed that such research creation of embryos would constitute crossing a "major moral boundary" (p. 132). Yet decades of research on human IVF beginning in the 1930s required investigation of various methods of laboratory fertilization, followed by study of cleaving fertilized eggs to determine their normality before transfer to a woman was even considered (Soupart and Strong; Edwards and Steptoe).

Commentators agree that there is no ontological or intrinsic distinction between surplus embryos remaining after infertility treatment and research embryos developed specifically for study. Arguments that support a moral distinction must identify other morally relevant factors. The concept of respect is often invoked, as is the notion of *intent.*

Respect for the special status of the embryo seems to require that embryos be treated as entities of intrinsic value. When embryos are created purely for research purposes, they become instruments for purposes that have nothing to do with the embryos themselves. In Kantian terms, the embryos are used solely as means for the welfare of others rather than as ends in themselves. The practice of creating research embryos thus results in treating embryos as commodities, equivalent to mere cells or tissues.

In contrast, the intent to procreate justifies the development of embryos in the laboratory. Even when a large number of eggs is fertilized in an IVF procedure, each fertilized egg has an equal chance of being transferred to a woman and developing into a human being. Thus each zygote is equally respected for its procreative potential.

It is only because some of the embryos cannot be transferred (because of the decision of the progenitors, or because there simply are too many of them) that they become surplus embryos and are destined for destruction. It is arguably permissible to derive some good from the inevitable destruction of these embryos by using them in research. In doing so, one may be said to be choosing the *lesser evil.*

These arguments have been countered by a number of considerations.

It may be true that respect for the special status of the human embryo requires that it be treated differently from mere human tissue. But the concept of respect is vague and undetermined, so that a wide range of concrete interpretations is plausible. The claim that respect precludes all creation of research embryos gives heavy weight to one interpretation of the concept at the expense of any countervailing considerations. Research projects that include the development of embryos may promise significant benefits for relieving the suffering of living human beings. These benefits could outweigh a particular interpretation of respect.

While procreative intent may justify the creation of embryos in the laboratory, it is plausible that other sorts of purposes could provide equally valid justifications. The treatment of infertility, an elective medical procedure, may even hold lesser moral significance than the development of cures for life-threatening or significantly disabling diseases and trauma outcomes. Hence such goals may also justify the creation of embryos.

Moreover, surplus embryos do not appear purely by chance. Clinicians frequently make a decision to fertilize large numbers of eggs in order to optimize the chances of establishing a pregnancy. The initial intent is not to give every zygote the opportunity for implantation, but to achieve one or more pregnancies and births, as desired by the progenitors. A later decision to direct unused embryos to research cannot be justified by the principle of the lesser evil, since the existence of surplus embryos should have been anticipated. This situation was deliberately caused and could have been avoided. Thus it is invalid to invoke the principle of the lesser evil to justify use of surplus embryos in research, while maintaining that any creation of research embryos is prohibited.

Parthenogenesis

A potentially non-controversial process for developing morulas and blastocysts for research is the activation of oocytes without use of sperm or transfer of somatic cell nuclei. Such activation can be achieved through electrostimulation or chemicals in a process called parthenogenesis. The resulting cleaving eggs, called *parthenotes,* may develop much like normal embryos at least to the blastocyst stage. Although no human parthenotes have progressed this far, in February 2002 scientists announced that they had developed monkey parthenote blastocysts and established stable stem cell lines from them (Cibelli, et al.).

Scientists believe "there is a profound and intrinsic biological barrier that prevents mammalian parthenotes from developing to advanced fetal stages" (Human Embryo Research Panel, p. 20). On this assumption, parthenogenic morulas or blastocysts lack the intrinsic potential to become human beings. If this potential is a defining aspect of the human embryo and the basis for its special moral status, then human parthenotes are not human embryos and should not arouse the same sorts of moral concerns. Thus they may offer an attractive alternative for research.

CAROL A. TAUER

SEE ALSO: *Abortion: Medical Perspectives; Children: Healthcare and Research Issues; Cloning; Feminism; Fetal Research; Infants; Infanticide; Maternal-Fetal Relationship; Moral Status; Reproductive Technologies: Ethical Issues; Research Policy: Risk and Vulnerable Groups; Research, Unethical;* and other *Embryo and Fetus* subentries

BIBLIOGRAPHY

Annas, George J.; Caplan, Arthur; and Elias, Sherman. 1996. "The Politics of Human-Embryo Research—Avoiding Ethical Gridlock." *New England Journal of Medicine* 334: 1329–1332.

Ashley, Benedict. 1976. "A Critique of the Theory of Delayed Hominization." In *An Ethical Evaluation of Fetal Experimentation: An Interdisciplinary Study,* ed. Donald G. McCarthy and Albert S. Moraczewski. St. Louis, MO: Pope John XXIII Medical-Moral Research and Education Center.

Ashley, Benedict, and Moraczewski, Albert. 2001. "Cloning, Aquinas, and the Embryonic Person." *National Catholic Bioethics Quarterly* 1(2): 189–201.

Braude, Peter; Bolton, Virginia; and Moore, Stephen. 1988. "Human Gene Expression First Occurs Between the Four- and Eight-Cell Stages of Preimplantation Development." *Nature* 332: 459–461.

Buckle, Stephen; Dawson, Karen; and Singer, Peter. 1990. "The Syngamy Debate: When Precisely Does an Embryo Begin?" In *Embryo Experimentation: Ethical, Legal and Social Issues,* ed. Peter Singer, Helga Kuhse, Stephen Buckle, et al. Cambridge, Eng.: Cambridge University Press.

Callahan, Daniel. 1995. "The Puzzle of Profound Respect." *Hastings Center Report* 25(1): 39–40.

Charo, R. Alta. 1995. "The Hunting of the Snark: The Moral Status of Embryos, Right-to-Lifers, and Third World Women." *Stanford Law and Policy Review* 6: 11–37.

Cibelli, Jose B.; Grant, Kathleen A.; Chapman, Karen B.; et al. 2002. "Parthenogenetic Stem Cells in Nonhuman Primates." *Science* 295: 819.

Coughlan, Michael J. 1990. *The Vatican, the Law and the Human Embryo.* Iowa City: University of Iowa Press.

Davis, Dena S. 1995. "Embryos Created for Research Purposes." *Kennedy Institute of Ethics Journal* 5(4): 343–354.

Edwards, Robert, and Steptoe, Patrick. 1980. *A Matter of Life: The Story of a Medical Breakthrough.* New York: William Morrow and Company.

Ethics Advisory Board, U.S. Department of Health, Education, and Welfare. 1979. "Report and Conclusions: HEW Support of Research Involving Human In Vitro Fertilization and Embryo Transfer." *Federal Register* 44: 35033–35058.

Evans, Donald, ed. 1996. *Conceiving the Embryo: Ethics, Law and Practice in Human Embryology.* The Hague, Netherlands: Martinus Nijhoff Publishers.

Ford, Norman M. 1989. *When Did I Begin?* Cambridge, Eng.: Cambridge University Press.

Ford, Norman M. 2001. "The Human Embryo as Person in Catholic Teaching." *National Catholic Bioethics Quarterly* 1(2): 155–160.

Green, Ronald M. 1994. "At the Vortex of Controversy: Developing Guidelines for Human Embryo Research." *Kennedy Institute of Ethics Journal* 4(4): 345–356.

Green, Ronald M. 2001. *The Human Embryo Research Debates.* New York: Oxford University Press.

Human Embryo Research Panel, National Institutes of Health. 1994. *Report of the Human Embryo Research Panel,* vol. 1. Washington, D.C.: National Institutes of Health.

Howard Hughes Medical Institute. 2002. "A Global Struggle to Deal with Human ES Cells." Sidebar in "Are Stem Cells the Answer?" *Howard Hughes Medical Institute Bulletin,* March: 10–17.

Keenan, James. 2001. "Casuistry, Virtue, and the Slippery Slope: Major Problems with Producing Human Life for Research Purposes." In *Cloning and the Future of Human Embryo Research,* ed. Paul Lauritzen. New York: Oxford University Press.

King, Patricia A. 1997. "Embryo Research: The Challenge for Public Policy." *Journal of Medicine and Philosophy* 22(5): 441–455.

Khushf, George. 1997. "Embryo Research: The Ethical Geography of the Debate." *Journal of Medicine and Philosophy* 22(5): 495–519.

Knowles, Lori P. 2000. "International Perspectives on Human Embryo and Fetal Tissue Research." In *Ethical Issues in Human Stem Cell Research,* vol. 2: *Commissioned Papers.* Rockville, MD: National Bioethics Advisory Commission.

Lakshmi, Rama. "India Plans to Fill Void in Stem Cell Research." *Washington Post,* August 28, 2001, p. A7.

Lauritzen, Paul, ed. 2001. *Cloning and the Future of Human Embryo Research.* New York: Oxford University Press.

Leggett, Karby, and Regalado, Antonio. "Fertile Ground: As West Mulls Ethics, China Forges Ahead in Stem-Cell Research." *Wall Street Journal,* March 6, 2002, p. A1.

Mahoney, John. 1984. "The Beginning of Life." In *Bio-ethics and Belief.* London: Sheed and Ward.

McCarthy, Donald G., and Moraczewski, Albert S., eds. 1976. *An Ethical Evaluation of Fetal Experimentation: An Interdisciplinary Study.* St. Louis, MO: Pope John XXIII Medical-Moral Research and Education Center.

McCormick, Richard A. 1991. "Who or What Is the Preembryo?" *Kennedy Institute of Ethics Journal* 1(1): 1–15.

Mirkes, Renee. 2001. "NBAC and Embryo Ethics." *National Catholic Bioethics Quarterly* 1(2): 163–187.

Moreno, Jonathan D., and London, Alex John. 2001. "Consensus, Ethics, and Politics in Cloning and Embryo Research." In *Cloning and the Future of Embryo Research,* ed. Paul Lauritzen. New York: Oxford University Press.

Mori, Maurizio 1996. "Is the Human Embryo a Person? No." In *Conceiving the Embryo: Ethics, Law and Practice in Human Embryology,* ed. Donald Evans. The Hague, Netherlands: Martinus Nijhoff Publishers.

National Bioethics Advisory Commission. 1997. *Cloning Human Beings: Report and Recommendations.* Rockville, MD: National Bioethics Advisory Commission.

National Bioethics Advisory Commission. 1999 and 2000. *Ethical Issues in Stem Cell Research,* vols. 1, 2, 3. Rockville, MD: National Bioethics Advisory Commission.

National Commission for the Protection of Human Subjects of Biomedical and Behavioral Research. 1975. *Research on the Fetus: Report and Recommendations.* Washington, D.C.: U.S. Department of Health, Education, and Welfare.

Porter, Jean. 2002. "Is the Embryo a Person? Arguing with the Catholic Traditions." *Commonweal* 129(3): 8–10.

Rahner, Karl. 1972. "The Problem of Genetic Manipulation." In *Theological Investigations,* vol. 9. New York: Seabury.

Robertson, John A. 1995. "Symbolic Issues in Embryo Research." *Hastings Center Report* 25(1): 37–38.

Rock, John, and Menkin, Miriam F. 1944. "In Vitro Fertilization and Cleavage of Human Ovarian Eggs." *Science* 100: 105–107.

Ryan, Maura A. 2001. "Creating Embryos for Research: Weighing Symbolic Costs." In *Cloning and the Future of Embryo Research,* ed. Paul Lauritzen. New York: Oxford University Press.

Shapiro, Harold T. 1997. Letter of transmittal to the President. In *Cloning Human Beings: Report and Recommendations of the National Bioethics Advisory Commission.* Rockville, MD: National Bioethics Advisory Commission.

Singer, Peter, and Dawson, Karen. 1990. "Embryo Experimentation and the Argument from Potential." In *Embryo Experimentation: Ethical, Legal and Social Issues,* ed. Peter Singer, Helga Kuhse, Stephen Buckle, et al. Cambridge, Eng.: Cambridge University Press.

Singer, Peter; Kuhse, Helga; Buckle, Stephen; et al., eds. 1990. *Embryo Experimentation: Ethical, Legal and Social Issues.* Cambridge, Eng.: Cambridge University Press.

Soupart, Pierre, and Strong, Patricia Ann. 1974. "Ultrastructural Observations on Human Oocytes Fertilized in Vitro." *Fertility and Sterility* 25(1): 11–44.

Steinbock, Bonnie. 2001. "Respect for Human Embryos." In *Cloning and the Future of Embryo Research,* ed. Paul Lauritzen. New York: Oxford University Press.

Tauer, Carol A. 1997a. "Bringing Embryos into Existence for Research Purposes." In *Contingent Future Persons,* ed. Nick Fotion and Jan C. Heller. Dordrecht, Netherlands: Kluwer Academic Publishers.

Tauer, Carol A. 1997b. "Embryo Research and Public Policy: A Philosopher's Appraisal." *Journal of Medicine and Philosophy* 22(5): 423–439.

Tauer, Carol A. 2001. "Responsibility and Regulation: Reproductive Technologies, Cloning, and Embryo Research." In *Cloning and the Future of Embryo Research,* ed. Paul Lauritzen. New York: Oxford University Press.

U.S. 45 Code of Federal Regulations 46: 201–207. 2001. "Additional Protections for Pregnant Women, Human Fetuses and Neonates Involved in Research." *Federal Register* 66: 56778–56780.

Van Blerkom, Jonathan. 1994. "The History, Current Status and Future Direction of Research Involving Human Embryos." In *Papers Commissioned for the Human Embryo Research Panel,* vol. 2. Bethesda, MD: National Institutes of Health.

Warnock, Mary. 1985. *A Question of Life; The Warnock Report on Human Fertilisation and Embryology.* Oxford: Basil Blackwell.

Wertz, Dorothy. 2002. "Embryo and Stem Cell Research in the USA: A Political History." *Trends in Molecular Medicine* 8(3): 143–146.

INTERNET RESOURCES

Canada. House of Commons. Assisted Human Reproduction Act, Bill C–13. Introduced May 9, 2002 as Bill C–56. Available from <www.parl.gc.ca>.

Dyer, Claire. "Pro-Lifers Lose Cloning Battle." *The Guardian* March 14, 2003. Available from <www.guardian.co.uk/uk_news/story/0,3604,913835,00.html>.

Grafton, Brigitte. 2002. "Survey on the National Regulations in the European Union Regarding Research on Human Embryos." Available from <europa.eu.int/comm>.

Hatch, Orrin G. 2001. "Testimony Before the Senate Appropriations Committee Subcommittee on Labor-HHS-Stem Cell Research," July 18. Available from <hatch.senate.gov>.

Howard Hughes Medical Institute. 2002. "A Global Struggle to Deal with Human ES Cells." Sidebar in "Are Stem Cells the Answer?" Available from <www.hhmi.org/bulletin>.

Manier, Jeremy. "U.S. Quietly OKs Fetal Stem Cell Work; Bush Allows Funding Despite Federal Limits on Embryo Work." *Chicago Tribune,* July 7, 2002. Available from <www.chicagotribune.com>.

Osborn, Andrew. "MEPs Vote Against Stem Cell Research." *The Guardian* April 11, 2003. Available from <www.guardian.co.uk/international/story/0,3604,934363,00.html>.

President's Council on Bioethics. 2002. *Human Cloning and Human Dignity: An Ethical Inquiry.* Available from <www.bioethics.gov>.

United Kingdom. Human Fertilisation and Embryology Act 1990 (amended 2001.) Available from <www.hmso.gov.uk>.

U.S. Public Law 103–43. 1993. The NIH Revitalization Act of 1993. "Part II—Research on Transplantation of Fetal Tissue." Available from <ohrp.osophs.dhhs.gov>.

III. STEM CELL RESEARCH AND THERAPY

In this entry we review the ethical and legal issues that arise in the context of stem cell research and therapy. Stem cells have attracted both immense scientific interest and equal ethical and legal concern because of their capacity to "specialize" and become virtually any part of the organism into which they are introduced. Thus if introduced into the brain they become brain cells, if into the cardiovascular system they become cells of that type and so on. They also appear to be able to trigger cell regeneration and colonize damaged tissue effecting "repair" in situ. Thus if such cells are made compatible with the genome of a host using cloning techniques they could in principle repair and regenerate damaged tissue and halt or even cure many diseases. This holds out both great promise and causes great unease in equal measure. Here we examine both the scientific promise and the extent to which ethical and legal safeguards may be appropriate.

Ethical Issues

The ethical aspects of human stem cell research raise a wide variety of important and controversial issues. Many of these issues have to do with the different sources from which stem cells may be obtained. Stem cells are at present obtained from adults, umbilical cord blood, and fetal and embryonic tissue. Although there are widely differing views regarding the ethics of sourcing stem cells in these ways, there is general consensus that embryos are the best source of stem cells for therapeutic purposes—a consensus that may of course change as the science develops. If spare embryos or aborted fetuses may be used as sources for stem cells, there is a further question: Should embryos or fetuses be deliberately produced in order to be sources of stem cells, whether or not they are also intended to survive stem cell harvesting and grow into healthy adults?

The European Group on Ethics in Science and New Technologies, which advises the European Commission, has highlighted the women's rights issues involved in stem cell research. It is particularly worth bearing in mind that women, as the most proximate sources of embryonic and fetal material and hence also of cord blood, may be under special pressures and indeed risks if these are to be the sources of stem cells.

The issue of free and informed consent, both of donors and recipients, raises special problems. Because embryos and fetuses can hardly consent to their role in sourcing stem cells, the question of who may give consent for the use of fetal or embryonic material is important, particularly because the usual basis for parental consent is hardly appropriate. This basis involves a judgment about what is in the best interests of the individual, and because, in most cases, the individual in question will not survive, the test is irrelevant (Harris, 2002a). Competent risk–benefit assessment is vital, and particular attention needs to be paid to appropriate ethical standards in the conduct of research on human subjects. Other issues concern the anonymity of the donors, the security and safety of cell banks, and the confidentiality and privacy of the genetic information and the tissue the banks contain. Finally, there are issues of remuneration for those taking part and of the transport and security of human tissue and genetic material and information across borders both within the European Union (EU) and worldwide. While these issues are important, they are well understood in biomedical ethics, and with the exception of the issue of consent, they do not raise special issues in connection with stem cell research and therapy (U.K. Human Genetics Commission).

Before considering the ethics of such use in detail, it is important to first explore the possible therapeutic and research uses of stem cells and also the imperatives for research and therapy.

WHY EMBRYONIC STEM CELLS? Embryonic stem cells were first grown in culture in February 1998 by James A. Thomson of the University of Wisconsin. In November of that year Thomson and his colleagues announced in the journal *Science* that such human embryonic stem cells formed a wide variety of recognizable tissues when transplanted into mice. Roger A. Pedersen, writing in 1999, noted potential applications of these stem cells:

Research on embryonic stem cells will ultimately lead to techniques for generating cells that can be employed in therapies, not just for heart attacks, but for many conditions in which tissue is damaged.

If it were possible to control the differentiation of human embryonic stem cells in culture the resulting cells could potentially help repair damage caused by congestive heart failure, Parkinson's disease, diabetes, and other afflictions. They could prove especially valuable for treating conditions affecting the heart and the islets of the pancreas, which retain few or no stem cells in an adult and so cannot renew themselves naturally.

Stem cells, then, might eventually enable us to grow tailor-made human organs. Furthermore, using cloning technology of the type that produced Dolly the sheep, these organs could be made individually compatible with their designated recipients. In addition to tailor-made organs or parts of organs, such as heart valves, it may be possible to use embryonic stem cells to colonize damaged parts of the body, including the brain, and to promote the repair and regrowth of damaged tissue. These possibilities have long been theoretically understood, but it is only now with the isolation of human embryonic stem cells that their benefits are being seriously considered.

Stem cells for therapy. It is difficult to estimate how many people might benefit from the products of stem cell research should it be permitted and prove fruitful. Most sources agree that the most proximate use of human embryonic stem cell therapy would for Parkinson's disease, a common neurological disease that has a disastrous effect on the quality of life of those afflicted with it. In the United Kingdom around 120,000 individuals have Parkinson's, and the Parkinson's Disease Foundation estimates that the disease affects between 1 million and 1.5 million Americans. Another source speculates that "the true prevalence of idiopathic Parkinson's disease in London may be around 200 per 100,000" (Schrag, Ben-Shlomo, and Quinn). Untold human misery and suffering could be stemmed if Parkinson's disease became treatable. If treatments become available for congestive heart failure and diabetes, for example, and if, as many believe, tailor-made transplant organs will eventually be possible, then literally millions of people worldwide will be treated using stem cell therapy.

When a possible new therapy holds out promise of dramatic cures, caution is of course advised, if only to dampen false hopes of an early treatment. For the sake of all those awaiting therapy, however, it is equally important to pursue the research that might lead to therapy with all vigor. To fail to do so would be to deny people who might benefit the possibility of therapy.

Immortality

Finally we should note the possibility of therapies that would extend life, perhaps even to the point at which humans might become in some sense "immortal." This,

albeit futuristic dimension of stem cell research raises important issues that are worth serious consideration. Many scientists now believe that death is not inevitable that that the process whereby cells seem to be programmed to age and die is a contingent "accident" of human development which can in principle and perhaps in fact be reversed and part of that reversal may flow from the regenerative power of stem cells. Immortality has been discussed at length elsewhere but we should, before turning to the ethics of stem cell research and therapy note one important possible consequence of life extending procedures.

Human Evolution and Species Protection

Human Embryonic Stem Cell research in general, but the immortalizing properties of such research in particular raises another acute question. If we become substantially longer lived and healthier, and certainly if we transformed ourselves from "mortals" into "immortals" we would have changed our fundamental nature. One of the common defining characteristics of a human being is our mortality. Indeed in English we are "mortals"—persons; not "immortals" or Gods, demi-gods or devils. Is there then any moral reason to stay as we are simply because it is "as we are"? Is there something sacrosanct about the human life form? Do we have moral reasons against further evolution whether it is "natural" Darwinian evolution, or evolution determined by conscious choice?

One choice that may confront us is as to whether or not to attempt treatments that might enhance human functioning, so-called "enhancement therapies." For example it may be that because of their regenerative capacities stem cells inserted into the brain to repair damage might in a normal brain have the effect of enhancing brain function. Again it would be difficult if the therapies are proved safe in the case of brain damaged patients to resist requests for their use as enhancement therapies. What after all could be unethical about improving brain function? We don't consider it unethical to choose schools on the basis of their (admittedly doubtful) claims to achieve this, why would a more efficient method seem problematic?

We should not of course attempt to change human nature for the worse and we must be very sure that in making any modifications we would in fact be changing it for the better, and that we can do so safely, without unwanted side-effects. However if we could change the genome of human beings, say by adding a new manufactured and synthetic gene sequence which would protect us from most major diseases and allow us to live on average twenty five per cent longer with a healthy life throughout our allotted time, many would want to benefit from this. In high-income countries human beings now do live on average twenty five per cent longer than they did 100 years ago and this is usually cited as an unmitigated advantage of "progress." The point is sometimes made that so long as humans continued to be able to procreate after any modifications, which changed our nature, we would still be, in the biological sense, members of the same species. But, the point is not whether we remain members of the same species in some narrow biological sense but whether we have changed our nature and perhaps with it our conception of normal species functioning.

THE ETHICS OF STEM CELL RESEARCH. Stem cell research is of ethical significance for three major reasons:

1. It will for the foreseeable future involve the use and sacrifice of human embryos.

2. Because of the regenerative properties of stem cells, stem cell therapy may always be more than therapeutic—it may involve the enhancement of human functioning and indeed the extension of the human lifespan.

3. So-called therapeutic cloning, the use of cell nuclear replacement to make the stem cells clones of the genome of their intended recipient, involves the creation of cloned pluripotent (cells that have the power to become almost any part of the re-sulting organism—hence pluri-potent)and possibly totipotent cells (cells which have the power to become any part of the resulting organism including the whole organism), which some people find objectionable.

In other venues, John Harris has discussed in detail the ethics of genetic enhancement (Harris, 1992, 1998a) and the ethics of cloning (Harris, 1997, 1998b, 1999b). The focus of this entry, however, is on objections to the use of embryos and fetuses as sources of stem cells.

Because aborted fetuses and preimplantation embryos are currently the most promising sources of stem cells for research and therapeutic purposes, the recovery and use of stem cells for current practical purposes seems to turn crucially on the moral status of the embryo and the fetus. There have, however, been a number of developments that show promise for the recovery and use of adult stem cells. It was reported in 2002 that Catherine Verfaillie and her group at the University of Minnesota had successful isolated adult stem cells from bone marrow and that these seemed to have pluripotent properties (capable of development in many ways but not in all ways and not capable of becoming a new separate creature), like most human embryonic stem cells have. Simultaneously, *Nature Online* published a paper from

Ron McKay at the U.S. National Institutes of Health showing the promise of embryo-derived cells in the treatment of Parkinson's disease.

Such findings indicate the importance of pursuing both lines of research in parallel. The dangers of abjuring embryo research in the hope that adult stem cells will be found to do the job adequately is highly dangerous and problematic for a number of reasons. First, it is not yet known whether adult cells will prove as good as embryonic cells for therapeutic purposes; there is simply much more accumulated data about and much more therapeutic promise for embryonic stem cells. Second, it might turn out that adult cells will be good for some therapeutic purposes and embryonic stem cells for others. Third, whereas scientists have already discovered that virtually any gene in embryonic stem cells can be modified or replaced, this has not yet been established to hold for adult stem cells. Finally, it would be an irresponsible gamble with human lives to back one source of cells rather than another and to make people wait and possibly die while what is still the less favored source of stem cells is further developed. This means that the ethics of embryonic stem cells is still a vital and pressing problem and cannot for the foreseeable future be bypassed by a concentration on adult stem cells.

RESOLVING THE ETHICS OF RECOVERING STEM CELLS FROM EMBRYOS. There are three more or less contentious ways of resolving the question of whether it is ethically permissible to use the embryo or the fetus as a source of material, including stem cells, for research and therapy. The three methods involve: (1) solving the vexing question of the moral status of the embryo; (2) invoking the principle of waste avoidance; and (3) showing that those who profess to accord full moral status to the embryo either cannot consistently do so or do not in fact believe (despite what they profess) that it has that status. Regarding the first of these, it is difficult to determine whether there will ever be sufficiently convincing arguments available for this question to be finally resolved in the sense of securing the agreement of all rational beings to a particular view of the matter (Harris, 1985, 1999a). Putting aside this contentious issue, then, the other two issues will be discussed below.

The principle of waste avoidance. This widely shared principle states that it is right to benefit people if we can, that it is wrong to harm them, and that faced with the opportunity to use resources for a beneficial purpose when the alternative is that those resources will be wasted, we have powerful moral reasons to avoid waste and do good instead.

That it is surely better to do something good than to do nothing good should be reemphasized. It is difficult to find arguments in support of the idea that it could be better (more ethical) to allow embryonic or fetal material to go to waste than to use it for some good purpose. It must, logically, be better to do something good than to do nothing good, just as it must be better to make good use of something than to allow it to be wasted.

It does not of course follow from this that it is ethical to create embryos specifically for the purposes of deriving stem cells from them. Nevertheless, in all circumstances in which "spare" embryos have been produced that cannot, or will not, be used for reproduction, because they have no chance of developing into normal adult human beings, it must be ethical to use such embryos as sources of stem cells or therapeutic material or for research purposes.

Does anyone really believe that embryos are moral persons? One way in which stem cell research and therapy using human embryos might be successfully defended is to draw a distinction between what people say and what they do, or rather to point out that there may be an inconsistency between the beliefs and values of people as revealed by their statements on the one hand and by the way they behave on the other. Although many people, including most so-called pro-life or right-to-life supporters, are prone to make encouraging noises about the moral importance of embryos, and even sometimes talk as if embryos have, and must be accorded, the same moral status as human adults, such people very seldom, if ever, behave as if they remotely believe any such thing. Taking for the moment as unproblematic the idea, made famous by the Greek philosopher Socrates (c. 470–399 B.C.E.), that "to know the good is to do the good," many pro-life advocates do not behave consistently with their professed beliefs about what is good. A few examples must suffice.

One would expect that those who give full moral status to the embryo, who regard it as a person, would both protect embryos with the same energy and conviction as they would their fellow adults and mourn an embryo's loss with equal solemnity and concern. This, however, they do not do. It is true that some extreme pro-life advocates in the United States have taken to murdering obstetricians who perform abortions, but those same individuals are almost always inconsistent in some or all of the following ways.

For every live birth, up to five embryos die in early miscarriages. Although this fact is widely known and represents massive carnage, pro-life groups have not been active in campaigning for medical research to stem the tide of this terrible slaughter. Equally well known is that, for the same reasons, the menstrual flow of sexually active women often contains embryos. Funeral rights are not usually routinely performed over sanitary towels, although they often contain embryos. In the case of spare embryos created by assisted reproductive technologies, there has not been the creation of a group of pro-life women offering their uteruses as homes for these surplus embryos. In his 1992 book, *Wonderwoman and Superman,* John Harris had to invent a fictitious quasi-religious order of women, "The Sisters of the Embryo," who would stand ready to offer a gestating uterus to receive unwanted embryos because (surprisingly given the large numbers of pro-life women available) there has never been such a movement. Indeed, anyone engaging in unprotected intercourse runs substantial risk of creating an embryo that must die, and yet few people think that this fact affords them a reason either to refrain from unprotected intercourse or to press for medical research to prevent this tragic waste of human life.

Finally, it is notorious that many pro-life supporters, including many Catholics, are prepared to permit abortions in exceptional circumstances, for example, to save the life of the mother or in the case of rape. In the former situation, however, the right course of action for those who believe the embryo has full moral status is to give equal chances to the embryo and the mother (perhaps by tossing a coin) in cases where one may survive but not both. In the case of rape, because the embryo is innocent of the crime and has therefore done nothing to compromise its moral status, the permitting of abortion by those who give full status to the embryo is simply incoherent (Richards).

These cases provide reasons for thinking that even if the views of those who believe the embryo to have the same moral status as normal adult human beings cannot be conclusively shown to be fallacious, it can at least be shown that these views are inconsistent with practice and that the "theory" is therefore not really believed by those who profess it or indeed that it is not actually compatible with the lives that human beings must, of necessity, lead.

Legal and Regulatory Issues

A draft United Nations (UN) convention to prohibit human reproductive cloning seeks to augment the advisory regulatory approach enshrined in the Universal Declaration on the Human Genome and Human Rights. The latter was developed by the United Nations Educational, Scientific and Cultural Organization (UNESCO), adopted unanimously by its 186 states on November 11, 1997, and adopted by the UN General Assembly on March 10, 1999 (via Resolution 53/152). Article 11 of the UNESCO Declaration states (in part): "Practices which are contrary to human dignity, such as reproductive cloning of human beings, shall not be permitted." The limitations of this provision were revealed in a report by the director-general of UNESCO. The report concluded that "this prohibition concerns the reproductive cloning of human beings and should not be interpreted as prohibiting other applications of cloning" (UNESCO, 1999, p. 13).

The Council of Europe's Convention for the Protection of Human Rights and Dignity of the Human Being with regard to the Application of Biology and Medicine (1997; known as the Convention on Human Rights and Biomedicine), to which the United Kingdom is not a signatory, does provide some form of protection for the human embryo. Thus, Article 18(1) provides the following: "Where the law allows research on embryos in vitro, it shall ensure adequate protection of the embryo," and Article 18(2) states, "The creation of human embryos for research purposes is prohibited." Under Article 36, countries—such as the United Kingdom—that have a preexisting law may make a reservation to the convention based on that existing law. Those countries that have no preexisting law on the embryo and that sign the convention will be hindered or prohibited from sanctioning embryo research, unless they formally withdraw from the convention, pass the new permissive law, and then re-sign (as has happened with Finland and Greece).

In the United Kingdom, the appending of the Human Rights Act of 1998, which brought U.K. domestic law closer to the provisions of the Convention on Human Rights and Biomedicine, has provoked some commentators to focus on the provisions of Article 2 as having potentially significant effect on domestic abortion law and hence the status of the embryo in law. Article 2 stipulates the following: "Everyone's right to life shall be protected by law." Whether this will afford any greater degree of recognition to the fetus, let alone to the embryo, is unlikely.

No European consensus exists on abortion, (or, as Table 1 shows, on embryo research), and the European Commission and the European Court of Human Rights have been reluctant to pronounce substantively on whether the protection in Article 2 of the convention extends to the fetus. In the light of these differing laws, a state will have what is called under European human rights legislation a wide "margin of appreciation" with regard to the convention on the issue of abortion, and hence, it is thought, on the status of the embryo (Decision Reports of the European Commission of Human Rights, Application 17004/90 H v Norway 73 DR 155 (1992) E Com HR.).

The European Court of Human Rights has yet to rule on whether the term *everyone* includes a fetus. In *Open Door*

Counselling & Dublin Well Woman v. Ireland, the European Commission had recognized the possibility that Article 2 might in certain circumstances offer protection to a fetus, but they took the point no further.

THE UNITED KINGDOM POSITION. Important distinctions must be drawn in the law's treatment of human cloning. The first distinction is between *reproductive cloning,* which is designed to result in the birth of a live human being genetically identical to another, and *therapeutic cloning,* in which an embryo is cloned for research purposes and will not be permitted to develop into a fetus or a live birth. The second essential distinction is that between two different cloning techniques: The first of these (when applied to *human* cloning) involves replacing the nucleus of an embryonic cell with a nucleus taken from another human embryonic or adult cell, and it is known as cell nuclear replacement (CNR).

The HFE Act of 1990. The Human Fertilisation and Embryology Act of 1990 (HFE Act) contains a clear prohibition on the first technique. Section 3(3)(d) states that a license granted under the act "cannot authorise ... replacing a nucleus of a cell of an embryo with a nucleus taken from a cell of any person, embryo or subsequent development of an embryo." CNR, on the other hand, is not *expressly* prohibited by the act, nor is "embryo splitting," a process that can occur naturally at a very early stage of embryonic development, forming identical twins, but which can also be done in vitro to produce identical, cloned embryos. The form of CNR whereby the nucleus of an oocyte is replaced with a nucleus from an *adult* cell was beyond the bounds of scientific credibility when the 1990 legislation was being debated and drafted.

The legal status of CNR in the United Kingdom is, therefore, unclear. The regulatory framework of the HFE Act rests on a definition in section 1(1)(a), in which an embryo is defined as "a live human embryo where fertilisation is complete." This definition's emphasis on the process of fertilization (an emphasis repeated throughout the act) raises the possibility that embryos created by CNR fall outside the scope of the act and that accordingly their creation and use is unregulated. In their 1998 report, *Cloning Issues in Human Reproduction,* the Human Genetics Advisory Commission (HGAC) and the Human Fertilisation and Embryology Authority (HFEA) argued for a *purposive* rather than a *literal* interpretation of the definition. Through such an approach, organisms created by CNR would fall within the statutory definition of *embryo* on the basis that Parliament clearly intended to regulate the creation and use of embryos outside the human body, and that excluding organisms created by

TABLE 1

Legislation on Reproductive/Therapeutic Cloning, Embryo Research, and Stem Cell Research, 2003

Country	Reproductive Cloning Allowed	Therapeutic Cloning (SCNT*) Allowed	(General) Research on Embryos Allowed	Stem Cell Research on Spare Embryos Allowed	Legislative Source(s)
Argentina	No				Decree No. 200 of March 1997: A Prohibition of Human Cloning Research
Australia (federal)	No	No	Yes	Yes	Research Involving Human Embryos Act of 2002; Prohibition of Human Cloning Act of 2002 (Embryos created before April 5, 2002, may be used for stem cell embryo research; Subject to license)
Austria	No	Possibly	No	No	Reproductive Medicine Law of 1992 (Embryos may be created for (Cf. Import) reproductive purposes only)
Brazil			Yes	Yes	Law 8974/95, Normative Instruction by National Technical Committee of Biosecurity
Canada	No	No	Yes	Yes	CIHR Guidelines; Bill C-13, An Act Respecting Assisted Human Reproductive Technologies and Related Research (Surplus embryos only; Subject to license)
Costa Rica		No	No	No	Decree no. 24029-S. A Regulation on Assisted Reproduction, February 3, 1995
Denmark	No	No	No*	No	Act no. 460 of June 10, 1997, on Assisted Procreation *as interpreted by the Danish Council of Ethics
Finland			Yes		Medical Research Act no. 488, April 9. 1999
France	No	No	Yes	Yes	Projet de loi relatif á la bioéthique, tel qu'adopte par l'Assemblée nationale le 22 jan. 2002 (Subject to licence)
Germany	No	No	No	Yes	Embryo Protection Law of 1990; Stem Cell Act of 2002 (Imported stem cell lines created before January 1, 2002; Subject to licence)
Iceland	No	No	Yes	No	Ministry of Health and Social Security, Regulation No. 568/1997 on Artificial Fertilization
Ireland	No	No	No	No	Constitution of Ireland, Article 40, para. 3
Israel	No	Yes	Yes	Yes	Prohibition of Genetic Intervention Law (1999); (Five year moratorium); Bioethics Advisory Committee of the Israel Academy of Sciences and Humanities (Section 8—surplus embryos only)
Japan	No	Yes	Yes	Yes	The Law concerning Regulation Relating to Human Cloning Techniques and Other Similar Techniques (Article 3); The Guidelines for Derivation and Utilization of Human Embryonic Stem Cells (Surplus and created embryos; Subject to license)
Netherlands	No	Yes	Yes	Yes	Act Containing Rules Relating to the Use of Gametes and Embryos (Embryos Act), October 2001
Norway	No	No	No	No	Norwegian Law on Assisted Reproduction and Genetics, 1994
Peru	No	No	No	No	General Law No. 26842 of 9 July 1997 on Health
Russia	No				Law of Reproductive Human Cloning, April 19, 2002
Spain			Yes	Yes	Law no 42/1988 of 28 December 1988 on the Donation and Use of Human Embryos and Fetuses or Their Cells, Tissues, or Organs
Sweden		No	Yes		Law 115 of March 14, 1991, Act Concerning Measures for the Purposes of Research or Treatment in connection with Fertilized Human Oocytes, as interpreted by the Swedish Research Council's Guidelines for Research—Ethical Review of Human Stem Cell Research, December 4, 2001; Swedish Council on Medical Ethics, Statement of Opinion on Embryonic Stem Cell Research, January 17, 2000
Switzerland	No	No?	No	Yes/No?	Constitution fédérale de al Confédération suisse, 1999
United Kingdom	No	Yes	Yes	Yes	Human Reproductive Cloning Act of 2001 (extends to Northern Ireland); Human Fertilisation and Embryology Act of 1990 (Subject to license)
United States		Yes**	Yes**	Yes**	**No federal law to date; no federal funds for embryo research nor for creation of stem cell lines after August 9, 2001

SOURCE: Compiled from various sources by Authors.

CNR from the definition in the HFE Act would frustrate this legislative intention.

It is important here to immediately observe three things:

1. CNR is not specifically prohibited by the HFE Act.
2. The same is true of embryo splitting.
3. The HFEA gave careful consideration to embryo splitting as an additional possible form of infertility treatment in 1994, when its potential use at the two- or four-cell embryonic stage was discussed. After considering the social and ethical issues involved, the HFEA decided to ban embryo splitting as a possible fertility treatment. The HFEA, however, did not make a similar prohibition with respect to CNR research.

Is somatic CNR specifically covered by the wording of section 3(3)(d) of the HFE Act? And, as CNR does not involve fertilization, does section ("No person shall bring about the creation of an embryo … except in pursuance of a licence") 3(1) apply either? Is CNR regulated at all by the HFE Act? At least from a moral point of view, and taking what could be called a purposive or result-oriented approach, it may be possible to reconcile the CNR embryo with embryos created in vitro. From this, it would follow that there is no particular difficulty in accepting the view with which the HFEA works—that the creation of embryos through CNR is *already* brought within the scheme of the HFE Act by an extended interpretation of section 1.

Section 1(1)(a) reads in full: "In this Act, *except where otherwise stated* (a) embryo means a live human embryo where fertilisation is complete" (emphasis added). The emphasized words make it plain that the legislators could have provided otherwise for embryos created other than by in vitro fertilization to be included within the statute, but evidently they did not. To read the statute as providing for embryos created by CNR is to read it as providing that an embryo means a live human embryo where fertilization is complete, *unless the context otherwise requires.*

The Quintavalle *case.* In the early 2000s, a legal challenge by the Pro-Life Alliance, a U.K. lobbying group, tested the question of whether the HFE Act can be interpreted purposively to include organisms produced by CNR. In the High Court (*Regina [on the Application of Quintavalle] v. Secretary of State for Health*, 2001), the claimant submitted simply that an embryo that has not been produced by fertilization cannot be "an embryo where fertilization is complete" in terms of section 1(1)(a) of the HFE Act. The Secretary of State for Health argued for a purposive construction of this section, whereby the definition would be expanded to include embryos produced other than by

fertilization. The judge decided that such a purposive approach would "involve an impermissible rewriting and extension of the definition" (*Quintavalle*, 2001, para. 62). In immediate response to this, the government introduced the Human Reproductive Cloning Act of 2001, under which it is an offense to place, in a woman, a human embryo that has been created by any method other than fertilization.

In the Court of Appeal (*Regina [on the Application of Quintavalle] v. Secretary of State for Health*, 2002), the Secretary of State continued to argue that section 1(1)(a) must be given a "strained" construction in order to give effect to the obvious intention of Parliament. The claimant disagreed that the intentions of Parliament with regard to CNR can be thought to have been clear when the technique was unheard of at the time the HFE Act was enacted. Furthermore, the claimant pointed out, had Parliament known of the CNR technique, they may well have decided to include it in the prohibition on cloning included in section 3(3)(d).

In upholding the appeal, the court placed particular emphasis on two considerations. First, it observed the dictum of Lord Wilberforce, in his dissenting judgment in the case of *Royal College of Nursing of the United Kingdom v. Department of Health and Social Security* (1981), that:

> Where a new state of affairs, or a fresh set of facts bearing on policy, comes into existence, the courts have to consider whether they fall within the Parliamentary intention. They may be held to do so, if they fall within the same genus of facts as those to which the expressed policy has been formulated. (*Royal College of Nursing*, p. 822)

The court decided, regarding "genus of facts," that the fact that an embryo was created by fertilization had not been a factor of particular relevance to the desirability of regulation when the HFE Act was envisaged, and that, furthermore, the embryo created by CNR is "morphologically and functionally indistinguishable" (*Quintavalle*, 2002, p. 639) from the embryo created by fertilization. The relevant point was taken to be the capacity to develop into a human being, which is shared by both.

The second point the court emphasized related to the policy of the HFE Act. Rejecting the argument that Parliament's intention was undiscoverable and that CNR, if possible at the time, may have been prohibited under s3(3)(d), the court decided that the rationale behind that prohibition was

> to prevent the production artificially of two or more genetically identical individuals. This policy would be put in jeopardy if the creation and use

of embryos by cell nuclear replacement were unregulated. It would be furthered by making the production of embryos by cell nuclear replacement subject to the regulatory regime under the Act, for it is inconceivable that the licensing authority would permit such an embryo to be used for the purpose of reproduction. (*Quintavalle*, 2002, pp. 641–642)

In the final appeal to the House of Lords (*Regina [on the Application of Quintavalle] v. Secretary of State for Health* 2003), the decision of the Court of Appeal was unanimously sustained. In his leading judgment Lord Bingham upheld the Court of Appeal's endorsement of the dictum in *Royal College of Nursing,* saying that this "may now be treated as authoritative" (*Quintavalle*, 2003, para. 10). Indeed, following the House of Lords' judgment in *Quintavalle,* the passage in question can be regarded as enshrining a new rule of statutory interpretation.

The House of Lords' decision (and the Court of Appeal ruling that it upheld) is highly contestable, on several grounds. First, the clarity of the statutory language in section 1(1)(a) casts doubt on either court's freedom to use a purposive approach to interpreting it; moreover, the 2001 act prohibiting human reproductive cloning was in force when the appeal was considered, so the court's view that a purposive approach was necessary to prevent the production of genetically identical individuals is surprising. Second, embryos produced by the process prohibited in section 3(3)(d) would *also* be "morphologically and functionally indistinguishable," in the words of the Court of Appeal, from embryos produced by fertilization, just as are embryos produced by CNR, and yet Parliament adopted a different regulatory approach to *their* creation and use. This being so, the assumption that Parliament intended to treat all "morphologically and functionally indistinguishable" embryos alike seems mistaken. Finally, in its consideration of *genus,* the House of Lords seems to have replicated the Court of Appeal's erroneous conflation of the term's legal application (to facts) and its scientific sense.

The current research purposes specified in the HFE Act relate only to research that could be envisaged at that time. It is nevertheless difficult to argue that they were based on immutable moral criteria, and indeed the existence in the HFE Act of the power to broaden the research purposes in due course supports this view. Additional research purposes were in fact added by important new regulations that were enacted in 2001, as is discussed below. In all types of embryo research under consideration it has to be accepted that the embryo cannot itself receive any benefit. The embryo is used instrumentally—as a means to an end—and will be destroyed. This is, in any event, an inevitable outcome for all spare embryos whether donated for research under the currently allowed research purposes or no longer required for treatment. If the arguments of the Warnock Committee (established in 1982 by the U.K. government to report and advise on developments in human fertilization and embryology, in its report published in 1984), are accepted, the issue to be considered is one of balance: whether the research has the potential to lead to significant health benefits for others and whether the use of embryos at a very early stage of their development in such research is necessary to realize those benefits.

*The post-*Quintavalle *situation.* So far as CNR research within the United Kingdom is concerned, the legislation now draws a line at the point of implantation by prohibiting the placing in a woman of "a human embryo which has been created otherwise than by fertilisation." Until the Court of Appeal reversed the High Court decision, a decision confirmed by the House of Lords, it would not have been unlawful to do CNR work preparatory to implantation. After the reversal, however, research involving CNR embryos is lawful only when authorized by a license granted by the HFEA, and so long as the Human Reproductive Cloning Act remains in place it is inconceivable that the HFEA would license research directed at human reproductive cloning.

A license authorizing specific research under the HFE Act may be granted by the HFEA for a maximum period of three years. Any research license may be made subject to conditions imposed by HFEA and specified in the license, and any authority to bring about the creation of an embryo, keep or use an embryo, or mix human sperm with a hamster or other specified animal's egg may specify how those activities may be carried out. Each research protocol must be shown to relate, broadly, to one of the existing categories of research aim, and then again only if the authority is satisfied that the research is "necessary for the purposes of the research" (Schedule 2, para. 3[5]). These research aims are:

- Promoting advances in the treatment of infertility
- Increasing knowledge about the causes of congenital disease
- Increasing knowledge about the causes of miscarriage
- Developing more effective techniques of contraception
- Developing methods for detecting the presence of gene or chromosome abnormalities in embryos before implantation
- Increasing knowledge about the creation and development of embryos and enabling such knowledge to be applied

The Human Fertilisation and Embryology (Research Purposes) Regulations of 2001 extended these original purposes. These regulations provided for three further purposes for which research licenses may be authorized:

(a) increasing knowledge about the development of embryos;

(b) increasing knowledge about serious disease, or

(c) enabling any such knowledge to be applied in developing treatments for serious disease.

THE EUROPEAN DIMENSION. The Council of Europe's Convention on Human Rights and Biomedicine (1997), along with its Additional Protocol on the Prohibition of Cloning Human Beings (1998), which covers only *reproductive* human cloning, is an important document. Ten of the fifteen EU countries have now signed the convention, despite what some have seen as its (almost necessary) limitations.

The protocol makes what was implicit in the convention explicit by declaring that "[a]ny intervention seeking to create a human being genetically identical to another human being, whether living or dead, is prohibited" (Article 1[1]). Because "genetically identical" is defined as "sharing with another the same nuclear gene set" (Article 1[2]), somatic CNR is included within this prohibition. The term *human being* is not defined in the convention, and because *human being* is unlikely to be interpreted to include embryonic human life, some countries, in signing the convention and its protocol, have added their own interpretative statements. For example, the Netherlands, in doing so, stated that "[i]n relation to Article 1 of the Protocol, the Government of the Kingdom of the Netherlands declares that it interprets the term 'human beings' as referring exclusively to a human individual, i.e., a human being who has been born."

In its report titled "Ethical Aspects of Human Stem Cell Research and Use," however, the European Group on Ethics in Science and New Technologies advised that, at present, "the creation of embryos by somatic cell nuclear transfer ['therapeutic cloning'] for research on stem cell therapy would be premature" because there are alternative sources of human stem cells.

EXAMPLES OF OTHER JURISDICTIONS' LEGAL APPROACHES. In the United States, regulation of human cloning and embryo research has been undertaken or debated at both the national and state levels. At the federal level, there is a rigid separation between the public and private sectors. Little if any regulation applies to research involving the use of human embryos if it is funded by the private sector, although the U.S. Food and Drug Administration has asserted jurisdiction over reproductive cloning whenever safety issues are raised.

Federal attempts to regulate cloning have the support of President George W. Bush, who, on April 10, 2002, called on the U.S. Senate to endorse the Human Cloning Prohibition Act, which would ban all human cloning in the United States, including the cloning of embryos for research. This bill was nearly identical to the bipartisan legislation that passed the U.S. House of Representatives by more than a 100-vote margin in 2001.

This announcement supplemented the one issued on August 9, 2001, regarding stem cell research. In the latter, Bush resolved that federal funding of research using the more than sixty existing stem cell lines from genetically diverse populations around the world that have already been derived would be permitted, but that he would not sanction or encourage the destruction of additional human embryos. Henceforth, federal funds could be used only for research on existing stem cell lines that were derived: (1) with the informed consent of the donors; (2) from excess embryos created solely for reproductive purposes; and (3) without any financial inducements to the donors. In order to ensure that federal funds are used to support only stem cell research that is scientifically sound, legal, and ethical, the U.S. National Institutes of Health was charged with examining the derivation of all existing stem cell lines and creating a registry of those lines that satisfy these criteria. A further result was that federal funds cannot be used for: (1) the derivation or use of stem cell lines derived from newly destroyed embryos; (2) the creation of any human embryos for research purposes; or (3) the cloning of human embryos for any purpose.

In Canada, a similar approach was taken in February 2002. In Australia, the Research Involving Embryos and Prohibition of Human Cloning Act of 2002 was introduced into Federal Parliament in June 2002. There are three main elements to the bill: a ban on human cloning, a ban on certain other practices relating to reproductive technologies, and a system of regulatory oversight for the use of excess embryos created through assisted reproductive technologies that would otherwise have been destroyed. The legislation would establish a system of licensing, administered by the National Health and Medical Research Council.

JOHN M. HARRIS
DEREK MORGAN
MARY FORD

SEE ALSO: *Abortion: Medical Perspectives; Cloning; Feminism; Fetal Research; Human Dignity; Infants; Infanticide;*

Maternal-Fetal Relationship; Moral Status; Reproductive Technologies: Ethical Issues; Research Policy: Risk and Vulnerable Groups; Research, Unethical; Transhumanism and Posthumanism; and other *Embryo and Fetus* subentries

BIBLIOGRAPHY

Brownsword, Roger. 2002. "Stem Cells, Superman, and the Report of the Select Committee." *Modern Law Review* 65(4): 568–587.

Council of Europe. 1997. *Convention for the Protection of Human Rights and Dignity of the Human Being with regard to the Application of Biology and Medicine: Convention on Human Rights and Biomedicine.* Strasbourg, France: Author.

Council of Europe. 1998. *Additional Protocol to the Convention for the Protection of Human Rights and Dignity of the Human Being with regard to the Application of Biology and Medicine, on the Prohibition of Cloning Human Beings.* Strasbourg, France: Author.

de Rijk, M. C.; Launer, L. J.; Berger, K.; et al. 2000. "Prevalence of Parkinson's Disease in Europe: A Collaborative Study of Population-Based Cohorts." *Neurology* 54(11, suppl. 5): S21–S23.

Harris, John. 1985. *The Value of Life.* London: Routledge and Kegan Paul.

Harris, John. 1992. *Wonderwoman and Superman: The Ethics of Human Biotechnology.* Oxford: Oxford University Press.

Harris, John. 1997. "'Goodbye Dolly?' The Ethics of Human Cloning." *Journal of Medical Ethics* 23(6): 353–360.

Harris, John. 1998a. *Clones, Genes, and Immortality: Ethics and the Genetic Revolution.* Oxford: Oxford University Press.

Harris, John. 1998b. "Cloning and Human Dignity." *Cambridge Quarterly of Healthcare Ethics* 7(2): 163–167.

Harris, John. 1999a. "The Concept of the Person and the Value of Life." *Kennedy Institute of Ethics Journal* 9(4): 293–308.

Harris, John. 1999b. "Genes, Clones, and Human Rights." In *The Genetic Revolution and Human Rights: The Oxford Amnesty Lectures, 1998,* ed. Justine Burley. Oxford: Oxford University Press.

Harris, John. 2002a. "Law and Regulation of Retained Organs: The Ethical Issues." *Legal Studies* 22(4): 527–549.

Harris, John. 2002b. "The Use of Human Embryonic Stem Cells in Research and Therapy." In *A Companion to Genethics: Philosophy and the Genetic Revolution,* edited by Justine Burley and John Harris. Oxford: Basil Blackwell.

Human Genetics Advisory Commission (HGAC) and the Human Fertilisation and Embryology Authority (HFEA). 1998. *Cloning Issues in Human Reproduction,* London: Author.

Open Door Counselling & Dublin Well Woman v. Ireland. 15 EHRR 244 (1992).

Pedersen, Roger A. 1999. "Embryonic Stem Cells for Medicine." *Scientific American* 280(4): 68–73.

Plomer, Aurora. 2002. "Beyond the HFE Act 1990: The Regulation of Stem Cell Research in the UK." *Medical Law Review* 10(2): 132–164.

Regina (on the Application of Quintavalle) v. Secretary of State for Health. WL 1347031 (2001).

Regina (on the Application of Quintavalle) v. Secretary of State for Health. Q.B. 628 (2002).

Regina (on the Application of Quintavalle) v. Secretary of State for Health. UKHL 13 (2003).

Richards, Janet Radcliffe. 1980. *The Sceptical Feminist: A Philosophical Enquiry.* London: Routledge and Kegan Paul.

Royal College of Nursing of the United Kingdom v. Department of Health and Social Security. A.C. 800 (1981).

Schrag, Anette, Ben-Shlomo, Yoav, and Quinn, Niall P. 2000. "Cross Sectional Prevalence Survey of Idiopathic Parkinson's Disease and Parkinsonism in London." *British Medical Journal* 321(7252): 21–22.

Thomson, James A.; Itskovitz-Eldor, Joseph; Shapiro, Sander S.; et al. 1998. "Embryonic Stem Cell Lines Derived from Human Blastocysts." *Science* 282(5391): 1145–1147.

U.K. Human Genetics Commission (HGC). 2002. *Inside Information: Balancing Interests in the Use of Personal Genetic Data.* London: United Kingdom Department of Health.

United Nations Educational, Scientific and Cultural Organization (UNESCO). Division of the Ethics of Science and Technology. 1999. *Global Report on the Situation World-Wide in the Fields Relevant to the Universal Declaration on the Human Genome and Human Rights.* BIO-503/99/CIB—6/2.

INTERNET RESOURCES

Decree no. 200 of March 1997: A Prohibition of Human Cloning Research. Available from <infoleg.mecon.gov.ar/txtnorma/42213.htm>.

Decree no. 24029-S. A Regulation on Assisted Reproduction, February 3, 1995. Available from <www.netsalud.sa.cr/ms/decretos/dec5.htm>.

Ministry of Health and Social Security, Regulation No. 568/1997 on Artificial Fertilization. Available from <htr.stjr.is/interpro/htr/htr.nsf/pages/lawsandregs0002>.

Parkinson's Disease Foundation. "Parkinson's Disease: An Overview." Available from <www.pdf.org/AboutPD/>.

Swedish Council on Medical Ethics. "Statement of Opinion on Embryonic Stem Cell Research, January 17, 2000." Available from <www.smer.gov.se>.

The Swedish Research Council's Guidelines for Research—Ethical Review of Human Stem Cell Research, December 4, 2001. Available from <www.vr.se/index.asp>.

United Kingdom Human Genetics Commission (HGC). 2002. *Inside Information: Balancing Interests in the Use of Personal Genetic Data.* Available from <www.hgc.gov.uk/insideinformation/>.

United Nations Educational, Scientific and Cultural Organization (UNESCO). 1997. "The Universal Declaration on the Human Genome and Human Rights." Available from <www.unesco.org/ibc/index.html>.

IV. RELIGIOUS PERSPECTIVES

Even for those who are not actively religious, nascent human life evokes awe and a sense of being in the presence of primal powers of creation. In the procreation of all species, from plants to domestic pets, religious consciousness often senses the divine at play in the natural. In human procreation in particular, human beings not only observe but also participate in that power, and by conceiving and giving birth humans play a small but profoundly personal role in creation.

There is little wonder, then, that for millennia, religious texts have spoken of human procreation with tones of wonder. In the Hebrew Scriptures, Psalm 139 reads in part:

> For thou didst form my inward parts,
> thou didst knit me together in my mother's womb.
> I praise thee, for thou art fearful and wonderful.
> Wonderful are thy works!
> Thou knowest me right well;
> my frame was not hidden from thee,
> when I was being made in secret,
> intricately wrought in the depths of the earth.
> Thy eyes beheld my unformed substance … (Psalms
> 139:13–16a)

In ancient Hebrew thought, procreation is the realm of divine prerogative. The protracted struggle for monotheism is in part a rejection of the idea, probably widespread in the ancient world, that fertility is itself divine. Hebrew monotheism could not tolerate lesser gods, such as fertility. In the name of one God, the prophets insisted that though mysterious, fertility is one of many processes of nature entirely under God's control. Various forms of polytheism in the ancient world saw these processes as deities in themselves, often female, and the success of monotheism is in some respects a desacralization and a defeminization of these processes. But such a desacralization goes only so far. For the ancient Hebrew monotheist, the one supreme God is intimately and personally present in these processes, making them anything but merely natural.

From Creation to Procreation

As an arena of divine presence, nascent life must be held in respect, for if it is God's work, its development must not be thwarted nor its condition questioned. According to the prophet Isaiah, God declares:

> Woe to you who strive with your Maker,

> earthen vessels with the potter!
> Does the clay say to the one who fashions it, "What
> are you making"?
> or "Your work has no handles"?
> Woe to anyone who says to a father, "What are you
> begetting?"
> Or to a woman, "With what are you in labor?"
> (Isa. 45:9–10)

Because procreation is the work of God, it is unseemly to question how or when it occurs, much less speculate about God's competence in making humankind.

Ancient biblical culture is also characterized by the command to propagate (Genesis 1:28) and thus by a strongly reinforced desire for children. In addition to any innate yearning or social pressure for offspring, the infertile in biblical culture no doubt feared being seen as disobedient, and several biblical stories contain impassioned pleas for children. The most notably such plea is that of postmenopausal Sarah, the wife of Abraham, who according to the story subsequently gives birth to Isaac from whom all Israel descends. That God can cause this to happen against nature is taken as evidence of God's supremacy over nature.

In view of the involvement of God in procreation and of the command to populate the earth, it is somewhat surprising that Hebrew Scripture says little or nothing about the moral status of human life in utero. Exodus, chapter 21, discusses the legal consequences that follow from an accidental miscarriage: "When men strive together, and hurt a woman with child, so that there is a miscarriage, and yet no harm follows, the one who hurt her shall be fined, according as the woman's husband shall lay upon him; and he shall pay as the judges determine. If any harm follows, then you shall give life for life …" (Exod. 21: 22–23).

While the text leaves much unsaid, it does prescribe different penalties for causing a miscarriage (a fine) and for causing the women's death (a capital offense), suggesting that these are offenses of a substantially different magnitude. Strictly speaking the scope here is limited to miscarriage or unintentional abortion, so its applicability to an intended abortion is subject to debate.

Early Judaism

In Judaism at the beginning of the common era, this text was interpreted in various ways. In most interpretations, developing life was not generally regarded as possessing the legal status of a person, but abortion was nonetheless opposed, in part because of its interference with creation, in part because it violated the command to reproduce, and in part because it deprived the family (in particular the father) of something of value in the birth of another child. Generally speaking, Judaism objected to the widespread acceptance of abortion (and even of infanticide) in the ancient world, even if it did not see abortion as a highly serious offense.

In the translation of this Hebrew text into Greek, a significant mistranslation occurred. Where the original says "no harm," the translators substituted "no form," thereby introducing into religious debate the distinction between the unformed and the formed fetus. The widely influential Jewish scholar Philo (c. 20 B.C.E.–c. 50 C.E.), for instance, distinguished between formed and unformed fetus, and early Christianity picked up this distinction.

Christian Origins

The New Testament itself takes no position on abortion or on the status of embryonic or fetal life, although some scholars feel that negative references to *pharmakeia* in several passages specifically refer to abortifacient drugs and not to medicine generally. As in Judaism, the core Scriptures of Christianity ignore the moral questions of fetal life and of abortion. But to say that because the New Testament does not address abortion, it says nothing *theological* about fetal life, is wrong. Two of the four Gospels (Matthew and Luke) devote substantial attention to the miraculous conception not just of Jesus but also of his forerunner, John the Baptist. According to the story, John's mother Elizabeth is too old to conceive, but in keeping with a tradition that goes back to Sarah, she conceives because of God's involvement and for the sake of God's purposes. Mary, the mother of Jesus, is Elizabeth's cousin, and in the story of the "virgin birth" (or more precisely the "virginal conception") the tradition of miraculous conceptions reaches its culmination. God is so immediately involved in the details of this human conception that a human sperm is replaced by a miracle. The virgin birth is often the subject of theological puzzlement by scholars but is widely, if only sentimentally, affirmed by many ordinary Christians to this day. One must not underestimate the significance of this tradition in forming Christian attitudes toward embryonic and fetal life.

Not unexpectedly, therefore, as Christianity developed and distinguished itself from Judaism, it opposed abortion more strongly than Judaism or than the teachings of the New Testament itself. In some early post–New Testament writings, abortion is equated with murder. For instance, an early writing known as the *Didache* comments on abortion by listing it among the commandments: "You shall not commit murder … you shall not murder a child by abortion nor kill that which is born" (2:2). This text not only prohibits abortion, but, by identifying it with murder, also

implies that fetal life is fully human or personal. Another early text, the *Letter of Barnabas,* uses essentially the same terms: "Thou shalt not kill the fetus by an abortion or commit infanticide" (19:5). These texts, critically important in shaping the early Christian conscience, expressed agreement in considering abortion as murder and as elevating its prohibition to the status of commandment. Furthermore, the claim that God is fully present in the human life of Jesus, even in utero, at once divided Christian from Jew and drove the Christian to a new consciousness of the value of nascent life.

Form and Soul

Even so, early Christian writers often retained the distinction between the formed and unformed fetus, implying that the unformed fetus possesses a lesser status than one that is fully formed. One of the first Latin Christian theologians, Tertullian, who lived around 200 C.E., opposed abortion but implied in his writings that there is a distinction of significance between the formed and unformed embryo. In chapter 37 of his treatise *On the Soul,* Tertullian wrote: "The embryo therefore becomes a human being in the womb from the moment that its form is completed."

One way to defend the distinction between formed and unformed is to hold that the human soul is added to the developing fetus when it attains a recognizably human shape. The metaphysics of the fourth century B.C.E. Greek philosopher Aristotle, which links soul and form, was often used here for support. Thus, what begins as an empirical question—does the fetus have a human shape?—becomes entwined with a religious and metaphysical question of whether the fetus has a soul, and at what stage this is so. The joining of the soul to the developing organism, a process called ensoulment, thus became a subject of intense religious debate among Christian theologians.

This debate was never resolved and in fact quickly became entangled in conflicting Christian views of the human soul, its origin, and the nature of its relationship to the human body, all set against the backdrop of competing philosophical options. In this regard Tertullian held a view peculiar among Christians that the soul is not a spiritual but a material substance and is transmitted sexually rather than created by God. Most other theologians of the early church saw the soul as a spiritual substance. In contrast, however, to philosophical views that accepted a dualism of soul and body, Christian theologians generally agreed that body and soul, though metaphysically distinct, are functionally inseparable. In death, the soul is not freed from the body, as the Greek philosopher Plato (c. 428–c. 347 B.C.E.) contended, but awaits the resurrection of the body in order that both soul and body might be transformed together into a glorified mode of immortal existence. Speculation about ensoulment, therefore, was always grounded on this insistence on the unity of soul with body.

Unity of Soul and Body

The widely influential Gregory of Nyssa (c. 335–c. 394), for instance, held so strongly to the unity of soul and body that he could not imagine the body developing at all without the soul being present. In a work called *On the Making of Man,* Gregory wrote: "As man is one, the being consisting of soul and body, we are to suppose that the beginning of his existence is one, common to both parts so that it is not true to say either that the soul exists before the body, or that the body exists without the soul, but that there is one beginning of both" (chap. 29). According to Gregory, at every stage of human development, from inception to resurrection, body and soul function as one.

In the same work, Gregory elaborates on the development of the soul with the body:

> For as the body proceeds from a very small original to the perfect state, so also the operation of the soul, growing in correspondence with the subject, gains and increases with it. For at its first formation there comes first of all its power of growth and nutriment alone, as though it were some root buried in the ground; for the limited nature of the recipient does not admit of more; then, as the plant comes forth to the light and shows its shoot to the sun, the gift of sensibility blossoms in addition, but when at last it is ripened and has grown up to its proper height, the power of reason begins to shine forth like a fruit, not appearing in its whole vigour all at once, but by care increasing with the perfection of the instrument, bearing always as much fruit as the powers of the subject allow. (chap. 29)

In Gregory's view, there is no moment or process of ensoulment subsequent to conception. Existence and ensoulment are one.

Augustine's Options

As Gregory of Nyssa profoundly influenced the development of Greek Christianity and thus of the subsequent Orthodox Churches, so Augustine (354–430) deeply shaped Western or Latin Christianity, which at the Reformation (beginning about 1520) became Catholicism and Protestantism. Augustine, whose influence can scarcely be exaggerated, accepted the distinction between the formed and unformed fetus. In addition he tended to be more dualistic

in his thinking, and he therefore accepted greater discontinuity between soul and body than did Gregory or other Eastern theologians.

Although Augustine was not generally indecisive on theological and moral matters, he remained undecided throughout his life on the question of the origin of the human soul and the way it is joined with the human body. One possibility (called *creationism*) is that God creates the soul at around the time of conception or somewhat later and joins it to the developing body. By allowing separate origins for the soul and the body, this view makes possible the idea that for a time, the body develops without a human soul being present, something Gregory flatly rejected. The other possibility that Augustine considered (called *traducianism*) is that soul and body come into existence together, that is to say, at conception, when both are transmitted together from one generation to the next. Tertullian accepted traducianism, and perhaps for that reason, other Western theologians see it as degrading the soul by making it material rather than spiritual in substance.

Both Augustine's indecision and his speculations remain influential in Western Christianity. Concerning the pastoral question of whether the results of miscarriage or abortion will share in the general human destiny of immortality, Augustine wrote in the *Enchiridion:*

> … with respect to the resurrection of the body … comes the question about abortive fetuses, which are indeed "born" in the mother's womb, but are never so that they could be "reborn." For, if we say that there is a resurrection for them, then we can agree that at least as much is true of fetuses that are fully formed. But, with regard to undeveloped fetuses, who would not more readily think that they perish, like seeds that did not germinate? (23:84–85)

Here Augustine accepts the distinction between formed and unformed and uses it in the ultimate theological context—the question of what is human in the resurrection. He also uses it to clarify his opposition to abortion. For him, destroying the formed fetus is murder, whereas destroying the unformed fetus is a lesser offense.

When it comes to the deeper theoretical question of the beginning of human life, Augustine admits his uncertainty in the *Enchiridion:*

> On this score, a corollary question may be most carefully discussed by the most learned men, and still I do not know that any man can answer it, namely: When does a human being begin to live in the womb? Is there some form of hidden life, not yet apparent in the motions of a living thing? To

deny, for example, that those fetuses ever lived at all which are cut away limb by limb and cast out of the wombs of pregnant women, lest the mothers die also if the fetuses were left there dead, would seem much too rash. (23:86)

The Development of Catholic Thought

In time creationism, with its dualistic tendencies, became the majority view in the Western or Latin church, and it was often combined with the idea that the soul was not joined to the body until formation. The reintroduction of Aristotle into Western thought brought new subtleties to the discussion. Thomas Aquinas, whose integration of Aristotle into Christian theology in the thirteenth century was at first controversial but was subsequently seen as authoritative for Catholics, combined creationism with the view that the soul undergoes transition. At its beginning, the embryo does not have a human soul, merely the kind of soul common to all forms of life and responsible for growth and development. Only when fetal development advances to a stage that resembles human form is it possible for the human soul to be present. The human or intellectual soul is immaterial and must be created by God, who joins it to the developing fetus. At that moment of ensoulment, the fetus becomes human or attains hominization, and its moral claim to life is absolute.

Thomas's position is dependent upon an empirical observation of Aristotle, who concluded that the human soul is present at forty days after conception for males and ninety for females. Because the soul was thought to animate the body, "quickening," or the feeling of fetal movement, was taken as a sign that ensoulment had occurred. Until 1869, the Catholic Church recognized a distinction between the ensouled and the unensouled fetus, insisting on a higher penalty for the destruction of the former.

Into the Modern Era

Protestantism, which in its various forms became separate from the Catholic Church in the sixteenth century, tended to take a more strict view against abortion than the Catholics, opposite to the modern situation. This is perhaps because of the Protestant return to early church standards and its rejection of much of the previous thousand years of church tradition, particularly in philosophical theology. Early followers of Martin Luther and John Calvin (leaders of the Reformation) held views that resembled those of Gregory of Nyssa more than those of Thomas Aquinas. In time, however, theological and philosophical considerations reentered Protestant discussion, along with both an encounter with new scientific discoveries in biology and embryology and a general tendency in Protestantism to accommodate

contemporary culture whenever reasonably possible. As a result, by the twentieth century, Protestantism was largely tolerant of abortion even while discouraging its members from obtaining one for less than urgent reasons.

During this same period, Catholic teaching moved in the opposite direction. Scientific discoveries (and in some cases, misinterpretation of data, such as the view that the earliest embryo is fully shaped like a tiny human being) led Catholic theologians to challenge their own previous view of delayed hominization and to propose in its place a new theory of immediate hominization. This idea gained popularity after 1700, until, in 1869, Catholic canon law removed the distinction between the ensouled and the unensouled fetus, thereby implying but not asserting that immediate hominization is the correct view. The key point, however, is that the abortion of an unformed fetus is to be regarded as the moral equivalent of the abortion of a formed fetus, and therefore abortion is murder at any stage. With this development, Catholic moral teaching became absolute, whereas Catholic theology remained somewhat open to various perspectives on the metaphysical status of the embryo. As a result, Catholic morals and theology developed somewhat independently, based in part on the claim that moral certainty does not require doctrinal clarity.

Current Catholic Teaching

In 1987 the Catholic Church provided guidance on reproductive medicine and embryo research in *Donum vitae* (Respect for human life). *Donum vitae* poses and then answers a key question: "how could a human individual not be a human person? The Magisterium has not expressly committed itself to an affirmation of a philosophical nature, but it constantly reaffirms the moral condemnation of any kind of procured abortion" (Congregation for the Doctrine of the Faith, 1987, part I, no. 1). In other words, immediate hominization is not affirmed doctrinally but its implications are fully asserted morally, not just for abortion some weeks into a pregnancy but in regard to the embryo at the earliest moment. *Donum vitae* insists:

> The human being must be respected—as a person—from the very first instant of his existence.... Thus the fruit of human generation, from the first moment of its existence, that is to say from the moment the zygote has formed, demands the unconditional respect that is morally due to the human being in his bodily and spiritual totality. The human being is to be respected and treated as a person from the moment of conception; and therefore from that same moment his rights as a person must be recognized, among which in the first place

is the inviolable right of every innocent human being to life. (Congregation for the Doctrine of the Faith, 1987, part I, no. 1)

Again asserting moral certainty while avoiding doctrinal conclusiveness, the Catholic Church in 1974 issued its *Declaration on Procured Abortion,* which states: "This declaration expressly leaves aside the question of the moment when the spiritual soul is infused. There is not a unanimous tradition on this point and authors are as yet in disagreement" (Sacred Congregation, p. 13). This statement almost invites debate on dogma while shutting the door to reconsideration of moral teaching.

Dogma and Debate

The discussion of the theology of nascent human life has been vigorous among Catholic scholars and some Protestants. Recent scientific discoveries in genetics and embryology have been considered in the debate, particularly relating to whether the human embryo prior to about fourteen days can be said to be an individual. There is general agreement, according to a 1984 article by Carol A. Tauer, that "the stage of individual has been seen as a morally relevant marker because it appears that only individuals can be wrongfully killed or otherwise injured" (p. 5).

While genetics and embryology support the idea that the newly conceived embryo is a genetically unique human life, three other biological considerations have been raised to argue against the idea that the early embryo is an individual: The embryo might divide into two (twinning); an embryo might join with another genetically unique embryo to form a chimera, which then continues to develop as one human individual; and as many as 75 percent of all human conceptions fail to survive. In a 1990 article, Thomas A. Shannon and Allan B. Wolter argued that "something human and individual is not a human person until he or she is a human individual, that is, not until after the process of individual is completed. Neither the zygote nor the blastocyst is an ontological individual, even though it is genetically unique and distinct from the parents" (p. 613).

A related question is whether the embryo, which lacks most human qualities, nonetheless typically anticipates their development and thus must be said to possess them potentially, or to have potentiality. If so, does that potentiality confer a status to the embryo as one who must be regarded morally as already possessing what is only its potential? Furthermore, if the embryo is out of the body (and thus unable to actualize its potential), does it possess a lower status? Or if the embryo is somehow biologically incapable of developing, either because of a natural or technologically

induced impairment, does it likewise lack whatever value potentiality confers? These questions remain open.

Given that Catholic theologians hold various views on the individuation or personhood of the embryo, how can Catholic moral certainty be possible? Much depends, of course, on the conclusion one draws from the variety of views. One might conclude that when various views are held, one should err on the side of caution, give the embryo the benefit of any doubt, and treat it as if it were a human person. Others conclude that in light of the evidence, it cannot be a human person and that therefore, aside from the authority of the church, there is no obligation to treat it as such.

Protestant Perspectives

Protestants, in the late-twentieth century, were generally supportive of the right of women to choose an abortion, even though they adopted a cautious approach of limiting to the most serious reasons the circumstances under which this right could be exercised. For instance, the Presbyterian Church (U.S.A.), in a 2000 publication, outlined a position similar to that of other traditional denominations:

> The considered decision of a woman to terminate a pregnancy can be a morally acceptable, though certainly not the only or required, decision. Possible justifying circumstances would include medical indications of severe physical or mental deformity, conception as a result of rape or incest, or conditions under which the physical or mental health of either woman or child would be gravely threatened. (p. 431)

This is not to suggest that the members of these denominations are in strong agreement with the official position, and in fact there is some reason to believe that support for these positions is eroding. In addition, the character of Protestantism has been changing in the United States, with the rapid growth of evangelical, independent, and charismatic churches that often criticize traditional denominations for being too accommodating to secular culture on matters such as abortion. As a result, even those who fully support the right of women to choose an abortion as a matter of public policy are recognizing that at the same time, they must acknowledge the moral value of what is lost. Furthermore, some African-American Christians are suspicious of abortion for the additional reason that it appears to them to be a way to limit their numbers.

Prominent Protestants have also stood in opposition to abortion. Karl Barth, often seen as the most important Protestant theologian of the twentieth century, objected to abortion, while Stanley Hauerwas, perhaps the most influential Protestant theologian in the United States at the beginning of the twenty-first century, is also critical of abortion along with other accommodations to modern culture.

Whether tolerating abortion under limited circumstances or condemning it in almost all cases, contemporary Protestants tend to agree among themselves that questions of ensoulment are too dualistic for Christian faith, at least in its Biblical roots. They see human life, as a whole and from beginning to end, as a gift of God that we dare not refuse lest we reject our own humanity. In some respects the views of recent Protestants have more in common with those of Gregory of Nyssa than with recent Catholic debate, and thus Protestants agree with Orthodox theologian John Breck's assessment that Orthodoxy would "take issue with the Catholic Church's doctrine of ensoulment, at least as it has been expressed in Aristotelian and Thomistic terms … [as] dualistic to Orthodox ears" (p. 140). While Orthodoxy has no doubt about when the unitary gift of human life begins (that is, at conception), Protestants by virtue of their institutional structure and communal ethos will surely continue to disagree, some siding with Orthodoxy and practically with Catholicism, others siding with Judaism and Islam.

Special notice should be paid to the perspective of the Church of Jesus Christ of Latter Day Saints, commonly known as the Mormons. While dependent in many ways upon the views of Christianity and Judaism, and sharing scriptures with these traditions, Mormonism develops a somewhat distinct view. Mormons have tended to be restrictive if not prohibitive on abortion, although not necessarily seeing it as murder. Furthermore, as Lester E. Bush observes, Mormonism does not hold to a dogma on the embryo or the fetus, but tends to see each human person or soul as the dynamic interplay between the biological and the spiritual. Somewhere in the process of fetal development, usually at quickening or at birth but not at conception, spirit is present and thus the developing life is a person deserving absolute protection. Given the size of the Latter Day Saints, these views have considerable political significance in the United States.

Judaism, Islam, and Buddhism

Judaism is generally tolerant of the public policy of choice in abortion but teaches that abortion should be chosen only for compelling reasons. It does not regard abortion as murder, however, and it is open to the prospect of using human embryos in research and therapy because it regards the embryo outside the body as having no legal standing. In fact, even in the body, the embryo's status for the first forty days,

according to the Talmud, is "as if it were simply water" (Dorff, 2002). As a result, Judaism is supportive not just of in vitro fertilization but of more recent developments such as preimplantation genetic diagnosis.

Islam bases its understanding of developing human life on the section in the Koran (23:12–16) that describes human creation as beginning with a tiny drop from which the larger and more complex structure of the fetus is fashioned by God the creator, who breathes life into what is formed. Islam thus sees each human life as created by God through a developmental process. Islamic scholars sometimes distinguish between the ensouled and the unensouled fetus, often arriving at the end of the fourth month as the point in fetal development when abortion is no longer permissible for any reason.

Other Islamic scholars argue that recent scientific discoveries demonstrate that the embryo is alive from the earliest moment and thus deserves full protection, but the more common and traditional view is to accord legal status as a person only after the form is recognizable and movement is voluntary. When it comes to the use of genetic or reproductive technology, Islam is guided primarily by the general context in which the technology is applied rather than by the technology considered abstractly. If reproductive technology serves the goal of health within the context of marriage, it is permitted; if not, it is rejected.

Detailed theological and moral discussion of topics such as abortion, the beginning of life, and embryo research is far more characteristic of the Western monotheisms (particularly Christianity) than of the other great religions. In Buddhism, however, rich conceptual and practical traditions have made it possible for some countries such as Japan to address abortion without the divisiveness characteristic of the West. The first of the Five Precepts of Buddhism is the prohibition against taking life, including embryonic life. While there is some traditional debate in Buddhism about when reincarnate life is present in the developing fetus, for the most part Buddhists agree that abortion is always wrong. At the same time, what is wrong is also sometimes necessary, but that does not make the act less wrong or the loss less tragic. On the one hand, there is the moral teaching, quoted by James Hughes as follows: "It is the woman carrying the fetus, and no one else, who must in the end make this most difficult decision and live with it for the rest of her life. As Buddhists, we can only encourage her to make a decision that is both thoughtful and compassionate" (Hughes, p. 191). But on the other hand, in Japan in particular, fetal loss of any sort is mourned and observed with ritual and remembrance (mizuko) far more than in the Christian West. Similar traditions are found in Thailand and Vietnam. Far from legitimizing abortion through religious sanction, these rituals help to maintain the Buddhist prohibition against taking even fetal life even in a social context that occasionally requires just this act.

New Technologies

Religious ideas about nascent human life were developed long before modern science opened up the fields of genetics or embryology and prior to technology making the embryo an object of manipulation. These new developments bear on religious understandings, and religious perspectives are likewise brought to bear in assessing the legitimacy of various technological options, such as in vitro fertilization, prenatal genetic testing, preimplantation genetic diagnosis, cloning, and embryonic stem cells.

The responses of various religious traditions to these developments are largely outgrowths of classic positions and thus predictable. Catholic teaching objects to any attempt to move procreation outside its natural context and thus opposes in vitro fertilization. Because of its uncompromising objection to abortion, *Donum vitae* objects to prenatal genetic diagnosis unless limited to healing the individual: "But this diagnosis is gravely opposed to the moral law when it is done with the thought of possibly inducing an abortion" (part I, no. 2). Judaism, Islam, and Protestantism generally permit in vitro procedures and also allow, with practical reservations, prenatal genetic diagnosis.

Preimplantation genetic diagnosis, which involves in vitro fertilization followed by a genetic test of the embryos to determine the most healthy for implantation, is likewise rejected by Catholic teaching but accepted by others, although the cost factor raises religious concerns for social justice.

Cloned Embryos

Reproductive cloning is widely condemned by religious institutions and by nearly all religious scholars, but use of the cloning technique (somatic cell nuclear transfer) to create embryos for research purposes is permitted under some religious grounds while being strongly condemned under others. Catholic teaching clearly forbids any form of embryo research that destroys the embryo, cloned or otherwise. According to the Pontifical Academy for Life, "The ablation of the inner cell mass (ICM) of the blastocyst, which critically and irremediably damages the human embryo, curtailing its development, is a gravely immoral act and consequently is gravely illicit."

In similar terms, the conservative Protestant Southern Baptist Convention, at its national meeting in 1999, stated: "[we] reaffirm our vigorous opposition to the destruction of innocent human life, including the destruction of human embryos." The opposite position, however, is taken by the Presbyterian Church (U.S.A.), which declared in 2001: "With careful regulation, we affirm the use of human stem cell tissue for research that may result in the restoring of health to those suffering from serious illness. We affirm our support for stem cell research, recognizing that this research moves to a new and challenging frontier."

On this, the Presbyterian position (shared by some other similar denominations) is substantially indistinguishable from that of Judaism. An example of the latter is found in a joint statement offered by the heads of the various branches of Judaism in the United States. This statement begins by stressing the God-given human role in mending the creation: "The Torah commands us to treat and cure the ill and to defeat disease wherever possible; to do this is to be the Creator's partner in safeguarding the created" (Union of Orthodox Jewish Congregations of America and the Rabbinical Council of America, 2002). To this end, humans are permitted to use human embryos in research, for "our tradition states that an embryo in vitro does not enjoy the full status of human-hood and its attendant protections. Thus, if cloning technology research advances our ability to heal humans with greater success, it ought to be pursued since it does not require or encourage the destruction of life in the process" (Union of Orthodox Jewish Congregations of America and the Rabbinical Council of America, 2002). Reproductive cloning, however, is opposed, and therefore careful oversight of research must be in place.

At the beginning of the twenty-first century, it appears possible to create human embryos by nuclear transfer, embryo splitting, or by a process usually called parthenogenesis by which researchers induce an egg to start dividing like an embryo without fertilization. In each of these processes, something like an embryo comes into existence without fertilization or conception in the usual sense. If an embryo strictly speaking is the result of conception, then these entities are not embryos. One cannot imagine, however, that those who hold passionately to the slogan that "life begins at conception" will not modify their rhetoric to say that life begins at conception or anything that replaces conception.

A deeper issue is whether these entities, even if implanted, have the biological potential to develop into a human life. In some cases, probably most, it will turn out that they lack this potential. If so, will they be seen as embryo-like but as sub-embryos, morally speaking? Surely, some out of religious conviction will defend their status as "one of us" or as fully human. In time, however, technology may find even more ways to create entities that function in some ways like embryos but in other ways fail as their biological equivalent, and so religious, moral, and policy distinctions are inevitable.

Conclusion

Far from being relics of a prescientific era, the religions today, even in their disagreements, serve to focus both our awe at the mysteries of our humanity and our anxieties about our future. Religious traditions, which are anything but changeless, will probably continue to adapt to our changing knowledge of ourselves and our growing powers to modify our nature. In so doing, through doctrinal argument and moral warning, they will perhaps shed some light on our biological origins and on our technological destiny.

RONALD COLE-TURNER

SEE ALSO: *African Religions; Bioethics, African-American Perspectives; Buddhism, Bioethics in; Christianity, Bioethics in; Daoism, Bioethics in; Eugenics and Religious Law; Islam, Bioethics in; Jainism, Bioethics in; Judaism, Bioethics in; Medical Ethics, History of Europe; Mormonism, Bioethics in; Native American Religions, Bioethics in; Reproductive Technologies; Sikhism, Bioethics in; Transhumanism and Posthumanism;* and other *Embryo and Fetus* subentries

BIBLIOGRAPHY

Anees, Munawar A. 1989. *Islam and Biological Futures: Ethics, Gender, and Technology.* London: Mansell.

Augustine. 1955. *Enchiridion.* In "Confessions and Enchiridion," tr. and ed. Albert C. Outler. *Library of Christian Classics,* vol. 7. Chap. 23: 84–85. Philadelphia: Westminster Press.

Breck, John. 2000. *The Sacred Gift of Life: Orthodox Christianity and Bioethics.* Crestwood, NY: St. Vladimir's Seminary Press.

Bush, Lester E. 1985. "Ethical Issues in Reproductive Medicine: A Mormon Perspective," *Dialogue: A Journal of Mormon Thought* 18(2): 41ff.

Cahill, Lisa Sowle. 1993. "The Embryo and the Fetus: New Moral Contexts." *Theological Studies* 54(1): 124–142.

Cole-Turner, Ronald, and Waters, Brent, ed. 2003. *God and the Embryo: Religious Voices on Stems and Cells and Cloning.* Washington, D.C.: Georgetown University Press.

Congregation for the Doctrine of the Faith. 1974. *Declaration on Procured Abortion.* Washington, D.C.: United States Catholic Conference.

Dorff, Elliot N. 1998. *Matters of Life and Death: A Jewish Approach to Modern Medical Ethics.* Philadelphia: Jewish Publication Society.

Ford, Norman M. 1988. *When Did I Begin? Conception of the Human Individual in History, Philosophy, and Science.* Cambridge, Eng.: Cambridge University Press.

Gorman, Michael J. 1982. *Abortion and the Early Church: Christian, Jewish, and Pagan Attitudes in the Greco-Roman World.* New York: Paulist Press.

Gregory of Nyssa. 1994. *On the Making of Man.* In *Nicene and Post-Nicene Fathers,* Series II, vol. 5, ed. Philip Schaff and Henry Wace. Peabody, MA: Hendrickson Publishers.

Hughes, James. 1999. "Buddhism and Abortion: A Western Approach." In *Buddhism and Abortion,* ed. Damien Keown. Honolulu: University of Hawaii Press.

Johnson, Mark. 1995. "Delayed Hominization: Reflections on Some Recent Catholic Claims for Delayed Hominization." *Theological Studies* 56(4): 743–763.

Mackler, Aaron L., ed. 2000. *Life and Death Responsibilities in Jewish Biomedical Ethics.* New York: Louis Finkelstein Institute, Jewish Theological Seminary of America.

McCormick, Richard A. 1981. *How Brave a New World: Dilemmas in Bioethics.* Washington, D.C.: Georgetown University Press.

Noonan, John T., ed. 1970. *The Morality of Abortion: Legal and Historical Perspectives.* Cambridge, MA: Harvard University Press.

Peterson, James C. 2001. *Genetic Turning Points: The Ethics of Human Genetic Intervention.* Grand Rapids, MI: W. B. Eerdmans.

Presbyterian Church (U.S.A.). 2000. "Do Justice, Love Mercy, Walk Humbly (Micah 6:8)." In *Presbyterian Social Witness Policy Compilation,* comp. The Advisory Committee on Social Witness Policy. Louisville, KY: Author.

Rahner, Karl. 1972. "The Experiment with Man" and "The Problem of Genetic Manipulation," In *Theological Investigations,* vol. 9, tr. Graham Harrison. New York: Seabury Press.

Ramsey, Paul. 1970. *Fabricated Man: The Ethics of Genetic Control.* New Haven, CT: Yale University Press.

Shannon, Thomas A., and Wolter, Allan B. 1990. "Reflections on the Moral Status of the Pre-embryo." *Theological Studies* 51(4): 603–626.

Tauer, Carol A. 1984. "The Tradition of Probabilism and the Moral Status of the Early Embryo." *Theological Studies* 45(1): 3–33.

Williams, George Huntston. 1970. "Religious Residues and Presuppositions in the American Debate on Abortion." *Theological Studies* 31(1): 10–75.

INTERNET RESOURCES

Congregation for the Doctrine of the Faith. 1974. "Declaration on Procured Abortion." Vatican. Available from <www.vatican.va/roman_curia/congregations/cfaith/documents/rc_con_cfaith_doc_19741118_declaration-abortion_en.html>.

Congregation for the Doctrine of the Faith. 1987. "Respect for Human Life (*Donum vitae*)," Vatican. Available from <www.cin.org/vatcong/donumvit.html>.

Dorff, Elliot N. 2002. "Embryonic Stem Cell Research: The Jewish Perspective," In *United Synagogue Review* Available from <www.uscj.org/item15_803_809.html>.

Pontifical Academy For Life. 2000. "Declaration on the Production and the Scientific and Therapeutic Use of Human Embryonic Stem Cells," Vatican. Available from <www.vatican.va/roman_curia/pontifical_academies/acdlife/documents/rc_pa_acdlife_doc_20000824_cellule-staminali_en.html>.

Presbyterian Church (USA) General Assembly. 2001. "Overture 01–50. On Adopting a Resolution Enunciating Ethical Guidelines for Fetal Tissue and Stem Cell Research—From the Presbytery of Baltimore." Louisville, KY: Author. Available from <www.pcusa.org/ga213/business/OVT0150.htm>.

Southern Baptist Convention. 1999. "Resolution: On Human Embryonic and Stem Cell Research."(Notation: Approved by the messengers to the Southern Baptist Convention, June 16, 1999.) Available from <www.sbcannualmeeting.org/sbc99/res7.htm>.

Union of Orthodox Jewish Congregations of America and the Rabbinical Council of America. 2002. "Cloning Research, Jewish Tradition & Public Policy: A Joint Statement," Washington, D.C.: Author. Available from <www.ou.org/public/Publib/cloninglet.htm>.

EMOTIONS

. . .

In bioethics, as in ethics more generally, there is much debate about the significance of emotions in an account of moral character. Intuitively speaking, emotions are important because as moral beings we care not only about how we act but also about how we feel—what our moods are, as well as our attitudes and affects. Within the practice of healthcare, the emotions of compassion and empathy seem to have a particularly important place in a full description of decent and ethical treatment of a patient. The general point is not that emotion is internal and action external, because both action and emotion have exterior moments that point to deeper interior states, commonly thought of as character. Rather, emotions are important as modes of sensitivity that record what is morally salient and that then communicate those concerns to self and others. Thus, to grieve, pity, show empathy, or love is to focus on an aspect of self or other and to grasp information to which purer cognition or thought may not have access. Generally put, different emotions are sensitive to different kinds of salience. In the case of grief, what is salient is that humans suffer and face loss; in the case of pity, that they sometimes fail through blameless ignorance, duress, sickness, or accident; in the case of empathy, that they need the expressed support and union of others who can understand and identify with them; and in the case

of love that they find certain individuals attractive and worthy of their time and attention.

In relations in which caring for others is definitive, emotional sensitivity plays a powerful role. In choosing physicians, for example, people tend to value medical skill and ability deeply, but value character and judgment as well. And part of what people look for in character and judgment is not just reliable and principled action but also a certain range of emotional responsiveness. Medical care ministered without human gesture may simply not be received in the same way as that conveyed through compassion and empathy. A physician's sensitivity to a patient's needs, worries, and fears is often also relevant to diagnosis, just as the physician's communication of emotions may be relevant to how a patient confronts illness and recovery. As in any relationship, emotional interaction is part of the exchange. In more intimate friendships, we hope that loved ones will be able to respond to our joy and suffering in more than merely intellectual ways and that they will communicate feelings through spontaneous affect and gesture as well as more deliberate action.

What Are Emotions?

In general terms, then, emotional sensitivity is a moral feature of personal interaction. But what are emotions? It is useful to first review some alternative views.

The first is the commonsense view in which emotion is thought to be an irreducible quality of feeling or sensation. It may be caused by physical states, but the emotion itself is the sensation we feel when we are in that state. It is a felt affect, a distinctive feeling, but not something dependent upon thought content or appraisals of situations. This view quickly appears faulty, however, when one realizes that on this view emotions become no more than private states—sensations such as itches and tickles that have little to do with what the emotions are about and how a person construes or represents those affairs.

A second view, associated with the American psychologist and philosopher William James and Danish physiologist Carl Lange is that emotions are an awareness of bodily changes in the musculature and viscera. We are afraid because we tremble or flee, not the other way around; likewise, we are angry because of the knots in our stomachs. This view, though rather counterintuitive, nonetheless captures the idea that emotions, more than other mental states, seem to have conspicuous physiological and kinesthetic components. These often dominate children's and adults' reports of their emotional experiences. They dominate the literary world, too. Consider in this vein the lines of the Greek poet Sappho composed around 600 B.C.E.:

When I see you, my voice fails,
my tongue is paralyzed,
a fiery fever runs through my whole body
my eyes are swimming,
and can see nothing
my ears are filled with a throbbing din
I am shivering all over …

Literary history, social convention, and perhaps evolution conspire to tell us this is love. But even here it is not hard to imagine that what is described could be dread or awe or perhaps, mystical inspiration. Even well-honed physiological feelings do not easily identify specific emotions. An awareness of our skin tingling or our chest constricting or our readiness to flee or fight do not specify just what emotion we are feeling. Many distinct emotions share these features, and without contextual clues and thoughts that dwell on those clues, we are in the dark about what we are experiencing (Schacter and Singer). The chief burden of the work of the American physiologist Walter B. Cannon was to show that many physiological affects are virtually identical across manifestly different states. While more current research suggests a tighter fit between specific emotions and specific autonomic system responses (such as skin temperature and heart rate), visceral responses such as these nevertheless have slow response times, too slow to determine what emotion one is actually feeling at a given time (LeDoux). So Cannon's general insight about the indeterminacy of the "feel" of an emotion still holds, though for different reasons than the ones he offered.

A third view with some kinship to the James-Lange view holds that emotions are felt action tendencies (Arnold). They are modes of readiness to act or, in the different idiom of psychoanalysis, discharge impulses. Supporting this view is the tendency of people to describe emotions in terms of dispositions to concrete behavior, for example, "I felt like hitting him," "I could have exploded," "I wanted to spit," and "I wanted to be alone with him, wrapped in his embrace." Nevertheless, the action tendency view seems at best a partial account of emotion. The basic issue here is not that some emotions such as apathy, inhibition, and depression seem to lack activation modes—while others are more a matter of the rich movement of thought so well depicted, for example, in Henry James's novels. It is rather that emotions are about something (internal or external) that people represent in thought. As such, emotions have propositional or cognitive content. They are identified by that content, by what we dwell on, whether fleetingly or with concentrated attention.

According to a fourth and most plausible view, emotions are constituted by appraisals or cognitive evaluations. (This is the view the fourth-century B.C.E. Greek philosopher

Aristotle developed in the *Rhetoric,* and a view the Stoics put forth in more radical form. It is the clear favorite of most philosophers of the late twentieth and early twenty-first centuries—for a sampling, see de Sousa, 1987; Stocker; Goldie; Nussbaum, 2001. It is also the reigning view in cognitive psychology—see Lazarus; Oatley; Frijda; Scherer, and for an important criticism, see Zajonc.) Such an account need not exclude other features of emotion, such as awareness of physiological and behavioral responses or a particular phenomenological feel. But these, when present, are dependent on the appraisals of circumstances that capture what the emotion is about. Moreover, it is compatible with this view that emotions have complex neuropsychological structures that can be investigated by science.

To be more precise, an appraisal, on this view, is a belief or evaluation about the goodness or badness of some perceived or imagined event. Anger requires an evaluation that one has been unjustly slighted by another, fear that there is present harm or danger, grief that something valuable has been lost, love that one values a person as supremely important in one's life. On the Aristotelian view, the evaluation is experienced with pleasure or pain, and in some, but not all, cases with a reactive desire, not unlike the earlier mentioned action tendency. According to Aristotle, "Anger is a desire [*orexis*] accompanied by pain toward the revenge of what one regards as a slight toward oneself or one's friends that is unwarranted" (*Rhetoric,* 1378a30–32).

The appraisals constitutive of emotions can be weaker than strict beliefs (P. Greenspan). Thus, many of the thoughts that ground emotions are not judgments to which we would give assent, but are rather thoughts, perceptions, imaginings, and construals (*phantasiai,* Aristotle would say) that we dwell on in compelling ways, though without concern about "objective truth." Familiar sorts of examples illustrate the point. Juan may fear spiders, even though he knows that most spiders he is likely to encounter are harmless; or Clarissa may know that Joe is a no-good lover for her, but she still finds herself yearning for him. In these cases emotions have thought contents or appraisals, though ones that are at odds with more circumspect judgment. They are mental states that seem to lag behind what a person is ready to grasp through belief.

On an Aristotelian view, appraisals constitutive of emotions have a qualitative flavor—a feeling of pleasure or pain. The flavor may be intense or mild, present to consciousness or hidden somewhere as background noise. So, for example, a patient reflecting on her illness may have fears that all may not turn out well, even though she never feels any strong or noticeable tension when she focuses on that thought. Some emotions may be felt as a mix of both pleasure and pain. Even a quick "flash" of emotion, such as a "twinge" of envy, can seem to oscillate quickly from one affective pole to another, from pain at another's good fortune to pleasure at being in a position to slight that person.

Aristotle suggests that many emotions have a motivational aspect, that is, they involve a reason or motive for action. Again, recognition of the diversity and variety of emotions is crucial here. Some emotions, such as calmness, confidence, and equanimity do not in an obvious way involve desires for action. In contrast, anger often involves a desire for revenge, just as envy seems to involve a desire to thwart others from having various goods. These sorts of desires can go on to constitute a motive or reason for full-fledged action, although often we train ourselves not to act, and not to take as a motive for action all our impulses and desires. In some cases, we act out our emotions only in our minds, as when out of anger, we slay the object of our anger in our fantasy life. Here impulses and urgings are present, but they are not taken up as reasons for action.

At yet other times we do externally act out our emotions but in a way in which that emotion still seems to fall short of constituting a full-fledged reason or motive for action. In anger, we sometimes act impulsively, slamming doors and storming out of rooms. This is a venting, a way of letting out tension, not a strategy for sweet revenge. Defiling a photograph of an ex-lover comes closer to the mark, for here at least there is symbolic aim. Nevertheless, these cases of anger do not really aim at effective revenge. They are reactive more than purposeful. And yet, they seem to be voluntary. They are certainly not the involuntary responses of the viscera. Like stroking a patient's brow or tousling a child's hair, emotion motivates the action. These two actions are likely done out of compassion and affection. But it seems strained, at least in some of these cases, to say that one does these actions in order to show compassion or affection—which is the common pattern a demand for reasons often takes. The gesture just expresses compassion or affection. The explanation stops there. It is not like drinking in order to slake thirst, in which drinking strategically promotes that end (Hursthouse).

Emotions and the Brain

In recent years neurophysiologists have turned to an analysis of emotions and the underlying brain structures of specific emotions and emotional pathologies. Two of the leading researchers in this field are Joseph E. LeDoux and Antonio R. Damasio.

In his 1996 book, *The Emotional Brain,* LeDoux makes three central points. First, he contends that emotions form a two-track response system. One track involves the "low road," or fast route where information travels directly from the thalamus, a subcortical "relay station" in the brain that mediates between external stimuli and specialized parts of the brain that process information, to the amygdala, a small region in the forebrain which generates the behavioral, autonomic and endocrine responses which make up an emotional reaction. The other track involves a "high road," or slow route where information takes a detour through the cortex, the more recently evolved part of the brain which supports higher cognitive functioning, including thinking, reasoning and consciousness. The first, subcortical pathway is a primitive survival mechanism, fast but "quick and dirty" and often filled with errors. It is the basis of the human fear response not only to snakes but also to slimy, bent sticks that look like snakes. The second cortical pathway is slower, but more precise, correcting for errors in overreaction and adding the advantages of conscious judgment and more fine-tuned discernment. The very slowness that makes it a poor defense mechanism suits it well for leisurely appraisal.

LeDoux notes, secondly, that memories of emotional situations are laid down by a two-track memory system. One system involves implicit or procedural memory, another explicit or declarative memory. So LeDoux asks us to imagine being in a horrific car accident, in which the horn gets stuck on. Later, when you hear a horn your body may automatically have a conditioned fear response—you break out in sweats, have a fast heartbeat, and so on. Procedural memory is at work, bringing information directly from the auditory system to the amygdala and opening the floodgates of emotional arousal. But in hearing the horn you also may remember the accident, consciously remembering the intersection where it happened, who was with you at the time, where you were headed, and so on. The two kinds of memories are of the same event, though one is emotion drenched, the other, cool and calm. Research by Larry R. Squire and Daniel Schacter, among others, suggests that the two memory systems are physically housed in different parts of the brain, though the memories, in normal cases, are "seamlessly fused" as one conscious, unified experience of the moment. The fusion results in memories that are "emotional." In those moments when we have arousal without declarative memory, we may experience intense emotions without knowing why. (This may be one explanation of the notion of "objectless" emotions.) Conversely, declarative memories without the emotional arousal of implicit memory may be experienced as emotionally flat.

In his third point, LeDoux focuses on our primitive fear response, suggesting that the brain system responsible for this mechanism can bypass higher, cognitive brain systems. But this leaves to the side questions about more complex, socially constructed emotions, such as indignation, compassion, pity, or shame. Do they operate solely through the high road, or do they have low-road counterparts, which they routinely correct and educate? Again, are memories of feeling compassion or indignation marked by a two-tier system—the fusion of an awareness of a present arousal with a conscious evaluation of the situation that invoked arousal? These sorts of questions raise a more general concern about how to generalize from LeDoux's important study of the fear defense mechanism to the wide array of emotions that characterize people's waking and dreaming lives.

In his 1994 book, *Descartes' Error,* Damasio argues that a wide range of emotional behavior is not primarily subcortical but is a function of the frontal lobe of the brain, typically associated with reasoning and decision making. Indeed, Damasio's research suggests that the prefrontal cortex is involved in both emotional arousal and rational decision making and that the emotion centers and the reasoning centers in the frontal lobe are intimately related. Damasio begins his account with the famous case of Phineas Gage, a mid-nineteenth-century railroad worker whose frontal lobe was pierced by an iron tamping rod in an accident that occurred while Gage was blasting stone to make way for a straight rail track. To the surprise of his doctors at the time, Gage's severe brain injury (the rod exited the front of his brain and landed more than a hundred feet away) affected not just his reasoning capacities, but his emotional character as well. A calm and polite man prior to the injury, Gage became irreverent and foul mouthed, obstinate and capricious, and full of plans quickly hatched and soon abandoned. A similar pattern had been repeated in others with prefrontal lobe damage. While patients were able to generate emotional responses that travel subcortical, "low-road" paths ("primary emotions," as Damasio calls them), they could not generate "secondary emotions" that require evaluation of stimuli (LeDoux's "high-road" emotional responses). On the basis of a series of related experiments, Damasio concludes that prefrontally damaged patients are unable to have normal, automatic emotional responses. Though they may understand abstractly the emotional significance of some stimuli (such as the punitive side of the risky moves they repeatedly make), they fail to correct their strategies, Damasio argues, because they seem unable to pair that understanding with a mechanism to reenact, in this case, a negative emotional response. They lack what Damasio calls a "somatic marker" mechanism that stamps the appraisal with its appropriate emotional flavor.

Both LeDoux's and Damasio's work shed important light on the interdependence of emotion and reason in emotional behavior—LeDoux through his notion of "high-road" emotional pathways that stand ready to correct "quick and dirty" subcortical responses, Damasio through his analysis of prefrontal responses that embody pairings between representations of situations and appropriate emotional dispositions.

Control and Responsibility

Emotions are reactive responses. But in what sense are we human beings able to choose their emotional responses? How, if at all, can the will intervene in emotional behavior?

Aristotle is once again helpful here. Both action and emotion, he holds, are subject to choice in the following sense. We choose to develop a state of character that stabilizes certain dispositions toward action and emotion. Accordingly, how one feels (and acts) may be less a matter of choice at the moment than the indirect effect of choice over time. In the case of emotion, especially, there are few shortcuts. For unlike action, emotion does not seem to engage choice (or will) in each episode. At a given moment, we may simply not be able to will to feel a certain way however skilled we are at posing appropriate emotional, facial expressions, such as a polite smile or a look of interest.

Common parlance includes many expressions presuming that emotions are "up to us" in various ways. We exhort ourselves and others by such phrases as "pull yourself together," "snap out of it," "put on a good face," "lighten up," "be cheerful," "think positive," and "keep a stiff upper lip." In many of these cases, what the person is being implored to do is to take on the semblance of an emotion with the hope that it might "take hold" and rub off on the person's inner state. Practice as if you believe and you will believe. Or, as de Sousa put it, "earnest pretense is the royal road to sincere faith" (de Sousa, 1988, p. 324; also see Ekman; and Tomkins on posed expressions and facial feedback mechanisms). Similarly, we can sometimes fuel the flames of a sincerely felt emotion by allowing it bodily expression. To weep may intensify our grief or make us more conscious of its presence. The James-Lange theory, and its notion of proprioceptive feedback from the expression of emotion, may be in the background here. There are other sorts of actions a person might take that are not a matter of body language or putting on a new face. A person may try to talk herself out of love, but discover that only when she changes locales do the old ways begin to lose their grip. Other times, it is more trial by fire: staying put and exposing herself to what is painful in order to become inured. The latter process involves desensitization.

Sometimes changing one's mood may be more a matter of mental or perceptual strategy. It may be a matter of bringing oneself to focus on different objects and thoughts—trying to see things under a new gestalt or recomposing the scene. Exhortation and persuasion play an important role here. A patient depressed by the possibility of relapse might be reminded of the favorable statistics and the steady progress she has made to date. Seeing things in a new light, with new emphases and stresses, helps to allay the fear. In a different vein, anger at a child may subside when one focuses less on minor annoyances and more on admirable traits. One may work on a more forgiving attitude in general by choosing to play down others' perceived faults or foibles. In certain cases, experiencing emotions is a matter of giving inner assent—of allowing oneself to feel angry or giving the green light to a new interest or love. It is as if something grabs hold, and then it is our turn to have some influence.

Mental training can of course follow a more methodical and introspective model. An individual can learn to take more careful note of the onset of certain emotions and of the movement of mind from one perceived object of importance to another. So Buddhists speak of a watchful mindfulness, an intensification of consciousness such that through awareness and knowledge, one comes to be more in charge (Thera).

There are other methods of effecting emotional change that depend upon so-called "deep" psychology. In psychoanalysis the recapitulation of patterns of emotional response through transference onto an analyst is intended to be a way of seeing at a detached level. The patient relives an emotional experience at the same time as he watches and interprets it. This is the putative advantage of an empathetic, clinical setting: A patient can come to see an emotional pattern in a detached way, free from judgment and accusation and from the crippling emotions that those stances often involve. In some cases, a patient tries to relieve the pain of present disabling emotions, such as anger, anxiety, or shame by coming to see their roots in primitive conflicts and frustrations that may have long been repressed. The goal is not to remove the patient from the vulnerabilities of emotion, but rather to make possible a way of experiencing emotions, including shame and anger, that is less crippling and self-destructive.

More Radical Extirpation or Removal of Emotions

Because emotions are valued as modes of attention, motivation, communication, and knowledge, we tend to put up with their messiness while at the same time attempting their reform. But there are venerable traditions in which moderating emotions through transformation and education is viewed as an inadequate therapy and an inadequate way of training moral character and agency. The Stoic view, which influenced later Kantian views and bears rough similarities to certain Eastern traditions, argues that the surges and delusions of emotion warrant their extirpation. Investment in objects and events we cannot control is the source of our suffering, and modification of our beliefs about these values is the source of our cure. In Stoic theory, virtue comes to be rooted in reason alone, for it is reason alone that is most appropriate to our nature and under our true dominion.

The attraction of the Stoic view rests in its powerful description of the anguish of the engaged emotional life. Many emotions (though not all) lead to attachment, but objects of attachment are never perfectly stable. Abandonment, separation, failure, and loss are the constant costs of love, effort, and friendship. The more tightly we cling to our investments, the more dependent we become upon what is uncontrolled and outside our own mastery. Self-reproach and persecution are often responses to lack of control. In our relations with others, the same clinginess of emotions can lead to stepping beyond what is appropriate, just as it can lead to exclusionary preferences and partialities. Provincialism can grow out of stubborn preference for what is familiar and comfortable according to class lines or other restrictive values.

This is a reasonable portrait of some moments of the life lived through emotion. Detachment and watchful awareness directed toward the emotions are important therapeutic stances in such a life. In addition, detachment and watchful awareness should be directed toward reason itself and its own tendencies toward egoism and imperious control. This is clearly at odds with Stoic practice though more in line with Eastern practices such as Buddhism. But it is difficult to see how a thoroughgoing rejection of the emotions can be compatible with what is a human life. Emotions, for all their selectivity, intensity, and stirring, enable us, through those very vulnerabilities, to attend, see, know, and experience in a way that pure cognition cannot. Some of that way of knowing and being known anguishes beyond words. Poetry and literature can only begin to express the reality. But even if at times unruled by reason's measure, emotion must not, on that account, be an outlawed feature of human life. Nor must it be an outlawed feature of morality. How we care for others, and what we notice and reveal, depends greatly on the subtlety, fineness, and often deep truth of our emotional readings of the world.

Conclusion

From the above, it should be clear that emotions play an expanded role within bioethics and within the moral practices of healthcare professionals. Emotional sensitivity is important for discerning the complexity of situations and for appreciating the competing needs and interests of various parties. A simple matter of noticing a patient's distress or displeasure, perhaps by attending to her facial expressions and bodily gestures, could figure importantly in assessing a case. But by the same token, it is important to communicate emotions and not just record those of others. Conveying compassion to a patient can be a significant part of therapeutic treatment and, in general, be an important part of establishing a relationship in which medical counsel can be trusted and followed. Again, emotions figure in deliberation of choices. Compassion toward a patient can ground a reason for telling a patient the true nature of her condition in a tone that respects the patient's fragile, emotional state. The relevant choice a caretaker faces may not be whether to withhold or not withhold the truth, but rather how to tell the truth in a way that respects both a patient's autonomy and feelings. It is here that healthcare providers' own feelings of compassion and sympathy can importantly ground the specific choices she makes. Finally, healthcare providers, as morally responsible agents, need to have ready access to their own emotions, so that emotions help rather than hinder effective care. In cases, for example, in which fears and prejudice cloud more circumspect judgment, healthcare providers must recognize such fears and prejudice as emotional impediments standing in the way of delivering quality care. In general, a reflective stance toward one's own emotions becomes an important part of caring for others.

NANCY SHERMAN (1995)
REVISED BY AUTHOR

SEE ALSO: *Care; Compassionate Love; Conscience; Grief and Bereavement; Life, Quality of; Narrative; Pain and Suffering; Psychoanalysis and Dynamic Therapies; Women, Historical and Cross-Cultural Perspectives*

BIBLIOGRAPHY

Aristotle. 1984. *The Complete Works of Aristotle: The Revised Oxford Translation,* 2 vols., ed. Jonathan Barnes. Princeton, NJ: Princeton University Press.

Arnold, Magda B. 1960. *Emotion and Personality,* 2 vols. New York: Columbia University Press.

Calhoun, Cheshire, and Solomon, Robert C., comps. 1984. *What Is an Emotion? Classic Readings in Philosophical Psychology.* New York: Oxford University Press.

Cannon, Walter B. 1929. *Bodily Changes in Pain, Hunger, Fear, and Rage,* 2nd edition. New York: Appleton. Excerpted in *What Is an Emotion?,* comp. Cheshire Calhoun and Robert C. Solomon. New York: Oxford University Press, 1984.

Cicero. 1943. *Tusculan Disputations,* tr. John Edward King. Cambridge, MA: Harvard University Press.

Damasio, Antonio R. 1994. *Descartes' Error: Emotion, Reason, and the Human Brain.* New York: Avon Books.

Davis, Wayne. 1987. "The Varieties of Fear." *Philosophical Studies* 51: 287–310.

de Sousa, Ronald. 1987. *The Rationality of Emotions.* Cambridge, MA: MIT Press.

de Sousa, Ronald. 1988. "Emotion and Self-Deception." In *Perspectives on Self-Deception,* ed. Brian McLaughlin and Amelie O. Rorty. Berkeley: University of California Press.

Ekman, Paul. 1992. "Facial Expressions of Emotion: New Findings, New Questions." *Psychological Science* 3(1): 34–38.

Fridja, Nico. 1986. *The Emotions.* Cambridge, Eng.: Cambridge University Press.

Goldie, Peter. 2000. *The Emotions: A Philosophical Exploration.* Oxford: Clarendon Press.

Gordon, Robert. 1987. *The Structure of Emotions.* Cambridge, Eng.: Cambridge University Press.

Greenspan, Patricia S. 1988. *Emotions and Reasons: An Inquiry into Emotional Justification.* New York: Routledge.

Greenspan, Stanley. 1989. *The Development of the Ego.* Madison, CT: International Universities Press.

Griffiths, Paul. 1997. *What Emotions Really Are.* Chicago: University of Chicago Press.

Herman, Barbara. 1985. "The Practice of Moral Judgment." *Journal of Philosophy* 82(8): 414–436.

Hursthouse, Rosalind. 1991. "Arational Actions." *Journal of Philosophy* 88(2): 57–68.

James, William. 1884. "What Is an Emotion?" *Mind* 9: 188–204. Excerpted in *What Is an Emotion?* comp. Cheshire Calhoun and Robert C. Solomon. New York: Oxford University Press, 1984.

Lazarus, Richard S. 1984. "On the Primacy of Cognition." *American Psychologist* 39(2): 124–129.

LeDoux, Joseph E. 1996. *The Emotional Brain: The Mysterious Underpinnings of Emotional Life.* New York: Simon and Schuster.

Nussbaum, Martha C. 1987. "The Stoics on the Extirpation of the Passions. " *Apeiron* 20(2): 130–175.

Nussbaum, Martha C. 1990. *Love's Knowledge.* New York: Oxford University Press.

Nussbaum, Martha C. 2001. *Upheavals of Thought: The Intelligence of Emotions.* Cambridge, Eng.: Cambridge University Press.

Oatley, Keith. 1992. *Best Laid Schemes: The Psychology of Emotions.* Cambridge, Eng.: Cambridge University Press.

Parrot, W. Gerrod. 1988. "The Role of Cognition in Emotional Experience." In *Recent Trends in Theoretical Psychology,* ed. William J. Baker, Leendert P. Mos, Hans V. Rappard, and Hendrikus J. Stam. New York: Springer-Verlag.

Rorty, Amelie Oksenberg. 1980. *Explaining Emotions.* Berkeley: University of California Press.

Schacter, Daniel. 1996. *Searching for Memory.* New York: Basic.

Schacter, Stanley, and Singer, Jerome. 1962. "Cognitive, Social, and Physiological Determinants of Emotional States." *Psychological Review* 69: 379–399. Excerpted in *What Is an Emotion?*

comp. Cheshire Calhoun and Robert C. Solomon. New York: Oxford University Press, 1984.

Scherer, Klaus R. 1993. "Studying the Emotion-Antecedent Appraisal Process: An Expert System Approach." *Cognition and Emotion* 7(3–4): 325–355.

Sherman, Nancy. 1989. *The Fabric of Character: Aristotle's Theory of Virtue.* New York: Oxford University Press.

Sherman, Nancy. 1990. "The Place of Emotions in Kantian Morality." In *Identity, Character, and Morality,* ed. Owen Flanagan and Amelie Oksenberg Rorty. Cambridge, MA: MIT Press.

Sherman, Nancy. 1997. *Making a Necessity of Virtue: Aristotle and Kant on Virtue.* Cambridge, Eng.: Cambridge University Press.

Solomon, Robert. 1976. *The Myth and Nature of Human Emotions.* New York: Doubleday.

Solomon, Robert C., ed. 2003. *What Is an Emotion: Classic and Contemporary Readings,* 2nd edition. New York: Oxford University Press.

Squire, Larry R. 1987. *Memory and Brain.* New York: Oxford University Press.

Stocker, Michael. 1996. *Valuing Emotions.* Cambridge, Eng.: Cambridge University Press.

Thera, Nyanaponika. 1986. *The Vision of Dhamma.* London: Rider.

Tomkins, Silvan S. 1962–1992. *Affect, Imagery, Consciousness,* 4 vols. New York: Springer.

Zajonc, Robert B. 1980. "Feeling and Thinking: Preferences Need No Inferences." *American Psychologist* 35(2): 117–123.

EMPIRICAL METHODS IN BIOETHICS

• • •

The period since 1970 has seen the development and maturation of the field of bioethics into a major area of scholarly inquiry. Scholarship in bioethics has traditionally relied on the discipline of moral philosophy and has taken a normative or prescriptive stance. However, bioethics is primarily a field of *practical* and *applied* study as well as a theoretical one. As such, to be relevant and useful to the providers and consumers of healthcare, bioethics must address questions and recommend solutions in the real world. Empirically-based studies provide an understanding of public and professional attitudes, practices, and the implications and intersections of practice and policy. These studies can provide information about the level at which purported problems actually exist and can be described and quantified. Similarly, they can measure the success or failure of public policies designed to help solve bioethics problems.

Employing the qualitative and quantitative methodologies of the social sciences and public health, bioethics scholars, often in collaboration with clinicians and scientists, have shed light on important bioethics questions such as:

- Patient and family preferences for treatment at the end of life;
- Nature and quality of communication between patients and physicians;
- Attitudes and understanding of informed consent by investigators and research subjects;
- Competency and the robustness of individual's stated wishes about end of life treatment;
- Why policy and legislative initiatives have failed to increase consent rates to organ donation;
- Impact of new genetic information on individuals, families, and society;
- Equity in allocation of scarce resources such as dialysis and organ transplantation;
- Disparities in the provision of care to ethnic minorities.

Research Methods

The methods used by researchers engaged in the empirical study of bioethics range from the quantitative to the qualitative, and often combine the two to provide a richer description of phenomenon and to answer research questions. Empirical research methods of all types comprise those that can be used to describe valid and reliable inquiries into phenomenon, including human behavior. Quantitative methods are used to answer hypotheses or to provide generalizable descriptions of populations and the incidence and prevalence of behaviors and problems within a population. Traditional quantitative methods in the social sciences include controlled experiments to compare the effects of an intervention on a sample population and measurement of subject characteristics. These measurements can include characterizing attitudes, behaviors, or physical characteristics. They are distinguished by the use of measurement tools that can provide reliable and replicable descriptions, usually in the form of numeric signifiers. Examples of such measurements are the use of psychometric tools to measure cognitive traits (e.g., anxiety, coping style, depression) and attitudes (trust in the healthcare system, fatalism). Psychometric techniques can also be sued to the measurement of physical traits such as health status (using measurements like the SF–36 or activities of daily living). Most of these measurements take place within structured interviews (either interviewer-administered or self-administered) in which the responses of subjects are strictly prescribed. The phrasing of questions is regimented and the respondent is provided with what are called forced choice responses in which information is produced as standardized coded information. Aside from obtaining information directly from subjects, another major source of quantitative data is secondary sources, such as administrative databases (such as the Medicare database) and medical records. The advantages of quantitative methods are that they enable collection of data from large sample sizes in standardized ways that permit comparisons across various populations and time periods. They also allow for controlled interventions or controlled introduction of conditions to subjects. These methods have allowed the documentation of racial and gender disparities in the provision of healthcare services.

Bioethics researchers have generally used qualitative methods in the generation of hypotheses rather than in the testing of hypotheses. Deduction characterizes qualitative methods, whereas induction characterizes research using quantitative methods. Qualitative methods permit detailed, and sometimes more accurate, observation of behaviors and contribute to the understanding of underlying social and cultural characteristics associated with specific patterns of behaviors. Moreover, qualitative methods allow discovery of subjects' perspectives rather than imposing a pre-existing framework. Qualitative methods can allow researchers to access areas of investigation not amenable to quantitative research, and to explore areas that have been little researched in the past. For example, how infertile couples have experienced new reproductive technologies and how they have incorporated traditional understandings of parenthood into their conceptual models of the rights and obligations of parents.

Qualitative methods include a variety of techniques. Subject interviews that incorporate wholly or partly open-ended questions are commonly used. These allow respondents to provide answers to questions in their own words, and allow interviewers to probe or follow up on information provided by respondents. More formative interviewing, in which the interviewer uses a guide to begin discussion about the research topic but does not structure the questions that follow, can also be used. In this type of interview, the subject creates a narrative and engages in a dialogue with the interviewer that informs the researcher about the topic under investigation. A similar technique, the focus group, uses six to twelve informants gathered to discuss a particular

issue. For example, a study of the social and ethical consequences of genetic testing for Huntington's Disease might gather individuals from families affected by Huntington's Disease to discuss their attitudes, preferences, and intentions about genetic testing.

Qualitative methods can also include direct observation of healthcare situations and populations. For example, studies of informed consent to clinical trials have included directly observing and audio- or videotaping the consent conversation. Conversations can be examined as narratives and themes explored, or behaviors can be coded to extract quantitative data. For example, a trained observer can use 0, 1 coding to measure whether certain behaviors (e.g., explaining that trial participation is voluntary) occur or not. Participant observation—in which the observer actually participates in and observes the daily activities of a setting of interest (for example, observing a primary care setting to understand how or when advance directives are discussed with elderly patients)—can also generate a variety of data types. Personal diaries in which individuals are asked to keep records of activities and behaviors are another technique.

Historically, social sciences researchers have strictly divided themselves into researchers using quantitative methods (i.e., psychologists) or qualitative methods (i.e., anthropologists). However, in recent years there has been a blurring of these distinctions and an increasing enthusiasm for multimethod research. Whereas qualitative research begins by acknowledging that there is a range of different ways of making sense of the world, and approaches its subject matter in a naturalistic, interpretive way, quantitative research overlays hypothesized paradigms on the research phenomena of interest and collects data that can help determine the distributions of characteristics and behaviors in populations and settings. For example, quantitative studies have established how frequently dying patients are treated with futile therapies, but have not been especially successful in explaining why.

Conclusion

Ultimately, scholarship in bioethics can benefit from the methodologies of both the humanities and the empirical sciences. Normative bioethics provides a framework and guideposts for suggesting how healthcare services ought to be delivered, and what the fiduciary responsibilities of clinicians to patients are. However, normative bioethics is unable to describe and explain how these play out in real life. Moreover, the value placed in the principles of bioethics and the use made of these principals by actors in healthcare settings can only be illuminated using empirical methods. In the final analysis, the best empirical research in bioethics will always be based on a sophisticated understanding of the historical, philosophical, and cultural contexts of the delivery and consumption of healthcare services. Similarly, philosophical debate can often be enriched by an awareness of empirical data.

LAURA A. SIMINOFF

SEE ALSO: *Anthropology and Bioethics; Medicine, Anthropology of; Medicine, Sociology of; Organ Transplants, Sociocultural Aspects of; Public Health: Methods; Public Policy and Bioethics; Research Ethics Committees; Research Methodology; Research Policy; Research, Unethical*

BIBLIOGRAPHY

Appleton, Jane V. 1995. "Analysing Qualitative Interview Data: Addressing Issues of Validity and Reliability." *Journal of Advanced Nursing* 22: 993–997.

Cummings, Kenneth Michael; Becker, M. H.; and Maile, M. C. 1980. "Bringing the Models Together: An Empirical Approach to Combining Variables Used to Explain Health Actions." *Journal of Behavioral Medicine* 3(2): 123–145.

Looker, E. Dianne; Denton, Margaret A.; and Davis, Christine K. 1989. "Bridging the Gap: Incorporating Qualitative Data into Quantitative Analyses." *Social Science Research* 18: 313–330.

Pope, Catherine, and Mays, Nick. 1995. "Reaching the Parts Other Methods Cannot Reach: An Introduction to Qualitative Methods in Health and Health Services Research." *British Medical Journal* 311: 42–45.

Scrimshaw, Susan C. M.; Carballo, Maneul; Ramos, Laura; and Blair, Betty A. 1991. "The AIDS Rapid Anthropological Assessment Procedures: A Tool for Health Education Planning and Evaluation." *Health Education Quarterly* 18(1): 111–123.

ENDANGERED SPECIES AND BIODIVERSITY

• • •

Although projections vary, reliable estimates are that about 20 percent of Earth's species may be lost within a few decades, if present trends go unreversed. These losses will be about evenly distributed through major groups of plants and animals in both developed and developing nations, with special concerns over tropical forests (Ehrlich and Ehrlich; Wilson).

The United Nations at the 1992 Earth Summit in Rio de Janeiro launched the Convention on Biological Diversity, signed by 153 nations that are "concerned that biological diversity is being significantly reduced by certain human activities" and who are "conscious of the intrinsic value of biological diversity and of the ecological, genetic, social, economic, scientific, educational, cultural, recreational and aesthetic values of biological diversity," and "conscious also of the importance of biological diversity for evolution and for maintaining life sustaining systems of the biosphere" (United Nations, Preamble).

The U.S. Congress has lamented the lack of "adequate concern [for] and conservation [of]" species, and has sought to protect species through the Endangered Species Act, as well as through the Convention on International Trade in Endangered Species (U.S. Congress, Sec. 2(a) (1)). About five hundred species, subspecies, and varieties of fauna have been lost since 1600 in what is now the continental United States. The natural rate would have been about ten (Opler). In Hawaii, of sixty-eight species of birds unique to the islands, forty-one are extinct or virtually so. Half of the twenty-two hundred native plants are endangered or threatened. A candidate list for all states contains over two thousand taxa (species and significant subspecies and forms) considered to be endangered, threatened, or of concern, three categories used to rank degree of jeopardy (U.S. Fish and Wildlife Service). Human-caused extinctions threaten to approach and even exceed the catastrophic extinction rates of the geological past.

Even where species are not endangered, almost all inhabited lands are impoverished of their native fauna and flora, owing to development, loss of habitat, hunting, collection, trade in fauna and flora, toxic pollutants, introduction of exotic species, and other disturbances produced by humans. Sustainable biodiversity, the use of biotic resources so as to leave them unimpaired for future generations, is an increasing concern. Another concern is the loss of wetlands, permanently or periodically flooded or wet areas, which at the end of the twentieth century in many areas are less than 10 percent of their original area. There is hardly a forest, grassland, or desert system in the developed world that is not impoverished of its once-native fauna and flora. Old-growth or pristine forests have been cut rapidly, as have tropical rain forests. Island ecosystems, often with species peculiar to that location and found nowhere else, are particularly at risk.

In the conservation of endangered species and biodiversity, bioethics in principle and in practice involves an unprecedented mix of science and conscience, especially since the species and ecosystem levels seldom figured in earlier ethical deliberations. A rationale for saving species that centers on their worth to persons is anthropocentric; a rationale that includes their intrinsic and ecosystemic values, in addition to or independently of persons, is naturalistic.

On an anthropocentric account, the duties involved are to persons; there are no duties to endangered species, though duties may concern species. Persons have a strong duty of nonmaleficence—not to harm others—and a weaker, though important, duty of beneficence—to help others. Many endangered species—which ones we may not now know—are expected to have agricultural, industrial, and medical benefits. They may be of scientific value, serve as indicators of ecosystem health, or provide genetic breeding stock for improvement of cultivated plants. Humans ought to conserve their global resources, a matter of prudence and enlightened self-interest in general, but a matter of moral concern when some persons threaten the benefits of these resources for other persons. Nonrenewable resources may have to be mined and consumed, but biological resources can be perennially renewable.

A developing concern between the species-rich, often underdeveloped countries and the developed countries, which are frequently responsible in part for environmental degradation, is who should bear the costs of saving species relative to benefits gained. Historically, native plant species, seeds, and germ plasm have been considered not to be owned by any nation. Developing nations are claiming ownership by the country of origin, arguing that these resources cannot be used by those in other nations without negotiating compensation. At the same time, developing nations claim that their biological resources are being conserved for the benefit of other nations, and that the developed nations ought to pay developing nations not only for new conservation measures put into effect there but also for the lost opportunity costs of development in such conserved areas.

The Convention on Biological Diversity states: "States have sovereign rights over their own biological resources" (United Nations, Preamble) and continues, "Recognizing the sovereign rights of States over their natural resources, the authority to determine access to genetic resources rests with the national governments and is subject to national legislation" (Art. 15). Nevertheless, the problem of reconciling biodiversity as a common heritage of humankind with biodiversity as a national resource remains unresolved. States may control access to biodiversity, but this does not imply ownership. The United States refused to sign the Convention over questions of ownership, both of the wild biodiversity and of beneficial technology derived from it.

On the harm side, the loss of a few species may have no evident results now, but the loss of many species imperils the resilience and stability of the ecosystems on which humans depend. The danger increases with subtractions from the ecosystem, a slippery slope into serious troubles. Many species that have no direct value to humans are part of the biodiversity that keeps ecosystems healthy. On the benefits side again, there are less tangible benefits. Species that are too rare to play roles in ecosystems can have recreational and aesthetic value—even, for many persons, religious value. Species can be curiosities. They can be clues to understanding natural history. Destroying species is like tearing pages out of an unread book, written in a language humans hardly know how to read, about the place where they live. Humans need insight into the full text of natural history.

Such anthropic reasons are pragmatic and impressive. They are also moral, since persons are benefited or hurt. But can all duties concerning species be analyzed as duties to persons? Many endangered species have no resource value, nor are they particularly important for the other reasons given above. Are there worthless species? As curiosities and relics of the past, perhaps all species can be given an umbrella protection by saying that humans ought to preserve an environment adequate to match their capacity to wonder. Nature is a kind of wonderland. But this introduces the question of whether preserving resources for wonder is not better seen as preserving a remarkable natural history that has objective worth—an evolutionary process that has spontaneously assembled millions of species. A naturalistic account values species and speciation directly.

A further rationale is that humans of decent character will refrain from needless destruction of all kinds, including destruction of any species. Such a prohibition seems to depend, however, on some value in the species as such, for there need be no prohibition against destroying a valueless thing. The deeper problem with the anthropocentric rationale is that its justifications are less than fully moral, fundamentally exploitive, and self-serving, even if subtly so. This is not true intraspecifically among humans, when out of a sense of duty an individual defers to the values of other persons. But it is true interspecifically, since *Homo sapiens* treats all other species as resources. Ethics has always involved partners with entwined destinies. But ethics has never been very convincing when pleaded as enlightened self-interest (that one ought always to do what is in one's intelligent self-interest), including class self-interest, even though in practice altruistic ethics often needs to be reinforced by self-interest. To value all other species only in terms of human interests is rather like a nation's arguing all its foreign policy in terms of national self-interest. Neither seems to be completely moral.

It is safe to say that in the decades ahead, the quality of life will decline in proportion to the loss of biotic diversity, though it is often thought that one must sacrifice that diversity to improve human life. So there is a sense in which humans will not be losers if we save endangered species. Humans who protect endangered species will, if and when they change their value priorities, be better persons for their admiring respect for other forms of life. But this should not obscure the fact that humans can be short-term losers. Sometimes we do have to make genuine sacrifices, at least in terms of what we presently value, to preserve species. If, for instance, Americans wish to save the spotted owl, they will have to pay higher prices for timber and accept some job losses and relocations.

Dealing with a problem correctly requires an appropriate way of thinking about it. On the scale of evolutionary time, humans appear late and suddenly. Even later and more suddenly they increase the extinction rate dramatically. What is offensive in such conduct is not merely the loss of resources but also the maelstrom of killing and insensitivity to forms of life. What is required is not prudence but principled responsibility to the biospheric Earth.

There are problems at two levels when considering duties to species; one is about facts (a scientific issue), and one is about values (an ethical issue). First, what sort of biological entity is a species? Indeed, do species exist at all? No one doubts that individual organisms exist, but species can have a more controversial factual reality. Taxonomists regularly revise species designations and routinely put after a species the name of the "author" who, they say, "erected" the taxon. If a species is only a category or class, boundary lines may be arbitrarily drawn, and the species is nothing more than a convenient grouping of its members, an artifact of taxonomists. Some natural properties are used—reproductive structures, bones, teeth. But which properties are selected and where the lines are drawn vary with taxonomists.

If this approach is pressed, species can become a conventional concept, a mapping device, that is only theoretical, something like the lines of longitude and latitude. Sometimes endangered species designations have altered when taxonomists have decided to lump or split previous groupings. To whatever degree species are artifacts of taxonomists, duties to save them seem unconvincing. No one proposes duties to genera, families, orders, phyla; biologists concede that these do not exist in nature.

On a more realist account, a biological species is not just a class; it is a living historical form (Latin *species,* a natural kind), propagated in individual organisms, that flows dynamically over generations. Species are dynamic natural kinds, historically particular lineages. A species is a coherent, ongoing form of life expressed in organisms, encoded in gene flow, and shaped by the environment. In this sense, species are objectively there as living processes in the evolutionary ecosystem—found, not made, by taxonomists. The claim that there are specific forms of life historically maintained in their environments over time does not seem arbitrary but, rather, as certain as anything else we believe about the empirical world, even though at times scientists revise the theories and taxa with which they map these forms.

Species are not so much like lines of latitude and longitude as like mountains and rivers, phenomena objectively there to be mapped. The edges of such natural kinds will sometimes be fuzzy, to some extent discretionary. We can expect that one species will slide into another over evolutionary time. But it does not follow from the fact that speciation is sometimes in progress that species are merely made up, instead of found as evolutionary lines articulated into diverse forms, each with its more or less distinct integrity, breeding population, gene pool, and role in its ecosystem (Rojas).

Having recognized what a species is, the next question is why species ought to be protected. The naturalistic answer is that humans ought to respect these dynamic life forms preserved in historical lines, vital informational processes that persist genetically over millions of years, overleaping short-lived individuals. It is not *form* (species) as mere morphology, but the *formative* (speciating) process that humans ought to preserve, although the process cannot be preserved without its products. Endangered "species" is a convenient and realistic way of tagging this process, but protection can be interpreted (as the Endangered Species Act permits) in terms of subspecies, variety, or other taxa or categories that point out the diverse forms of life.

A consideration of species is both revealing and challenging because it offers a biologically based counterexample to the focus on individuals—typically sentient and usually persons—so characteristic in Western ethics. In an evolutionary ecosystem, it is not mere individuality that counts; the species is also significant because it is a dynamic life form maintained over time by an informed genetic flow. The individual represents (re-presents) a species in each new generation. It is a token of a type, and the type is more important than the token. A biological identity—a kind of value—is here defended. The dignity resides in the dynamic form; the individual inherits this, exemplifies it, and passes it on.

A species lacks moral agency, reflective self-awareness, sentience, and organic individuality. Some have been tempted to say that species-level processes cannot count morally. But each ongoing species defends a form of life, and these diverse species are, on the whole, good kinds. Such speciation has achieved all the planetary richness of life. All ethicists say that in *Homo sapiens* one species has appeared that not only exists but also ought to exist. A naturalistic ethic refuses to say this exclusively of a late-coming, highly developed form, and extends this duty more broadly to the other species—though not with equal intensity over them all, in view of varied levels of evolutionary achievement. Only the human species contains moral agents, but conscience ought not to be used to exempt every other form of life from consideration, with the resulting paradox that the sole moral species acts only in its collective self-interest toward all the rest.

Extinction shuts down the generative processes. The wrong that humans are doing, or allowing to happen through carelessness, is stopping the historical gene flow on which the vitality of life is based, and which, viewed at another level, is the same as the flow of natural kinds. Every extinction is an incremental decay in this stopping of life. Every extinction is a kind of superkilling. It kills forms (species) beyond individuals. It kills "essences" beyond "existences," the "soul" as well as the "body." It kills collectively, not just distributively. We do not merely lament the loss of potential human information; we lament the loss of biological information, present independently of instrumental human uses of it. A shutdown of the life stream on Earth is the most destructive event possible. Each human-caused extinction edges us further in this direction; already the rate may be catastrophic.

A consideration of species strains any ethic fixed on individual organisms, much less on sentience or persons. But the result can be biologically sounder, though it revises what was formerly thought to be logically permissible or ethically binding. When ethics is informed by this kind of biology, it is appropriate to attach duty dynamically to the specific form of life. The species line is the more fundamental living system, the whole of which individual organisms are the essential parts. The species, too, has its integrity, its individuality; and it is more important to protect this than to protect individual integrity. The appropriate survival unit is the appropriate level of moral concern.

A species is what it is inseparably from the environmental niche into which it fits. Particular species may not be essential in the sense that the ecosystem can survive the loss of individual species without adverse effect. But habitats are essential to species, and an endangered species typically means an endangered habitat. Species play lesser or greater roles in their habitats. This leads to an enlarged concern for the preservation of species in the system. It is not merely *what* they are, but *where* they are that one must value correctly. This limits the otherwise important role that zoos and botanical gardens can play in the conservation of species. They can provide research, a refuge for species, breeding programs, aid for public education, and so forth, but they cannot simulate the ongoing dynamism of gene flow over time under the selection pressures in a wild ecosystem. They amputate the species from its habitat.

Extinction is a quite natural event, but there are important theoretical and practical differences between natural and anthropogenic (human-caused) extinctions. Artificial extinction, caused by human encroachments, is radically different from natural extinction. Relevant differences make the two as morally distinct as death by natural causes is from murder. Though harmful to a species, extinction in nature is seldom an evil in the system. It is, rather, the key to tomorrow. The species is employed in, but abandoned to, the larger historical evolution of life. There are replacements. Such extinction is normal turnover in ongoing speciation.

Anthropogenic extinction differs from evolutionary extinction in that hundreds of thousands of species will perish because of culturally altered environments that are radically different from the spontaneous environments in which such species are naturally selected and in which they sometimes go extinct. In natural extinction, nature takes away life when it has become unfit in habitat, or when the habitat alters, and typically supplies other life in its place. Artificial extinction shuts down tomorrow, because it shuts down speciation. Natural extinction typically occurs with transformation, either of the extinct line or of related or competing lines. Artificial extinction is without issue. One opens doors; the other closes them. In artificial extinctions, humans generate and regenerate nothing; they only dead-end these lines.

Through evolutionary time nature has provided new species at a net higher rate than the extinction rate; hence the accumulated global diversity. There have been infrequent catastrophic extinction events, anomalies in the record, each succeeded by a recovery of previous diversity. Although natural events, these extinctions so deviate from the normal trends that many paleontologists look for causes external to the evolutionary ecosystem—supernovas or collisions with asteroids. Typically, however, the biological processes that characterize Earth are both prolific and have considerable powers of recovery after catastrophe. Uninterrupted by accident, or even interrupted so, they steadily increase the numbers of species.

An ethicist has to be circumspect. An argument may commit what logicians call the genetic fallacy in supposing that present value depends upon origins. Species judged today to have intrinsic value may have arisen anciently and anomalously from a valueless context, akin to the way in which life arose mysteriously from nonliving materials. But in an ecosystem, what a thing is differentiates poorly from the generating and sustaining matrix. The individual and the species have their value inevitably in the context of the forces that beget them. There is something awesome about an Earth that begins with zero and runs up toward five to ten million species in several billion years, setbacks notwithstanding.

Several billion years' worth of creative toil, several million species of teeming life, have been handed over to the care of the late-coming species in which mind has flowered and morals have emerged. On the humanistic account, such species ought to be saved for their benefits to humans. On the naturalistic account, the sole moral species has a duty to do something less self-interested than count all the products of an evolutionary ecosystem as human resources; rather, this host of species has a claim to care in its own right. There is something Newtonian, not yet Einsteinian, as well as something morally naive, about living in a reference frame where one species takes itself as absolute and values everything else relative to its utility.

In addition to the deeper ethical principles at issue in conservation of species, questions of pragmatic strategy arise. One strategy proposed when there are limited resources is to sort jeopardized species into three groups: those that are probably going extinct even if we try hard to save them, those that will probably survive without our help, and those that will probably go extinct unless we intervene. This strategy is called triage. An alternative, or complementary, strategy is to focus more on endangered ecosystems than on single species, an approach that may result both in more effective management and in more efficient use of resources. Another strategy discourages claiming biodiversity as a national resource while thinking of conservation in other nations in terms of foreign policy, for if biodiversity is the common heritage of humankind, all nations share duties to protect it.

HOLMES ROLSTON III (1995)
BIBLIOGRAPHY REVISED

SEE ALSO: *Animal Welfare and Rights: Ethical Perspectives on the Treatment and Status of Animals; Environmental Ethics; Environmental Policy and Law; Hazardous Wastes and Toxic Substances; Native American Religions; Sustainable Development*

BIBLIOGRAPHY

Cairns, J. Jr. 1997. "Defining Goals and Conditions for a Sustainable World." *Environmental Health Perspectives* 105(11): 1164–1170.

Czech, Brian, and Krausman, Paul R. 2001. *The Endangered Species Act: History, Conservation Biology, and Public Policy* Baltimore, MD: Johns Hopkins University Press.

Ehrlich, Paul, and Ehrlich, Anne. 1981. *Extinction: The Causes and Consequences of the Disappearance of Species.* New York: Random House.

Heywood, V. H.; Watson, R. T.; United Nations Environment; and Dowdeswell, Elizabeth, eds. 1996. *Global Biodiversity Assessment* New York: Cambridge University Press.

Kinzig, Ann P.; Pacala, Stephen W.; and Tilman, David, eds. 2001. *The Functional Consequences of Biodiversity: Empirical Progress and Theoretical Extensions.* Princeton, NJ: Princeton University Press.

Norton, Bryan G., ed. 1986. *The Preservation of Species: The Value of Biological Diversity.* Princeton, NJ: Princeton University Press.

Opler, Paul A. 1976. "The Parade of Passing Species: A Survey of Extinctions in the U.S." *The Science Teacher* 43(9): 30–34.

Perlman, Dan L., and Osborne, Edward. 2000. *Conserving Earth's Biodiversity.* Washington, D.C.: Wilson Island Press.

Pimm, S. L., and Raven P. 2000. "Biodiversity. Extinction by Numbers." *Nature* 403(6772): 843–845.

Polasky, Stephen, ed. *The Economics of Biodiversity Conservation (International Library of Environmental Economics and Policy).* Burlington, VT: Ashgate Publishing Company.

Rojas, Martha. 1992. "The Species Problem and Conservation: What Are We Protecting?" *Conservation Biology* 6(2): 170–178.

Rolston, Holmes, III. 1985. "Duties to Endangered Species." *Bioscience* 35: 718–726.

Rolston, Holmes, III. 1988. "Life in Jeopardy: Duties to Endangered Species." Chap. 4 in *Environmental Ethics: Duties to and Values in the Natural World.* Philadelphia: Temple University Press.

Shouse, Ben. 2002. "Endangered Species Act. Cherished Concepts Faltering in the Field." *Science* 296(5571): 1219–1221.

Stokstad, E. 2002. "Endangered Species. Fur Flies Over Charges of Misconduct." *Science* 295(5553): 250–251

The Stanford Environmental Law Society. *The Endangered Species Act (Stanford Environmental Law Society Handbook).* 2001. Palo Alto, CA: Stanford University Press.

Tilman, D. 2000. "Causes, Consequences and Ethics of Biodiversity." *Nature* 405(6783): 208–211.

Torrence, P. F. 1995. "The Endangered Species Act." *Science* 269(5232): 1803–1804.

United Nations Environment Program. 1992. *Convention on Biological Diversity,* 5 June 1992.

United States Congress. 1973. Endangered Species Act of 1973. 87 Stat. 884. Public Law 93–205.

United States Fish and Wildlife Service. 1990. List in 55 *Federal Register* (35)(February 21): 6184–6229.

Vogel, G. 2000. "Endangered Species. Migrating Otters Push Law to the Limit." *Science* 289(5483): 1271–1273.

Wilson, Edward O., ed. 1988. *Biodiversity.* Washington, D.C.: National Academy Press.

ENHANCEMENT USES OF MEDICAL TECHNOLOGY

• • •

In bioethics, one frequently encounters the belief that there is an important moral distinction between using biomedical tools and products to combat human disease and attempting to use them to "enhance" human traits. Thus, people argue that using biosynthetic human growth hormone to treat an inborn growth-hormone deficiency is praiseworthy, but that the use of the same product to increase the height of a short but hormonally normal child is not (Daniels, 1992). Similarly, while the use of human gene-transfer techniques to treat disease enjoys widespread support from secular and religious moral authorities, a line is usually drawn at using the same protocols to attempt to improve upon otherwise healthy traits (Anderson; Baird).

Even those unwilling to condemn the enhancement uses of biomedicine outright generally concur that ethics demands that therapeutic applications of these tools be given priority for research and development (Walters and Palmer). As a result, this distinction has been enshrined in policies at both professional and governmental levels, and it continues to inform much of the public discussion of new biomedical advances (Parens, 1998). The distinction is explicated in several different ways, however, which have different merits as moral boundary markers for medical research and practice. In fact, it often seems in danger of evaporating entirely under conceptual critiques even before the question of its moral merits is entertained.

Professional Domain Approaches

One approach to the enhancement/treatment distinction is to define it in terms of the accepted limits of professional medical practice. Under this view, *treatments* are any interventions that physicians and their patients agree are useful and proper, while *enhancements* are simply interventions that are considered to fall beyond a physician's professional purview. Thus, physician-prescribed physical therapy to improve muscle strength would be considered legitimate

medical treatment, while weight lifting under a coach's supervision to achieve a particular physique would be considered an enhancement. This view resonates well with a number of contemporary social-scientific critiques of biomedicine, which suggest that medicine has no natural domain of practice beyond that which it negotiates with society (Good). It also provides a simple normative lesson for professionals concerned about their obligations in specific cases. Given medicine's fundamentally patient-centered ethos, one takes one's cues from the patient's value system, and thus negotiates toward interventions that can help achieve the patient's vision of human flourishing (Engelhardt).

Unfortunately, these same features also deny this approach the ability to be of help to those attempting to use the treatment/enhancement distinction in order to regulate biomedical research. Some argue that medicine's lack of an essential domain of practice means that a coherent distinction between medical and nonmedical services can never be drawn in the first place (Davis). Others accept the distinction between treating and enhancing, but question traditional values of medicine by arguing that privileging treatment over enhancement is itself wrong (Silvers). Still others argue that, for psychological and economic reasons, a professional medical line between treatment and enhancement will be impossible to maintain in practice (Gardner). To the extent that useful "upper-boundary" concepts are required at the policy level—for societies making healthcare research allocation decisions, for example—this impotence is an important weakness.

The Normalcy Approach

Fortunately, another approach to interpreting the treatment/enhancement distinction is framed explicitly as a policy tool for separating legitimate healthcare needs from luxury services. The most developed exposition of this view is Sabin and Daniel's endorsement of what they call the "normal function" standard for determining the limits of "medically necessary" (and therefore socially underwritten) health services (p. 13). Sabin and Daniels argue that an appropriate boundary between medically necessary treatments and optional enhancements can be drawn by thinking about how to provide medical services fairly within a population. Following Daniels' earlier work, they construe healthcare as one of society's means for preserving equality of opportunity for its citizens, and they define "healthcare needs" as those services that allow individuals to enjoy the portion of the society's "normal opportunity range" to which their full array of skills and talents would give them access. This is done by restoring or improving the patient's abilities to the range of functional capacities typical for members of his or her reference class (e.g., age and gender) within the human species. Any interventions that would expand an individual's range of functional capacities beyond the range typical for his or her reference class would be deemed a medically unnecessary enhancement. Others have used similar understandings of human malady to help explicate a distinction between "negative" (e.g., therapeutic) and "positive" (e.g., enhancing) human genetic engineering (Berger and Gert).

The advantage of the normal-function approach is that it provides one relatively unified goal for healthcare, toward which the burdens and benefits of various interventions can be relatively objectively titrated (measured against one another), balanced, and integrated. The normal-function approach comes close to accurately reconstructing the rationale behind many actual "line drawing" judgments by healthcare coverage plans and professional societies (Brock et al.). Unfortunately, this approach also faces conceptual challenges in an important way. The first serious problem is that of prevention. While efforts at generic "health promotion" straddle the border of biomedicine, efforts to prevent the manifestation of specific maladies in individuals are always accepted as legitimate parts of biomedicine, and thus are automatically located on the treatment side of the enhancement boundary. On the other hand, one of the ways one can prevent a disease is to strengthen the body's ability to resist it long before any diagnosable problem appears. These forms of prevention attempt to elevate bodily functions above the normal range for the individual (and in some cases the species), and to that extent seem to slide into enhancement (Juengst). If human gene–transfer protocols like these are acceptable as forms of preventive medicine, how can it be claimed that healthcare practitioners should be "drawing the line" at enhancement?

Disease-Based Approaches

Probably the most common rejoinder to the problem of prevention is to distinquish the problems to which prevention efforts respond. Treatments are interventions that address the health problems created by diseases and disabilities ("maladies" in the helpful language of Clouser, Culver, and Gert). Enhancements, on the other hand, are interventions aimed at healthy systems and normal traits. Thus, prescribing biosynthetic growth hormone to rectify a diagnosable growth-hormone deficiency is legitimate treatment, while prescribing it for patients with normal growth-hormone levels would be an attempt at "positive genetic engineering," or enhancement (Berger and Gert). Thus, to justify an intervention as appropriate medicine means to be able to identify a pathological problem in the patient. If no medically recognizable malady can be diagnosed, the intervention cannot be "medically necessary," and is thus suspect as an enhancement.

This interpretation has the advantages of being simple, intuitively appealing, and consistent with a good bit of biomedical behavior. Maladies are both objectively observable phenomena and the traditional target of medical intervention. They can be discovered through diagnosis, and it will be clear when one has gone beyond medicine when no pathology can be identified (Juengst). This interpretation is used by professionals working at the boundary, like cosmetic surgeons, to justify their services in terms of relieving "diagnosable" psychological suffering rather than satisfying the aesthetic tastes of their clients (Morgan), and it is also used when insurance companies insist on being provided with a diagnosis before providing coverage for surgery.

However, this interpretation does also face at least two major difficulties. The first problem that any disease-based interpretation of the enhancement boundary faces is, of course, biomedicine's infamous nosological elasticity. It is not that hard to coin new maladies for the purposes of justifying the use of enhancement interventions. By interpreting the boundary of medicine in terms of maladies, this approach puts the power for drawing that boundary squarely in the profession's hands, with the corresponding potential for abuse.

The more important problem, however, is that no matter where the line is drawn, most biotechnological interventions that could become problematic as enhancement interventions would not have to cross that line in order to be developed and approved for clinical use, because they will also have legitimate therapeutic applications. In fact, most biosynthetic biologicals and gene-transfer protocols with potential for enhancement uses will first emerge as therapeutic agents. General cognitive-enhancement interventions, for example, are likely to be approved for use only in patients with neurological diseases (Whitehouse et al.). However, to the extent that they are in high demand by individuals who are merely suffering the effects of normal aging, the risk of unapproved, or "off-label," uses of these products will be high (Mehlman). This last point is critical for policy purposes, because it suggests that the real challenge to regulation in this area may not be the development of enhancement interventions or "enhancement research," but downstream off-label uses of gene therapies for nonmedical enhancement purposes. The policy problem then becomes controlling access and use of the technologies, not their research and development. This presents another set of challenges for the law, since the novelty of enhancement technologies will make it difficult for judges and juries to ascertain the reasonableness of physician behavior (Mehlman).

These realities have pressed those who would use the treatment/enhancement distinction for policy purposes to articulate the moral dangers of genetic enhancement more clearly. After all, personal improvement is praised in many spheres of human endeavor, and biomedical interventions such as cosmetic surgery are well accepted, at lease in American society, as means to achieving personal improvement goals.

The Moral Dangers of Enhancement

There are two lines of thought that have emerged from this work. The first focuses on the idea that biomedical enhancements are a form of social cheating. In this view, taking the biomedical shortcut erodes the specific social practices that make the analogous human achievement valuable in the first place. Thus, some argue that it defeats the purpose of the contest for the marathon runner to gain endurance chemically rather than through training, and it misses the point of meditation if one can gain Nirvana through psychosurgery. In both cases, the value of the improvements lie in the achievements they reward as well as the benefits they bring. The achievements (successful training or disciplined meditation) add value to the improvements because they are understood to be admirable social practices in themselves. Wherever a biomedical intervention is used to bypass an admirable social practice, then, the improvement's social value (the value of a runner's physical endurance or a mystic's visions) is weakened accordingly. To preserve the value of the social practices considered to be "enhancing," it may be in society's interest to impose a means-based limit on biomedical enhancement efforts.

Interpreting enhancement interventions as those that short-circuit admirable human practices has special utility for policy analysis. To the extent that biomedical shortcuts allow specific accomplishments to be divorced from the admirable practices they were designed to signal, the social value of those accomplishments will be undermined. Not only will the intrinsic value be diminished for everyone that takes the shortcut, but the resulting disparity between the enhanced and unenhanced will call the fairness of the whole game—be it educational, recreational, or professional—into question. If the extrinsic value of being causally responsible for certain accomplishments is high enough (like professional sports salaries), the intrinsic value of the admirable practices that a particular institution was designed to foster

may start to be called into question (Murray). For institutions interested in continuing to foster the social values for which they have traditionally been the guardians, a choice will have to be made. Either they must redesign the game (of education, sports, etc.) to find new ways to evaluate excellence in the admirable practices that are not affected by available enhancements, or they must prohibit the use of the enhancing shortcuts. Which route an institution should take depends on the possibility and practicality of taking either, because ethically they are equivalent.

Unfortunately, some of the social games people can play (and cheat at) do not turn on participants' achievements at all, but on traits over which individuals have little control, such as stature, shape, and skin color. The social games of stigmatization, discrimination, and exclusion use these traits in the same manner that other practices use achievements: as intrinsically valuable keys to extrinsic goods. It is becoming increasingly possible to seek biomedical help in changing these traits in order to short-circuit these games as well. The biomedical interventions involved, such as skin lighteners or stature increasers, are enhancements because they serve to improve the recipient's social standing, but only by perpetuating the social bias that inspired their use. When *enhancement* is understood in this way, it warns of still another set of moral concerns.

What makes the provision of human growth hormone to a short child a morally suspicious enhancement is not the absence of a diagnosable disease or the "species atypical " hormone level that would result—it is the intent to improve the child's social status by changing the child, rather than by changing her social environment, that is questionable (White). Such enhancement interventions are almost always wrongheaded, because the source of the social status they seek to improve is, by definition, the social group and not the individual. Attempting to improve that status in the individual amounts to a moral mistake akin to "blaming the victim": it misattributes causality, is ultimately futile, and can have harmful consequences. This is the interpretation of enhancement that seems to be at work when people argue that to use Ritalin to induce cooperative behavior in the classroom inappropriately "medicalizes" a social problem. In such cases, the critics dispute the assumption that the human need in question is one that is created by, and quenchable through, the human body, asserting instead that both its source and solution really lie in quite a different sphere of human experience.

This interpretation of the enhancement concept is useful to those interested in the ethics of personal improvement because it warns of a number of moral pitfalls beyond the baseline considerations that the enhancement/treatment distinction provides. Attempting to improve social status by changing the individual risks being self-defeating (by inflating expectations), futile (if the individual's comparative gains are neutralized by the enhancement's availability to the whole social group), unfair (if the whole group does not have access to the enhancement), or complicit with unjust social prejudices (by forcing people into a range of variation dictated by biases that favor one group over others). For those faced with decisions about whether to attempt to enhance themselves or their children through gene transfer, this way of understanding enhancement is much more illuminating than attempts to distinquishing it from medical treatment, because it points to the real values at stake. Ideally, gene transfer should not make an existing social problem worse, even if exacerbating injustice would further one's own interests.

On the other hand, protecting these values is difficult in a pluralistic society, because it means developing ways to police individuals' complicity with suspect social norms (Little). Under the historical shadow of state-sponsored eugenics programs, the U.S. government is unlikely to promulgate lists of acceptable and unacceptable enhancements, even if the intent of the lists are to protect the interests of those who are unenhanced.

Policy Implications

Clearly, all of the ways of understanding enhancement as a moral concept reviewed here have limitations. However, all these interpretations do seem to be alive and well and mixed together in the literature on the topic. It is not possible to cleanly assign the different interpretations of enhancement to different spheres of ethical analysis. But there do seem to be some rough correlations that might be made. Thus, the interpretations that contrast enhancement interventions with treatments seem most useful where it is the limits of medicine's expertise that are at issue. Whether medicine's boundary is defined in terms of concepts of disease, or in sociological terms as the scope of medical practice, or in terms of some theory of the human norm, this interpretation at least provides tools to draw that boundary. Moreover, all other considerations being equal, the line that it draws is the boundary of medical obligation, not the boundary of medical tolerance. Using this tool, enhancement interventions such as cosmetic surgery can still be permissable for physicians to perform, but it is also permissable to deny them to patients.

This has important implications for social policymaking about healthcare coverage, to the extent that society relies on medicine's sense of the medically necessary to define the limits of its obligations to underwrite care. Again, all other considerations being equal, this interpretation of the concept suggests that few enhancement interventions should be actively prohibited by society or foregone by individuals, even when they are not underwritten as a part of healthcare, since there is nothing intrinsically wrong with seeking self-improvements beyond good health.

In contrast, the interpretations of enhancement that focus on the misuse of biomedical tools in efforts at self-improvement seem the most relevant to issues of personal, rather than professional, ethics. Concerns about the authenticity of particular accomplishments are moral challenges to the individual, but find little purchase in the professional ethics of biomedicine, with its focus on the physical safety and efficacy of its tools. The primary policy implications of this interpretation are for the social institutions charged with fostering particular admirable practices, for enhancement interventions that offer biomedical shortcuts to achievement force reassessments of the values these institutions stand for, as well as the practices designed to foster them.

Finally, at the other end of the spectrum, enhancement interventions that seem to commit the moral mistake of trying to address social problems through the bodies of the potentially oppressed do seem to mark a stronger set of moral boundaries for all concerned. For biomedicine, this concept marks an epistemic limit beyond which medical approaches to problem solving are not only unnecessary, but conceptually wrong-headed. For individuals, parents, and society, these kinds of enhancement interventions risk either backfiring (by exacerbating the social problems they are intended to address) or being futile (if they merely result in a shift of the normal range for a given social trait).

ERIC T. JUENGST

SEE ALSO: *Aging and the Aged: Anti-Aging Interventions; Genetic Engineering, Human; Human Dignity; Human Nature; Responsibility; Technology; Transhumanism and Posthumanism*

BIBLIOGRAPHY

Anderson, W. French. 1989. "Human Gene Therapy: Why Draw a Line?" *Journal of Medicine and Philosophy* 14: 681–693.

Baird, Patricia. 1994. "Altering Human Genes: Social, Ethical and Legal Implications." *Perspectives in Biology and Medicine* 37: 566–575.

Berger, Edward, and Gert, Bernard. 1991. "Genetic Disorders and the Ethical Status of Germ-Line Gene Therapy." *Journal of Medicine and Philosophy* 16: 667–685.

Clouser, Danner; Culver, Charles; and Gert, Bernard. 1981. "Malady: A New Treatment of Disease." *Hastings Center Report* 11: 29–37.

Daniels, Norman. 1986. *Just Health Care.* Cambridge, Eng.: Cambridge University Press.

Daniels, Norman, 1992. "Growth Hormone Therapy for Short Stature: Can We Support the Treatment/Enhancement Distinction?" *Growth, Genetic and Hormones* 8(Suppl. 1): 46–48.

Davis, Kathy. 1995. *Reshaping the Female Body: The Dilemma of Cosmetic Surgery.* New York: Routledge.

Engelhardt, H. T. 1990. "Human Nature Technologically Revisited." *Social Philosophy and Policy* 8: 180–191.

Gardner, Willam. 1995. "Can Enhancement Be Prohibited?" *Journal of Medicine and Philosophy* 20: 65–84.

Good, Byron. 1994. *Medicine, Rationality, and Experience: An Anthropological Perspective.* New York: Cambridge University Press.

Juengst, Eric. 1997. "Can Enhancement Be Distinguished from Prevention in Genetic Medicine?" *Journal of Medicine and Philosophy* 22: 125–142.

Little, Margaret. 1997. "Suspect Norms of Appearance and the Ethics of Complicity." In *In the Eye of the Beholder: Ethics and Medical Change of Appearance,* ed. I. de Beaufort, M. Hilhorst, and S. Holm. Stockholm: Scandanavian University Press.

Mehlman, Maxwell. 1999. "How Will We Regulate Genetic Enhancement?" *Wake Forest Law Review* 34: 671–617.

Morgan, Katherine. 1991. "Women and the Knife: Cosmetic Surgery and the Colonization of Women's Bodies." *Hypatia* 6: 25–53.

Murray, Thomas. 1983. "Drugs, Sports, and Ethics." In *Feeling Good and Doing Better: Ethics and Nontherapeutic Drug Use,* ed. T. Murray, W. Gaylin, and R. Macklin. Clifton, NJ: Humana Press.

Parens, Eric. 1997. "The Goodness of Fragility: On the Prospect of Genetic Technologies Aimed at the Enhancement of Human Capabilities." *Kennedy Institute of Ethics Journal* 5: 141–153.

Parens, Eric. 1998. *Enhancing Human Traits: Ethical and Social Implications.* Washington, D.C.: Georgetown University Press.

Sabin, J., and Daniels, Norman. 1994. "Determining 'Medical Necessity' in Mental Health Practice." *Hastings Center Report* 24: 5–13.

Silvers, Anita. 1994. "'Defective Agents': Equality, Difference, and the Tyranny of the Normal." *Journal of Social Philosophy* 25: 154–175.

Walters, L., and Palmer, J. 1996. *The Ethics of Human Gene Therapy.* Oxford: Oxford University Press.

White, Gladys. 1993. "Human Growth Hormone: The Dilemma of Expanded Use in Children." *Kennedy Institute of Ethics Journal* 3: 401–409.

Whitehouse, Peter; Juengst, Eric; Murray, Tom; and Mehlman, Maxwell. 1997. "Enhancing Cognition in the Intellectually Intact." *Hastings Center Report* 27(3): 14–22.

ENVIRONMENTAL ETHICS

• • •

I. OVERVIEW

The magnitude and urgency of contemporary environmental problems—collectively known as the environmental crisis—form the mandate for environmental ethics: a reexamination of the human attitudes and values that influence individual behavior and government policy toward nature. The principal approaches to environmental ethics are "anthropocentrism," or the human-centered approach; "biocentrism," or the life-centered approach; and "ecocentrism," or the ecosystem-centered approach. Variously related to these main currents of environmental ethics are "ecofeminism" and "deep ecology." Moral "pluralism" in environmental ethics urges that we endorse all of these approaches and employ any one of them as circumstances necessitate.

Anthropocentrism

An anthropocentric environmental ethic grants moral standing exclusively to human beings and considers nonhuman natural entities and nature as a whole to be only a means for human ends. In one sense, any human outlook is necessarily anthropocentric, since we can apprehend the world only through our own senses and conceptual categories. Accordingly, some advocates of anthropocentric environmental ethics have tried to preempt further debate by arguing that a non-anthropocentric environmental ethic is therefore an oxymoron. But the question at issue is not, "Can we apprehend nature from a nonhuman point of view?" Of course we cannot. The question is, rather, "Should we extend moral consideration to nonhuman natural entities or nature as a whole?" And that question, of course, is entirely open.

In the mainstream of the Western cultural tradition, only human beings have been treated morally. Thus—at least for those working in that tradition—anthropocentrism is the most conservative approach to environmental ethics. Nevertheless, anthropocentric environmental ethicists have had to assume a more reactive than proactive posture and devote considerable effort to defending traditional Western moral philosophy against calls by bolder thinkers to widen the purview of ethics to encompass nonhuman natural entities and nature as a whole.

John Passmore and Kristin Shrader-Frechette were among the first to advocate a strictly anthropocentric approach to environmental ethics. Shrader-Frechette finds it "difficult to think of an action which would do irreparable harm to the environment or ecosystem, but which would not also threaten human well-being" (Shrader-Frechette, p. 17). Since many of the anthropocentric ethics in the Western canon censure behavior that threatens human well-being (utilitarianism, most directly), she argues that there is therefore no need to develop a newfangled non-anthropocentric environmental ethic.

Some of the damage that people have done to the environment certainly does threaten human well-being. Global warming and the depletion of the ozone layer are notorious examples. But it is easy to think of other instances of environmental vandalism that do not materially threaten human well-being. David Ehrenfeld asks us to contemplate the probable demise of the endangered Houston toad, a victim of urban sprawl, that "has no demonstrated or conjectural resource value to man" (p. 650). But, as Ehrenfeld points out, the Houston toad is not unique in this respect. Thousands of other species in harm's way are nondescript "non-resources."

To morally censure the extinction of such species and other kinds of environmental destruction that do not materially threaten human well-being, must we abandon anthropocentrism? Amplifying the work of Mark Sagoff (1988) and Eugene C. Hargrove (1989), Bryan Norton (1987), the leading contemporary apologist for anthropocentric environmental ethics, argues that we should enlarge our conception of human well-being instead. In addition to goods (energy, foods, medicines, raw materials for manufacture) and services (crop pollination, oxygen replenishment, water purification), an undegraded natural environment contributes to human well-being in important psychological, spiritual, and scientific ways. Scenery unmarred by strip mines or clear cuts and undimmed by dirty air is important to human aesthetic satisfaction. Clean air and water, open spaces and green belts, complex and diverse landscapes, national parks and wilderness playgrounds are important human "amenities." Experiencing the solitude of wilderness and the otherness of wild things is an important aspect of human religious experience. Even if no one will be materially worse off after the extinction of "non-resource"

species before science has a chance to discover and study them, important subject matter for pure, disinterested human knowledge will nevertheless have been irredeemably lost. Norton also suggests that contact with and care for the integrity of the natural environment can also be "transformative"; it can make better people of us.

Additionally, Norton argues that we should, as a matter of intergenerational justice, ensure that future human beings will be able to enjoy bountiful natural resources, a whole and functioning ecosystem, the full spectrum of environmental amenities, and the opportunity to partake of the psycho-spiritual experiences afforded by nature and to explore ecology and taxonomy intellectually. If we make our conception of human well-being both wide and long, he thinks that we may ground an adequate and effective environmental ethic without sailing off into the unfamiliar and treacherous waters of non-anthropocentrism.

The principal reason Norton offers for preferring an anthropocentric approach to environmental ethics is pragmatic. Anthropocentrism and non-anthropocentrism, he argues, support the same environmental policies. Norton (1991) calls this practical equivalence of anthropocentrism and non-anthropocentrism the "convergence hypothesis." Why then advocate non-anthropocentrism? Most people, including most environmentalists, he claims, accept the familiar and venerable idea that human beings are ends-in-themselves deserving moral standing. On the other hand, the suggestion that all living beings (and species and ecosystems) ought to be granted a similar status is unfamiliar and controversial. If we rest environmental ethics on as broad and firm a foundation as possible, we can best ensure its rapid implementation. Indeed, Norton suggests that the vigorous philosophical effort to develop non-anthropocentric approaches to environmental ethics has actually done the beleaguered environment a disservice. The environmental movement, as a result, has been divided over purely intellectual issues that have little if any practical import.

Norton's empirical claim that most people and even most environmentalists are anthropocentrists is supported only anecdotally. But opinion polls and the outcome of political contests suggest that most people probably have narrower allegiances—to self-interest, to institutional interests, to class interests, or to national interests—than to present and future collective or general human interests, very broadly construed. On the other hand, a growing minority of environmentalists seem to doubt the philosophical foundations of anthropocentrism. Are human beings really created in the image of God—the idea upon which anthropocentrism in Western religious ethics is founded? Are we uniquely self-conscious, rational, autonomous (some of the foundations of anthropocentrism in Western moral philosophy)? Must every being possess such characteristics to qualify for moral treatment? One may agree with the convergence hypothesis—that practical environmental goals are as well served by anthropocentric as by non-anthropocentric environmental ethics—but disagree that anthropocentrism is philosophically defensible. Hence, the question of the philosophical merits—the truth, as it were, of anthropocentrism—remains open.

Norton's convergence hypothesis, furthermore, overlooks an important difference between the way anthropocentric and non-anthropocentric environmental ethics support the same environmental policies. Suppose, as non-anthropocentrists variously argue, that the environment is "intrinsically" as well as "instrumentally" valuable—that is, that the environment is valuable for its own sake as well as for all the benefits, tangible and intangible, that it provides human beings. Warwick Fox decisively argues that such a supposition would shift the burden of proof from those who would disinterestedly preserve the environment to those who would destroy it for personal gain:

> If the nonhuman world is only considered to be instrumentally valuable then people are permitted to use and otherwise interfere with it for whatever reasons they wish…. If anyone objects to such interference then, within this framework of reference, the onus is clearly on the person who objects to justify why it is *more useful* to humans to leave that aspect of the nonhuman world alone. If, however, the nonhuman world is considered intrinsically valuable then the onus shifts to the person who would want to interfere with it to justify why they should be allowed to do so; anyone who wants to interfere with any entity that is intrinsically valuable is morally obliged to be able to offer *sufficient justification* for their actions. (Fox, 1993, p. 101)

Norton, for example, might object to lumber companies cutting down redwood forests because the remaining redwood forests are of greater benefit to present and future human generations as amenities than as raw material for decks and hot tubs. But to preserve the remaining redwood forests, Norton would have to persuade a court to issue an injunction preventing lumber companies from harvesting redwoods, based on the assertion that the trees, while living, are more useful to human beings as psycho-spiritual and transformative resources than cut down and sawed up as consumptive resources. If, on the other hand, the trees were regarded as being intrinsically valuable, then a lumber company would have to make a case in court that the utility of redwood forests as raw material is so enormous as to justify their destruction. Thus, although Norton may be

correct in claiming that a long and wide anthropocentric environmental ethic supports the same policies as non-anthropocentric environmental ethics—in the case at hand, the policy of preserving redwood forests—he cannot correctly claim that it would do so as forcefully.

Biocentrism

At first, theories of environmental ethics that morally enfranchise both individual living beings and natural wholes, such as species and ecosystems, were called "biocentric." Then, Paul W. Taylor (1986) commandeered the term to characterize his militantly individualistic theory of environmental ethics. Not only in deference to Taylor's influence and authority, but in deference to the literal sense of the term ("life-centered"), "biocentrism" in this discussion refers to theories of environmental ethics that morally enfranchise living beings only. Since species and ecosystems are not, per se, living beings, a biocentric theory would not accord them any moral standing.

Although animal welfare ethics and environmental ethics are by no means the same, biocentrism is launched from a platform provided by animal welfare ethics. Both attempt to extend our basic anthropocentric ethics—which, generally speaking, prohibit harming human "others" or violating their rights—to a more inclusive class of individuals: animal welfare ethics to various kinds of animals, biocentric environmental ethics to all living beings.

Peter Singer and Tom Regan, the principal architects of contemporary animal welfare ethics, exposed anthropocentric ethics to a dilemma. If the criterion for moral standing is pitched high enough to exclude all nonhuman beings, it will also exclude some human beings; but if it is pitched low enough to include all human beings, it will also include a large and diverse group of nonhuman animals.

An anthropocentrist may follow such philosophers as René Descartes and Immanuel Kant and proffer some highly esteemed and peculiarly human capacity—such as the capacity to reason, to speak, or to be a moral agent—as the qualification a being must possess to deserve ethical consideration. However, if practice is to be consistent with theory, anthropocentrism, so justified, should permit people who cannot reason or speak or who are not morally accountable for their behavior—human infants, the severely retarded, and the abjectly senile, for example—to be treated in the same ways that it permits animals to be treated: used as experimental subjects in painful biomedical research, hunted for sport, slaughtered and processed into dog food, and so on. To obviate these repugnant implications, Singer (1975) suggests that we follow Jeremy Bentham, the founder of utilitarian ethics, and settle upon sentience, the capacity to experience pleasure and pain, as a less hypocritical—and arguably a more relevant—qualification for moral consideration. That standard would secure the ethical standing of the so-called marginal cases, since irrational, unintelligent, or irresponsible people are all capable of experiencing pleasure and pain. But it would open membership in the moral community to all other sentient beings as well. If, as Bentham asserted, pleasure is good and pain is evil, and if, as Bentham also asserted, we should try to maximize the one and minimize the other irrespective of who experiences them, then animal pleasure and pain should count equally with human pleasure and pain in all our moral deliberations.

Singer vigorously advocates vegetarianism. Ironically, however, Singer's Benthamic animal welfare ethic is powerless to censure raising animals in comfort and slaughtering them painlessly to satisfy human dietary preferences. Indeed, one might even deduce from Singer's premises that people have a positive moral obligation to eat meat, provided that the animals bred for human consumption experience a greater balance of pleasure over pain during their short lives. For if everyone became a vegetarian, many fewer cows, pigs, chickens, and other domestic animals would be kept and thus many fewer animals would have the opportunity, for a brief time, to pursue happiness.

Recognizing these (and other) inadequacies of Singer's theory in relation to the moral problems of the treatment of animals, Tom Regan (1983) advocates a "rights approach." He argues that some individual animals have "inherent value" because they are, like ourselves, not only sentient but "subjects of a life"—beings that are self-conscious, experience desire and frustration, and that anticipate future states of consciousness—that from their point of view can be better or worse. Inherent value, in turn, may be the grounds for basic moral rights.

Neither Singer's nor Regan's prototype of animal welfare ethics will also serve as environmental ethics. For one thing, neither provides moral standing for plants and all the many animals that may be neither sentient nor, more restrictively still, subjects of a life—let alone for the atmosphere and oceans, species and ecosystems. Moreover, concern for animal welfare, on the one hand, and concern for the larger environment, on the other, often lead to contradictory indications in practice and policy. Examples follow: Advocates of animal liberation and rights frequently oppose the extermination of feral animals competing with native wildlife and degrading plant communities on the public ranges; they characteristically demand an end to hunting and trapping, whether environmentally benign or necessary; and they may prefer to let endangered plant species become extinct, rather than save them by killing sentient or subject-of-a-life animal pests.

On the other hand, animal welfare ethics and environmental ethics lead to convergent indications on other points of practice and policy. Both should resolutely oppose "factory farming": animal welfare ethics because of the enormous amount of animal suffering and killing involved; environmental ethics because of the enormous amount of water used and soil eroded in meat production. Both should staunchly support the preservation of wildlife habitat: animal welfare ethics because nature reserves provide habitat for sentient subjects; environmental ethics because many other forms of life, rare and endangered species, and the health and integrity of ecosystems are accommodated as well.

Despite the differences, animal welfare ethics may be regarded as "on the way to becoming" full-fledged environmental ethics, according to Regan (1983, p. 187). Animal welfare ethicists went the first leg of the philosophical journey by plausibly lowering the qualifying attribute for moral consideration. Albert Schweitzer (1989), Kenneth Goodpaster (1978), Robin Attfield (1983), and Paul Taylor (1986) variously suggest pitching it lower still—from being sentient to being alive.

Schweitzer, writing long before the efflorescence of contemporary animal welfare and environmental ethics literature, appears to ground his "reverence for life" ethic in the voluntarism of Arthur Schopenhauer:

> Just as in my own will-to-live there is a yearning for more life … so the same obtains in all the will-to-live around me, equally whether it can express itself to my comprehension or whether it remains unvoiced.

> Ethics consists in this, that I experience the necessity of practising the same reverence for life toward all will-to-live, as toward my own. (Schweitzer, 1989, pp. 32–33)

Contemporary biocentrism appears to have been inspired by Joel Feinberg's observations about the moral importance of interests and the range of entities to which interests may be attributed. The foundational role of the concept of "conation" (an often unconscious striving, reified by Schopenhauer as the "will-to-live") in Feinberg's characterization of interests unifies contemporary Anglo-American biocentric environmental ethics with Schweitzer's version. According to Feinberg:

> A mere thing, however valuable to others, has no good of its own … [because] mere things have no conative life: no conscious wishes, desires, and hopes; or urges or impulses; or unconscious drives, aims, and goals; or latent tendencies, directions of growth, and natural fulfillments. Interests must be compounded somehow out of conations; hence

mere things have no interests, *A fortiori,* they have no interests to be protected by legal or moral rules. Without interests a creature can have no "good" of its own the achievement of which can be its due. Mere things are not loci of value in their own right, but rather their value consists entirely in their being objects of other beings' interests. (Feinberg, pp. 49–50)

The clear implication of this passage is that the "insuperable line," as Bentham called the boundary separating beings who qualify for moral consideration from those who do not, falls between living beings and nonliving things, not between sentient animals and insentient animals and plants. Why? Because even plants have "unconscious drives, aims, and goals; or latent tendencies, directions of growth, and natural fulfillments." Feinberg, nevertheless, goes on to deny that plants have interests of their own. His reasons for doing so, however, appear to be less clear and decisive than his derivation of interests from conations and his argument that beings who have interests deserve moral consideration.

Kenneth Goodpaster (1978) argues that all living beings, plants as well as animals, have interests. And he argues, appealing to Feinberg as an authority, that beings who have interests deserve "moral considerability"—a term that Goodpaster uses to indicate precisely the ethical status of moral patients (those on the receiving end of an action), as distinct from moral agents (those who commit an act). Goodpaster agrees with Singer that their sentience is a sufficient condition for extending moral considerability to animals, but he disagrees that it is a necessary one, because sentience evolved to serve something more fundamental—life: "Biologically, it appears that sentience is an adaptive characteristic of living organisms that provides them with a better capacity to anticipate, and so avoid, threats to life.... [T]he capacities to suffer and enjoy are ancillary to something more important, rather than tickets to considerability in their own right" (p. 316).

Goodpaster's life-principle ethic is modest. All living beings are morally considerable, but all may not be of equal moral "significance." He leaves open the question of how much weight we should give to a plant's interests when they conflict with a sentient creature's or with our own. Paul Taylor (1986) has struck a much stronger and bolder stance and argued that all living beings are of equal "inherent worth."

Taylor bases a living being's inherent worth on the fact that it has a good of its own, quite independent of our anthropocentric instrumental valuation of it and quite independent of whether the organism is sentient or cares. Light, warmth, water, and rich soil are good for a sprig of poison ivy, though poison ivy may not be good for us. Unlike machines and other purposeful artifacts that we design to serve our own ends, organisms are ends-in-themselves. Most generally, they strive to reach a state of maturity and to reproduce. Therefore, just as we insist that others not interfere with our own striving and thriving, so, Taylor urges, expressly patterning his reasoning on Kant's, we should respect the striving and thriving of all other "teleological centers of life." Kant argued that we should respect, as individuals-in-themselves, all rational, autonomous beings equally. And Taylor argues that we should respect equally all living beings because they too are ends-in-themselves.

Because biocentrism is concerned exclusively with biological individuals, not biological wholes, it is an approach to environmental ethics that seems at once so restrictive that it would be impossible to practice, and an approach that has scant relevance to the set of problems constituting the environmental crisis. How can we do anything at all, if, before we act, we are obliged to consider the interests of each and every living being that we might affect? Why should we feel compelled to do so for the sake of the environment? Environmental concern focuses primarily on the spasm of abrupt massive species extinction and the loss of biodiversity generally, on rapid global warming and the erosion of stratospheric ozone, on soil erosion, water pollution, and the like; not on the welfare of individual grubs, bugs, and shrubs.

Schweitzer and Goodpaster frankly acknowledge the difficulty in practicing biocentrism. Schweitzer writes, "It remains a painful enigma how I am to live by the rule of reverence for life in a world ruled by creative will which is at the same time destructive will" (1989, p. 35). And Goodpaster writes:

> The clearest and most decisive refutation of the principle of respect for life is that one cannot *live* according to it, nor is there any indication in nature that we were intended to. We must eat, experiment to gain knowledge, protect ourselves from predation.... To take seriously the criterion being defended, all these things must be seen as somehow morally wrong. (p. 310)

Both reasonably suggest that we can at least respect the interests of other living beings when they do not conflict with our own. According to Goodpaster, biocentrism is not suicidal. It requires only that we use living beings considerately and sensitively. Schweitzer thinks that biocentrism permits us to injure or destroy other forms of life, but only when doing so is necessary and unavoidable.

Taylor's egalitarianism renders the practicability problem of biocentrism virtually insurmountable (Wenz). Starting with any individual's right to self-defense, he rationalizes our annihilating disease organisms with medicines and goes on from there to defend our killing and eating other living beings to feed ourselves. But the satisfaction of any "nonbasic" human interest, according to Taylor, must be forgone if it violates the basic interests of another teleological center of life. So it would seem that strict adherence to biocentric egalitarianism would require one to live a life of sacrifice that would make a monk's life appear opulent.

Writing before the advent of the environmental crisis, Schweitzer was not intending to address its problems. He seems genuinely concerned, rather, with the welfare of individual living beings. Thus, it would be unfair and anachronistic to criticize his reverence-for-life ethic for being largely irrelevant to the set of problems constituting the environmental crisis. Taylor, on the other hand, represents his biocentric ethic as an environmental ethic. And he is clearly aware that contemporary environmental concerns focus on such things as species loss and ecosystem deterioration. But he remains antagonistic to the holistic environmental ethics crafted in response to such concerns. He prefers to think of the extinction of species and destruction of ecosystems in anthropocentric, rather than in biocentric or ecocentric terms. Goodpaster, on the other hand, invokes "concern felt by most person about 'the environment'" as a reason for trying to extend moral considerability to all living beings (p. 309). He seems, moreover, to be aware that to actually reach the concern felt by most persons about the environment, biocentrism would have to "admit of application to … systems of entities heretofore unimagined as claimants on our moral attention (such as the biosystem itself)" (p. 310). Having once mentioned systems of entities, however, Goodpaster lavishes all his attention on individual living beings and has nothing at all to say about how biocentrism might actually admit of application to species, ecosystems, and the biosphere as a whole.

Biocentrism may be not only irrelevant to actual environmental concerns, it could aggravate them. Biocentrism can lead its proponents to a revulsion toward nature—giving an ironic twist to Taylor's title, *Respect for Nature*—because nature seems as indifferent to the welfare of individual living beings as it is fecund. Schweitzer, for example, comments that

> the great struggle for survival by which nature is maintained is a strange contradiction within itself. Creatures live at the expense of other creatures. Nature permits the most horrible cruelties.… Nature looks beautiful and marvelous when you view it from the outside. But when you read its pages like a book, it is horrible. (1969, p. 120)

Ecocentrism

Though the term "ecocentrism" is a contradiction of the phrase "ecosystem-centered," ecocentrism would provide moral considerability for a spectrum of nonindividual environmental entities, including the biosphere as a totality, species, land, water, and air, as well as ecosystems. The various ecologically informed holistic environmental ethics that may appropriately be called ecocentric are less closely related, theoretically, than either the anthropocentric or biocentric families of environmental ethics.

Lawrence E. Johnson has attempted to generate an environmental ethic that reaches species and ecosystems by a further extension of the biocentric approach. He does this not by making the criterion for moral considerability more inclusive but by attributing interests to species and ecosystems. Extensively developing the line of thought that Feinberg (1974) tentatively and ambiguously initiated, Johnson concludes that we should "give *due* respect to all the interests of all beings that have interests, in proportion to their interests" (p. 118). As this, his summary moral principle, suggests, Johnson follows Goodpaster in allowing that all interests are not equal and thus that all interested beings, though morally considerable, are not of equal moral significance. Johnson, however, provides no principle or method for hierarchically ordering interests and the beings who possess them; nor does he provide an ethical procedure for adjudicating conflicts of interest between people, animals, and plants, and, more difficult still, between all such individuals and environmental wholes.

In arguing that species have interests, Johnson exploits the fact that some biologists and philosophers of biology regard species not as classes of organisms but as spatially and temporally protracted individuals. To plausibly assign them interests, in other words, Johnson assimilates species to individual organisms. During the first quarter of the twentieth century, ecosystems (though then they were not so denominated) were represented in ecology as supraorganisms. Johnson adopts this characterization of ecosystems, as doing so allows him to attribute interests to ecosystems by assimilating them to individual organisms, just as in the case of species. Finally, Johnson points out that James Lovelock (1979) has suggested that the Earth as a whole is an integrated living being (named Gaia); if so, it (she) too may have interests and thus may be morally considerable. Adopting nonstandard, obsolete, or highly controversial scientific models of species, ecosystems, and the biosphere is the price Johnson pays to purchase moral considerability for these natural wholes. His attempt to add an ecocentric dimension to his essentially biocentric approach to environmental ethics is thus seriously compromised.

Holmes Rolston's ecocentric environmental ethic, like Johnson's, is launched from a biocentric platform. Rolston (1988) endorses the central tenet of biocentrism that each living being has a good of its own and that having a good of its own is the ground of a being's intrinsic value. And upon the existence of intrinsic value in nature he founds our duties to the natural world in all its aspects.

Rolston's biocentrism, in sharp contrast to Taylor's, is inegalitarian. Rolston finds more intrinsic value in beings that sense their own good, that feel hurt when harmed, than in those that lack consciousness. And Rolston finds the most intrinsic value of all in normal adult human beings because we are rational and fully self-conscious as well as conative and sentient.

Rolston avoids the scientifically suspect route that Johnson takes to enfranchise ethically such environmental wholes as species and ecosystems. Rolston argues instead that since the most basic telos of a teleological center of life is to be "good of its kind" and to reproduce its species, then its kind or species is its primary good. Species per se do not have a good of their own, but as the most basic good of beings that do have a good of their own, they too can be said to possess intrinsic value. The myriad natural kinds or species, however, evolved not in isolation but in a complex matrix of relationships—that is, in ecosystems. Thus, though not themselves teleological centers of life, either, some intrinsic value rubs off on ecosystems in Rolston's theory of environmental ethics. Rolston coins a special term, "systemic value," to characterize the value of ecosystems.

Systemic value does not seem to be entirely parallel, logically or conceptually speaking, to intrinsic value in Rolston's theory of environmental ethics. Rather, it seems that a necessary condition for the existence of the things that he believes do have intrinsic value—beings with a good of their own and the goods (their kinds or species) that such beings strive to actualize and perpetuate—is the existence of their natural contexts or matrices. Like the moon that shines by a borrowed light, systemic value seems to be a kind of reflected intrinsic value. Rolston finds a similar sort of derivative intrinsic value, "projective value," in elemental and organic evolutionary processes going all the way back to the Big Bang, since such processes eventually produced (or "projected") living beings with goods of their own.

Rolston's theory of environmental ethics hierarchically orders intrinsically valuable individuals in a familiar and conventional way. Human beings are at the pinnacle of the value hierarchy, followed by the higher animals, and so on, pretty much as in the Great Chain of Being envisioned by many Western philosophers of yore. Rolston is prepared to invoke his hierarchical arrangement of intrinsically valuable kinds of beings to resolve biocentric moral conundrums. For example, he expressly argues that it is morally permissible for people to kill and eat animals and for animals to kill and eat plants. Though such a hierarchical ordering of intrinsically

valuable beings jibes with tradition and uncultivated common sense, it may not always jibe with, and hence may not adequately justify, our considered environmental priorities. Most environmentalists, faced with the hard choice of saving a sensitive, subjective dog or an unconscious, merely conative thousand-year-old redwood tree, would probably opt for the tree—and not only because redwoods are becoming rare. Pressed for good reasons for making this choice, Rolston might answer that an environmentally ethical agent is perfectly free, in reaching a decision to give priority to the redwood over the dog, to add to their intrinsic value the way standing redwoods are valued anthropocentrically and the way they serve the systemic value of ecosystems. The ethical agent can legitimately add the redwood's economic value to its systematic value, intrinsic value, aesthetic value, or religious value. How the intrinsic value of species and the systemic value of ecosystems fits into Rolston's value hierarchy is not entirely clear. Is a plant species more or less intrinsically valuable than a specimen of *Homo sapiens*, or than a specimen of *Ovis aries* (domestic sheep)?

According to Regan (1981) the very possibility of an environmental ethic turns on constructing a plausible theory of intrinsic (or "inherent") value in nature. He argues that anthropocentric environmental ethics are "management ethics," ethics for the "use" of the environment, not environmental ethics proper. Regan sets clear and stringent conditions for such value: first, it must be strictly objective, independent of any valuing consciousness; second, it must attend some property or set of properties that natural entities possess; and third, it must be normative, it must command ethical respect or moral considerability.

Rolston's basing a being's intrinsic value on its having a good of its own seems to meet the first two of these conditions, but possibly not the third. Before consciousness evolved, living beings had goods of their own; they could be harmed if not hurt; they had interests, whether they cared or not. The move, however, from the hardly disputable fact that living beings objectively possess goods of their own to the assertion that they have objective intrinsic value may turn on an ambiguity in the meaning of "good."

The word "good" has a teleological as well as a normative sense. All living beings have goods of their own in the teleological sense. They have, in other words, ends that were not imposed upon them—as the goods or ends of machines and other artifacts are—by beings other than themselves. But it is still possible to ask if such teleological goods generate normative goods. At this point in the argument, the smallpox and AIDS viruses are usually invoked as examples of organisms that have goods of their own in the teleological sense of the term, but organisms that one would be loath to say are good in the normative sense of the term.

However this particular conceptual issue may be resolved, another, moral general one casts a very large and dark shadow on Rolston's claim of finding objective intrinsic value in nature. While Rolston is very careful not to buck prevailing scientific opinion on the sort of reality possessed by species, ecosystems, and evolutionary processes, his argument that intrinsic value exists objectively in nature does buck more general assumption of modern science. From the modern scientific point of view, nature is value-free. Goodness and badness, like beauty and ugliness, are in the eye of the beholder. According to this entrenched dogma of modern science, there can be no valuees without valuers. Nothing under the sun—no rational self-conscious person, no sentient animal, no vegetable, no mineral—has value of any kind, either as a means or an end, unless it is valued by some valuing subject.

The crisp objective/subjective distinction in modern science, however, has been undermined by the Heisenberg Uncertainty Principle in quantum physics, as the observation of subatomic entities unavoidably affects their state of being. Therefore, the modern scientific worldview has become problematic. Seizing upon this circumstance, J. Baird Callicott (1989), among others, has broached a value theory for environmental ethics that is neither subjective nor objective. Just as experimental physicists actualize the potential of an electron to be at a particular place by observing it, so, Callicott suggests, the potential value of an entity, both instrumental and intrinsic, is actualized by a valuer appreciating it.

Although it may eventually give way to a postmodern scientific worldview, the modern scientific worldview continues to reign supreme. The "land ethic" sketched by Aldo Leopold (1949) has been the moral inspiration of the non-anthropocentric wing of the contemporary popular environmental movement, in part because Leopold respects the subjectivity of value required by the modern scientific world view without at the same time reducing nature to natural resources.

Callicott (1987) claims that Leopold's ecocentric environmental ethic may be traced to the eighteenth-century moral philosophy of David Hume and Adam Smith, who think that feelings lie at the foundations of value judgments. While feelings fall on the subjective side of the great subject/object divide, Hume and Smith also point out that our feelings may be altruistic or other-oriented as well as selfish. Hence we may value others for their own sakes, as ends-in-themselves. Further, Hume and Smith note that in addition to sympathy for others, respectively, we also experience a "public affection" and, accordingly, value the "interests of society even on their own account."

In *The Descent of Man,* Charles Darwin (1874) adopted the moral psychology of Hume and Smith and argued that the "moral sentiments" evolved among human beings in conjunction with the evolution of society, growing in compass and refinement along with the growth and refinement of human communities. He also developed the incipient holism of Hume and Smith, flatly stating that primeval ethical affections centered on the tribe not its individual members.

Leopold, building directly on Darwin's theory of the origin and evolution of ethics, points out that ecology represents human beings to be members not only of multiple human communities but also of the "biotic community." Hence, "the land ethic simply enlarges the boundaries of the community to include soils, waters, plants, and animals, or collectively: the land.... It implies respect for ... fellow members and also respect for the community as such" (Leopold, p. 204).

Animal welfare ethicists and biocentrists claim that Leopold's ecocentrism is tantamount to "environmental fascism." Leopold wrote—and his exponents affirm—that "a thing is right when it tends to preserve the integrity, stability, and beauty of the biotic community [and] wrong when it tends otherwise" (pp. 224–225). If this is true, then not only would it be right deliberately to kill deer and burn bushes for the good of the biotic community, it would also be right to undertake draconian measures to reduce human overpopulation—the underlying cause, according to conventional environmental wisdom, of all environmental ills.

Providing for the possibility of moral consideration of wholes, however, does not necessarily disenfranchise individuals. The land ethic is holistic as well as (not instead of) individualistic, although in the case of the biotic community and its nonhuman members holistic concerns may eclipse individualistic ones. Nor does the land ethic replace or cancel previous socially generated human-oriented duties—to family and family members, to neighbors and neighborhood, to all human beings and humanity. Human social evolution consists of a series of additions rather than replacements. The moral sphere, growing in circumference with each stage of social development, does not expand like a balloon—leaving no trace of its previous boundaries. It adds, rather, new rings, new "accretions," as Leopold called each emergent social-ethical community. The discovery of the biotic community simply adds several new outer orbits of membership and attendant obligation. Our more intimate social bonds and their attendant obligations remain intact. Thus we may weigh and balance our more recently discovered duties to the biotic community and its members with our more venerable and insistent social obligations in ways that are entirely familiar, reasonable, and humane.

Ecofeminism

The term "ecofeminism" is a contraction of the phrase "ecological feminism," which may be understood as an analysis of environmental issues and concerns from a feminist point of view and, vice versa, as an enrichment and complication of feminism with insights drawn from ecology. Ecofeminism is both an approach to environmental ethics and an alternative feminism.

An axiom of ecofeminism is that, both historically and globally, men have dominated women and "man" has dominated nature. Further, many male-centered, culture-defining texts, such as the epics of Homer and Hesiod, the works of the ancient philosophers, and so forth, have associated women with nature and personified the Earth and nature generally as female (Griffin). The domination of women and nature appears to stem from a single source: patriarchy (literally, father-rule). Criticize and overcome patriarchy, the principal ideological force responsible for the domination of women, and one will at the same time have criticized and overcome the principal ideological force responsible for the degradation and destruction of nature. According to Marti Kheel, "for deep ecologists, it is the anthropocentric worldview that is foremost to blame.... Ecofeminists, on the other hand, argue that it is the androcentric worldview that deserves the primary blame" for the environmental crisis (p. 129).

Some environmentalists suspect such an analysis to be a thinly disguised ploy to divert the energies of the environmental movement into the feminist movement. Deep ecologist Warwick Fox (1989), for example, argues that a feminist environmental ethic focused on abolishing patriarchy is too self-serving, simplistic, and facile to be taken seriously as a panacea for environmental ills. Other movements, he points out, can make, and have made, the same implausible claim: If we only abolish the ideology of racism, capitalism, imperialism, and so on, then we will usher in the millennium and all will be right with the world, natural as well as social.

Karen J. Warren (1990) does not follow Kheel and blame the domination and subordination of nature by "man" on the domination and subordination of women by men. Rather, she argues, both forms of "oppression" are "twin" expressions of hierarchically ordered "value dualisms" reinforced with a "logic of domination." Critiques of anthropocentrism and androcentrism are mutually illuminating and complementary. A person opposed to the one ought to be opposed to the other—because subordination, domination, and oppression are wrong, whether of women by men or of nature by "man." Environmentalists should also be feminists and feminists, environmentalists. Ecofeminism is the union of the two.

An ecofeminist approach seeks to correct an alleged "male bias" in environmental ethical theory—a selection of concepts and methodology that ignores, discounts, or denigrates women's issues, concerns, and experience. Alison M. Jagger has suggested that modern Western ethics, "Enlightenment moral theory," is thoroughly male-biased since it portrays moral agents as being "disembodied, asocial, autonomous, unified, rational, and essentially similar to all other" agents (p. 367). In short, it abstracts, generalizes, universalizes. Intimately associated with this "Cartesian" moral psychology are such commonplaces of modern Western ethics as universal application of abstract principles and rules, impartiality, objectivity, rights, and the victory of synoptic and dispassionate reason over myopic and prejudicial feelings. Warren argues, accordingly, that "ecofeminism … involves a shift *from* a conception of ethics as primarily a matter of rights, rules, or principles predetermined and applied in specific cases to entities viewed as competitors in the contest of moral standing, *to* a conception of ethics as growing out of … defining relationships … and community" (pp. 141–142). She notes further that "ecofeminism makes a central place for [the more feminine, less male] values of care, friendship, trust, and appropriate reciprocity—values that presuppose that our relationships to others are central to our understanding of who we are" (p. 143).

It is surprising that ecofeminists have not warmly endorsed the Aldo Leopold land ethic, which grounds morality in such sentiments as love, sympathy, and fellow-feeling. The *locus classicus* for an environmental ethic growing out of "defining relationships" and "community" is found in Leopold's *A Sand County Almanac* (1949). Marti Kheel, however, castigates Leopold's land ethic, arguing that it epitomizes male bias. Leopold endorses hunting, historically a predominantly male activity, as a means not only of ecological management but also of experiencing our defining relationships with nature and cultivating a "love and respect" for "things natural, wild, and free."

Deep Ecology

Just as there are Democrats (with a capital "D," members of one of the two major political parties in the United States) and democrats (with a lower-case "d," persons, irrespective of party affiliation, who agree with Winston Churchill that democracy is the worst form of government except for all the others), so there are Deep Ecologists (with a capital "D" and "E") and deep ecologists (with a lower-case "d" and "e"). The latter, such as Aldo Leopold, think that ecology has profound philosophical implications that it transforms our understanding of the world in which we live and what it means to be a human being. Deep Ecologists, on the other hand, endorse the eight-point "platform" of Deep Ecology that Arne Naess co-authored with George Sessions (Devall and Sessions). Moreover, they downplay the importance of environmental *ethics*, and advocate "Self-[with a capital 'S'] realization," instead. In short, deep ecology is a philosophical orientation; Deep Ecology is an ideology.

Ethics per se, Deep Ecologists allege, assumes "social atomism," a conception of each individual self as externally related to all other selves and to unselfconscious nature (Fox, 1990). Therefore, Deep Ecologists suppose that an ethical act on the part of an atomic moral agent involves grudgingly considering the interests of other morally considerable beings equally and impartially with his or her own. But for people actually and consistently to behave ethically—as thus characterized—is as rare as it is noble. Therefore, even if environmental ethics could be broadly infused, environmental destruction and degradation would be little abated.

However, the metaphysical implications of ecology undermine the social atomism upon which ethics is supposedly premised. We human beings are internally, not externally, related to one another and to non-human natural entities and nature as a whole. "Others" cannot be cleanly and neatly distinguished from ourselves. Our relationships, natural as well as social, with "them" are mutually defining. We are embedded in communities, biotic as well as human. If we could only realize that the environing world is ultimately indistinguishable from ourselves, then we could enlist the powerful and reliable motive of self-interest in the effort to reverse environmental degradation and destruction (Naess).

The process of Deep Ecological Self-realization is experiential as well as intellectual. Through practice as well as study, we should cultivate a palpable sense of identification with the world. Nature-protecting behavior will flow from experiential identification with nature. Warwick Fox (1990) has suggested that Deep Ecology should actually be renamed "transpersonal ecology," since, as in transpersonal psychology, the goal of Self-(with a capital "S") realization involves self-(with a lower-case "s") transcendence.

Deep Ecology's suspicions about the efficacy of environmental ethics seems to be based upon a narrow characterization of ethics that excludes sentiment-based communitarian ethics like the Leopold land ethic and its ecofeminist correspondents. Ecofeminists have also sharply criticized Deep Ecology because it seems to "totalize" and "colonize" the "other" (Cheney; Plumwood). With the important exception of Naess, Deep Ecologists either explicitly or implicitly claim that the integrated, systemic ecological world view is true and regard other ways of constructing nature and the relationship of people to nature to be false. A

cornerstone of feminism is openness to the experience of women, experience that is quite varied. The experience of all or even of most women may not jibe well with Deep Ecological Self-realization. Hence the Deep Ecologists' often doctrinaire assertions about how the world is really and truly organized and how we *ought* to experience it are anathema to most ecofeminists.

Pluralism

The term "pluralism" in ethics characterizes two things equally well.

What we might call "social pluralism" is the view that diverse and often mutually inconsistent ethical outlooks should be respected and that there may not be any single moral principle or set of principles, however basic, that all moral agents must acknowledge. Human rights, for example, may be widely acknowledged in the West, but not in other parts of the world; hence, from a social pluralist's point of view, for Western governments to try to impose standards of human rights upon non-Western societies is inappropriate.

Personal pluralism, on the other hand, is the view that a single moral agent may endorse a variety of different moral principles, some of which may be mutually inconsistent, and employ one or another in different morally charged situations. For example, in resolving ethical questions about diet, a personal pluralist might apply Singer's principle that one should not cause sentient beings unnecessary suffering and therefore decide not to eat factory-farmed meat. In resolving ethical questions about abortion, he or she might apply Schweitzer's reverence-for-life principle and vote for an anti-abortion candidate for public office. And, in resolving ethical questions about species conservation, the same person might embrace Leopold's principle that one should preserve the integrity, stability, and beauty of the biotic community and help save an endemic plant species by shooting the feral goats or pigs threatening it.

Social pluralism appears attractive because it seems to imply inclusiveness and tolerance. In extremis, however, social pluralism is vulnerable to the same sort of criticism that ethical relativism, in extremis, has attracted. A social pluralist recognizes no universal ethical values or principles, he or she has no means of ethically challenging any one else's sincerely held moral beliefs. Further, if there are no universal ethical values or principles upon which to base agreement, then radical and intractable differences of moral outlook are irreconcilable. How then can they be resolved except by coercion?

Personal pluralism arose in environmental ethics because finding a single moral principle that could guide our actions in respect to other people, animals, plants, species, ecosystems, the atmosphere, the oceans, and the biosphere proved difficult (Stone). Moreover, our inherently rich and complicated moral lives may be distorted if reduced to a single master principle of action and we are frequently misled if we try rigorously to follow one (Brennan). According to Mary Midgley (1992), we may read the history of Western ethical theory, from Plato and Aristotle to Singer and Leopold, not as a series of formulations of and justifications for competing master principles of action, but as a series of illuminating insights into human ethical experience that can deepen our moral reflection and help us to make wise practical choices.

Proponents and critics alike of personal pluralism have noted some obvious problems. An agent who has a variety of principles and their theoretical justifications at the ready, with no faithful commitment to any of them required, may be tempted to choose the most convenient or self-serving. But all ethics, whether pluralistic or unitary, assume good will on the part of moral agents. A more difficult problem is how to select which principle to apply when more than one is relevant at some moment of decision, and when those that are relevant indicate different and incompatible courses of action. But to demand an algorithmic solution to this problem is to beg the question against personal pluralism.

Moral principles, however, do not exist in an intellectual vacuum (Callicott, 1990). They are often derived from and are always associated with a complex of supporting ideas—usually an ethical theory, which is in turn supported by a moral philosophy. In choosing to act upon a moral principle, a personal moral pluralist thus also endorses—whether consciously or not—the ethical theory and ultimately the moral philosophy supporting it. But the ethical theories and moral philosophies supporting such popular principles as the Christian golden rule, the Aristotelian golden mean, the Kantian categorical imperative, the utilitarian greatest-happiness principle, and so on, offer radically different visions of nature and human nature. Are we morally autonomous rational ends-in-ourselves for whom nature exists only as means, as Kant argues; or are we vessels of pleasure and pain, equal in this morally relevant respect to all other sentient animals, as Singer holds? How can we be both at once?

Communitarianism

A communitarian moral philosophy might provide a coherent sense of self and world without compromising the richness and complexity of our moral lives or attempting to derive all ethical actions from a single principle. Suppose that ethics, as Darwin argued, is correlative to society; that at this stage of human social evolution, we are simultaneously members of many communities or societies, including families, neighborhoods, towns or cities, nation-states, the global human community, the mixed human-domestic animal community, and the biotic community; and that a spectrum of different and not always compatible duties and obligations grow out of our various social relationships—for example, to provide our children with affection, to watch our neighbors' houses when they are away on vacation, to donate old clothes to the Salvation Army, to pay our taxes, to relieve world hunger, to boycott factory-farmed meat, and to help preserve biodiversity.

Right and wrong behavior in respect to family and family members, humanity and human beings, the biotic community and wild animals and plants, grows out of the very different kinds of communal relationships that we bear in these very different cases. Hence what is right in the context of one kind of community (feeding domestic animals, who are members of the "mixed community," for example) may be wrong in another (feeding wild animals, who are members of the biotic community). A multiplicity of community-generated principles guides our actions, but this multiplicity is united and coordinated by a single general understanding of how our various duties arise and to whom they apply. A coherent moral outlook like this certainly does not automatically determine the best course of action when one's multiple duties conflict. But one can at least hope rationally to decide, in circumstances of hard choice, which of several relevant but conflicting duties is the most pressing because they can all be expressed in comparable and commensurable terms.

J. BAIRD CALLICOTT (1995)
BIBLIOGRAPHY REVISED

SEE ALSO: *Animal Welfare and Rights; Environmental Health; Environmental Policy and Law; Population Ethics;* and other *Environmental Ethics* subentries

BIBLIOGRAPHY

Attfield, Robin. 1983. *The Ethics of Environmental Concern.* New York: Columbia University Press.

Benson, John. 2001. *Environmental Ethics: An Introduction With Readings.* London: Routledge.

Brennan, Andrew. 1992. "Moral Pluralism and the Environment." *Environmental Values* 1(1): 15–33.

Callicott, J. Baird. 1987. *Companion to A Sand County Almanac: Interpretive and Critical Essays.* Madison: University of Wisconsin Press.

Callicott, J. Baird. 1989. *In Defense of the Land Ethic: Essays in Environmental Philosophy.* Albany: State University of New York Press.

Callicott, J. Baird. 1990. "The Case Against Moral Pluralism." *Environmental Ethics* 12(2): 99–124.

Callicott, J. Baird, and Hayden, Tom. 1997. *Earth's Insights: A Survey of Ecological Ethics from Mediterranean Basin to the Australian Outback,* reprint edition. Berkeley: University of California Press.

Callicott, J. Baird, and Nelson, Michael P., eds. 1998. *The Great New Wilderness Debate.* Atlanta: University of Georgia Press.

Carrick, Paul. 1999. "Environmental Ethics and Medical Ethics: Some for End-of-life Care, Part I." *Cambridge Quarterly of Healthcare Ethics* 8(1): 107–17

Carrick, Paul. 1999. "Environmental Ethics and Medical Ethics: Some for End-of-life Care, Part II." *Cambridge Quarterly of Healthcare Ethics* 8(2): 250–256.

Cheney, Jim. 1987. "Eco-Feminism and Deep Ecology." *Environmental Ethics* 9(2): 115–145.

Darwin, Charles. 1874. *The Descent of Man and Selection in Relation to Sex.* London: John Murray.

Desjardins, Joseph. 1998. *Environmental Ethics: Concepts, Policy, and Theory.* New York: WCB/McGraw-Hill.

Devall, Bill, and Sessions, George. 1985. *Deep Ecology: Living as if Nature Mattered.* Salt Lake City, Utah: G. M. Smith.

Ehrenfeld, David W. 1976. "The Conservation of Non-Resources." *American Scientist* 64(6): 648–656.

Feinberg, Joel. 1974. "The Rights of Animals and Unborn Generations." In *Philosophy and Environmental Crisis,* pp. 43–68, ed. William T. Blackstone. Athens: University of Georgia Press.

Fox, Michael W., and Rollin, Bernard E. 2001. *Bringing Life to Ethics: Global Bioethics for a Humane Society.* Albany: State University of New York Press.

Fox, Warwick. 1989. "The Deep Ecology-Ecofeminism Debate and Its Parallels." *Environmental Ethics* 11(1): 5–25.

Fox, Warwick. 1990. *Toward a Transpersonal Ecology: Developing New Foundations for Environmentalism.* Boston: Shambala.

Fox, Warwick. 1993. "What Does the Recognition of Intrinsic Value Entail." *Trumpeter* 10(3): 101.

Goodpaster, Kenneth E. 1978. "On Being Morally Considerable." *Journal of Philosophy* 75: 308–325.

Griffin, Susan. 1978. *Woman and Nature: The Roaring Inside Her.* New York: Harper & Row.

Hargrove, Eugene C. 1989. *Foundations of Environmental Ethics.* Englewood Cliffs, NJ: Prentice Hall.

Jaggar, Alison M. 1992. "Feminist Ethics." In *Encyclopedia of Ethics,* pp. 361–370, ed. Lawrence C. Becker and Charlotte B. Becker. New York: Garland Publishing.

Johnson, Lawrence E. 1991. *A Morally Deep World: An Essay on Moral Significance and Environmental Ethics.* Cambridge, Eng.: Cambridge University Press.

Kheel, Marti. 1990. "Ecofeminism and Deep Ecology: Reflections on Identity and Difference." In *Reweaving the World: The Emergence of Ecofeminism,* pp. 128–137, ed. Irene Diamond and Gloria Feman Orenstein. San Francisco: Sierra Club Books.

Light, Andrew, and Rolston, Holmes III., eds. 2003. *Environmental Ethics: An Anthology.* Oxford: Blackwell Publishers Ltd.

Leopold, Aldo. 1949. *A Sand County Almanac and Sketches Here and There.* New York: Oxford University Press.

Lovelock, James. 1979. Gaia: *A New Look at Life on Earth.* Oxford: Oxford University Press.

Midgley, Mary. 1992. "Beasts Versus the Biosphere." *Environmental Values* 1(2): 113–121.

Naess, Arne. 1989. *Ecology, Community and Lifestyle: Outline of an Ecosophy,* tr. David Rothenberg. Cambridge, Eng.: Cambridge University Press.

Norton, Bryan G. 1987. *Why Preserve Natural Variety?* Princeton, NJ: Princeton University Press.

Norton, Bryan G. 1991. *Toward Unity Among Environmentalists.* New York: Oxford University Press.

Passmore, John. 1974. *Man's Responsibility for Nature: Ecological Problems and Western Traditions.* New York: Charles Scribner's Sons.

Plumwood, Val. 1993. *Feminism and the Mastery of Nature.* London: Routledge.

Potter, Van Rensselaer. 1971. *Bioethics: Bridge to the Future,* ed. Carl P. Swanson. Prentice-Hall Biological Science Series. Englewood Cliffs, NJ: Prentice-Hall.

Regan, Tom. 1981. "The Nature and Possibility of an Environmental Ethic." *Environmental Ethics* 3(1): 19–34.

Regan, Tom. 1983. *The Case for Animal Rights.* Berkeley: University of California Press.

Rolston, Holmes, III. 1988. *Environmental Ethics: Duties to and Values in the Natural World.* Philadelphia: Temple University Press.

Sagoff, Mark. 1988. *The Economy of the Earth: Philosophy, Law, and the Environment.* Cambridge, Eng.: Cambridge University Press.

Schmidtz, David, and Willott, Elizabeth, eds. 2001. *Environmental Ethics: What Really Matters, What Really Works.* New York: Oxford University Press.

Schweitzer, Albert. 1969 (1966). *Reverence for Life,* tr. Reginald H. Fuller. New York: Harper & Row.

Schweitzer, Albert. 1989. "The Ethic of Reverence for Life," tr. John Naish. In *Animal Rights and Human Obligations,* 2nd edition, pp. 32–37, ed. Tom Regan and Peter Singer. Englewood Cliffs, NJ: Prentice Hall.

Shrader-Frechette, Kristen S. 1981. *Environmental Ethics.* Pacific Grove, CA: Boxwood Press.

Shrader-Frechette, Kristin. 1995. "Practical Ecology and Foundations for Environmental Ethics." *Journal of Philosophy* 92(12): 621–635.

Singer, Peter. 1975. *Animal Liberation: A New Ethics for Our Treatment of Animals.* New York: New York Review.

Stone, Christopher D. 1987. *Earth and Other Ethics: The Case for Moral Pluralism.* New York: Harper & Row.

Taylor, Paul W. 1986. *Respect for Nature: A Theory of Environmental Ethics.* Princeton, NJ: Princeton University Press.

Varner, Gary E. 2002. *In Nature's Interests?: Interests, Animal Rights, and Environmental Ethics (Environmental Ethics and Science Policy Series).* New York: Oxford University Press.

Warren, Karen J. 1990. "The Power and Promise of Ecofeminism." *Environmental Ethics* 12(2): 125–146.

Wenz, Peter S. 1988. *Environmental Justice.* Albany: State University of New York Press.

Zimmerman, Michael; Callicott, J. Baird; Sessions, George; Warren, Karen J. and Clark, John., eds. 2000. *Environmental Philosophy: From Animal Rights to Radical Ecology,* 3rd edition. Englewood Cliffs, NJ: Prentice-Hall.

II. DEEP ECOLOGY

Deep ecology is a comprehensive worldview of humans in harmony with nature, an "ecosophy" ("ecowisdom") that responds to ecological crisis. It is also a movement to translate this worldview into radical societal reform. Supporters of the deep ecology movement contrast their position with "shallow" reform movements, holding that every living being has intrinsic or inherent value that gives it the right to flourish, independent of its usefulness for humans. All life is interrelated, and living things, humans included, depend on the support of others. For supporters of deep ecology, who tend to oppose the degradation of nature except to satisfy vital needs, the long-range integrity and health of the ecosystems of Earth are of fundamental ethical importance.

The ecological crisis has deep roots in misguided, anthropocentric attitudes about the dominion of humans on Earth. These exploitative, consumptive attitudes, according to the position of deep ecology, cannot be overcome without significant social changes, including changes in the lifestyles of those who live in the rich countries. Such changes can emerge only from a philosophical or religious basis that nurtures a sense of personal responsibility, not simply to persons living now but also to future human generations as well as fauna and flora. The current human population is already too large in many countries; further human population increases will lower the quality of life for both humans and nonhuman forms of life. A smaller human population is desirable and can be achieved by reduced birthrates over several centuries.

The position of the deep ecology movement can be illuminated by contrasting it with the position of so-called shallow ecology. The shallow position considers it unnecessary or even counterproductive to take up philosophical or religious questions to solve the ecological crisis. Its supporters argue that reforms of existing practices are needed, but reforms of basic principles are unnecessary. Those who advocate the shallow position do not find intrinsic value in nonhuman life forms, nor do they find the consumptive economic system problematic. Humans ought to exploit nature, though prudently. High standards of living are not objectionable, and can be raised even further by concentrating on investment in science and technology. Attempts should be made to bring less-developed nations up to this standard.

The deep ecology movement's historic forebears include Henry David Thoreau and John Muir. Aldo Leopold and Rachel Carson, also of the United States, are more recent pivotal figures. In 1962 Carson's book *Silent Spring* set off an ecological alarm. Starting with practical issues related to pesticides, Carson probed the philosophical assumptions underlying this attack on pests that stood in the way of human progress. In Europe such ecological concerns joined with the peace and social justice movements to create the first wave of the "green movement." Australians also became involved. In eastern Europe, ecologists were judged hostile to state-sponsored industrial development, and were banned. In the Third World, long-term ecological sustainability often had to take second place to short-term economic survival.

The deep ecology movement argues for ecological sustainability, human development that conserves the richness and diversity of life forms on Earth. This position, often said to be biocentric (centered on life) rather than anthropocentric (centered on human life only), includes what Leopold called "the land": the whole community of life on the landscape—rivers, mountains, canyons, forests, grasslands, and estuaries. Reforestation, for example, does not mean large tree plantations, producing timber and fiber for humans. Such plantations, which lack the biodiversity, complexity, health, and integrity of spontaneous natural ecosystems, are not genuine biological communities.

Those who advocate deep ecology and the more shallow reformers must learn to cooperate. Some strengths of each approach can be combined; some weakness of each, offset. The former sometimes become lost in utopian visions of a "green world"; the latter may be too absorbed in ad hoc, short-range solutions. The former can press for, and practice, more modest standards of living and support higher prices for nonvital products. Those who are less "deep" can be more pragmatic, willing to respond to what is currently politically realizable reform. Through such cooperation the supporters of both movements may help avoid crises likely to occur if ecologically responsible policies are forced too soon and too fast on populations that are not prepared for them. The deep premises of argumentation add to the utilitarian arguments, which are shallow in relation to philosophical and religious premises, needing more depth of analysis of the problem.

The discussions surrounding deep ecology have implications for the medical area of bioethics as well. "Rich life, simple means," an aphorism of the deep ecology movement, suggests for medical bioethics a strengthening of preventive medicine and a reduced reliance on technically advanced treatments, especially if they require large investments of resources and energy. Medical bioethics can learn from ecological bioethics the need for a moral vision that can reorder its priorities.

ARNE NAESS (1995)

SEE ALSO: *Animal Welfare and Rights; Endangered Species and Biodiversity; Future Generations, Obligations to; Jainism, Bioethics in; Native American Religion, Bioethics in; Population Ethics; Population Policies; Value and Valuation; Xenotransplantation* and other *Environmental Ethics* subentries

BIBLIOGRAPHY

Devall, Bill, and Sessions, George. 1985. *Deep Ecology.* Salt Lake City: Gibbs M. Smith.

Fox, Warwick. 1990. *Towards a Transpersonal Ecology: Developing New Foundations.* Boston: Shambhala.

Leopold, Aldo. 1949. *A Sand County Almanac: And Sketches Here and There.* New York: Oxford University Press.

Naess, Arne. 1989. *Ecology, Community and Lifestyle,* tr. and rev. David Rothenberg. Cambridge, Eng.: Cambridge University Press.

Pepper, David. 1984. *The Roots of Modern Environmentalism.* London: Croom Helm.

Snyder, Gary. 1974. *Turtle Island.* New York: New Directions.

The Trumpeter: Canadian Journal of Ecosophy. Victoria, B.C.: Author.

III. LAND ETHICS

After graduating from the Yale Forest School, Aldo Leopold (1887–1948) joined the U.S. Forest Service in 1909 and served for fifteen years. He resigned to pursue his interest in wildlife ecology and management; in 1933 he was named Professor of Game Management and inaugurated a doctoral program in the subject at the University of Wisconsin. Over the course of his multifaceted career, Leopold came to believe that human harmony with nature could be achieved

only if, in addition to governmental management and regulation, private citizens (and property owners in particular) acquired a "land ethic." Such an ethic would make ecosystems and their parts direct beneficiaries of human morality: "A land ethic changes the role of Homo sapiens from conqueror of the land community to plain member and citizen of it. It implies respect for his fellow-members, and also respect for the community as such" (Leopold, 1949, p. 204).

Leopold is routinely called a modern American "prophet." *A Sand County Almanac,* his slender book of literary and philosophical essays, has become the "bible" of the contemporary environmental movement in the United States. And his land ethic is the environmental ethic of choice among most American environmentalists and conservationists, both amateur and professional. It rests upon secular scientific, not sectarian or supernatural religious, foundations. It is less rigidly doctrinaire than deep ecology's eight-point ethical "platform." Unlike ecofeminism, it focuses directly on the human-nature relationship, unrefracted by the alleged historical oppression of women by men. And, in sharp contrast to Western ethical paradigms, it has a holistic dimension that can ground environmental policy and law respecting endangered species and biodiversity.

In the foreword to *A Sand County Almanac,* Leopold (1949, pp. viii–ix) identifies the central eco-axiological theme: "That land is a community is the basic concept of ecology, but that land is to be loved and respected is an extension of ethics. That land yields a cultural harvest is a fact long known, but latterly often forgotten. These essays attempt to weld these three concepts." Its forty-odd essays document two decades of Leopold's reflective intimacy with the natural world; they span the North American continent from Mexico to Canada and from the Southwest to the Midwest; and they range in style from pastoral vignettes to didactic sermonettes. Part One introduces the basic ecological concept of a biotic community (or ecosystem) personally and experientially through artful seasonal sketches of Leopold's beloved 120 acres of Wisconsin River bottomland. The regional sketches of Part Two develop the community concept in ecology more intellectually, generally, and abstractly. The prescriptive essays of Part Three frankly and forcefully explore the ethical and aesthetic implications of the community concept in ecology. The final essay, "The Land Ethic," is the book's philosophical climax and consummation.

The Biological Paradigm

Though liberally educated, Leopold was primarily a student of biology, not of philosophy. Hence his thinking about ethics was influenced more by Charles Darwin than by Immanuel Kant and Jeremy Bentham, the fountainheads of the two major modern paradigms in ethics—deontology and utilitarianism, respectively—both of which proceed somewhat as follows: I demand that others dutifully respect my rights (in the deontological tradition) or take full account of how the consequences of their actions affect my interests (in the utilitarian). To defend that demand, I identify a characteristic I possess that arguably justifies my claim to moral rights or to consideration of my interests. According to Kant, it is rationality; according to Bentham, sentience. If I am to be consistent in my moral reasoning, then I must acknowledge that those who possess the same morally enfranchising property are entitled to the same regard from me as I demand of them. In short, the prevailing modern paradigms reach the moral standing of others starting from one's claim against others of one's own moral standing.

In sharp contrast, the biological paradigm, the paradigm in which Leopold works, starts with altruism, not egoism. Human beings are bonded to their fellows through sympathetic feelings and what David Hume and Adam Smith call the moral sentiments. The prehuman ancestors of Homo sapiens, whose survival and reproductive success greatly depended upon communal living, sympathy, and the other moral sentiments, were strengthened by natural selection and ever more broadly cast through social expansion. With the evolution of the powers of speech and reflection, forms of behavior that accorded with altruistic and social sensibilities were articulated in codes of conduct. As clans merged into tribes, tribes into nations, and so on, such codes were extended to each emergent social whole and its members. Leopold (1949, p. 202) comments that "Ethics, so far studied only by philosophers, is actually a process in ecological evolution." And he alludes to natural selection when he defines an ethic from a biological point of view "as a limitation on freedom of action in the struggle for existence." That he built directly and self-consciously upon this scenario of ethics arising out of community membership, which Darwin had fully articulated in the Descent of Man, therefore, seems certain. To the evolutionary foundation laid by Darwin, Leopold adds crucial material from ecology—the "community concept," especially—in order to erect his land ethic.

In Leopold's (1949, p. 203) own words: "All ethics so far evolved rest upon a single premise: that the individual is a member of a community of interdependent parts." That is Darwin's account of the origin and development of ethics in a nutshell. Ecology "simply enlarges the boundaries of the community to include soils, waters, plants, and animals, or collectively: the land" (p. 204). When this novel ecological insight is added to Darwin's classic evolutionary account of ethics, Leopold believes that the land ethic follows. Therefore, he writes, "A thing is right when it tends to preserve the integrity, stability, and beauty of the biotic community. It is wrong when it tends otherwise" (pp. 224–225).

Most contemporary environmental philosophers follow another path to an environmental ethic. They work well within either deontology or utilitarianism, and proceed to extend ethical standing to nonhuman beings by lowering the qualifications for moral rights or for consideration of interests. "Animal liberation" follows from Bentham's first principles virtually without modification, if we acknowledge that most animals are sentient. And "animal rights" follows from Kant's first principles if we acknowledge that while few, if any, animals may be rational, many have sufficiently robust mental capacities to support claims of rights on their behalf. Of course, animal welfare ethics are not the same as environmental ethics. But, taking the next step along these parallel paths, other philosophers have variously argued that all things having interests, broadly construed, or goods of their own—that is, all living beings—deserve, if not rights, then either dutiful respect (according to the deontologists) or moral consideration (according to the utilitarians).

From Facts to Values

To most moral philosophers, the biological paradigm seems to be more a scientific theory about ethics than a normative theory of ethics. And Leopold's facile move from an ecological "is" (that Homo sapiens is a plain member and citizen of the biotic community) to an environmental "ought" (that therefore we ought to preserve the integrity, stability, and beauty of the biotic community) seems to commit the naturalistic fallacy—the fallacy (named by G. E. Moore, but attributed to David Hume) of deducing prescriptive statements about our moral obligations and ethical values exclusively from descriptive statements about the way things in fact are.

The two major modern philosophical paradigms, on the other hand, seem strained to the breaking point when one attempts to extend rights or entitlements to an entire species or to whole ecosystems, let alone "soils and waters." The Leopold land ethic, grounded in feeling and community, better accords with the holistic focus of contemporary environmental concerns. Environmentalists and conservationists are not too concerned about the well-being of individual grubs, bugs, and shrubs. They are concerned, rather, about what pollution is doing to Earth's atmosphere, fresh waters, and oceans; about what fragmentation is doing to ecosystems; about endangered species and biological diversity.

Contemporary environmental philosophers thus face a theoretical dilemma. Cling to the modern paradigm and remain out of phase with the more holistic character of genuine environmental concerns, or give up the intellectual security and familiarity of the modern paradigm, follow Leopold's application of the biological paradigm to environmental concerns, and work to solve the daunting problem of deriving environmental ethical values from facts about human moral psychology, evolutionary biology, and ecology.

Ironically, Hume himself may provide the key to bridging the lacuna between "is" and "ought," fact and value, and thus clear the way for environmental philosophers to embrace the biological paradigm of ethical theory that the land ethic extends. "Reason," our tool for determining facts, according to Hume (1960, p. 469), "in a strict and philosophical sense can have influence on conduct only after two ways: either when it excites a passion [such as the love and respect that Leopold identifies with ethics] by informing us of the existence of something which is a proper object of it; or when it discovers the connexion of causes and effects, so as to afford us means of exerting any passion." Dispassionate, descriptive evolutionary biology, a product of what Hume calls "reason," has discovered that human beings and other extant forms of life are descended from common ancestors. Evolutionary biology thus discloses a previously unknown fact: that we are literally kin to "our fellow-voyagers ... in the odyssey of evolution," as Leopold (1949, p. 109) characterizes them. The discovery of the fact excites the passions—love and respect—we feel for our kin. Equally dispassionate and descriptive ecological biology has discovered the existence of the biotic community, of which we are no less members than of our various human communities. And the discovery of that fact excites the passions—loyalty and patriotism in this case—that we feel for the social wholes to which we belong. Thus may we move from facts to values, from "ises" to "oughts," in the land ethic, after a manner, according to Hume, that is so strict and philosophical.

J. BAIRD CALLICOT (1995)

SEE ALSO: *Animal Welfare and Rights; Endangered Species and Biodiversity; Environmental Health; Environmental Policy and Law; Life; Virtue and Character;* and other *Environmental Ethics* subentries

BIBLIOGRAPHY

Callicott, J. Baird. 1987. *Companion to A Sand County Almanac: Interpretive and Critical Essays.* Madison: University of Wisconsin Press.

Callicot, J. Baird. 1989. *In Defense of the Land Ethic: Essays in Environmental Philosophy.* Albany: State University of New York Press.

Flader, Susan L. 1974. *Thinking like a Mountain: Aldo Leopold and the Evolution of an Ecological Attitude Toward Deer, Wolves, and Forests.* Columbia: University of Missouri Press.

Hume, David. 1967 (1739). *A Treatise of Human Nature,* ed. L. A. Selby-Bigge. Oxford: Clarendon Press.

Leopold, Aldo. 1933. *Game Management.* New York: Scribner's.

Leopold, Aldo. 1949. *A Sand County Almanac, and Sketches Here and There.* New York: Oxford University Press.

Leopold, Aldo. 1953. *Round River: From the Journals of Aldo Leopold,* ed. Luna B. Leopold. New York: Oxford University Press.

Leopold, Aldo. 1991. *The River of the Mother of God and Other Essays by Aldo Leopold,* eds. Susan L. Flader and J. Baird Callicott. Madison: University of Wisconsin Press.

Meine, Curt. 1988. *Aldo Leopold: His Life and Work.* Madison: University of Wisconsin Press.

Potter, Van Rensselaer. 1971. *Bioethics: Bridge to the Future.* Prentice-Hall Biological Science Series, ed. Carl P. Swanson. Englewood Cliffs, NJ: Prentice-Hall.

Potter, Van Rensselaer. 1988. *Global Bioethics: Building on the Leopold Legacy.* East Lansing: Michigan State University Press.

IV. ECOFEMINISM

"Environmental ethics" refers to a wide range of normative positions, from traditional Western, utilitarian, rights- and justice-based ethics to nontraditional and non-Western ethics. Feminist concerns in environmental ethics span this broad range of positions. However, one feminist position is distinctive: ecological feminism.

"Ecofeminism" is expressly committed to making visible the nature and significance of connections between the treatment of women and the treatment of nonhuman nature, or "women-nature connections." Ecofeminism claims that understanding women-nature connections is essential to any adequate feminism or environmental ethic.

Varieties of Ecofeminism

Just as there is not one feminism, so there is not one ecofeminism. "Ecofeminism" is a term that refers collectively to various environmental perspectives with roots in different feminisms: liberal feminism, traditional Marxist feminism, radical feminism, socialist feminism, and Third World feminism. These roots give rise to different, sometimes competing, ecofeminist positions on the nature and resolution of contemporary environmental problems. What makes them ecofeminist is their explicit focus on "women-nature connections."

Consider the range of women-nature connections explored by ecofeminism (see Warren, 1993). Some ecofeminists discuss *historical* connections: for example, the role rationalism has played in Western philosophy and science in justifying the inferiorization of what is associated with female nature (Plumwood). They argue that to the extent that either the concept or the ascription of reason historically has been applied only to (some) human males, rationalism has been male-gender-biased. The male-gender bias arises from the mistaken assumption that women (and, typically, men of color) are incapable of the impartial, objective, abstract, universalizable reason by virtue of which rational men are both distinguished from and superior to nonrational "nature" (see Warren, 1989). These ecofeminists argue that philosophical conceptions of the human self, ethics, and culture that rely on Western historical conceptions of reason will thereby be male-gender biased (see Warren, 1989).

Some ecofeminists discuss *conceptual* women-nature connections: for example, the way women and nature have been conceived as inferior to male-identified reason and culture. Many ecofeminists claim that the twin dominations of women and nature grow out of and reflect oppressive ways of thinking. These are characterized at least minimally by value dualisms (mind/body, reason/emotion, man/woman, culture/nature), value hierarchies (assigning greater status, value, or prestige to what is "up" in "up-down" hierarchies), conceptions of power as power of "ups" over "downs," conceptions of privilege that systematically favor the "ups," and a logic of domination (the assumption that superiority justifies subordination) (Warren, 1990). On this view, oppressive patriarchal conceptual frameworks sanction behaviors that maintain the domination of women and nature.

Ecofeminists discuss *empirical* women-nature connections: for example, Third World women as managers of domestic households, primary gatherers of food and fuel (typically wood), and collectors and distributors of water (see Warren, 1992). These women must walk further for fuel and suffer greater exposure to contaminated water; in Western countries, poor women, men, and children of color face increased health risks associated with radioactive waste and hazardous waste incinerators (Warren, 1992; Commission for Racial Justice, 1987). Development policies and practices do not recognize the distinct gendered division of labor experienced by Third World women, or the gender, race, and class factors that contribute, even if unconsciously and unintentionally, to the subordination of women and people of color cross-culturally.

Ecofeminists also are interested in *epistemological* and *methodological* women-nature connections. At least 80 percent of the farmers in Africa are women, and women grow about 60 percent of the world's food (see Warren, 1992). A study in Sierra Leone showed that while local men could name an average of eight products of nearby bushes and trees, local women could identify thirty-one (see Warren, 1992). Such data suggest that women often have "indigenous technical knowledge" (ITK) or farming and forestry due to their gendered-role responsibilities in these areas (see Warren, 1992). Consequently, issues of epistemology and methodology in framing environmental ethics, policy, and decision making must ask not simply "What is known?" but "Who has the requisite knowledge and expertise?" According to ecofeminism, what women know as household managers of domestic economies, forests, and agriculture is important to the development of environmental ethics.

Symbolic associations between women and nature appear in art, literature, religion, and philosophy. This is especially evident in the sexist, naturist, and ageist language used to describe women and nonhuman nature. Women are characterized frequently as cows, sows, foxes, chicks, bitches, beavers, dogs, mares, dingbats, old bats, pussycats, birdbrains, harebrains, and serpents. They are pets, dolls, babes, childlike, whiny, "domesticated creatures." Nature is raped, mastered, mined, penetrated, domesticated, manipulated, conquered, and controlled by "the man of science." Virgin timber is felled, cut down; land that lies fallow is barren and useless (not "impotent" and "sterile"). (Similarly, men of color are disproportionately described in the subordinating language of the "downs" as animals, studs, dicks, weasels, wolves, unruly and dangerous "savages" driven by "animalistic instinct"; as docile, wimpy, sissy, childish, or childlike, and not fully rational; as childlike, simple [nonrational] "slaves" who need the guidance and protection of the paternalistic master, the "up.") In a patriarchal context, whatever is woman-, animal-, nature-, or even child-identified has historically been inferior ("down") to what is man-, male-, human-, adult-, or culture-identified. Thus language that feminizes animals and nature, animalizes and naturalizes women (and some men), or describes women, nature, and some men as domesticated pets or children, serves to reflect and reinforce their inferiorization.

What, then, about the allegedly positive connotations of "Mother Nature" or "Mother Earth"? Ecofeminists disagree about whether such female-gendered language truly liberates or merely reinforces harmful gender stereotypes (see Roach). However, all ecofeminists agree that within a patriarchal context, where gendered language has functioned historically to elevate that which is associated with men and male culture, its uncritical continued use in the prefeminist present is problematic.

Finally, there are *political* ("*praxis*") women-nature connections. The term "ecofeminism," coined by Françoise d'Eaubonne in 1974, has always referred to grass-roots activism by local women interested in bringing together feminist environmental concerns. Whether it is the Chipko women in India, who are attempting to save trees from commercial fiber producers by hugging the trees, or Native American women, who are protesting the dumping of uranium mining residue on their lands, or the thousands of women from various cultures who gathered to develop strategies for policy and community organizing to combat water pollution, soil erosion, deforestation, and desertification at planning sessions, conferences, and seminars in conjunction with the Earth Summit in Rio de Janeiro in 1992, ecofeminism has always been grounded in grass-roots, local community political organizing (see Lahar). Properly understood, then, ecofeminist ethics is largely a theoretical response to such grass-roots political concerns involving women's lives globally.

Contributions of Ecofeminism

One might summarize ecofeminism's contributions to environmental ethics as threefold: First, ecofeminism challenges male-gender bias wherever and whenever it occurs. Second, ecofeminism offers a corrective lens to oppressive male-gender bias by self-consciously attempting to develop environmental analyses and positions that are not male-gender-biased. Third, ecofeminism offers a transformative perspective in environmental ethics, one that builds on but goes beyond both feminisms that do not have an adequate environmental component and environmental ethics that does not have a distinctly feminist component.

Ecofeminism does this by using a feminist lens to form different insights about women-nature connections; those environmental ethics that do not include (eco)feminist insights are viewed by ecofeminists as either antifeminist or nonfeminist. Nonfeminist environmental ethics, unlike antifeminist environmental ethics, is not ipso facto male-biased; its claims and conclusions might be quite compatible with and supportive of ecofeminist ethics. What an explicitly (eco)feminist environmental ethic does is overtly challenge androcentric (male-centered) bias in the way environmental ethics is conceived and practiced. For this reason, many ecofeminists criticize other environmental ethics (e.g., deep ecology, traditional Western ethics) for either their androcentric bias or their inattention (however inadvertent or unintentional) to important historical and empirical data about women-nature connections. Ecofeminists

insist that within the intellectual traditions of the past few thousand years and at least of Western cultures, anthropocentrism (human-centeredness) has functioned historically as androcentrism (male-centeredness); failure to see this results in a gender blindness that is harmful to the framing of an environmental ethic or philosophy.

Similarly, ecofeminist conceptual concerns challenge the dominant notions of reason, knowledge, and objectivity, as well as the dominant notions of the human self that underlie them, that have been a mainstay of Western philosophical and environmental ethics. What ecofeminists seek is the development of different, nonoppressive notions of each that change or expand how the notions of reason, knowledge, objectivity, and the human self are conceived. In this vein, many ecofeminists challenge the extension of rights by animal-rights ethics to some nonhuman animals because those rights are based on historically intact, unrevised (and hence problematic) notions of the human self as moral agent (claimant, right holder, interest carrier) separate from and superior to lower plant and inorganic life.

Ecofeminist epistemological concerns raise related issues about the underrepresentation of women's voices in environmental ethics. Such concerns prompt ecofeminists to criticize, for example, land ethicists for their apparent lack of interest in gender issues. Ecofeminist concerns about gendered language and nature symbols (e.g., Mother Earth) challenge those environmental ethics (e.g., stewardship ethics) that uncritically adopt or perpetuate gender-exclusive or gender-problematic language and symbol systems (see Adams). Ecofeminist political concerns about unequal distributions of power and privilege in maintaining systems of domination (e.g., domination over women and nature) challenge any environmental ethic uncorrected by feminism to pay more attention to power and privilege in discussions of environmental ethics (see Warren, 1990).

Concluding Remarks

In conclusion, ecofeminist ethics is a self-consciously feminist-biased ethics insofar as it consciously, intentionally, and explicitly adopts a feminist perspective as the organizing lens through which any environmental ethic is constructed. Despite their critics (see Biehl; Fox), ecofeminists argue that in contemporary patriarchal society, the label "feminist" *does* add something important to the nature and description of environmental ethics; in a nonpatriarchal context, "feminist" concerns may well be unnecessary and the label "feminist" may drop away (see Warren, 1990). But for now, ecofeminist ethics reminds us that in contemporary patriarchal culture, there are important ways in which the domination of nature and the domination of women are linked, and that failure to acknowledge such links perpetuates the mistaken view that feminism does not contribute anything significant to any environmental or biocentric ethics.

KAREN J. WARREN (1995)
BIBLIOGRAPHY REVISED

SEE ALSO: *Care: Contemporary Ethics of Care; Endangered Species and Biodiversity; Environmental Health; Environmental Policy and Law; Ethics: Normative Ethical Theories; Feminism; Hazardous Wastes and Toxic Substances; Women, Historical and Cross-Cultural Perspectives;* and other *Environmental Ethics* subentries

BIBLIOGRAPHY

Adams, Carol J., ed. 1993. *Ecofeminism and the Sacred.* New York: Continuum.

Adams, Carol J., ed.1994. *Ecofeminism and the Sacred,* reprint edition. New York: Continuum.

Biehl, Janet. 1991. *Rethinking Ecofeminist Politics.* Boston: South End.

Caldecott, Leonie, and Leland, Stephanie, eds. 1983. *Reclaim the Earth: Women Speak out for Life on Earth.* London: Women's Press.

Cheney, Jim. 1987. "Eco-Feminism and Deep Ecology." *Environmental Ethics* 9(2): 115–145.

Cook, Julie. 1998. "The Philosophical Colonization of Ecofeminism." *Environmental Ethics* 20(3): 227–246.

Crittenden, Chris. 1998. "Subordinate and Oppressive Conceptual Frameworks: A Defense of Ecofeminist Perspectives." *Environmental Ethics* 20(3): 247–263.

Crittenden, Chris. 1999. "Deep Ecology and Ecofeminism." In *Philosophical Dialogues: Arne Naess and the Progress of Ecophilosophy,* pp. 255–269, ed. Nina Witoszek and Andrew Brennan. Lanham, MD: Rowman & Littlefield.

D'Eaubonne, Françoise. 1974. *Le feminisme ou la mort.* Paris: Pierre Horay.

Diamond, Irene, and Orenstein, Gloria Feman, eds. 1990. *Reweaving the World: The Emergence of Ecofeminism.* San Francisco: Sierra Club.

Fox, Warwick. 1989. "The Deep Ecology-Ecofeminism Debate and Its Parallels." *Environmental Ethics* 11(1): 5–25.

Gaard, Greta. 1997. "Ecofeminism and Wilderness." *Environmental Ethics* 19(1): 5–24.

Gray, Elizabeth Dodson. 1981. *Green Paradise Lost.* Wellesley, MA: Roundtable.

Griffin, Susan. 1978. *Woman and Nature: The Roaring Inside Her.* New York: Harper & Row.

Hawkins, Ronnie Zoe. 1998. "Ecofeminism and Nonhumans: Continuity, Difference, Dualism, and Domination." *Hypatia* 13(1): 158–197.

Heresies #13. 1981. H, no. 1. Special issue, "Feminism and Ecology."

Howell, Nancy R. 1997. "Ecofeminism: What One Needs to Know." *Zygon* 32(2): 231–241.

King, Ynestra. 1981. "Feminism and the Revolt of Nature." *Heresies* #13 4(1):12–16.

Lahar, Stephanie. 1991. "Ecofeminist Theory and Grassroots Politics." *Hypatia* 6(1): 28–45.

Mellor, Mary. 1997. *Feminism and Ecology.* New York: New York University Press.

Merchant, Carolyn. 1980. *The Death of Nature: Women, Ecology, and the Scientific Revolution.* New York: Harper & Row.

Merchant, Carolyn. 1989. *Ecological Revolutions: Nature, Gender, and Science in New England.* Chapel Hill: University of North Carolina Press.

Merchant, Carolyn, ed. 1984. "Women and Environmental History." *Environmental Review* 8(1). Special issue.

Murphy, Patrick, ed. 1988. "Feminism, Ecology, and the Future of the Humanities." *Studies in the Humanities* 15(2) Special issue.

Murphy, Patrick D. 1995. *Literature, Nature, and Other Ecofeminist Critiques.* Albany: State University of New York Press.

"Nature." 1991. *Woman of Power: A Magazine of Feminism, Spirituality, and Politics.* 9(Spring). Special issue.

New Catalyst. 1987–1988. "Woman/Earth Speaking: Feminism and Ecology." no. 10.

Ortner, Sherry. 1974. "Is Female to Male as Nature is to Culture?" *In Woman, Culture, and Society,* pp. 67–87, ed. Michelle Zimbalist Rosaldo. Stanford, CA: Stanford University Press.

Plant, Judith, ed. 1989. *Healing the Wounds: The Promise of Ecofeminism.* Philadelphia: New Society.

Plumwood, Val. 1991. "Nature, Self, and Gender: Feminism, Environmental Philosophy, and the Critique of Rationalism." *Hypatia* 6(1): 3–27.

Roach, Catherine. 1991. "Loving Your Mother: On the Woman-Nature Relationship." *Hypatia* 6(1): 46–59.

Ruether, Rosemary Radford. 1975. *New Woman/New Earth: Sexist Ideologies and Human Liberation.* New York: Seabury.

Ruether, Rosemary Radford. 1997. "Ecofeminism: First and Third World Women." *American Journal of Theology and Philosophy* 18(1): 33–45.

Salleh, Ariel Kay. 1984. "Deeper Than Deep Ecology: The Eco-Feminist Connection." *Environmental Ethics* 6(4): 339–345.

Sandilands, Catriona. 1999. *The Good-Natured Feminist: Ecofeminism and the Quest for Democracy.* Minneapolis, MN: University of Minnesota Press.

Shiva, Vandana. 1988. *Staying Alive: Women, Ecology and Development,* ed. Noël Sturgeon. London: Zed. Ecofeminist Newsletter.

United Church of Christ. Commission for Racial Justice. 1987. *Toxic Wastes and Race in the United States: A National Report on the Racial and Socio-Economic Characteristics of Communities with Hazardous Waste Sites.* New York: Author.

Warren, Karen J. 1987. "Feminism and Ecology: Making Connections." *Environmental Ethics* 9(1): 3–20.

Warren, Karen J. 1989. "Male-Gender Bias and Western Conceptions of Reason and Rationality: A Literature Overview." *Newsletter on Philosophy and Feminism* 88(2): 48–53. Special Issue. "Gender, Reason, and Rationality."

Warren, Karen J. 1990. "The Power and the Promise of Ecological Feminism." *Environmental Ethics* 12(2): 125–146.

Warren, Karen J. 1992. "Taking Empirical Data Seriously: An Ecofeminist Philosophical Perspective." In *Human Values and the Environment: Conference Proceedings,* pp. 32–40. Madison: Wisconsin Academy of Sciences, Arts and Letters.

Warren, Karen J. 1993. Introduction to ecofeminism section. In *Environmental Philosophy: From Animal Rights to Radical Ecology,* ed. Michael E. Zimmerman, J. Baird Callicott, John Clark, George Sessions, and Karen J. Warren. Englewood Cliffs, NJ: Prentice-Hall.

Warren, Karen J. 2000. *Ecofeminist Philosophy: A Western Perspective on What it is and Why it Matters.* Totowa, NJ: Rowman & Littlefield Publishing.

Warren, Karen J., ed. 1991. "Ecological Feminism." *Hypatia* 6(1). Special issue.

Warren, Karen J., ed. 1996. *Ecological Feminist Philosophies (A Hypatia Book).* Bloomington: Indiana University Press.

Warren, Karen, and Erkal, Nisvan, eds. 1997. *Ecofeminism: Women, Culture, Nature.* Bloomington: Indiana University Press.

ENVIRONMENTAL HEALTH

• • •

Environmental health is "the segment of public health that is concerned with assessing, understanding, and controlling the impacts of people on their environment and the impacts of the environment on them" (Moeller, p. 1). The importance of environmental health has received increasing attention since the early 1990s as the connections between health and environment have come to be better understood and environmental challenges to health have become more pronounced.

Environmental health problems arise from poor air quality, lack of clean water, unhygienic living conditions, dangerous workplaces, unsafe food, careless disposal and treatment of wastes, and toxic pollution. A number of longer-range and more globally dispersed problems also pose significant challenges to health, including global climate change, depletion of the ozone layer, acid rain, nitrogen loading, loss of biodiversity, deforestation, loss of topsoil, increased pressure on resources as a result of changing patterns of consumption, and a rapid increase in the human population (McMichael, 2001; McCally, 2002).

The Global Environmental Health Picture

Although health around the world improved on average over the last half century—due mainly to improvements in environmental health fundamentals such as access to clean water, nutritious food, and adequate sanitation, alongside public health basics such as prenatal care and immunizations—it is likely that these gains will be lost if the environmental foundation for health continues to deteriorate. Billions of people already suffer from the effects of degraded environments: At the beginning of the twenty-first century fully one-third of the global burden of disease was attributed to environmental factors (Murray and Lopez).

Lack of clean water for drinking, inadequate sanitation, and lack of hygiene affect a third to a half of the world's population and are responsible for 7 percent of all death and disease globally. Chemical agents, particularly in the form of air pollution, are considered major causative factors in increased rates of bronchitis, heart disease, and cancer. The incidence of asthma is mushrooming. Certain forms of cancer are on the rise. The health of people around the world is diminished by exposure to toxic substances such as lead, mercury, arsenic, cadmium, and dioxins. As local and global ecosystems show increasing signs of stress, human health is likely to become far less stable and far more difficult to maintain. Children are hit especially hard by environmental health problems: The World Health Organization estimates that environmental hazards kill at least 3 million children under age five each year (United Nations Environment Programme).

There is a broad international consensus that the earth's ecosystems are under considerable strain, and global environmental decline will be the defining public health context in the twenty-first century (McMichael, 2001). According to an international report, the overall health of the earth's natural systems declined by 37 percent in the 1990s (World Wildlife Fund), fueled largely by population growth combined with unsustainable levels of consumption and production, which have increased in aggregate even more quickly than have human numbers.

Environmental Health in the United States

Concern with environmental health in the United States has long focused almost exclusively on the problem of toxic pollution, and concern about toxins has shaped the American regulatory, legislative, and philosophical approach to environmental health. Since the publication of *Silent Spring* (Carson) the country has been alerted to the mortal danger of exposing human beings and other life-forms to many products and by-products of an industrialized lifestyle. Although the negative effects of environmental pollution on human health cannot be denied, the existence and magnitude of danger associated with particular processes and products remain controversial.

One reason for the controversy is that powerful interests typically have a stake in denying that their industries create health hazards. Nuclear industries deny that low-level radiation causes cancer. Cigarette manufacturers deny a causal link between passive smoking and cancer. Manufacturers of asbestos products take a similar stand about asbestos, as do manufacturers of agricultural pesticides in regard to their products.

A second reason for the continued controversy is that because causal connections between human health and environmental pollution are inherently difficult to establish, the affected industries can hire competent scientists to dispute claims of environmental hazards to human health. In general, three types of evidence can be used to show that an environmental constituent is a health hazard, but none can establish that connection beyond dispute (Luoma).

First, nonhuman animals can be exposed to a suspected health hazard and the effect can be observed. This cannot prove anything conclusively about human exposure because human beings are biochemically different from nonhuman animals. Also, to establish a connection quickly and at minimal cost, nonhuman animals often are exposed to doses much larger than those to which human beings are expected to be exposed. The effect of a small dose on human beings cannot be established conclusively from evidence about the effects of much larger doses on nonhuman animals.

A second method of investigation is to expose human beings over short periods to mild doses of materials suspected of causing serious health problems when exposure is considerably greater or more prolonged. The problem here is that some substances may be so toxic that it would violate human rights to expose people deliberately even to mild doses. Other substances, in contrast, may not have a deleterious effect at low levels of exposure but may be toxic at higher concentrations or over longer periods. In these cases public health hazards may be underestimated or missed entirely.

Third, in epidemiological studies a substance is tested by comparing the rate of disease in one population with that in another in an attempt to correlate differences between the two populations' rates of disease with differences in their rates of exposure. However, it is difficult to establish in that way a connection between a specific suspected toxin and illness or death because under normal conditions people are exposed constantly to many suspected toxins of various strengths for varying periods. It therefore is difficult to isolate the effect of any single substance. Also, the effect of exposure, if there is one, is often weak. In a small population, for example, few additional cancers can be expected to result from exposure to low-level radiation. In addition, the cancer effect is long delayed and spread out in the population over a forty-year period, making it difficult to detect at any specific time (Stewart). Finally, radiation exposure and cancer exist in the human population in any case, and so it is impossible to determine that any given cancer is caused by exposure to low-level radiation or that the low-level radiation in question is related, for example, to a nuclear industry (Stewart).

Basically the same considerations apply when the issue is the effect of exposure to passive smoking, asbestos, or agricultural pesticides. Thus, controversies can continue for decades. Nevertheless, the weight of evidence supports the claim that the exposure of human beings to chemicals and other products and by-products of industrial civilization is often harmful to human health.

The Problem of Toxins in the United States

"Since the 1950s, age-standardized cancer incidence rates in the U.S. have increased by 43.5 percent" (Epstein, 1992, p. 233). Death from cancer has increased at a similar rate. The best attempts to isolate the causes of cancer have resulted in the conclusion that environmental factors account for 60 to 90 percent of cancers. The rest are attributable to inherited tendencies and internal biochemical malfunctions (Epstein, 1987).

Studies have shown cancer effects from doses of radiation that previously were thought to be safe. In one study a distinguishing fact about children who died of cancer before age ten compared with both those who died of other causes and those who survived to age ten is that the cancer victims' mothers received on average twice as many X rays while pregnant (Stewart). Another study showed a strong statistical association between a father's exposure to external radiation while working at a nuclear-waste reprocessing plant before a child was conceived and that child's chance of contracting leukemia (Gardner).

Radiation is not the only risk factor for cancer: Pesticides and other chemicals are implicated as well. A study showed that the mammary adipose tissue of women with breast cancer contained significantly more residues of chemicals associated with pesticides than did the mammary tissue of women with nonmalignant tumors (Falck et al.). Another study revealed that among white male scientists and engineers those who were members of the American Chemical Society had significantly more deaths from leukemia and lymphatic cancer (Arnetz et al.). A study of men from Iowa and Minnesota showed a link between elevated environmental chemical exposures that resulted from living near a factory and two types of cancer: non-Hodgkin's lymphoma and leukemia (Linos et al.). Non-Hodgkin's lymphoma also has been linked to the use of certain pesticides (Weber). Foundry workers in Denmark who were exposed to elevated levels of silica dust, metallic fumes, carbon monoxide, and several organic chemicals had markedly elevated rates of lung cancer (Sherson et al.). Occupational exposure to asbestos is considered responsible for 8,000 to 12,000 deaths each year in the United States (Rauber).

Typically, years intervene between exposure to environmental contaminants and an associated cancer or death. However, in some cases the connection between environmental pollution and human mortality is more direct. The "U.S. Office of Technology Assessment estimates that the mix of sulphates and particulates in ambient air may cause 50,000 premature deaths in the United States each year—about 2 percent of annual mortality" (Postel, 1986, p. 34). Toxic chemicals released into the air in 1988 were estimated by the U.S. Environmental Protection Agency (EPA) to cause "up to 3,000 cases of fatal cancer yearly as well as birth defects, lung disease, nervous system disorders, liver damage, and other health problems" (U.S. General Accounting Office, p. 8). When all types and sources of air pollution are considered, the American Lung Association puts the toll at 120,000 premature deaths per year (French).

There is increasing evidence that indoor air is often a health hazard. Radon in homes is believed to be a leading cause of cancer. The "sick building" syndrome is also a concern; it is the phenomenon of buildings inducing illnesses of various sorts in a large percentage of the people who spend considerable amounts of time in them. For example, chemicals in materials used to build and decorate the Dupage County Judicial and Office Facility in Wheaton, Illinois, were considered responsible for a variety of employee illnesses. As a result, a nearly new building was evacuated temporarily.

Scientists have been concerned particularly about exposure to heavy metals such as lead and mercury. Although exposure to lead has been reduced greatly, pockets of the population still are exposed to lead in peeling household paint, and everyone is exposed to lead in outdoor air pollution and food. The health effects of lead are well documented and include serious and irreversible impairment of children's neurobehavioral development (Brooks et al.). Mercury contamination also has been of particular concern. As with lead, the health effects of mercury are relatively well understood, largely because of several large-scale exposures, including the Minimata Bay disaster, in which a whole Japanese village was poisoned after eating mercury-laced fish. Methylmercury is absorbed readily by fish in polluted aquatic environments. When humans eat contaminated fish, the methylmercury is absorbed readily into the bloodstream and tissues. Mercury can cause tremors, dementia, and congenital neurological deformities (Brooks et al.).

Beginning in the 1990s, concern has intensified about a group of chemicals called persistent organic pollutants (POPs). Those chemicals include the polychlorinated biphenyls (PCBs); pesticides such as DDT, chlordane, aldrin, and heptachlor; and industrial by-products such as dioxins. POPs are fat-soluble and accumulate in the fatty tissues of animals, where they persist for long periods. Research suggests that POPs are "endocrine disruptors": They mimic hormones and may play a significant and largely unacknowledged role in altering reproduction and development. Endocrine disruptors have long concerned wildlife biologists, who believe that declines in avian and amphibian populations are linked to POPs in the environment (Colborn, Dumanoski, and Myers). The way in which these chemicals affect humans is unknown, although some research has connected exposure to POPs with diminished sperm quality and quantity, impaired sexual function, increased testicular cancer, hypospadias, and cryptorchidism (Solomon and Schettler).

Environmental Racism

The risks of contracting environmentally influenced diseases and deaths are not distributed evenly across the population in the United States. Geographically, the people at greatest risk are those who live near sources of industrial pollution such as factories and certain types of mines and those who live near deposits of toxic waste. For example, it seems that a geometrically increasing cancer rate for people in some communities in Cape Cod, Massachusetts, is due to toxic deposits from the nearby Otis Air Force Base (Hallowell). By 1989, 14,401 sites of toxic contamination had been noted in 1,579 military installations around the United States (Renner). When cancer rates are plotted on a map of the nation, the places that show the highest rates are areas of industrial production such as Chicago, Detroit, northern New Jersey, and the lower Mississippi valley.

There is also a disparate impact on minority communities that is referred to as environmental racism. "Three out of every five African Americans and Hispanics live in a neighborhood with a hazardous waste site, and … race is the most significant variable in differentiating communities with such sites from the communities without them" (Steinhart, p. 18). "Probably the greatest concentration of hazardous-waste sites in the United States is on the predominantly black and Hispanic South Side of Chicago" (Russell, p. 25). With 28 million pounds of toxics poured into that area annually, the U.S. Environmental Protection Agency (EPA) estimates that the risk of cancer is 100 to 1,000 times the normal risk (Lavelle). According to the federal Centers for Disease Control, "lead poisoning endangers the health of nearly 8 million inner-city, largely black and Hispanic children" all over the United States (Russell, p. 24). Rural minority groups suffer disproportionately as well: "2 million tons of radioactive uranium tailings have been dumped on Native American lands; reproductive organ cancer among Navajo teenagers is seventeen times the national average" (Russell, p. 24).

Environmental racism is international as well as domestic. Toxic waste from industrial countries has been deposited in Africa (Jacobson). Some corporations in industrial countries continue to manufacture pesticides that are considered too dangerous for use in their own countries. Those pesticides are sold to farmers in the Third World, resulting in 10,000 to 40,000 poisonings per year (Postel, 1988). The Bhopal accident, in which 2,000 people were poisoned by a chemical leak from a factory in India, highlights the fact that environmental safeguards in the Third World are sometimes inadequate. The company that owns the factory is based in the United States, where it maintains higher standards of safety in its factories.

The Legal Structure

According to traditional Anglo-American jurisprudence, when one person injures another person, the injured party can sue in court to recover damages. The legal rules governing those proceedings constitute the law of torts. This body of law is largely unhelpful, however, when injuries are due to most forms of environmental pollution because it is difficult to prove that a harm such as a case of cancer resulted from a particular emission of radioactivity or a certain dumping of toxic waste. Also, it would be inefficient for each injured

party to sue individually, as was done traditionally, when the activity in question is alleged to affect many people, possibly thousands. Finally, tort actions can take place only after harm is done, and it is preferable to use the law to avoid harms when possible. Thus, the major role of government in the area of environmental health lies in the regulatory process.

In 1970 the National Environmental Policy Act was signed into law to "fulfill the responsibilities of each generation as trustee of the environment for succeeding generations." The EPA, which was established soon afterward, required that most federally funded projects be accompanied by an environmental impact statement so that the deleterious effects of those projects could be recognized and possibly ameliorated. Subsequent legislation has given the EPA the authority, for example, to regulate processes that pollute the air and water (the Clean Air Act and the Clean Water Act); locate, authorize, and fund the cleanup of hazardous wastes (the Resource Conservation and Recovery Act, which established the Superfund); and control the use of pesticides (the Federal Insecticide, Fungicide, and Rodenticide Act). States have their own EPAs that perform similar functions.

The U.S. EPA is not the only agency with the responsibility to oversee activities that can affect environmental health. The U.S. Department of Energy (DOE) oversees the disposal of nuclear waste, the U.S. Department of Agriculture (USDA) helps determine consumer exposure to pesticide residues in food, and the U.S. Department of Labor protects the health of workers through the Occupational Safety and Health Administration (OSHA). In addition, most states have administrative agencies with similar responsibilities for intrastate activities.

Because Congress has authorized those agencies and the many subagencies through which they operate to protect the public, courts are reluctant to intervene, making private lawsuits particularly difficult. If an agency is operating within its congressional mandate and arguably is doing its job in a reasonable fashion, the courts usually will protect both the agency and those in compliance with its standards from private lawsuits seeking compensation for environmentally related illnesses. Thus, the protection of environmental health depends much more directly on the actions of those agencies than on the concerns of private citizens and their elected representatives.

Enforcement Problems

As was noted above, the protection of human health from environmental contamination in the United States is largely the responsibility of the EPA and other federal and state agencies. Unfortunately, the performance of those agencies is sometimes disappointing. The EPA's regulation of pesticides exemplifies the general problem. The EPA regulates pesticides under the Federal Insecticide, Fungicide, and Rodenticide Act. The general public is exposed to pesticides primarily through residues in food and contamination of the groundwater that serves as a major source of drinking water. The EPA recognized in 1988 that "forty-six pesticides … contaminate groundwater solely as a result of normal agricultural use" (Fultz, p. 3). However, a registered chemical can remain in use for up to fifteen years after it is discovered in groundwater before a decision is made about its continued use. An example is atrazine, a pesticide that is in widespread agricultural use (Fultz). For pesticides that already have been found to be toxic, the EPA has not lowered acceptable exposure through residues in food in light of additional exposure through drinking water.

Not all pesticides in widespread use are registered with the EPA, resulting in the continued exposure of the public through food and water to pesticides that have not been tested for their "potential to cause birth defects, cancer, and other chronic health effects" (Fultz, p. 5). Exemption from the registration requirement is given in so-called emergencies for one year at a time, but some exemptions have been granted for more than a decade, during which time people have been exposed to pesticides of unknown toxicity (Guerrero, 1991b). Also, the EPA continues to emphasize the control of point sources of water pollution such as factories and municipal sewer systems instead of nonpoint sources such as agricultural runoff despite evidence that nonpoint sources pose a greater water pollution problem (Guerrero, 1991b). This may be due to the fact that the USDA promotes the use of many pesticides to increase crop yields even though those chemicals constitute health hazards.

Unfortunately, the EPA's inadequate protection of public health from the dangers of pesticides is typical. Similar stories can be told about surface-water pollution, hazardous waste management and cleanup, enforcement of the Clean Air Act, and U.S. Department of Energy (DOE) decisions about the disposal of nuclear waste: "The National Research Council estimated that only 2 percent of at least 60,000 chemicals that are used widely have been comprehensively studied for toxic effects" (Ziem and Davidoff, p. 88).

In addition to poor funding, a general reason for inadequate protection is that agencies tend to establish such close ties to the industries they are charged with regulating that they identify with industry perspectives and needs. An agency's capture by industry results partly from industry offers of future high-paying employment to regulatory personnel who are "reasonable." Another factor may be pressure on an agency by the legislators who are responsible for approving its budget. Those legislators may depend on the regulated industry for campaign contributions (Sanjour).

Conscientious federal employees who try to regulate effectively are relegated to tasks that have little impact. Employees who blow the whistle on an agency's failure to do its job must go before the presidentially appointed Merit System Protection Board, which may be more interested in protecting the president and "the system" than in protecting the whistle-blower (Sanjour).

There is also the appearance of racism in the EPA's enforcement efforts: "Penalties under hazardous waste laws at sites having the greatest white population were about 500 percent higher than penalties at sites with the greatest minority population" (Lavelle, p. S2). This disparity can be accounted for only by race, not by income. There is a similar disparity of 46 percent in penalties concerning nontoxic waste, air pollution, and water pollution. It takes 20 percent longer for toxic waste sites in minority areas to be placed on the priority list for cleanup, and the cleanup in minority areas is more likely than that in white areas to consist only of containment of the waste rather than treatment that removes its toxicity.

Environmental racism also appears to affect government regulation of international trade. For example, pesticides banned in the United States because of their toxicity to human beings can be manufactured and then sold abroad. Some return as residues on imported food.

Decisional Frameworks

How should decisions about environmental health be made? Advocates of free trade and free markets suggest that market mechanisms can protect public health adequately. However, from the perspective of firms competing for customers, environmental protection seldom makes sense. A manufacturer's plastic toys, for example, seldom are more attractive to customers because the water and air used in its manufacturing processes were purified before being released into the environment. Similarly, catalytic converters on automobiles add to cost but do not improve cars in most customers' eyes. Without government mandates requiring all the producers in an industry to protect the environment, the cost of such protection impairs the competitiveness, or reduces the profits, of conscientious firms that act alone. Thus, the free market discourages the protection of environmental health in the absence of government-mandated regulations such as those administered by OSHA and the EPA.

The EPA and other government agencies have been faulted for their failure to oppose the market-driven activities of private enterprise with sufficient vigor. Three kinds of reforms may be ameliorative. First, agency personnel could be barred for five years from employment, directly or indirectly, by companies that their agency regulates. This would encourage greater independence of agency personnel from the perspectives of regulated companies. Second, campaign finance reform could help diminish the influence of financial interests on the regulatory process. Third, whistle-blowers could be given special job and financial protection (Sanjour).

What decisional framework should those agencies employ? Some libertarians, who stress the importance of individual rights, maintain that any environmental pollution that may harm anyone should be disallowed. The government should "enjoin anyone from injecting pollutants into the air, and thereby invading the rights of persons and property. Period" (Rothbard, p. 5). However, this purist approach seems unrealistic because it would disallow, for example, most manufacturing and almost all uses of fossil fuels, including use in automobiles. Polluting the environment in ways that are potentially harmful to human health is too ingrained in industrial ways of life to be eliminated entirely.

Pointing to the benefits of industrialization—air-conditioning in the summer, heating in the winter, rapid transportation, and sophisticated medical interventions—some people maintain that pollution should be allowed until the risks to people outweigh the benefits. According to this view, government agencies such as the EPA should use risk-benefit analysis to determine permissible kinds and levels of pollution (Ruckelshaus).

Critics maintain, however, that risk-benefit analysis favors continued pollution over health-related concerns. First, current levels of pollution often are assumed to be acceptable and are used as precedents for future decisions. Second, whereas the benefits of current pollution practices are assumed, risks must be proved scientifically, a task that is difficult. Third, risk-benefit analysis depends largely on subjective judgments of "experts" whose opinions may reflect employers' interests (Winner).

Some people suggest avoiding subjectivity by using cost-benefit analysis (CBA), in which all the costs and benefits of proposed pollution-controlling regulations are expressed in monetary terms. The alternative with the highest net benefit should be chosen. Costly health hazards thus would be taken into account. The EPA usually allows environmental impact statements to employ CBA, and the Nuclear Regulatory Commission uses CBA regularly.

However, there are many problems with CBA. First, the costs and benefits associated with the length and quality of human life, which are affected by environmental health, cannot be translated reliably into monetary terms. Second, subjectivism remains because there is great uncertainty in projections of health hazards (Shrader-Frechette). Third, by employing money as its standard, CBA takes into account views and desires only insofar as they are expressed in monetary terms. The opportunity for that expression is proportional to the money at people's disposal. Using CBA, then, agencies would give protection to people not equally but in proportion to their wealth or income. In regard to the actions of government agencies CBA denies equal protection of the law. Fourth, using normal economic techniques, CBA discounts the future, making a present cost or benefit larger than an otherwise equivalent but future cost or benefit. This biases public policy toward the short term. If the duty to avoid or minimize harming people is based on human rights, harming future generations is morally equivalent to harming contemporaries. CBA discounts the lives and well-being of future generations (Wenz).

Alternative Frameworks

Instead of CBA, the following are possible rules of thumb. First, the burden of proof should be reversed from that employed in risk-benefit analysis. Before a potentially harmful addition is made to the environment, its safety should be demonstrated. At the beginning of the twenty-first century, for example, potentially carcinogenic pesticides can be used widely for ten to fifteen years before investigations are completed. Products are withdrawn then only if they are demonstrated to harm public health. The burden to demonstrate its safety should be on those who want to expose people to a new chemical.

Second, the people at greatest risk should be given the greatest voice in decisions about creating or using potentially hazardous substances (Shrader-Frechette). For example, corporate officials and owners interested in manufacturing processes that create toxic wastes would retain a significant voice in regulatory decisions if they could and would store the wastes near themselves and their families.

Third, through subsidies the government should encourage sustainable agriculture, integrated pest management, mass transit, energy conservation, and other practices and products that reduce the introduction of health hazards into the environment.

Fourth, when the indirect costs of a product can be calculated reliably, those costs should over time be added as a tax to the consumer price of that product. For example, the price of gasoline should reflect the costs associated with the deleterious health effects of smog. Only then will consumers be guided by accurate information about how much a product actually costs them. Such information generally improves the results of reliance on market mechanisms.

Fifth, agencies should discourage practices that hide the existence or severity of environmental health problems. Storage of nuclear wastes underground so that the continuing health hazard is not noticed and the war on cancer that lulls people into thinking a cure is near lead the public to underestimate its jeopardy. This should be avoided in part because an informed public is central to addressing problems of pollution. In the absence of an objective formula for balancing alleged benefits against alleged harms to determine the acceptability of pollution, an informed public must be the ultimate judge of government decisions related to environmental health.

PETER S. WENZ (1995)
REVISED BY JESSICA PIERCE

SEE ALSO: *Environmental Ethics; Environmental Policy and Law; Future Generations, Reproductive Technologies and Obligations to; Hazardous Wastes and Toxic Substances; Occupational Safety and Health; Public Health; Sustainable Development*

BIBLIOGRAPHY

Arnetz, Bengt B.; Raymond, Lawrence W.; Nicolich, Mark J.; et al. 1991. "Mortality among Petrochemical Science and Engineering Employees." *Archives of Environmental Health* 46(4): 237–248.

Brooks, Stuart M.; Gochfeld, Michael; Herzstein, Jessica; et al., eds. 1995. *Environmental Medicine.* St. Louis: Mosby.

Bryant, Bunyan. 1995. *Environmental Justice: Issues, Policies, and Solutions.* Washington, D.C.: Island Press.

Carson, Rachel. 1962. *Silent Spring.* Boston: Houghton Mifflin.

Chivian, Eric. 2001. "Environment and Health: 7. Species Loss and Ecosystem Disruption—The Implications for Human Health." *Canadian Medical Association Journal* 164(1): 66–69.

Chivian, Eric; McCally, Michael; Hu, Howard; et al. 1993. *Critical Condition: Human Health and the Environment.* Cambridge, MA: MIT Press.

Clapp, Richard. 2000. "Environment and Health: 4. Cancer." *Canadian Medical Association Journal* 163(8): 1009–1012.

Colborn, Theo; Dumanoski, Dianne; and Myers, John P. 1996. *Our Stolen Future: Are We Threatening Our Fertility, Intelligence, and Survival—A Scientific Detective Story.* New York: Dutton.

Daily, Gretchen, ed. 1997. *Nature's Services: Societal Dependence on Natural Ecosystems.* Washington, D.C.: Island Press.

De Gruijl, Frank R., and van der Leun, Jan C. 2000. "Environment and Health: 3. Ozone Depletion and Ultraviolet Radiation." *Canadian Medical Association Journal* 163(7): 851–855.

Epstein, Samuel S. 1987. "Losing the War against Cancer." *Ecologist* 17(2–3): 91–101.

Epstein, Samuel S. 1992. "Profiting from Cancer: Vested Interests and the Cancer Epidemic." *Ecologist* 22(5): 233–240.

Falck, Frank, Jr.; Ricci, Andrew, Jr.; Wolff, Mary S.; et al. 1992. "Pesticides and Polychlorinated Biphenyl Residues in Human Breast Lipids and Their Relation to Breast Cancer." *Archives of Environmental Health* 47(2): 143–146.

French, Hilary F. 1991. "You Are What You Breathe." In *The World Watch Reader on Global Environmental Issues,* ed. Lester R. Brown. New York: W. W. Norton.

Frumkim, Howard. 2001. "Beyond Toxicity: Human Health and the Natural Environment." *American Journal of Preventive Medicine* 20(3): 234–240.

Fultz, Keith O. 1991. *EPA Should Act Promptly to Minimize Contamination of Groundwater by Pesticides.* GAO/T–RCED–91–46. Washington, D.C.: U.S. General Accounting Office.

Gardner, Martin J. 1991. "Father's Occupational Exposure to Radiation and the Raised Level of Childhood Leukemia Near the Sellafield Nuclear Plant." *Environmental Health Perspectives* 94: 5–7.

Grifo, Fransesca, and Rosenthal, Joshua, eds. 1997. *Biodiversity and Human Health.* Washington, D.C.: Island Press.

Guerrero, Peter F. 1991a. "Greater EPA Leadership Needed to Reduce Nonpoint Source Pollution," testimony. GAO/T–RCED–91–34. Washington, D.C.: U.S. General Accounting Office.

Guerrero, Peter F. 1991b. "Pesticides: EPA's Repeat Emergency Exemptions May Provide Potential for Abuse," testimony. GAO/T–RCED–91–83. Washington, D.C.: U.S. General Accounting Office.

Haines, Andrew; McMichael, Anthony J.; and Epstein, Paul. 2000. "Environment and Health: 2. Global Climate Change and Health." *Canadian Medical Association Journal* 163(6): 729–734.

Hallowell, Christopher. 1991. "Water Crisis on the Cape." *Audubon,* July–August, pp. 65–74.

Jacobson, Jodi L. 1989. "Abandoning Homelands." In *State of the World, 1989: A Worldwatch Institute Report on Progress toward a Sustainable Society,* ed. Lester R. Brown. New York: W. W. Norton.

Kolpin, Dana W.; Furlong, Edward T.; Meyer, Michael T.; et al. 2002. "Pharmaceuticals, Hormones, and Other Organic Wastewater Contaminants in U.S. Streams, 1999–2000: A National Reconnaissance." *Environmental Science and Technology* 36(6): 1202–1211.

Last, John. 1998. *Public Health and Human Ecology,* 2nd edition. Stamford, CT: Appleton & Lange.

Lavelle, Marianne. 1992. "Unequal Protection: The Racial Divide in Environmental Law." *National Law Journal,* September 21, pp. S1–S12.

Linos, Athena; Blair, Aaron; Gibson, Robert W.; et al. 1991. "Leukemia and Non-Hodgkin's Lymphoma and Residential Proximity to Industrial Plants." *Archives of Environmental Health* 46(2): 70–74.

Luoma, Jon R. 1988. "The Human Cost of Acid Rain." *Audubon,* July, pp. 16–25.

McCally, Michael. 2000. "Environment and Health: An Overview." *Canadian Medical Association Journal* 163(5): 533–535.

McCally, Michael, ed. 2002. *Life Support: The Environment and Human Health.* Cambridge, MA: MIT Press.

McMichael, Anthony J. 1993. *Planetary Overload: Global Environmental Change and the Health of the Human Species.* Cambridge, Eng., and New York: Cambridge University Press.

McMichael, Anthony J. 1994. "Global Environmental Change and Human Health: New Challenges to Scientist and Policy Maker." *Journal of Public Health Policy* 15(4): 407–419.

McMichael, Anthony J. 1995. "Global Climate Change and Health." *Lancet* 346: 835.

McMichael, Anthony J. 2001. *Human Frontiers, Environments, and Disease: Past Patterns, Uncertain Futures.* Cambridge, Eng., and New York: Cambridge University Press.

McMichael, Anthony, ed. 1996. *Climate Change and Human Health.* Geneva: World Health Organization.

McMichael, Anthony J.; Woodward, Alistair J.; and van Leeuwen, Ruud E. 1994. "The Impact of Energy Use in Industrialized Countries upon Global Population Health." *Medicine and Global Survival* 1: 23–32.

Moeller, Dade. 1997. *Environmental Health,* rev. edition. Cambridge, MA: Harvard University.

Mohnen, Volker A. 1988. "The Challenge of Acid Rain." *Scientific American* 259(2): 30–38.

Mortimer, Nigel. 1991. "Nuclear Power and Carbon Dioxide: The Fallacy of the Nuclear Industry's New Propaganda." *Ecologist* 21(3): 129–132.

Murray, Christopher J. L., and Lopez, Alan D., eds. 1996. *The Global Burden of Disease Study: A Comprehensive Assessment of Mortality and Disability from Diseases, Injuries, and Risk Factors in 1990 and Projected to 2020.* Cambridge, MA: Harvard School of Public Health on behalf of the World Health Organization and the World Bank, distributed by Harvard University Press.

Mutz, Kathryn M.; Bryner, Gary C.; and Kenney, Douglas S., eds. 2002. *Justice and Natural Resouces: Concepts, Strategies, and Applications.* Washington, D.C.: Island Press.

Patz, Jonathan A.; Epstein, Paul R.; Burke, Tom A.; and Balbus, John M. 1996. "Global Climate Change and Emerging Infectious Diseases." *Journal of the American Medical Association* 275: 217–223.

Pierce, Jessica, and Jameton, Andrew. 2003. *The Ethics of Environmentally Responsible Health Care.* New York: Oxford University Press.

Pimentel, David; Tort, Maria; D'Anna, Linda; et al. 1998. "Ecology of Increasing Disease: Population Growth and Environmental Degradation." *Bioscience* 48(10): 817–826.

Pope, C. Arden, III; Burnett, Richard T.; Thun, Michael J.; et al. 2002. "Lung Cancer, Cardiopulmonary Mortality, and Long-Term Exposure to Fine Particulate Air Pollution." *Journal of the American Medical Association* 287(9): 1132–1141.

Pope, C. Arden; Schwartz, Joel; and Ransom, Michael R. 1992. "Daily Mortality and PM10 Pollution in Utah Valley." *Archives of Environmental Health* 47(3): 211–217.

Postel, Sandra. 1986. *Altering the Earth's Chemistry: Assessing the Risks.* Worldwatch Paper 71. Washington, D.C.: Worldwatch Institute.

Postel, Sandra. 1988. "Controlling Toxic Chemicals." In *State of the World, 1988: A Worldwatch Institute Report on Progress toward a Sustainable Society,* ed. Lester R. Brown. New York: W. W. Norton.

Rauber, Paul. 1991. "New Life for White Death." *Sierra,* September–October, pp. 62–65, 104–105, 110–111.

Renner, Michael. 1991. "Assessing the Military's War on the Environment." In *State of the World, 1991: A Worldwatch Institute Report on Progress toward a Sustainable Society,* ed. Lester R. Brown. New York: W. W. Norton.

Rothbard, Murray. 1970. "The Great Ecology Issue." *The Individualist* 2(2): 1–8.

Ruckelshaus, William D. 1983. "Science, Risk, and Public Policy." *Science* 221(4615): 1026–1028.

Russell, Dick. 1989. "Environmental Racism." *Amicus Journal* 11(2): 22–32.

Sanjour, William. 1992. "In Name Only." *Sierra,* September–October, pp. 74–77, 95–103.

Sherson, David; Svane, Ole; and Lynge, Elsebeth. 1991. "Cancer Incidence among Foundry Workers in Denmark." *Archives of Environmental Health* 46(2): 75–81.

Shrader-Frechette, Kristin S. 1991. *Risk and Rationality: Philosophical Foundations for Populist Reforms.* Berkeley: University of California Press.

Solomon, Gina M., and Schettler, Ted. 2000. "Environment and Health: 6. Endocrine Disruption and Potential Human Health Impacts." *Canadian Medical Association Journal* 163(11): 1471–1476.

Speidel, Joseph. 2000. "Environment and Health: 1. Population, Consumption and Human Health." *Canadian Medical Association Journal* 163(5): 551–556.

Steingraber, Sandra. 1998. *Living Downstream.* New York: Vintage.

Steinhart, Peter. 1991. "What Can We Do about Environmental Racism?" *Audubon,* May, pp. 18–21.

Stetson, Marnie. 1992. "Saving Nature's Sunscreen." *Worldwatch* 5(2): 34–36.

Stewart, Alice. 1993. "Low Level Radiation—The Effects on Human and Nonhuman Life." In *Poison Fire/Sacred Earth,* ed.

Sibylle Nahr and Uwe Peters. Munich: World Uranium Hearing.

Thornton, Joe. 2000. *Pandora's Poison: Chlorine, Health, and a New Environmental Strategy.* Cambridge, MA: MIT Press.

United Nations Development Programme, United Nations Environment Programme, World Bank, and World Resources Institute. 2000. *A Guide to World Resources 2000–2001: People and Ecosystems: The Fraying Web of Life.* Washington, D.C.: World Resources Institute.

United Nations Environment Programme. 2002. *Global Environment Outlook 3.* London: Earthscan.

United Nations Environment Programme, United Nations Children's Fund, and World Health Organization. 2002. *Children in the New Millennium: Environmental Impact on Health.* Geneva: World Health Organization.

U.S. General Accounting Office. 1991. *Air Pollution: EPA's Strategy and Resources May Be Inadequate to Control Air Toxics: Report to the Chairman.* GAO/RCED–91–143. Washington, D.C.: U.S. General Accounting Office.

Weber, Peter. 1992. "A Place for Pesticides?" *Worldwatch* 5(3): 18–25.

Wenz, Peter S. 1988. *Environmental Justice.* Albany: State University of New York Press.

Winner, Langdon. 1986. *The Whale and the Reactor: A Search for Limits in an Age of High Technology.* Chicago: University of Chicago Press.

World Wildlife Fund. 2002. *Living Planet Report 2002.* Gland, Switzerland: World Wide Fund for Nature.

Ziem, Grace E., and Davidoff, Linda L. 1992. "Illness from Chemical 'Odors': Is the Health Significance Understood?" *Archives of Environmental Health* 47(1): 88–91.

INTERNET RESOURCE

World Resources Institute. 2000. *World Resources 2000–2001: People and Ecosystems: The Fraying Web of Life.* Elsevier Science. Available from <http//:www.wristore.com>.

ENVIRONMENTAL POLICY AND LAW

• • •

Among the many purposes of environmental law, two stand out: the protection of personal and property rights and the preservation of places. Laws controlling pollution serve primarily the first goal; they constrain the risks people can impose on others. Statutes that pursue the second purpose seek to preserve national forests, landscapes, and landmarks; to protect historical districts; to maintain biodiversity; and to defend the integrity of ecological systems, such as rivers and wetlands.

These two sorts of statutes emerge from two foundational traditions in the political culture of the United States, the first of which draws on the values of property and autonomy; the second, on those of community and diversity. The first tradition, which is associated with libertarianism and individualism, would protect each person from involuntary risks and harms. The second tradition, which is associated with Madisonian republicanism, suggests that Americans may use the representative and participatory processes of democracy to ask and answer moral questions about the goals of a good society. Americans, most of whom are immigrants or descended from immigrants, find in the natural environment a common heritage—a res publica—that unites them as a nation. Environmental laws, then, may regard shared nature as having a cultural shape, form, or value we are responsible to maintain for its own sake and for future generations.

Pollution-control law may be understood in ethical rather than economic terms insofar as it protects the separateness and inviolability of persons rather than satisfies their interests or preferences. Land-use law preserves the ecological and historical character but not necessarily the economic product of landscapes. Environmental law thus responds to intrinsic values, namely, the autonomy of persons and the integrity of places.

This entry provides a brief account of the three stages—aspiration, recrimination, and collaboration—that characterize the historical development of environmental law in the United States since the passage of the National Environmental Policy Act of 1969. It then describes some of the normative and conceptual problems that are most likely to affect the future of environmental policy.

Aspiration: 1980–1990

During the 1970s, when politicians discovered that being in favor of the environment won votes, Congress enacted, among other statutes, the Clean Air Act of 1970, the Occupational Safety and Health Act of 1970 (OSHA), the Endangered Species Act (CAA) of 1972, the Safe Drinking Water Act of 1974, the Toxic Substances Control Act of 1976, and the Resource Conservation and Recovery Act of 1976. These laws were aspirational—one might say, demagogic—because they set lofty but often vague and unrealistic goals, calling, for example, for *safe* thresholds for pollutants for which no such thresholds exist. The Ocean Dumping Act of 1972 prohibited ocean dumping—but did not say where the wastes should go instead. The Clean Water Act of 1972 required the restoration and maintenance of the "chemical, physical, and biological integrity of the Nation's waters." There is still no agreement on what these words mean.

The rhetorical objectives of laws enacted during the 1970s, which are strong enough to warm the heart of the most ardent environmentalist, soon became fictions as deadlines passed, violations were not monitored or prosecuted, and the agencies fought uphill political and legal battles to make whatever gains they could, given their limited resources. On those rare occasions when the regulatory agencies threatened to enforce a statute to its full extent, Congress could be counted on to weaken it. In 1973, when a court ordered the Environmental Protection Agency (EPA) to bring California into compliance with the Clean Air Act, for example, administrator William Ruckelshaus responded with gasoline rationing, since nothing less draconian would do the job. Congress intervened by extending deadline after deadline; they, too, passed unmet.

Some might regard the aspirational and draconian goals of environmental statutes as cynical: By promising environmentalists the moon, these statutes provided scant direction about how to solve conflicts on earth. OSHA requires the workplace to be as safe from hazards as *feasible,* but the government has regulated only about one hazardous substance per year. The Fish and Wildlife Service avoided drastic effects in applying the Endangered Species Act by failing to list species and by approving inadequate plans to protect those that were listed. This was often as much as was politically possible given the opposition of those who would rather "shoot, shovel, and shut up" than to dedicate their property to zoological ideals. The draconian wording of the statutes at least gave agencies a strong legal foothold when they could muster the political will to act.

The late and unlamented Delaney Clause of the Food, Drug and Cosmetic Act prohibited in prepared food any trace of a pesticide that can be shown to induce cancer when administered in massive doses to laboratory animals. It was rarely enforced. New methods of detection showed that every box, bottle, or can of food contains a trace of some carcinogen, so defined. Rather than close down the food industry, officials used dodges, such as a *de minimis* risk exemption, to skirt the law. Political factors—a congressional or presidential election, for example—did wonders in softening regulations in key districts; industry and other interest groups, moreover, knew how to use campaign contributions and their friends in Congress to chasten agency zeal in applying the law.

Retrospective Liability and Criminalization: 1980–1989

By 1981 environmental regulation had reached an impasse. Congress had announced the good news that the environment would be pollution-free and that the nation would preserve its scenic wonders and biological resources. Regulatory agencies then had to announce the bad news: what it would cost and who would have to pay for it. Many who bore the costs blamed the messenger; EPA and other agencies came under fire for policies that required great outlays to achieve sometimes minor improvements. When President Ronald Reagan announced a program of regulatory rescission and appointed Anne Gorsuch at EPA and James Watt at the Department of the Interior, it seemed that the goals of the 1970s would be abandoned, in view of the ideological commitments and managerial styles of these appointees.

By 1981 however, the constituency of the environmental movement had changed. At first enlisting primarily upper-middle class, well-educated suburbanites, environmentalism had become a populism, including lower-middle-class Americans in the heartland who resented the effects of global markets on their communities. Social-science surveys showed overwhelming support among all economic and social groups for the strictest regulation, regardless of cost. Because of the strength of environmentalism among his own supporters, President Reagan found himself obliged to replace the head of the EPA and the secretary of the interior, and to accept a new barrage of environmental statutes that appealed to a populist not to a technocratic constituency.

During the 1980s, Congress intensified top-down *command-and-control* regulation by enacting, for example, the Comprehensive Environmental Response, Compensation, and Liability Act of 1980, which makes the buyer of a contaminated property liable for the entire cleanup even though it did not contribute to the contamination. Other statutes—such as the Resource Conservation and Recovery Act Amendments of 1984, the Superfund Amendments and Reauthorization Act of 1986, and the Oil Pollution Act of 1990—likewise addressed not just present hazards but also the remediation of past ones. Some of these statutes included criminal penalties or made polluters jointly and severally liable for the entire cost of a cleanup, regardless of fault. Thus, any company whose name appeared on a manifest at a poorly operated waste dump might find itself legally liable to pay the entire cost of a gold-plated remediation.

Laws of this kind take a moralistic or retributivist approach, associated with populist crusades, in regulating pollution. In response, industries backed away from investments entirely, for example, where they were most needed in inner city neighborhoods, or they hired lawyers to avoid or spread liability rather than engineers to clean up or prevent pollution. It took about a dozen years for industry to deal with Superfund in some way other than litigation; eventually, public officials and industry lawyers learned to paper transactions needed to get some decontamination. EPA and state agencies began to allow industries to develop polluted properties—so-called *brownfields*—without incurring open-ended liabilities for perfect cleanups. EPA began to experiment with case-by-case negotiation to turn confrontation into compromise. Half way measures—often enshrined in consent decrees, supplemental environmental provisions, prospective purchaser agreements, habitat conservation plans, negotiated rulemakings, and many other instruments—kept the perfect environment the laws envisioned from becoming an implacable enemy of the good environment that patient case-by-case conflict-resolution could achieve.

The Contractual State

With the Clinton administration, the ethos of environment policy changed again. Large-scale polluters, such as smelters and refineries, had largely been controlled, but small sources, such as automobiles, trucks, lawn mowers, bakeries, cleaners, gas stations, and other modest businesses cumulatively added massively to pollution problems. Global threats, such as climate change, habitat loss, and fisheries depletion, implicated the average consumer, for example, those who drive gas-guzzling cars. Programs to *reinvent regulation* proposed to bring into the public sector innovations—such as information sharing, technology benchmarking, incentives, systems-thinking, and collaborative engagement—that had been introduced successfully in private enterprise.

EPA established several *banking, offset,* and *pollution trading* regimes that allowed firms to avail themselves of the cheapest ways to reduce pollution and gave them incentives to develop more efficient control technologies. Markets for trading pollution allowances, which capped total emissions at reduced levels, lowered lead and, especially, sulfur dioxide emissions, which were halved in a decade. Environmentalists could purchase and thus retire emission *allowances,* which sold at surprisingly low prices. EPA through Project XL engaged corporations in collaborative and negotiated rulemaking. Federal and state agencies also inspired decentralized community and individual action by providing information; for example, EPA's Green Lights program encouraged a transition from energy-intensive incandescent bulbs to far more efficient compact fluorescent ones. Similarly, toxic release inventories, eco-labeling, right-to-know regulations, and environmental certification programs illustrate other ways information can initiate local, decentralized improvements.

With the greater and easier availability of information, individuals and firms have begun to internalize environmental norms. Frustration with agency inaction, moreover, has led citizen and industry groups to try to collaborate to resolve their conflicts. Successful habitat conservation plans—the most famous concerns the desert tortoise—emerged from *civil society,* that is, from negotiation among concerned groups. Environmentalists and ranchers, usually at each other's throats, joined to petition the government to establish a market in tradable grazing rights that environmentalists can retire by buying them from ranchers. Officials have initiated successful stakeholder negotiations as well, for example, to protect visibility in the Grand Canyon, although agency intransigence and turf-mindedness—the Forest Service has opposed stakeholder governance of national forests, as in Quincy, California—can also undermine collaborative agreements.

In trying to decentralize decision making through collaboration, negotiation, information, incentive-formation, and so on, regulatory agencies have gotten ahead of legislation. Since 1990, Congress has enacted no major new environmental regulatory statutes nor significantly amended old ones. Since 1970, only two environmental statutes—the Right-to-Know Act of 1986 and the SO_2 trading program in 1990 CAA Amendments—depart from the standard top-down, command-and-control, one-size-fits-all approach. The trend toward more reflexive, adaptive, and collaborative approaches to conflict-resolution remains tenuous and vulnerable, since it lacks a statutory basis.

Economic Theory and the Environment

In the 1970s, economists described pollution and other environmental concerns as economic problems—external costs of production—that arise because markets fail to internalize in the prices of goods the costs of all the resources they consume. It soon became obvious, however, that public officials were no better able than private actors to gather and process the information needed to set *optimal* levels of pollution. Since the government confronts the same or greater information and bargaining costs as private parties, it is no more able than they to determine what people are willing to pay (or to accept) to gain or allow various outcomes. The government has confronted prohibitive costs when it has sought to measure the environmental losses caused by an episode of pollution—and defend those measurements.

In the early 1990s, for example, the government spent $30 million to commission experts to assess the damages associated with the discharge of DDT and PCBs into the Los Angeles Harbor. Tens of millions of dollars have funded Contingent Valuation (CV) studies of the non-use value of various environmental goods, such as the losses associated with the EXXON *Valdez* oil spill. EXXON commissioned Nobel laureates and other economists to debunk that study. Economists, like lawyers, take sides; economic estimates and valuations themselves become goods people are willing to pay for. No CV study, however expensive, has ever stood up as credible evidence in litigation.

Chastened by the transaction and information costs that bedevil official efforts to "get the prices right" or second-guess market outcomes, economists have turned to recommending ways that the government can create voluntary arrangements, such as markets in tradable rights and allowances, stakeholder negotiations, and governance committees, as ways to get to consensual and in that sense optimal outcomes. The question "what is the efficient allocation?" has given way to the question "what is the appropriate institution?" for governing resources such as watersheds and forests. When the government agency itself tries to govern, it becomes the object of *rent-seeking*, for example, zero-sum jockeying by opposing interest groups, which hire their own lawyers, economists, toxicologists, ecologists, and other experts. When these interest groups deal directly with each other by trading rights or by collaborating on decisions, they immensely reduce the transaction and information costs that tend otherwise to stymie environmental progress.

A Look Ahead

For thirty years, Congress and the executive branch have engaged in what psychologists call enabling behavior. Like an alcoholic and his or her spouse, Congress and the executive agencies may quarrel, but at a deeper level they have been in league with each other. By letting deadlines pass, accepting *reasonable progress* in lieu of compliance, substituting *reduced risk* for statutory *zero risk* standards, and otherwise failing to enforce legislation, agencies such as EPA spared Congress the unpleasantness of making hard choices and allowed it to parade itself as the defender of nature, personal rights, purity, and so on. Congress in turn gave the

agencies autonomy—the ability to work the law as they liked—within the tolerance of the courts.

In the spirit of the civil rights movement, environmentalists enforced landmark legislation by confrontation and litigation, primarily by suing EPA and other agencies for evading draconian statutes, such as the Delaney Clause. In 1992, the Ninth Circuit Court held that the EPA exceeded its statutory authority by allowing a *de minimis* risk standard in conflict with the language of the Delaney Clause. (*Les v. Riley*, 1992). The decision implied that food must be absolutely free of chemical additives, including pesticide residues, as the law requires, even if as a result no food could be produced or sold in the United States.

Congress responded by repealing the Delaney Clause and enacting a more flexible policy, the Food Quality Protection Act of 1996, in its place. This result whet the appetite of industry groups who hoped that if environmentalists prevailed in other suits, Congress might be forced to repeal other aspirational statutes. Industry lawyers began to argue that the CAA, for example, taken literally, prohibited all air pollution—and thus nearly all economic activity—or, if, taken in any other way, delegated the entire burden of lawmaking to executive agencies and derivatively to the courts. This would involve an unconstitutional delegation of legislative authority to other branches of government.

When in 1997, EPA tightened the air quality standards for particulate matter and ozone, the D.C. Circuit Court, in *American Trucking Association v. Whitman* (1999), in response to an industry legal challenge, remanded the regulation to EPA on the grounds that neither the statute nor EPA's interpretation of it provided an *intelligible principle* necessary to channel the authority Congress delegated to the executive agencies. In reviewing this decision in 2001, the Supreme Court refused to declare the CAA unconstitutional on the grounds that it delegated the tough tradeoffs—and thus legislative authority—to the agencies. The Court and others recognized, however, that EPA has yet to determine a stopping point for regulation, that is, a point at which emissions are safe enough.

Some commentators argue that EPA should regulate emissions to the *knee of the curve*, referring to a graph in which the x-axis represents pollution reduction and the y-axis represents cost. The idea is that the government should require firms to reduce pollution to the point at which the costs of controlling the *next* unit increase exponentially or go asymptotic. In addition, agencies can encourage new technologies that may push the knee of the curve ever farther out along the pollution-control or the x-axis.

Other commentators argue that the most efficient controls on big sources of pollution are mostly in place, and it is small polluters, indeed, individual households, that hold the key to reducing pollution by becoming more energy-efficient. The reluctance of Americans to replace incandescent with fluorescent bulbs, to drive cars with greater fuel economy, to install better thermostats, windows, insulation, and so on, indicates the extent of the problem. Throughout the 1970s and 1980s, Americans blamed others—particularly large corporations—for their environmental woes, but it is apparent that the behavior of individuals has to change. The motto of the environmental movement has become more and more pertinent since cartoonist Walt Kelly's Pogo coined it: "We have met the enemy, and he is us."

The International Perspective

The other motto, "Think globally; act locally," recognizes that environmental problems have important global dimensions, particularly because carbon dioxide and other *greenhouse* gasses threaten to cause climate change. To some extent the international community has dealt successfully with environmental threats; for example, the Montreal Protocol, an international accord signed in 1987, initiated controls on the production of chemicals that damage stratospheric ozone. And conventions aimed at preserving endangered species and controlling the harvest of common resources—whales, for example—have long exerted influence on the international community.

To an even greater extent, however, international environmental conventions and the institutions—called *regimes*—set up to implement them meet many of the same problems of enforcement that are familiar in domestic contexts. Many of the conventions—such as those that ban pollution in the North Sea—are hortatory or idealistic. Politicians enact these protocols under pressure from the *green* movement, but because of the very great costs involved, they make slow progress in enforcing them. Nongovernmental organizations take the lead in litigating, harassing, and otherwise reminding officials of their responsibilities under the protocols they signed.

In 1997, industrialized nations, including Japan, the United States, and members of the European Union, promised at Kyoto that by 2012 they would cut to significantly less than 1990 levels, and permanently limit their production of, CO_2 and other greenhouse gases. Developing countries such as China, India, Indonesia, and Malaysia, believing that the welfare of their people depends more on the growth of their economies than on the stability of the

atmosphere, refused to join the effort to lower emissions. These countries, because of rapid economic and population growth, are likely to surpass the industrialized nations in their greenhouse emissions within about fifteen years, and will by themselves emit more than enough greenhouse gases to destabilize the atmosphere. Partly for this reason, but also because of the costs involved, the U.S. Senate said that it would never ratify the climate treaty unless developing nations commit to *substantial participation.* President George W. Bush later brushed off the Kyoto Treaty entirely.

Environmental organizations have begun to turn their attention to international problems, particularly global climate change. Little has been said, however, about exactly how the United States should lower its emissions—whether by converting from coal-fired to nuclear energy, for example. Ethical debate has centered on a U.S. proposal to allow nations to sell credits for their *excess* reductions to other nations, who would then count them toward meeting their own targets. The United States, for example, might assist Russia to convert inefficient coal-burning electric utilities to cleaner and more efficient gas-fired power plants. The Russians would receive the new technology at little or no cost, and the United States would be able to take credit for the reduction in emissions from the Russian plants. It costs a lot less to achieve a 50 percent reduction from the dirtiest industries in Russia or India than a 10 percent reduction in industries that are already technologically advanced.

Critics have condemned pollution-trading because it "turns pollution into a commodity to be bought and sold," and thereby "removes the moral stigma that is properly associated with it" (Sandel). Yet CO_2, unlike toxic agents or carcinogens, should not be stigmatized. Under a safe global cap—let us say, the levels accepted at Kyoto—CO_2 emissions are not harmful or objectionable. If wealthy countries buy allowances by providing poorer countries with more efficient technologies, moreover, this does not necessarily indicate disrespect or arrogance, but might be looked at as partnership, if wealthy countries do not use less efficient technology at home than they subsidize abroad.

Some commentators have proposed a general requirement that ties CO_2 emissions to economic product, with the idea that wealthy countries can get credit for helping others reach the carbon-efficiency per dollar economic output achieved by the most efficient economies. The ethical impasse that stymies carbon *trading* strategies lies in finding a fair principle on which to distribute initial allowances—namely, whether to *grandfather* present levels or establish per-capita quotas. A global cap on greenhouse gases, in other words, must be translated into an initial set of permits nations can use or trade. This problem has proven intractable. As economist Tom Schelling has said, "Global emissions trading is an elegant idea, but I cannot seriously envision national representatives sitting down to divide up rights in perpetuity worth a trillion dollars" (Passell).

The greatest threat to the global environment remains war—especially in view of the proliferation of nuclear weapons. Environmental protocols, regimes, and conventions, when successful, bring nations closer together and teach them to cooperate with and to trust each other. Insofar as environmental protection encourages a sustainable peace, it will lay the surest foundation for environmental protection and sustainable development.

MARK SAGOFF (1995)
REVISED BY AUTHOR

SEE ALSO: *Endangered Species and Biodiversity; Environmental Ethics; Environmental Health*

BIBLIOGRAPHY

Ackerman, Bruce A. 1974. *The Uncertain Search for Environmental Quality.* New York: Free Press.

Ackerman, Bruce A., and Hassler, William T. 1981. *Clean Coal/Dirty Air: Or How the Clean Air Act Became a Multibillion-Dollar Bail-out for High-Sulfur Coal Producers and What Should Be Done About It.* New Haven, CT: Yale University Press.

American Trucking Association v. Whitman (175 F3d 1027 (DC Cir 1999), rev. in part as *Whitman v American Trucking Associations, Inc,* 531 US 457 (2001).

Farber, Daniel A. 1999. "Taking Slippage Seriously: Noncompliance and Creative Compliance in Environmental Law." *Harvard Environmental Law Review* 23.

Freeman, Jody. 2000. "The Contracting State." *Florida State University Law Review* 28(Fall): 155–204.

Kennedy, Duncan. 1981. "Cost Benefit Analysis." *Stanford Law Review* 33: 387–421.

Les v. Riley, 968 F.2d 985, 990 (9th Cir. 1992).

Melnick, R. Shep. 1983. *Regulation and the Courts: The Case of the Clean Air Act.* Washington, D.C.: Brookings Institution.

Orts, Eric W., and Deketelaere, Kurt, eds. 2001. *Environmental Contracts: Comparative Approaches to Regulatory Innovation in the United States and Europe.* Boston: Kluwer Law International.

Passell, P. 1997. Trading on the Pollution Exchange; Global Warming Plan Would Make Emissions a Commodity. New York Times, October 24, Section D, page 1, column 2.

Rosenbaum, Walter A. 1991. *Environmental Politics and Policy,* 2nd edition. Washington, D.C.: Congressional Quarterly Press.

Ruff, Larry. 1970. "The Economic Common Sense of Pollution," *The Public Interest* 19(Spring): 69–85.

Sandel, M. 1997. "It's Immoral to Buy the Right to Pollute." *New York Times,* Dec. 15, Sec. A., p. 23.

Stewart, Richard B. 2001. "A New Generation of Environmental Regulation?" *Capital University Law Review* 21: 29–141.

Vig, Norman J., and Axelrod, Regina S., eds. 1999. *The Global Environment: Institutions, Law, and Policy.* Washington, D.C.: Congressional Quarterly Press.

Vig, Norman J., and Kraft, Michael E., eds. 1994. *Environmental Policy in the 1990s: Toward a New Agenda,* 2nd edition. Washington, D.C.: Congressional Quarterly Press.

EPIDEMICS

• • •

Epidemics may be defined as concentrated outbursts of infectious or noninfectious disease, often with unusually high mortality, affecting relatively large numbers of people within fairly narrow limits of time and space. They probably emerged in human populations with the "Neolithic Revolution," roughly eight to ten thousand years ago, as humans began to domesticate animals, practice agriculture, and settle into towns and villages, with a corresponding increase in the density of population. This entry will cover the history of epidemics with particular reference to their implications for bioethics, beginning with a survey of ancient and medieval times, moving on to responses to epidemics before the nineteenth century, then examining in more detail the impact of cholera and the bacteriological revolution. It will conclude with a discussion of the epidemiological transition and its aftermath, the emergence of new epidemics in the late twentieth century, and the ethical implications of the data surveyed. The focus will be mainly but not exclusively on Europe and North America, where historical source material is richest, and scholarly and scientific studies are most numerous.

Ancient and Medieval Times

Hippocratic texts indicate the presence of tuberculosis, malaria, and influenza in the population of ancient Greece, and the historian Thucydides provides the first full description of a major plague, the precise nature of which remains uncertain, in Athens (430–429 B.C.E.), in his history of the

Peloponnesian War. The increase in trade brought about by the growth of the Roman Empire facilitated the transmission of disease, and there were massive epidemics in the Mediterranean (165–180 c.e. and 211–266 c.e.). The "plague of Justinian" (542–547 c.e.), which was said to have killed ten thousand people per day in Constantinople, is the first recorded appearance of bubonic plague (McNeill). In Europe and Asia, diseases such as measles and smallpox gradually became endemic, affecting virtually all parts of the population on a regular basis, with occasional epidemic outbursts. Periodic epidemics of bubonic plague continued, most seriously in the fourteenth century, when perhaps as much as one-third of Europe's population perished.

When Europeans arrived in the Americas, from 1492 on, they brought many of these diseases to native American populations for the first time, with devastating effects. The importation of African slaves introduced malaria and yellow fever by the seventeenth century (Kiple, 1984). The merging of the disease pools of the Old and New Worlds was completed by what appeared to be the transmission of syphilis to Europe from the Americas at the end of the fifteenth century, though the subject remains disputed by historians, some arguing that it was a recurrence or mutation of a disease that already existed on the Continent (Crosby).

Responses to Epidemics before the Nineteenth Century

The ancient Greeks and Romans commonly, though not universally, believed that epidemics were brought into human communities from outside. Thucydides, for example, described the plague that struck Athens during the Peloponnesian War as having arrived by sea. This belief was the basis of official reactions to epidemics in medieval Europe. Following the closure of the port at Venice to all shipping for thirty days as the plague threatened in 1346, regulations imposed in Marseilles in 1384, and in other ports thereafter, prescribed the biblical period of isolation for a "quarantine" (forty days) outside the harbor for any ship thought to have called previously at a place infected with the plague. In 1423 the Venetians set up a hospital where plague victims were isolated, and by 1485 the city had a sanitary authority armed with wide-ranging powers during epidemics. In some epidemics, as in the Great Plague of London in 1665, victims were compulsorily isolated in their own houses, which were marked with a red cross to warn the healthy not to enter. Compulsory screening was not an issue before the late nineteenth century, however, because diseases were recognized as such only after the onset of obvious symptoms, and the concept of the asymptomatic carrier did

not exist. In addition to these measures, the authorities in many medieval towns, working on the theory that epidemics were spread through the contamination of the atmosphere, ordered the fumigation of the streets to try to clear the air. Doctors and priests were expected to attend to the sick; and those who fled, as many did, are strongly criticized in the chronicles of these events.

Popular reactions to epidemics included not only flight from infected areas and evasion of public health measures, but also attacks on already marginalized and stigmatized minorities. As bubonic plague spread in Europe in 1348–1349, for example, rumors that the Jews were poisoning water supplies led to widespread pogroms. Over nine hundred Jews were massacred in the German city of Erfurt alone (Vasold). Such actions reflected a general feeling, reinforced by the church, that plagues were visited upon humankind by a wrathful Deity angered by immorality, irreligion, and the toleration of infidels. A prominent part in these persecutions was played by the flagellants, lay religious orders whose self-flagellating processions were intended to divert divine retribution from the rest of the population. Jews were scapegoated because they were not part of the Christian community. Drawing upon a lengthy tradition of Christian anti-Semitism, which blamed the Jews for the killing of Christ, the people of medieval Europe regarded Jews at such times as little better than the agents of Satan (Delumeau).

State, popular, religious, and medical responses such as these remained essentially constant well into the nineteenth century. The medical understanding of plague continued throughout this period to draw heavily on humoral theories, so that therapy centered on bloodletting and similar treatments designed to restore the humoral balance in the patient's body. They were of limited effectiveness in combating bubonic plague, which was spread by flea-infested rats. The isolation and hospitalization of victims also therefore did little to prevent the spread of plague. Nevertheless, the disease gradually retreated from western Europe, for reasons that are still imperfectly understood. The introduction of more effective quarantines with the emergence of the strong state in the seventeenth and eighteenth centuries was almost certainly one of these reasons, however, and helped prevent the recurrence of epidemics in the seventeenth and eighteenth centuries (Vasold).

State intervention also played a role in reducing the impact of smallpox, the other major killer disease of the age after bubonic plague. Its spread was first reduced by inoculation, before compulsory programs of cowpox vaccination brought about a dramatic reduction in the impact of the disease in nineteenth-century Europe. Despite the imperfections of these new methods, which sometimes included accidentally spreading the disease, vaccination programs in particular may be regarded as the first major achievement of the "medical policing" favored by eighteenth-century absolutist monarchies such as Prussia. Police methods that paid scant attention to the liberties of the subjects were used to combat the spread of epidemics. They included the use of troops to seal off infected districts, quarantines by land and sea, and the compulsory isolation of individual victims. Most of these measures had little effect, however, either because of lack of medical knowledge or because poor communications and lack of police and military manpower prevented them from being applied comprehensively (Rosen).

The Impact of Cholera

These theories and practices were brought into question above all by the arrival in Europe and North America of Asiatic cholera. The growth of the British Empire, especially in India, improved communications and trade, and facilitated the spread of cholera from its base in the Ganges delta to other parts of Asia and to the Middle East. Reaching Europe by the end of the 1820s, the disease was spread further by unsanitary and overcrowded living conditions in the rapidly growing towns and cities of the new industrial era. At particular moments of political conflict, above all in the European revolutions of 1830 and 1848, the Austro-Prussian War of 1866, and the Franco-Prussian War of 1870–1871, it was carried rapidly across the continent by troop movements and the mass flight of affected civilian populations (Evans, 1988).

Cholera epidemics affected the United States in 1832, 1849, and 1866, on each occasion arriving from Europe in the aftermath of a major conflict. State, popular, and medical responses in 1830–1832 were unchanged from earlier reactions to epidemics. Quarantine regulations were imposed, military cordons established, victims isolated, hospitals prepared. In Prussia, the breaching of such regulations was made punishable by death. But the opposition that such measures aroused among increasingly powerful industrial and trading interests, and the feeling among many liberals that the policing of disease involved unwarranted interference with the liberty of the individual, forced the state to retreat from combating cholera by the time of the next epidemic, in the late 1840s. In addition, medical theories of contagion were brought into disrepute by the failure of quarantine and isolation to stop the spread of the disease in Europe. Until the 1880s, many doctors thought that cholera was caused by a "miasma" or vapor rising from the ground

under certain climatic circumstances. It could be prevented by cleaning up the cities so as to prevent the source of infection from getting into the soil (Evans, 1987). This was a contributory factor in the spread of sanitary reform in Europe and the United States during this period. But its importance should not be overestimated. Boards of health established in American cities in the midst of the cholera epidemics of 1832 and 1849 were short-lived and of limited effectiveness, and even in 1866 the more determined official responses had less to do with the impact of cholera than with the changed political climate (Rosenberg).

The fact that cholera affected the poorest sectors of society most profoundly was the result above all of structural factors such as unsanitary and overcrowded living conditions, unhygienic water supplies, and ineffective methods of waste disposal. But state and public responses to epidemics in the nineteenth century, at least in the decades after the initial impact of cholera, were primarily voluntaristic. Religious and secular commentators blamed cholera on the alleged immorality, drunkenness, sexual excess, idleness, and lack of moral fiber of the victims. Fast days were held in eleven New England states in 1832, in the belief that piety would divert God's avenging hand. Once again, the socially marginal groups of industrial society, from vagrants and the unemployed to prostitutes and beggars—or, in the United States in 1866, the newly emancipated slaves and the newly arrived Irish immigrants—were blamed (Rosenberg).

The rise of the medical profession, with well-regulated training and a code of ethics, ensured that doctors were more consistently active in treating victims of epidemics in the nineteenth century than they had been in previous times. Partly as a result, there were popular attacks on the medical profession in Europe during the epidemic of 1830–1832. Angry crowds accused doctors of poisoning the poor in order to be able to reduce the burden of support they imposed on the state or, in Britain, in order to provide fresh bodies for the anatomy schools (Durey). As late as 1892, doctors and state officials were being killed in cholera riots in Russia (Frieden). There were also disturbances in the United States, where a hospital was burned down in Pittsburgh and a quarantine hospital on Staten Island, in New York City, was destroyed by rioters fearing the spread of yellow fever. However, in most of Europe, public disturbances caused by epidemics had largely ceased by the middle of the nineteenth century. Fear of disorder was another reason for the state's withdrawal from policing measures (Evans, 1988). In Europe, too, religious responses to epidemics had become less important by the end of the century as religious observance declined. In 1892, however, as cholera once more threatened America's shores, it fed nativist prejudice and led to the introduction of harsh new restrictions on immigration.

The Bacteriological Revolution

Cholera was only the most dramatic of a number of infectious diseases that took advantage of urbanization, poor hygiene, overcrowding, and improved communications in the nineteenth century (Bardet et al.). Typhus, typhoid, diphtheria, yellow fever, tuberculosis, malaria, and syphilis continued to have a major impact, and even smallpox returned on a large scale during the Franco-Prussian War of 1870–1871. Treatment continued to be ineffective. But the rapid development of microscope technology in the last quarter of the century enabled medical science to discover the causative agents of many infectious diseases in humans and animals. Building on the achievements of Louis Pasteur, Robert Koch identified the tubercle bacillus in 1882 and the cholera bacillus in 1884. These discoveries marked the triumph of bacteriology and completed the swing of medical opinion back from belief in "miasmas" as causes of epidemics toward a contagionist point of view.

From the 1880s, states once more imposed quarantine and isolation, backed by preventive disinfection. The greater effectiveness of state controls, compared with the earlier part of the century, was combined with the more precise focus on eliminating bacterial organisms. Once the role of victims' excretions in contaminating water supplies with the cholera bacillus became known, it was possible to take preventive action by ensuring hygienic water supplies and safe waste disposal. By the outbreak of World War I in 1914, the role of the human body louse in spreading typhus, and that of the mosquito in transmitting malaria and yellow fever, had been identified. Mosquito control programs were launched by the U.S. Army in Cuba following the Spanish-American War of 1898, and subsequently in the Panama Canal Zone, in order to reduce the incidence of yellow fever cases to an acceptable level. Regular delousing reduced typhus among armies on the western front in Europe during World War I. The Japanese army prevented casualties from typhoid and smallpox by a campaign of systematic vaccination during the war with Russia in 1904–1905 (McNeill; Cartwright).

The bacteriological revolution thus inaugurated an age of sharply increased state controls over the spread of disease. Laws were introduced in many countries making the reporting of infectious diseases compulsory. The growth of a comprehensive, state-backed system of medical care, working through medical officers, medical insurance plans, and the like, made comprehensive reporting easier. Hospital building programs in the second half of the nineteenth century facilitated the isolation of victims in hygienic conditions where they could be prevented from spreading the disease. The greater prestige of the medical profession in most industrialized countries by the late nineteenth and early twentieth century ensured that doctors were no longer attacked, and that the necessity of compulsory reporting and isolation was widely accepted by the public. However, a bacteriological understanding of disease causation also involved a narrowing of focus, in which increased emphasis was placed on the compulsory reporting of cases, followed by their isolation, at the expense of broader measures of public health and environmental improvement (Porter).

The Epidemiological Transition

Lower death rates from diseases such as cholera, typhoid, and tuberculosis were only partially the consequence of bacteriologically inspired state preventive measures, and the disease burden from acute infectious disease began to decline rapidly. The provision of clean, properly filtered water supplies and effective sewage systems reflected growing municipal pride and the middle-class desire for cleanliness. It made epidemics such as the outbreak of cholera that killed over eight thousand people in Hamburg, Germany, in little over six weeks in the autumn of 1892 increasingly rare. Just as important were improvements in personal hygiene, which again reflected general social trends as well as the growing "medicalization" of society in western Europe and the United States. Such developments reinforced the stigmatization of poor and oppressed minorities as carriers of infection, since they were now blamed for ignoring official exhortations to maintain high standards of cleanliness, even though their living conditions and personal circumstances frequently made it difficult for them to do so. Particular attention was focused on working-class women, who were held responsible by official and medical opinion for any lack of hygiene in the home (Evans, 1987).

The development of tuberculin by Koch in 1890 made possible the compulsory screening of populations even for asymptomatic tuberculosis. This was increasingly implemented after 1900, in conjunction with the forcible removal of carriers to sanatoria, although this was more effective in isolating people than in curing them. Educational measures also helped reduce the spread of the disease. The development and compulsory administration in many countries of a preventive vaccine against tuberculosis from the 1920s aroused resistance among the medical community, not least because by creating a positive tuberculin reaction in noncarriers, it made it impossible to detect those who truly had the disease, except where symptoms were obvious. These measures had some effect in reducing the impact of the disease. However, although the precise causes of the retreat of tuberculosis remain a matter of controversy among historians, the long-term decline of the disease from the middle of the nineteenth century was probably more the result of improvements in housing, hygiene, environmental sanitation, and living standards than of direct medical intervention. The introduction of antibiotics such as strep-tomycin after World War II proved effective in reducing to insignificant levels mortality from a disease that had been the most frequent cause of death or disability among Americans aged fifteen to forty-five (Dubos and Dubos).

Similarly, official responses to syphilis centered, especially in Europe, on the forcible confinement of prostitutes to state-licensed brothels or locked hospital wards, where they were subjected to compulsory medical examination. Before World War I, New York, California, and other states had introduced compulsory reporting of cases of venereal disease, and official concern for the health of U.S. troops led to the jailing of prostitutes. Measures such as these had no discernible effect on infection rates, which rose sharply during the war. They also represented a serious restriction on the civil liberties of an already stigmatized group of women, while the men who were their customers, and equally active in the sexual transmission of disease, were regarded as irresponsible at worst, and were not subjected to similar measures. The development of Salvarsan (arsphenamine) by Paul Ehrlich in 1910 introduced the possibility of an effective treatment for syphilis. But here again there was resistance, both within the medical community and from outside, from those who considered that an increase in sexual promiscuity would be a result. This view became even more widespread following the use of penicillin on a large scale during World War II (Brandt).

Epidemics of the Late Twentieth Century

In the West, epidemic infectious disease was regarded by the second half of the twentieth century as indicating an uncivil-ized state of mind, and was ascribed above all to nonwhite populations in parts of the world outside Europe and North America. This reflected structural inequalities in the world economy, as the great infections became increasingly con-centrated in the poor countries of the Third World. By the middle of the twentieth century, however, rapidly increasing life expectancy was bringing rapid growth of noninfectious cardiac diseases, cancer, and other chronic conditions that posed new epidemic threats to an aging population in the affluent West. Under increasing pressure from the medical profession, the state responded not only with education initiatives but also with punitive measures directed toward habits, such as cigarette smoking, that were thought to make such conditions more likely. The arsenal of sanctions gov-ernments employed included punitive taxation on tobacco

and the banning of smoking, under threat of fines and imprisonment, in a growing number of public places. Increas-ingly, institutions in the private sector also adopted these policies. They raised the question of how far state and nonstate institutions could go in forcing people to abandon pleasures that were demonstrably harmful to their own health. At the same time, they contrasted strongly with the reluctance of many states and companies to admit responsi-bility for cancer epidemics caused by factors such as nuclear weapons testing, the proximity of nuclear power stations to human populations, or the lack of proper precautions in dealing with radioactivity in industrial production.

In the 1980s, the identification of a new epidemic, known as acquired immune deficiency syndrome (AIDS), once more raised the ethical problems faced by state and society, and by the medical profession, in the past. Lack of medical knowledge of the syndrome and the danger of infection from contact with blood or other body fluids, posed the question of whether the medical profession had a duty to treat AIDS sufferers in the absence of any cure. The evidence of the overwhelming majority of past epidemics, for which there was also no known cure, seems to be, however, that medical treatment, even in the Middle Ages, could alleviate suffering under some circumstances, and was therefore a duty of the practitioner. In a condition that could prove rapidly fatal, the ethics of prolonged tests of a drug such as AZT, in which control groups were given placebos, was contested by AIDS sufferers anxious to try anything that might possibly cure the condition, or at least slow its progress.

If this was a relatively novel ethical problem, then the question of compulsory public-health measures was a very old one. Like the sufferers in many previous epidemics, AIDS victims tended to come from already stigmatized social groups: gays, drug abusers and prostitutes, Haitians and Africans. The ability to screen these high-risk groups for the presence of the causative agent, the HIV retrovirus, even at the asymptomatic stage, raised the possibility of compul-sory screening measures, quarantine, and isolation. On the other hand, individuals publicly identified as HIV-positive generally found it difficult or impossible to stay employed, to obtain life or health insurance, or to avoid eviction from their homes. In the absence of adequate supportive meas-ures, public-health intervention reinforces existing discrimi-nation against these groups, as in many past epidemics.

An alternative state response has consisted of neglect, on the assumption that AIDS is unlikely to affect the heterosexual, non-drug-abusing, nonpromiscuous majority of the voting public. It is noticeable that, generally, politi-cians have invested resources in public education and other preventive measures only when they have believed that the majority population is at risk. These problems have been raised again by the recent resurgence of tuberculosis in Western countries, among the HIV-positive but also among the poor and the homeless. Drug-resistant strains of the disease have become common, and the transient, jobless, and destitute have neither the means nor the stability of lifestyle to complete the lengthy course of drugs that is necessary to effect a cure. The compulsory isolation of victims and their forcible subjection to a course of treatment is not a satisfactory long-term solution to the problem, since reinfection is likely upon release, unless the social and personal circumstances of the affected groups undergo a dramatic improvement.

Conclusion: Ethical Implications

The history of epidemics suggests that society's responses have usually included scapegoating marginal and already stigmatized groups and the restriction of their civil rights. From the Jews massacred during the Black Death in medieval Europe, through the beggars and vagrants blamed for the spread of cholera in the nineteenth century, to the prostitutes arrested for allegedly infecting troops with syphilis during World War I, and the minorities whose life-styles were widely regarded as responsible for the spread of AIDS in the 1980s and 1990s, such groups have frequently been subjected to social ostracism and official hostility in times of epidemic disease. Frequently, though not invariably, they have been the very people who have suffered most severely from the disease they were accused of spreading. Doctors have sometimes been reluctant to treat them; the state has often responded with punitive measures.

At no time have public-health measures to combat epidemics been politically uncontested. Nineteenth-century feminists, for example, campaigned vigorously against the state's restriction of the civil liberties of prostitutes in the name of disease control. The fact that their male customers were left free to spread sexually transmitted diseases unhampered by the attentions of the state implied an official endorsement of different standards of morality for men and for women, and it was this major structural element of the social value system that the feminists were seeking to change. Without such change, not only was medical intervention ethically indefensible, but there would never be any likelihood of effective control of sexually transmitted diseases. Similarly, many nineteenth-century epidemics, such as cholera or tuberculosis, were spread by poor nutrition, overcrowded housing, and inadequate sanitation. Social reformers therefore regarded major improvements in these areas as more important than direct medical intervention through measures such as compulsory hospitalization.

Epidemics are frequently caused by social and political upheavals. In the past, movements of large masses of troops and civilians across Europe, from the Crusades to the Crimean War, brought epidemics in their wake. In the early 1990s, a major cholera epidemic broke out in Peru as the result of the flight of thousands of peasants from their mountain settlements, driven out by the pitiless armed conflict between the army and the "Shining Path" guerrillas, to the narrow coastal strip, where they lived in makeshift shantytowns with no sanitation. Economic crisis and the dismantling of welfare measures for the homeless, the mentally disturbed, and the destitute in many Western countries in the 1980s contributed to a massive increase in the transient population on the streets of the great cities. Discrimination against AIDS sufferers by landlords and employers has added to this problem. By the early 1990s there were an estimated ninety thousand homeless on the streets of New York City, half of whom were HIV-positive and several thousand of whom were suffering from tuberculosis. Any long-term solution to these epidemics must be more than merely medical, as must any explanation of their occurrence. Public-health measures are thus inevitably political in their implications, since they can be considered and administered only with reference to the wider social and cultural context within which the disease they seek to prevent or control has originated.

RICHARD J. EVANS (1995)
BIBLIOGRAPHY REVISED

SEE ALSO: *AIDS; Bioethics, African-American Perspectives; Bioterrorism; Care; Communitarianism and Bioethics; Human Rights; Literature and Healthcare; Medical Ethics, History of Europe; Narrative; Public Health, History; Public Health, Philosophy; Sexual Behavior, Social Control of*

BIBLIOGRAPHY

Bardet, Jean-Pierre; Bourdelais, Patrice; Guillaume, Pierre; Lebrun, François; and Queétel, Claude, eds. 1988. *Peurs et terreurs face à la contagion: Cholera, tuberculose, syphilis: XIXe-XXe siécles.* Paris: Fayard.

Benatar, Soloman R. 2002. "The HIV/AIDS Pandemic: A Sign of Instability in a Complex Global System." *Journal of Medicine and Philosophy* 27(2): 163–177.

Brandt, Allan M. 1987. *No Magic Bullet. A Social History of Venereal Disease in the United States Since 1880,* rev. edition. New York: Oxford University Press.

Cartwright, Frederick F. 1972. *Disease and History.* London: Hart-Davis.

Cliff, Andrew; Haggett, Peter; and Smallman-Raynor, Matthew. 1998. *Deciphering Global Epidemics: Analytical Approaches to the Disease Records of World Cities, 1888–1912.* New York: Cambridge University Press.

Crosby, Alfred W. 1972. *The Columbian Exchange: Biological and Cultural Consequences of 1492.* Westport, CT: Greenwood.

Delumeau, Jean. 1990. *Sin and Fear: The Emergence of a Western Guilt Culture, 13th–18th Centuries.* New York: St. Martin's Press.

Dubos, René, and Dubos, Jean. 1987. *The White Plague. Tuberculosis, Man and Society.* New Brunswick, NJ: Rutgers University Press.

Durey, Michael. 1979. *The Return of the Plague: British Society and the Cholera.* Dublin: Gill & Macmillan.

Evans, Richard J. 1987. *Death in Hamburg: Society and Politics in the Cholera Years 1830–1910.* Oxford: Clarendon Press.

Evans, Richard J. 1988. "Epidemics and Revolutions: Cholera in Nineteenth-Century Europe." *Past and Present* (120): 123–146.

Frieden, Nancy M. 1977. "The Russian Cholera Epidemic, 1892–93, and Medical Professionalization." *Journal of Social History* 10: 538–559.

Gayle, Helene. 2000. "An Overview of the Global HIV/AIDS Epidemic, with a Focus on the United States." *AIDS* 14 (Supplement 2): S8–S17.

Gostin, Lawrence O.; Ward, John W.; and Baker, A. Cornelius. 1997. "National HIV Case Reporting for the United States. A Defining Moment in the History of the Epidemic." *New England Journal of Medicine* 337(16): 1162–1167.

Guillemin, Jeanne. 2000. "Anthrax: The Investigation of a Deadly Outbreak." *New England Journal of Medicine* 343(16): 1198.

Hays, J. N. 1998. *The Burdens of Disease: Epidemics and Human Response in Western History.* Piscataway, NJ: Rutgers University Press.

Kiple, Kenneth F. 1984. *The Caribbean Slave: A Biological History.* Cambridge, Eng.: Cambridge University Press.

Kiple, Kenneth F. 1993. *The Cambridge World History and Geography of Human Disease.* Cambridge, Eng.: Cambridge University Press.

Lachmann, Peter J. 1998. "Public Health and Bioethics." *Journal of Medicine and Philosophy* 23(3): 297–302.

Lederberg, Joshua. 2000. "Infectious History." *Science* 288(5464): 287–293.

Markel, Howard. 1999. *Quarantine!: East European Jewish Immigrants and the New York City Epidemics of 1892* Baltimore: Johns Hopkins University Press.

McNeill, William H. 1979. *Plagues and Peoples.* Harmondsworth, Eng.: Penguin.

Oldstone, Michael B. A. 1998. *Viruses, Plagues, and History.* New York: Oxford University Press.

Porter, Dorothy. 1993. "Public Health." In *Companion Encyclopedia of the History of Medicine,* ed. W. F. Bynum and Roy Porter. London: Routledge.

Rosen, George, comp. 1974. *From Medical Police to Social Medicine: Essays on the History of Health Care.* New York: Social History Publications.

Rosenberg, Charles E. 1987. *The Cholera Years: The United States in 1832, 1849, and 1866,* rev. edition. Chicago: University of Chicago Press.

Rosenberg, Charles E. 1992. *Explaining Epidemics: And Other Studies in the History of Medicine.* New York: Cambridge University Press.

Tuohey, John F. 1995. "Moving From Autonomy to Responsibility in HIV-Related Healthcare." *Cambridge Quarterly of Healthcare Ethics* 4(1): 64–70.

van Niekerk, Anton A. 2002. "Moral and Social Complexities of AIDS in Africa." *Journal of Medicine and Philosophy* 27(2): 143–162.

Vasold, Manfred. 1991. *Pest, Not und schwere Plagen: Seuchen und Epidemien von Mittelalter bis heute.* Munich: C. H. Beck.

Watts, Sheldon. 1999. *Epidemics and History: Disease, Power and Imperialism.* New Haven, CT: Yale University Press.

ETHICS

• • •

I. TASK OF ETHICS

Ethics as a philosophical or theoretical discipline is concerned with tasks that concern ordinary, reflective individuals. Since its origins in classical and preclassical times, it has sought to understand how human beings should act and what kind of life is best for people. When Socrates and Plato dealt with such questions, they presupposed or at the very least hoped that they could be answered in "timeless" fashion, that is, with answers that were not dependent on the culture and circumstances of the answerer, but represented universally valid, rational conclusions.

In fact, however, the history of philosophical or theoretical ethics is intimately related to the ethical views and practices prevalent in various societies over the millennia. Although philosophers have usually sought to answer ethical questions without regard to (and sometimes in defiance of) some of the standards and traditions prevalent around them, the history of ethics as a philosophical discipline bears interesting connections to what has happened in given philosophers' societies and the world at large. Perhaps the clearest example of this lies in the influence of Christianity on the history of theoretical ethics.

Philosophical/theoretical ethics, of course, has had its own influence on Christianity, for example, Aristotle's influence on the philosophy of Thomas Aquinas and on the views and practices of the church. Nonetheless, to compare the character of the pre-Christian ethics of Socrates, Plato, Aristotle, the Stoics, the Epicureans, and other schools of ancient ethical thought with the kinds of ethics that have flourished in the academy since Christianity became a dominant social force is to recognize that larger social and historical currents play significant roles in the sphere of philosophical ethics.

Socrates, Plato, and Aristotle, for example, do not discuss kindness or compassion, moral guilt, or the virtue of self-denial, or selflessness. Christianity helped to bring these notions to the attention of philosophy and to make philosophers think that issues framed in terms of them were central to their task. By the same token, a late-twentieth-century revival of interest in ancient approaches to ethics may reflect the diminishing force and domination of Christian thinking in the contemporary world.

But if the concepts that ethics focuses on can change so profoundly, one may well wonder whether a single discipline of ethics can be said to persist across the ages, or even whether such a thing as "the task" of philosophical ethics can be said to endure. Socrates, and later Plato, were perhaps the first philosophers to make a self-conscious attempt to answer general ethical questions on the basis of reason and argument rather than convention and tradition. But was the task they accepted really the same as that of contemporary ethics? This issue needs to be addressed before the task of ethics can be described.

Despite the fact that the concepts and problems of physics have varied over the last few centuries, it is still possible to speak of the history of a single discipline called physics. Moreover, we might say that the task of physics has been and remains that of developing physical concepts for the explanation and description of physical phenomena. Something similar can be said about theoretical ethics. Over the millennia, thoughtful people and philosophers have asked what kind of life is best for the individual and how one ought to behave in regard to other individuals and society as a whole. Although different concepts have been proposed to assist in the task of answering these questions, the questions themselves have retained an identity substantial enough to allow one to speak of the task of philosophical ethics without doing an injustice to the history of ethics.

The History of Ethical Theories

There has been a good deal less variation in philosophical concepts between those Plato employed and those we employ than there has been in regard to physical concepts within the field of physics. Concepts in philosophical ethics are the instruments with which philosophers address perennial ethical questions, and the distinctive contribution of any given theoretical approach to ethics resides in how (and how well) it integrates such concepts into an overall ethical view.

The concepts of ethics fall into two main categories. The first category comprises notions having to do with morality, virtue, rationality, and other ideals or standards of conduct and motivation; the second, notions pertaining to human good or well-being and the "good life" generally. Notice that morality is only one part, albeit a major one, of the first category. Claims and ideals concerning how it is rational for us to behave are not necessarily "moral" within our rather narrow modern understanding of that notion. Prudence and far-sightedness, for example, are rational, but their absence is not usually regarded as any kind of moral fault; and since these traits are also usually regarded as virtues, it seems we have room for virtues that are not specifically moral virtues. In addition, questions about human well-being and about what kind of life is best to have are less clearly questions of morality, narrowly conceived, than of ethics regarded as an encompassing philosophical discipline. The two categories mentioned above basically divide the concepts of ethics understood in this broad sense, and all major, substantive ethical theories attempt to say something about how these two classes of concepts relate to one another. Since modern views employ concepts and ask specific questions that are more familiar to contemporary readers, these views will be discussed first.

DEONTOLOGY. Modern deontology treats moral obligations as requirements that bind us to act, in large measure, independent of the effects our actions may have on our own good or well-being, and to a substantial extent, even independent of the effects of our actions on the well-being of others. The categorical imperative of Immanuel Kant (1724–1804), in one of its main formulations, tells us that we may not use or mistreat other people as a means either to our own happiness or to that of other people, and various forms of moral intuitionism make similar claims (1964). Intuitionists typically differ from Kant in holding that there are several independent, fundamental moral requirements (e.g., to keep promises, not to harm others, to tell the truth). But they agree with Kant that moral obligation is not just a matter of good consequences for an individual agent or for sentient beings generally. Thus even though deontologists such as Kant and, in the twentieth century, W. D. Ross, have definite views about human well-being, they do not think of moral goodness and moral obligation as rooted in facts about human well-being (or the well-being of sentient beings generally); and here a comparison with Judeo-Christian religious thought seems not inappropriate.

The Ten Commandments are not a product of rational philosophy; they have their source in religious tradition and/or divine command. They do, however, represent a kind of answer to the question about how one should behave toward others; that is, they ask the question that philosophical ethics attempts to answer. Moreover, the way the Ten Commandments answer this question is somewhat analogous to the way moral principles are conceived by deontologists such as Kant and the intuitionists.

In religious thinking, the Ten Commandments are not morally binding through some connection to the well-being or happiness of individuals or even the larger community; they are binding because God has commanded them, and deontology seeks to substitute for the idea of a deity, the idea of requirements given by reason itself or of binding obligations perceivable by moral insight. The deontologist typically holds that one's own well-being and that of others are taken into account and given some weight by the set of binding moral requirements, but that these are not the only considerations that affect what we ought to do generally or on particular occasions. For deontologists, the end does not always justify the means, and certain kinds of actions—torture, betrayal, injustice—are wrong for reasons having little to do with good or desirable consequences.

CONSEQUENTIALISM. The contrast here is with so-called consequentialists, for whom all moral obligation and virtue are to be understood in terms of good or desirable consequences. Typically, this has meant framing some conception of human or sentient good or well-being and claiming that all morality is derivative from or understandable in terms such as "good" or "well-being." Thus Jeremy Bentham, Henry Sidgwick (1981), and other utilitarian consequentialists regard pleasure or the satisfaction of desire as the sole, intrinsic human good, and pain or dissatisfaction as the sole,

intrinsic evil or ill, and they conceive our moral obligations as grounded entirely in considerations of pleasure and pain. The idea that one should always act to secure the greatest good of the greatest number is simply a way of saying that whether an act is right or wrong depends solely on whether its overall and long-term consequences for human (or sentient) well-being are at least as good as those of any alternative act available to a given agent. And since classical utilitarianism conceives human good or well-being in terms of pleasure or satisfaction, it holds that the rightness of an action always depends on whether it produces, overall and in the long run, as great a net balance of pleasure over pain as could have been produced by performing any of its alternatives.

This utilitarian moral standard is rather demanding, because it says that anything less than the maximization of overall human good or pleasure is wrong, and that means that if I fail to sacrifice my own comfort or career when doing so would allow me to do more overall good for humanity, then I act wrongly. But apart from the fact of how much it demands—there is nothing, after all, in the Ten Commandments or in the obligations defended by deontologists that requires such extreme sacrifice—what is most distinctive about utilitarianism is its claim that moral right and wrong (and moral good and evil) are totally, not merely partially, concerned with producing desirable results. The end, indeed, does justify the means, according to utilitarianism, and thus one might even be justified in killing, say, one innocent person in order to preserve the lives of two others.

Most deontologists would regard this as the most implausible, vulnerable feature of utilitarian and other consequentialist moral conceptions. But the utilitarian can point out that if you do not make human or sentient happiness the touchstone of all morality, but rely instead on certain "given" intuitions about what morally must or must not be done, you have given yourself a formula for preserving all the moral prejudices that have come down to us from the past. We require, Bentham argued, some external standard by which not only the state of individuals and society, but also all our inherited moral beliefs and intuitions can be properly evaluated. Bentham claimed that judging everything in terms of pleasure and pain can enable us to accomplish this goal. Historically, utilitarianism was conceived and used as a reformist moral and political doctrine, and that is one of its main strengths. If overall human happiness is the measure of moral requirement and moral goodness, then aristocratic privilege and the political disenfranchisement of all but the landed and wealthy are clearly open to attack, and Bentham and his "radical" allied did, in fact, make use of utilitarian ideas as a basis for making reforms in the British political and legal system.

But not all the reformist notions and energies lie on the side of consequentialism. The version of Kant's categorical imperative that speaks of never treating people merely as means, but always (also) as ends in themselves, was based on the idea of the fundamental dignity and worth of all human beings. Such a notion is clearly capable of being used—and, in fact, has been used—in reformist fashion to defend political and civil rights.

The debate between deontology and consequentialism has remained fundamentally important in philosophical ethics. Although there are other forms of consequentialism besides utilitarianism and other forms of deontology besides Kantian ethics, the main issue and choice has been widely regarded as lying between utilitarianism and Kant. This may be partly explained by the interest contemporary ethics has shown in understanding ethical and political issues as fundamentally interrelated; for both utilitarianism and Kantianism can claim to be "on the side of the angels" in regard to the large questions of social-political choice and reform that have exercised us in the modern period and may well continue to do so.

In the ancient world, the philosophical interest in ethics was also connected to larger political and social issues; both Plato (ca. 430–347 B.C.E.) and Aristotle sought to embed their ideas about personal morality within a larger picture of how society or the state should operate. Moreover, Plato was a radical and a reformer, though the *Republic* takes a direction precisely opposite to that of both utilitarianism and Kantianism. Plato was deeply distrustful of democratic politics and of the moral and political capacities of most human beings. His *Republic* (1974) advocates the rule of philosophers who have been specially trained to understand the nature of "the Good" over all those who have not attained such mystic/intellectual insight. Nor does Aristotle defend democracy. In somewhat milder form, he prefers the rule of virtuous individuals over those who lack—and lack the basic capacity for—virtue. If the ancient world contains any roots of democratic thinking, they lie in Stoicism, which emphasized the brotherhood of man (which seems to leave women out of account), but also spoke of the divine spark in every individual (including women). (Kant took the idea that all human beings have dignity, rather than mere price, from the Stoic Seneca [4 B.C.E.–C.E. 65].)

VIRTUE ETHICS. All schools of ancient ethics defended one or another form of "virtue ethics." That is, they typically conceived what was admirable about individuals in terms of traits of character, rather than in terms of individual obedience to some set of moral or ethical rules or requirements. Ancient ethics was also predominantly eudaimonistic.

Eudaimonia is the ancient Greek word for being fortunate or doing well in life, and eudaimonism is the view that our first concern in ethics is with the nature and conditions of human happiness/well-being and in particular our own happiness/well-being. This does not mean that all ancient ethics was egoistic, if by that term one refers to views according to which the moral or rational agent should always aim at his or her own (greatest) good or well-being. Aristotle is a clear example of an ethical thinker whose fundamental orientation is eudaimonistic, but who is far from advocating that people should always aim at their own self-interest.

For Aristotle, the question to begin with in ethics is the question of what is good for human beings. But Aristotle argues that human good or happiness largely consists in being actively virtuous, thus tying what is desirable in life to what is admirable in life in a rather distinctive way. For Aristotle, the virtuous individual will often aim at the good of others and/or at certain noble ideals, rather than seek to advance his or her own well-being, so egoism is no part of Aristotelianism.

But certainly most interpreters have regarded the Epicureans as having a basically egoistic doctrine. Epicureanism resembled utilitarianism in treating pleasure and the absence of pain as the sole conditions of human well-being. Rather than urge us to seek the greatest good of the greatest number, however, the Epicureans argued that virtue consisted in seeking one's own greatest pleasure/absence of pain. (Given certain pessimistic assumptions, the Epicureans thought this was best accomplished by minimizing one's desires and simplifying one's life.)

Although there are some notable modern egoists (e.g., Hobbes, Spinoza, and Nietzsche), most recent moral philosophers have assumed that there are fundamental, rational reasons for being concerned with something other than one's own well-being. Moreover, the eudaimonistic assumption that questions about individual happiness or well-being are the first concern of ethics has, in modern times, given way to a more basic emphasis on questions like, "How ought I to act?" and "What obligations have I?" The Jewish and Christian religious traditions seem to have made some difference here. In both traditions, God's commandments are supposed to have force for one independent of any question of one's own well-being (assuming that one is to obey because God has commanded, and not just because one fears divine punishment). For most Christians, moreover, Jesus sacrificing himself for our redemption places a totally non-egoistic motive at the pinnacle of the Christian vision of morality. So the notions that one should always be concerned with one's own well-being, and that ethics is chiefly about how one is to conceive and attain a good life, are both profoundly challenged by any moral philosophy that takes Judaism or Christianity, understood in the above fashion, seriously.

Recent Developments

Twentieth-century philosophical ethics bears the imprint of much of the history of the discipline, and many of the more current, prominent approaches to the subject represent developments of historically important views. But earlier in the twentieth century, ethics, at least in Britain and in the United States, veered away from its past in the direction of what has come to be called metaethics. The move toward metaethics and away from traditional ethical theory resulted, in part, from the influence of a school of philosophy called logical positivism. The positivists held up experimentally verifiable science as the paradigm of cognitively meaningful discourse and claimed that any statement that was not empirically confirmable or mathematically demonstrable lacked real content. Since it is difficult to see how moral principles can be experimentally verified or mathematically proved, many positivist ethicists began to think of ethical claims as cognitively meaningless and refused to advance substantive moral views, turning instead to the analysis of ethical terms and ethical claims. Issues about the meaning of moral terms have a long history in philosophical ethics, but the idea that these metaethical tasks were the main task of philosophical ethics gained a prevalence in the early years of the twentieth century that it had never previously had.

In the latter half of the twentieth century, substantive or normative ethics (that is, ethics making real value judgments rather than simply analyzing such judgments) once again came to the fore and tended to displace metaethics as the center of interest in ethics. In particular, there was a resurgence of interest in Kantian ethics and utilitarianism, followed by a renewal of interest in the kind of virtue ethics that dominated the philosophical landscape of ancient philosophy.

The revival and further development of Kantian ethics received its principal impetus from John Rawls and younger philosophers influenced by him. Rawls's principal work, *A Theory of Justice* (1971) represents a sustained attack on utilitarianism and seeks to base its own positive conception of morality and social justice on an understanding of Kant's ethics that bypasses the controversial metaphysical assumptions Kant was thought to have made about absolute human freedom and rationality. Other Kantian ethicists (Christine Korsgaard, Onora O'Neill, and Barbara Herman), however, have sought to be somewhat truer to the historical Kant while developing Kant's doctrines in directions fruitful for contemporary ethical theorizing.

Meanwhile, the utilitarians responded to Rawls's critique with reinvigorated forms of their doctrine, and, in particular, Derek Parfit's Reasons and Persons (1984) seeks to advance the utilitarian tradition of ethical theory within a philosophical perspective that fully takes into account the insights of the Rawlsian approach.

Finally, virtue ethics has been undergoing a considerable revival. In a 1958 article, Elizabeth Anscombe argued that notions like moral obligation are bankrupt without the assumption of God (or someone else) as a lawgiver, whereas concepts of character excellence or virtue and of human flourishing can arise, without such assumptions, from within a properly conceived moral psychology. This challenge was taken up by philosophers interested in exploring the possibility that the notions of good character and motivation and of living well may be primary in ethics, with notions like right, wrong, and obligation taking a secondary or derivative place or perhaps even dropping out altogether. Such virtue ethics does not, however, abandon ethics' traditional task of telling us how to live, since, in fact, ideals of good character and motivation can naturally lead to views about how it is best to treat others and to promote our own character and happiness. Rather, the newer virtue ethics sought to learn from the virtue ethics of the ancient world, especially of Plato, Aristotle, and the Stoics, while making those lessons relevant to a climate of ethical theory that incorporates what has been learned in the long interval since ancient times.

More recently, however, a radical kind of virtue ethics without precedent in the ancient world has developed out of feminist thought and in the wake of Carol Gilligan's groundbreaking *In a Different Voice* (1982). Gilligan argued that men tend to conceive of morality in terms of rights, justice, and autonomy, whereas women more frequently think of morality in terms of caring, responsibility, and interrelation with others. And at about the same time as Gilligan wrote, Nel Noddings in *Caring: A Feminine Approach to Ethics and Moral Education* (1984) articulated and defended the idea of a feminine morality centered on caring.

The ideal of caring Noddings has in mind is particularistic: It is not the universally directed benevolence of the sort utilitarianism sometimes appeals to, but rather caring for certain particular people (e.g., one's friends and family) that she treats as the morally highest and best motivation. Actions then count as good or bad, better or worse, to the extent that they exhibit this kind of caring. Clearly, Nodding's view offers a potential answer to the traditional question of how one should live, but since the answer seems to be based on fundamental assumptions about what sorts of inner motivation are morally good or bad, it is a form of virtue ethics. Of course, her view can be stated in terms of the principle "Be caring and act caringly." But if we focus on conforming to the principle instead of on the needs of the individuals we care about, we risk falling short of what the principle itself recommends. It is the state or process of sensitive caring, rather than attention to principle, that generates what Noddings would take to be satisfying answers to moral questions and appropriate responses to particular situations.

Enriched by such feminine/feminist possibilities, ethical theory has been actively and fertilely involved with the perennial task(s) of ethics. But because few of the traditional questions have been answered to the satisfaction of all philosophers, one may well wonder whether philosophy will ever be able fully to answer those questions or even whether philosophers have, over the centuries, made real or sufficient progress in dealing with them. But it is also possible to attack the tradition(s) of philosophical ethics in a more radical fashion.

Modern Challenges to Philosophical Ethics

Some modern intellectual and social traditions have questioned the notion that ethics can validly function as a distinct sphere of rational inquiry. One example of such questioning was the widespread view, earlier in the twentieth century, that ethics should confine itself to the metaethical analysis of concepts and epistemological issues (and possibly to the sociological description of the differing ethical mores of different times and places) rather than continue in its traditional role of advocating substantive ethical views. (Metaethics has undergone something of a revival, but largely in a form regarded as compatible with substantive ethical theorizing.)

Historically, various forms of religion and religious philosophy have also posed a challenge to the autonomy and validity of traditional ethics. The claims of faith and religious authority can readily be seen as overriding the kind of rational understanding that typifies traditional philosophical inquiry. Thus, Thomas Aquinas believed strongly in the importance of the ethical issues raised by Aristotle and in Aristotle's rational techniques of argument and analysis; but he also permitted his Christian faith to shape his response to Aristotle and did not fundamentally question the superiority of faith to reason. He believed, however, that reason and philosophy could accommodate and be accommodated to faith and religious authority.

EXISTENTIALISM. But more radical religionists have questioned the importance of reason and have even prided themselves in flying in the face of reason. Religious views that stress our dependent, finite, sinful creatureliness can lead one to view philosophical ethics as a rather limited and even perverse way to understand the problems of the human condition. In modern times this religion-inspired critique of ethics and the philosophical received a distinctive existentialist expression in the writings of Blaise Pascal (1966) and Søren Kierkegaard (1960, 1983).

It is very difficult to give a completely adequate characterization of existentialism as a philosophical movement or tendency of thought. It cuts across the distinction between theism and atheism, and some of the most prominent existentialists have, in fact, been atheists. But the earlier theistic existentialism that one finds in Pascal and, more fully developed, in Kierkegaard is principally concerned with attacking rationalistic Western philosophy and defending a more emotional and individualistic approach to life and thought. Plato and Aristotle, for example, sought rationally to circumscribe the human condition by treating "man" as by his very essence a "rational animal" and prescribing a way of life for human beings that acknowledged and totally incorporated the ideal of being rational. But for Pascal, the heart has reasons that reason cannot know, and Kierkegaard regarded certain kinds of rationally absurd religious faith and love as higher and more important than anything that could be circumscribed and understood in rational, ethical, or philosophical terms.

The atheistic Nietzsche (1844–1900) also attacked philosophical ethics and rational philosophy generally by attempting to deflate their pretensions to being rational. Nietzsche saw human life as characterized by a "will to power," that is, a desire for power over other individuals and for individual achievement, and in *The Genealogy of Morals* (1956) he argued that Judeo–Christian ethics, as well as philosophical views that reflect the influence of such ethics, are based in debilitating and poisonous emotions rather than having their source in rational thought or enlightened desire. What comes naturally to man is, he thought, an aristocratic morality that is comfortable with power and harsh in regard to failure, and the idea that the meek and self-sacrificing represents the highest form of human being he took to be the frustrated and angry response of those who have failed to attain power, but are unwilling to admit even to themselves how they really feel.

Nietzsche clearly expressed an antipathy to the whole tradition of philosophical ethics, and even if he did defend an iconoclastic ethics "of the superman," his writings point the way to an attitude like that of the more recent existentialist Jean-Paul Sartre (1905–1980). In his *Being and Nothingness* (1956), Sartre argued that all ethics is based in error and illusion, and he attempted instead to describe the human condition in nonjudgmental, nonmoral terms. Sartre argued that human beings are radically free in their choice of actions and values, and he claimed that all value judgments, because they purport to tell us what we really have to do, involve a misunderstanding, which he called "bad faith," of just how free we actually are. At the end of his book, Sartre proposed to write a future book on ethics, but also set out, in compelling fashion, the reasons for thinking that any future ethics is likely to fall into error and illusion about the character of human freedom. Here, as in *Being and Time* of Martin Heidegger (1889–1976) which had a decisive influence on Sartre's existentialism, the existentialist philosopher is essentially critical of the role ethical thinking plays in philosophy and in life generally and says, in effect, that if we face the truth about our own radical freedom, we must stop doing ethics. Ethics may think of itself as a rational enterprise, but for Sartre, it was mainly a form of self-deception.

MARXISM. Existentialism has had a great influence on Western culture, but Marxism has probably had a much greater influence, and Karl Marx's writings (*Capital and the German Ideology*), like those of some of the existentialists, attempt to accustom us to the idea of taking ethics less seriously than practitioners of philosophical ethics have tended to do. According to Marx (1818–1883) (and Friedrich Engels), philosophical ethics and philosophy generally are best understood as expressions of certain class interests, as ideological tools of class warfare, rather than as independently and timelessly valid methods of inquiry into questions that can be settled objectively and rationally.

For example, intellectual, philosophical defenses of property rights can be seen as expressing and asserting bourgeois class interests against a resentful and increasingly powerful proletariat. All philosophy, according to such a view, is merely the expression of underlying economic forces and struggles. A truly liberated view of human history requires us stop moralizing and start understanding and harnessing the processes of history, using the tools of Marx's own "scientific socialism." While Marx believed that a "really human morality" might emerge under communism, philosophical ethics is seen more as a hindrance than as a means to enlightened understanding of human society.

PSYCHOANALYSIS. In addition, psychoanalysis, as a movement and style of thought, has often been taken to argue against traditional ethics as an objective discipline with a valid intellectual task of its own. The psychoanalytic account of moral conscience threatens to undercut traditional ethical views and traditional views of ethics by making our own ethical intuitions and feelings seem illusory. In a manner partly anticipated by Nietzsche, Sigmund Freud's original formulation of psychoanalytic theory (e.g. in The Interpretation of Dreams and Introductory Lectures on Psychoanalysis) treat conscience and guilt as forms of aggression directed by the individual against himself (Freud). (Freud [1856–1939] tended to focus on the development of conscience in males.) Rather than attack parental figures he feared, the individual psychologically incorporates the morality of these seemingly threatening figures. If conscience is a function of hatred against one or more parental figures, then its true nature is often obscured to those who have conscience. According to classic psychoanalysis, the very factors that make us redirect aggression in such a fashion also make it difficult consciously to acknowledge that conscience has such a source.

If moral thought has this dynamic, then much of moral life and moral philosophy is self-deluded. However, for some more recent psychoanalysts, not all forms of ethical thinking are illusory. Followers of the British psychoanalyst Melanie Klein (1975) have said that various ethical ideals can and do appeal to us and guide our behavior, once "persecutory guilt" of the kind based in aggression redirected against the self is dissolved through normal maturation or through psychotherapy. Moreover, the analyst Erik Erikson (1964) gave a developmental account of basic human virtues that has clear, ethical significance.

In the end, perhaps it should not be surprising that many attempts to undermine ethics eventually reintroduce something like familiar ethical notions and problems. We have to live with one another, and the problems of making life together possible and, if possible, beneficial are problems that will not and cannot go away. Even if a given society and generation has settled on a particular solution to the problems of living together, new historical developments can make these solutions come unstuck, or at least force people to reconsider their appropriateness. And even if different societies and cultures have different moral standards, it is possible to overestimate the differences. For example, however much aggression societies may allow toward outsiders and enemies, no society has a moral code that permits people, at will, to kill members of that society. Moreover, the very fact of moral differences among different societies indicates a need for cooperative and practical ethical thinking that will enable people either to resolve or live with the differences.

APPLIED ETHICS. This is a point where the need for applied ethics most clearly comes into view. Whether it is in medicine, science, biotechnology, business, or the law, people have to come together to solve problems, and ethics or ethical thinking can play a role in generating cooperative solutions. If existentialism, religion, Marxism, and psychoanalysis all in varying degrees question the need for philosophical ethics, the practical problems of contemporary life seem to indicate some new ways and to highlight some old ways in which philosophical ethics has validity and value.

The explosive development of new knowledge and techniques in medicine and biology has made bioethics one of the central areas of practical, moral concern. And those seeking to solve moral problems in this area naturally appeal to philosophical ethics. To take just one controversial area, the question of euthanasia engages the ideas and energies of different ethical theories in different ways and often with differing results. Thus, the Kantian may focus on issues concerning the autonomy of the dying patient and the right to life, whereas utilitarians will stress issues about the quality of life and the effects of certain decisions on families and society as a whole, and defenders of an ethics of caring will perhaps see less significance in larger social consequences and focus on how a medical decision will affect those most intimately and immediately affected by it.

Applied ethics in our contemporary sense is not new: Socrates' discussion of the duty of obedience to unjust laws in the Crito and Henry David Thoreau's of civil disobedience are only two of countless historical instances of what we would call applied ethics. Today, we think, civilization is more complicated and our problems are more complex. Still, in facing those problems, bioethicists, business ethicists, and other applied ethicists typically look to philosophical ethics, to substantive theories like utilitarianism and virtue ethics and Kantianism, and to the criticisms each makes of the others, for some enlightenment on practical issues.

MICHAEL A. SLOTE (1995)

SEE ALSO: *Autonomy; Cancer, Ethical Issues Related to Diagnosis and Treatment; Care; Coercion; Communitarianism and Bioethics; Dementia; Emotions; Feminism; Justice; Life; Principalism; Virtue and Character;* and other *Ethics* subentries

BIBLIOGRAPHY

Anscombe, G. E. M. 1958. "Modern Moral Philosophy." *Philosophy* 33: 1–19.

Aristotle. 1962. *Nicomachean Ethics,* tr. Martin Ostwald. New York: Macmillan.

Bentham, Jeremy. 1982. *An Introduction to the Principles of Morals and Legislation.* New York: Methuen.

Erikson, Erik H. 1964. *Insight and Responsibility.* New York: W. W. Norton.

Freud, Sigmund. 1989. *A General Selection from the Works of Sigmund Freud.* New York: Anchor.

Gilligan, Carol. 1982. *In a Different Voice: Psychological Theory and Women's Development.* Cambridge, MA: Harvard University Press.

Kant, Immanuel. 1964. *Groundwork of the Metaphysic of Morals,* 3rd edition; tr. Herbert H. Paton. New York: Harper and Row.

Kierkegaard, Søren. 1960. *Kierkegaard's Concluding Unscientific Postscript,* tr. Walter Lowrie. Princeton, NJ: Princeton University Press.

Kierkegaard, Søren. 1983. *Fear and Trembling: Repetition,* tr. by Howard V. Hong and Edna H. Hong. Princeton, NJ: Princeton University Press.

Klein, Melanie. 1975. *Love, Guilt, and Reparation and Other Works, 1921–1963.* New York: Delacorte Press.

Long, A. A., and Sedley, D. N. eds. 1989. *The Hellenistic Philosophers,* 2 vols. New York: Cambridge University Press. See especially vol. 1, sections "Epicureanism" and "Stoicism."

Marx, Karl. 1977. *Selected Writings of Karl Marx,* ed. David McLellan. Oxford: Oxford University Press.

Nietzsche, Friedrich. 1956. *The Birth of Tragedy and The Genealogy of Morals,* tr. Francis Gaffing. Garden City, NY: Doubleday.

Noddings, Nel. 1984. *Caring: A Feminine Approach to Ethics and Moral Education.* Berkeley: University of California Press.

Parfit, Derek. 1984. *Reasons and Persons.* Oxford: Clarendon Press.

Pascal, Blaise. 1966. *Pensées.* Harmondsworth, Eng.: Penguin Books.

Plato. 1974. *Republic,* tr. by G. M. A. Grube. Indianapolis, IN: Hackett Publishing.

Rawls, John. 1971. *A Theory of Justice.* Cambridge, MA: Harvard University Press.

Ross, W. D. 1930. *The Right and the Good.* Oxford: Clarendon Press.

Sartre, Jean-Paul. 1956. *Being and Nothingness: An Essay on Phenomenological Ontology,* tr. Hazel E. Barnes. New York: Philosophical Library.

Sidgwick, Henry. 1981 (1907). *The Methods of Ethics,* 7th edition. Indianapolis, IN: Hackett Publishing.

II. MORAL EPISTEMOLOGY

Moral epistemology is the systematic and critical study of morality as a body of knowledge. It is concerned with such issues as how or whether moral claims can be rationally justified, whether there are objective moral facts, whether moral statements strictly admit of truth or falsity, and whether moral claims are universally valid or relative to historically particular belief systems, conceptual schemes, social practices, or cultures.

The subdiscipline of moral epistemology is hardly a recent arrival on the philosophical scene. Plato's *Republic,*

Aristotle's *Nicomachean Ethics*, Hume's *Treatise on Human Nature*, Kant's *Critique of Practical Reason*, and Hegel's *Phenomenology of Spirit* all grapple with moral-epistemological themes and issues. However, the lion's share of explicit, self-conscious reflection on moral-epistemological problems has taken place in the twentieth century, reflecting Western philosophy's more general preoccupation with the problem of knowledge since the time of Kant. This entry describes and critically evaluates some of the major options in moral epistemology taken during that period.

Intuitionism

When one describes a person as "good," or when one says of an action that it is "the right thing to do" under the circumstances, is one pointing out an objective feature of the person or action, or is one expressing one's own subjective reaction? Is one stating something that could be either true or false? Is one making a claim that could be supported by reasons or evidence, and that would warrant the assent of any rational human being? Or is one merely giving voice to one's own attitudes or feelings? Much of the contemporary debate in moral epistemology turns on the answer to these questions.

Intuitionists, chief among whom were G. E. Moore and W. D. Ross, insist that moral terms such as "good" and "right" name objective properties, refer to real aspects of real things, events, activities, and persons, and claim that we have access to these properties by a form of direct insight or perception. Because of this, moral statements are genuine propositions capable of being assigned a truth value of "true" or "false." To use a technical, philosophical term, morality is "cognitive." Intuitionists, while drawing an analogy between sensory intuition and moral intuition, also generally insist that moral intuition is different in kind from sense perception. While sense perception acquaints us with objective facts, moral intuition acquaints us with equally objective values.

According to G. E. Moore's *Principia Ethica* (1903), "good" is a simple, unanalyzable concept. Like the property concept "yellow," "good" cannot be defined except by pointing out instances of the concept, which enables one to grasp its unitary meaning. Unlike "yellow," which denotes a property intuited by our ordinary sensory apparatus, "good" names a nonnatural property, which, despite the fact that it is not empirically given, is nonetheless just as objective and real as is the property "yellow." W. D. Ross, in *The Right and the Good*, expands Moore's table of simple, objective moral properties to include "duty," or "rightness," and the degrees of rightness that attach to conflicting prima facie duties in different circumstances.

Intuitionists like Moore do not deny that there is moral knowledge; in fact, they affirm it emphatically. But for both Moore and Ross, our knowledge of what is ultimately good or right is not inferred or deduced but immediately given; we do not need to define, rationalize, or justify it. Thus a physician, deciding to remove an irreversibly brain-dead patient from a respirator, might give reasons for her decision by citing the beneficial consequences (e.g., an end to the patient's fruitless suffering) that might be achieved, or by insisting that the duty to preserve life is trumped by the higher duty to preserve a patient's dignity. But as to why these consequences are good, or why these putative duties are duties, the intuitionist physician can rightfully appeal only to her perception of the basic quality of goodness or rightness in them. Look and you too shall see.

The very immediacy of moral knowledge poses a serious problem for the intuitionist, namely, how moral argument and moral disagreement are possible. According to Moore, one either "sees" that something is good or one doesn't, and if one doesn't, there's little to be done except to look again. But what if two or more competent moral agents persistently "see" different values in the same circumstances? Who is "seeing" what is really there, and who is "seeing" a moral illusion? The intuitionist faces the difficulty of accounting for genuine moral disagreement—disagreement not about the empirical, factual issues of how to bring about the greatest good or do one's duty, but the evaluative issue of what sorts of things are genuine, intrinsic goods or actual obligations. This faculty of moral intuition is therefore curious. It is supposed to yield insight into objective properties of things, outcomes, deeds, and institutions, yet it lacks any public criterion against which claims like "X is good" or "Y is the morally right thing to do" might be checked and rationally validated.

Emotivism

A number of thinkers influenced by logical positivism, most notably A. J. Ayer and Charles L. Stevenson, rejected intuitionism and with it the conviction that moral discourse was objective and cognitive. The resulting theory, emotivism, denied that "good" or "right" named any sort of objective, intuitable property. Rather, to say of something that it is "good" or "evil," "right" or "wrong," is to express a subjective attitude or emotional response toward it. For example, the proposition, "You ought not to have lied to that patient," asserts nothing more than "you lied to that patient"; the "ought" merely notes an attitude of disapproval on the part of the speaker. Emotivists emphasize the imperative quality of moral utterance. To say lying is wrong is, in effect, to issue the command, "Do not lie." To place ethical discourse in a recognizable context, the effort on the part of agents is to influence the behavior of others and to persuade them to adopt different beliefs. If emotivists like Ayer and Stevenson are right about the meaning of moral statements, the demand to account for "moral knowledge" is senseless, since all moral discourse is inherently noncognitive, nonrational, and subjective.

Perhaps this is an acceptable price to pay to make the phenomenon of moral disagreement intelligible. An intuitionist would be vexed by disagreements such as the following:

(1a) Active, involuntary euthanasia is morally acceptable under certain conditions, versus

(1b) Active, involuntary euthanasia is always immoral, under any and all conditions.

Yet what for the intuitionist is an epistemological dilemma, for the emotivist is not a dilemma at all. The proponent of (1a) is "commending" the permissibility of involuntary, active euthanasia under certain conditions rather than asserting a true-or- false proposition; she is expressing a "pro-attitude" toward (1a), and trying to persuade others to do so as well. The proponent of (1b) is doing precisely the same thing, expressing an "anti-attitude." The disagreement is one of subjective attitude and feeling and does not concern anything objective; there is no deep, moral truth under dispute.

But perhaps it might be premature to claim that the ability to make sense of moral disagreement thereby vindicates emotivism. One serious difficulty with emotivism is that it narrows the human significance of moral discourse by flatly denying that whenever one makes a moral claim, one places oneself in the position of having to back up that claim by citing what one takes to be good reasons in its behalf.

Universal Prescriptivism

Universal prescriptivism is a compromise between emotivism and the commonsense conviction that morality is a rational enterprise. Its chief exponent, R. M. Hare, argues in *The Language of Morals* (1952) that moral imperatives carry certain inexorable rational constraints. If I make the moral judgment, "Active, involuntary euthanasia is wrong," I am in effect declaring that one ought not to perform active, involuntary euthanasia on someone, and thus commanding, "Do not perform active, involuntary euthanasia," where the ought command is issued to anyone in the relevant situation, including me, the speaker. So while moral judgments have an imperative or prescriptive component—like Moore, Hare rejects naturalism—they exhibit a universality that binds the speaker's deeds to her claims, and enables the

speaker to use reason to draw further moral conclusions on the basis of prescriptions that function as premises in deductive arguments.

In affirming the role of deductive reason in ethics, Hare's universal prescriptivism challenges the emotivist's assumption that only indicative premises are beyond suspicion in valid argumentation. For surely the following argument is a valid deduction:

(2a) I ought not to lie to my patients and thus intentionally mislead them.

(2b) My patient Bill asked me to tell him about his medical condition.

(2c) I ought not to lie to Bill about his condition.

All its premises are meaningful, and since the major premise is prescriptive, the taboo against deducing an "ought" from an "is" is not violated. Furthermore, (2a) itself could be justified by being a valid conclusion drawn from more general prescriptions:

(2d) I ought not to be unjust.

(2e) To lie to one's patients and thus intentionally mislead them is unjust.

(2f) I ought not to lie to my patients and thus intentionally mislead them.

However, there cannot be an infinite hierarchy of such deductions. For the prescriptivist, one's ultimate prescriptive or evaluative premises are chosen rather than deduced: One cannot ground one's moral convictions in premises more basic. The foundations for moral reasoning cannot themselves have a foundation; they reflect one's basic stance or attitude toward persons and things. No "ought" can be derived from an "is." One's moral first principles, being prescriptions, cannot be rooted in indicative soil.

This might lead one to wonder whether universal prescriptivism is more a refinement of emotivism than a genuine advance on it. It seems to push the point where ethical discourse is a matter of attitude and criterionless choice back to the most general evaluation the agent wishes to make. For example, substitute the following premise for (2a) above:

(2a1) I ought not to lie to my patients and thus intentionally mislead them *unless* I have ample reason to judge that doing so will confer some psychological or medical benefit to them.

If a physician were to judge that some such benefit were to be obtained from intentional deception, then the conclusion that one may intentionally deceive a patient will follow, in direct contradiction to (2c) and (2f). Given the initial moral orientation, certain principles for action are validated, but the original moral orientation cannot itself be validated; it can only be accepted, endorsed, chosen. Since this nonrational, inaugural choice provides the basis for all subsequent moral reasoning, the content of an agent's morality appears to be ultimately arbitrary, even if it is not arbitrary in all its detail.

Hare disagrees. In *Freedom and Reason* (1963) he argues that universal prescriptivism sets limits on the kinds of fundamental moral choices an agent can make. Consider the following:

(3a) Certain people ought to be persecuted because, and only because, their skin is black.

If moral imperatives using "ought" are, as Hare claims, universal prescriptions, then the agent uttering these words is, or ought to be, committing himself to the proposition that if his skin were black he, too, ought to be persecuted. It is clear that few individuals who make such assertions, apart from those Hare dubs "fanatics," would assent to the latter claim. Yet it is entailed by the universal prescription (3a); hence, the morality of any agent who asserts (3a) and refuses to extend it to cover himself is, for that very reason, rationally inadequate.

Of course, there is no possibility of genuine argument with a genuine "fanatic": The fanatic's assertion of ultimate principles or fundamental commitments, however odious or bizarre they may be, can only be met with counterassertion and not counterreasoning. Hare seems willing to accept this lack of logical resources against fanaticism. Nevertheless it seems reasonable to ask universal prescriptivists such as Hare whether, by cutting off rational argument at fundamental principles, they are granting too much to fanatics by ruling out any way in which their convictions can be criticized, rather than their unpleasant characters. The fanatic may be vile and depraved, but by universal prescriptivist standards, he is not necessarily defective in reason.

Naturalism

Intuitionists, emotivists, and prescriptivists all agree that "facts" are distinct from "values"—that an "ought" cannot be deduced from an "is." G. E. Moore coined the term, "the naturalistic fallacy," to describe the frequent attempts on the part of philosophers to define "the good" by deducing it from some matter of fact about human beings and their desires. A number of philosophers have challenged this no-ought-from-an-is doctrine by providing counterexamples to it, in effect denying that the naturalistic fallacy is a fallacy.

Philippa Foot (1959), for example, has cited "rude" and "courageous" as concepts whose evaluative meaning cannot be pried from their descriptive meaning. The criteria for identifying someone as "rude" or "courageous" are factual. If someone fits a given description, one has warrant for saying that he or she is rude or courageous; thus, the proposition "She is rude/courageous" is cognitive. But to describe someone as rude is to evaluate that person negatively. Consider the absurdity of saying: "You're rude, cowardly, and abusive, but that isn't meant as a put-down." So, according to Foot, valid moral arguments can draw evaluative conclusions from factual premises.

Peter Geach (1956) makes an analogous point in his analyses of "good." To say that a thing is good is to say something concerning the kind of thing it is. "Good" does not mean precisely the same thing in the following sentences: "That car is good"; "that watch is a good watch"; and "Mohandas Gandhi was good." To say of each one of these that it is good is to employ criteria determined by the kind of thing being evaluated. But this is to say, again against the emotivist and the prescriptivist, that the criteria that fix the meaning of evaluative terms such as "good" are not ultimately matters of choice, but rather matters of fact. To know a good watch, one needs to know what a watch is and what it is for; to know a good person, one, likewise, must know what a human being is and those ends at which humans aim in their actions.

Finally, John Searle (1964) accuses noncognitivists of harboring an arbitrarily constricted notion of what constitutes a "fact." Human institutions are part of what is the case, and these "institutional facts" can appear in descriptive premises in valid deductive arguments that generate evaluative conclusions. For example, to acknowledge the institution of promising is to grant that under certain circumstances, when one utters the words, "I promise to do X," one places oneself under an obligation to do X, and therefore is obliged to do X, and therefore one ought to do X. Because institutional facts are determined by the rules guiding the aims and actions of participants, one can deduce values from them.

Naturalists sketch a picture of moral language in which moral concepts are understood by deriving them from nonmoral, "naturalistic" ones, upon which moral knowledge rests. A robust naturalism in bioethics, then, would show no qualms about defining "the good" or "the right" in a medical context by appealing to certain key facts about human beings (e.g., their pain, dignity, mortality, etc.) and about the social and institutional setting for these facts.

At this point, however, the prescriptivist can offer a rebuttal that is difficult to answer on the naturalist's own terms without begging an important question. The prescriptivist concedes that moral language necessarily has a factual or descriptive component, but insists that it also makes ineliminable reference to the agent's desires, aims, and wishes. These can be more or less rational depending on whether their satisfaction interferes with or complements other sets of desires, aims, and wishes, but no desire can be judged rational or irrational per se. These basic desires and attitudes might differ from person to person; there is no escaping the fundamental choice behind all evaluations and prescriptions. So when the naturalist claims to have deduced an "ought" from an "is," either the major premise harbors an implicit prescription (e.g., "One ought to honor institutions like promise-keeping") or the argument is not a strict deduction.

Naturalists might reply that the "natural" premises to which they appeal and that ground moral judgment and description are rooted not in the desires or aims of individuals but in general facts about human nature of which it is the philosopher's job to remind us. For example, Aristotle understood *eudaimonia,* or "human flourishing," to be the good for a human being, because it was a result of acting in accord with one's rational human nature; Thomas Aquinas defined the good in terms of human creatures' reestablishing a right relation to God; and John Stuart Mill's psychological theories stand behind his definition of the good as pleasure seeking and pain avoidance. Aristotle, Thomas Aquinas, and Mill all pursued ethics in the context of what might be called "philosophical anthropology." Yet this simply elevates the naturalist's dispute with the prescriptivist to a higher level of abstraction. The prescriptivist could deny that there is any fact of the matter that might constrain the choice between philosophical anthropologies, while the naturalist could just as adamantly insist upon it. Thus naturalism might provide a coherent, consistent alternative to prescriptivism, but only by accepting philosophical stalemate at a higher level.

Rationalism

One possible avenue around the prescriptivist/naturalist impasse would be to repudiate the naturalistic fallacy, yet insist that moral principles are justified by examining the nature of rationality itself. This sort of moral epistemology owes much to Kant. A number of notable philosophers, inspired by Kant yet eager to avoid his dubious treatment of the self, have endeavored to ground moral knowledge in the reflective exercise of reason by actual human agents.

The most ambitious of these attempts is clearly that of Alan Gewirth, who in *Reason and Morality* tries to prove the fundamental principle of morality by analyzing the bare concept of rational agency. Every rational agent, Gewirth argues, must presuppose certain generic goods—namely,

freedom and a degree of well-being—that make the exercise of his or her agency possible. If the agent must claim these generic goods as necessary, he or she must also claim them as rights. But since these goods flow from the generic features of agency, he or she must also concede that all other agents must claim them as rights, and that there is a corresponding obligation to acknowledge and respect them. Hence, the Principle of Generic Consistency (PGC)—"Act in accord with the generic rights of your recipients as well as yourself" (1978, p. 135)—is the fundamental, categorical principle of morality, from which all other concrete moral norms and precepts can be derived, and which can be denied only on pain of logical self-contradiction.

Many of Gewirth's critics (e.g., Nielsen; MacIntyre, 1984; Arrington) have questioned a crucial move in his dialectical "proof" of the PGC: Acknowledging that there exist necessary goods of rational agency need not entail recognizing them as one's rights. If these critics are correct, Gewirth's foundational moral principle is not necessarily true. If it is only contingently true, Gewirth's claim to a proof of the one fundamental principle of morality has not been vindicated.

In contrast to Gewirth's "hard" rationalism, other moral rationalists adopt a "soft" rationalism that proceeds not from unassailable premises about rational agency, but from contingent truths about what all rational agents would, in fact, choose under ideal conditions. For example, John Rawls, in *A Theory of Justice* (1971), maintains that in a hypothetical "original position," where the specific identities, desires, and advantages of rational agents are deliberately obscured behind a perspective of impartiality—a "veil of ignorance"—rational agreement would be secured regarding two specific principles of justice, equal liberty and equal distribution of goods, except in those cases where an unequal distribution of goods would work to the benefit of the worst-off social group.

"Soft" rationalism proceeds from assumptions about the rational choices individuals would make in imagined, empirical situations; thus it lends itself well to concrete application in such fields as legal, business, and medical ethics. For example, Robert M. Veatch, in *A Theory of Medical Ethics* (1981), argues that the responsibilities of medical professionals are set in an implicit "triple contract" involving those professionals, their patients, and society at large; specifically, medical rights and obligations are fixed by determining what sorts of agreements would be rational for all three interested parties to agree upon.

There are serious difficulties with these "soft" forms of moral rationalism. Rawls's "original position" suggests that individuals could and should be able to abstract themselves from their specific, contingent identities when formulating and justifying the principles of justice. But, as Michael Sandel (1982) and Charles Taylor (1985) have argued, this project faces formidable epistemological difficulties. It presupposes that "the self" is prior to its ends, that one's identity as a pure, rational chooser is separable from and more basic than one's identity as, say, an American, a Christian, a physician, and so on—and that it can and must draw upon rational resources that are neutral with respect to the ends and desires connected with these identities. Yet it is questionable whether such an "unencumbered" self would have any rational resources upon which to draw or any concrete intentions upon which to act; whether, indeed, the contracting chooser in the "original position" could ever be more than a philosophical fiction. Thus it seems as if moral rationalism—if it is to remain on epistemologically solid ground—must compromise its purity by admitting that the contingencies of time, place, and personal identity do make at least some difference in determining which choices and which sets of moral beliefs will be accepted as rational.

Realism and Antirealism

Another way to get around the prescriptivist/naturalist standoff would be to insist with the naturalist that there are objective moral truths, but to question whether such truths can be deduced from more basic facts concerning human nature or human institutions. On this "realist" account of moral knowledge (so called because it affirms objective moral realities independent of the knowing subject), moral discourse is less a matter of reason than of careful perception and insight, of developing the capacity to discriminate moral facts and to describe them accurately and adequately. To the extent that moral knowledge rests on "seeing" moral properties, moral realism suggests Moore's intuitionism. Yet, unlike Moore, moral realists claim no special faculty of moral intuition, insist that moral properties are observable in precisely the same way as are empirical properties, and hold that moral judgments and observations are fallible and revisable.

This renewed form of moral realism has been advanced by a number of British philosophers (Platts; McDowell, 1979; Lovibond) influenced by Donald Davidson's theory of meaning and Ludwig Wittgenstein's critique of reductionism in the philosophy of language. From Davidson they have borrowed the idea that to know what any sentence means is to be able to specify the conditions under which it is true. From Wittgenstein they have taken the conviction that there is no way to establish a ground for language that is independent of and cognitively superior to actual language in use. Taken together, these Davidsonian and Wittgensteinian commonplaces work to deflate all forms of noncognitivism.

The noncognitivist needs to rely on a contrast between two kinds of utterances—those that carry truth values and those that do not—and thus insists on two kinds of "meaning" and two kinds of discourse. One kind of discourse can accurately represent facts (usually assumed to be science), and the other does not represent facts, but expresses attitudes and imposes those attitudes on a world plastic enough to accept them (art, poetry, morality). But since determining the meaning of any linguistic statement is inseparable from determining whether that which it asserts is true or false, the noncognitivist cannot plausibly draw the required contrast between first-rate, fact-picturing discourse and second-rate, value-projecting discourse. To know what any expression means is to know what would make it true, and this ability neither demands nor supports any assumptions about the superior cognitive reliability of any one form of discourse (scientific) over any other (commonsense, literary, or moral).

The moral realist argues that there are moral facts just as there are scientific facts, and does not expect moral facts to be reducible to or deducible from any other kind of fact. Moral properties are "supervenient" upon nonmoral properties. One discerns a moral property by enumerating a number of nonmoral properties standing in relation to each other, from which the moral property "emerges" without being strictly entailed by them. "Supervenience" becomes clearer when one turns from examining "thin," abstract moral concepts ("good," "right," "duty") to "thick" moral concepts (concrete, specific concepts, like "courage," "loyalty," or "mercifulness"). To know, for example, that a physician's treatment of an end-stage cancer patient with larger than usual doses of painkillers was merciful involves knowing a great number of facts concerning cancer, pain, the special needs of the terminally ill in general and of this patient in particular, and so on. While one does not infer the moral property of being merciful from these nonmoral facts, the property is a function of them; one perceives the moral fact that this act is merciful in and through perceiving the aforementioned nonmoral facts.

"Seeing" the moral facts in the associated nonmoral facts is a complex skill, demanding discipline, practice, and attentiveness to matters of minute detail. For the moral realist, becoming a morally competent bioethicist is largely a matter of acquiring and honing a certain sensibility, akin to that of understanding a work of art or literature, whereby one comes to notice the moral goods and obligations in the context of medical practice, and to disclose and explicate them in descriptive speech.

A number of moral epistemologists (e.g., Mackie) have complained that the realists' account of supervenience is incoherent. If the supervenient moral properties of a person change (for example, if someone ceases to be courageous or just), it is necessary that other, nonmoral properties also have changed (fleeing from every danger; ceasing to give others their due). Yet if that person possesses all the nonmoral dispositions associated with a moral property (steadfastness in the face of danger; a consistent willingness to keep promises), it cannot be inferred that he or she necessarily possesses the associated moral properties (the person might not be courageous or just, "despite appearances"). Supervenience is supposedly a logical relation between properties, yet because it cannot be interpreted as a form of inference, it becomes an inexplicable fact.

John Mackie subscribes to a form of moral antirealism or "projectivism" that allows for cognitive expressions in moral discourse—that is, the truth or falsity of moral beliefs, the validity or invalidity of moral arguments—yet understands them in an equivocal sense, as a disguised, second-level reflection upon first-level moral judgments and attitudes. The moral idiom forces us to speak as if there were moral facts, but such "facts" are ultimately projections of our attitudes. To insist that moral judgments are more than expressions of attitude would be to reintroduce supervenience, with all its difficulties. Moral antirealists would not exactly deny, then, that moral knowledge is a result of coming to "see things" and describe them in a certain way; they would, however, deny that such descriptions bear more than an instrumental function. The physician who "sees" that a particular act toward a patient is merciful is indeed "seeing" something, but that something is a function of the physician's subjective attitude projected outward toward the patient.

This may not be cause for genuine worry on the realist's part. He or she could, of course, stand firm and endorse the reality of objective moral facts—the instantiation of "thick," descriptive moral properties such as "courage," "patience," and "mercifulness"—in the face of the logically peculiar notion of supervenience. Perhaps supervenience is an inexplicable logical and epistemological fact. So what? Supervenience is a feature of ordinary moral discursive practice, one that morally competent speakers can handle without much trouble. The difficulties that antirealist moral epistemologists claim to have uncovered are more a matter of their a priori prejudices (perhaps their epistemological "scientism") than their discovery of a defect in moral language and moral practice.

The realist, like Wittgenstein, confidently affirms that ordinary moral language is in good working order as it is.

The antirealist, of course, can reply that such "folk" moral philosophy is untidy, plagued with logical ambiguities and desperately in need of philosophical reinterpretation. Thus the clashes between moral realists and moral antirealists recapitulate the earlier standoff between prescriptivists and naturalists. What is at issue is not whether values can be derived from facts, but whether it even makes sense to speak of emergent "moral facts" alongside nonmoral ones.

Against Epistemology

Virtually all the various schools of moral epistemology considered seem to employ an ahistorical approach to moral discourse, argument, and judgment. Both prescriptivists and naturalists confidently speak of "*the* language of morals," presupposing that "morality" has a singular essence lurking under all the various "moralities" of human history. Their dispute only concerns what this "essence" might be. Rationalists, realists, and antirealists also claim their particular moral epistemologies for morality per se, as opposed to the morality characteristic of a particular time, place, or community; these epistemologies are seen as perennial options for anyone who wishes to think about ethics.

The assumption that "epistemology" studies the invariant universal structures of human knowledge, entitling it to "legislate" over all knowledge claims, has been the target of sustained philosophical attack in the latter half of the twentieth century by Ludwig Wittgenstein, Martin Heidegger, and John Dewey, among others. Richard Rorty's landmark *Philosophy and the Mirror of Nature* (1979) was one of the first works to point out the affinities between the projects of Wittgenstein, Heidegger, and Dewey. Rorty showed that all three undermined the pretense of "epistemologically oriented philosophy" to have attained a timeless, ahistorical, necessary vantage point in its judgments about knowledge by pointing out, in different ways, how knowledge claims are situated and justified in shared practical and social contexts and are unintelligible apart from such contexts. From Rorty's perspective, the different approaches of moral epistemologists are less important than their common goal of discovering the foundations of moral reason and showing how these foundations might (or might not) be "justified" to any rational person. But Rorty insists that the epistemological assumptions undergirding their "common goals" are baseless. Among those assumptions are the idea that there are moral truths available to human rationality as such, or that "morality," like "knowledge" and "being," is a concept with a unique, stable core meaning. Rorty's Wittgensteinian, Heideggerian, and Deweyan case against foundationalist philosophy thus makes a new, antifoundationalist and self-consciously historical approach to moral knowledge all the more appealing.

Relativism and the Feminist Critique of Objectivity

Antifoundationalism in moral philosophy has taken a number of different forms. One of them, relativism, has once again emerged as a serious option in moral epistemology. The doctrine associated with the ancient Sophists—that objectivity, truth, and knowledge are matters of adhering to sociocultural convention rather than of attaining insight into nature—has been revived and expressed in more sophisticated ways by Gilbert Harman (1975), Bernard Williams (1985), Joseph Margolis (1991), and David Wong (1984). Wong, for example, maintains that the concept of "an adequate moral system" is relative to particular places and times: There is no single, universally valid moral system available, even as an unattainable ideal. Within each extant system, there are resources available for evaluating and criticizing rival systems binding on all who share its standpoint. Wong is neither a subjectivist nor a noncognitivist. There is, however, no standpoint outside all such systems from which judgment could be passed upon each of them indifferently. For Wong, the collapse of epistemological foundationalism, and the acknowledgment that our "moral systems" are not the deliverances of pure, universal human reason but are products of historical contingencies, supports a form of relativism that is less concerned about specific judgments of right or wrong than with the assessment of moral systems or cultures on the widest scale.

Many critics of contemporary relativism have argued that it retains most of the self-referential inconsistencies that plagued its earlier incarnations. Can the relativist maintain that the relativistic thesis is "true" or "reasonable" without begging the question? (See Putnam.) Other critics argue that the historical contingency of moral beliefs and their lack of necessary epistemic foundations does not imply relativism, since it does not preclude the possibility of one moral system being more rationally adequate than its competitors (see Stout).

Yet this response elicits a further question: Whose conception of "rationality" is being employed when someone judges a moral system superior or inferior? Several important feminist philosophers have responded to this question by noting that, generally, the "rationality" employed and championed by moral philosophers has been "rationality" as understood and defined by men, who are ideologically biased by their place in a patriarchal social system and who tend to exclude the experiences and judgments of women (Tong; Code; Tuana). The idea that reason and objectivity could be "gendered" concepts has led some feminists to conclude that men and women evince different kinds of moral knowing, and to champion a feminine "ethic of care" as against a masculine "ethic of principles" (Gilligan), just as it has led others to reject those very "feminine virtues"

as yet another aspect of women's oppression by men (Bartky; Puka). Whatever the ultimate outcome of these debates, contemporary feminism has done much to reinforce the antifoundationalist and historicist critique of "objectivity" and "rationality" as universal, unproblematic features of human thought and discourse. But does that critique undermine the idea of "moral knowledge" as such?

Historicism, Virtue, and Tradition

One systematic moral philosopher who disagrees with that sentiment, and who has used the insights of historicism and antifoundationalism in rethinking and recovering a workable notion of "moral knowledge," is Alasdair MacIntyre. *After Virtue* (1984) begins by noting both the interminable and arbitrary character of contemporary moral arguments and the vehemence with which they are conducted, and asks what might account for the powerlessness of contemporary moral philosophy to resolve moral conflict and secure agreement. MacIntyre attempts to answer this question by pursuing a historical inquiry into the succession of moral theories and the social contexts in which they arose. MacIntyre maintains that the intractability of moral disagreement is one aspect of the "emotivist culture" of late modernity that provides no solid basis for making shared, rational moral judgments and thus renders the idea of genuine moral knowledge unintelligible.

Most modern moral theory and practice has dispensed with the Aristotelian idea of a human *telos,* an "end" proper to human beings as such. Modern social and political orders have ceased to define their mission as that of articulating a shared vision of the good life and communally pursuing it, since it is assumed that there is no good-defining end to seek. Then what can moderns claim to "know" when they make ethical assertions, decisions, and judgments? MacIntyre dubs the standard modern response to this question "the Enlightenment project": the task of finding the universal rules or standards that guide conduct yet swing free from any substantive conception of a good life, and are justifiable by appealing to rationality.

All attempts to fulfill the ambitions of the Enlightenment project have failed, according to MacIntyre, by their own standards of success. Kantians, Utilitarians, Humeans, Intuitionists, and so on, all presuppose that there is something universally known or grasped (the Categorical Imperative, the principle of utility, the sentiment of benevolence, the self-validating property of goodness or rightness) that provides an adequate ground for moral judgment and action. Upon closer inspection, however, both the prescriptive force and the specific content of such moral foundations seem arbitrary and local rather than necessary and universal.

If this is so, the epistemological universalism of the Enlightenment project functions as a mask, concealing the manipulative, will-driven ambitions of its disciples under guise of the objectivity of universal principle. Friedrich Nietzsche thus stands as both the fruition and the ruin of the Enlightenment project. His achievement is to have revealed that behind the rhetoric of objective, universal rational foundations, the morality of the modern West is yet another arbitrary upsurge of "will to power," and its impending collapse is testament to its own timid denial of this hard truth.

While MacIntyre insists that Nietzsche is certainly right about modern moral theory and practice, he has not thereby shown that all morality falls victim to the same disease. If the history of moral beliefs and moral theories can reveal the bankruptcy of the Enlightenment project and the moral nihilism of Nietzsche's "genealogical" critique of morality, it can also show how the moral philosophies they displaced can succeed where they themselves failed. MacIntyre contends that contemporary Aristotelians can draw upon epistemological resources that both Enlightenment rationalists and Nietzschean skeptics lack.

First, Aristotelians begin thinking about morality with a systematic conception of the virtues, a set of character traits that enable human agents to perfect their natures and thus realize, however imperfectly, their ultimate end. Duties and obligations—what one ought to do—begin to make sense only against the background of belief about what one ought to be. Since virtue is intrinsically connected to a conception of well-being or human flourishing shared by members of a moral community, one can establish a sound, rational motive for being moral, without reducing what one ought to prefer or desire, in light of one's true end, to what one empirically happens to prefer or desire.

Second, by understanding moral behavior as action that proceeds from a character perfected by these virtues, one eliminates the need for thinking of morality as exclusively, or even primarily, a matter of conscientious rule-following. Hence one evades the difficulty afflicting most forms of moral rationalism, that of specifying substantial moral principles, rather than empty generalities, to putatively compel the rational assent of anyone whosoever. For Aristotelians, as MacIntyre understands them, there is no moral knowledge apart from moral education and training, education not so much in assimilating precepts and norms, but in acquiring the skilled moral wisdom (*phronesis*) to express the proper responses and sentiments in the proper way at the proper times.

Finally, Aristotelianism, for MacIntyre, can make sense of the ways in which traditions of rational inquiry and communal practice can sustain a conception of the virtues while subjecting it to both internal scrutiny and external challenge. Most moral epistemologists make the false assumption that morality names a universal phenomenon rooted in universal human reason. If MacIntyre is right, there is no morality except as rooted in particular communities with their own particular traditions concerning the nature of the virtues and their role in promoting human well-being. This might seem to lend comfort to those moral and political conservatives who take reason and tradition to be polar opposites, and who denigrate the former and deify the latter. Yet only by participating in the common life and practices of a tradition can we come to recognize moral reasons as reasons. By dialectically examining and testing these reasons against those of rival traditions of thought and practice, we can confirm or deny their adequacy and provisionally justify our confidence in them. Traditions are the primary bearers of moral reasons; the internal evolution of traditions and the conflicts between alternative traditions indicates the way in which moral knowledge is embodied in time and history, and how moral knowers can yet transcend historical limitations.

Conclusion

The virtue-centered historicism exemplified by MacIntyre might seem, at first, to be yet another item on the menu of moral epistemologies, yet another intellectual position for ethicists to choose and then defend. But it would be a mistake to view it in this way. Moral epistemology, as a historicist like MacIntyre conceives of it, differs from moral epistemology as most moral epistemologists have conceived of it. MacIntyre denies the ability to transcend all traditional allegiances and to spell out the conditions for moral knowledge in general and as such. As MacIntyre suggests, the moral system it would be rational to adopt depends on who one is and how one understands oneself; there is no moral system that is rational without qualification (1988). This is certainly not to suggest a radical moral relativism, since one's initial loyalties, convictions, and self-understandings are precisely what are to be tested by inquiry and comparative criticism. One must begin inquiring somewhere, however, and the only available starting points are within the assumptions and ways of life of the specific traditions one happens to inhabit.

Thus, for historicists like MacIntyre, Rorty, Stanley Hauerwas, and Jeffrey Stout, moral epistemology can no more escape the gravitational pull of human practice and human history than can any other form of inquiry. Since they cannot be detached from the changing, finite traditions that give them rational legitimacy, it may be more accurate to speak of moral epistemologies in the plural rather than a singular moral epistemology.

The implications of historicism for bioethics are, if anything, even more profound. Since claims to moral knowledge are always made within specific traditions of thought and practice, the claims made by bioethicists about informed consent, active and passive euthanasia, paternalism and autonomy will inevitably reflect these particular traditions and will preclude appeal to any neutral ground transcending these traditions to bioethics as such. "Bioethics as such," like "rationality as such," is a post-Enlightenment fiction. Each moral tradition—whether Christian, Jewish, Islamic, or secular—will provide resources for bioethical reflection, but the individual bioethicist cannot escape reflecting and theorizing as a member of his or her tradition, as opposed to being a disengaged, impersonal spectator on "universal values." From the vantage point of historicism, bioethical inquiry and debate need to be reconfigured as conflict among and reconciliation between these traditions, which give moral thought and action their lease on life.

MICHAEL J. QUIRK (1995)
BIBLIOGRAPHY REVISED

SEE ALSO: *Authority in Religious Traditions; Autonomy; Care; Communitarianism and Bioethics; Conscience; Conscience, Rights of; Consensus, Role and Authority of; Feminism; Medicine, Art of; Natural Law; Principalism; Profession and Professional Ethics; Utilitarianism; Virtue and Character;* and other *Ethics* subentries

BIBLIOGRAPHY

Arrington, Robert L. 1989. *Rationalism, Realism, and Relativism: Perspectives in Contemporary Moral Epistemology.* Ithaca, NY: Cornell University Press.

Ayer, A. J. 1946. *Language, Truth, and Logic.* New York: Dover.

Audi,-Robert. 1997. *Moral Knowledge and Ethical Character.* New York: Oxford University Press.

Bartky, Sandra Lee. 1990. "Feeding Egos and Tending Wounds: Deference and Disaffection in Women's Emotional Labor." In *Femininity and Domination: Studies in the Phenomenology of Oppression,* pp. 99–119. London: Routledge.

Bernstein, Richard J. 1983. *Beyond Objectivism and Relativism: Science, Hermeneutics, and Praxis.* Philadelphia: University of Pennsylvania Press.

Blackburn, Simon. 1971. "Moral Realism." In *Morality and Moral Reasoning,* ed. John Casey. London: Methuen.

Bloomfield, Paul. 2000. "Virtue Epistemology and the Epistemology of Virtue."

Bloomfield, Paul. 2001. *Moral Reality.* New York: Oxford University Press.

Code, Lorraine. 1991. *What Can She Know? Feminist Theory and the Construction of Knowledge.* Ithaca, NY: Cornell University Press.

Dancy, Jonathan. 1991. "Intuitionism." In *A Companion to Ethics,* pp. 411–414, ed. Peter Singer. Oxford: Basil Blackwell.

Fins, Joseph J.; Miller, Franklin G.; and Bacchetta, Matthew D. 1998. "Clinical Pragmatism: Bridging Theory and Practice." *Kennedy Institute of Ethics Journal* 8(1): 37–42.

Foot, Philippa. 1959. "Moral Beliefs." *Proceedings of the Aristotelian Society* 59: 83–104.

Foot, Philippa. 1978. *Virtues and Vices: And Other Essays in Moral Philosophy.* Berkeley: University of California Press.

Geach, Peter T. 1956. "Good and Evil." *Analysis* 17(2): 33–42.

Gewirth, Alan. 1978. *Reason and Morality.* Chicago: University of Chicago Press.

Gewirth, Alan. 1982. *Human Rights: Essays on Justification and Applications.* Chicago: University of Chicago Press.

Gilligan, Carol. 1982. *In a Different Voice: Psychological Theory and Women's Development.* Cambridge, MA: Harvard University Press.

Goldman, Alan H. 1988. *Moral Knowledge.* London: Routledge & Kegan Paul.

Grimshaw, Jean. 1991. "The Idea of a Female Ethic." In *A Companion to Ethics,* pp. 491–499, ed. Peter Singer. Oxford: Basil Blackwell.

Hare, R. M. 1952. *The Language of Morals.* Oxford: Oxford University Press.

Hare, R. M. 1957. "Geach: Good and Evil." *Analysis* 17, no. 5:103–11.

Hare, R. M. 1963. *Freedom and Reason.* Oxford: Clarendon Press.

Hare, R. M. 1964. "The Promising Game." *Revue Internationale de Philosophie* 70: 398–412.

Harman, Gilbert. 1975. "Moral Relativism Defended." *Philosophical Review* 84(1): 3–22.

Hauerwas, Stanley. 1979. *The Peaceable Kingdom: A Primer in Christian Ethics.* Notre Dame, IN: University of Notre Dame Press.

Hauerwas, Stanley. 1986. *Suffering Presence: Theological Reflections on Medicine, the Mentally Handicapped, and the Church.* Notre Dame, IN: University of Notre Dame Press.

Lovibond, Sabina. 1983. *Realism and Imagination in Ethics.* Minneapolis, MN: University of Minnesota Press.

Jaggar, Alison M. 2000. "Ethics Naturalized: Feminism's Contribution to Moral Epistemology." *Metaphilosophy* 31(5): 452–468.

MacIntyre, Alasdair C. 1966. *A Short History of Ethics.* New York: Macmillan.

MacIntyre, Alasdair C. 1984. *After Virtue: A Study in Moral Theory.* 2d ed. Notre Dame, Ind.: University of Notre Dame Press.

MacIntyre, Alasdair C. 1988. *Whose Justice? Which Rationality?* Notre Dame, IN: University of Notre Dame Press.

MacIntyre, Alasdair C. 1990. *Three Rival Versions of Moral Enquiry: Encyclopaedia, Genealogy, and Tradition.* Notre Dame, IN: University of Notre Dame Press.

Mackie, John L. 1977. *Ethics: Inventing Right and Wrong.* New York: Penguin.

Margolis, Joseph. 1991. *The Truth About Relativism.* Oxford: Basil Blackwell.

McDowell, John. 1979. "Virtue and Reason." *Monist* 62(3): 331–50.

McDowell, John. 1988. "Values and Secondary Qualities." In *Essays on Moral Realism*, ed. Geoffrey Sayre-McCord. Ithaca, NY: Cornell University Press.

McNaughton, David. 1988. *Moral Vision: An Introduction to Ethics.* Oxford: Basil Blackwell.

Moore, G. E. 1903. *Principia Ethica.* Cambridge: Cambridge University Press.

Nielsen, Kai. 1984. "Against Ethical Rationalism." In *Gewirth's Ethical Rationalism: Critical Essays with a Reply by Alan Gewirth*, pp. 59–82, ed. Edward Regis, Jr. Chicago: University of Chicago Press.

Pigden, Charles R. 1991. "Naturalism." In *A Companion to Ethics*, pp. 421–431, ed. Peter Singer. Oxford: Basil Blackwell.

Platts, Mark de Bretton. 1979. *Ways of Meaning: An Introduction to a Philosophy of Language.* London: Routledge & Kegan Paul.

Puka, Bill. 1990. "The Liberation of Caring: A Different Voice for Gilligan's 'Different Voice.'" *Hypatia* 5(1): 58–82.

Putnam, Hilary. 1981. *Reason, Truth, and History.* Cambridge: Cambridge University Press.

Rawls, John. 1971. *A Theory of Justice.* Cambridge, MA: Harvard University Press.

Rawls, John. 1985. "Justice as Fairness: Political not Metaphysical." *Philosophy and Public Affairs* 14(3): 223–251.

Regis, Edward, Jr., ed. 1984. *Gewirth's Ethical Rationalism.* Chicago: University of Chicago Press.

Rorty, Richard. 1979. *Philosophy and the Mirror of Nature.* Princeton, NJ: Princeton University Press.

Ross, W. D. 1930. *The Right and the Good.* Oxford: Clarendon Press.

Sandel, Michael. 1982. *Liberalism and the Limits of Justice.* Cambridge, Eng.: Cambridge University Press.

Sayre-McCord, Geoffrey, ed. 1988. *Essays on Moral Realism.* Ithaca, NY: Cornell University Press.

Searle, John R. 1964. "How to Derive 'Ought' from 'Is.'" *Philosophical Review* 73(1): 43–58.

Sinnott-Armstrong, Walter, and Timmons, Mark, eds. 1996. *Moral Knowledge?: New Readings in Moral Epistemology.* New York: Oxford University Press.

Stevenson, Charles L. 1944. *Ethics and Language.* New Haven, CT: Yale University Press.

Stevenson, Charles L. 1963. *Facts and Values: Studies in Ethical Analysis.* New Haven, CT: Yale University Press.

Stout, Jeffrey. 1989. *Ethics After Babel: The Languages of Morals and Their Discontents.* Boston: Beacon Press.

Taylor, Charles. 1985. "The Nature and Scope of Distributive Justice." In *Philosophy and the Human Sciences.* vol. 2 of *Philosophical Papers.* Cambridge, Eng.: Cambridge University Press.

Tong, Rosemarie. 1989. *Feminist Thought: A Comprehensive Introduction.* Boulder, CO: Westview.

Tuana, Nancy. 1992. *Woman and the History of Philosophy.* New York: Paragon House.

Veatch, Robert M. 1981. *A Theory of Medical Ethics.* New York: Basic Books.

Williams, Bernard. 1985. *Ethics and the Limits of Philosophy.* Cambridge, MA: Harvard University Press.

Wong, David B. 1984. *Moral Relativity.* Berkeley: University of California Press.

Wong, David B. 1991. "Relativism." In *A Companion to Ethics*, pp. 442–450, ed. Peter Singer. Oxford: Basil Blackwell.

III. NORMATIVE ETHICAL THEORIES

The concept of normative ethics was invented early in the twentieth century to stand in contrast to the concept of metaethics. In ethical theories prior to the twentieth century, it is impossible to discern any sharp distinction between what have come to be called metaethics and normative ethics. In the first half of the twentieth century, however, this distinction began to structure ethics as an intellectual discipline and it continues to be influential at the end of the twentieth century even though crucial theoretical supports for it have disappeared.

Normative ethics was regarded as that branch of ethical inquiry that considered general ethical questions whose answers had some relatively direct bearing on practice. The answers had to be general rather than particular in order to distinguish normative ethics from casuistry; they had to have a bearing on practice in order to distinguish normative ethics from metaethics. Casuistry was understood in its classical sense as the study of particular cases, while metaethics was understood originally as the inquiry into the semantics of ethical language.

G. E. Moore's classic proposal for the structure of ethics distinguished three key questions: (1) What particular things are good? (2) What kinds of things are good? and (3) What is the meaning of "good"? The first question is the central question of casuistry, while the second question falls within normative ethics, and the third, within metaethics (although Moore used neither the term "metaethics" or "normative ethics" in his early work). Normative ethics as a field of inquiry, then, is positioned somewhat precariously between the detail of casuistry and the abstractness of metaethics.

The character of normative ethics was also strongly influenced in the first half of the twentieth century by the almost universal acceptance of the principle of moral neutrality. This principle, accepted by virtually all mainstream Anglo-American moral philosophers from the 1930s to the 1960s, asserted that the results of metaethical investigations were logically independent of normative ethics. When coupled with the original understanding of metaethics as an account of the meaning of key ethical terms, it implied that such semantic investigations were logically irrelevant to inquiries about how to live. Under the influence of this principle, normative ethics was largely abandoned by Anglo-American moral philosophers in favor of a single-minded pursuit of metaethical inquiry. And since the metaethical views most in favor during this period were various forms of noncognitivism (e.g., emotivism and prescriptivism), it was regularly asserted that normative ethics should be relegated to preachers, novelists, and other nonphilosophers. The widely accepted noncognitivist views held that there was no cognitive content to normative ethical judgments since these judgments were primarily expressions of attitudes (as emotivists held) or primarily expressions of prescriptions (as prescriptivists held). But if normative judgments had no cognitive content—if, that is, they were primarily the expression of noncognitive attitudes or imperatives—then it was unclear why moral philosophers should be concerned with examining them. Normative ethics was regarded as largely a matter of exhortation and was removed from the standard repertoire of strictly philosophical concerns.

This sharp distinction between metaethical and normative inquiry, however, together with the relegation of normative ethics to nonphilosophical inquiry, was too unstable to last. Philosophers increasingly recognized that the principle of moral neutrality was not a theoretically neutral presupposition of ethical inquiry but rather drew a considerable amount of its support from the prevailing noncognitivist view. When these noncognitivist views were severely challenged in the late 1950s and 1960s (by, among others, Philippa Foot, Kurt Baier, Stephen Toulmin, and Alan Gewirth), the sharp distinction between metaethics and normative ethics was blunted; this opened the way to a resurgence of interest in normative ethics, expressed by new attempts to reformulate and to defend classical ethical views. Although a complete historical explanation of the remarkably sudden return of philosophers in the 1960s and 1970s to the classical questions of normative theory will no doubt be extremely complex, the decline of noncognitivism and the concomitant rejection of a sharp distinction between normative ethics and metaethics surely contributed to it. Classical Kantian theory was developed in a creative and persuasive manner by John Rawls and his student, Thomas Nagel, along with Alan Donagan, Alan Gewirth, and others. Utilitarianism received new attention from, among others,

Richard Hare and his students Derek Parfit and Peter Singer. The classical Aristotelian/Thomist view was reformulated and defended by Elizabeth Anscombe, Peter Geach, Alasdair MacIntyre, and like-minded moral philosophers.

What was revived under the label "normative ethics," however, was not identical to what had previously been neglected by moral philosophers as normative ethics. The watershed in ethical theory in the 1960s changed not only the interests of moral philosophers but also changed their conception of their discipline. The task of metaethics was expanded from the narrow one of clarifying the semantics of ethical terms to a much broader investigation of the whole range of metaphysical, epistemological, and semantic questions associated with ethical inquiry. Metaethics came to be concerned not only with questions about the meaning of ethical terms and judgments, but also with metaphysical questions about the nature of ethical properties and epistemological questions about how claims to ethical knowledge are to be appraised. Normative ethics in turn came to be understood as that pole of ethical theory that stood closest to practice. Whereas previously the distinction that most clearly structured ethical inquiry was the distinction between metaethics and normative ethics, the crucial distinction increasingly came to be that between ethical theory and applied ethics.

Ethical theory was distinguished from applied ethics by being both more general and more abstract, and also by being less driven by a concern that its results would have some immediate consequences for action or policy. Within ethical theory, however, elements coexisted that, according to earlier views, would have been sharply distinguished as metaethical and normative. Ethical theory inquired into the epistemological and metaphysical features of ethics as well as into the most general truths about how we should live. Also, the new conception of ethical theory held that these two kinds of inquiry were continuous; it was not possible to pursue either kind without attending to its implications for the other. Ethical theory had become a seamless web with areas of greater or less practical relevance, roughly corresponding to those areas earlier distinguished as the normative and the metaethical.

One consequence of these complex historical developments is that it has become much more difficult to give a precise characterization of normative ethics than it would have been at an earlier time. Nevertheless, certain common assumptions about the nature of normative ethics, as well as a widely shared taxonomy of the varieties of normative theory, have persisted through these developments in the concept of normative ethics. The common assumptions include the claim that the central task of normative ethics is to define and to defend an adequate theory for guiding conduct. The received taxonomy divides normative theories into three basic types: virtue theories, *deontological* theories, and *consequentialist* theories. The following section will examine these three types of normative theory with the aim of exploring their distinctive features.

Types of Normative Theory

The basis for distinguishing the three types of normative theory lies in three universal features of human actions. This recourse to the features of actions should not be surprising, since the aim of normative theory is to guide action. Every human action involves (1) an agent who performs (2) some action that has (3) particular consequences. These three features may be set out as follows:

$$P \qquad \longrightarrow \qquad +++++++$$
$$\text{Agent} \qquad \text{Action} \qquad \text{Consequences}$$

If Jones tells a lie to Smith that causes Smith to miss his train, then Jones is the agent, his telling a lie is the action, and Smith's missing the train is one of the consequences of the action. Difficulties arise, of course, in many cases in determining whether someone is an agent in a particular case (e.g., if Jones is insane when he shoots the president, is he really the agent of any action?); or the nature of the particular action performed (e.g., if Jones is cutting down a tree, believing reasonably that he is the only one in the forest, but Smith wanders by and the tree falls on him, causing his death, does a killing take place or merely a death?); or what the consequences of a particular action may be (e.g., if Jones tells Smith "Take the stuff," but Smith understands him to say "Take the snuff," with the consequence that he takes the snuff and due to a hitherto undiscovered allergy becomes ill, is his illness a consequence of Jones's action in saying "Take the stuff"?). These are difficult questions, of course, and they have been much discussed in contemporary action theory in philosophy. In the typical case of human action, however, agent, action, and consequences can be identified, and the typical case provides the basis for the widely shared taxonomy of normative theories.

Ethical or broadly evaluative judgments can also be classified using a taxonomy drawing on these features of human action. Some ethical judgments are primarily evaluations of agents, such as "Jones is a compassionate doctor" or "Smith is a conscientious nurse." In these cases the object evaluated is a particular person, and he or she is evaluated as a possible or actual agent of an action. Some other ethical judgments are primarily about actions in the narrow sense, such as "Jones has a duty to tell the patient the truth about the diagnosis" or "The direct killing of the innocent is always wrong." In these cases, the primary object of ethical evaluation is an action—the thing done or to be done. This action

may be characterized either as required ("X must be done") or as permitted ("X would be right to do") or as forbidden ("A would be wrong to do"). More concrete characterizations of actions are also possible, such as "X was a vicious action" or "X was a heroic action." In all of the cases, however, the action is the primary object of evaluation.

A third class of ethical judgments is primarily about states of affairs or objects that are neither agents nor actions, such as "Health is more important than money" or "Human suffering is a terrible thing." Ethical judgments like these do not, directly at least, evaluate either agents or actions. However, the objects evaluated in them, may be, and frequently are, the possible consequences of actions. Thus, this last class of judgments can also be matched to one of the three basic features of human action.

Normative theories may have any of three basic structures, and the differences among these structures are determined by which of the three kinds of practical judgments is taken as basic by a particular theory. *Virtue* theories take judgments of agents or persons as most basic; *deontological* theories take judgments of actions as most basic; and *consequentialist* theories take judgments of the possible consequences of an action as more basic. The sense in which a theory takes a judgment of a certain kind as most basic will become clear in the discussion of each type of theory.

VIRTUE THEORIES. Normative theories that regard judgments of agents or of character as most basic are called virtue theories because of the central role played in them by the notion of a virtue. In the context of these theories, a virtue is understood as a state of a thing "in virtue of which" it performs well or appropriately. In this broad understanding of virtue not only human beings possess virtues but also certain inanimate objects—a virtue of a knife, for example, will be a sharp blade. Indeed, anything that can be said to have a function or role attached to it because of the kind of thing it is may be said to possess virtues, at least potentially.

A virtue theory takes judgments of character or of agents as basic in that it regards the fundamental task of normative theory as depicting an ideal of human character. The ethical task of each person, correspondingly, is to become a person who has certain dispositions to respond in a characteristic way to situations in the world. Differences among persons may be of quite different kinds. Some people are shorter or fatter than others, some more or less intelligent, some better or worse at particular tasks, and some more courageous, just, or honest than others. These differences can be classified in various ways: physical versus mental differences, differences in ability versus differences in performance, and so on. Those features of human beings on which virtue theories concentrate in depicting the ideal human being are states of character. Such theories typically issue in a list of virtues for human beings. These virtues are states of character that human beings must possess if they are to be successful as human beings.

Typically, a virtue theory has three goals:

1. to develop and to defend some conception of the ideal person
2. to develop and to defend some list of virtues necessary for being a person of that type
3. to defend some view of how persons can come to possess the appropriate virtues.

Virtually all ancient moral philosophers developed normative ethical theories of this sort. The ethical theories of Plato and Aristotle, in particular, provide models of this kind of normative ethical theory. As a consequence, the particular disputes that occurred among ancient philosophers centered on questions that one would expect to arise within a virtue perspective. What are human virtues? How are they acquired? Are they essentially states of knowledge? Can one know that a certain trait of character is a virtue without possessing it? Is it possible to have one, or a few, of the virtues without possessing all of them? Are all human virtues of the same type or are there fundamentally different kinds? Are human virtues a matter of nature or of convention? And, most important of all, what is the correct list of moral virtues? Much of the discussion of ethics in ancient Greece centered on a particular short list of virtues—justice, temperance, courage, and wisdom—that came to be called the *cardinal virtues.* After the introduction of Christianity into Europe, these four virtues were joined by faith, hope, and charity—the so-called *Christian virtues*—to form the seven virtues; these, together with the seven deadly vices, dominated medieval thinking about ethics.

One can also see how questions of human character are basic according to virtue theories by seeing how questions about (1) which actions one ought to perform and (2) which consequences one ought to bring about are subordinated to questions of human character. For a virtue theory the question "Which actions ought one to perform?" receives the response "Those actions that would be performed by a perfectly virtuous agent." Similarly, those states of affairs one is required to bring about in the world as a consequence of one's actions are those states of affairs valued by a perfectly virtuous person. Of course, particular actions may also be required by one's particular virtues. For example, someone who possesses the virtue of honesty may be required by the virtue itself to tell the truth in certain cases. Or someone may be required to pursue certain consequences by certain virtues. For example, an agent who has the virtue of benevolence may be required to pursue the happiness or well-being of others. But these requirements are derivative from the virtues, and the fundamental ethical question thus remains a question about the correct set of virtues for human beings.

DEONTOLOGICAL THEORIES. Deontological normative theories take moral judgments of action as basic, and they regard the fundamental ethical task for persons as one of doing the right thing—or, perhaps more commonly, of avoiding doing the wrong thing. While virtue theories guide action by producing a picture of ideal human character and a list of virtues constitutive of that character, deontological theories characteristically guide action with a set of moral principles or moral rules. These rules may refer to particular circumstances and have the following form:

Actions of type T are never (always) to be performed in circumstance C.

Or, they may be absolute in that they forbid certain actions in all circumstances and have the following form:

Actions of type T′ are never to be performed.

The essential task of a deontological theory, then, is twofold:

1. to formulate and to defend a particular set of moral rules
2. to develop and to defend some method of determining what to do when the relevant moral rules come into conflict.

One must qualify, however, the claim that deontological theories make rules fundamental in ethics. What is fundamental, in fact, are actions themselves and their moral properties. This emphasis on actions can take either of two forms: A normative theory may guide action by requiring agents to perform certain kinds of action that can be specified by a rule or other general action guide. Alternatively, one might regard normative theories as requiring particular actions that in their "particularity" elude specification by a rule. This difference has led some moral philosophers to distinguish two forms of deontological normative theories: *rule deontological theories,* which guide action in the first manner, and *act deontological theories,* which guide action in the second. Virtually all influential deontological theories, however, have taken a rule form and, for this reason, this discussion will continue to emphasize the centrality of rules.

Just as a virtue theory subordinates judgments of actions and consequences in a characteristic way, a deontological theory subordinates judgments of character and consequence. The state of character ethically most important in a deontological view is *conscientiousness*—that state of character that disposes persons to follow rules punctiliously, whatever the temptations may be to make an exception in a particular case. Conscientiousness does not have value in itself, but it has value derivatively because it is the most important state of character for ensuring that persons follow rules and, hence, that they do what is right. In a similar way, the consequences of actions that deontologists are most concerned with are the consequences of particular rule-followings. Not all of an agent's practical life, however, need be reduced to rule-following. An agent may have certain personal ideals or particular projects that exist apart from moral rules. These personal ideals or personal projects may be pursued, according to the deontologist, but their pursuit is permitted only if it does not violate the moral rules. Moral rules define the limits of practical pursuits and projects. They are the moral framework within which nonmoral matters can go on. And this is the sense in which moral rules with their emphasis on judgments of actions are basic, according to the deontological view.

Just as virtue theory has its historical roots in the moral philosophy of ancient Greece, deontological theories have affinities with legalistic modes of thought characteristic of Judaic and later Roman thought. The Decalogue (Ten Commandments), although it functions in a religious context, provides a model of a set of rules of conduct that are basic in much the same way rules function in a deontological theory. One is required to follow the rules in the Decalogue because they are the commandments of God, and reasons can be given why it is appropriate to do what God tells one to do. When a deontological theory is deployed in a secular context, however, this reason for rule-following is necessarily absent. Nor can deontologists require that rules be followed because doing so is necessary to become persons of a certain sort or because doing so is necessary to bring about certain consequences. If they took the first route, their view would become a *virtue* theory; if they took the second route it would become a *consequentialist* theory. For a view to be genuinely deontological, it must claim that an agent's fundamental ethical task is to perform certain actions and that the value of this task cannot be dependent on the value of either virtues or consequences.

The most profound attempt to defend this view was anticipated in ancient moral philosophy by the Stoics and was developed in its most persuasive form by the modern German philosopher Immanuel Kant. The Stoics claimed that moral rules are expressions in the human realm of laws of nature and that rational creatures are required to follow these rules because, as creatures, they are parts of nature and, as such, obligated to bring their action in line with natural forces. Human beings differ from other objects of nature by possessing both freedom and reason. Since they are free, they may act against nature; since they have reason, however, they can understand natural laws and choose to bring their action

in line with such forces. Kant's view agrees with the Stoic view in broad outline, but he develops the notions of freedom and reason far beyond the Stoic view. Kant's ultimate answer to questions about how we discover the correct set of moral rules is that only by following the dictates of reason can we be genuinely free.

CONSEQUENTIALIST THEORIES. Consequentialist normative theories take judgments of the value of the consequences of actions as most basic. According to these theories, one's crucial ethical task is to act so that one will bring about as much as possible of whatever the theory designates as most valuable. If a particular consequentialist theory designates, for example, that pleasure is the only thing valuable in itself, then one should act so as to bring about as much pleasure as possible. The goals of a consequentialist theory itself are threefold:

1. to specify and to defend some thing or list of things that are good in themselves
2. to provide some technique for measuring and comparing quantities of these intrinsically good things
3. to defend some practical policy for those cases where one is unable to determine which of a number of alternative actions will maximize the good thing or things.

Like deontological theories, consequentialist theories can be divided into act and rule varieties. *Act consequentialism* requires agents to perform the particular action that in a particular situation is most likely to maximize good consequences. *Rule consequentialism* requires agents to follow those moral rules the observance of which will maximize good consequences. The difference between these two forms of consequentialism, however, is not as straightforward as it may at first seem. It is particularly difficult to precisely characterize rule consequentialism. Is the agent supposed to follow those rules that, if followed by everyone, would maximize good consequences, or rather those rules that will maximize goodness, regardless of how other agents act? There are a number of similar difficulties in characterizing rule consequentialism, and these difficulties have led some moral philosophers to deny that there is a genuine distinction here at all. They have argued, indeed, that when any form of rule consequentialism is rigorously characterized it will be found to degenerate into a form of act consequentialism.

For consequentialists, the distinction between instrumentally good things and *intrinsically* good things is also of special importance. Instrumentally good things are good only insofar as they play some role in bringing about intrinsically good things. If, in a particular case, something that is ordinarily instrumentally good does not stand in the appropriate relation to an intrinsically good object, then its goodness evaporates. Its goodness is merely dependent. Intrinsically good things, on the contrary, are good not because of any relation in which they may stand to other things. Their goodness is independent because it is constituted by the kind of thing the good thing is. Thus, a particular consequentialist theory may hold that only pleasure is intrinsically good, but that other things, including types of action and states of character, are instrumentally good. The virtue of honesty, for example, might be regarded as instrumentally good by such a theory since honesty is likely to contribute to maximizing human happiness. Even if honesty is typically instrumentally good, however, situations may arise in which one could maximize pleasure by acting deviously rather than honestly. In such cases, a consequentialist theory (complications about rule versions of the theory aside) would hold that one should perform the devious action. According to this view, there is nothing about honesty in itself that is good.

Consequentialist theories find their fullest expression in modern thought, especially in the thought of the British utilitarians Jeremy Bentham, John Stuart Mill, and Henry Sidgwick. Drawing on earlier work in the British empiricist tradition, the classic utilitarians claimed that the only intrinsically good thing is human happiness, which they understood as constituted by pleasure and the absence of pain. The utilitarian maxim, "Act always in such a way as to promote the greatest happiness to the greatest number," has been the paradigmatic consequentialist moral principle and has inspired many more recent consequentialists.

There was much disagreement among classical utilitarians, however, about the details of their view. Can pleasures be distinguished qualitatively as well as quantitatively? What role should rules and virtues play within the practical thought of a utilitarian? How can the flavor of the absolute prohibitions associated with justice and the inviolability of the person be preserved within a utilitarian framework? These questions, along with other similar ones, were answered differently by different utilitarians. They were at one, however, in aspiring to formulate and defend a particular version of consequentialism.

The distinction above between the instrumentally and intrinsically good makes it possible to specify more clearly what a consequentialist theory is and to overcome certain difficulties of definition that may creep in. If a consequentialist theory is characterized as one that specifies some object, state of affairs, or property that should be maximized, one might ask whether the object or state of affairs referred to in this definition might be either a state of character or the performance of certain actions. If so, then the distinctions between a

consequentialist theory, on the one hand, and a deontological theory or a virtue theory, on the other, seems to be in jeopardy. If the intrinsically valuable things specified by a consequentialist theory can include actions or states of character, then virtue theories and deontological theories would seem to be mere species of consequentialism, distinguished from other forms of consequentialism by the type of thing they specify as intrinsically valuable. Virtue theories would be consequentialist theories that specify states of character as intrinsically valuable; deontological theories would be consequentialist theories that specify the performance of certain actions as valuable. If deontological and virtue theories are merely varieties of consequentialism, however, there are not three basic structures but rather one basic structure with a number of varieties.

One might deal with this difficulty by defining a consequentialist theory as one that specifies what is intrinsically good but includes neither states of affairs nor actions, but this seems arbitrary. In addition, although this solution no longer allows that deontological theories and virtue theories are varieties of consequentialism, it does not make it possible to understand how these three types of theory exhibit different structures. One can see that there are different structures here, however, by looking more closely at the differences among these theories. Suppose that a particular consequentialist theory specifies certain virtues as the only intrinsically valuable things. Suppose, more specifically, that a particular consequentialist theory, C, specifies that the virtue of justice is the only intrinsically valuable thing. One can also suppose that a virtue theory, V, specifies the good for human beings such that it is constituted solely by the virtue of justice. Are these two theories practically equivalent? If virtue theories are a mere variety of consequentialism, they should be. If they are not, then virtue theories are not a mere variety of consequentialist theory.

One can see that these two theories are not practically equivalent by considering the practical requirements each imposes on an agent. C requires that an agent act in such a way that he or she will maximize the number of just persons. Since consequentialist theories require that agents maximize whatever is intrinsically valuable, and since the only intrinsically valuable thing according to C is the virtue of justice, agents are required by this theory to maximize justice. V, however, need not have this consequence. What V requires of an agent is that he or she develop those virtues that are constitutive of being a good human being. V requires, then, merely that an agent develop justice. There is nothing in V itself that requires an agent to try to bring about justness in others. A virtue theory more complicated than V may include a virtue—perhaps benevolence—that requires agents to promote the well-being of others as well as themselves.

But this requirement to maximize the number of people who possess virtues is not a requirement derived from the nature of a virtue theory itself. It can be derived only from some particular virtue that may—or may not—be a component of a particular virtue theory.

One can arrive at this same point by considering an agent who finds herself in a situation where she can maximize the number of just persons only by becoming herself unjust. In order to make others just, she must become unjust. One example of such a case might be a politician who believes that the best way to make the citizens of her country just is to acquire political power and to exercise it in ways that only she can succeed in doing. Also, suppose she knows that only by renouncing justice herself, by being prepared to act unjustly, can she acquire political power. Thus it is only by becoming unjust that she can most efficiently make others just.

What do C and V have to say to this agent? It is clear that C would approve the renunciation of justice on her part if that would maximize the number of persons who possess justice. The loss of this particular agent's own justice to the sum of justice in the world is more than offset by the gain in the number of persons who are just. The sacrifice is worth it. But what would V require? It is equally clear that V does not require the agent to sacrifice her own justice. Virtue theories hold that an agent's own character plays a special role in his or her practical thinking that it does not play in a consequentialist theory. A virtue theory gives agents reasons to act because it is supposed that each person wants to be a flourishing and fulfilled human being. An agent's own life and character then will have a certain primacy according to a virtue theory. Virtues are not just intrinsically valuable things that should be inculcated in as many agents as possible. They are states of character that each agent must acquire in order to succeed as a human being. Thus, V will not necessarily require that this agent become unjust even if this would maximize the amount of justice in the world.

Similar conclusions follow with regard to a comparison between consequentialist theories and deontological theories. Consider a particular consequentialist teleological theory, C', that specifies that the only intrinsically valuable things are acts of truth-telling, and a particular deontological theory, D, that specifies that the only moral rule is one that enjoins truth-telling in all cases. Are these two theories practically equivalent? Again it is useful to consider a case in which maximizing a particular good requires the renunciation of it by an agent. Suppose that an agent finds himself in a situation in which he can most efficiently produce the maximum ratio of truth-tellings to lyings by himself telling a lie. Perhaps he has discovered that, by telling others that whenever they tell a lie their life is shortened by three weeks,

he can most efficiently promote truth-telling. But he also knows that this is a lie. What should he do?

It seems clear that C' would require him to act in whatever way will maximize the number of truth-tellings, and, if this requires him to lie, so be it. Although his lie may be intrinsically bad, its badness will be more than outweighed by the intrinsically good states of affairs it brings about. The person who accepts D, however, believes that there is a moral rule enjoining everyone always to tell the truth. This rule gives him a reason to act, because he is committed to doing the right thing. He is not committed primarily to bringing about as many right or dutiful actions as possible; rather, he is committed to doing the right thing. Just as a virtue theory holds that an agent stands in a more intimate relation to his own character than he does to the characters of other persons, a deontological theory holds that an agent stands in a more intimate relation to his own actions than he does to the actions of others. The action of an agent who follows a moral rule will have a different moral significance for a deontologist than the action of an agent who brings it about that someone else follows a moral rule. For a deontologist, it is not as important that there be rule-followings as that he or she follow moral rules. D need not then require, or even permit, that the agent tell a lie if this is necessary to maximize truth-telling, and hence C' and D, like C and V, are not practically equivalent. If they are not practically equivalent, however, then deontological normative theories, like virtue theories, are not mere varieties of consequentialism.

Deeper Differences among Normative Theories

This comparison of virtue, deontological, and consequentialist normative theories suggests that the differences among them are deeper than might at first appear. Indeed it suggests that while they certainly differ with regard to which of the three kinds of practical judgments they take as most basic, there are other, and more fundamental, differences among them. To accept one of these normative theories is to accept a particular attitude toward the relation of an agent to his or her character and actions. If one adopts a virtue theory, one's own character comes to have an especially important place in one's practical thinking. It is of the first importance that one become a person of a certain sort. This view need not imply, as it may seem to, that one is committed to an egoistic or selfish life. One may be guided by a virtue theory to pursue a life dominated by generosity and concern for others. One may, indeed, strive to become completely selfless in the sense of always putting the needs of others ahead of one's own needs. But even if this is one's goal, it is also true that one's own character forms the primary focus of one's practical life. The apparent combination here of concern for self and concern for others may appear paradoxical, but it is surely not incoherent. Some of the greatest moral heroes—for example, Gandhi, Jesus, and Albert Schweitzer—seem to have combined these two concerns in their lives.

In a similar way, if one adopts a deontological theory, one's own actions come to play an especially important role in one's practical thinking. It makes a difference to one that one's actions are wrong. It is more important practically to an agent that he or she has told a lie than that a lie has been told. In cases where one's telling a single lie will prevent three others from telling lies, one will not decide what to do by simple arithmetic. Of course, a deontologist will not expect that others will have the same concern for her lie as she will have for it. She may recognize that for someone else, his telling a lie will have a different practical significance for him than *her* telling a lie will have for him. And just as she may not be prepared to tell one lie to prevent him from telling two, she will not expect him to tell one lie to prevent her from telling two. Indeed, she will recognize that from his point of view, his telling one lie is worse in an important sense than her telling two, just as from her point of view her telling one lie is worse than his telling two.

The special significance given to one's actions by a deontological theory need not imply that a deontologist is egoistic or, in the ordinary sense of the term, self-centered. In this way the deontologist is in a situation similar to that of the virtue theorist. The particular moral rules that one is required to follow may give the needs and interests of others parity with one's own, or, more likely, they may require one to put others ahead of oneself. What they cannot require is that one take up a particular attitude toward the rules themselves. The rules cannot, as it were, define their own condition of application—nor can they specify how they relate to one's faculty of practical decision making at the deepest level.

To a consequentialist, giving this special significance to one's character or one's actions may seem confused and possibly morally corrupt. Of course, consequentialists may be concerned with questions of character, but character cannot be their central normative focus. According to consequentialism, what is of primary ethical importance is that the amount of the intrinsically valuable be maximized. Determining the most effective means for maximization involves straightforward questions of efficiency. These questions may be neither simple nor easily answered, but structurally they are straightforward: Which of the possible courses of action will most likely maximize the amount of goodness in the world? In canvassing the possible means to

this end, the consequentialist requires an agent to throw his own character and actions into the same category with other possible means. The kind of character one should develop depends upon the kind of character that will contribute most to the relevant goal. The actions one should perform depend similarly on consequentialist goals. For a consequentialist, one must put a certain distance between oneself—considered as the agent who must make practical choices—and one's own character and actions. One's character and actions have the same role in one's practical thinking as would any other possible means—one's wealth, for example, or influence—that are in a more usual sense external. More important, one's own character and actions have no more special role in practical thinking than do the character and actions of others. All are regarded as possible means to maximize intrinsically good things, and one's own actions and character may have special significance only insofar as they may be more easily—because more directly—manipulated by oneself.

One might think, however, that one feature of the agent's character cannot be treated as a mere means, even by a consequentialist. For any consequentialist theory, it will surely be important that persons have those states of character that dispose them to pursue or to favor intrinsically good things. It might be argued that this state of character cannot be treated by the theory as a mere means. But this argument underestimates the resources within consequentialism for distancing an agent from his or her character. Suppose an agent holds a consequentialist normative theory, C", according to which the only intrinsically good things are states of human pleasure. Suppose also that this agent has a character such that he is disposed always to act in ways he believes will maximize human pleasure. This argument suggests that this agent will not be prepared to sacrifice for the goal of maximal pleasure his own disposition to pursue this goal. But why should this be the case? One might think that a case could never arise in which an agent could contribute most to maximizing pleasure by changing his character to that of someone unconcerned with maximizing pleasure. But this view is surely wrong. Suppose the agent discovers an empirical law according to which human pleasure is maximized only if agents are disposed not to pursue human pleasure but to pursue knowledge. But if this is true—and it is surely possibly true—the agent should act to change as many persons' characters as possible from pleasure-seeking to knowledge-seeking characters. Nor is there any reason why, on consequentialist grounds, this agent should make an exception in his or her own case. So even those features of human character that lead an agent to pursue the maximization of intrinsically good things are not given a special place by consequentialists. Every feature of the character of an agent may be regarded as a possible means to the maximization of the relevant goal.

This feature of consequentialist theories was first emphasized by Henry Sidgwick, the greatest of modern utilitarians. Sidgwick was convinced that if the utilitarian goal of human happiness was to be maximized, then it was necessary that most persons not be utilitarians. Indeed, he thought that what was probably required was that most persons hold deontological views and have their character shaped in accordance with such views. He proposed then, for utilitarian reasons, that utilitarianism be propagated as an esoteric view, and that only a few of the most able and intelligent members of society have their characters shaped in accord with it. These bearers of the esoteric view, in turn, would mold the characters of those less able and enlightened in accord with a deontological perspective. Had Sidgwick's enlightened few become convinced that maximal human happiness required that they, too, acquire "deontological characters," simple consistency would have required them to change their own characters appropriately. In this way, consequentialism might require that agents strive to bring about a world in which no one, not even oneself, has the kind of character that would dispose one to strive at the most basic practical level for consequentialist goods.

Justifying Normative Theories

The question of how, if at all, one can rationally choose among these three normative theories is a question taken up under the topic of moral epistemology. It is important to note here, however, that these normative theories emerge in Western thought as components in comprehensive philosophical theories developed by Plato, Aristotle, Aquinas, Kant, Mill, and other major philosophers. They are embedded in rich and complex worldviews in ways that make it difficult to discuss them in isolation from their theoretical and historical settings.

The tendency within contemporary ethical theory is to discuss the merits of these views in purely ethical terms and to ignore to a large extent their larger theoretical settings. Thus, consequentialism is frequently attacked because it is alleged to countenance the judicial punishment of the innocent if that is required for achieving some good end. In arguments like this one, the alleged ethical implications of a normative theory are appealed to in order to evaluate the theory. Similarly, deontologists may be criticized for holding that certain actions are morally forbidden even if performing them in a particular case might prevent an enormous tragedy. It is now a matter of record that these arguments have been unsuccessful in producing agreement within

normative ethics. Nevertheless, the same slightly tired arguments continue to be made.

The lesson from the history of these views would seem to be, however, that if any of them is to be adequately defended, or successfully criticized, its theoretical setting must be taken into account. Each of these theories has complex relations with particular philosophical accounts of rationality, explanation, nature, intention, the law, the passions, and other topics of central philosophical interest. A more adequate account of them, if possible here, would have to take these theoretical entanglements into account. Certainly any serious attempt to choose rationally among them would have to locate them in this larger theoretical setting.

Normative Ethics and Practice

The raison d'être for normative ethics, as we have seen, is to guide action, and the theories explored above have been developed with such guidance in mind. There is general disagreement, however, about exactly how these normative theories are to relate to the resolution of particular normative problems. It is not easy to demonstrate how the debate between consequentialists and deontologists is related to more concrete disagreements about physician-assisted suicide or recombinant DNA research. Part of the difficulty arises from the fact that each of the three normative theories embodies a particular conception of how it relates to concrete normative problems. There is no theory-independent criterion of how normative theories are to guide action, since each theory embodies a view about its own application. In this way normative theories double back on themselves with regard to their action-guiding function.

An illustration of this doubling-back phenomenon is found in current debates about the relation of virtue theories to practice. Virtue theories are frequently criticized because they do not yield concrete action guides in the way that consequentialist and deontological theories appear to do. The moral advice to "Be just" lacks the action-guiding bite of either a moral rule that requires an agent to perform certain actions or a consequentialist conception that specifies some good to be maximized. But this objection fails to take account of the distinctive way in which virtue theories purport to guide action. A central claim of virtue theories is that the action-guiding function of a normative theory is not to resolve concrete puzzles about action. Edmond Pincoffs, a leading contemporary virtue theorist, coined the useful term "quandary ethics" precisely to designate what virtue theories are against: a conception of normative ethics as guiding action by giving a particular solution to quandaries about action. If one supposes that the only way in which a normative theory can guide action is by resolving particular moral quandaries, then one is unlikely to take virtue theories seriously.

Virtue theories offer, however, an alternative account of the action-guiding function of normative theories. They claim that an adequate normative theory will prescribe something like a training program to make agents ethically "fit." This program may not specify exactly how one is to act in particular cases, because these decisions are best left to the prudential decisions of a "morally fit" agent in the concrete decison-making situation. Thus, virtue theories double back on themselves and specify how they are to relate to practice. Both deontological and consequentialist theories also contain such self-referential accounts of their own application.

An important implication of this doubling-back phenomenon is that one cannot assess the adequacy of normative theories by invoking a well-defined criterion for "successful" action-guiding without begging the question. To have such a well-defined criterion is already to have taken a position on some of the fundamental questions in normative ethics.

This difficulty is actually even more serious than this first point suggests. It is not just that each of the three normative theories embodies a well-defined criterion of how normative theory should relate to practice. Also, there are a number of different models of how general ethical thinking should relate to concrete practice. Some of these models have loose affinities with some of the normative theories, but there is not a fixed or necessary connection between them. Indeed, the conflicts among the normative theories cut across, in complex ways, the conflicts among these models for relating normative theory to practice. A representative collection of these models would include: (1) deductivism, (2) dialectical models, (3) principlism, (4) casuistical models, and (5) situation ethics. These models have been for the most part badly defined in the current literature, and the differences among them and their relations to traditional normative theories tend to be matters of dispute.

DEDUCTIVISM. The deductivist model regards the action-guiding function of ethical theory to be the development of highly abstract and general first principles that, together with some factual description of a particular morally problematic situation, will entail concrete action guides. According to this model, moral principles developed and defended within normative ethical theory will play the role of premises in deductive arguments for ethical judgments about particular cases. This model of application is particularly attractive to some deontologists and consequentialists. It is related to more general accounts of justification in contemporary epistemology that suggest that all justification must come from some set of foundational claims in the area in question.

It also makes large demands on the justificatory resources of a normative theory, since all of the justification for the principles must come from the theory itself. There is no "bottom up" justification from particular moral beliefs to general principles, as will be found in some of the other models.

DIALECTICAL MODELS. Partly because of worries about the foundationalist character of deductivism, some moral theorists understand the relation between normative theory and practice in a dialectical way. Instead of supposing that justification is exclusively "top down," they suppose that there is dialectical interplay between the principles in a normative theory and particular moral judgments. Normative principles may be modified if they fail to fit our deeply held particular moral beliefs, just as our particular beliefs may be modified in order to fit principles. Whether agents modify principles or particular judgments will depend upon their degree of commitment to each and to the other beliefs they might hold. Just as the deductivist model has affinities with foundationalist theories in epistemology, the dialectical model is inspired by coherentist epistemological theories, which suggest that justification in general is to be understood as a function of how large sets of propositions "hang together" or cohere. The most influential form of the dialectical model is John Rawls's "method of reflective equilibrium," which he uses to support his deontological normative theory.

PRINCIPLISM. Some philosophers have wanted to downplay the importance of normative theory for resolving concrete ethical problems. They emphasize, for example, that consequentialist and deontological normative theories in most cases mandate the same actions, and that it is only in exceptional cases that differences seem to emerge. And they add that the exceptional cases are likely to be so difficult to resolve that both consequentialists and deontologists disagree among themselves about what normative theory requires. They conclude that general ethical reflection should focus on what they call "middle-level" principles, that is, not the most general principles in any normative theory but those that are likely to be acceptable to adherents of different normative theories. They hope that agreement may be easier to achieve in practical matters if the premises for practical arguments are not sought at the deepest level of normative theory. This model has been especially influential in bioethics and has been developed and defended by Tom Beauchamp and James Childress (1989). The middle-level principles they propose are labeled autonomy, beneficence, nonmaleficence, and justice. Their claim is that these principles, when suitably refined, are likely to be acceptable to both rule consequentialists and deontologists.

CASUISTICAL MODEL. Some philosophers have understood genuinely practical and action-guiding thinking in a way that makes it even more remote from the disputes among the classical normative theories. They propose that the appropriate model for practical reflection is found in the case-based approach popular in late medieval and early modern moral thought. According to this approach, ethical reflection should focus on certain paradigm cases of morally good action or morally bad action. Arguments from these paradigm cases to more problematic cases may be made by exploring similarities and differences between the two. This approach rejects attempts to formulate the goodness or badness of paradigm cases in abstract and general principles, and emphasizes analogical as opposed to deductive reasoning. Albert Jonsen and Stephen Toulmin (1988) have been the leading advocates of this model in recent normative ethics.

SITUATION ETHICS. Some might suggest that situation ethics is not so much a model for practical thinking as a rejection of any model. It claims that one should approach the resolution of particular moral problems by eschewing all general action guides in favor of concentrated attention to the details of the particular situation. In some of its versions it may look a bit like the casuistical model; but in its most radical formulations it would mandate that even paradigm cases should play no central role in particular reflection because they could deflect the agent's attention from the particular features of the case under consideration. Among contemporary thinkers, Joseph Fletcher has been the most prominent advocate of this view, although his early commitment to situation ethics developed later into a more general commitment to consequentialism. In his formulation of situation ethics, he suggests that reflection on particular cases should be guided by the general principle, "Do the loving thing!" However, he is insistent that this principle does not play the role of a premise in any deductive practical argument.

These five models represent different ways of thinking about how ethical reflection might be brought to bear on particular moral problems. They range from deductivism, in which successful ethical reflection requires premises drawn from an adequate normative theory, to situation ethics, which eschews any dependence on normative theory. The other three theories occupy the middle ground between these two extremes. In contemporary ethics there is no consensus on which of these models is most adequate. Each has its defenders and its critics, and there is a lively discussion in the contemporary literature about their respective merits.

When this disagreement about the correct approach to concrete ethical reflection is added to the disagreement among classical normative theories, it is easy to see why contemporary applied ethics involves conflicts of such depth and complexity. One is confronted not only with competing normative theories, but also with competing conceptions of how such theories would relate to concrete ethical problems. These two different levels of disagreement indeed tend to reinforce one another, since particular disagreements at each level tend to be tied to particular disagreements at the other.

Normative Theories and Bioethics

The revival of normative ethics in the 1960s was associated with a general renewed interest, across Western culture, in applied ethics and especially in bioethics. Rational reflection on the difficult ethical issues associated with the expanded technological resources of the biological sciences demanded a theoretical structure of some richness, and the classical normative theories provided that structure.

The conflicts between deontological and consequentialist theories have been particularly salient in discussions within bioethics. Indeed, some general discussions of bioethics and many popular textbooks treat these two options as if they are the only possible theoretical perspectives. Part of the explanation for this is surely that so many of the ethical problems in medical practice, as well as in the biological sciences more generally, involve questions about whether actions that are generally regarded as morally problematic can be justified in cases where they appear to promise great benefits. Examples of this kind of conflict are plentiful in contemporary bioethics: Can information obtained by a physician in a doctor-patient encounter be revealed to a third party without the patient's consent, if doing so will prevent some great harm? Can physicians lie to their patients in cases where doing so will increase the effectiveness of therapy and decrease the chances of severe depression? Can physicians override the religious objections of patients to certain therapies when it is clear that these therapies will provide important benefits to the patients?

Moral difficulties like these have been at the center of contemporary discussions in bioethics from its inception. They lend themselves to an analysis that regards them as embodying a general conflict between the thought that some actions (e.g., revealing confidential information, lying, or paternalistic interference) are simply not to be done and the thought that one should be prepared to do whatever is necessary so that things go as well as they can. This conflict in turn seems very close to the fundamental issues at stake between the deontologist and the consequentialist.

Until recent years, virtue theories have been conspicuously absent from most discussions of bioethics. The renewed interest in these approaches is associated with their revival within moral philosophy generally. But there are also features of contemporary bioethics that explain the attention they receive. First, a kind of impasse has developed between consequentialist and deontological approaches to some bioethical problems, and bioethicists have turned to virtue theories with the hope that they can avoid this impasse. Second, there is a new interest in questions about the character of the various agents (e.g., physicians, nurses, researchers, and technicians) who work in settings where bioethical issues arise. This interest in character is partially a reflection of impatience with "quandary ethics." It also, however, grows out of the search for new models of moral education. Molding and shaping character has seemed to many a more attractive goal for moral education than the goal of inculcating rules. Shaping character indeed seems especially important in bioethics, where change is endemic and rules become outdated quickly.

Finally, virtue theories seem to be attracting more attention within bioethics because of the strong analogies between the notion of health and overall biological fitness, on the one hand, and, on the other, the more general notion of human flourishing that lies at the heart of virtue theories. For those who think that bioethical issues are best approached by getting clear on the goals of the biomedical sciences, this analogy is likely to lead them to take virtue theories seriously.

In spite of the recent revival of virtue ethics both within bioethics and within moral philosophy more generally, however, the dominant argumentative strategies in bioethics continue to be drawn from the deontological and consequentialist traditions. Nevertheless, each of the three traditions is now represented in the contemporary bioethical discussion by competent and enthusiastic advocates, and it seems certain that the central problems within bioethics will continue to be discussed in terms contributed by these normative traditions.

W. DAVID SOLOMON (1995)
BIBLIOGRAPHY REVISED

SEE ALSO: *Care; Casuistry; Communitarianism and Bioethics; Contractarianism and Bioethics; Double Effect, Principle or Doctrine of; Emotions; Obligation and Supererogation; Human Rights; Natural Law; Principalism; Utilitarianism; Virtue and Character;* and other *Ethics* subentries

BIBLIOGRAPHY

Alora, Angeles Tan, and Lumitao, Josephine M., eds. 2001. *Beyond Western Bioethics: Voices from the Developing World.* Washington, D.C.: Georgetown University Press.

Anscombe, G. E. M. 1958. "Modern Moral Philosophy." *Philosophy* 33: 1–19.

Beauchamp, Tom L., and Childress, James F. 1989. *Principles of Biomedical Ethics,* 3rd edition. New York: Oxford University Press.

Beauchamp, Tom L., and Walters, LeRoy, eds. 1999. *Contemporary Issues in Bioethics (Fifth Edition).* Belmont, CA: Wadsworth Publishing Company.

Brandt, Richard. 1979. *A Theory of the Good and the Right.* Oxford: Clarendon Press.

Broad, Charlie D. 1930. *Five Types of Ethical Theory.* London: Routledge & Kegan Paul.

Curran, Charles E. 1999. *The Catholic Moral Tradition Today: A Synthesis.* Washington, D.C.: Georgetown University Press.

Donagan, Alan. 1977. *The Theory of Morality.* Chicago: University of Chicago Press. A defense of a comprehensive deontological normative theory.

Dwyer, Judith A., ed. 1999. *Vision and Values: Ethical Viewpoints in the Catholic Tradition.* Washington, D.C.: Georgetown University Press.

Fletcher, Joseph. 1966. *Situation Ethics: The New Morality.* Philadelphia: Westminster.

Foot, Philippa. 1978. *Virtues and Vices; And Other Essays in Moral Philosophy.* Berkeley: University of California Press.

Frankena, William K. 1973. *Ethics,* 2nd edition. Englewood Cliffs, NJ: Prentice-Hall.

Gomez-Lobo, Alfonso. 2002. *Morality and the Human Good: An Introduction to Natural Law Ethics.* Washington, D.C.: Georgetown University Press.

Jonsen, Albert R., and Toulmin, Stephen E. 1988. *The Abuse of Casuistry: A History of Moral Reasoning.* Berkeley: University of California Press.

Kavanaugh, John F. 2002. *Who Counts as Persons? Human Identity and the Ethics of Killing.* Washington, D.C.: Georgetown University Press.

Kittay, Eva Feder, and Meyers, Diana T., eds. 1987. *Women and Moral Theory.* Totowa, NJ: Rowman and Littlefield.

MacIntyre, Alasdair C. 1981. *After Virtue: A Study in Moral Theory.* Notre Dame, IN: University of Notre Dame Press.

Macklin, Ruth. 1999. *Against Relativism: Cultural Diversity and the Search for Ethical Universals in Medicine.* New York: Oxford University Press.

McGee, Glenn, ed. 1999. *Pragmatic Bioethics.* Nashville, TN: Vanderbilt University Press.

Moore, G. E. 1903. *Principia Ethica.* Cambridge: Cambridge University Press.

Moser, Paul K., and Carson, Thomas L., eds. 1997. *Morality and the Good Life.* New York: Oxford University Press.

Nagel, Thomas. 1970. *The Possibility of Altruism.* Oxford: Clarendon Press.

Oderberg, David S., and Laing, Jacqueline A., eds. 1997. *Human Lives: Critical Essays on Consequentialist Bioethics.* New York: Macmillan.

Parfit, Derek. 1984. *Reasons and Persons.* Oxford: Clarendon Press.

Pellegrino, Edmund D. 2000. "Bioethics at Century's Turn: Can Normative Ethics Be Retrieved?" *Journal of Medicine and Philosophy* 25(6): 655–675.

Rawls, John. 1971. *A Theory of Justice.* Cambridge, MA: Harvard University Press.

Ross, W. D. 1930. *The Right and The Good.* Oxford: Clarendon Press.

Scheffler, Samuel, ed. 1988. *Consequentialism and Its Critics.* Oxford: Oxford University Press.

Sidgwick, Henry. 1907. *The Methods of Ethics.* 7th edition. London: Macmillan.

Smart, John Jameson Carswell, and Williams, Bernard A. 1973. *Utilitarianism: For and Against.* Cambridge, Eng.: Cambridge University Press.

Sugarman, Jeremy, and Sulmasy, Daniel P., eds. 2001. *Methods in Medical Ethics.* Washington, D.C.: Georgetown University Press.

Thomasma, David C. 2000. "Medical Ethics: Its Branches and Methods." *Philosophical Inquiry* 22(4): 7–23.

Tong, Rosemarie P. 1993. *Feminine and Feminist Ethics.* Belmont, CA: Wadsworth Publishing Company.

Wildes, Kevin William. 2000. *Moral Acquaintances: Methodology in Bioethics.* Notre Dame, IN: University of Notre Dame Press.

Williams, Bernard A. 1985. *Ethics and the Limits of Philosophy.* Cambridge, MA: Harvard University Press.

IV. SOCIAL AND POLITICAL THEORIES

Every social and political theory is entangled with ethics. The great political philosopher Jean-Jacques Rousseau proclaimed that the person who would separate politics from ethics will fail to understand both. Despite the efforts of practitioners of "value-free social science," the concepts and categories with which political theorists work—order, freedom, authority, legitimacy, justice—are part and parcel of competing ethical frameworks. It is very difficult to talk about justice without talking about fairness. What is fair is an ethical question that cannot be adjudicated without some reference to what is good for human beings or what kind of good human beings may strive to attain. Terms that circulate within ordinary discourse, such as "fairness" and "freedom," are also central themes within social and political thinking. The implication for bioethics is straightforward. No matter how strenuously the bioethicist may hope to isolate his or her perspective from metaphysical, ontological, epistemological, and civic imperatives, social and political theory frames and penetrates all bioethical considerations.

The human sciences cannot be value-free. In Charles Taylor's words, "they are moral sciences in a more radical sense than the eighteenth century understood" (p. 51).

There are, according to Taylor, inescapable epistemological arguments for what might be called an interpretive approach to the human sciences, for human beings are self-defining animals. These self-definitions, in turn, take place within a context that shapes our understanding of self and other as well as our appreciation of human possibilities and the need for constraint. We are caught in conceptual webs. It is the task of social and political theory to make more explicit the nature of the frameworks within which we think and act, and hence, the context within which bioethical imperatives make themselves felt, whether as advances in human freedom, triumphs of human control, or dangerous new forms of oppression. Based on an interpretive approach to political theory, this entry will demonstrate why political theory must be normative and will go on to rehearse contemporary debates in social and political theory using the public/private distinction and the women's movement as illustrative examples.

Why Social and Political Theory Must be Normative

Terms of ordinary discourse serve as a conceptual prism through which we view different human relationships, activities, and forms of life. Most of the time we take such terms for granted. We are all shaped by ways of life that are built upon basic notions and rules. Political theorists concern themselves with the ways in which a society's constitutive understandings either nourish or deplete human capacities for purposive activity. It is, therefore, one task of the political theorist to examine critically the resources of ordinary language, revealing latent meanings, nuances, and shades of interpretation others may have missed or ignored. When we examine our basic assumptions, we enhance our ability to sift out the most important issues (Elshtain, 1981).

Society's understanding of the terms "public" and "private," for example, are always defined and understood in relationship to each other. One version of private means "not open to the public," and public, by contrast, is "of or pertaining to the whole, done or made in behalf of the community as a whole." In part these contrasts derive from the Latin origin of "public," *pubes,* the age of maturity when signs of puberty begin to appear: Then and only then does the child enter, or become qualified for, public activity. Similarly, *publicus* is that which belongs to, or pertains to, "the public," the people. But there is another meaning: public as open to scrutiny; private as that not subjected to the persistent gaze of publicity. The protection of privacy is necessary, or so defenders of constitutional democracy have long insisted, in order to prevent government from becoming all-intrusive, as well as to preserve the possibility of different sorts of relationships—both mother and citizen, friend and official.

Our involvement in one of a number of competing ethical or normative perspectives is inescapable. It is influenced by what we take to be the appropriate relationship between public and private life, for this also defines our understanding of what politics should or should not attempt to define, regulate, or even control. There is widespread disagreement over the respective meaning of public and private within societies. Brian Fay sees the public and the private as part of a cluster of "basic notions" that serve to structure and give coherence to all known ways of life. The boundaries between the public and the private help to create a moral environment for individuals, singly and in groups; to dictate norms of appropriate or worthy action; and to establish barriers to action, particularly in areas such as the taking of human life, regulation of sexual relations, promulgation of familial duties and obligations, and the arena of political responsibility. Public and private are embedded within a dense web of meanings and intimations and are linked to other basic notions: nature and culture, male and female, and each society's "understanding of the meaning and role of work; its views of nature; … its concepts of agency; its ideas about authority, the community, the family; its notion of sex; its beliefs about God and death and so on" (p. 78). The content, meaning, and range of public and private vary within each society and turn on whether the virtues of political life or the values of private life are rich and vital or have been drained, singly or together, of their normative significance.

The social and political theorist recognizes that no idea or concept is an island unto itself. Basic notions comprise a society's intersubjectively shared realm. "Intersubjectivity" is a rather elusive term referring to shared ideas, symbols, and concepts that reverberate within a society and help to constitute a way of life. The philosopher Ludwig Wittgenstein claims that when we first "begin to believe anything, what we believe is not a single proposition, it is a whole system of propositions. (Light dawns gradually over the whole.)" (p. 21e). Similarly, when we use a concept, particularly one of the bedrock notions integral to a way of life, we do not do so as a discrete piece of "linguistic behavior" but with reference to other concepts, contrasts, and terms of comparison.

As with the concepts of public and private, there are no neatly defined and universally accepted limits on the boundaries of politics. Politics, too, is essentially contested. An essentially contested concept is internally complex or makes reference to several dimensions, which are, in turn, linked to other concepts. Such a concept is also open-textured, in that the rules of its application are relatively flexible, and it is appraisive or normative. For example, one political theorist might claim that a given social situation is unjust. Another might argue that to label the situation unjust only inflames matters, because he or she believes that certain underlying cherished social institutions and relations should not be tampered with or eliminated in the interest of attaining a political or ideological goal. In another example, the feminist political theorist who believes that being born female in and of itself constitutes an injustice on the "biological" level may want to eliminate all sex differences and a public/private distinction as well, for she will see in distinctions themselves a ploy to oppress women (Firestone). Other feminist thinkers may find this view reprehensible, as it deepens rather than challenges societal devaluation of female bodies and a woman's central role in reproduction. This latter group sees injustice in inequalities that are socially and politically, not biologically, constituted. The point is not to eliminate a public/private distinction but to push for parity in male and female participation in both realms.

Boundary shifts in our understanding of "the political" and hence, of what is public and what is private, have taken place throughout the history of Western life and thought. Minimally, a political perspective requires that some activity called politics be differentiated from other activities. If all conceptual boundaries are blurred and all distinctions between public and private are eliminated, no politics can, by definition, exist (Elshtain, 1981). The relatively open-textured quality of politics means that innovative and revolutionary thinkers are often those who declare politics to exist where politics was not thought to exist before. Should their reclassifications remain over time, the meaning of politics—indeed of human life itself—may be transformed. Altered social conditions may also provoke a reassessment of old, and a recognition of new, "political" realities. Sheldon Wolin observes, "The concepts and categories of a political philosophy may be likened to a net that is cast out to capture political phenomena, which are then drawn in and sorted in a way that seems meaningful and relevant to the particular thinker" (p. 21). Thus each social and political theorist must be clear about what rules he or she is employing to sort the catch and to what ends and purposes.

Bioethical Issues in the Concepts of Public and Private

In the history of Western political thought, public and private imperatives, concepts, and symbols have been ordered in a number of ways, including the demand that the private world be integrated fully within the public arena; the insistence that the public realm be "privatized," with politics controlled by the standards, ideals, and purposes emerging from a particular vision of the private sphere; or, finally, a continued differentiation or bifurcation between the two spheres. Bioethics is deeply implicated in each of these broad, general theoretical tendencies that often touch on the private and the public, as in a case, for example, where a couple decides to conceive a child through artificial insemination by donor (AID). What happens to a society's view of the family and intergenerational ties if more couples resort to artificial insemination? What is the effect on the psychosocial development of donor children? What are the responsibilities, if any, of the donor father beyond the point of sperm donation for a fee? Do contractual agreements suffice to "cover" not just the legal but also the ethical implications of such agreements? Does society have a legitimate interest in such "private" choices, given the potential social consequences of private arrangements? Should such procedures be covered by health insurance, whether public or private?

Questions such as these pitch us into the world of social and political theory and the ways particular ideals are deeded to us. Thus, the social-contract liberal endorses a different cluster of human goods than the virtue theorist or the communitarian. Political and social theory yield ethical debates about these competing ideals of human existence. Moral rules—and whether they are to be endorsed or overridden—are inescapable in debating human existence and the human imperative to create meaning. "Public" and "private" and the relations of politics to each exist as loci of human activity, moral reflections, social and historic relations, the creation of meaning, and the construction of identity.

The ways in which our understanding of public, private, and politics plays itself out at present is dauntingly complex. Contemporary society is marked by moral conflicts. These conflicts have deep historical roots and are reflected in our institutions, practices, laws, norms, and values. For example, the continuing abortion debate in the United States taps strongly held, powerfully experienced moral and political imperatives. These imperatives are linked to concerns and images evoking what sort of people we are and what we aspire to be. The abortion debate will not "go away" because it is a debate about matters of life and death, freedom and obligation, and rights and duties.

Perhaps the intractability of many of the debates surrounding bioethics can best be understood as flowing from a central recognition that language itself has become a preoccupation for theorists and ethicists because of our growing concern for establishing norms, limits, and meanings in the absence of a shared ethical consensus. A persistent theme of contemporary social and political theory is that language helps to constitute social reality and frames available forms of action. We are all participants in a language community and hence share in a project of theoretical and moral self-understanding, definition, and redefinition. Our values, embedded in language, are not icing on the cake of social reasoning but are instead part of a densely articulated web of social, historical, and cultural meanings, traditions, rules, beliefs, norms, actions, and visions. A way of life, constituted in and through language, is a complex whole. One cannot separate attitudes toward surrogacy contracts, in vitro fertilization (IVF), use of fetal tissue for medical experimentation, sex selection as a basis for abortion, or genetic engineering to eliminate forms of genetically inherited "imperfection," from other features of a culture. These bioethical dilemmas do not take place in isolation but emerge from within a culture and thus engage in the wider contests over meaning that culture generates.

Contemporary Debates in Social and Political Theory

Current debate in social and political theory has focused on the question of whether to buttress or to challenge the liberal consensus that came to prevail in modern Western industrial societies. These broad, competing schools of thought are known as liberalism, civic republicanism, and communitarianism. A social movement informed by one or more of these traditions will exhibit conflicting tendencies and posit incompatible claims.

Liberalism comes in many different forms. Some liberal thinkers stress the individual and his or her rights, often downplaying notions of duty or obligation to a wider social whole. They assume, optimistically, that each individual's pursuit of self-interest will result in "good" for the society as a whole. Those whose analyses begin with the free-standing individual as the point of reference and the "good" of that individual as their normative ideal are often called individualists. In the nineteenth century, this standard of individualism was most cogently articulated by John Stuart Mill in his classic work, *On Liberty* (1859).

By contrast, communitarians begin not with the autonomous individual but with a social context out of which individuals emerge. They argue that the pursuit of individual self-interest is more likely to yield a fragmented society than a "good" and fair one. Communitarians insist that rights, while vital, are not the individual's alone. Instead, individual rights necessarily flow from rights recognized by others within a community of a particular sort in which responsibilities are also cherished, nourished, and required of individuals (Bellah et al.).

FEMINISM. The contemporary women's movement and the way in which it reflects, deepens, and extends features of these traditions illustrate the range of social and political debate. There is no single ethics or moral theory of feminism. Liberalism, with its vibrant individualist strand, has been attractive to feminist thinkers. The language of rights is a potent weapon against traditional obligations, particularly those of family duty or any social status declared "natural" on the basis of ascriptive characteristics. To be free and equal to men became a central aim of feminist reform. The political strategy that followed was one of inclusion. Since women, as well as men, are rational beings, it followed that women as well as men are bearers of inalienable rights. It followed further that there was no valid ground for discrimination against women as women. Leading proponents of women's suffrage in Britain and the United States undermined arguments that justified legal inequality on the basis of sex differences. Such feminists, including the leading American suffragists Susan B. Anthony and Elizabeth Cady Stanton, claimed that denying a group of persons basic rights on the grounds of difference could not be justified unless it could be shown that the difference was relevant to the distinction being made. Whatever differences might exist between the sexes, none, in this view, justified legal inequality and the denial of the rights and privileges of citizenship.

Few early feminists pushed this version of liberal individualist universalism to its most radical conclusion of arguing that there were no bases for exclusion of adult human beings from legal equality and citizenship. Nineteenth-century proponents of women's suffrage were also heirs to a civic-republican tradition that stressed the need for social order and shared values, emphasized civic education, and pressed the importance of having a propertied stake in society. Demands for the inclusion of women often did not extend to all women. Some women, and men, would be excluded by criteria of literacy, property ownership, disability or, in the United States, race. Thus liberal feminism often incorporated the civic-republican insistence on citizenship as a robust, civically demanding, and limited privilege rather than a legalistic and universalistic standing.

At times, feminist theory turned liberal egalitarianism on its head by arguing in favor of women's civic equality on grounds of difference, an argument that might be called neo-Aristotelianism. Ronald Beiner writes,

> The basic conception of neo-Aristotelianism is that moral reason consists not in a set of moral principles, apprehended and defined through procedures of detached rationality, but in the concrete embodiment of certain human capacities in a moral subject who knows those capacities to be constitutive of a consummately desirable life. (p. 75)

Thus greater female political participation was promoted in terms of women's moral supremacy or characteristic forms of virtue. These appeals arose from and spoke to women's social location as mothers, using motherhood as a claim to citizenship, public identity, and civic virtue (Kraditor). To individualist, rights-based feminists, however, the emphasis on maternal virtue as a form of civic virtue was a trap, for they were, and are, convinced that only liberalism, with its more individualistic construal of the human subject, permits women's equality and standing.

The diverse history of feminism forms the basis for current feminist discourse and debate. These debates are rife with ethical imperatives and moral implications. Varieties of liberal, socialist, Marxist, and utopian feminism abound. Sexuality and sexual identity have become highly charged arenas of political redefinition. Some feminists see women as universal victims, some as a transhistorical sex class, others as oppressed "nature." A minority want separation from "male-dominated" society. Others want full integration into that society, hence its transformation toward liberal equality. Others insist that the feminist agenda will not be completed until "women's virtues," correctly understood, triumph. Feminism, too, is an essentially contested concept.

Divisions among feminists over such volatile matters as AIDS, IVF, surrogate embryo transfer, surrogate motherhood, sex selection—the entire menu of real or potential techniques for manipulating, controlling, and altering human reproduction—are strikingly manifest. One broad general tendency in feminist theory might be called noninterventionist. Noninterventionists see reproductive technologies as a strengthening of arrogant human control over nature and thus over women as part of the "nature" that is to be controlled. Alternatively, the prointerventionist stance foresees technological elimination of males and females themselves. Prointerventionists celebrate developments that promise control over nature.

The prointerventionists, who welcome and applaud any and all techniques that further sever biological reproduction from the social identity of maternity, are heavily indebted to a stance best called ultraliberalism. This theory is driven by a vision of the self that exists apart from any social order. This view of the self, in turn, is tied to one version of rights theory that considers human beings as self-sufficient, promoting a view of society that sees itself organized around contractual agreements between individuals.

THE SOCIAL-CONTRACT MODEL. The contract model has its historical roots in seventeenth-century social-contract theory, and it incorporates a view of society constituted by individuals for the fulfillment of individual ends, with social goods as aggregates of private goods. Critics claim that this vision of self and society ignores aspects of community life, such as reciprocal obligation and mutual interdependence, thereby eroding the bases of authority in family and polity alike.

The pervasiveness of the individualist position is further evident in the prointerventionist stance on bioethical innovations in the area of reproduction. In this view, new reproductive technologies present no problem as long as they can be wrested from male control (Donchin). Women, having been oppressed by "nature," can overthrow those shackles by seizing the "freedom" offered by technologies that promise deliverance from biological "tyranny." Strong prointerventionists go so far as to envisage forms of biological engineering that would make possible the following: "One woman could inseminate another, so that men and nonparturitive women could lactate and so that fertilized ova could be transplanted into women's or even into men's bodies" (Jaggar, p. 132). The standard of evaluation concerning these technologies is self-sufficiency and control, paving the way for invasive techniques that break women's links to biology, birth, and nurturance, the vestiges of our animal origins and patriarchal control.

The prointerventionist position owes a great deal to Simone de Beauvoir's feminist classic, *The Second Sex*. Beauvoir argues that the woman's body does not "make sense" because women are "the victim of the species." The female, simply by being born female, suffers an alienation grounded in her biological capacity to bear a child. Women are invaded by the fetus, which Beauvoir describes as a "tenant" and a parasite upon the mother. Men, by contrast, are imbued with a sense of virile domination that extends to reproductive life. The life of the male is "transcended" in the sperm. Beauvoir's negative appraisal of the female body extends even to the claim that a woman's breasts are "mammary glands" that "play no role in woman's individual economy: they can be excised at any time of life" (p. 24). If to this general repudiation of female embodiment one adds strong individualism, the prointerventionist stand becomes clearer.

Opposed to the radical prointerventionist stance is the noninterventionist voice associated with feminism in a less individualist, more communitarian frame. The noninterventionists ponder the nature of the many choices the new reproductive technology offers. They wonder whether amniocentesis is really a free choice or merely a coercive procedure with only one "correct" outcome: to abort if the fetus is defective. They speculate whether new reproductive technologies are an imposition upon women who see themselves as failures if they cannot become pregnant. Furthermore, noninterventionists reassess the values identified with mothering and encourage the growth and triumph of values

they consider to be strongly, if not exclusively, female. They insist that technological progress is never neutral, stressing that "progress" requiring the invasion and manipulation of women's bodies must always be scrutinized critically and may need to be rejected.

Strong noninterventionists claim that women want nothing to do with new reproductive technologies. In the words of one, "The so-called new technology does not bring us and our children any kind of qualitative or quantitative improvement in our lives, it solves none of our basic problems, it will advance even more the exploitation and humiliation of women; therefore we do not need it" (Mies, p. 559). As with the prointerventionist posture, there are noninterventionists who maintain a critical stance but do not condemn all reproductive technologies outright. Moderate prointerventionists support some but not all of the technological possibilities presented by contemporary reproductive science.

These differences played themselves out in the quandaries confronted by feminists with the Baby M surrogacy-motherhood case, a situation in which biological motherhood and social parenting were severed—as feminists, especially strong individualist feminists, had long claimed they could or should be (*Baby M, In re*, 1988). It was also a case in which everyone presumably freely agreed to a contract. Baby M was born to Mary Beth Whitehead, who had contracted with a couple, the Sterns, to be artificially inseminated with Mr. Stern's sperm. She was to relinquish the baby on birth for $10,000. Ultimately, she could not give the baby up and refused the money. The Sterns sued on breach of contract grounds.

Although liberal feminism emphasizes contractarian imperatives, many liberal feminists, including such popular leaders of the women's movement as the liberal Betty Friedan, saw in the initial denial of any claim by Mary Beth Whitehead, the natural mother, to her child, "an utter denial of the personhood of women—the complete dehumanization of women. It is an important human rights case. To put it at the level of contract law is to dehumanize women and the human bond between mother and child" (Barron). Friedan implies an ethical limitation to freedom of choice and contract.

Clearly, feminist debates concerning reproductive technology and surrogacy inexorably lead feminists back into discussions of men, women, children, families, and the wider community. Once again we see that bioethical capabilities and possibilities cannot be severed from wider cultural and social surroundings, including our understanding of the human person and his or her private and public needs, identities, and commitments. One broad frame, the social contract, has been noted; it either assumes or promotes the image of the self-sufficient self and goods as the properties of individuals.

THE SOCIAL-COMPACT MODEL. A second model of social theory, that of the social compact, or social covenant, offers a more rooted and historical picture of human beings than that of the social contract. Compact, or covenant, theory does not recognize primacy of rights and individual choice as the self-evident starting point. The compact self is a historical being who acknowledges that he or she has a "variety of debts, inheritance, rightful expectations, and obligations" and that these "constitute the given of my life, the moral starting point" (MacIntyre). Modern uprootedness is construed as a problem in the social compact. To be cut off from a wider community as well as from the past, as required by strong individualist modes, is to deform present relationships. The argument here is not that the compact self is totally defined by particular ties and identities, but that without a beginning that recognizes our essential sociality, there is no beginning at all.

The world endorsed in the social-compact model is in tension with the dominant individualist mindset. For this reason, individualists sometimes claim that communitarians, who endorse a social-compact idea, express little more than nostalgia for a simpler past. But the compact defenders argue, in turn, that the past presents itself as the living embodiment of vital traditional conflicts. The social compact makes room for rebellion against one's particular place as one way to forge an identity with reference to that place. But there is little space in the compact frame for social revolt to take a form that excises all social ties and relations if the individual "freely chooses" to do so, a possibility the contractarian must admit. It follows that the familial base of the social compact is opaque to the standpoint of contract theory, given its individualist foundation. This difference about the family, the social institution that first introduces the child into the world, is the focus of political theory debates that bear important implications for bioethics.

The Family as a Theoretical Battleground

Given their individualist starting point, contractarians tend to devalue women's traditional roles and identities as mothers and familial beings. Proponents of the social-compact model, by contrast, understand women's contributions as wives, mothers, and social benefactors as vital to the creation and sustenance of life itself and, beyond that, of any possibility for a "good life." The compact theorist argues that community requires that an important segment or significant number of its members be devoted to the task of caring for the young, the vulnerable, and the elderly. Historically, the work of care has been seen by ethicists, political theorists, and political leaders, including many prominent women, as the mission of women. They worry that in a world of individualism, an ethic of care will be repudiated or replaced by modes of intervention less tied to concrete knowledge and concern of those being cared for (Ruddick; Tronto). They also advocate a reevaluation of families that gives conceptual weight to the "private realm" by showing that this sphere is central to social and political life. They insist that our understanding of justice must include a notion of what it means to be a caring society and to honor the work of care.

The compact theorist regrets the lack of a descriptive vocabulary that aptly and richly conveys what we mean when we talk about families and what makes caring commitments different from contractual agreements. The intergenerational family, for example, necessarily constitutes human beings in a particular web of relationships in a given time and place. Stanley Hauerwas, for example, claims that, "Set out in the world with no family, without a story of and for the self, we will simply be captured by the reigning ideologies of the day." We do not choose our relatives—they are given—and as a result, Hauerwas continues, we know what it means to have a history. Yet we continue to require a language to "help us articulate the experience of the family and the loyalty it represents.... Such a language must clearly denote our character as historical beings and how our moral lives are based in particular loyalties and relations. If we are to learn to care for others, we must first learn to care for those we find ourselves joined to by accident of birth."

Political theorists have grappled with the issue of the family's relationship to the larger society from the beginning: Where does the family fit in relation to the polity? In his work *Republic,* Plato eliminates the family for his ideal city. The ruler-philosophers he calls Guardians must take "the dispositions of human beings as though they were a tablet ... which, in the first place, they would wipe clean." Women must be held "in common." A powerful, all-encompassing bond between individuals and the state must be achieved such that all social and political conflict disappears, and the state comes to resemble a "single person," a fused, organic entity. All private loyalties and purposes must be eliminated.

Plato constructs a meritocracy that requires that all considerations of sex, race, age, class, family ties, tradition, and history be stripped away in order to fit people into their appropriate social slots, performing only that function to which each is suited. Children below the ruler class can be shunted upward or downward at the will of the Guardians, for they are so much raw material to be turned into instruments of social "good." A system of eugenics is devised for the Guardians. Children are removed from mothers at birth and placed in a child ghetto, tended to by those best suited for the job. No private loyalties of any kind are allowed to emerge: Homes and sexual attachments, devotion to friends, and dedication to individual or group aims militate against single-minded devotion to the city. Particular ties are a great evil. Only those that bind the individual to the state are good.

No doubt the modern reader finds this rather extreme. Many contemporary theorists contend that Plato constructed his utopia in an ironic mode. Whether Plato meant it or not, his vision is instructive, for it helps us to think about the relation of the family to wider civic loyalties and obligations. Plato aspired to "rational self-sufficiency." He would make the lives of human beings immune to the fragility of messy existence. The idea of self-sufficiency was one of mastery in which the male citizen was imbued with a "mythology of autochthony that persistently, and paradoxically, suppressed the biological role of the female and therefore the family in the continuity of the city" (Nussbaum).

Moral conflicts, for Plato, suggest irrationalism. If one cannot be loyal both to families and to the city, loyalty to one must be made to conform to the other. For Plato, then, "Our ordinary humanity is a source of confusion rather than of insight … [and] the philosopher alone judges the right criterion or from the appropriate standpoint" (Nussbaum). Hence the plan of *Republic,* which aims to purify and to control human relations and emotions. Later strong rationalists and individualists take a similar tack: They hold that all relationships that are not totally voluntary, rationalistic, and contractual are irrational and suspect. Because the family is the ultimate example of embedded particularity, ideal justice and order will be attained only when "the slate has been wiped clean" and human beings are no longer limited by familial obligations.

Yet a genuinely pluralist civic order would seem to require diversity on the level of families as well as other institutions which, in turn, promote and give rise to many stories and visions of virtue. This suggests the following questions for social and political theory: In what ways is the family issue also a civic issue with weighty public consequences? What is the relationship between democratic theory and practice and intergenerational family ties and commitments? Do we have a stake in sustaining some models of adults in relation to children compared to others? What do families, composed of parents and children, do that no other social institution can? How does current political rhetoric support family obligations and relations?

Equality among citizens was assumed from the beginning by liberals and democrats; indeed, the citizen was, by definition, equal to any other citizen. Not everyone, of course, could be a citizen. At different times and to different ends and purposes, women, slaves, and the propertyless were excluded. But these exclusions were slowly dropped. Whether the purview of some or all adults in a given society, liberal and democratic citizenship required the creation of persons with qualities of mind and spirit necessary for civic participation. This creation of citizens was seen as neither simple nor automatic by early liberal theorists, leading many to insist upon a structure of education in "the sentiments." This education should usher into a moral autonomy that stresses self-chosen obligations, thereby casting further suspicion upon all relations, practices, and loyalties deemed unchosen, involuntary, or natural.

Within such accounts of civic authority, the family emerged as a problem. For one does not enter a family through free consent; one is born into the world unwilled and unchosen by oneself, beginning life as a helpless and dependent infant. Before reaching "the age of consent," one is a child, not a citizen. This vexed liberal and democratic theorists, some of whom believed, at least abstractly, that the completion of the democratic ideal required bringing all of social life under the sway of a single democratic authority principle.

COMMUNITARIAN VERSUS INDIVIDUALIST VIEWS OF FAMILY: MILL AND TOCQUEVILLE. In his tract *The Subjection of Women,* John Stuart Mill argued that his contemporaries, male and female alike, were tainted by the atavisms of family life with its illegitimate, or unchosen, male authority, and its illegitimate, or manipulative and irrational, female quests for private power (1970). He believed that the family can become a school in the virtues of freedom only when parents live together without power on one side and obedience on the other. Power, for Mill, is repugnant: True liberty must reign in all spheres. But what about the children? Mill's children emerge as blank slates on which parents must encode the lessons of obedience and the responsibilities of freedom. Stripped of undemocratic authority and privilege, the parental union serves as a model of democratic probity (Krouse).

Mill's paean to liberal individualism is an interesting contrast to Alexis de Tocqueville's observations of family life in nineteenth-century America, a society already showing the effects of the extension of democratic norms and the breakdown of patriarchal and Puritan norms and practices. Fathers in Tocqueville's America were at once stern and forgiving, strong and flexible. They listened to their children and humored them. They educated as well as demanded obedience, promulgating a new ethic of child rearing. Like the new democratic father, the American political leader did not demand that citizens bow or stand transfixed in awe. The leader was owed respect and, if he urged a course of action upon his fellow citizens following proper consultation and procedural requirements, they had a patriotic duty to follow.

Tocqueville's discerning eye perceived changing public and private relationships in a liberal, democratic society. Although great care was taken "to trace two clearly distinct lines of action for the two sexes," women, in their domestic sphere, "nowhere occupied a loftier position of honor and importance," Tocqueville claimed. The mother's familial role was enhanced in her civic vocation as the chief inculcator of democratic values in her offspring. Commenting in a civic-republican vein, Tocqueville notes, "No free communities ever existed without morals and, as I observed …, morals are the work of women."

Clearly, Tocqueville rests in the social-covenant or communitarian camp; Mill, in the social-contract or individualist domain. In contrast to Mill, Tocqueville insisted that the father's authority in a liberal society was neither absolute nor arbitrary. In contrast to the patriarchal authoritarian family where the parent not only has a "natural right" but acquires a "political right" to command his children, in a democratic family the right and authority of parents is a natural right alone. This natural authority presents no problem for democratic practices as Tocqueville construed democracy, in contrast to Mill. Indeed, the fact that the "right to command" is natural, not political, signifies its special and temporary nature: Once the child is self-governing, the right dissolves. In this way, natural, legitimate paternal authority and maternal moral education reinforce a political order that values flexibility, freedom, and the absence of absolute rule, but requires order and stability as well.

Popular columnists and "child experts" in Tocqueville's America emphasized kindness and love as the preferred technique of child nurture. Obedience was still seen as necessary—to parents, elders, God, government, and the conscience. But the child was no longer construed as a depraved, sin-ridden, stiff-necked creature who needed harsh, unyielding instruction and reproof. A more benign view of the child's nature emerged as notions of infant depravity faded. The problem of discipline grew more, rather than less, complex. Parents were enjoined to get obedience without corporal punishment and rigid methods, using affection, issuing their commands in gentle but firm voices, insisting quietly on their authority lest contempt and chaos reign in the domestic sphere (Elshtain, 1990).

FAMILY AUTHORITY AND THE STATE. In Tocqueville's image of the democratic family, children were seen both as ends and as means to a well-ordered family and polity. A widespread moral consensus reigned in the America of that era, a kind of Protestant civic religion. When this consensus began to erode under the force of rapid social change (and there are analogues to the American story in all modern democracies), certainties surrounding familial life and authority as a secure locus for the creation of democratic citizens were shaken as well. Tocqueville suggested that familial authority, though apparently at odds with the governing presumptions of democratic authority, is nonetheless part of the constitutive background required for the survival and flourishing of democracy.

Family relations, so this politico-ethical argument goes, could not exist without family authority. These relations and responsibilities, in turn, remain the best way to create human beings with a developed capacity to give ethical allegiance to the principles of democratic society. Because democratic citizenship relies on the self-limiting freedom of responsible adults, a mode of child rearing that builds on basic trust, loyalty, and a sense of commitment is necessary. Family authority structures the relationship between adult providers, nurturers, educators, and disciplinarians, and dependent children, who slowly acquire capacities for independence. Modern parental authority is shared by mother and father.

What makes family authority distinctive is its sense of stewardship: the recognition that parents undertake continuing obligations and responsibilities. Certainly in the modern West, given the long period of childhood and adolescence we honor and recognize, parenting is an ongoing task. The authority of the parent is special, limited, and particular. Parental authority, like any form of authority, may be abused, but unless it exists, the activity of parenting itself is impossible. The authority of parents is implicated in moral education required for the creation of a democratic political morality. The intense loyalties, obligations, and moral imperatives nurtured in families may clash with the requirements of public authority, for example, when young men refuse to serve in a war they claim is unjust because war runs counter to the religious beliefs of their families. This, too, is vital for democracy. Keeping alive a potential locus for revolt, for particularity, for difference, sustains democracy in the long run. It is no coincidence, this argument concludes, that all twentieth-century totalitarian orders aimed to destroy the family as a locus of identity and meaning apart from the state. Totalitarian politics strives to require that individuals identify only with the state rather than with specific others, including family and friends.

Family authority within a democratic, pluralistic order, however, does not exist in a direct homologous relation to the principles of civil society. To establish an identity between public and private lives and purposes would weaken, not strengthen, democratic life overall. For children need particular, intense relations with specific adult others in order to learn to make choices as adults. The child confronted prematurely with the "right to choose" is likely to be less capable of choosing later on. To become a being capable of posing alternatives, one requires a sure and certain place from which to start. In Mary Midgley's words: "Children … have to live *now* in a particular culture; they must take some attitude to the nearest things right away." The social form best suited to provide children with a trusting, determinate sense of place and ultimately a "self" is a family in which parents provide ongoing care, protection, and concern.

The stance of the democratic political and social theorist toward family authority resists easy characterization. It involves a rejection of any ideal of political and familial life that absorbs all social relations under a single authority principle. Families are not democratic polities. The family helps to hold intact the respective goods and ends of exclusive relations and arrangements. Any further erosion of that ethical life embodied in the family bodes ill for democracy. For this reason, theorists representing the communitarian or social-covenant perspective are often among the most severe critics of contemporary consumerism, violence in streets and the media, the decline of public education, the rise in numbers of children being raised without fathers, and so on. They insist, against their critics, that a defense of the family—by which they mean a normative ideal of mothers and fathers in relation to children and to a wider community—can help to sustain a variety of ethical and social commitments, including providing a strong example of adults working together to create a home. Because democracy itself turns on a generalized notion of the fraternal bond between citizens (male and female), it is vital for children to have early experiences of trust and mutuality. The child who emerges from such a family is more likely to be capable of acting in the world as a complex moral being, one part of, yet somewhat detached from, the immediacy of his or her own concerns and desires.

Toward an Ethical Polity

All political and social theorists, whatever their particular philosophic frameworks and normative commitments, agree that social and political theories always embody some ideal of a preferred way of life. Although a handful of postmodern or deconstructive contemporary theorists disdain all normative standards, most social and political thinkers insist that no way of life can persist without a widely shared cluster of basic notions. Those who locate ethical concerns at the heart of their theories hope for a world in which private and public lives bearing their own intrinsic purpose are allowed to flourish. A richly complex private sphere requires freedom from some all-encompassing public imperative for survival. But in order for the private sphere to flourish, the public world itself must nurture and sustain a set of ethical imperatives, including a commitment to preserve, protect, and defend human beings in their capacities as private persons, and to allow men and women alike to partake in the good of the public sphere with participatory equality (Elshtain, 1981). Such an ideal seeks to keep alive rather than to eliminate tension between diverse spheres and competing ideals and purposes. There is always a danger that a too strong and overweening polity will overwhelm the individual, as well as a peril that life in a polity confronted with a continuing crisis of legitimacy may decivilize both those who oppose it and those who would defend it.

The prevailing image of the person in an ethical polity is that of a human being with a capacity for self-reflection. Such persons can tolerate the tension between public and private imperatives. They can distinguish between those conditions, events, or states of affairs that are part of a shared human condition—grief, loss through death, natural disasters, and decay of the flesh—and those humanly made injustices that can be remedied. Above all, human beings within the ethical polity never presume that ambivalence and conflict will one day end, for they have come to understand that ambivalence and conflict are the wellspring of a life lived reflectively. A clear notion of what ideals and obligations are required to animate an authentic public life, an ethical polity, must be adumbrated: authority, freedom, public law, civic virtue, the ideal of the citizen, all those beliefs, habits, and qualities that are integral to a political order.

Much of the richest theorizing of democratic civil society since 1980 has come from citizens of countries who were subjected for forty years or more to authoritarian, even totalitarian regimes. They pose alternatives both to collectivism and to individualism by urging that the associations of civil society be recognized as subjects in their own right. They call for a genuinely pluralist law to recognize and sustain this associative principle as a way to overcome excessive privatization, on the one hand, and overweening state control, on the other. Solidarity theorist Adam Michnik insists that democracy

> entails a vision of tolerance, and understanding of the importance of cultural traditions, and the realization that cherished human values can conflict with each other…. The essence of democracy

as I understand it is freedom—the freedom which belongs to citizens endowed with a conscience. So understood, freedom implies pluralism, which is essential because conflict is a constant factor within a democratic social order. (p. 198)

Michnik insists that the genuine democrat always struggles with his or her own tradition, eschewing the hopelessly heroic and individualist notion of going it alone. Michnik positions himself against contemporary tendencies to see any defense of tradition as necessarily "conservative"; indeed, he criticizes all rigidly ideological thinking that severs every political and ethical concern between right and left, proclaiming that "a world devoid of tradition would be nonsensical and anarchic. The human world should be constructed from a permanent conflict between conservatism and contestation; if either is absent from a society, pluralism is destroyed" (p. 199).

A second vital political-ethical voice is that of Vaclav Havel, a playwright, dissident, political theorist, and, in the years following the "tender revolution" of 1989, the president of a then-united Czechoslovakia. In his essay, "Politics and Conscience," he writes:

We must trust the voice of our conscience more than that of all abstract speculations and not invent other responsibilities than the one to which the voice calls us. We must not be ashamed that we are capable of love, friendship, solidarity, sympathy and tolerance, but just the opposite: we must see these fundamental dimensions of our humanity free from their "private" exile and accept them as the only genuine starting point of meaningful human community. (pp. 153–154)

To this end, he favors what he calls "anti-political politics," defined not as the technology of power and manipulation, of cybernetic rule over humans or as the art of the useful, but politics as one of the ways of seeking and achieving meaningful lives, of protecting them and serving them. "I favor politics as practical morality, as service to the truth, as essentially human and humanly measured care for our fellow humans. It is, I presume, an approach which, in this world, is extremely impractical and difficult to apply in daily life. Still, I know no better alternative" (p. 155). This is the voice of an ethical polity. Were this voice to prevail, the way in which our ethical dilemmas are adjudicated, including those emerging from bioethics, would be rich and complex enough to enable us to see the public and civic consequences of our private choices, even as it would guard against severe intrusion into intimate life from the outside.

Ethical dilemmas are inescapably political and political questions are unavoidably ethical. Bioethical matters can never be insulated from politics, nor should they be. But the way in which such matters are addressed will very much turn on the social or political theories to which the ethicist, the medical practitioner, the patient or consumer, and the wider, interested community are indebted.

JEAN BETHKE ELSHTAIN (1995)
BIBLIOGRAPHY REVISED

SEE ALSO: *Coercion; Consensus, Role and Authority of; Communitarianism and Bioethics; Contractarianism and Bioethics; Human Rights; Justice; Medicine, Sociology of; Natural Law; Paternalism;* and other *Ethics* subentries

BIBLIOGRAPHY

Baby M, In re. 109 N.J. 396, 537 A.2d 1277 (1988).

Barron, James. 1987. "Views on Surrogacy Harden After Baby M Ruling." *New York Times* April 2, pp. A1, B2.

Beauvoir, Simone de. 1968. *The Second Sex,* tr. Howard Madison Parshley. New York: Bantam.

Beiner, Ronald. 1990. "The Liberal Regime." *Chicago-Kent Law Review* 66(1): 73–92.

Bellah, Robert N.; Sullivan, William; Tipton, Stephen; Marsden, Richard; and Swidler, Ann. 1985. *Habits of the Heart. Individualism and Commitment in American Life.* Berkeley: University of California Press.

Cohen, Andrew Jason. 2000. "Does Communitarianism Require Individual Independence?" *Journal of Ethics* 4(3): 283–305.

Donchin, Anne. 1986. "The Future of Mothering: Reproductive Technology and Feminist Theory." *Hypatia* 1(2): 121–137.

Elshtain, Jean Bethke. 1981. *Public Man, Private Woman: Women in Social and Political Thought.* Princeton, NJ: Princeton University Press.

Elshtain, Jean Bethke. 1984. "Reflections on Abortion, Values, and the Family." In *Abortion: Understanding Differences,* 47–72, ed. Sidney Callahan and Daniel Callahan. New York: Plenum.

Elshtain, Jean Bethke. 1990. *Power Trips and Other Journeys: Essays in Feminism as Civic Discourse.* Madison: University of Wisconsin Press.

Elshtain, Jean Bethke, ed. 1982. *The Family in Political Thought.* Amherst: University of Massachusetts Press.

Etzioni, Amitai, ed. 1998. *The Essential Communitarian Reader.* Totowa, NJ: Rowman & Littlefield.

Fay, Brian. 1975. *Social Theory and Political Practice.* London: Allen and Unwin.

Field, Martha A. 1988. *Surrogate Motherhood: The Legal and Human Issues.* Cambridge, MA: Harvard University Press.

Firestone, Shulamith. 1970. *The Dialectic of Sex.* New York: Bantam Books.

George, Robert P., ed. 2001. *Natural Law, Liberalism, and Morality: Contemporary Essays.* New York: Oxford University Press.

Hauerwas, Stanley. 1981. "The Moral Value of the Family." In *A Community of Character: Toward a Constructive Christian Social Ethic*. Notre Dame, IN: Notre Dame University Press.

Havel, Vaclav. 1986. *Living in Truth*. London: Faber and Faber.

Jaggar, Alison M. 1983. *Feminist Politics and Human Nature*. Totowa, NJ: Rowman and Allanheld.

Kraditor, Aileen S. 1971. *The Ideas of the Woman Suffrage Movement* 1890–1920. Garden City, NY: Doubleday.

Krouse, Richard W. 1982. "Patriarchal Liberalism and Beyond: From John Stuart Mill to Harriet Taylor," In *The Family in Political Thought*, pp. 145–172, ed. Jean Bethke Elshtain. Amherst: University of Massachusetts Press.

Kuczewski, Mark G. 1997. *Fragmentation and Consensus: Communitarian and Casuist Bioethics*. Washington, D. C.: Georgetown University Press.

Kuczewski, Mark G. 2001. "The Epistemology of Communitarian Bioethics: Traditions in the Public Debates." *Theoretical Medicine and Bioethics* 22(2): 135–150.

MacIntyre, Alasdair C. 1981. *After Virtue: A Study in Moral Theory*. Notre Dame, IN: Notre Dame University Press.

May, Thomas. 1999. "Bioethics in a Liberal Society: Political, Not Moral." *International Journal of Applied Philosophy* 13(1): 1–19.

May, Thomas. 2002. *Bioethics in a Liberal Society: A Political Framework for Bioethics Decision Making*. Baltimore: Johns Hopkins University Press.

Michnik, Adam. Interviewed by Eric Blair. 1988. "Towards a Civil Society: Hopes for Polish Democracy." *Times Literary Supplement*. February 19–25, pp. 188, 198–199.

Midgley, Mary. 1978. *Beast and Man: The Roots of Human Nature*. Ithaca, NY: Cornell University Press.

Mies, Mark. 1985. "'Why Do We Need All This?' A Call Against Genetic Engineering and Reproductive Technology." *Women's Studies International Forum* 8(6): 553–560.

Mill, John Stuart. 1970 (1869). *The Subjection of Women*. Cambridge, MA: MIT Press.

Mill, John Stuart. 1989 (1859). *On Liberty*, ed. Alburey Castell. Arlington Heights, IL: H. Davidson.

Nussbaum, Martha C. 1986. *The Fragility of Goodness: Luck and Ethics in Greek Tragedy*. Cambridge, Eng.: Cambridge University Press.

Pateman, Carole. 1988. *The Sexual Contract*. Stanford, CA: Stanford University Press.

Plato. 1986. *Republic*, tr. Allan Bloom. New York: Basic Books.

Rothman, Barbara Katz. 1989. *Recreating Motherhood: Ideology and Technology in Patriarchal Society*. New York: W. W. Norton.

Ruddick, Sara. 1989. *Maternal Thinking: Toward a Politics of Peace*. Boston: Beacon Press.

Savulescu, Julian. 1997. "Liberal Rationalism and Medical Decision–Making." *Bioethics* 11(2): 115–129.

Shanley, Mary Lyndon. 1989. *Feminism, Marriage, and the Law in Victorian England,* 1850–1895. Princeton, NJ: Princeton University Press.

Strike, Kenneth A. 2000. "Liberalism, Communitarianism and the Space between: In Praise of Kindness." *Journal of Moral Education* 29(2): 133–147.

Taylor, Charles. 1971. "Interpretation and the Sciences of Man." *Review of Metaphysics* 25(1): 3–51.

Tocqueville, Alexis de. 1980 (1851). *Democracy in America,* ed. Phillips Bradley. New York: Knopf.

Tronto, Joan C. 1993. *Moral Boundaries: A Political Agreement for an Ethic of Care*. New York: Routledge.

Wall, Steven. 1998. *Liberalism, Perfectionism and Restraint*. New York: Cambridge University Press.

Wittgenstein, Ludwig. 1969. *On Certainty,* ed. G. E. C. Anscombe and G. H. von Wright. New York: Harper.

Wolin, Sheldon S. 1960. *Politics and Vision: Continuity and Vision in Western Political Thought*. Boston: Little, Brown.

V. RELIGION AND MORALITY

In the minds of many people, religion and morality are closely connected. Even in secular discussions of ethics, law, and medicine, the presumption remains strong that religious beliefs are an important source of moral guidance, and that religious authorities have a significant influence in shaping attitudes toward biomedical research, new technologies, and medical interventions at the beginning and end of life. Both those who hold religious beliefs and those who do not expect that such beliefs will make a significant difference in the moral lives of their adherents.

When this commonplace assumption about the connection between religion and morality is subjected to examination, however, problems emerge. Although moral virtues and behaviors characteristic of Christian love or Buddhist compassion may be clearly associated with a specific religion, the human possibilities they describe are often familiar and admired, even among those who do not share the religious beliefs. Persons outside of a community of faith may display its characteristic virtues, and those who reject a particular religion may realize its moral ideals better than most of its adherents. For example, Christian writers often turn to Gandhi as the modern model of the love that Jesus preached, while Gandhi valued the life of Jesus as an example of the harmlessness he sought to encourage. This recognition of specific moral virtues in persons outside the community of belief in which those virtues are defined and taught is so common today as to be unremarkable, but it challenges the assumption that specific moral beliefs and practices can be tied to specific religious commitments.

The assumption that religion and morality are somehow related thus gives way to questions about exactly what forms this relationship may take and how it is understood. What claims are persons making when they relate a moral judgment to a religious belief, and how are we to understand the similar judgments that others make on nonreligious grounds? How will these different moral and religious orientations relate to the findings of the biomedical sciences? How should the providers of medical services relate to the diversity of these religious and moral orientations in a complex, pluralistic society?

Types of Relationships

A first step toward answering these questions is to identify the variety of relationships between religion and morality that are found in the world's moral and religious traditions (Little and Twiss). In general, religion is an authoritative source of moral norms and a primary motivation for conformity to moral requirements. Significant variations on this general idea do, however, exist. Is religion the only source of the moral norms, or may those norms, or some of them, be discovered or created in other ways? Is the authoritative source the will of a divine lawgiver, or an intrinsic goodness in the nature of things themselves? Is the motive for moral action a religious love of the good for its own sake, or the hope for an ultimate compensation for the hardships that moral behavior sometimes requires?

Answers to these questions differ, both among different religious traditions and among different schools of thought within a single tradition. The major monotheistic traditions—Judaism, Christianity, and Islam—often represent key moral norms as direct commands of God. In the religions that originated in India—Hinduism, Jainism, and Buddhism—by contrast, the central concept is *karma,* a cosmic moral order that fixes inescapable consequences for any action (Green). Protestant Christianity has often stressed the word of God, the direct divine command that is independent of any human knowledge or wisdom, while Roman Catholic moral theology has relied more on the concept of "natural law," a moral order established by God, but knowable by human reason and apparent in the workings of the natural order (Gustafson).

While it would be possible to explore the relationships between religion and morality by surveying major religious traditions individually, that approach would quickly become a volume unto itself, and it would still do scant justice to the nuances and variety within each tradition. For present purposes, we must limit consideration to a typology of relationships that can be observed in a number of traditions, especially as these traditions come into contact with one another and with the forces of modern technological change. Examples of each type can be identified in a variety of religious traditions, but readers who seek a comprehensive understanding of morality in, for instance, Buddhism or Islam will need to consult other sources, some of which are identified in the bibliography for this entry.

The wide variety of possible relationships between religion and morality may be organized in three prominent types that have received most serious attention from modern scholars: (1) cosmic unity, in which moral obligations derive from a natural or metaphysical order that is understood in religious terms; (2) logical independence, in which moral norms, despite their historical connections to religion, do not depend directly on religion for their validity, and in which religious values must be sharply distinguished from judgments of moral worth; and (3) cultural interdependence, in which neither religion nor morality can be understood apart from the communities in which they have developed and in which their practices have become intertwined.

This typology is derived from modern Western scholarship and reflects particularly the development of religion in modern, secular societies. Each of the types, however, has roots in earlier developments in Western theology and philosophy, and most have parallels in other, non-Western religious and cultural communities. While the emphasis in what follows will be on the modern West, much will be relevant to modern and modernizing cultures in other parts of the world, and analogies to the relationship between religion and morality in other cultural settings may illuminate both those settings and the West's.

COSMIC UNITY. Many cultures have conceived moral and natural orders as an undifferentiated unity. The rewards and punishments associated with moral action are as much a part of reality as the forces of wind and water or the patterns of growth and development observed in plants and animals. To put the matter another way, both the observable patterns of nature and the system of moral requirements are part of a larger order that encompasses all reality, seen and unseen. This unity, expressed both in myths and poetry and in speculative metaphysics, comes into question as science and philosophy develop, but it remains a powerful influence, even in modern, secular societies.

Sometimes, the power that requires moral conduct is thought of in impersonal terms, as a force to be reckoned with by humans and by more powerful beings as well. Early Greek philosophers and poets understood justice (*diké*) in these terms. Justice keeps gods and humans from exceeding their limits, and those who ignore justice risk disaster for the whole community (Adkins). In ancient China, *dao* was a pervasive force that both regulated the order of natural events and set the standard for human conduct (Girardot). Similar concepts appear in other traditions.

In the Hebrew scriptures, the ultimate power is a personal God who is not subject to higher forces, but who addresses human beings in terms of moral commandments (Deut. 5:1–21). This God is also the creator of the natural forces with which humans must reckon. A somewhat later strand of the tradition represents wisdom (*hokmah*) as the pervasive, unifying power by which God both shapes the material world and directs the conduct of good persons (Prov. 8:1–31).

These early conceptions of a moral order inherent in the order of things often gave way to an understanding of laws and obligations as purely human creations, having power only so far as they are enforced. The development of these skeptical ideas often coincided with the breakdown of traditional social patterns, or with the discovery of other peoples and cultures who lived by quite different rules. Both Greek and Roman philosophers, however, retained the notion that some requirements are not conventional, but natural. However much Greece and Persia otherwise may have differed, some moral requirements remained the same in both places (Aristotle).

This idea provided theologians with the basis for a concept of "natural law," through which God's commandments could be known by all rational persons. Thus, the same minimal requirements of morality apply to everyone, whether or not they share the same ideas about God. Both Judaism and Islam developed philosophical systems that transmitted the Hellenistic notion of natural law to the Christian West, and for a brief time in the Middle Ages, teachers in all three traditions could debate the relationship between God's will and the created order in a shared philosophical framework (Jacobs). In medieval Christian theology, natural law related all rational beings to God. Natural law was seen to be the way a finite, rational being participates in the eternal law by which God orders the universe.

The ever-present possibility of elevating a particular aspect of nature to the level of equality with God led, however, to widespread suspicion of natural law ideas among moral and religious reformers. The main line of development in Jewish ethics centered on observance of a code of law based on scripture and rabbinic interpretation, rather than on a rationalist moral philosophy (Lichtenstein). In Islam, the philosophical movement evolved in a more mystical direction, focused on the identity of the human spirit with the spiritual character of all reality, rather than on the moral requirements of a natural order (Rahman). In

Western Christianity, the Protestant Reformation challenged all forms of religious legalism, including the precepts of natural law.

During the seventeenth century, however, a new group of legal and political theorists seized upon the concept of natural law as the key to understanding the relationships between nations as well as persons. While the religious significance of the natural law was not necessarily rejected, it was the universality of the obligation, not its divine origin, that attracted these jurists to the idea. In both legal and theological treatments of natural law, however, these highly articulated systems of moral thought share with the earliest myths of cosmic unity the notion that some moral requirements are inescapable because they are part of the structure of reality itself. Since World War II, renewed interest in theories of natural law as a starting point for an international recognition of basic human rights testifies to the continuing significance of this way of relating moral requirements to religious beliefs about the origin and end of the world in which the moral life is lived (Maritain).

The idea of a comprehensive order that encompasses both moral and religious requirements thus appears both in the most ancient religious traditions and in modern Western theories of natural law. Although reformers in many theistic traditions have sought to restore religious morality to a direct dependence on the will of God, the underlying idea that what God wills is also supported by the natural order that God has created never entirely disappears, even when the human ability to know God's will through the natural order is contested.

LOGICAL INDEPENDENCE. The fact that religion and morality are closely related in the history of Western thought does not, of itself, establish that their connection is important for contemporary moral decisions. The historical relationships might be viewed as accidental or contingent, subject to change without altering the basic requirements of morality. The links between religion and morality might even be points of confusion that obscure important features of both religious and moral truths. For some thinkers, then, it is important to establish the distinction between religious and moral evaluations, even though these may be commonly confused in practice, or integrally related in some more comprehensive system of ideas. Failure to make the distinction between religion and morality runs the risk of subordinating both to prevailing cultural practices, which may themselves be morally questionable.

By the eighteenth century, European philosophers had begun to advance theories about the historical development of religion that were not based on the history presented in the Bible. Religion could thus be given a "natural history," as opposed to the sacred history revealed in scripture. David Hume's "The Natural History of Religion" postulated a primitive connection between fear of the awesome power of natural forces and dread of punishment for moral transgressions. Such fear may continue to serve as a useful inducement to moral conformity, but it leads only to confusion if the source of the moral imperatives is sought in a supernatural power. Against those who worried that a distinction between religion and morality would lead to a decline in moral standards, Hume argued that a sound logical connection between moral requirements and the public good was the only secure basis for morality. A utilitarian calculation of the line of conduct that will produce the largest social benefits is the final source of moral norms, and respect for that public good is the only secure ground of moral motivation.

In addition to the possibility that the connection between religion and morality is simply a residue of primitive superstitions, philosophers noted another point that seemed not only to distinguish religion from morality, but also to give a logical priority to morality. Religious traditions frequently praise a divine center and origin of moral goodness, or point to the lives of exemplary religious figures as examples to be followed. To recognize that goodness seems, however, to require a moral judgment that precedes the religious assent. We can only praise God or emulate the saints for moral goodness if we have an idea of what is morally good, by which we measure even these supreme examples. "Even the Holy One of the gospel," wrote Immanuel Kant, "must first be compared with our ideal of moral perfection before we can recognize him as such" (p. 76).

Clearly, whether one begins with Hume's "natural history" of religion or Kant's rational foundation for moral judgments, morality and religion cannot be simply identical. The Christian natural law tradition used reason to discern God's will in the order of the created world. In Kant and Hume, reason formulates its requirements independently, on the basis of social utility or of logical necessity. The resulting standard of morality is then applied to religion, which may or may not measure up.

This separation of moral requirements from religious belief does not, however, imply that religion has no connection to morality. Many who accepted a rational morality, the requirements of which did not depend on faith, continued to value religion as a motive for the moral life. Love of a God who is perfect in goodness, and reverence for saints who have upheld the requirements of morality in the face of severe temptations, provide powerful motives for people to live up to moral expectations in more ordinary circumstances. Indeed, Kant argued that some conception of God is ultimately required to make sense of the sacrifices that all moral action

requires of us. The logical independence of morality from religion does not require that religion be abandoned, but it does require that moral actions be undertaken precisely because we are convinced that they are morally right, and not because we believe that God commands us to do them.

These philosophical developments coincided with important historical changes in European religious life. By the end of the seventeenth century, the normative requirement of religious conformity was rapidly being replaced by practices of religious toleration and, eventually, by a civic commitment to religious freedom. The logical separation of religion from morality became a sociological necessity as well, if citizens who were no longer united in their religious beliefs were to acknowledge moral obligations to one another. In the United States, especially, the idea developed that a variety of quite different religious beliefs could support a common moral consensus (Frost). Because morality and religion are independent, diversity of religious beliefs need not lead to moral conflict, and moral order does not require religious agreement.

In other cases, where the break with traditional forms of religious and social life was sharper, or where the conflict between religious groups was more intense, public moral expectations were reformulated in nonreligious terms. Where cooperation between religion and government proved difficult, or where the moral consensus between different religious groups was obviously lacking, the concept of a "secular state" provided the necessary basis for social unity. A secular state not only refuses to privilege one or another religious perspective among its people, it resolutely excludes religious considerations from the formation of policy and regulations. Religion and religious morality become private considerations, subject to regulation for the public good.

This understanding first emerges clearly in the French Revolution, but the idea of a secular state has also provided hope for civil unity for many twentieth-century leaders in countries deeply divided by religious strife or torn by controversy over modernizations that undermine traditional forms of religious life. In the United States, where the prevailing model has been the religious consensus on moral expectations, elements of the secular state concept have nonetheless been invoked to curb sectarian religious practices that differ sharply from those of the majority, or to exclude religious arguments from controversial questions of policy. Judicial limitation of a parent's power to withhold medical care from children on religious grounds and political arguments that Roman Catholic opposition to abortion violates the constitutional separation of church and state are two instances in which the apparent lack of religious consensus has prompted arguments for policies of a secular state.

The logical separation of morality from religion, then, provides an important intellectual starting point for the ordering of societies divided by religious differences or seeking to modernize in the face of opposition by traditional religious groups. The distinction between religion and morality does not, by itself, prescribe a role for religion in public life. Religion may be one element in a powerful moral consensus that differs from the religious morality of a traditional society, or it may be virtually excluded from influence by a secular state that defines public morality in terms of a utilitarian calculation of the public good.

CULTURAL INTERDEPENDENCE. Although the logical separation of morality from religion is a premise for much of Western European and North American thought in ethics, law, politics, and even theology, its relevance to other points in history and other parts of the world is less clear. The modern Western distinction between religion and morality is missing from many highly developed religious and cultural systems, which assign duties to persons on the basis of their position in society without obvious distinctions between what modern Westerners differentiate into moral requirements, common courtesy, religious obligations, and patriotic duties.

This is most clear in the traditional societies of India, China, and Japan. Hinduism recognizes few duties that correspond to the universal moral obligations of modern Western ethics. Specific persons owe duties to specific others, based on the place each occupies in a social, moral, and religious hierarchy, so that traditional Hinduism can hardly exist outside of the social system in which it originates. In China, a Confucian system of philosophical morality was tied to the details of the education and duties of an elite corps of governing intellectuals, while in Japan, the traditional religion of the people centered on the cults of specific ancestors and the spirits of specific places. Hinduism and, to a certain extent, Confucianism demonstrated in the nineteenth century that they could be reinterpreted in more universal philosophical terms, but the reconstruction of State Shinto in Japan during the same time period suggests that the unitary system of religion, state, and morals can also be adapted to the demands of modernizing societies (Hardacre).

While the interdependence of religion and culture is most clearly seen in these highly developed national traditions, the missionary religions that have moved across large parts of the world also illustrate this interdependence, precisely in their adaptability to very different cultural settings. Christianity presents very different appearances in Moscow and in Dallas. Buddhism in Tokyo is distinctively Japanese, as it is distinctively Thai in Bangkok. The same might be said for Islam in Cairo and in Kuala Lumpur. Nor are these variations simply the result of a constant teaching consciously applied to different situations. Religious traditions develop by interacting with the economic life and productive systems by which their adherents meet their material needs, as well as by the inner logic of their spiritual teachings. The modern sociological study of religion rests on this awareness of the nonreligious forces that operate on religious communities and the unintended consequences that religious beliefs have in the world of economic life (Weber).

Those who view religion from this perspective identify important changes that religions undergo in modern, technological societies. The institutions of religion no longer occupy the central positions of power and authority they once held. Wider knowledge of the world and more exposure to other cultures lead to an awareness of other religions beside one's own. These changes mark what sociologists call secularization, but the interactions of religion and culture are no less real in that context than they were when religion had a more dominant position.

Secularization may reduce the power of religions institutions and leaders, but it does not produce a neutral culture free of religious influences. A "secular" society is shaped in part by the historical interactions between the religion and culture that have shaped the particular place in which the society now exists. A modern economy influenced by a Confucian past differs significantly from one that has developed out of European Protestantism. The process of secularization, therefore, does not provide a neutral, universal standpoint from which to settle questions of morality and policy.

Since the 1970s, social scientists, philosophers, and theologians have widely accepted this contextualization of their work and have sought to explore its implications for their systematic thought (Stout). What was believed to be universal and rational is now widely seen to be particular. Notions of objectivity, tables of individual rights and duties—even, perhaps, the idea of rationality itself—are shaped by particular cultural starting points.

Where supposed neutrality and rational authority have been used to suppress religious conflict, the continuing influence of religion on culture sometimes results in violent rejection of the secular state and its institutions. Fundamentalist movements throughout the Islamic world and among Hindus in India reject modern secular culture as an alien Western imposition and reassert an identity of religion, morality, and culture. In the United States and elsewhere, renewed interest in the religions of indigenous peoples includes a rediscovery of their distinctive understandings of health and healing, which link religion, morality, and medicine in ways unfamiliar to modern medical science (Sullivan).

The implications of this reassertion of the cultural integrity of religion and morality are, however, variously construed by authors reflecting on modern pluralistic societies. One view suggests that the loss of community and the rise of social disorder is a direct result of the attempt to exclude from public discussion the religious values that are the only available foundation for morality. The social achievements that people in the United States most prize, including their individual rights and political freedoms, are simply the fruit of the Christian moral traditions that gave rise to them. If we hope to continue to enjoy them, we must restore those moral traditions in which they originate to a central role in shaping the life of society (Neuhaus).

Another point of view suggests, by contrast, that the public life of a pluralistic society can no longer provide a forum for genuine moral convictions, which always have a particular religious basis. If we seek to develop persons of moral character, we must do it within religious communities that have a distinctive identity. It may then be possible to translate some of these religious values into public policy through political action, but it will not be possible to offer a public argument for the values at stake. They can only be understood in a community where the way of life in which they originate is cherished and enacted (Hauerwas).

An understanding of the cultural interdependence of religion and morality thus calls into question both the cosmic order that sustains religion's requirements everywhere and the universal, rational morality that is characteristic of modern understandings of the independence of morality from religion. In this emphasis on cultural specificity that is sometimes called "postmodern," everything depends on the relationship between religion and morality in a particular place and time. Those who hold this view agree on the importance of the interaction of morality and religion. They differ over whether this interaction should take the form of cultural hegemony by a particular religious tradition, in order to provide the necessary foundation for public order, or should be practiced in small communities of shared faith, who venture into politics and public policy only for limited purposes and confine their virtues to their separated life.

Implications for Bioethics

Perhaps the most striking result of this survey is the diversity of relationships between religion and morality that are held in different religious traditions and, indeed, within the same religious tradition, in different historical and cultural settings. In a pluralistic society, where researchers often work in global networks and medical-care providers deal with patients and families from many communities, many different understandings of morality and religion will impinge on their work, raising new issues in bioethics.

Questions of patient autonomy and appropriate respect for the human subjects of biomedical research become even more difficult when the parties have not only different religious beliefs about the nature of the human being, but also different understandings of how these beliefs appropriately relate to moral decisions that doctor and patient, researcher and subject, primary parties and review committees must make together. Conflicts may arise, for example, when medical personnel appeal for decisions on clinical or scientific grounds to patients and families whose beliefs do not admit nonreligious reasons for decisive personal choices. It is important in the first instance simply to be aware of this diversity of moral and religious perspectives and alert to their relevance to professional choices. Even specialists who are well trained in bioethics often uncritically accept the viewpoint that morality is logically independent of religion, because that is the position of the moral philosophy that has provided much of the theoretical framework for contemporary bioethics. Without awareness of the other possibilities this entry has surveyed, significant moral issues may be overlooked until they become the subject of public controversy or undermine the relationship of trust between medical-care providers and patients.

Investigations of the cultural interdependence of religion and morality may make us aware of serious moral claims. What a patient believes about ritual purity or about the fate of the soul after death deserves more than just respectful interest. It may determine what it means to treat that patient as a free person with an inherent dignity. In any case, the cultural specificity of all moral and religious perspectives should also alert us to the limitations of the claims of biomedical science.

Cultural interdependence opens up possibilities for serious conflicts between cultural perspectives in medical and scientific institutions. Often, research and clinical personnel do not share the commitments of universities or hospitals that have religious sponsorship. An ethical commitment to scientific objectivity or clinical autonomy, which is easy to sustain when religion and morality are believed to be logically distinct, may come into conflict with the view that sustaining a distinctive religious culture within the institution is the only way to sustain it as a moral community. Alternatively, religious views that stress the importance of distinctive moral communities may withdraw from the more complex, pluralistic world of the medical center or research institute, thus eliminating a possibly important mediating influence between the narrowly focused aims of medical practice and the values of ordinary Jews, Catholics, Muslims, or Baptists who happen for the moment to be patients in a medical facility.

The increasing cultural complexity of biomedical science and its institutions prompts the search for a core of morality that would provide the basis for policy decisions, without requiring unanimity on the religious reasons for those moral requirements. Logical independence of this common morality from particular religious commitments seems to be required, whether the morality is to be founded on a universal moral logic or, less ambitiously, on the necessary requirements of medical practice. Although the idea of a completely neutral, secular medical ethics may no longer be plausible, a standard of "secular arguments" for policy choices seems to some observers to solve the problem of moral and religious difference. By insisting that arguments for or against specific policy choices must be made for reasons accessible to all parties in the debate, we eliminate public choices based on specific religious convictions. Arguments for or against a program of acquired immunodeficiency syndrome (AIDS) education and prevention on ground of its effect on community health are acceptable. Arguments for or against it on grounds that it conforms to the requirements of a specific religious teaching are not.

While the standard of "secular arguments" or "publicly accessible reasons" is appealing, it presupposes a very large area of public moral consensus. Although some such consensus does exist, its scope is unclear, and there is no guarantee that it is actually broad enough to resolve the difficult bioethical issues that divide society today. In short, it may be that a strictly defined "secular argument" will be insufficient to yield a determinate solution to the problems, that some appeal to the religious convictions or other private views of the participants will be necessary if we are to settle the questions at all (Greenawalt).

Efforts to define an independent system of morality, in which bioethical issues could be resolved without reference to the diversity of religious moral positions, are thus subject to a variety of problems. The issues range from attacks on the supposed neutrality and objectivity of secular scientific inquiry, to the criticism that if it should achieve this neutrality, it would be unable to provide determinate solutions to policy questions that have been posed to medicine and science.

Another possibility, however, is to accept the unity of religious and moral discourse and ask whether biomedical science and clinical practice might participate in it. Physicians and other providers of medical services have ideas about human flourishing based on long experience with patients and clients. Scientific research may confirm or disprove widespread convictions about the best means to achieve and sustain a good life, and it may provide new evidence of causal links between choices and outcomes. Discussion of the human good typically takes quite different forms from the highly structured discourse of the biomedical sciences, but those sciences clearly do have a contribution to make to it.

Beliefs that hold that there is a cosmic unity of religion and morality, a single reality in which religious and moral truths make sense together, offer the clearest opportunities for biomedical participation. This openness is most apparent in contemporary formulations of natural law theory, which explicitly make use of biomedical knowledge as part of the determination of what is natural and what the conditions for human flourishing are. Even where religious traditions have not developed systematic statements, however, their narratives and rituals make implicit claims about the constraints that the world imposes on human life, and about what human beings must do to live well within those limits (Lovin and Reynolds).

Where these myths, narratives, hymns, and rites are taken to be rivals to a scientific account of reality, there will inevitably be conflicts between the biomedical sciences the religious ideas about morality. But religious discourse is never simply an objective account of the way things are. It is always also an orientation of human life within that world of facts, and the physician's or the medical researcher's account of those facts may have a place in that orientation. Such an understanding neither separates religion from morality, nor links them both to a specific cultural system, but regards morality as an orientation of human life within a reality that is susceptible both to scientific examination and to the imaginative and liberating comprehension that religion offers.

Those who seek to join a discussion of the human good in which both religious wisdom and scientific discovery have a place must acknowledge that there are other views, religious and scientific, that will reject that collaboration. A moral realism that links religion, science, and morality may provide the best framework for biomedical researchers and clinicians to explain the ethical implications of their work in terms that many religious traditions can accept.

ROBIN W. LOVIN (1995)

SEE ALSO: *African Religions; Bioethics, African-American Perspectives; Buddhism, Bioethics in; Christianity, Bioethics in; Daoism, Bioethics in; Eugenics and Religious Law; Islam, Bioethics in; Jainism, Bioethics in; Judaism, Bioethics in; Medical Ethics, History of Europe; Mormonism, Bioethics in; Native American Religions, Bioethics in; Reproductive*

Technologies; Sikhism, Bioethics in; Transhumanism and Posthumanism; and other *Ethics* subentries

BIBLIOGRAPHY

Adkins, Arthur W. H. 1985. "Cosmogony and Order in Ancient Greece." In *Cosmogony and Ethical Order: New Essays in Comparative Ethics,* pp. 39–66, ed. Robin W. Lovin and Frank E. Reynolds. Chicago: University of Chicago Press.

Aristotle. 1962. *Nicomachean Ethics,* tr. Martin Ostwald. Indianapolis, IN: Bobbs-Merrill.

Frost, J. William. 1990. *A Perfect Freedom: Religious Liberty in Pennsylvania.* Cambridge, Eng.: Cambridge University Press.

Girardot, Norman J. 1985. "Behaving Cosmogonically in Early Taoism." In *Cosmogony and Ethical Order: New Essays in Comparative Ethics,* pp. 67–97, ed. Robin W. Lovin and Frank E. Reynolds. Chicago: University of Chicago Press.

Green, Ronald M. 1978. *Religious Reason: The Rational and Moral Basis of Religious Belief.* New York: Oxford University Press.

Greenawalt, Kent. 1988. *Religious Convictions and Political Choice.* New York: Oxford University Press.

Gustafson, James M. 1978. *Protestant and Roman Catholic Ethics: Prospects for Rapprochement.* Chicago: University of Chicago Press.

Hardacre, Helen. 1989. *Shinto and the State, 1868–1988.* Princeton, NJ: Princeton University Press.

Hauerwas, Stanley. 1981. *A Community of Character: Toward a Constructive Christian Social Ethic.* Notre Dame, IN: University of Notre Dame Press.

Hume, David. 1927. "The Natural History of Religion." In *Hume: Selections,* pp. 253–283, ed. Charles W. Hendel. New York: Scribner's.

Jacobs, Louis. 1978. "The Relationship Between Religion and Ethics in Jewish Thought." In *Contemporary Jewish Ethics,* pp. 41–58, ed. Menachem Marc Kellner. New York: Sanhedrin Press.

Kant, Immanuel. 1964. *The Moral Law; or Kant's Groundwork of the Metaphysics of Morals,* tr. Herbert J. Paton. New York: Harper and Row.

Lichtenstein, Aharon. 1978. "Does Jewish Tradition Recognize an Ethic Independent of Halakha?" In *Contemporary Jewish Ethics,* pp. 102–123, ed. Menachem Marc Kellner. New York: Sanhedrin Press.

Little, David, and Twiss, Sumner B. 1978. *Comparative Religious Ethics: A New Method.* New York: Harper and Row.

Lovin, Robin W., and Reynolds, Frank E. 1985. "In the Beginning." In *Cosmogony and Ethical Order: New Essays in Comparative Ethics,* pp. 1–35, ed. Robin W. Lovin and Frank E. Reynolds. Chicago: University of Chicago Press.

Maritain, Jacques. 1951. *Man and the State.* Chicago: University of Chicago Press.

Neuhaus, Richard J. 1984. *The Naked Public Square: Religion and Democracy in America.* Grand Rapids, MI: William B. Eerdmans.

Rahman, Fazlur. 1979. *Islam,* 2nd edition. Chicago: University of Chicago Press.

Stout, Jeffrey. 1988. *Ethics after Babel: The Languages of Morals and Their Discontents.* Boston: Beacon Press.

Sullivan, Lawrence E. 1988. *Icanchu's Drum: An Orientation to Meaning in South American Religions.* New York: Macmillan.

Weber, Max. 1958. *The Protestant Ethic and the Spirit of Capitalism,* tr. Talcott Parsons. New York: Scribner's.

ETHICS COMMITTEES AND ETHICS CONSULTATION

• • •

The dominant mechanism for dealing with clinical ethics problems in healthcare at the beginning of the twenty-first century is the ethics committee. Present in various capacities since the 1960s, ethics committees in their contemporary form emerged in the late 1970s and 1980s in response to the growing need for a formal means to address ethical issues in clinical settings (Fost and Cranford). Early ethics committees were typically staffed by physicians and convened on an *ad hoc* basis. Indeed, in the period immediately following *In re Quinlan* (1976), ethics committees functioned largely as prognosis committees for difficult end-of-life cases in acute care settings. A 1983 study indicated that only about 1 percent of all U.S. hospitals had ethics committees, a figure that is consistent with this very limited function (Youngner, Jackson, Coulton, et al.). As awareness of the value-laden nature of clinical decision making grew, so did the role and number of ethics committees. Just four years later, a 1987 study suggested the presence of ethics committees in over 60 percent of U.S. hospitals (Fleetwood, Arnold, and Baron). In 1998–1999, the University of Pennsylvania Ethics Committee Research Group (ECRG) conducted the most comprehensive study of ethics committees to date and found that approximately 93 percent of U.S. hospitals have ethics committees (McGee, Caplan, Sanogle, et al.). Around the same time, an Agency for Healthcare Research and Quality (AHRQ) study of ethics consultation in U.S. hospitals, a standard function of ethics committees today, found ethics consultation services in all U.S. hospitals with 400 beds or more, all federal hospitals, and all hospitals that are members of the Council of Teaching Hospitals (Fox). Though there has been no systematic study of the presence of ethics committees outside of hospital settings, it should be noted that ethics committees are present in many other healthcare settings, such as long term care, hospice, and even home care.

Contemporary ethics committees are usually standing committees with multidisciplinary representation, including medicine, nursing, social work, law, pastoral care, healthcare administration, and various specialty areas (McGee, et al.). The primary functions of contemporary ethics committees are ethics education, policy formation and review, and ethics consultation, in decreasing order of time commitment (McGee, et al.).

Education

In re Quinlan gave impetus to the development of early ethics committees. Since, as mentioned above, these committees were largely staffed by physicians and primarily concerned with prognosis issues in end-of-life situations, the educational needs of ethics committee members were rather narrowly focused. Encouraged, among others, by a President's Commission (1983), professional societies such as the American Medical Association (1985), and accrediting bodies such as the Joint Commission on the Accreditation of Healthcare Organizations (JCAHO, 1992), ethics committees evolved to become the primary mechanism through which clinical ethics issues are formally addressed. Educational efforts of a thriving ethics committee should include self education, education of health professionals and staff, and community outreach. Of these, self education is critical as it is an important precondition of both sound policy formation and review and ethics consultation. Consistent with this, the 1999 ECRG study indicated "self education" as the single activity to which ethics committees devoted the highest percentage of time (McGee, et al.).

Though physicians and nurses make up the largest majority of ethics committee membership, most ethics committees are multidisciplinary with members from social work, pastoral care, legal, and administration, among others (McGee, et al.). This broad spectrum of health professionals brings valuable experience and perspective in dealing with clinical ethical issues, which are inevitably complex and multilayered. The vast majority of ethics committee members, however, have no formal education or training in clinical ethics; thus self education is an important ethics committee activity (Fox; McGee, et al.). Indeed, in the 1999 ECRG study mentioned above, half of all ethics committee chairs reported "feeling inadequately prepared to address" the issues they face (McGee, et al.). This is not surprising, given that ethics committees face an array of complex clinical ethics issues, including informed consent and refusal of treatment, decision capacity or competence, confidentiality and privacy, minors and decision making, and a host of issues related to end of life decision making. To deal with

these and other clinical ethics issues, ethics committees need to have a sustained self-education program.

Ethics committees have used a variety of means to meet this need. Ethics committees at academic medical centers, for example, often have members who are bioethics faculty at their respective centers or departments who are able to offer (or arrange for) ethics education for the committee. Some ethics committees that are part of large integrated systems may have access to system-supported centers or departments of clinical ethics that themselves offer ethics education for committee members. A notable example of this is the Veterans Health Administration (VHA), which has established a National Center for Ethics in Health Care, in part to assist in meeting the educational needs of ethics committee members throughout the VHA network (Glover and Nelson). Ethics committees without access to these types of resources might identify one or two members willing to do formal education and training in clinical ethics through the completion of a clinical bioethics degree, fellowship, or certificate program. Other ethics committees avail themselves of sustained continuing ethics education offered through regional ethics networks such as the University of Pittsburgh's Consortium Ethics Program (Pinkus), the Midwest Ethics Committee Network of the Medical College of Wisconsin (Kuczewski), or the West Virginia Network of Ethics Committees (Moss). These efforts foster partnerships to bring the bioethics resources often present in primarily academic settings to serve the broader healthcare community (Glover and Nelson).

Policy Formation and Review

A second important function of ethics committees is policy formation and review. The type and number of policies that are formulated or reviewed by the ethics committee will vary depending on the nature of the institution, and the authority and responsibility of the ethics committee. For example, a medical-staff-level ethics committee at a major academic medical center may have input on a large number of ethics-related policies. In addition to any policy governing the ethics committee itself, these might include policies governing informed consent, end-of-life decisions (e.g., advance directive and life-sustaining treatment policies), brain death, organ donation and transplant, disclosure of medical mistakes, and so forth. Indeed, the policy formation and review function of ethics committees has developed to the point where a number of "model policy" manuals are available as resources for ethics committees that may be struggling to establish themselves (Aspen Health and Administration Development Group). In addition to these more traditional ethics policy areas, ethics committees are increasingly being asked to give input on organizational ethics issues, especially when these issues may have an impact on patient care (Schyve, Emanuel, Winslade, et al.). The JCAHO ethics standards, for example, extend to organizational ethics issues (e.g., marketing, billing, financial incentives for clinicians, and so forth) and explicitly acknowledge the interdependence of patient rights and organizational ethics (see JCAHO, 2002).

Ethics Consultation

Ethics consultation, perhaps the best known and most discussed function of ethics committees, commands only about 20 percent of ethics committee effort, with the average number of consults ranging from twelve to twenty-three per year (McGee, et al.). Though variously defined, ethics consultation is "… a service provided by an individual or a group to help patients, families, surrogates, healthcare providers, or other involved parties address uncertainty or conflict regarding value-laden issues that emerge in healthcare" (American Society for Bioethics and Humanities, p. 3). Clinical ethics consultation focuses on ethical issues that arise in specific clinical cases and on policy consultation regarding patient care issues. As noted above, partly due to the rise of managed care in the United States, the 1990s brought a growing awareness of the important relationship between clinical and organizational ethics, thereby raising the visibility of organizational ethics consultation. The mid-to late-1990s also saw the first national level effort in the United States to set voluntary standards for ethics consultation when the American Society for Bioethics and Humanities (ASBH) released its report *Core Competencies for Health Care Ethics Consultation*. The report was the result of a two year effort by a national task force on standards for bioethics consultation which functioned as a consensus panel.

The prevalence of ethics consultation is hard to gauge. Ellen Fox's AHRQ supported study of ethics consultation in U.S. hospitals found that approximately 81 percent of all U.S. hospitals have an ethics consultation service of some kind; ethics consultation services were found to be present in 100 percent of hospitals with 400 beds or more, federal hospitals, or hospitals that are members of the Council of Teaching (Fox). The same study estimated that each year in U.S. hospitals, approximately 35,000 individuals are involved in performing over 15,000 ethics consultations. The predominant model for ethics consultation is a small team approach (68%), as opposed to a full committee (23%) or an individual consultant (9%). Of those doing ethics consultation, 36 percent are physicians, 30 percent are nurses, 11

percent are social workers, 10 percent are chaplains, and 10 are administrators, while less than 1 percent are philosophers or theologians. Only 5 percent of those doing ethics consultation were reported to have completed a fellowship or degree program in bioethics or to have had any formal education or training for ethics consultation other than direct supervision (Fox).

From its inception in the late 1960s and early 1970s through the present, ethics consultation has raised a number of controversial questions (LaPuma and Schiedermayer; Singer, Pellegrino, and Siegler; Fletcher, Quist, and Jonsen). Some of these questions are directly attributable, no doubt, to the fact that ethics consultation emerged in part to address highly-charged and conflicted issues such as withholding or withdrawing life-sustaining treatment (see also *In re Quinlin*). Other questions, however, are endemic to the practice of ethics consultation. These include both practical and theoretical questions such as: What types of issues are involved in ethics consultation? Is ethics consultation best done by individuals, teams or committees? What is an appropriate approach to ethics consultation? What types of skills and knowledge are important for doing ethics consultation? Should those doing ethics consultation be required to be certified or accredited in some way? How might ethics consultation be evaluated?

In order to see the controversial and complex nature of these questions, it will be helpful to consider a case that is fairly representative of the types of cases that are brought to ethics consultation services, the Case of Mr. Jones:

> Mr. Jones, an 82 year old man, came to the ER with a gangrenous leg. He had fallen in his apartment and was unable to contact family or friends. Mr. Jones was discovered by his niece, his closest living relative, two days later. Mr. Jones, who was otherwise healthy, needed to have his leg amputated in order to save his life (without amputation he was likely to die from septicemia). Mr. Jones adamantly refused amputation and expressed a deep desire to die "in one piece." Mr. Jones' niece was devastated by his refusal of amputation and wanted the healthcare team to save her uncle's life. Mr. Jones' niece felt responsible for his condition since she was supposed to check-in on him everyday, but she had missed a day due to illness. Members of the healthcare team were split over whether Mr. Jones' refusal of treatment should be honored. The attending physician believed that the team had a moral obligation to go ahead with amputation since it was a "straightforward, relatively low risk, procedure that could save Mr. Jones' life." He argued that the procedure was

"ordinary," not "extraordinary," and therefore obligatory. He emphatically stated "I became a doctor to save life, not to watch people die because they are afraid!" Other members of the healthcare team, especially several nurses, thought Mr. Jones' wishes should be respected. Some worried, however, that Mr. Jones might be depressed and was trying to kill himself by refusing amputation. An ethics consultation was called to resolve the conflict. (Aulisio, 1999, p. 211)

TYPES OF ISSUES. Clinical ethics consultation typically involves any of a range of clinical ethics issues, including informed consent, decision capacity, surrogate decision making, confidentiality and privacy, and a variety of issues surrounding end of life care (ASBH). The best current data suggests that a number of different types of cases are brought to ethics consultation and that these cases themselves may involve a variety of issues. For example, the ECRG study by McGee, et al. lists research trials, new technologies, patient autonomy and competency, cost containment, distribution of goods, improving communications, clinician competency, and end-of-life decision making as among the most common issues raised in ethics consultation. Among these, the largest percentage by far fall into three categories: patient autonomy and competence (38%±25%); improving communications (35%±26%); and end of life (7%±21%).

The case of Mr. Jones, however, illustrates well how a single case can (and often does) raise multiple issues, and the problem of categorizing cases. The case surely raises questions about patient autonomy and competence, as some members of the healthcare team fear that Mr. Jones may be depressed and "trying to kill himself" by refusing amputation. The case also raises questions about end-of-life decision making: Should Mr. Jones, even if competent and well informed, be allowed to refuse a life saving intervention? What is an appropriate role for family members or loved ones in end-of-life (or other) decisions? When are health professionals obliged to accede to patient wishes? Are health professionals ever permitted to override patient wishes or refuse to participate in certain patient decisions? Lastly, the case might just as easily be categorized as an "improving communications" case. Mr. Jones, for example, may simply not understand that he will die without the amputation due to septicemia, because he is confused by technical medical terminology or because he mistook probabilistic language as uncertainty on the part of his doctors.

In addition to the multiple issues that might be raised in a single case, the actual practice of ethics consultation differs from mere case analysis in important ways. As the 1998 ASBH report states, "The actual cases that give rise to these questions frequently also have complex interpersonal and affective features, such as guilt over a loved one's sickness or impending death, disagreement among healthcare providers, possible conflicts of interest, or distrust of the medical system. Increasingly, ethical issues regarding clinical care are raised or complicated by organizational factors" (ASBH, p. 3).

Even from a distance, one can discern these features in the case of Mr. Jones. His niece's feeling of guilt is a powerful factor in the case, as are divisions among members of the healthcare team. These factors are compounded by the time pressures of a real case, i.e., that a decision must be made and soon.

INDIVIDUALS, TEAMS, OR COMMITTEES. Though nearly always conducted under the auspices of an ethics committee, ethics consultation may be done by individual consultants, small groups or teams, or a full ethics committee. Which of these models is best is a matter of some controversy (Rushton, Youngner, and Skeel). Consultation by ethics committee was the dominant model following the *Quinlan* case and the rise of ethics committees in general. If ethics consultations are rare and called only in crisis situations, consultation by a full committee may be practical; however, the more active the consult service the more cumbersome full committee consults will be. Full committee consults also tend to be more formal and adversarial (Rushton, et al.). In contrast, consultation by an individual ethics consultant, though possibly present in a few U.S. healthcare institutions as early as the late 1960s or early 1970s, grew in popularity through the early 1990s at least in part as an alternative to full committee consults. Criticized by some as anti-democratic, the individual consultant model, though efficient, is impractical for many institutions because of the knowledge, skill and time demands it places on one person (Rushton, et al.). A small ethics consult team that functions as an extension of the ethics committee is probably the best model for most institutions. Not surprisingly, in U.S. hospitals today, as noted above, the predominant model for ethics consultation is a small team (Fox).

APPROACHES TO ETHICS CONSULTATION. A number of different approaches to ethics consultation can be found in the literature (Agich; ASBH; Rubin and Zoloth-Dorfman; Zaner). These range from those focused primarily on conflict resolution through facilitation or negotiation, to those that emphasize consensus building, to more directive approaches aimed at guiding participants to the morally "right" solution. One of the challenges for proponents of ethics consultation over the years has been to carve out a role for it that is consistent with societal values. In the United States, this means creating a model of ethics consultation that is consistent with the defining characteristic of a liberal society: that no particular set of substantive moral values should be politically privileged. For example, in the case of Mr. Jones, all involved parties have a right to their moral views and those moral views are widely divergent. Indeed, it is arguably the convergence of these features with the complex and value-laden nature of medical decision making that creates the need for ethics consultation in contemporary clinical settings (Aulisio, 2003).

In the case of Mr. Jones, the intersection of these factors leads to a value conflict that raises a question regarding the role of ethics consultation. Whether or not it is "right" to amputate Mr. Jones's leg depends, in part, on the individual set of values through which the decision is assessed. Mr. Jones's niece and the attending physician think that the morally right course is to amputate Mr. Jones's leg, but for different reasons. Mr. Jones, because he values "dying whole," considers the morally right course to be one that allows him to keep his bodily integrity, even if it ultimately leads to his death. According to the case vignette, "an ethics consultation was called to resolve the conflict," but how should the conflict be resolved? The ethics consultants themselves will bring their own moral values to the case. Should they help resolve the case based on whether their moral values are more in line with those of the doctor, nurse, niece, or patient? Do they get to play the role of the moral sage, adjudicating on who is morally right—that is, who has the correct values? What is the role of ethics consultation in such a case?

The most strident critics of ethics consultation have made much of this problem, claiming that ethics consultation is at odds with democratic values (Ross; Scofield). Democratic values alone, however, would leave ethics consultation susceptible to a tyranny of the majority, in which the morally appropriate course might be determined, for example, by a vote. The deeper question is whether there is an appropriate role for ethics consultation that is consistent with the rights of individuals to live by their values (that is, consistent with a liberal society) (May). The 1998 ASBH report recognized the importance of societal context in informing a proper role for ethics consultation when it stated that:

> ... societal values frame the context in which ethics consultation occurs and, therefore, shape the appropriate role for ethics consultation in contemporary healthcare settings. Individuals, for example, do not give up the right to live by their own moral values when they become patients or take up the

practice of healthcare. These rights set boundaries that must be respected in ethics consultation, and they often suggest who has decision-making authority in different types of cases. Discussions of these boundaries, not surprisingly, comprise a large portion of the bioethics literature (e.g., explorations of informed consent, autonomy, confidentiality, privacy, resource allocation, and conscientious objection). Indeed, helping to identify the implications of these rights and who has decision-making authority in particular cases is an important role for healthcare ethics consultation in our society (p. 4).

Though a full characterization of any approach to ethics consultation is well beyond the scope of this entry, it should be noted that the ASBH report does go on to endorse what it terms an "ethics facilitation" approach to ethics consultation that is intended to be consistent with the societal context described above. "Ethics facilitation," according to the report, aims at "identifying and analyzing the nature of the value uncertainty" that underlies the request for consultation and "facilitating the building of consensus" among involved parties (pp. 6–7). This approach is contrasted with what the report terms "pure facilitation" and "authoritarian" approaches to ethics consultation, which risk running afoul of appropriate boundaries for ethics consultation and displacing those with legitimate decision-making authority. The "ethics facilitation" approach aims at consensus building but in deference to the decision-making authority of involved parties. Indeed, when a consensus cannot be reached, the report recommends that

> ... the proper course of action can sometimes be determined by answering the question "Who should be allowed to make the decision?" Societal values often indicate who should be allowed to make the decision in the absence of consensus. As several of the cases above underscore, the right of a competent and well informed patient to refuse treatment typically establishes decision-making authority even if some family members or healthcare providers disagree with the decision. Similarly, the right of conscientious objection typically gives a healthcare provider the authority to refuse to participate in a procedure that would seriously violate his or her conscience even if a patient and/or family wants the provider to participate (p. 8).

It is important to note that, at a general level, the ethics facilitation approach as characterized in the ASBH report is far more concerned with who has the right to decide than with who is right, and with building a consensus that respects legitimate decision-making authority. In the case of

Mr. Jones, this would require establishing whether he is competent and well informed. If so, his moral and political right to accept or refuse treatment is firm and, thus, any consensus will have to respect his decision-making authority (this does not preclude compromises or even a change of heart on his part). It is also important to highlight the general nature of the ethics facilitation approach and its potential compatibility with many different consult models and methodologies. Attempts to offer normative characterizations of ethics consultation, with their attendant methodological questions, will undoubtedly continue to receive attention in the coming years.

SKILLS AND KNOWLEDGE. Just as there is some disagreement about broad approaches to ethics consultation and more particular methodological issues regarding how ethics consultations should be done, there is also some disagreement about the skills and knowledge required to do ethics consultations. Some emphasize the importance of a strong clinical background such as medicine or nursing, while others emphasizes the importance of formal education and training in ethics, or, more commonly, bioethics (LaPuma and Schiedermayer; Baylis). Despite the disagreements in emphasis, there are some broad areas of agreement regarding core skills and knowledge for ethics consultation. The ASBH Task Force tried to capture these in its 1998 report, *Core Competencies for Ethics Consultation.*

The 1998 ASBH report articulated the broad skill areas as including interpersonal, process, and ethical assessment. Ethical assessment skills are those involved in identifying and analyzing the ethical issues that arise in specific clinical cases. This might include the ability to distinguish the ethical from other (e.g., legal, medical, psychiatric) dimensions of the case, identify relevant values, clarify key concepts, and justify a range of morally acceptable options given the contextual features of the case. Certain types of process skills, such as the ability to facilitate meetings and build consensus, are likewise central to helping to resolve ethical conflicts in actual cases. Finally, certain types of interpersonal skills are critical to nearly every aspect of ethics consultation. For example, the ability to listen well and to communicate interest, respect, support, and empathy to involved parties will be important throughout the consult process.

With respect to important knowledge areas for those doing ethics consultation, the 1998 ASBH report emphasized the importance of advanced knowledge in three areas as they relate to ethics consultation: moral reasoning and ethical theory; bioethical issues and concepts; and local healthcare institution's relevant policies. The report identified six additional areas in which those doing ethics consultation should have basic knowledge: clinical context, relevant health law; knowledge of local healthcare institution, beliefs and perspectives of patient and staff population, relevant codes of ethics and professional conduct, and guidelines of accrediting organizations.

It is important to underscore that the skill and knowledge can be distributed across a small team or even a full committee, depending on the model for ethics consultation employed. As noted above, over 90 percent of U.S. hospitals employ a team or committee approach, while less than 10 percent employ an individual consultant. The "core competency" recommendations are fair less onerous when considered against this backdrop. Individual ethics consultants, however, may need to supplement their professional backgrounds in order to satisfy these recommendations. This is discussed in the ASBH report and elsewhere (Baylis).

Conclusion

There are, of course, a plethora of other issues that must be addressed as ethics committees and ethics consultation continue to evolve and develop. These include questions concerning how their activities might be evaluated, legal liability for committees and consultants, and the ever-present question of whether committees or consultants should be certified or accredited in some form. Some of the data considered above, however, suggest a more immediate and pressing concern. Recall that contemporary ethics committees are usually standing committees with multidisciplinary representation, including medicine, nursing, social work, law, pastoral care, healthcare administration, and various specialty areas, and that half of all ethics committee chairs reported "feeling inadequately prepared to address" the issues they face (McGee, et al.). Even more concerning, recall that only 5 percent of those doing ethics consultation were reported to have completed a fellowship or degree program in bioethics, or to have had any formal education or training for ethics consultation other than direct supervision (Fox). Perhaps the single biggest challenge in the immediate future, then, will be helping to ensure that ethics committee members and ethics consultants have adequate education and training to carry out the important work that is entrusted to them.

MARK P. AULISIO

SEE ALSO: *Casuistry; Clinical Ethics; Consensus, Role and Authority of; Healthcare Institutions; Hospital, Modern*

History of the; Long-Term Care; Managed Care; Organizational Ethics in Healthcare; Surrogate Decision-Making

BIBLIOGRAPHY

Agich, George J. 2001. "The Question of Method in Ethics Consultation." *The American Journal of Bioethics* 1(4): 31–41.

American Society for Bioethics and Humanities (SHHV-SBC Task Force on Standards for Bioethics Consultation). 1998. *Core Competencies for Ethics Consultation: The Report of the American Society for Bioethics and Humanities.* Glenview, IL: American Society for Bioethics and Humanities.

Aspen Health and Administration Development Group. 1998. *Medical Ethics Policies, Protocols, and Guidelines.* Gaithersburg, MD: Aspen Publishers.

Aulisio, Mark P. 1999. "Ethics Consultation: Is it Enough to Mean Well?" *Healthcare Ethics Committee Forum* 11(3): 208–217.

Aulisio, Mark P. 2003. "Meeting the Need: Ethics Consultation in Health Care Today." In *Ethics Consultation: From Theory to Practice,* ed. Mark P. Aulisio, Robert M. Arnold, and Stuart J. Youngner. Baltimore: Johns Hopkins University Press.

Baylis, Françoise E., ed. 1994. *The Health Care Ethics Consultant.* Totowa, NJ: Humana Press.

Fleetwood, Janet E.; Arnold, Robert M.; and Baron, Richard J. 1989. "Giving Answers or Raising Questions?: The Problematic Role of Institutional Ethics Committees." *Journal of Medical Ethics* 15(3): 137–142.

Fletcher, John C.; Quist, Norman; and Jonsen, Albert R., eds. 1989. *Ethics Consultation in Health Care.* Ann Arbor, MI: Health Administration Press.

Fost, Norman, and Cranford, Ronald. 1985. "Hospital Ethics Committees: Administrative Aspects." *Journal of the American Medical Association* 253(18): 2687–2692.

Fox, Ellen. 2002. "Ethics Consultation in U.S. Hospitals: A National Study and Its Implications." Abstract and Presentation at the Annual Meeting of the American Society for Bioethics and Humanities, Baltimore, MD.

Glover, Jacqueline J., and Nelson, William. 2003. "Innovative Educational Programs: A Necessary First Step in Improving Quality in Ethics Consultation." In *Ethics Consultation: From Theory to Practice,* ed. Mark P. Aulisio, Robert M. Arnold, and Stuart J. Youngner. Baltimore: Johns Hopkins University Press.

Joint Commission for Accreditation of Healthcare Organizations. 1993. "Patient Rights." In *1992 Accreditation Manual for Hospitals.* Chicago: Author.

Joint Commission for Accreditation of Healthcare Organizations. 2002. "Patient Rights and Organizational Ethics Standard." *Accreditation Manual for Hospitals.* Chicago: Author.

Judicial Council of the American Medical Association. 1985. "Guidelines for Ethics Committees in Health Care Institutions." *Journal of the American Medical Association* 253(18): 2698–2699.

Kuczewski, Mark G. 1999. "When Your Healthcare Ethics Committee 'Fails to Thrive.'" *Healthcare Ethics Committee Forum* 11(3): 197–207.

La Puma, John, and Schiedermayer, David L. 1991. "Ethics Consultation: Skills, Roles, and Training." *Annals of Internal Medicine* 114(2): 155–160.

May, Thomas. 2002. *Bioethics in a Liberal Society: The Political Framework of Bioethics Decision Making.* Baltimore: Johns Hopkins University Press.

McGee, Glen; Caplan, Arthur L.; Sanogle, Joshua P.; and Asch, David A. 2001. "A National Study of Ethics Committees." *American Journal of Bioethics* 1(4): 60–64.

Quinlan, In re. 355 A.2d 647 (N.J. 1976).

Moss, Alvin H. 1999. "The Application of the Task Force Report in Rural and Frontier Settings." *The Journal of Clinical Ethics* 10(1): 42–48.

Pinkus, Rosa Lynn. 1999. "The Consortium Ethics Program: Continuing Ethics Education for Community Healthcare Professionals." *Healthcare Ethics Committee Forum* 11(3): 233–246.

Ross, Judith Wilson. 1993. "Why Clinical Ethics Consultants Might Not Want to Be Educators." *Cambridge Quarterly of Healthcare Ethics* 2(4): 445–448.

Rubin, Susan, and Zoloth-Dorfman, Laurie. 1994. "First-Person Plural: Community and Method in Ethics Consultation." *The Journal of Clinical Ethics* 5(1): 49–54.

Rushton, Cynda; Youngner, Stuart J.; and Skeel, Joy. "Models for Ethics Consultation: Individual, Team, or Committee." In *Ethics Consultation: From Theory to Practice,* ed. Mark P. Aulisio, Robert M. Arnold, and Stuart J. Youngner. Baltimore, MD: Johns Hopkins University Press.

Schyve, Paul M.; Emanuel, Linda L.; Winslade, William.; and Youngner, Stuart J. "Organizational Ethics: Promises and Pitfalls." In *Ethics Consultation: From Theory to Practice,* eds. Mark P. Aulisio, Robert M. Arnold, and Stuart J. Youngner. Baltimore: Johns Hopkins University Press.

Scofield, Giles. 1995. "Ethics Consultation: The Most Dangerous Profession, A Reply to Critics." *Cambridge Quarterly of Healthcare Ethics* 4(2): 225–228.

Singer, Peter A.; Pellegrino, Edmund D.; and Siegler, Mark. "Ethics Committees and Consultants." *The Journal of Clinical Ethics* 1(4): 263–267.

U.S. President's Commission for the Study of Ethical Problems in Medicine and Biomedical Research. 1983. *Deciding to Forgo Life-Sustaining Treatment: A Report on the Ethical, Medical, and Legal Issues in Treatment Decisions.* Washington, D.C.: Superintendent of Documents.

Youngner, Stuart J.; Jackson, David L.; Coulton, Claudia; Juknialis, Barbara; et al. 1983. "A National Survey of Hospital Ethics Committees." *Critical Care Medicine* 11(11): 902–905.

Zaner, Richard M. 1993. "Voices and Time: The Venture of Clinical Ethics." *The Journal of Medicine and Philosophy* 18(1): 9–31.

EUGENICS

• • •

I. HISTORICAL ASPECTS

The word "eugenics" was coined in 1883 by the English scientist Francis Galton, a cousin of Charles Darwin and a pioneer in the mathematical treatment of biological inheritance. Galton took the word from a Greek root meaning "good in birth" or "noble in heredity." He intended the term to denote the "science" of improving human stock by giving the "more suitable races or strains of blood a better chance of prevailing speedily over the less suitable" (Kevles, p. ix).

The idea of eugenics dated back at least to Plato, and discussion of actually achieving human biological melioration had been boosted by the Enlightenment. In Galton's day, the science of genetics had not yet emerged: Gregor Mendel's 1865 paper, the foundation of that discipline, was not only unappreciated but also generally unnoticed by the scientific community. Nevertheless, Darwin's theory of evolution taught that species did change as a result of natural selection, and it was well known that through artificial selection farmers and flower fanciers could obtain permanent breeds of animals and plants strong in particular characters. Galton thus supposed that the human race could be similarly improved—that through eugenics, human beings could take charge of their own evolution.

The idea of human biological improvement was slow to gather public support, but after the turn of the twentieth century, eugenics movements emerged in many countries. Eugenicists everywhere shared Galton's understanding that people might be improved in two complementary ways—to use Galton's language, by getting rid of the "undesirables" and by multiplying the "desirables" (Kevles, p. 3). They spoke of "positive" and "negative" eugenics. Positive eugenics aimed to foster greater representation in a society of people whom eugenicists considered socially valuable. Negative eugenics sought to encourage the socially unworthy to breed less or, better yet, not at all.

How positive or negative ends were to be achieved depended heavily on which theory of human biology people brought to the eugenics movement. Many eugenicists, particularly in the United States, Britain, and Germany, believed that human beings were determined almost entirely by their germ plasm, which was passed from one generation to the next and overwhelmed environmental influences in shaping human development. Their belief was reinforced by the rediscovery, in 1900, of Mendel's theory that the biological makeup of organisms was determined by certain "factors," which were later identified with genes and were held to account for a wide array of human traits, both physical and behavioral, "good" as well as "bad."

In the first third of the twentieth century, eugenics drew the support of a number of leading biologists, not only in the United States and western Europe but also in the Soviet Union, Latin America, and elsewhere. Many of these biologists came to the creed from the practice of evolutionary biology, which they extrapolated to the Galtonian idea of taking charge of human evolution. One of the most influential was Charles B. Davenport, the head of the Station for Experimental Evolution, a part of the Carnegie Institution of Washington and located at Cold Spring Harbor, New York, where Davenport established the Eugenics Record Office. Other eugenic enthusiasts included, in the United States, the biologists Raymond Pearl, Herbert S. Jennings, Edwin Grant Conklin, William E. Castle, Edward M. East, and Herman Muller; in Britain, F. A. E. Crew, Ronald A. Fisher, and J. B. S. Haldane; and in Germany, Fritz Lenz, who held the chair of racial hygiene in Munich, and Otmar von Verschuer.

Some eugenicists, notably in France, assumed that biological organisms, including human beings, were formed primarily by their environments, physical as well as cultural. Like the early-nineteenth-century biologist Jean Baptiste Lamarck, they contended that environmental influences might even reconfigure hereditary material. Environmentalists were mainly interested in positive eugenics, contending that more attention to factors such as nutrition, medical care, education, and clean play would, by improving the young, better the human race. Some urged that the improvement should begin when children were in the womb, through sound prenatal care. The pregnant mother should avoid toxic substances, such as alcohol. She might even expose herself, for the sake of her fetus, to cultural enrichment, such as fine plays and concerts.

Individuals with good genes were assumed to be easily recognizable from their intelligence and character. Those with bad genes had to be ferreted out. For the purpose of identifying such genes, in the early twentieth century eugenics gave rise to the fist programs of research in human heredity, which were pursued in both state-supported and private laboratories established to develop eugenically useful knowledge. The Eugenics Record Office at Cold Spring Harbor was typical of these institutions; so were the Galton Laboratory for National Eugenics at University College (London), whose first director was the statistician and population biologist Karl Pearson, and the Kaiser Wilhelm Institute for Anthropology, Human Heredity, and Eugenics in Berlin, which was directed by the anthropologist Eugen Fischer. Staff at or affiliated with these laboratories gathered information bearing on human heredity by examining medical records or conducting extended family studies. Often they relied on field workers to construct trait pedigrees in selected populations—say, the residents of a rural community—on the basis of interviews and the examination of genealogical records. An important feature of German eugenic science was the study of twins.

However, social prejudices as well as dreams pervaded eugenic research, just as they did all of eugenics. Eugenic studies claimed to reveal that criminality, prostitution, and mental deficiency (which was commonly termed "feeble-mindedness") were the products of bad genes. They concluded that socially desirable traits were associated with the "races" of northern Europe, especially the Nordic "race," and that undesirable ones were identified with those of eastern and southern Europe.

Eugenics entailed as many meanings as did terms such as "social adequacy" and "character." Indeed, eugenics mirrored a broad range of social attitudes, many of them centered on the role in society of women, since they were indispensable to the bearing of children. On the one hand, positive eugenicists of all stripes argued against the use of birth control or entrance into the work force of middle-class women, on grounds that any decline in their devotion to reproductive duties would lead to "race suicide." On the other hand, social radicals appealed to eugenics to justify the sexual emancipation of women. They contended that if contraception were freely available, women could pursue sexual pleasure with whomever they wished, without regard to whether a male partner was eugenically promising as a father. If and when a woman decided to become pregnant, then her choice of the father could focus on the production of a high-quality child. Sex for pleasure would thus be divorced from sex for eugenic reproduction.

In practice, little was done for positive eugenics, though eugenic claims did figure in the advent of family-allowance policies in Britain and Germany during the 1930s, and positive eugenic themes were certainly implied in the "Fitter Family" competitions that were a standard feature of eugenic programs held at state fairs in America during the 1920s. In the interest of negative eugenics, germ-plasm determinists insisted that "socially inadequate" people should be discouraged or prevented from reproducing themselves by urging or compelling them to undergo sterilization. They also argued for laws restricting marriage and immigration to their countries, in order to keep out genetically undesirable people.

In the United States, eugenicists helped obtain passage of the Immigration Act of 1924, which sharply reduced eastern and southern European immigration to the United States. By the late 1920s, some two dozen American states had enacted eugenic sterilization laws. The laws were declared constitutional in the 1927 U.S. Supreme Court decision of *Buck v. Bell*, in which Justice Oliver Wendell Holmes delivered the opinion that three generations of imbeciles are enough. The leading state in this endeavor was California, which as of 1933 had subjected more people to eugenic sterilization than had all other states of the union combined (Kevles).

At the time, a number of biologists, sociologists, anthropologists, and others increasingly criticized eugenic doctrines, contending that social deviancy is primarily the product of a disadvantageous social environment—notably, for example, of poverty and illiteracy—rather than of genes, and that apparent racial differences were not biological but cultural, the product of ethnicity rather than of germ plasm. In 1930, in the papal encyclical *Casti connubii,* the Roman Catholic church officially opposed eugenics, along with birth control. By the 1930s, a coalition of critics had helped bring a halt in most countries to the attempts of eugenicists to gain significant social and political influence. An exception to this tendency was Germany, where eugenics reached its apogee of power during the Nazi regime. Hundreds of thousands of people were sterilized for negative eugenic reasons and scientific authority joined with social hatred to send millions of the "racially unfit" to the gas chambers. Verschuer trained doctors for the SS in the intricacies of racial hygiene, and he analyzed data and specimens obtained in the concentration camps. In the years after World War II, eugenics became a dirty word.

In the 1930s, attempts to sanitize eugenics had been made by various British and American biologists. They wanted to maintain Galton's idea of human biological improvement while rejecting the social prejudice that had pervaded the conception. They realized that sound eugenics would have to rest on a solid science of human genetics, one that scrupulously rejected social bias and weighed the respective roles of biology and environment, of nature and nurture, in the making of the human animal. They succeeded in laying the foundation for such a science of human genetics, and that field made great strides in the following decades.

The advances in human genetics boosted the new field of genetic counseling, which provided prospective parents with advice about what their risk might be of bearing a child with a genetic disorder. In the 1950s, the early years of such counseling, some geneticists had sought to turn the practice to eugenic advantage—to reduce the incidence of genetic disease in the population, and by extension to reduce the frequency of deleterious genes in what population geneticists were coming to call the human gene pool. To that end, some claimed that it was the counselor's duty not simply to inform a couple about the possible genetic outcome of their union but also to instruct them whether to bear children at all. By the end of the 1950s, however, the informal standards of practice in genetic counseling were strongly against eugenically oriented advice—that is, advice aimed at the welfare of the gene pool rather than of the family. The standards had it that no counselor had the right to tell a couple not to have a child, even for the sake of the couple's welfare.

At first, genetic counseling could draw only on family histories and could tell parents nothing more than the odds that they might conceive a child with a recessive or dominant disease or abnormality. Since the 1960s, as the result of amniocentesis and advances in human biochemical and chromosomal genetics, genetic counseling has become coupled to technical analyses that can identify whether a prospective parent actually carries a deleterious gene and can determine prenatally whether a fetus truly suffers from a selection of genetic and chromosomal diseases or disorders. If the fetus is found to be at such a disadvantage, the parents have the option to abort—at least in countries where abortion is legal, which in 1993 included the United States, Great Britain, and France.

Reproductive selection on a genetic basis—by screening of parents, abortion of fetuses, or both—has found support among liberal religious groups, secular ethicists, and many feminists. They regard it as enlarging women's freedom to control their lives and as contributing to family well-being. However, reproductive selection has been contested by the Roman Catholic church and fundamentalist Protestants, mainly because of their opposition to abortion for any reason. Some feminists have interpreted such selection as yet another among several recent innovations in reproductive technology—for example, in vitro fertilization—that threaten to reduce women to mere reproductive machines in a patriarchal social order. Others have pointed to the heavy emotional and familial burdens placed upon women by prenatal diagnosis that reveals a fetus with a genetic disease or disorder. Genetic selection also has raised apprehensions among some members of minority groups and among disabled persons that it will lead to a revival of negative eugenics that may affect them disproportionately. Handicapped people and their advocates have attacked the attitude that a newly conceived child with a genetic affliction merits abortion, calling it a stigmatization of the living who have the ailment and the expression of a eugenics mentality (Stanworth; Rothman, 1986, 1989; Duster; Cowan).

The Human Genome Project

These fears have been exacerbated by the Human Genome Project, the multinational effort, begun in the late 1980s, to obtain the sequence of all the DNA in the human genome. Once the complete sequence is obtained, it will in principle be easy to identify individuals with deleterious genes of a physical (or presumptively antisocial) type, and the state may intervene in reproductive behavior so as to discourage the transmission of these genes in the population. Such a policy could work special injury upon certain minority groups—for example, people of African origin, since the recessive gene for sickle-cell anemia occurs among them with comparatively high frequency. It could also threaten the disabled, since the only "therapy" currently available for most genetic or chromosomal diseases or disorders is abortion, and since identifying such fetuses as candidates for the procedure stigmatizes people who have been born with the handicap. In 1988, China's Gansu Province adopted a eugenic law that would—so the authorities said—improve population quality by banning the marriages of mentally retarded people unless they first submit to sterilization. Such laws have been adopted in other provinces and in 1991 were endorsed by Prime Minister Li Peng.

Negative eugenic intentions appeared to lie behind a July 1988 proposal from the European Commission for the creation of a human genome project in the European Community. Called a health measure, the proposal was entitled "Predictive Medicine: Human Genome Analysis." Its rationale rested on a simple syllogism—that many diseases result from interactions of genes and environment; that it would be impossible to remove all the environmental culprits from society; and that, hence, individuals could be better defended against disease by identifying their genetic predispositions to fall ill. According to the summary of the proposal: "Predictive Medicine seeks to protect individuals from the kinds of illnesses to which they are genetically most vulnerable and, where appropriate, to prevent the transmission of the genetic susceptibilities to the next generation." In the view of the European Commission, the genome proposal would make Europe more competitive—indirectly, by helping to slow the rate of increase in health expenditures; directly, by strengthening its scientific and technological base (Commission of the European Community).

Economics may well prove to be a powerful incentive to a new negative eugenics. In the United States, the more that healthcare becomes a public responsibility, paid for through the tax system, and the more expensive this care becomes, the greater the possibility that taxpayers will rebel against paying for the care of those whose genetic makeup dooms them to severe disease or disability. Even in countries with national health systems, public officials might feel pressure to encourage, or even to compel, people not to bring genetically affected children into the world—not for the sake of the gene pool but in the interest of keeping public health costs down.

However, a number of factors are likely to offset a broad-based revival of negative eugenics. Eugenics profits from authoritarianism—indeed, almost requires it. The institutions of political democracy may not have been robust enough to resist altogether the violations of civil liberties characteristic of the early eugenics movement, but they did contest them effectively in many places. The British government refused to pass eugenic sterilization laws. So did many American states; and where they were enacted, they were often unenforced. Awareness of the barbarities and cruelties of state-sponsored eugenics in the past has tended to set most geneticists and the public at large against such programs. Moreover, persons with handicaps or diseases are politically empowered, as are minority groups, to a degree that they were not in the early twentieth century. They may not be sufficiently empowered to counter all quasi-eugenic threats to themselves, but they are politically positioned, with allies in the media, the medical profession, and elsewhere, including the Roman Catholic church, to block or at least to hinder eugenic proposals that might affect them.

The European Commission's proposal for a human genome project provoked the emergence of an antieugenic coalition in the European Parliament that was led by Benedikt Härlin, a member of the West German Green Party. The Greens had helped impose severe restrictions on biotechnology in West Germany and raised objections to human genome research on grounds that it might lead to a recrudescence of Nazi biological policies. Guided by Härlin, the European Parliament's Committee on Energy, Research and Technology raised a red flag against the genome project as an enterprise in preventive medicine. It reminded the European Community that in the past, eugenic ideas had led to "horrific consequences" and declared that "clear pointers to eugenic tendencies and goals" inhered in the intention of protecting people from contracting and transmitting genetic diseases or conditions. The application of human genetic information for such purposes would almost always involve decisions—fundamentally eugenic ones— about what are "normal and abnormal, acceptable and unacceptable, viable

and non-viable forms of the genetic make-up of individual human beings before and after birth." The Härlin Report also warned that the new biological and reproductive technologies could make for a "modern test tube eugenics," a eugenics all the more insidious because it could disguise more easily than its cruder ancestors "an even more radical and totalitarian form of 'biopolitics'" (European Parliament, Committee on Energy, Research, and Technology, pp. 23–28).

The Härlin Report urged thirty-eight amendments to the European Commission's proposal, including the complete excision of the phrase "predictive medicine" from the text. As a result of the report, which won support not only from German Greens but also from conservatives on both sides of the English Channel, including German Catholics, the European Commission produced a modified proposal that accepted the thrust of the amendments and even the language of a number of them. The new proposal called for a three-year program of human genome analysis as such, without regard to predictive medicine, and committed the European Community in a variety of ways—most notably, by prohibiting human germ line research and genetic intervention with human embryos—to avoid eugenic practices, prevent ethical missteps, and protect individual rights and privacy. It also promised to keep the European Parliament and the public fully informed via annual reports on the moral and legal basis of human genome research. Formally adopted in June 1990, the European Community's human genome program will cost 15 million ECU (about $17 million) over three years, with some one million ECU devoted to ethical studies (Kevles and Hood).

In the United States, apprehensions of the ethical dangers in the Human Genome Project found expression in the Congress across the political spectrum—from liberals who had long been concerned about governmental intrusion into private genetic matters to conservatives who worried that the Human Genome Project might foster increased practice of prenatal diagnosis and abortion. Among the Americans most sensitive to the eugenic hazards and the ethical challenges inherent in the project were a number of its leading scientific enthusiasts, particularly James D. Watson, the first head of the National Center for Human Genome Research, who considered it both appropriate and imperative that the American genome program stimulate study and debate about its social, ethical, and legal implications. In 1988, Watson announced that such activities would be eligible for roughly 3 percent of the National Center's budget. He told a 1989 scientific conference on the genome: "We have to be aware of the really terrible past of eugenics, where incomplete knowledge was used in a very cavalier and rather awful way, both here in the United States and in Germany. We have to reassure people that their own DNA is private and that no one else can get at it" (Kevles and Hood, pp. 34–35).

Human Genetics in a Market Economy

Despite the specter of eugenics that some see in the Human Genome Project, many observers hold that its near-term ethical challenges lie neither in private forays into human genetic improvement nor in some state-mandated program of eugenics. They lie in the grit of what the project will produce in abundance: genetic information. These challenges center on the control, diffusion, and use of that information within the context of a market economy.

The advance of human genetics and biotechnology has created the capacity for a kind of individual eugenics— families deciding what kinds of children they wish to have. At the moment, the kinds they can choose are those without certain disabilities or diseases, such as Down syndrome or Tay-Sachs disease. Although most parents would now probably prefer just a healthy baby, in the future they might be tempted by the opportunity—for example, via genetic analysis of embryos—to have improved babies, children who are likely to be more intelligent or more athletic or better-looking (whatever such terms might mean). People may well pursue such possibilities, given the interest that some parents have shown in choosing the sex of their child or that others have shown in the administration of growth hormone to offspring they think will grow up too short. In sum, a kind of private eugenics could arise from consumer demand.

Many commentators have noted that the torrent of new human genetic information will undoubtedly pose challenges to social fairness and equity. They have emphasized that employers may seek to deny jobs to applicants with a susceptibility—or an alleged susceptibility—to disorders such as manic depression or illnesses arising from features of the workplace. For example, around 1970, it came to be feared that people with sickle-cell trait—that is, who possess one of the recessive genes for the disease—might suffer the sickling of their red-blood cells in the reduced-oxygen environment of high altitudes. Such people were unjustly prohibited from entering the Air Force Academy, were restricted to ground jobs by several major commercial air carriers, and often were charged higher premiums by insurance companies. Life and medical insurance companies may well wish to know the genomic signatures of their clients, their profile of risk for disease and death. Even national health systems might choose to ration the provision of care on the basis of genetic propensity for disease, especially to families at risk for bearing diseased children (U.S. Congress, Office of Technology Assessment; Kevles).

In response to these threatening prospects, many analysts have contended that individual genomic information should be protected as strictly private. However, legal and insurance analysts have pointed out that insurance, and insurance premiums, depend on assessments of risk. If a client has a high genetic medical risk that is not reflected in the premium charged, then that person receives a high payout at low cost to himself or herself but at high cost to the company. The problem would be compounded if the person knows the risk—while the company does not—and purchases a large amount of insurance. In either case, the company would have to pass its increased costs to other policyholders, which is to say that high-risk policyholders would be taxing low-risk ones. Thus, insisting on a right to privacy in genetic information could well lead—at least under the largely private system of insurance that now prevails in the United States—to inequitable consequences.

American legislatures have already begun to focus on the genuine social, ethical, and policy issues that the Human Genome Project raises, particularly those concerning the use of private human genetic information. In the fall of 1991, a U.S. House of Representatives subcommittee held hearings on the challenge that such information posed to insurability. About the same time, the California state legislature passed a bill banning employers, health service agencies and disability insurers from withholding jobs or protection simply because a person is a carrier of a single gene associated with disability. Although California Governor Pete Wilson vetoed the bill, it was a harbinger of the type of public policy initiatives that the genome project no doubt will increasingly call forth. The Human Genome Project, like most of human and medical genetics, is less likely to foster a drive for a new eugenics than it is to pose vexing challenges to public policy and private practices for the control and use of human genetic information.

DANIEL J. KEVLES (1995)
BIBLIOGRAPHY REVISED

SEE ALSO: *Eugenics and Religious Law; Genetics and Human Behavior; Genetics and Human Self-Understanding; Genetics and Racial Minorities; Holocaust; Human Nature; Judaism, Bioethics in; Minorities as Research Subjects; Race and Racism;* and other *Eugenics* subentries

BIBLIOGRAPHY

Adams, Mark B., ed. 1990. *The Wellborn Science: Eugenics in Germany, France, Brazil, and Russia.* New York: Oxford University Press.

Allen, G. E. 1999. "Genetics, Eugenics and the Medicalization of Social Behavior: Lessons from the Past." *Endeavour* 23(1): 10–19.

Bernard, Jean. 1990. *De la biologie à l'éthique: Nouveaux pouvoirs de la science, nouveaux devoirs de l'homme.* Paris: Éditions Buchet-Chastel.

Childs, Donald J. 2002. *Modernism and Eugenics: Woolf, Eliot, Yeats, and the Culture of Degeneration.* Cambridge, Eng.: Cambridge University Press.

Commission of the European Community. 1988. *Proposal for a Council Decision Adopting a Specific Research Programme in the Field of Health; Predictive Medicine: Human Genome Analysis* (1989–1991). COM (88) 424 final-SYN 146. Brussels: Author.

Cooke, K. J. 1998. "The Limits of Heredity: Nature and Nurture in American Eugenics Before 1915." *Journal of History and Biology* 31(2): 263–278.

Coutts, Mary Carrington, and McCarrick, Pat Milmoe. 1995. "Eugenics." *Kennedy Institute of Ethics Journal* 5(2): 163–178.

Cowan, Ruth Schwartz. 1992. "Genetic Technology and Reproductive Choice: An Ethics for Autonomy." In *The Code of Codes: Scientific and Social Issues in the Human Genome Project,* pp. 244–263, ed. Daniel J. Kevles and Leroy Hood. Cambridge, MA: Harvard University Press.

Davis, Joel. 1990. *Mapping the Code: The Human Genome Project and the Choices of Modern Science.* New York: John Wiley.

Duster, Troy. 1990. *Backdoor to Eugenics.* New York: Routledge.

European Parliament, Committee on Energy, Research and Technology. 1988–1989. *Report Drawn up on Behalf of the Committee on Energy, Research and Technology on the Proposal from the Commission to the Council (COM/88424-C2–119/88) for a Decision Adopting a Specific Research Programme in the Field of Health: Predictive Medicine: Human Genome Analysis* (1989–1991). Rapporteur European Parliament Session Documents, 1988–89, 30.01.1989, Series A, Doc. A2–0370/88 SYN 146. Benedikt Härlin, rapporteur. Brussels: Author.

Farrall, Lyndsay A. 1979. "The History of Eugenics: A Bibliographical Review." *Annals of Science* 36(2): 111–123.

German Bundestag. 1987. *Report of the Commission of Enquiry on Prospects and Risks of Genetic Engineering. 10th Legislative Period, Paper 10/6775.* Bonn: Author.

Gillham, Nicholas Wright. 2001. *A Life of Sir Francis Galton: From African Exploration to the Birth of Eugenics.* New York: Oxford University Press.

Holtzman, Neil A. 1989. *Proceed with Caution: Predicting Genetic Risks in the Recombinant DNA Era.* Baltimore: Johns Hopkins University Press.

Kevles, Daniel J. 1986. *In the Name of Eugenics: Genetics and the Uses of Human Heredity.* Berkeley: University of California Press.

Kevles, Daniel J. 1995. *In the Name of Eugenics: Genetics and the Uses of Human Heredity.* Cambridge, MA: Harvard University Press.

Kevles, Daniel J., and Hood, Leroy, eds. 1992. *The Code of Codes: Scientific and Social Issues in the Human Genome Project.* Cambridge, MA: Harvard University Press.

Kline, Wendy. 2001. *Building a Better Race: Gender, Sexuality, and Eugenics from the Turn of the Century to the Baby Boom.* Berkeley: University of California Press.

Kuhl, Stefan. 2002. *The Nazi Connection: Eugenics, American Racism, and German National Socialism.* New York: Oxford Press.

Mazumdar, P. M. 2002. "'Reform' Eugenics and the Decline of Mendelism." *Trends in Genetics* 18(1): 48–52.

Müller-Hill, Benno. 1988. *Murderous Science: Elimination by Scientific Selection of Jews, Gypsies, and Others, Germany, 1933–1945,* tr. George F. Fraser. New York: Oxford University Press.

Nathanson J. A., and Grodin, M. A. 2000. "Eugenic Sterilization and a Nazi Analogy." *Annals of Internal Medicine* 132(12): 1008.

Paul, Diane B. 1998. *The Politics of Heredity: Essays on Eugenics, Biomedicine, and the Nature-Nurture Debate (Suny Series, Philosophy and Biology).* Albany: State University of New York Press.

Paul, D. B., and Spencer, H. G. 1995. "The Hidden Science of Eugenics." *Nature* 23; 374(6520): 302–304.

Proctor, Robert. 1988. *Racial Hygiene: Medicine Under the Nazis.* Cambridge, MA: Harvard University Press.

Rothman, Barbara Katz. 1986. *The Tentative Pregnancy: Prenatal Diagnosis and the Future of Motherhood.* New York: Viking.

Rothman, Barbara Katz. 1989. *Recreating Motherhood: Ideology and Technology in a Patriarchal Society.* New York: W. W. Norton.

Schneider, William H. 1990. *Quality and Quantity: The Quest for Biological Regeneration in Twentieth-Century France.* Cambridge, Eng.: Cambridge University Press.

Sofair, A. N., and Kaldjian, L. C. 2000. "Eugenic Sterilization and a Qualified Nazi Analogy: The United States and Germany, 1930–1945." *Annals of Internal Medicine* 132(4): 312–319.

Stanworth, Michelle, ed. 1987. *Reproductive Technologies: Gender, Motherhood and Medicine.* Minneapolis: University of Minnesota Press.

U.S. Congress. Office of Technology Assessment. 1990. *Genetic Monitoring and Screening in the Workplace.* Washington, D.C.: U.S. Government Printing Office.

Weindling, Paul. 1989. *Health, Race and German Politics Between National Unification and Nazism, 1870–1945.* Cambridge, Eng.: Cambridge University Press.

Wingerson, Lois. 1990. *Mapping Our Genes: The Genome Project and the Future of Medicine.* New York: Dutton.

II. ETHICAL ISSUES

To what extent are there continuities, parallels, and trajectories between past eugenic ideas and practices, and current and pending developments with genetic testing and screening, prospective gene therapies, and the increasing utilization of sperm banks and egg donations? To begin to answer these questions, it is imperative to distinguish between state-sanctioned eugenic programs on the one hand, and private, individualized, *personal* decisions that are socially patterned, on the other. In the former case eugenic goals are usually explicitly articulated, and thus easy to identify, examine, and oppose or support. In the latter the eugenic implications are often unarticulated and subterranean—only exposed by a review of statistical patterns of what are otherwise perceived as individual choices. In matters of public policy and market choices, emphasis upon individual intent can camouflage the collective eugenic force of personal decision-making.

One heuristically useful attempt to distinguish between different kinds of contemporary eugenic forms can be found in Philip Kitcher's *The Lives to Come* (1996). Kitcher makes a distinction between *laissez-faire eugenics,* a hands-off approach that presumes that everyone will make their own *individual choices*—and a *utopian eugenics,* where as a matter of public policy there is an attempt to make available to all sectors of a society the information and technology to make those choices. While no public policy can ever deliver such information and technology evenly across all sectors, this provides an analytic device for assessing the degree of success of such an attempted distribution. The major difficulty surfaces with an empirical problem generated by the molecular genetic revolution itself, the fracture of the public health consensus of what constitutes *the public good.* Allen Buchanan and his associates, in *From Chance to Choice* (2000), argue that an assessment of the consequences for the general public good are vital to a discussion of the treatment/enhancement distinction. Before 1960 it was possible to achieve consensus that the public good was well-served by an elimination or mitigation of such diseases as smallpox, cholera, tuberculosis, yellow fever, typhoid, and sexually transmitted diseases. However, with the discovery that genetic disorders are located in risk populations that do not place the general population at risk, a new set of issues and new kinds of eugenic concerns have been generated regarding who has control over genetic screening and testing.

While it is true that individuals make choices, they do so in a social and economic context that can be demonstrably coercive. While relatively obvious when looking at other societies, it is less understood when examining one's own—substantially obscured because individual choice is deeply embedded in the taken-for-granted assumptions about decision-making. For example, long before the advent of prenatal detection technologies, preference for a male child in India and China was so great that a notable fraction of the population practiced infanticide of newborn females. While sex selection does not qualify as a eugenic strategy (unless the purpose is to prevent a gender-linked disorder), the practice

in India and China does illustrate how and why a focus on individual choice can obscure the dramatically collective aspect of socially patterned individual choices.

Once technologies for prenatal determination of sex became available, the quest for *disclosure* of the sex of the fetus took a momentous turn for public policy in India. In 1971 India passed the Medical Termination of Pregnancy Act, which stipulates that a woman can be given an abortion only if there is a life-threatening situation, or grave injury to her physical or mental health. Amniocentesis use began in India in 1974, but there were early reports that the test was being used less to detect birth defects than to determine the sex of the fetus. In August 1994 the Indian Parliament passed a new law that stiffened the penalties for screening the fetus to determine the sex. However, there was a large loophole in the law that made it practically unenforceable—and the practice has continued at such a high rate that in 1994 *New York Times* reported that Haryana, a populous northern state, had an astonishingly low sex ratio of 874 females to every 1,000 males.

Individual Decision and Unexamined Group Patterns

It should be clear from the above examples of sex selection preferences in India that what appear to be individual familial choices may often be better understood as empirical social patterns reflective of the social and cultural hegemony. For example, in early 1994, *Nature* published "China's Misconception of Eugenics," an article that portrayed the Chinese government's policy of trying to prohibit couples with certain diseases from procreating as having a distinctively distasteful eugenic quality. While the article was forthright in denouncing the use of state power as the vehicle for discouraging procreation, it implied that a personalistic and individualistic decision to interrupt a pregnancy. Health Minister for China, Chen Minzhang, announced the plan to enforce a new law that would not only prohibit screening of the fetus for sex determination, but also ban marriages for people "diagnosed with diseases that may totally or partially deprive the victim of the ability to live independently, that are highly possible to recur in generations to come and that are medically considered inappropriate for reproduction"—as reported in the *New York Times* on November 14, 1993 in an article titled "China to Ban Sex-Screening of Fetuses."

The logical and empirical extension of the technology can be made explicit: Once it is possible to determine in time for the termination of a pregnancy whether the fetus has a condition that is regarded as a defect, who is entitled to make the decision about carrying to full term, or aborting? As noted, this should not be seen as a simple binary matter of voluntarism versus state power. There is considerable evidence to support the observation that what are characterized as personal or individual decisions in Western societies are upon closer inspection (just as with sex selection in India) actually very remarkably socially patterned.

In an influential treatise on reproductive choice titled *Children of Choice,* John Robertson acknowledged that social and economic constraints such as access to employment, housing and child care might play a role in the decision to have a child. However, the overarching theme, to which he returns again and again, is that reproduction "is first and foremost an individual interest" (p. 22). Because this is not reducible to an either/or formulation, it should be clearer why a continuum is a better analytic device for arraying an understanding of strategies and options—from individual choice to embedded but powerful social pressures (stigma and ridicule)—and from economic pressures (fear of loss of health insurance, or even of inability to obtain such insurance), and only then to the coercive power of the state to penalize.

When framed as individual choice, debate about a reproductive choice is set into the arena of individual rights: to have a child or not, then to have a male or female child, to have a child with Down Syndrome, cleft palate, or to choose to produce a clone. Such discussions of individual rights are typically de-contextualized from systemic concerns such as affordability. But amniocentesis is a relatively expensive procedure for the poor. The state often provides assistance to women seeking amniocentesis. In the 1980s California's Department of Maternal and Child Health noted with alarm that primarily wealthier women were getting state support for amniocentesis. Mindful of the state's eugenic history, officials embarked upon a program to try to get poorer women to accept the service. However, because the poor tend to have their children at an early age, this has become moot as a visible issue in the eugenics debate.

Continuity and Persistence of Eugenic Thought and Goals

During a time of rapid social change in which there are disruptions of the established order and the attendant challenges to authority and tradition, there is a special appeal of genetic explanations and eugenic solutions to the most privileged strata of society. The power of the state to control its population can be awesome, and thus when the state puts forward eugenic programs in a post-holocaust world, critics are well prepared to react with revulsion. The government of Singapore came under fire during the 1990s for its program to reward middle-class and wealthy families for having more children, while actively discouraging the poor from having large families. Far less attention has been given to the fact that 30,000 babies have been produced by sperm banks and egg donations in the United Kingdom alone, from people who are literally choosing what they consider to be *better human stock* (Maranto; Hill).

The industrial revolution and rapid urbanization wreaked havoc with traditional life and traditional social roles in both nineteenth-century Europe and the United States. Extended kinship systems that had been valued as an economic advantage on farmlands were often inverted and became economic liabilities when those families were forced off the land and moved to the teeming cities. Unemployment, homelessness, mental illness and a host of other social problems seemed to especially victimize the poor, whose visibility if not sheer numbers dominated the public sphere of urban life.

Cholera, yellow fever, typhoid, and tuberculosis were the scourge of city dwellers, and once again, the poor were the most likely victims. But as Sylvia Tesh noted in *Hidden Arguments* (1988), the poor were also the most likely to be blamed for causing the problems, typically characterized as living in unclean conditions. Hygiene came first as both an explanation for the better fortunes of the privileged and middle classes, and later—as a challenge to the poor.

As the wealthier families began to have fewer children, and to have the resources to hire the poor as servants to help them *clean up*—some observers began to notice what they thought was a disturbing pattern. The more well-to-do members of society were procreating less, while the poor were still having very large families. The dark Malthusian prediction about a population explosion took a particularly elitist turn. If people are to learn anything from the past, it is imperative to have a more complete understanding of the appeal and popularity of eugenics and why it was compelling to the full range of thinkers of all political persuasions at the beginning of the twentieth century. Very much like its sister concept *hygiene*—there was a strong association between cleanliness and order, progress and eugenics.

Just as hygiene was seen as the normal value of cleanliness to which all should aspire, eugenics was widely accepted and actively promoted by the major public figures of the period. University presidents, medical doctors, judges, academic scholars, writers, intellectuals, political figures on both the left and right of the political spectrum—all espoused the idea that the betterment of humankind would result from the practices and techniques that would prevent the procreation of *imbeciles* and *mental retards* and *criminals* and *prostitutes* and *homosexuals* and *alcoholics* and *gamblers.*

Contemporary Echoes of a Eugenic Past: The Genetic Screen

Genetic screening is one of the outgrowths of health screening for a number of public health problems, most notably tuberculosis. But unlike tuberculosis, genetic disorders tend to cluster in populations in which there have been centuries of in-breeding, because of cultural endogamy rules (who can marry whom), and/or because of long-term geographical residence of a population in which there has not been much physical mobility. In both circumstances, genes that cause diseases cluster in these populations, making those who are part of those populations at greater risk. Examples include cystic fibrosis, a disease affecting the lung's ability to accumulate liquids, primarily affecting persons of North-European descent; beta-thalassemia, a blood disease affecting persons living in the Mediterranean area; and sickle-cell anemia, a blood disorder primarily affecting persons with ancestors from West Africa, and in some areas of the Mediterranean.

In the last two decades of the twentieth century, many states began to offer postnatal genetic screening of all newborns. If the screen detects a high level of a particular chemical (alpha-feta protein) on the first go-round, the woman is offered a second test to determine if the fetus is likely to have anencephaly, which can produce a serious neural tube defect. In the most literal sense, to *screen* something means to prevent that something from getting past the screen. Thus, whether explicitly or implicitly, the institutionalization of genetic screening programs contains a strong residue of the old image of *cleaning* or *purifying* the gene pool. The social aspect of the eugenic implication is disguised by its being offered to individual women, or individual families. Thus the specter of state-sponsored screening of a particular group is diffused and obscured. However, as noted above, since genetic diseases tend to cluster in certain ethnic and racial groupings, individual decision-making (imposed or presumed) cannot mitigate the fact of systematically different outcomes for different groups.

Getting rid of *bad babies* with *genetic defects* is only half of the eugenic equation. There is also the idea of a positive eugenics, in which there is the active recruitment of some to procreate and selectively breed to increase some human trait or characteristic that is considered positive. Singapore actively encourages and rewards its wealthy and middle-class citizens to have more children. That is the group-approach to positive eugenics. On the individual level, contemporary residues of eugenic thinking can be seen in the emergence and increasing use of sperm banks with sperm donated by medical students, athletes, and Nobel laureates; the much higher cost of ova from young women from exclusive private colleges; and the exorbitant pricing of the ova from supermodels, which are offered on a website. Given a choice, there is evidence that some people will try to add a bit of height to their offspring with a growth hormone. Each of these developments indicates a lingering of a eugenic past.

Population/Group Taxonomy and the Relevance to Debates on Germ Line Intervention

The current discussions and debates about whether we should engage or support research that might alter the germ line rarely address the systematically eugenic potential that is a possible outcome. Germline is the term used to describe genetic changes that would influence inheritance across the generations, and is distinguished from genetic interventions that alter only the particular person undergoing gene therapy. Because bioethicists do not tend to formulate ethical concerns along dimensions of group stratification or access to political power on the part of *groups of individuals,* the discussion about the ethics of germ line intervention for group differentiation and social stratification is rare. An increased understanding of human genetics will enable the sorting of groups at higher and lower risk for certain diseases even more systematically than what was noted above.

If technology permitted entry into the germ line to eliminate either cystic fibrosis or sickle-cell anemia in an individual, that individual (or parent or guardian acting in behalf of that individual) might well make the individual choice. But a different order of ethical concern surfaces if one thinks about this more at the social and political level and less at the individual level. Zuni Indians are more likely to have cystic fibrosis than are persons of European ancestry, albeit a different mutation for cystic fibrosis than *Caucasians.* Yet the genetic test for cystic fibrosis is aimed at the Delta F508, the mutation most likely to be found in those of North-European ancestry. Quite simply, this is because genetic disease research is most likely to be aimed at those diseases that have the most politically powerful constituencies and/or for which there is a strong profit motive in the biotechnology industry. With more research dollars going into the Delta F508, than into the mutation which appears more frequently among the Zuni, individual Caucasians may come to believe that they are making an individual decision about altering the familial germ line. Stepping back to another level of analysis, social, political, and economic engines are driving molecular biology down certain research corridors of a particular group's genetic disorder and not others, and these have little to do with individual choice at the user end.

Parallel Massive Social Displacements: Late-Nineteenth and Late-Twentieth Centuries

Just as the twin shifts from agrarian to industrial and rural to urban dominated the shifting social demography of the late-nineteenth century in Europe and the United States, so the shift from industrial to service (or tertiary) and from urban to suburban dominated shifting social demography of the late-twentieth century. The United States has been in the vanguard of this development, and the massive economic displacement of African-American urban youth is the context for a renewed conception of biological thinking about social issues. At the beginning of the twenty-first century, the United States is heading down a subtly parallel road entertaining the connection between genes and social outcomes. This is being played out on a stage with converging preoccupations and tangled webs that interlace youth unemployment, crime and violence, race, and genetic explanations.

There is direct link between de-industrialization, youth unemployment, and ethnic or racial or immigrant minority status in the United States. In 1954 black and white youth unemployment rates in the United States were equal, with blacks actually having a slightly higher rate of employment in the age group from 16 to 19. By 1982 the black unemployment rate had nearly quadrupled in this age group, while the white rate had increased only marginally (Kasarda). Just as unemployment rates among African-American youth were skyrocketing during these three decades, so were their incarceration rates. This provides the context in which to review and interpret the clear pattern of the recent historical evolution of general prison incarceration rates by race. In the last half of the twentieth century, the incarceration rate of African Americans in relation to whites has gone up in a striking manner. In 1933 blacks were incarcerated at a rate approximately three times that of whites. By 1970 it was six times; and in 1995 it was seven times that of whites.

Genetic studies of criminality have a heavy dependency on incarcerated populations. Thus, for example, one of the more controversial issues in the *genetics* of crime is whether males with the extra Y chromosome, or XYY males, are more likely to be found in prisons than are XY males. The first major study suggesting a genetic link came from Edinburgh, Scotland. In 1965 Patricia Jacobs and her colleagues reported that while all of the 197 males in this account of prison hospital inmates were described as *dangerously violent,* seven had the XYY karotype. These seven males constituted about 3.5 per cent of the total. But since it was estimated that only about 1.3 per cent of all males has the XYY chromosomal make-up, the authors posited that the extra Y significantly increased one's chances of being incarcerated. Ever since a controversy has raged as to the meaning of these findings

and the methodology that produced them. The claim for a genetic link to crime is based entirely upon studies of incarcerated populations.

Yet, incarceration rates are a function of a full range of criminal justice decisions, a fact which research has long shown to be a function of social, economic and political factors (Cole; Mauer; Miller; Currie). At the beginning of the twenty-first century, forensic sciences are attempting to use DNA markers to identify *ethnic affiliation estimations* of suspects in criminal investigations (Lowe et al.; Shriver et al.). Just as health and hygiene were the vanguard for the late-nineteenth century screen for the *unfit,* so the genetic screen was first a health screen. However, the shift in use and focus to forensic science has already begun. The national DNA database, CODIS (acronym for COmbined DNA Identification System) contained, as of January 2000, genetic profiles of 210,000 convicts. It is coordinated by the Federal Bureau of Investigation (FBI), and all fifty states contribute to the databank.

The states are the primary venues for the prosecution of violations of the criminal law, and their autonomy has generated considerable variation in the use of DNA databanks and storage. Even as late as the mid-1980s, most states were only collecting DNA samples from sexual offenders. The times have changed quite rapidly. There has been active change in the inter-linking of state databases, and states are uploading an average of 3,000 offender profiles every month. Computer technology is increasingly efficient and extraordinarily fast, and it requires only 500 microseconds to search a database of 100,000 profiles.

As the United States increases the numbers of profiles in the national database, there will be researchers proposing to provide genetic profiles of specific offender populations. Twenty states authorize the use of databanks for research on forensic techniques. Based on the statutory language in several of those states, this could easily mean assaying genes or loci that contain predictive information (Kimmelman). The program of research for CODIS is increasing exponentially on an annual basis, and this data base is sitting there waiting to be tapped by researchers looking for *violence genes*—as evidenced by the spate of national interest over the monoamine oxidase A (MAOA) gene. In the latter part of 2002, Caspi and his associates published an article in *Science* that cemented the relationship between behavioral and molecular genetics. The authors claimed to have produced findings that a functional polymorphism in the MAOA gene affects the impact of early childhood maltreatment on the development of antisocial and violent behavior. The policy implications of the research were strongly suggested in the conclusions, and re-ignite an old debate about the prospects and dangers of early identification of children who are thought to be at risk for violent or antisocial behavior. As in the earlier forms of eugenics, early identification always carries with it the appendage of both treatment and prevention.

Conclusion

Eugenic thought, practice, and advocacy are best understood as existing along a continuum with degrees of activity. It is therefore misleading and obscuring the complexity of the range of reproductive options to suggest that either a society does or does not have eugenic practices. Most significantly the social setting in which eugenics flourishes or declines is as important as the knowledge base in genetics and biology. The oft cited post-World War II defeat of eugenic thought is actually therefore better framed as its mitigation, its submersion, muting, or transmogrification. These changes came about more because of the defeat of the Nazis, and less because of advances in scientific knowledge of the genetics of race. As early as the 1930s, German and U.S. scientists had conclusive evidence that the ABO blood system did not track along racial or ethnic lines, but this knowledge did not inhibit some of the most vicious racist eugenic practices ever promulgated and perpetrated.

The social and economic setting in the technologically developed part of the world since the mid-1980s is propitious for a strong resurgence of eugenic thinking and advocacy, similar in degree to the social transformations of early-twentieth century Europe and the United States. The decline of the welfare state, the increasing gap between rich and poor, and the erosion of safety nets for the poorest members of a society have set the stage. This is accompanied by transnational migrations of laborers in the increasingly global labor markets of major post-industrial nations. The entry and consignment of these workers to the bottom quartile of the economic order, with the highest rates of poverty, disease, and recorded crime and violence will fuel the re-insurgency of attempts to explain their behavior. The new forms of eugenic insurgency will be disguised, muted, and made more palpable as: (a) the neutral requirements of forensic techniques of ethnic estimation; (b) the convergence of molecular and behavioral genetics in explanations of violent and antisocial behavior; and (c) the over-arching framework of individual choice regarding reproductive options, whether to prevent the birth of a child with a genetic defect, or in the use of new technologies to enhance the prospect of the fetus for competitive advantage.

TROY DUSTER

SEE ALSO: *Eugenics and Religious Law; Genetic Engineering, Human; Genetics and Human Self-Understanding; Genetics and Racial Minorities; Harm; Holocaust; Human Nature; Judaism, Bioethics in; Minorities as Research Subjects; Race and Racism;* and other *Eugenics* subentries

BIBLIOGRAPHY

Adams, M. 1990. "Towards a Comparative History of Eugenics." In *The Wellborn Science. Eugenics in German, France, Brazil, and Russia,* ed. M. Adams. New York and Oxford: Oxford University Press.

Allen, Garland. 1986. "The Eugenics Record Office at Cold Spring Harbour, 1910–1940: An Essay in Institutional History." *Osiris* 2nd series, (2) 225–264.

Broberg, G., and Roll-Hansen, N., eds. 1996. *Eugenics and the Welfare State: Sterilization Policy in Denmark, Sweden, Norway, and Finland.* East Lansing: Michigan State University Press.

Buchanan, Allen; Brock, Dan W.; Daniels, Norman; and Wikler, Daniel. 2000. *From Chance to Choice: Genetics and Justice.* Cambridge, Eng.: Cambridge University Press.

Caspi, A.; McClay, J.; Moffitt, T. E.; et al. 2002. "Role of Genotype in the Cycle of Violence in Maltreated Children." *Science* 297: 851–854.

"China's Misconception of Eugenics." 1994. *Nature* 367: 1.

Cole, David. 1999. *No Equal Justice: Race and Class in the American Criminal Justice System.* New York: New Press.

Currie, Elliott. 1985. *Confronting Crime: An American Challenge.* New York: Pantheon.

Duster, Troy. 1990. *Backdoor to Eugenics.* New York and London: Routledge.

Duster, Troy. 1995. "Post-Industrialism and Youth Unemployment." In *Poverty, Inequality and the Future of Social Policy: Western States in the New World Order.* New York: Russell Sage.

Haller, Mark. 1963. *Eugenics: Hereditarian Attitudes in American Thought.* New Brunswick, NJ: Rutgers University Press.

Jacobs, P.; Brunton, A. M.; Melville, M.; et al. 1965. "Aggressive Behavior, Mental Subnormality, and the XYY Male." *Nature* 208: 1351–1352.

Juengst, Eric T. 1998. "Groups as Gatekeepers to Genomic Research: Conceptually Confusing, Morally Hazardous and Practically Useless." *Kennedy Institute of Ethics.* 8: 183–200.

Kasarda, John D. 1983. "Caught in the Web of Change." *Society* November: 41–47.

Kevles, Daniel J. 1985. *In the Name of Eugenics: Genetics and the Uses of Human Heredity.* New York: Alfred A. Knopf.

Kimmelman, Jonathan. 2000. "Risking Ethical Insolvency: A Survey of Trends in Criminal DNA Databanking." *Journal of Law, Medicine and Ethics.* 28: 209–221.

Kuhl, S. 1994. *The Nazi Connection: Eugenics, American Racism, and German National Socialism.* New York and Oxford: Oxford University Press.

Laughlin, H. H. 1914. *The Scope of the Committee's Work,* Bulletin No. 10A. Cold Springs Harbor, NY: Eugenics Records Office.

Lowe, Alex L.; Urquhart, Andrew; Foreman, Lindsey A.; and Evett, Ian. 2001. "Inferring Ethnic Origin by Means of an STR Profile," *Forensic Science International.* 119: 17–22.

Ludmerer, Kenneth M. 1972. *Genetics and American Society.* Baltimore, MD and London: The John Hopkins University Press.

Maranto, Gina. 2000. *Quest for Perfection: The Drive to Breed Better Human Beings.* Lincoln, NE: iUniverse.

Mauer, Marc. 1999. *Race to Incarcerate.* New York: New Press.

Miller, Jerome G. 1992. *Hobbling A Generation: Young African American Males in the Criminal Justice System of America's Cities.* Baltimore, MD: National Center on Institutions and Alternatives, Alexandria, Virginia.

Nelkin, Dorothy M., and Lindee, Susan. 1995. *The DNA Mystique: The Gene as a Cultural Icon.* New York: Freeman.

New York Times. 1993. "China to Ban Sex-Screening of Fetuses." November 14.

New York Times 1994. "India Fights Abortion of Female Fetuses." August 27.

Paul, Diane. 1984. "Eugenics and the Left." *Journal of the History of Ideas.* 45(4): 567–590.

Proctor, Robert. 1988. *Racial Hygiene: Medicine under the Nazis.* Cambridge, MA: Harvard University Press.

Proctor, Robert. 1999. *The Nazi War on Cancer.* Princeton, NJ: Princeton University Press.

Reilly, Philip. 1991. *The Surgical Solution: A History of Involuntary Sterilization in the United States.* Baltimore: Johns Hopkins University Press.

Robertson, John A. 1994. *Children of Choice: Freedom and the New Reproductive Technologies.* Princeton, NJ: Princeton University Press.

Roll-Hansen, N. 1988. "The Progress of Eugenics: Growth of Knowledge and Change in Ideology." *History of Science* 26(Part 3, No. 73): 295–331.

Shriver, Mark D.; Smith, Michael W.; Jin, Li; et al. 1997. "Ethnic-Affiliation Estimation by Use of Population-Specific DNA Markers." *American Journal of Human Genetics* 60: 957–964.

Silver, Lee M. 1997. *Remaking Eden.* New York: Avon Books.

Tesh, Sylvia N. 1988. *Hidden Arguments: Political Ideology and Disease Prevention Policy.* New Brunswick, NJ: Rutgers University Press.

U.S. Department of Justice, Office of Justice Programs. 1992. *Bureau of Justice Statistics,* January, Vol. 1., No. 3, NCJ-133097. Washington, D.C.: Author.

INTERNET RESOURCES

"Call to End Sperm Donor Anonymity." BBC News. Available from <news.bbc.co.uk/1/hi/health/2065329.stm>.

Hill, M. 2002. "Fertility Clinics Can Only Pass on Basic Information." BBC News. Available from <news.bbc.co.uk/1/hi/health/2065329.stm>.

EUGENICS AND RELIGIOUS LAW

• • •

I. Judaism

II. Christianity

III. Islam

IV. Hinduism and Buddhism

I. JUDAISM

The laws against incest and consanguinity in the Old Testament would seem to have a rationale in eugenics, although this is never specified in the biblical text. The traditional commentators, too, advert only to the natural repugnance against incest. In the Talmudic discussion as well as in the legal codes, the subject is treated as a sexual offense, involving a breach of morality rather than a eugenic error. (The Talmud is the repository of rabbinic exposition of biblical law and teaching, spanning more than five centuries. The legal codes are based on the Talmud and on subsequent development of the law, such as in Responsa, formal opinions rendered by rabbinic authorities in response to new case-law inquiries.)

Even bastardy is a moral rather than a eugenic category. The *mamzer* (in Jewish law, the product of an adulterous or incestuous liaison, not of a relationship between two persons who are not married to one another) is not legally ill-born; his or her status is compromised only legally and socially, rendered so in punitive or deterrent judgment against parents not free to have entered the relationship. But no difference obtains between the *mamzer* born of adultery—even a technical adultery, such as when the document of divorce for the mother's previous marriage was impugned—and the *mamzer* born of incest. Hence, no eugenic motive can be assigned here.

A man "maimed in his privy parts" bears the same legal disabilities as the *mamzer.* Thus, a man of "crushed testicles or severed member" is excluded from "the congregation of the Lord" (Deut. 23:2). This verse is interpreted to mean only that he may not enter into conjugal union with an Israelite woman. Thus, the castrated male is under the ban because the act of castration is forbidden. But one "maimed in his privy parts" as a result of a birth defect or disease, as opposed to one castrated by his own or another's deliberate assault, is free of this disability. The legal situations were thus analogized: "Just as the *mamzer* is the result of human misdeeds, so only the castrated one who is such as a result of human misdeeds is to be banned." Since that distinction is made in both cases, and since the banned *mamzer* and the castrated are permitted to marry, for example, another *mamzer* or a proselyte, it must be concluded that moral outrage and punitive judgment rather than eugenic considerations are operative.

Eugenics, in the sense of choosing a marriage partner with the well-being of progeny in mind, is more clearly present in Talmudic counsel and legislation. A man is counseled to choose a wife prudently, and guidance is offered in doing so in accordance with the intellectual and moral virtues of the prospective bride. And since, we are told, a son, for example, normally takes after his mother's brothers, a man should regard the maternal uncles in making his decision (Bava Batra, 110a). A hidden physical blemish in a spouse is grounds for invalidating a marriage, unless the other spouse can be presumed to have known of it in advance.

Heredity as a eugenic principle takes its legal model from rulings with respect to circumcision. A male infant whose two brothers died possibly as a result of this operation may not be circumcised. He is deemed to have inherited the illness (probably hemophilia) that proved fatal to his two brothers. The Talmud goes on to say that an infant whose two maternal cousins showed that weakness may not be circumcised either. That is, statistical evidence yielded by two sons from the same mother can also be reflected in two sisters of that mother (Yevamot, 64b). Coming from Talmudic times (before 500 c.e.), this is a remarkably early recognition that hemophilia is transmitted through maternal lineage—in itself a significant eugenic discovery.

The statistical evidence or the presumption of adverse hereditary factors in a third family member, when those factors are seen to exist in two others, thus becomes the basis of Talmudic laws of eugenics. With modern laboratory means to determine the presence of these factors, the principle of course operates even sooner, without waiting for statistical evidence in two members. The Talmud rules that one may not marry into a family of epileptics or lepers (Yevamot, 64b) or—by extension—a family in which tuberculosis or any similar disease appears in multiple members. This may be the first eugenic edict in any social or religious system.

The pure "heredity" underlying this recommendation is not unanimously agreed upon. While one view in the Talmud attributes the transmission of characteristics in the pre-Mendelian age to heredity, another view sees it as "bad luck." In a Responsum where the questioner considered abortion because the mother was epileptic, the rabbi responded that the latter of the two views stated above may be the right one, and that fear of bad luck is an inadequate warrant for abortion (Feldman, 1968).

In an earlier context, the Mishnah (the foundation layer of the Talmud) speaks of the faculties that a father bequeaths to his son: "looks, strength, riches, and length of years" (Eduyot, II, 9). Here, too, the commentaries align themselves on both sides: one sees the bequeathing of faculties as a natural hereditary process, the other sees them as divine reward for the father's virtues.

Two other Talmudic ideas with eugenic motifs are reflected in current practice. In the interests of fulfilling the injunction to "love one's wife as much as himself and honor her more than himself," a man is advised to seek his sister's daughter as a bride; his care for her will be the more tender due to his affection for his own sister. Yet in the thirteenth century, Rabbi Judah the Pious left a testamentary charge to his children and grandchildren that became a source of guidance to others on the level of precedent for subsequent Jewish law. In this famous testament, he advises against marriage with a niece because it may have adverse genetic results. Modern rabbinic authorities dismiss such fears as unjustified unless they are medically warranted.

A second point is a Talmudic notion that eugenic factors operate in intercourse during pregnancy. Conjugal relations, we are told, should be avoided during the first trimester as "injurious to the embryo"; but they are encouraged during the final trimester as desirable for both mother and fetus, for then the child is born "well-formed and of strong vitality" (Niddah, 31a). A medieval Jewish authority makes the matter a point of pride in comparative culture: the Talmud recommends coitus during the final trimester, whereas the Greek and Arab scholars say it is harmful. Do not listen to them, he says (Responsa Bar Sheshet, no. 447). Nonetheless, the Talmud prohibits the marriage of a pregnant or nursing widow or divorcee. In the case of a pregnant woman, the second husband, it is suggested, may be less considerate of a fetus fathered by another man and may inadvertently damage it through abdominal pressure during intercourse (Yevamot, 36a). In the nursing situation, the new father may fail to take the necessary steps to supplement the diet of his stepchild (it is assumed that a pregnancy diminishes the mother's milk). And a pregnant woman who feels an urgent physical or psychological need for food during the Yom Kippur fast is to be fed for the sake of her fetus's welfare as well as her own (Yoma, 82a).

More a matter of preaching than of law is the notion that defective children can be the result of immoral or inconsiderate modes of intercourse—an idea expounded but ultimately rejected by the Talmud (Nedarim, 20a). Yet in more modern times, the Hasidim (pietistic Jewish groups with a mystical orientation) maintain that spiritual consequences of the act are indeed possible; that if a man has pure and lofty thoughts during or preparatory to cohabitation, he can succeed in transmitting to the child of either sex an especially lofty soul. Hence dynastic succession of leadership, presuming the inheritance of that loftier soul, as opposed to democratic selection, obtains among Hasidic groups.

A study of biblical and Talmudic sources written by Max Grunwald in 1930, cited by Immanuel Jakobovits, discerns a broad eugenic motif. Grunwald writes that Judaism

> quite consciously strives for the promotion of the quantity of progeny by the compulsion of matrimony, the insistence on early marriage, the sexual purity of the marital partners and the harmony of their ages and characters, the dissolubility of unhappy unions, the regulation of conjugal intercourse, the high esteem of maternity, the stress on parental responsibility, the protection of the embryo, etc. To be sure, there can be no question here of a compulsory public control over the health conditions of the marriage candidates, but that would positively be in line with the principles of Jewish eugenics: the pursuit after the most numerous and physically, mentally, and morally sound natural increase of the people, without thinking of an exclusive race protection. (p. 154)

Although abortion is warranted primarily for maternal rather than fetal indications, screening of would-be parents for actual or potential defective genes, such as in Tay-Sachs disease, would, like premarital blood tests, be much in keeping with the Jewish traditional eugenic concern. Such genetic screening is, in fact, facilitated by a unique computerized system under the auspices of the New York-based Dor Yesharim (Generation of Upright [Descendants], from Psalms 112:2). Young men and women diagnosed as Tay-Sachs carriers are identified by code number. When marriage is contemplated, the couple is alerted to the fact that both are carriers, with one chance in four of a homozygous fetus, so that marriage plans may be reconsidered. Besides Tay-Sachs, which is fatal to the child by about age five, nonfatal disabilities have been added to Dor Yesharim's data base.

Although surrogate parenting and artificial insemination create social and family problems, the conceptional procedures that make them possible are in and of themselves acceptable when natural means are ineffective. In vitro fertilization, to assist in a conception that might otherwise be thwarted by blocked fallopian tubes or by sperm inadequacy, has been accorded full moral and legal sanction. Genetic engineering that alters the germ line has been ruled out by Jewish ethicists, but gene therapy, removing or correcting defective genes, would be a proper extension of the mandate to heal. The newly announced technology for cloning embryos has been greeted with more caution than hope—hope for improved procreational prospects for couples otherwise limited to one or no progeny, but caution against creating multiple embryos deprived of their distinctiveness as individuals. Safeguards are called for against the dangers of genetic mutation, or of political or profit-motive "baby farming" that could result from abuse of broader eugenic techniques.

DAVID M. FELDMAN (1995)

SEE ALSO: *Eugenics; Genetic Discrimination; Genetic Engineering, Human; Genetic Testing and Screening; Human Dignity; Judaism, Bioethics in; Medical Ethics, History of Near and Middle East: Israel; Population Ethics, Religious Traditions: Jewish;* and other *Eugenics and Religious Law* subentries

BIBLIOGRAPHY

Feldman, David M. 1968. *Birth Control in Jewish Law: Marital Relations, Contraception, and Abortion as Set Forth in the Classical Texts of Jewish Law.* New York: New York University Press.

Feldman, David M. 1991. "The Case of Baby M." In *Jewish Values in Health and Medicine,* pp. 163–169, ed. Levi Meier. Lanham, MD: University Press of America.

Jacobs, Louis. 1974. "Heredity." In *What Does Judaism Say About … ?,* pp. 165–166. New York: Quadrangle/New York Times.

Jakobovits, Immanuel. 1975. *Jewish Medical Ethics: A Comparative and Historical Study of the Jewish Religious Attitude to Medicine and Its Practice,* new edition. New York: Bloch Publishing Company.

Kolata, Gina. 1994. "Reproductive Revolution Is Jolting Old Views." *New York Times,* January 11, pp. A1, C12.

Rosner, Fred. 1986. *Modern Medicine and Jewish Ethics.* Hoboken, NJ: Ktav Publishing House.

Zevin, Shelomoh Yosef. 1957. *Le'Or Ha-Halakhah: Be-ayot u-verurim,* pp. 147–158, 2nd edition. Tel Aviv: Abraham Zioni.

II. CHRISTIANITY

The following is a revision and update of the first edition entry "Eugenics and Religious Law: Christian Religious Laws" by the same author. Portions of the first edition entry appear in the revised version.

Christian religious laws historically comprehend a large spectrum of rules to guide individual conduct and social relationships among the baptized. The laws most likely to have eugenic significance are the canons prohibiting the marriage of relatives. These regulations also form the basis for the modern civil law prohibitions against the marriage of relatives in both the Continental legal systems and the Anglo-Saxon statutory scheme. Though the principal justification given for such prohibitions in Christian law has been ethical and social, there is substantial evidence that they also may reflect considerations classified as eugenic in contemporary scientific research.

The ecclesiastical regulations that forbid marriage between persons closely related by consanguinity are among the most ancient canons of the Christian tradition. Penalties attached to the violation of religious exogamic laws have varied historically in their severity, as, indeed, have the ways of measuring the degrees of kinship and defining within which degrees the crime of incest shall be punished. But the core of the tradition of canon law remains constant and reflects an extreme reluctance to accept the marriages of close relatives as humanly or religiously feasible.

For Roman Catholics all marriages within the direct line of blood relationship, that is, between an ancestor and a descendant by parentage, and within the collateral line to the fourth degree, that is, to third cousins, are forbidden (*Code of Canon Law,* 1983, canon 1091). The definition of marriages within four degrees of relationship as incestuous dates to the Fourth Lateran Council in 1215 (c. 50). In the Greek Orthodox tradition, marriage in the direct line and in the collateral line to the sixth or seventh degree by the Roman method of computation is prohibited in canon 54 of the Synod in Trullo, 691/692 (Hefele). All Oriental Christians forbid marriages in the direct line; Armenians, Jacobites, and Copts prohibit it in the collateral line to the fourth degree, Melkites to the sixth degree, Serbs and Chaldeans to the third degree, and Ethiopians without distinction. Among Protestant reformers the restrictions of the medieval canon law were accepted by some, such as Phillip Melanchthon and Martin Chemnitz (Kemnitz); only the Old Testament regulations of Leviticus 18:6–18 by others, such as Martin Bucer and, perhaps, Martin Luther; and only the closest ties of direct parental relationship by still others, such as John Wycliffe. In the Anglican community, The Book of Common Prayer contains a table drawn up by Archbishop Matthew Parker based on Leviticus in naming relatives incapable of marriage (Wheatly). Most Protestant churches today follow the prohibitions of civil law regarding incest and kinship marriage (Acte for Kynges Succession; Acte for Succession of Imperyall Crowne; Concerning Precontracte and Degrees).

The sources of and commentaries upon the Christian laws record debate about the extent of the prohibition, the possibility of dispensation within certain close degrees of kinship, and the related question of the divine or natural law origin of the laws (e.g., Burchard of Worms, *Decretum,* bk. 7, "De Incesto"; Burchard of Worms, *Collection in 74 titulis* 65.281–284). They reveal, however, only the most sketchy discussion of the foundations of the regulations themselves.

The classical reasons given for the prohibition of consanguineous marriages are ethical and social. The first reason was called the *respectus parentelae,* namely, that such marriages would undermine the respect due to parents and consequently to all those who are closely related (Aquinas, 1948, *Summa theologiae* II–II, 154, 9). Second, they constitute a moral danger to family life arising from the possibility of early moral corruption of the young dwelling within the same household in which marriage could be allowed (ibid.; Sánchez 1605, 7.52.12, 7.53). Third, the prohibition of consanguineous marriages prevents the disruption of the family by sexual competition and forces the multiplication of friendships and the spread of charity (Augustine). These three reasons seem to have been sufficient to justify the laws, so that most scholars did not go beyond them to seek a further justification. Adhémar Esmein, for example, said the laws arose out of an instinctive repulsion for incest and were not reflective of any known adverse physical consequences. Some modern authors speculate that the reason for strict enforcement of prohibitions against incestuous marriages was to force the breakup of landed family estates (Duby).

It is only in comparatively modern times that an explicitly eugenic reason for the prohibition has received scientific attention. Writing in 1673, Samuel Dugard noted: "There is a *judgment* which is said often to accompany these Marriages, and that is *Want of Children* and a *Barrennesse"* (p. 53). "The Children are weak, it may be; grow crooked, or, what is worse, do not prove well; presently, Sir, it shall be said what better could be expected? an unlawfull Wedlock must have an unprosperous successe" (p. 51). Ambrosius J. Stapf's *Theologia moralis* in 1827 alluded to this possibility (p. 359). A fuller treatment is found in Dominic Le Noir's 1873 edition of St. Alphonsus's *Theologia moralis.* Edward Westermarck in 1889 and Eduard Laurent in 1895 spoke at length of a physiological justification of the canons to prevent indiscriminate inbreeding and the risk of a high incidence of deleterious genetic effects. Franz Wernz, in 1928 (n. 352 [70]), writing from a comprehensive knowledge of the canonical tradition, said the ancient writers also knew of the undesirable effects of excessive inbreeding. He noted reasons derived from contemporary medical science in the writings of Gratian (early twelfth century) (C.xx "Anglis permittitur, ut in quarta vel in quinta generatione cognibitur,"

c. 20, c. 35, q. 2), Pope Innocent III (1161–1216) (Schroeder), and Thomas Aquinas (*Commentum in libros IV Sententiarum,* dist. 40 and 41, q. 1, art. 4). Since the late nineteenth century nearly all commentators on the canonical rules speak of eugenic objections to marriages of blood relatives.

It is possible to find in the ancient ecclesiastical commentators an awareness of a eugenic foundation to the prohibition expressed in primitive and undifferentiated modes of speech. For example, a persistent belief was kept alive among theologians and canonists that children of incestuous relationships will die or will be greatly debilitated, or that the familial line will be cursed with sterility. Benedict the Levite (850?) wrote of these marriages: "From these are usually born the blind, the deaf, hunchbacks, the mentally defective, and others afflicted with loathsome infirmities" (*Capitularum collectio*). Furthermore, in the explanations of the name of the impediment (i.e., the impediment of consanguinity), if one traces their origins through medieval glossography to the *Etymologies* of Isidore of Seville (560?–636), there appears an awareness of a physiological factor in the blood bond of close relatives that must be weakened before marriage can be contracted safely.

The antecedents of the Christian canons in the Mosaic law (Lev. 18:6–18) and the Roman law (Burge) were taken as expressions of natural law by the canonists and were continued in the barbarian codes (*Pactum legis salicae* 13.11; *Leges visigothae* 4.1.1–7; *Codex Euriciani* 2). In his *Ecclesiastical History* (I, 27), where the Venerable Bede (673–735) notes these laws, he records a quotation from a letter of Pope Gregory I to Augustine of Canterbury, written in 601 (*Responsa Gregorii*). The reason given by Gregory for forbidding marriages of close relatives is, "We have learned from experience that from such a marriage offspring cannot grow up." This letter and this reason not only are later picked up and cited by Gratian ("Anglis permittatur," c. 2, c. 35, q. 5) and Thomas Aquinas (*Summa theologiae suppl.* 54, 3), but may be found in virtually all the canonical collections of the early Middle Ages. Though comment on this passage is rare, comment was, perhaps, unnecessary. The passage from Gregory seems clearly to say that experience teaches that children from forbidden consanguineous marriages are affected or unable to grow up. There is thought to be a physiological consequence to incest. In the light of this it seems probable that the labored argumentation over the question of how close the relationship must be for marriage to be forbidden by natural law must have been conducted in some awareness of a popular belief in the biological consequences of such unions. The fear of genetic anomalies or biological debilitation from indiscriminate inbreeding may not be perfectly articulated. It is difficult to imagine, however, that warning of some physiological dangers to offspring

may not have been intended in the frequent citation of Pope Gregory to sustain the severity of the prohibition.

Tomás Sánchez (1605), who wrote the greatest of the canonical commentaries on marriage, says that the most suasive ground for forbidding incestuous unions is that there is a sharing of the blood among close relatives and that the physical image of a progenitor (*imago, complexio, effigies, mores, virtus paterna*) passes to offspring, so that the blood must be weakened through successive generations before marriage should be contracted (7.50; 7.51.1–2). Thus, preventing marriages of close relatives to protect the offspring by allowing several generations to pass before procreation can be called a measure of eugenic foresight, however simple the scientific awareness to support it may have been.

In summary, a eugenic foundation to Christian religious laws forbidding the marriage of close relatives is clearly articulated and commented upon by modern scholars from the late eighteenth and nineteenth centuries. Evidence of this kind of awareness may be discovered earlier in the canonical sources, however, going back at least to the seventh century. It would seem consistent with the eugenic connotation of those laws rooted in antiquity, together with a Christian sense of responsibility for offspring that partly motivated them, to consider further eugenic restrictions on marriage in Christian communities today, in light of contemporary knowledge of genetics.

WILLIAM W. BASSETT (1995)

SEE ALSO: *Christianity, Bioethics in; Eugenics; Genetic Discrimination; Genetic Engineering, Human; Genetic Testing and Screening; Human Dignity; Human Rights; Population Ethics, Religious Traditions: Protestant Perspectives; Population Ethics, Religious Traditions: Roman Catholic Perspectives;* and other *Eugenics and Religious Law* subentries

BIBLIOGRAPHY

An Acte for the Establishement of the Kynges Succession. 1533–1534. 25 Hen. VIII, c. 22. *The Statutes of the Realm,* vol. 3, pp. 471–474, esp. 472–473.

An Acte for the Establishement of the Succession of the Imperyall Crowne of This Realme. 1536. 28 Hen. VIII, c. 7. *The Statutes of the Realm,* vol. 3, pp. 655–662, esp. pp. 658–659.

Aquinas, Thomas. 1878. *Commentum in libros IV sententiarum,* dists. 40 and 41, ques. 1, art 4, pp. 770–771. vol. 30 of *Opera omnia,* ed. Stanislai Eduardi Frette. Paris: Ludovicum Vivès.

Aquinas, Thomas 1948. "Utrum consanguinitas de iure naturali impediat matrimonium," ques. 54, art. 3. In vol. 4 of *Summa theologiae,* pp. 838–840, esp. "Sed contra," p. 839. Rome: Marietti, tr. the Fathers of the English Dominican Province under the title "Whether Consanguinity Is an Impediment to

Marriage by Virtue of Natural Law." In vol. 3 of *Summa Theologica: First Complete American Edition*, pp. 2758–2760, esp. "On the Contrary," p. 2759. New York: Benziger Brothers.

Aquinas, Thomas. 1948. "Utrum incestus sit species determinata luxuriae," ques. 154, art 9. In vol. 3 of *Summa theologiae*, pp. 722–723, Rome: Marietti, tr. the Fathers of the English Dominican Province under the title "Whether Incest Is a Determinate Species of Lust?" In vol. 2 of *Summa Theologica: First Complete American Edition*, pp. 1823–1824. New York: Benziger Brothers.

Augustine. 1844–1891. "De jure conjugiorum, quod dissimile a subsequentibus matrimoniis habuerint prima connubia." In *Patrologiae cursus completus: Series Latina*, vol. 41, cols. 457–460; comp. Jacques-Paul Migne. Paris: Garnier Fratres.

Augustine. 1950. "Of Marriage Between Blood-Relations, in Regard to Which the Present Law Could Not Bind the Men of Earliest Ages." *The City of God*, bk. 15, ch. 16, pp. 500–502, tr. Marcus Dods. New York: Modern Library.

Bede (Venerable Bede). 1969. *Bede's Ecclesiastical History of the English People*, bk. 1, ch. 27, pp. 78–102, esp. p. 85, ed. Bertram Colgrave and R. A. B. Mynors. Oxford: Clarendon Press. Facing Latin and English texts.

Benedict the Levite (Benedictus diaconi). 1844–1891. "Captularum collectio: Pertz monitum." In *Patrologiae cursus completus: Series Latina*, vol. 97, bk. 3, sec. 179, col. 820, comp. Jacques-Paul Migne. Paris: Garnier Fratres.

Bouchard, Constance B. 1981. "Consanguinity and Noble Marriage in the Tenth and Eleventh Centuries." *Speculum* 56(2): 268–287.

Brundage, James A. 1987. *Law, Sex, and Christian Society in Medieval Europe*. Chicago: University of Chicago Press.

Burchard of Worms. 1965 (1915). *Collectio in 74 titulis*. In *Anselmi episcopi Lucensis collectio una cum collectione minore*. Aalen: Scientia Verlage, tr. John Gilchrist under the title *The Collection in Seventy-four Titles: A Canon Law Manual of the Gregorian Reform*. Toronto: Pontifical Institute of Medieval Studies, 1980.

Burge, William. 1910. *The Comparative Law of Marriage and Divorce*, ed. Alexander W. Renton and George G. Phillimore. London: Sweet and Maxwell.

Code of Canon Law: A Text and Commentary. 1976. Canon 1976, secs. 1 and 2, pp. 487–489, ed. Timothy Lincoln Bouscaren and Adam C. Ellis. Milwaukee: Bruce. English text with commentary.

Code of Canon Law: Latin-English Edition. 1983. Washington, D.C.: Canon Law Society of America.

Concerning Precontracte and Degrees of Consanguinite. 1540. 32 Hen. VIII, c. 38. *The Statutes of the Realm*, vol. 3, p. 792.

Coussa, Acacio. 1948. *Epitome praelectionem de iure ecclesiastico orientali*, vol. 3, *De matrimonio*. Rome: Typis Monasterii Exarchici Cryptoferratensis.

Dauvillier, Jean-DeClercq Charles. 1936. *Le mariage en droit canonique oriental*. Paris: Recueil Sirey.

Duby, Georges. 1983. *The Knight, the Lady, and the Priest: The Making of Modern Marriage in Medieval France*. New York: Pantheon.

Dugard, Samuel. 1673. *The Marriages of Cousins German, Vindicated from the Censures of Unlawfullnesse, and Inexpediency, Being a Letter Written to His Much Honour'd T.D.* Oxford: Printed by Hen. Hall for Thomas Bowman. Attributed to Dugard although it is taken largely from Jeremy Taylor's *Ductor dubitantium*. Attributed to Simon Dugard in the British Museum Catalog.

Esmein, Adhémar. 1929. *Le mariage en droit canonique*, 2 vols, 2nd edition. Paris: Recueil Sirey.

Fleury, Jacques. 1933. *Recherches historiques sur les empêchements de parenté dans le mariage canonique dès origines aux fausses décrétales*. Paris: Recueil Sirey.

Goody, Jack. 1983. *The Development of the Family and Marriage in Europe*. Cambridge, Eng.: Cambridge University Press.

Gratian (Gratianus, The Canonist). 1554. *Decretum divi Gratiani, universi iuris canonici pontificias constitutiones & canonicas brevi compendio complectens*, pt. 2, causa 35, ques. 2, canon 20, p. 1217; ques. 5, canon 2, pp. 1218–1221. Lyons: I. Pideoius.

Gregory I. 1957. "Gregorius Augustino Episcopo." *Registrum epistolarum*, vol. 2, pp. 332–343, esp. pp. 335–336, 2nd edition, ed. Paulus Ewald and Ludovicus M. Hartman. Monumenta Germaniae Historica, vols. 1 and 2. Berlin: Weidmannos.

Hefele, Karl Joseph von. 1896. "The Quinsext or Trullan Synod, a.d. 692." In *A History of the Councils of the Church: From the Original Documents*, vol. 5, sec. 327, pp. 221–239, esp. canon 54, p. 231, 2nd edition, rev; ed. and tr. William R. Clark. Edinburgh: T. and T. Clark, 1896.

Herlihy, David. 1985. *Medieval Households*. Cambridge, MA: Harvard University Press.

Isidore of Seville. 1911. "De adfinitatibus et gradibus," "De agnatis et cognatis," "De conivgiis." *Etymologiarum sive originum, libri XX*, vol. 1, bk. 9, chs. 5–7, ed. Wallace Martin Lindsay. Oxford: Clarendon Press. See also *Patro-logia cursus completus: Series Latina*, vol. 82, cols. 353–368.

Laurent, Emile. 1895. *Mariages consanguins et dégénérescences*. Paris: A. Maloine.

Liguori, Alfonso Maria de' (Alfonsus Liguori). 1872–1874. "De matrimonio." *Theologia moralis*, vol. 3, bk. 5, tract. 6, pp. 661–858, esp. pp. 783–784, ed. Dominic Le Noir. 4 vols. Paris: Ludovicum Vivès.

Meyvaert, Paul. 1971. "Bede's Text of the Libellus Responsionem of Gregory the Great to Augustine of Canterbury." In *England Before the Conquest: Studies in Primary Sources Presented to Dorothy Whitelock*, pp. 15–33, ed. Peter Clemoes and Kathleen Hughes. Cambridge, Eng.: Cambridge University Press.

Patrologiae cursus completus. Series latina [Patrologia latina]. 1851–1894. 221 vols. Paris: Garnier Fratres Supplementum. Paris: Editions Garnier Frères.

Sánchez, Tomás. 1605. "De impedimentis." In his *Disputationum de sancto matrimonio sacramento*, vol. 3, bk. 7, dis. 50, pp. 332–336; dis. 51, pars. 1–2, pp. 336–337; dis. 52, par. 12, p. 352; dis. 53, pp. 352–354. 3 vols. in 4. vols. 1 and 2, Genoa: Iosephum Pavonem, 1602. vols. 3 and 4, Madrid: Ludouici Sanchez.

Schroeder, Henry Joseph. 1937 (1215). "The Twelfth General Council: Fourth Lateran Council." *Disciplinary Decrees of the General Councils: Text, Translation, and Commentary,* pp. 236–296, esp. canon 50, pp. 279–280. St. Louis: B. Herder. Latin text: "Canones Concilii Lateranensis IV (Oecumen XII): Anno 1215 habiti." *Disciplinary Decrees,* pp. 560–584, esp. canon 50, p. 578.

Stapf, Ambrosius Joseph. 1827. *Theologiae moralis,* vol. 2, sec. 312, p. 359. Innsbruck: Typis and Sumtibus Wagnerianis.

The Statutes of the Realm, Printed by Command of His Majesty King George the Third, in Pursuance of an Address of the House of Commons of Great Britain, from the Original Records and Authentic Manuscripts. 1963. Repr. 11 vols. in 12. London: Dawsons of Pall Mall.

Wahl, Francis X. 1934. *The Matrimonial Impediments of Consanguinity and Affinity: An Historical Synopsis and Commentary.* Washington, D.C.: Catholic University of America Press.

Wernz, Franz Xavier. 1928. *Ius decretalium,* vol. 4., rev. editon. Florence: Libraria Gaichetti.

Westermarck, Edward A. 1921. *The History of Human Marriage,* 3 vols., 5th edition, rev. London: Macmillan; New York: Allerton, 1922. Repr. New York: Johnson Reprint Corp., 1971.

Wheatly, Charles. 1759 (1710). "Of the Preface and Charge and the Several Impediments to Matrimony." In *A Rational Illustration of the Book of Common Prayer of the Church of England,* ch. 10, sec. 3, pp. 376–383, 8th edition. London: C. Hitch et al. A commentary.

III. ISLAM

The idea of eugenics is not well developed in the Islamic world. Both Islamic law and tradition generally condemn abortion, which is permitted only if the mother's life is endangered, so there is no genetic counseling that would lead to abortion. Both religious law and tradition do include references to a man's choosing an appropriate wife, but these concerns have been interpreted as moral and social, rather than eugenic.

Islamic religious-moral law, the Shari'a, deals with questions concerning laws of incest and consanguinity from the perspective of moral and social relationships rather than eugenic concerns. The general counsel of the Qur'an and the Prophetic traditions regarding marriage is promulgated in the laws that require a Muslim to marry within the community of believers. A Muslim is better than a non-Muslim as a spouse. "A woman may be married for four reasons: for her property, her status, her beauty, and her religion; so try to get one who is religious" (Muslim, tradition 3457). There is no law to suggest choosing a marriage partner with the intention of improving the progeny through the control of hereditary factors. With slight variations among the Sunni and Shiite schools, the law specifies that a woman may not marry a man who is not equal to her. The earliest ruling to require equality in matters of piety and freedom from physical defects detrimental to marriage is found among the Malikis (see al-Juzayri, for variations among the four schools of Sunni law).

In the Qur'an the main source for marriage law is book 4, verse 23. This prohibits marriage between persons closely related by blood, but this ban reflects ethical and social, rather than eugenic, considerations. Thus in Muslim jurisprudence a man and a woman may be forbidden to marry either because of blood relationship (e.g., a man may not marry his mother or either of his grandmothers, etc.) or relationships established through marriage (e.g., he may not marry the mother or grandmothers of his wife, etc.). Moreover, there are women whom a man may marry singly, but not be married to at the same time (e.g., two sisters, a woman and the sister of her mother or father). This latter prohibition seems to be more for psychological than for eugenic reasons.

Evidence that the Qur'an (or Shari'a) considers nurture, or the environment, to have impact on a child perhaps comparable to that of nature, or genetic inheritance, comes from the Book of Marriage, which prohibits marriage not only between a man and the woman who gave birth to him but also between a man and the foster mother who breastfed him at least a certain number of times.

The ruling seems to indicate similar consequences for foster relations established through suckling: "What is unlawful because of blood relations, is also unlawful because of corresponding foster suckling relations" (al-Bukhari, tradition 46; al-E'Amili, 7/281, tradition 2). In establishing unmarriageability, a foster mother who suckles an infant is regarded exactly as the infant's real mother.

There is further evidence of the Islamic tradition's lack of interest in eugenics. Islam abolished one of the four types of marriages among Arabs, the one described in Arab tradition in terms that may reflect eugenic concerns. The tradition says:

> The second type [of marriage] was that a man would say to his wife after she had become clean from her period, "Send for so-and-so [whose nobility is well established] and have sexual relations with him." Her husband would then keep away from her and would not touch her at all till her pregnancy became evident from that man with whom she was sleeping. After the pregnancy was established her husband would sleep with her if he wished. However, he allowed his wife to sleep with that person being desirous of the nobility of the

child (*najabat al-walad*). Such marriage was called "marriage seeking advancement" (*nikah al-istibda*). (al-Bukhari, 1986, sec. 37)

Islam, which insisted that faith in God was the main source of all human nobility, was uninterested in this practice, traditional in the Arab tribal culture, for the improvement of the human race through the control of hereditary factors.

Other traditions counsel the believers to choose a partner for breeding (*al-nutaf*) "bravery among the people of Khurasan" [in Iran], sexual potency among the Berber [in North Africa], and "generosity and envy among the Arabs" (al-'Amili, 7/29, tradition #6). The Islamic traditions (hadith literature) do reflect explicit knowledge of eugenics in choosing a marriage partner. The source of these eugenic considerations seems to be the Irano-Semitic culture, in which such interests were commonplace. Although these traditions were never used as authoritative precedents for legislation in the Shari'a, they express the popular piety connected with marital relations. For example, the Prophet is quoted saying, "Anyone wishing to follow my tradition should know that among my traditions is marriage. Seek children [through it].... Protect your children from the milk of the prostitute and the insane among women, because milk makes inroads [in the character of a child]" (al-'Amili, 1969, 7/4, tradition 6). Moreover, in the case of a person drinking wine, the Prophet regarded it permissible to annul the marriage contract, especially, if the person was alcoholic (literally, "sick" with alcohol) (al-'Amili). There also existed a warning against marrying fatuous individuals because their offspring would be a loss. However, it was acceptable to marry them for sexual reasons, as long as one did not seek children through such a union. These traditions reveal the concern about hereditary factors in the progeny.

Other traditions encourage marriages within one's own collateral line, to first cousins. The Prophet, who belonged to the Hashimite clan, at one time looked at the children of 'Ali and Ja'far, two brothers and his paternal cousins by relation, and said, "Our daughters for our sons, and our sons for our daughters" (al-'Amili, 7/49, tradition 7). This encouragement is contradicted by other traditions that recommend exogamous marriage and even intermarriage between Arab and non-Arab, and between a free person and a slave. There does not seem to be any awareness in these early traditions of deleterious genetic effects from excessive inbreeding. However, since 1970 there has been a growing debate among traditional Muslim jurists over the authenticity of the tradition that encourages endogamy indiscriminately. Certain injurious hereditary conditions have been detected in the fourth and fifth generations of some tribes in Muslim societies where endogamy is the norm.

Muslim traditions also speak about the negative impact on the fetus of "improper" modes of intercourse rejected by the Qur'an. Yet it was believed that special prayer when one intends to have intercourse with his wife keeps the devil away from what God has ordained to be created. The pure state of the parents' minds and bodies can be transmitted to the child through the invocation of the Divine Name before intercourse. In light of belief in the divine purpose and decree in the creation of offspring ("It is God who brought you forth from your mothers' wombs," Qur'an 16:78), either born with birth defects or normal, there does not seem to be any indication to support genetic diagnosis or screening that would justify abortion, which Islam permits primarily to safeguard the mother's health.

ABDULAZIZ SACHEDINA (1995)

SEE ALSO: *Abortion, Religious Traditions: Islamic Perspectives; Eugenics; Genetic Discrimination; Genetic Engineering, Human; Genetic Testing and Screening; Human Dignity; Islam, Bioethics in; Judaism, Bioethics in; Population Ethics, Religious Traditions: Islamic Perspectives;* and other *Eugenics and Religious Law* subentries

BIBLIOGRAPHY

SUNNI VIEWS

al-Bukhari, Muhammad ibn Isma'il. 1986. *Kitab al-nikah.* Vol. 4. In *Sahih al-Bukhari.* Beirut: 'Alam al-Kutub.

al-Juzayri, 'Abd al-Rahman. 1969. *al-Fiqh 'ala al-madhahib al-arba'a.* Vol. 4. Cairo: Dar al-Fikr al-'Arabi.

Muslim ibn al-Hajjaj al-Qushayri. 1956. *Kitab al-nikah.* In *Sahih al-Muslim.* Beirut: Dar Ihya' al-Turath al-'Arabi.

SHIITE VIEWS

al-'Amili, al-Shahid al-Thani. 1969. *Al-Rawdat al-bahiyya fi sharh al-lum'at al-dimashqiyya,* vol. 5. An-Najaf, Iraq: Matba'a al-Adab.

al-Hurr, al-'Amili, Muhammad ibn al-Hasan. 1968. *Wasa'il al-shi'a,* vol. 14. In *Kitab al-nikah.* Beirut: Dar Ihya' al-Turath al-'Arabi.

IV. HINDUISM AND BUDDHISM

Because reproduction is one of the most important concerns of human life, most religions concern themselves with the regulation of sexual activity, marriage, and production of children. Hinduism and Buddhism also guide their followers in these matters, but in ways very different both from each other and from Western religions.

Eugenics might be defined as controlling human reproduction to modify or benefit the species. Prior to the present innovation of genetic engineering, eugenics meant restrictions on who could reproduce and with which partner. The recent development of methods of altering the human genome has opened a new area of ethical discussion: the propriety of voluntarily altering the human genome. Eugenics has also been used to excuse genocide, but this aspect will not be discussed here since nothing in Hinduism or Buddhism allows rationalization of genocide.

Although Hinduism and Buddhism have highly developed ethical philosophies, neither religion produces set positions on such contemporary matters as eugenics, nor is it likely that they will, given the nature and organization of the two religions. In both religions, ethics are developed by the individual or the social community; there is no official body that produces ethical statements. Hence there are no official Hindu or Buddhist positions on issues that were not envisioned when their scriptures were composed over 2,000 years ago. However, both religions have ethical ideas or methods that can be applied to modern problems.

Hinduism has its beginnings in the two millennia before the Common Era; the historical Buddha, Shakyamuni, died about 500 B.C.E. In those remote times there were no concepts akin to those of modern genetics and hence there could be no ethical discussions of genetic manipulation. Rather than a single scripture analogous to the Judeo-Christian Bible or the Koran, Hinduism and Buddhism have vast collections of diverse canonical texts that have appeared over millennia. Hinduism does have several authoritative legal texts, the most important of which, *The Laws of Manu,* was composed from about 200 B.C.E. to 200 C.E. These texts codify religious law (*dharma*) but are not regarded as the only legal or ethical authority. Buddhist texts are concerned with spiritual development and give only very general precepts for regulation of lay life. However, it is possible to develop Hindu or Buddhist positions on eugenics.

Hinduism and Buddhism both arose in India and share many common beliefs, such as the doctrine of *karma* (discussed below), yet the differences between the two religions must not be underestimated. Generally speaking, Hinduism is a legalistic religion and pays great attention to regulating life in the world. Buddhism sees worldly life as secondary in importance; attainment of release from suffering in this or subsequent existences is its central concern.

Reproduction in Hindu Religious Law

Although Hinduism recognizes a final stage of life in which the individual is released from domestic and social obligations in order to be able to pursue enlightenment (*moksha*), in the earlier, householder stage, detailed rules define acceptable behavior. Among the most important are those that regulate reproduction. The intent of these rules is to maintain the hereditary caste distinctions. Here Hinduism's outlook is very similar to that of nineteenth- and early twentieth-century Western eugenics, which proposed controlling reproduction to prevent what were considered undesirable unions. Although the specific rules for regulating marriage and reproduction were different from those proposed by Western eugenics, the spirit is the same: to protect the human species from degeneration due to unsuitable matches. Hinduism does not define suitability for marriage according to scientific understanding of genetics, but by caste membership, which is hereditary, and by physical traits, which are correlated with astrology. Traditionally, prospective brides were inspected undressed and an elaborate system of body divination existed for interpreting body markings, particularly on erogenous areas. Manu states, "A man should not marry a girl who is a redhead or has an extra limb or is sickly or has not body hair or ... is too sallow ... He should marry a woman who does not lack any part of her body ... whose body hair and hair on the head is fine ..." (Manu, p. 44). There are also rules for selecting the sex of children (males are conceived on even-numbered nights) and in all cases, the social class of husband and wife must match.

These procedures amount to methods of selecting marriage partners according to biological suitability, although the biological traits selected for concern may not seem very appropriate today. Marriage is discouraged if partners are not biologically and astrologically suited. In India, marriages have been and still are arranged by parents on the basis of social, economic, and reproductive suitability. Romantic interest is at best a very secondary consideration. The entire basis of marriage in Hinduism is eugenic, but the factors felt to predispose favorably to suitable offspring are quite different from modern Western ones. Marriage in Hinduism exists to ensure offspring and perpetuate family distinction and caste separation. These laws were intended to regulate reproduction rather than sexuality. Sexual liaison outside of marriage and across caste, though not approved of, was not considered wrong so long as no offspring resulted.

Hinduism does not contemplate elimination of inferior castes, but simply limitation of physical contact between them and higher ones. The higher castes must preserve their purity, but all castes are necessary and have their place in the cosmos (Danielou). This contrasts with the extreme, modern racism, in which one group, which considers itself superior, aims at the elimination of others. There is no idea of altering the genetic or social situation of humanity as a whole. On the contrary, marriage rules attempt to maintain the status quo. Their rationale is not to improve the human species but to prevent its degeneration.

In general, Hinduism has not been opposed to attempts to control reproduction. Female infanticide has been extensively practiced in India. An innovation is the use of ultrasound machines by entrepreneurs; at village marketplaces a pregnant woman can find out whether she is carrying a boy or girl, with abortion elected in the instance of the latter. A similar practice exists in China. Although the practice of female infanticide can be explained in economic terms (a girl's parents must provide a dowry if she is to be married), it represents a practice of controlling reproductive outcome for family or social goals. Infanticide has not been viewed with the same opprobrium as in the West, although it is certainly not fair to imply that the Hindu religion condones such acts.

The Indian concept of karma, which is fundamental to all its philosophical and religious systems, has some similarities to modern genetics. It is a law of moral cause and effect. The literal meaning of karma is action, and the theory holds that one's present state is the result of personal and collective actions in this and previous lives. Actions, like genes, have effects that persist across lifetimes. Much of each individual's present circumstances are the result of previous actions carried across generations. Karma and scientific genetics seek to account for the human experience that the past tends to repeat itself in the present. Both offer an explanation of how an individual comes to have certain traits.

Buddhism and Human Reproduction

Buddhism, which abolishes the caste system, has no concern with the suitability of marriages. Indeed, its monastic nature has made Buddhism generally uninterested in family life and reproduction. Throughout Buddhist history, clergy were forbidden to solemnize marriages; this was seen as inappropriate involvement in worldly affairs. (Wedding ceremonies officiated by Buddhist monks are a recent innovation.) Nor does Buddhism have an elaborate ethical code for regulation of lay behavior. Throughout most of its 2,500-year history, Buddhism has been monastic; lay life was not considered conducive for progress toward enlightenment. However, the sangha, the order of monks and nuns, did try to inculcate simple moral understanding in the laity.

In the Theravada form of Buddhism, which most closely resembles early Buddhism, the laity is taught the Five Precepts, which call on the Buddhist to avoid (1) unnecessary killing, (2) taking what is not given, (3) sexual misconduct, (4) harmful speech, and (5) use of intoxicants. Although

Buddhist teachers will offer their particular interpretations of these principles, detailed rules are not given in any canonical text. Sexual misconduct, for example, is rarely defined and there is no position on contraception. Nor are there specific rules on suitability of marriage or sexual partners. The first precept might be interpreted as discouraging abortion; however, termination of pregnancy is not absolutely forbidden, though it is considered highly undesirable. Buddhism would see the ideal situation as one in which the partners are mindful of the consequences of their actions and avoid a situation in which abortion is a consideration. If carried out, abortion should use a method that minimizes any suffering. (For Buddhist analyses of the abortion issue see Taniguchi, 1987, and Redmond, 1991.) In Japan, where abortion is used as a method of family planning, Buddhist monks are involved in practices that women use to atone for abortion.

In contrast to the religious law of Judaism, Christianity, and Islam, the Buddhist precepts are very general, expressing morality in spirit rather than letter. Nothing in the five lay precepts can be construed to oppose genetic manipulation, provided that it is not harmful. Buddhism does not try to regulate lay behavior by detailed codes of laws, but rather by teaching *sati,* "mindfulness" and *ahimsa,* "harmlessness." The ultimate value in Buddhism is not living in accordance with a code of religious laws but being aware of the effects of one's actions so as to minimize harm. In general, a Buddhist would be concerned that genetic knowledge not be used in a way that causes suffering, but would not be opposed in principle to the acquisition or application of such knowledge. Buddhism places its highest value on knowledge, which it sees as the sole vehicle for enlightenment and release from suffering. Ignorance, not sin or disobedience, is the case of a human's unhappy state. Hence, Buddhism may be seen as favoring the acquisition and use of genetic knowledge, provided that it is applied in ways that help, rather than harm, living beings. Changing the genetic code so as to eliminate a disease in the offspring would be quite acceptable so long as it was carried out skillfully, that is, not harmfully. Partner selection for genetic or ethnic reasons is not supported by Buddhism, which abolished the Hindu caste system. However, such selection would not be ethically improper if it did not cause suffering to those involved.

Cosmology and Eugenics

There are two commonly held contemporary Western positions about eugenics that Hinduism and Buddhism see rather differently from most Western ethicists. One position is that since the world and everything in it, including human beings, are held to be created by God according to a divine plan, then altering the human genome is altering the very basis of God's creation, which is impermissible. Thus the Vatican's statement on reproductive technology holds that "no biologist or doctor can reasonably claim, by virtue of his scientific competence, to be able to decide on people's origin or destiny" (Vatican, Congregation for the Doctrine of the Faith, 1992, p. 84). A similar but secular argument holds that we should not alter nature. Although altering nature may not be inherently wrong, pragmatically such alterations are much more likely to do harm than good. The only safe course is stringently to restrict novel technologies such as genetic engineering.

Neither Hinduism nor Buddhism conceives of a creator God whose divine plan might be altered by genetic manipulation. (Although Brahma is considered the creator in Hinduism, the metaphysics of creation are quite different. Creation occurs from moment to moment and not according to a perfect plan.) Far from seeing the world as divine or perfect, both religions regard the world as inevitably a place of suffering. The fundamental virtue in both Hinduism and Buddhism is practicing *ahimsa,* or harmlessness, which means to avoid making living beings suffer. For example, the environment should not be harmed because living creatures are dependent on it. Since the universe was not created by divine plan, altering it is not considered a repudiation of God. In this context genetic manipulation is perfectly acceptable.

As to the second argument, that humans cannot handle their power over the genome, neither Hinduism nor Buddhism can be held to have a clear position on this. Evil is the result, respectively, of delusion, *moha,* or ignorance, *avidya.* Ethical ignorance is simply an aspect of more general spiritual ignorance, which clouds perception of the true nature of existence. However, Buddhism and Hinduism conceive of ethical ignorance somewhat differently. In Hinduism, it is necessary to be aware of the complex laws, or dharma, regulating human behavior. In Buddhism, ignorance is lack of awareness of the law of cause and effect, for example, of knowing how one's actions will affect oneself and others (Taniguchi, 1994). Mindfulness shows that an action harmful to another will cause suffering just as it would if done to oneself. A unique moral insight of Buddhism is that ethical behavior requires factual knowledge (Redmond, 1989)—for example, what effects behavior will have on others—as well as knowledge of ethical precepts. The way to this knowledge is through self-cultivation such as meditation, study of religious texts, and, especially, the influence of a teacher. Ethical behavior results from personal moral development rather than detailed moral legislation.

Karma and Eugenics

The concept of karma can be interpreted, or sometimes misinterpreted, so that it appears to oppose eugenics. Karma holds that misfortunes in this life are due to harmful actions in a former life (although there are also social sources of unfavorable karma). By this interpretation, if a child is born with a genetic disorder, then the misfortune is due to previous voluntary actions that harmed others and hence is deserved. Furthermore, this karma must be worked off; the suffering must be endured to expiate the previous wrongdoing. If the suffering is prevented, it will simply occur later. Thus, if a fetus with Down syndrome is aborted, the same individual will simply be reincarnated later with a similar affliction.

The idea that suffering should not be relieved, because karmically deserved, is widespread in India and Buddhist countries and is sometimes articulated by Buddhist teachers in the West. It is a misunderstanding of the Buddha's teaching, which was concerned to explain the way of release from suffering. Although Buddhism teaches compassion, some Buddhists, in common with some followers of other religions, find interpretations that rationalize evasion of the ethical obligation to be kind to others. It is not consistent with Buddhist teachings on compassion to refrain from relieving another's suffering on the grounds that it is due to the operation of karma.

Buddhism, although not opposed to eugenics if it is skillfully applied, does not require it. In contrast to Hinduism, it does not establish rules regarding reproductive behavior. Some contemporary Buddhists believe that each individual has his or her tasks in life and that, although these might be different for someone with a birth defect, others should not assume that such a life is therefore less worthy. This has affinities with the idea that we should not interfere with nature because we may not fully understand the effects of what we do.

Hinduism, then, requires a form of eugenics, and Buddhism is essentially neutral on eugenics as such, but would be greatly concerned to ensure that eugenic practice decreased suffering rather than increasing it. Neither religion sees eugenics as in itself improper, but both concern themselves with how it is carried out. However, Hinduism and Buddhism produce no set positions, and individual Hindus and Buddhists may have views different from those summarized here.

GEOFFREY P. REDMOND (1995)

SEE ALSO: *Buddhism, Bioethics in; Hinduism, Bioethics in; Medical Ethics, History of South and East Asia; Population*

Ethics, Religious Traditions: Buddhist Perspectives; Popula-tion Ethics, Religious Traditions: Hindu Perspectives; and other *Eugenics and Religious Law* subentries

BIBLIOGRAPHY

Danielou, Alain. 1993. *Virtue, Success, Pleasure, and Liberation: The Four Aims of Life in the Tradition of Ancient India.* Rochester, VT: Inner Traditions International.

Manu. 1991. *The Laws of Manu,* tr. and with an introduction and notes by Wendy Doniger, with Brian K. Smith. London: Penguin.

Redmond, Geoffrey P. 1989. "Application of the Buddhist Anatma Doctrine to the Problems of Biomedical Ethics." *Ninth Conference of the International Association of Buddhist Studies Abstracts.* Taipei, Taiwan: Institute for Sino-Indian Buddhist Studies.

Redmond, Geoffrey P. 1991. "Buddhism and Abortion." *News-letter on International Buddhist Women's Activities,* no. 26 (January–March), pp. 7–11.

Taniguchi, Shoyo. 1987. "Biomedical Ethics from a Buddhist Perspective." *The Pacific World. New Series* (3): 75–83.

Taniguchi, Shoyo. 1994. "Methodology of Buddhist Biomedical Ethics." *Religious Methods and Resources in Bioethics,* pp. 31–65, ed. Paul F. Camenisch. Dordrecht, Netherlands: Kluwer Academic Publishers.

Vatican. Congregation for the Doctrine of the Faith. 1992. "Instruction of Respect for Human Life in Its Origin and on the Dignity of Procreation." In *The Ethics of Reproductive Technology,* pp. 83–97, ed. Kenneth D. Alpern. New York: Oxford University Press.

EXPERT TESTIMONY

• • •

Courts frequently look to the testimony of expert medical witnesses to assist them in the search for legal truth. In addition to Egyptian and Biblical references to forensic medicine, physicians in Greece and Rome functioned as expert witnesses. A physician testifying at the inquest into Julius Caesar's death stated that he found twenty-three stab wounds on the corpse but only one wound, a wound in the throat, that could have caused death. The Institutes of Justinian (529–533 C.E.) and the codices of Charles V, the Lex Bambergensis (1507), also made provisions for expert medical testimony (Landé; Clements and Ciccone). In the United States, physicians are called on to testify as expert witnesses in a variety of civil and criminal matters. The civil issues range from workers' compensation to child custody,

from physical and emotional damages to malpractice. The issues in criminal cases range from cause of death to compe-tence to stand trial, from deoxyribonucleic acid (DNA) typing to the insanity defense. This entry traces how a physician becomes involved as a medical expert witness, what the requirements of the role are, and the ethical issues that may arise.

Courts of law distinguish between fact witnesses and expert witnesses. Fact witnesses may be required to testify if they have some direct knowledge about the issue before the court, but may not express opinions. Expert witnesses have knowledge that goes beyond that of the ordinary citizen and agree to undertake the role of expert witness and are permitted to express opinions.

The difference between a "fact" and an "opinion" is the degree of concreteness of the description, or the difference in the "nearness or remoteness of inference" (McCormick, p. 26). The courts and the public receive expert testimony with both admiration and suspicion. There is appreciation for the clarity provided, but fear that experts may control the legal outcome. This fear may be accentuated in a democratic society that mistrusts those with special knowledge. In 1986, the American Medical Association (AMA) took the position that "as a citizen and as a professional with special training and experience, the physician has an ethical obligation to assist in the administration of justice" (Council on Ethical and Judicial Affairs of the AMA, p. 138). The participation of the medical expert may be justified on the basis that a meaningful concept of justice requires empirical data on the function of the human organism in health and disease—data that the medical expert can provide (Ciccone and Clements).

The Expert-Witness Role

Expert-witness testimony in an adversarial legal system may lead to a battle of the experts, a battle that may be avoided if the court appoints an expert approved by both sides of a legal action. There are different models for the expert-witness role. In the first model, the court-appointed or "impartial expert" witness model, the expert witness is still subjected to cross-examination, yet has the implied endorsement of the court—the court would not hire an unqualified expert. However, the view that such an expert witness is neutral is a fallacy (American Academy of Orthopedic Surgeons) be-cause the expert is necessarily an advocate for his or her opinion. In the second, the objective "expert-model," the expert is hired by or appointed to one party, but the expert's role is limited to a comprehensive examination of the evidence and formulation of an opinion, if possible. In the third, the "consultant" model, the expert functions as a consultant to the attorney. The expert provides an accurate statement of the examination conducted, the findings of the examination, and the opinion and reasoning used to arrive at the opinion, and provides assistance with trial strategy and cross-examination (Appelbaum). The ethical hazard of this model is that the expert may identify with the attorney's position and become an advocate.

In each model, the medical expert is expected to provide a clinical evaluation and a review of the applicable data in light of the legal question posed and in the spirit of honesty and striving for objectivity—the expert's ethical and professional obligation. This includes a thorough, fair, and impartial review and should not exclude any relevant information in order to create a view favoring either the plaintiff or the defendant (American Academy of Psychiatry and the Law). The treating physician, whom the court may compel to testify as a fact witness regarding contact with a patient, is frequently sought to provide expert-witness testimony. The legal system assumes that the treating doctor is more credible than a nontreating doctor. The treating physician has a specific therapeutic focus—the patient's health—that may not allow service as an expert witness. The treating physician may encounter a conflict of interest (e.g., maintaining the patient's confidentiality versus providing the court with information).

When taking on the functions and obligations of the expert-medical-witness role, the treating physician may, out of loyalty to the patient's best interests, act as an advocate for the patient. This distorts the obligation of the expert witness. On the other hand, if the treating doctor's expert testimony does not have the effect of adequately supporting the patient's position, the doctor-patient relationship may deteriorate as a result. Hence, the role of physician as advocate for the patient may be inconsistent with the role of physician as expert witness and pose the ethical issue of conflict of role obligation. This conflict should be avoided. When this is not possible, self-awareness of the possible conflict and awareness by the court of the conflict may minimize its effects.

The Ethics of Being a Medical Expert Witness

Medical professionals who undertake the role of expert witness are generally expected to have an unrestricted license to practice medicine, to be knowledgeable and experienced in the area in which they are functioning as a medical expert, and to have knowledge of the legal system. At the initial contact by the court or an attorney, the expert clarifies the question being asked and explores the relevant information about the case. The discussion of the question also permits the expert to be explicit about limitations of the evaluation he or she can offer. The expert witness must know the law

that is relevant to the forensic question in the jurisdiction in which the expert may testify. The court or the attorney can provide the applicable statutes. Professional values require such obligations. In addition, legal consequences involving criminal and civil verdicts with ensuing penalties require this standard of obligation.

Medical experts can expect cooperation from the court or attorney in obtaining all the relevant legal, social, and medical documents. Medical experts should obtain consultations from others when there are important areas outside of the expert's knowledge. The medical expert must also be aware that the attorney may have a hidden agenda—understanding the hidden agenda may influence the expert's decision to accept or refuse the case. For example, when the evidence is not strong, is the prosecuting attorney's raising the question of competence to stand trial (CST) a way to keep the individual from being released? Is the defense attorney's request for an evaluation of CST a way to prolong the legal process so that prosecution witnesses may become difficult to locate, thereby weakening the district attorney's case? These are ethical questions the legal system must address, but medical experts who work with the legal system have a clinical obligation to avoid abuse of their role.

The individual who agrees to function as an expert witness is entitled to an expert witness fee, the terms of which should be clear and explicit at the time that the work is started. It is unethical for expert witnesses to make their fees contingent on the outcome of trials. In fact, there are advantages to the expert working with a retainer fee, against which the work of the forensic expert may be charged: (1) it diminishes whatever influence the examiner's concern for payment has on the quality of the work, and (2) if asked on cross-examination if the experts are being paid for their opinions, the experts are able to respond that in fact they were paid on a retainer basis for their time. Such arrangements avoid the ethical problem of experts being seen as "hired guns."

The informed consent of the individual to undergo a forensic medical evaluation should be obtained whenever possible. This includes a description of the purpose of the evaluation, the limits to confidentiality that may exist, and to whom a report will be made. The doctor-patient relationship includes, as one of its ethical requirements, the qualified obligation that the physician maintain confidentiality. The examinations conducted by the medical expert witness are usually outside the scope of the doctor-patient relationship; however, the bioethical obligations remain, and the physician must be aware of the bioethical obligation not to harm the individual unnecessarily by gratuitous disclosure of information. The disclosure of information must conform with the requirements of the law and the explanation made to the individual examined. In a legal context, the medical expert is bound not by rules of medical confidentiality, but by the rules of confidentiality that the legal circumstances require. It is expected that the medical expert witness will be aware of and abide by the specific rules of confidentiality applicable to work with the legal system. Informing the examinee may not be sufficient protection because the physician can create a relationship in which the examinee forgets the warning (Diamond). There are circumstances in medical-legal evaluations where consent is not required. The individual is then informed that the evaluation is legally required. However, if the individual chooses not to participate, the refusal will be included in any report or testimony.

Admission of Expert Testimony

The role of the expert witness is based on education, training, and experience that gives the expert knowledge in a particular discipline. The United States Supreme Court in *Daubert* v. *Merrell Dow Pharmaceuticals* (1993) described the limits of expert scientific testimony and endorsed the *Federal Rules of Evidence* (United States) that had broadened the admissibility of scientific testimony to include theories that were not widely held. The *Daubert* decision rejected the restrictive standard that permitted the judge to exclude expert testimony that the judge found was not "sufficiently established to have gained general acceptance in the particular field to which it belongs" (*Frye* v. *United States*, 1923). However, the U.S. Supreme Court also put limits on "the admissibility of purportedly scientific evidence" by requiring the trial judge to determine whether the reasoning or methodology underlying the testimony is scientifically valid and whether that reasoning or methodology properly can be applied to the facts in issue (*Daubert* v. *Merrell Dow Pharmaceuticals*, p. 2796). This gatekeeping function of the judge on expert scientific testimony may lead to judges who appoint their own experts to examine the experts put forward by opposing parties in the litigation.

Ethics and Medical Expert Testimony

The medical expert may be required to testify in perhaps one of ten cases that the expert is called upon to evaluate. It is this public role that causes the most discomfort and is the most sensationalized of all the expert's functions. The medical expert witness usually engages in this work as a part of a larger clinical practice. While some experts have given up clinical work, this is rare. Medical experts who have not actively engaged in their discipline or who have given it up may find their credibility questioned in court. Medical experts have the ethical obligation to inform the court or attorney hiring them of the status of their clinical practice.

Prior to entering the courtroom, experts assist the attorney as well as they can "but only within the requirement of medical ethics" (Stone, p. 27). Each of the three models carries the ethical obligation that the expert be honest and, even when assisting an attorney, not become an advocate. The medical expert who is called to testify should require full and complete preparation from the attorney. Preparation for testimony, which almost always includes at least one pretrial conference between attorney and expert, is essential to adequate work in the courtroom.

In court, medical expert witnesses are not advocates for either side in the litigation, but may advocate their opinion. The most effective role of the expert witness is that of teacher—that is, one who elucidates the nature of the evaluations and the reasoning used to arrive at his or her opinions. The expert should present credentials without exaggeration. The expert should be prepared to present specific perspectives or bias and identify value components that are always present in interpretations of the data. If the issue before the court presents an ethical dilemma for the expert, whether as a result of personal belief or from concerns about societal harm that his or her opinion may cause, the expert has the obligation to avoid involvement in such cases. The requirement of truthfulness on the part of the medical expert witness requires that relevant information not be kept secret (Rappeport). In addition, there are limitations that occur in medical examinations, and these limitations of reviewed materials (e.g., completeness of the examination or knowledge of that area of medicine) may require the expert to qualify an opinion or, at times, to decline to provide an opinion to a particular question.

The attorney who retained the medical expert will call and question the expert with direct examination. This usually begins with eliciting the expert's credentials; the questions present the expert's education, training, experience, and other information that chronicle the achievements of the expert to the court. Using the *Daubert* directives, the judge may rule to exclude the expert. Medical-expert witnesses are expected to present their testimony—avoiding jargon—with sufficient clarity so that those lacking expertise can understand the findings and follow the reasoning. The attorney who has retained the expert can be expected to emphasize his or her ability and the brilliance of the conclusions. The cross-examining attorney, both in speech and gesture, will often attempt to convey to the court that the expert witness lacks credibility and that his or her conclusions are worthless.

The expert may be presented a hypothetical question, which is a conflation of assumptions and proven facts into an organized account of a situation. The hypothetical question calls for expert witnesses to assume the information in the question to be fact. Then experts are asked if they have an opinion derived from those facts and, if they do, to state that opinion. The hypothetical question is used because there is a dispute about the facts, and the hypothetical question allows the court to hear the expert's opinion without deciding if the facts in evidence are true.

The expert witness has rights in the courtroom and may ask the judge to clarify when material that is asked for is privileged. The expert witness may ask for clarification of a question or refuse to answer questions the expert does not understand. Experts may and should say that they do not have a response to the question, if in fact they do not have one. Experts, when asked a yes or no question, can ask the judge whether the answer can be qualified. If on cross-examination this is not permitted, on subsequent redirect examination the attorney who retained the expert may ask for further clarification. The expert has a right to complete an answer and should protest if interrupted. Expert witnesses, as contrasted with fact witnesses, may refresh their recollections using written notes and records.

The courtroom, the most visible portion of the adversarial system with its "battle of the experts," is viewed by some critics as a three-ring circus. Even when expert witnesses agree substantially, small differences may be exaggerated by an attorney and held up as proof that the entire discipline has nothing to offer the courts. If expert witnesses are expected to provide absolute certainty, the witnesses will inevitably be clowns in the courtroom. However, the opinion of the expert witness, as with a medical diagnosis, is a probability statement and as such, is the best conclusion given the analysis of the data. This conclusion may certainly be open to question. Although the credibility of the expert witness is important, the courtroom belongs to the attorneys. The weight given to the testimony of the expert is markedly influenced by the courtroom skill of the attorneys involved. Do the faults of the legal system outweigh its benefits and is there an alternative, superior system for arriving at legal verdicts? This is a question better considered in an analysis of the adversarial system.

At a trial, the ultimate issue is the question about which the jury or judge must arrive at a verdict (e.g., did the defendant's negligence cause the injury to the plaintiff?). It has been suggested that the medical expert respond only to questions about the medical condition and avoid responding to the ultimate issue, which some have called either a leap in logic (American Psychiatric Association [APA] Statement on the Insanity Defense) or the application of medical reality to a legal procedure. It is contended that the ultimate issue is an issue of social and moral policy and, therefore, is beyond the province of scientific inquiry. While there are circumstances when the information does not permit the medical expert to arrive at an opinion, the fact that the question has been framed in a legal context may make it appropriate for the expert to express an opinion. This opinion need not usurp the role of the trier of fact.

Conclusion

Much of society's ambivalence toward expert witnesses is derived from society's unrealistic hopes and fears of expert witnesses. The hope that the expert will have secret skills, which provide special access to absolute truth, imbues the expert role with unrealistic authority and certainty. This expectation of expert witnesses is not consistent with the reality of scientific expertise that allows for probable conclusions. The fear that the expert will take over the legal process and subvert justice is also exaggerated. The legal system has rules of procedure that limit the influence of the expert witness. Functioning within the boundaries of science and governed by ethical guidelines, experts are not oracles whose conclusions are not open to question, but witnesses who can provide the legal system with useful information.

J. RICHARD CICCONE (1995)
BIBLIOGRAPHY REVISED

SEE ALSO: *Confidentiality; Conflict of Interest; DNA Identification; Law and Bioethics, Law and Morality; Malpractice, Medical*

BIBLIOGRAPHY

Agich, George J., and Spielman, Bethan J. 1997. "Ethics Expert Testimony: Against the Skeptics." *Journal of Medicine and Philosophy* 22(4): 381–403.

American Academy of Orthopedic Surgeons. 1992. "Orthopaedic Medical Testimony." In *Guide to the Ethical Practice of Orthopaedic Surgery*. Rosement, IL.: American Academy of Orthopaedic Surgeons.

American Academy of Psychiatry and the Law. 1987. "Ethical Guidelines for the Practice of Forensic Psychiatry." *Newsletter* 12(1):16–17.

American Psychiatric Association. 1983. "American Psychiatric Association Statement on the Insanity Defense." *American Journal of Psychiatry* 140(6): 681–688.

Appelbaum, Paul S. 1987. "In the Wake of Ake: The Ethics of Expert Testimony in an Advocate's Word." *Bulletin of the American Academy of Psychiatry and the Law* 15(1): 15–25.

Baylis, Françoise. 2000. "Expert Testimony by Persons Trained in Ethical Reasoning: the Case of Andrew Sawatzky." *Journal of Law Medicine and Ethics* 28(3): 224–231.

Brodsky, Stanley L. 1999. *The Expert Expert Witness: More Maxims and Guidelines for Testifying in Court*. Washington, D.C.: American Psychological Association (APA).

Ciccone, J. Richard, and Clements, Colleen D. 1987. "The Insanity Defense: Asking and Answering the Ultimate Question." *Bulletin of the American Academy of Psychiatry and the Law* 15(4): 329–338.

Cleary, Edward W., ed. 1986. *McCormick on Evidence.* St. Paul, MN: West Publishing.

Clements, Colleen D., and Ciccone, J. Richard. 1984. "Ethics and Expert Witnesses: The Troubled Role of Psychiatrists in Court." *Bulletin of the American Academy of Psychiatry and the Law* 12(2): 127–136.

Council on Ethical and Judicial Affairs of the American Medical Association. 1994. *Code of Medical Ethics: Current Opinions with Annotations.* Chicago: Author.

Daubert v. Merrell Dow Pharmaceuticals Inc. 113 S.Ct. 2786. U.S.L.W. #4805 (1993).

Diamond, Bernard L. 1959. "The Fallacy of the Impartial Expert." *Archives of Criminal Psychodynamics* 3: 221–236.

Dresser, Rebecca. 1999. "Science in the Courtroom. A New Approach." *Hastings Center Report* 29(3): 26–27.

Federal Rules of Evidence. 1994. 702, 28 U.S.C.A. St. Paul, MN: West Publishing.

Fletcher, John C. 1997. "Bioethics in a Legal Forum: Confessions of an "Expert" Witness." *Journal of Medicine and Philosophy* 22(4): 297–324.

Frye v. United States. 293 Fed. 1013 (D.C. Cir. 1923).

Gee, D. J., and Mason, J. K. 1995. *The Courts and the Doctor* (Oxford Medical Publications). New York: Oxford University Publishers.

Halleck, Seymour L.; Appelbaum, Paul S.; Rappeport, Jonas; and Dix, G. 1984. "Psychiatry in the Sentencing Process. A Report of the Task Force on the Role of Psychiatry in the Sentencing Process." In *Issues in Forensic Psychiatry: Insanity Defense, Hospitalization of Adults, Model Civil Commitment Law, Sentencing Process, Child Custody Consultation.* Washington, D.C.: American Psychiatric Press.

Kipnis, Ken. 1997. "Confessions of an Expert Ethics Witness." *Journal of Medicine and Philosophy* 22(4): 325–343.

Landé, Kurt E. 1936. "Forensic Medicine in Europe—Legal Medicine in America." *New England Journal of Medicine* 215(18): 826–834.

Lubet, Steven. 1999. *Expert Testimony: A Guide for Expert Witnesses and the Lawyers Who Examine Them.* Notre Dame, IN: National Institute for Trial Advocacy.

Malone, David M., and Zwier, Paul J. 2000. *Effective Expert Testimony* (Practical Guide series). Notre Dame, IN: National Institute for Trial Advocacy.

McCormick, Charles T. 1986. *Handbook of the Law of Evidence.* St. Paul, MN: West Publishing.

Menninger, Karl. 1969. *The Crime of Punishment.* New York: The Viking Press.

Morreim, E. Haavi 1997. "Bioethics, Expertise, and the Courts: An Overview and an Argument for Inevitability." *Journal of Medicine and Philosophy* 22(4): 291–295.

Rappeport, Jonas. 1981. "Ethics and Forensic Psychiatry." In *Psychiatric Ethics* pp. 285–276; eds. Sidney Block and Paul Chodoff. Oxford: Oxford University Press.

Sharpe, Virginia A., and Pellegrino, Edmund D. 1997. "Medical Ethics in the Courtroom: A Reappraisal." *Journal of Medicine and Philosophy* 22(4)(Aug): 373–379.

Stone, Alan A. 1981. "The Ethical Boundaries of Forensic Psychiatry: A View from the Ivory Tower." *Bulletin of the American Academy of Psychiatry and the Law* 12(3): 209–227.

West Information Publishing Group Staff. 2002. *Modern Scientific Evidence: The Law and Science of Expert Testimony,* 2nd edition. St. Paul, MN: West Group Publishing.

United States. 1975. Federal Rules of Evidence, Annotated. New York: M. Berder.

F

FAMILY AND FAMILY MEDICINE

• • •

Families have played a most important role in the history of medicine, tending the sick when doctors were unavailable or unavailing. Medicine and the family, the two ancient and in some respects rival systems of care for the very vulnerable, are each in part shaped by the other and rely upon the other for certain kinds of help. When illness or injury exhausts a family's capacity for care, the family looks to professional medicine for the necessary facilities and expertise; in turn, technological advances in medicine have driven the healthcare system to depend on families for what can be enormous sacrifices of time, money, caring labor, and even spare body parts on behalf of its patients. Recent developments in medicine have not only expanded the options for forming families—for example, through in vitro fertilization and contract pregnancy—but they have also had an impact on familial demographics: artificial means of birth control have helped reduce family size, while improvements in healthcare have extended longevity, though they have not eradicated the ills of old age.

Yet the most profound impact of contemporary medicine on the family may not be so much a function of new technologies as of new social practices. A characteristic of the social arrangement of healthcare in the twentieth century was the professionalization of care and the concomitant migration of care provision from home to hospital. If trends in the 1990s hold true, however, the twenty-first century may see a reversal of that process, with greater amounts of care—requiring greater skill, and more intensive investment of time, energy, and emotion—moving back into family contexts.

Bioethics has a rather checkered record of engagement with moral issues that arise where families and medicine meet. While new reproductive technologies have been the focus of bioethical attention from the start, the proper role of family interests in healthcare decision making has been addressed only by relatively few workers in the area, and bioethics has, as of yet, taken little notice of the moral questions involved in the "hospital to home" shift. The lack of attention to issues apart from those suggested by reproductive technologies is curious, both because of the practical exigencies involved (family members, for example, are and will continue to be much more influential than formal advance directives in making healthcare choices for the incompetent), and because the conceptual and moral questions involved in understanding the special character of these intimate associations are very challenging. What constitutes a family? How do various forms of family relationship translate into moral duties and prerogatives? What does "justice" mean in such contexts, and how should justice within families relate to broader concerns about justice in the allocation of healthcare resources in society?

With the turn of the twenty-first century, however, bioethicists have shown a greater willingness to take up these questions, and to consider in particular that the role of family members in the care of ill relatives may be morally more complex than simply that of serving as conduits of information about the treatment preferences of patients too ill to express them on their own. The pioneering work of scholars such as John Hardwig has helped to instigate broader bioethical reflection on how healthcare choices can affect the well being of other family members, and has pressed in particular the question whether the impact of patient care on families gives them a legitimate stake in the treatment decision-making process. While the notion that the interests of families should be considered along with patient interests in choosing among treatment options remains highly controversial among bioethicists, there is some evidence that healthcare providers are more receptive to this idea than are theorists. A 2003 study by Hardart and Truog reports that many physicians regard the interests of family members as pertinent to healthcare decision making, even in the absence of specific patient acknowledgement of those interests. A sizable minority went further, regarding family interests as of equal significance to those of patients. If these results are representative, then bioethicists will have a strong incentive to consider the role of families more carefully then they have yet done, and to address in particular the burdens on families that do not emerge primarily from clinical decision making, but rather from policies on the part of hospitals and insurers that send patients home "quicker and sicker."

There is other evidence that healthcare providers have been more sympathetic than bioethicists to the role that families play in the lives of so many patients. *Family medicine* or *family practice* is a distinct primary care specialty within medicine, but there is no comparably entrenched specialty within bioethics and little bioethical attention has been paid to family medicine's particular focus and problems. In addition to its treatment of the family from perspectives pertinent to bioethics, then, this entry also contains a brief discussion of the ethical dimensions of family medicine.

Families: Myth and History

The development of a mature "bioethics of the family" is significantly complicated by controversies concerning the nature and importance of this much-vaunted, much-maligned social institution. The dramatic shifts in the demographics of American families have rendered them suspect, as have public debates that underscore the family's role in sustaining practices hostile to women's interests and that identify families or *family values* as a particular focus of conservative political perspectives. Families have come to seem so fragile, their configurations so arbitrary compared with what they once were, and their value so contested, that offering them a special role in bioethical deliberation may seem a dubious enterprise.

Yet neither hostility nor sentimentality does justice to the moral character of these complex and puzzling entities. Nor is the notion that families are particularly unstable in today's world altogether accurate. American families have always been somewhat fragile and subject to rapid reconfigurations. African- and European-American families in the Chesapeake colonies of Virginia and Maryland, to take only one instance, were so vulnerable to malaria and other fatal illnesses that it was not at all unusual for an adult, whether slave or free, to bury three or even four spouses, or for half-orphaned children to be reared by relatives other than the surviving parent. In the matrilineal Iroquois societies of that same period, divorce was quite common. It is true that middle-class families gained a certain solidity when they underwent a shift around 1800 to a sentimental, child-centered model of domestic life, but this was achieved through an arguably unjust gendered division of labor, in which the middle-class father was increasingly absent from home and the mother's work was narrowed principally to unpaid domestic tasks. For many poor young nineteenth-century mothers—whether black, Latina, Irish, or east European—this arrangement was not an option, and the long hours spent working outside the home left the care of their children a somewhat haphazard business. Death in childbed and other premature deaths once threatened the family's integrity as much as the divorce rate, which has risen by a steady 3 percent in every decade since the Civil War, does now. In short, there is good reason to think that stress, turmoil, and identity crises have long been a feature of American families.

The "Culture of Divorce"

The long history of family fragility notwithstanding, however, sophisticated scholarship now identifies divorce as a source of instability particularly threatening to children's well being. Sociological and ethnographic studies appearing since the mid-1990s suggest that the fate of the "family of origin" is of systematic and enduring importance to many central features of children's lives, and that the damage ensuing from divorce has a strong tendency to reach well into adulthood, at least in contemporary American culture. Judith S. Wallerstein, Julia M. Lewis, and Sandra Blakeslee argue in *The Unexpected Legacy of Divorce* (2000) that divorce impairs children's ability to consolidate their identities as mature adults and to form their own enduring intimate relations, in a way that is apparently different and seemingly graver than other forms of familial disruption and reconfiguration. Some of this damage would seem to be a function of features that often attend divorce: the subsequent inability of parents to provide reliable, timely, and well-directed care, the tendency of noncustodial parents—particularly fathers—to attenuate or even abandon their connections to their children, economic losses leading to a reduced ability of custodial parents to spend time with children, and so forth. Some damage, however, apparently is attributable to divorce itself. Even when parents divorce relatively amicably, maintain continual and substantial engagement in their children's lives, do not require their children to "take care of them" emotionally in inappropriate ways, and are able to support their children's fiscal and emotional needs without interruption, children undergo losses in their expectations and abilities concerning the maintenance of their own long-term intimate relationships, and seem to suffer a measurable delay in their movement into adulthood. These decrements seem to be of a different and more severe character than the harms that affect children who have grown up in families where the parents were continually unhappy but did not divorce.

While many questions remain to be answered—for example, why these harms seem to be more pernicious in the United States than in, say, Scandinavia; and whether divorces in which care is taken to protect the children are worse on the whole than other ways in which families have come unglued throughout history—recent social scientific studies make it difficult to regard divorce as a feature of contemporary life that children can simply get over.

These results may have implications for bioethics as well as for healthcare practice and policy. Is the process of transferring ever more intensive forms of care from hospital to home made more morally suspect by the possibility that children with divorce in their pasts will be less willing to provide such attention with the consistency and quality required for good health outcomes? Is the role of family members as presumptive proxy decision makers cast under a cloud? Is the apparent willingness of many physicians and at least some bioethicists to recognize family interests as relevant to medical choices rendered more problematic by these data? And, given the emotionally complex, internally contested, and structurally protean character of people's affiliative and kinship patterns, what counts as a family anymore, anyway?

Defining *Family*

A measure both of the importance of families to our lives and of our ambivalence about them is that any discussion of the topic quickly elicits a demand for an explicit statement of what is meant by *family*. The most useful such account is perhaps a normative one, which identifies features of special moral significance in the clear paradigm cases. Those features can then be used to determine what counts as a family in the less clear cases. Ludwig Wittgenstein's notion of family resemblances may be pressed into service here: any social configuration that incorporates at least most of the morally significant features of, say, marital and parent-child relationships can be thought of as a family for purposes pertinent to healthcare. These features include longstanding, committed relationships; blood ties; emotional intimacy; shared histories; and shared projects that produce solidarity among family members. Other crucial features identify functions: families forge the selves of their youngest members and help maintain the selves of adults. Further, familial relationships go beyond the contractual and the voluntary; in them people incur responsibilities not of their own choosing.

Relationships within families will take on greater or lesser bioethical significance, depending on the familial question under consideration. If treatment decisions for a badly damaged neonate are at issue, *family* means the mother and father; if the issue at hand is pedigree testing for a genetic disorder, *family* means blood kinship; if the issue is determining the appropriate caregiver for a person with progressive dementia, *family* may mean spouse or child.

Family and the Law

Discussions in family law echo the question of how we are to define families. While there was for many years no basis in common law for family members to make treatment decisions for incompetent adults, for example, a number of court decisions in the 1980s as well as various legislative actions gave families explicit decisional authority in twenty states. By the turn of the century, thirty-five states plus the District of Columbia recognized the authority of family members to make many significant healthcare decisions, should their relatives become incompetent, without having an explicit advance directive. This legal trend makes it all the more necessary to know just who is entitled to count as family. A strictly biological definition does not capture what seems socially significant about single parenting, adoptive parenting, step-parenting, or contract pregnancy. The legal notion of marriage skips over *kith*—long-standing, committed relationships resembling kinship that might give, say, a neighbor or housemate moral authority to speak on behalf of a patient who is too ill to make treatment decisions. The law also fails to recognize gay and lesbian relationships, though these are often more significant than blood ties to the people within them. On the other hand, functionalist definitions of families require courts to determine whether a particular relationship closely enough approximates an accepted norm of *family* to count as one. This involves inquiry into such areas as sexual activity, management of finances, and degree of exclusivity and commitment—a profound intrusion into personal privacy.

When one compares the body of family law against the body of law dealing with, for example, commercial transactions, family law seems distinctly underdeveloped and lacking in detail. The reason for this, Lee Teitelbaum argues in

"Intergenerational Responsibility and Family Obligation: On Sharing," is that families, incorporating "diffuse, particularistic, and collective values and relations," tend to reflect a wide-ranging set of circumstances and goals, while law is better suited to consider individuals as abstracted from these particulars in public settings that can be assimilated into a formal, rational scheme (Teitelbaum, p. 789). There is a further problem. In "Bioethics and the Family," Carl Schneider points out that in the last few decades family law has increasingly eschewed moral discourse. The temptation is understandable: the problems within families are complex and often "reduce to unresolvable disputes over unverifiable beliefs" (Schneider, p. 822). But by avoiding the language of morality, family law has stripped itself of conceptual notions that might help resolve such bioethical perplexities as contract pregnancy and the family's role in decision making for incapacitated patients.

Challenges to an Ethics of Strangers

Bioethics, however, need not lie down with the law. Because it can achieve a high degree of particularity, it is better suited than the law to use a working definition of families that identifies morally relevant features and notes family resemblances (so to speak) among various small-scale human groups that include some such features. Roughly speaking, two approaches have been used to incorporate what is morally valuable about families into bioethics.

The first approach assumes the moral framework characteristic of the Enlightenment, with its stress on the impartial and the universalizable. Within this tradition, Nancy Rhoden has criticized the suspicion of the motives and interests of family members that has opened family decisions concerning nontreatment of incapacitated relatives to court review. Arguing in "Litigating Life and Death" (1988) that because family members "are in the best position to reproduce the preferences of an incompetent patient," Rhoden concludes that the burden of proof should be on the physician rather than the family to convince a court of law that an unwise decision has been made. Using the same moral framework but setting it in service of a more radical departure from current practice, Hardwig (1990) has attacked the exclusionary bias of the doctor-patient relationship, insisting that the interests of all those with a stake in a medical decision, not just the patient's, be honored impartially.

At the same time, the so-called personal turn in ethics explored by Bernard Williams, Lawrence Blum, Jeffrey Blustein, Margaret Urban Walker, and others has challenged the orthodox assumption that ethics has primarily to do with right conduct among strangers—an ethics that favors no one and whose dictates are universalizable. The personal turn might be said to have begun with Williams's germinal observation in "Persons, Character, and Morality" (1981) that impartialist dictates, if followed scrupulously, leave insufficient room for moral agents to pursue their own individual interests, desires, and projects—all the substance, in fact, that gives life its meaning, yet such meaning is what motivates one to go on. The task of Williams and others has been to construct moral accounts that honor the particular and the personal, but do so in a nonarbitrary way. Feminist ethical theory has devoted much attention to this task (see Hanen and Nielsen; Kittay and Meyers; Mahowald; Nussbaum; Walker).

In bioethics, one can see the direct impact of the personal turn in the writings of Ferdinand Schoeman. He has argued that a Kantian ethics for strangers, which insists that medical decisions for an incompetent person can be made only in accordance with what is in that person's best interests, provides an inadequate basis for understanding the parent-child relationship. That relationship, because it is intimate, permits parents to compromise the child's interests so as to promote the family's goals and purposes. Parents could, for example, permit a child to donate bone marrow to save a sibling's life, even though donating the marrow is not in the child's medical interests. In Schoeman's view, then, the family is seen as an entity with an integrity of its own that is greater than the sum total of the interests of its members (Schoeman, 1980, 1985).

Rhoden's attempt to vindicate the decisional authority of families and Hardwig's challenge to the patient-centered focus of conventional bioethics use the relatively straightforward strategy of applying impartialist standards to a context—the doctor-patient relationship—where they have not been applied before. Both writers are concerned with decision making, and more particularly with the locus of the decision. By contrast, the personal turn in bioethics, which is concerned with a more fine-grained understanding of the structures of interpersonal relationships and their importance for human action, is less well developed. But attention to the personal suggests certain moral features of family life that might be used to construct an ethics of the family.

Some Elements of an Ethics of the Family

Social critics from Plato through Shulamith Firestone have argued that the distinctive features of the family constitute moral liabilities, and that families ought to be altered or abolished. In *A Theory of Justice* (1971), John Rawls notes quite explicitly that the family is always a problem for egalitarian social theory. A more sympathetic approach would portray those features as morally valuable, but whatever one's basic stance toward families, they do possess features that require moral attention and analysis.

One rather marked characteristic of families is their tendency to favor their own over outsiders. A central question is whether this sort of bias can be adequately understood inside a universalizable, impersonal framework. For example, can the favoritism parents show their children be justified insofar, and only insofar, as it increases the overall utility? James Rachels has argued for a position he calls "partial bias," which allows the expression of particular regard for children (and presumably for one's intimates in general) in those cases where their needs are in conflict with similarly serious needs of others, but not otherwise. This approach, he suggests, allows the special goods of intimacy to flourish within the context of appropriate regard for the needs of all, impartially considered. It is, however, questionable whether a truly disinterested regard for the needs of others, in a world where resources are massively maldistributed, would leave any appreciable room for special regard for the needs of one's own, particularly for people living in affluence. But even if some measure of special attention to loved ones could be made consistent with general impartialist norms, unless family members favor their own to at least a slightly greater degree than impartialist considerations mandate, it would seem they express only an ersatz partiality, not true loyalty, love, or commitment. To feel the force of this point, consider the intuitive response to a father who, when his only daughter thanks him affectionately for taking her to a baseball game, tells her, "Oh, I would have had to do the same for any child of mine."

Rather than attempt, as Rachels does, to assimilate personal loyalty into an impartialist framework, a promising strategy might be to put less emphasis on individual integrity and the separateness of individuals, and attend a little more to the connections among individuals. A careful attention to these interconnections offers a basis for just dealings with others that takes account of the difference between strangers and intimates.

A second notable feature of families is that not all of its relationships fit comfortably under what has come to be modern ethics' most favored image of relationship: the contract. Children notoriously "didn't ask to be born," and no one chooses one's blood relations. This fact has important implications for any theory that bases duties solely on consent; indeed, families are perhaps the most plausible counterexample to such theories. It is sometimes claimed that parental duties toward children arise from the parents' having tacitly consented to the child's existence, first, by agreeing to have sexual intercourse and second, by choosing not to abort the fetus. But this analysis entails that where

intercourse was forced or good-faith efforts at contraception failed, and where abortion is for ethical, logistical, or economic reasons not an option, the parents are off the moral hook. Many will be reluctant to pay this dearly to retain the contract as the model of obligation. Ordinarily, responsibilities can arise from causal as well as contractual relationships. A proximate causal role in putting another in danger, for example, obligates one to stand ready to provide aid. This thought leads Hilde Lindemann Nelson and James Lindemann Nelson to suggest, in their 1995 work *The Patient in the Family,* that parental responsibility may stem from the fact that parents caused the child's existence and not from their having contracted for the child. In fact it can be maintained that intimate living as such creates expectations and other vulnerabilities, which, as Robert E. Goodin has argued, carry with them certain prima facie noncontractual duties (Goodin). Such an analysis would embrace family members other than parents in a web of moral but nonconsensual relationship.

A third feature of the ethics that typifies families is a less individualistic image of persons than is customary in impersonal ethics. Actions are often assessed in terms of their impact on the family overall, and there is a certain amount of collective responsibility for family members' well-being. A family of immigrants might, for example, devote its resources to settling other relatives in the new country, an enterprise that requires individual family members to subsume their own projects and goals to the familial one. While the communitarian feature of family ethics has often lent itself to abuse as repeated sacrifices are demanded of certain family members (particularly women) in service of an agenda set by its dominant members, it is also true that a family cannot function if its members are altogether unwilling to pull in common. An ethics of the family, in contrast to standard ethical theories, will concern itself with interests that are essentially held in common, as well as with individual interests.

A fourth distinguishing feature of what might emerge as an ethics of the family is that it is particularistic. Leo Tolstoy notwithstanding, happy families are not all alike. There are myriad differences among and within them—as there are, for that matter, among unhappy ones. Because familial relationships are not only intimate but also of long standing, family members can come to know each other in rich, particular detail and from a highly specific standpoint. This means that the principles governing their behavior toward one another can be fine-tuned to a pitch of precision that is impossible in other contexts such as law, where individual differences are perforce flattened out. What Iris Murdoch has called loving attention and Martha Nussbaum calls fine awareness would likely play an important role in any ethics of intimacy, whether among friends or within families. Attention to the particulars is what allows people involved in intimate relationships to focus on who they are together. This self-awareness, guided by general moral ideas such as justice, permits intimates to arrive at ethical decisions that are highly sensitive to circumstances and persons; the ethical work can be done "close up." Further, as these ethical deliberations become a part of the history of the relationship, their results can be used to guide future decisions that will be just as sensitive to the particulars.

Implications for Medicine

The primary health specialty of family medicine, or family practice, distinguishes itself by focusing on the healthcare needs of people from cradle to grave, and by explicitly acknowledging the ways in which illness or traumas that individuals confront resonate through the families of which they are a part. More than any other medical specialty, family practitioners have espoused the view that "the patient is the family," and they are typically trained to understand various family systems theories to gain a systematic perspective on how families can both suffer from, and contribute to, the ailments with which patients present. These skills and this orientation naturally lend themselves to dealing with ethical issues that involve patients and their families. While family practice physicians do not as a group dissent from the orthodox medical ethics doctrine that the interests of the patient always trump any inconsistent interests that individual relatives or the family as a whole might have, their interest in the family as an integral part of understanding both illness and caring can contribute to more nuanced and thoughtful ways of appreciating and ameliorating tensions between patient and family interests, as well as ways of supporting family contributions to the care of their relatives.

When a patient is incompetent to decide about his or her own medical treatment, or when competence is intermittent, physicians turn to the family for help, since families are presumed to know best what the patient would want and also to care about the patient's interests. Families are instructed to make their decision on the basis of what the patient would want—the "substituted judgment" standard established in the 1976 *In re Quinlan* case. If the patient was never competent, the family is expected to decide on the basis of what is best for her or him—the "best interests" standard. Tightly focused on the patient, either standard is open to challenge.

Linda L. Emanuel and Ezekiel J. Emanuel observe that the substituted judgment standard has been challenged on both theoretical and empirical grounds. An important theoretical objection is that reconstructing what a patient would want in highly specific circumstances from a general knowledge of the person's values requires a tremendous imaginative effort that may be beyond most people, while the empirical objections are that patients do not in fact discuss their preferences with family members, that family members are not good at assessing a patient's quality of life, and that proxies' selections are not much better than random chance in predicting patients' preferences for life-sustaining interventions. As Patricia White points out, people often do not know what they themselves would want if seriously ill.

The best interests standard is open to the objection that it cannot be seen as a patient's exercise, by proxy, of his or her right to refuse or consent to treatment, but instead gives the family power to exercise its own authority over the incompetent patient—something our society is reluctant to do because of the fear of abuse. While there are certainly instances of familial abuse of patients, one might question whether we ought to base social policy on the assumption that abuse is the possibility most to be feared. Yet if this objection to the best interests standard is unpersuasive, there is another that may be more convincing: the standard is not suitable to families because they are not, typically, a group of people each simply seeking to maximize his or her own self-interest. There is a collective character to family life that is not easily accommodated by the notion of individual best interests, and so the best interests standard is a code of conscience that from the family's point of view is distinctly second best. In fact, the standard is invoked primarily in adversarial situations where the family's solidarity has broken down, as in child custody disputes.

An ethics of the family might suggest that what family members owe each other is not the best, understood abstractly. If it were, parents would have a duty to find better parents for their children than they are themselves. Rather, what is owed is the good that inheres in this particular set of relationships. If this is right, then at the sickbed it is less important that a brother, lover, or daughter-in-law should correctly decide what is best for an incompetent patient than that the decision be made by this particular person, the one who stands as close to the patient as possible and so serves the patient as an extended self. Here, as well as where the patient is competent, decision making that recognizes morally salient features of family life might set the needs and desires of the patient into careful balance against the family's resources for care, bringing a nuanced understanding of all the relevant particulars to bear on the decision.

What, if anything, do adult children owe their frail elderly parents? Theories affirming a duty of reciprocity argue that parents gave their children life and cared for them when they needed care; in return, children owe their parents care when they are in need. The difficulty with such theories (held by Aristotle and Aquinas, and more recently by the Victorian jurist William Blackstone) is that they do not seem to recognize that parents have a duty to provide their children a decent minimum of goods and services. If parents are merely discharging their own obligations, it is hard to see why the child need respond with anything more than thanks. Following this line of reasoning, neither Jane English nor Norman Daniels can defend a duty of adult children to care for their parents. The child, not having contracted for the parental sacrifices made on his or her behalf, has no duty to reciprocate, since sacrifices that have not been requested require no return. A third view, shared by Blustein and Joel Feinberg, distinguishes between duties of indebtedness and duties of gratitude, and concludes that duties of gratitude are owed even for those actions that are included in the parents' own duties (Blustein, 1982; Feinberg). To discharge this duty of gratitude, children must help their parents when help is needed. And a fourth theory, developed by Nelson and Nelson (1992; 1995), bases a duty to parents in the parents' own moral duties, holding that the parental duty consists in part in encumbering the child with a loving relationship that in the child's maturity will be mutual. Once that mutuality is achieved, the mature relationship in turn generates the duty to care for parents in need.

Whatever the source of duties to frail elderly parents, the content of those duties is not easy to ascertain. If postindustrial societies do not set limits on the amount of increasingly costly medical care they offer the old as they leave this life, they may impoverish the young. Within a family, this dilemma might be played out in terms of nursing-home care for a grandparent versus a child's college fund. In "Moral Particularity" (1987), Walker has described such a decision as an opportunity for defining oneself morally, ratifying or breaking from a past course of action as one sets the course of one's future. Families, too, might be capable of strong moral self-definition of this kind.

Medical solutions to infertility are genetic solutions; there is an attempt to establish a genetic tie between the child and at least one parent. In a *genetic* contract pregnancy (in which the birth mother's egg is used to produce a child for people who have paid her to have the baby on their behalf), the importance of the maternal genes is played down, but the paternal genes—those of the contracting father—are considered crucial. In the far less common arrangement whereby the birth mother is hired to carry to term an embryo formed in vitro by the contracting couple's egg and sperm (this is called gestational contract pregnancy), the maternal genes regain their standard social meaning; the woman who is genetically linked to the child is regarded as its mother. By contrast, in artificial insemination by donor, the paternal genes are seen to carry no social responsibility for the child.

The model for all this is one of consumer choice, in which the infertile parties are at liberty to decide for themselves what weight to give genetic ties.

This model raises important questions about the moral significance of being a parent. If those who contribute genetically to a child can be said to cause that particular child to exist, and if an ethics of the family adopts a causal rather than a contractual model of responsibility, then the child's genetic parents would seem to have a prima facie obligation to remain in the child's life in an ongoing way. Even if they delegate much of their responsibility for rearing the child, it does not follow that they may put themselves totally out of power to keep the child from harm. Thus lesbian or gay couples, for example, might have a duty to foster a loving bond between the child and the biological parent of the opposite gender.

Medicine invites a consumer-choice approach not only in the matter of genetic ties but also in the matter of genetic screening. While it is reasonable to protect one's family by trying to avoid giving birth to a child with a serious genetic defect, the choices made possible by genetic screening can be a burden as well as a benefit. An important mechanism for drawing new members into the family—the pregnant woman's continual process of making friends with her fetus—is distorted and interrupted by amniocentesis, endoscopy, chorionic villus sampling, ultrasound, alpha-fetoprotein assays. Such screening, along with the new possibility of fetal surgery, prompts the question, not when the fetus becomes a person, but how and when the fetus joins the family. As Stanley Hauerwas and William Ruddick ask, when is a fetus a child? (Hauerwas; W. Ruddick, 1989). At what point in the process of family creation ought the pregnant woman to make specific sacrifices on the fetus's behalf, and to what extent should these sacrifices be socially imposed?

A major function of the family is the care of its sick and vulnerable members. Because the United States has not acknowledged a basic responsibility to provide a minimum of healthcare for all its citizens, and because healthcare institutions are greatly concerned to minimize their own costs, the burden of providing that care has fallen disproportionately on families—and within families, on women. The difficulty in achieving gender justice with respect to healthcare is not conceptual but political: how can we reconfigure our society—and our families—to eliminate the bias that sees unpaid care as a natural task for women?

A further allocation issue concerns the range of the family's care. To whom is it owed, and when is it discretionary? What about adult siblings? Cousins? Grandparents? A child's partner? Need and the person's role in the family's history are both relevant considerations, as are the family's resources. If, after all, familial caregiving is exhausted, no further care will be forthcoming. What limits may the family set on the care it owes to its own? What limits may the family set on individual members' sacrifices? More particularly, in light of the fact that women assume a greatly disproportionate amount of the burden of care, what steps should be taken both within families and in the larger society to achieve gender justice? An ethics of the family might offer guidance through the concept of familial integrity, understood as the particular way in which a given family strives to sustain a fruitful tension between intimacy and autonomy, and the way it engages in its characteristic projects and activities. Family integrity cannot, perhaps, be preserved at any price, but it is important to recognize that families as well as individuals can be destroyed unless justice forbids it.

Implementing an Ethics of the Family

Just as medical care is ethically inadequate when the focus is on the organ to be treated rather than on the person in whom the organ resides, so it is likely to be inadequate when no notice is taken of the families in which patients reside. An ethics that treats people as if they were unconnected and self-centered is not up to the task of promoting either justice or human flourishing. Primary care physicians—not only practitioners of family medicine but also pediatricians and internists—are often adept at seeing beyond the patient to the nest of relationships within which that patient lives. They, like nurses and social workers, although hampered by institutional pressures that push families into the background, tend to be attuned to these relationships even when they cannot give a formal moral account of them. That account has been slow in coming; the values of families remain much more diffuse and implicit than the well-articulated values of medicine. But the relationship between the two systems of care is beginning to receive systematic exploration.

As discussions continue regarding what that relationship should be in the twenty-first century, it may be concluded that taking families seriously requires major institutional changes. Hospitals might need to be restructured so that patients are not so estranged from their families; hospital ethics committees might have to take on a mediator's role for disputes among family members concerning patient care; the moral significance of families might have to be better reflected in case law; the conditions under which care is delivered will certainly have to be more hospitable to an ongoing relationship between patients and those who care for them; there will have to be a greater acknowledgment that families—the original providers of

primary care—are as essential a source of healthcare as medicine is. The practical difficulties in implementing an ethics of the family as it relates to healthcare, while daunting, are surely counterbalanced by the importance of the enterprise to the larger task of bioethics: thinking well and carefully about the concrete human realities—our differences, our similarities, our particularities, our intimacies—that have a direct bearing on health, whether within a medical or a familial setting.

HILDE LINDEMANN NELSON
JAMES LINDEMANN NELSON (1995)
REVISED BY AUTHORS

SEE ALSO: *Abortion; Abuse, Interpersonal; Adoption; Aging and the Aged; Care; Children; Cloning: Reproductive; Confidentiality; Dementia; Environmental Ethics: Ecofeminism; Fertility Control; Future Generations, Reproductive Technologies and Obligations to; Genetic Counseling, Ethical Issues in; Genetic Counseling, Practice of; Grief and Bereavement; Infants; Long-Term Care; Maternal-Fetal Relationship; Natural Law; Organ and Tissue Procurement: Ethical and Legal Issues Regarding Living Donors; Population Ethics; Psychiatry, Abuses of; Reproductive Technologies; Sexual Ethics*

BIBLIOGRAPHY

Aneshensel, Carol; Zarit, Stephen; and Whitlach, Carol. 1995. *Profiles in Caregiving: The Unexpected Career.* San Diego, CA: Academic Press.

Areen, Judith. 1987. "The Legal Status of Consent Obtained from Families of Adult Patients to Withhold or Withdraw Treatment." *Journal of the American Medical Association* 258(2): 229–235.

Areen, Judith. 1991. "Advance Directives under State Law and Judicial Decisions." *Law, Medicine and Health Care* 19(1–2): 91–100.

Arras, John, ed. 1995. *Bringing the Hospital Home: Ethical and Social Implications of High-Tech Home Care.* Baltimore: Johns Hopkins University Press.

Beauchamp, Tom L., and Childress, James F. 1989. *Principles of Biomedical Ethics,* 3rd edition. New York: Oxford University Press.

Blackstone, William. 1856. *Commentaries on the Laws of England,* Volume 1. Philadelphia: J. B. Lippincott.

Blum, Lawrence A. 1980. *Friendship, Altruism, and Morality.* New York: Routledge and Kegan Paul.

Blustein, Jeffrey. 1982. *Parents and Children: The Ethics of the Family.* New York: Oxford University Press.

Blustein, Jeffrey. 1993. "The Family in Medical Decisionmaking." *Hastings Center Report* 23(3): 6–13.

Brody, Elaine M. 1990. *Women in the Middle: Their Parent-Care Years.* New York: Springer.

Buchanan, Allen E., and Brock, Dan W. 1989. *Deciding for Others: The Ethics of Surrogate Decisionmaking.* Cambridge, Eng.: Cambridge University Press.

Card, Claudia, ed. 1991. *Feminist Ethics.* Lawrence: University Press of Kansas.

Charles, Casey. 2003. *The Sharon Kowalski Case: Lesbian and Gay Rights on Trial.* Lawrence: University Press of Kansas.

Daniels, Norman. 1988. *Am I My Parents' Keeper? An Essay on Justice Between the Young and the Old.* New York: Oxford University Press.

Emanuel, Ezekiel J., and Emanuel, Linda L. 1992. "Proxy Decision Making for Incompetent Patients: An Ethical and Empirical Analysis." *Journal of the American Medical Association* 267(15): 2067–2071.

English, Jane. 1979. "What Do Grown Children Owe Their Parents?" In *Having Children: Philosophical and Legal Reflections on Parenthood,* edited by Onora O'Neill and William Ruddick. New York: Oxford University Press.

Feinberg, Joel. 1966. "Duties, Rights, and Claims." *American Philosophical Quarterly* 3(2): 139–144.

Goodin, Robert E. 1985. *Protecting the Vulnerable: A Reanalysis of Our Social Responsibilities.* Chicago: University of Chicago Press.

Hanen, Marsha, and Nielsen, Kai, eds. 1987. *Science, Morality and Feminist Theory.* Calgary: University of Calgary Press.

Hardart, George, and Truog, Robert. 2003. "Attitudes and Preferences of Intensivists Regarding the Role of Family Interests in Medical Decision-Making for Incompetent Patients." *Critical Care Medicine* 31(7): 1895–1900.

Hardwig, John. 1990. "What About the Family?" *Hastings Center Report* 20(2): 5–10.

Hardwig, John. 2000. *Is There a Duty to Die? and Other Essays in Bioethics.* New York: Routledge.

Hastings Center. 1987. *Guidelines on the Termination of Life-Sustaining Treatment and the Care of the Dying.* Briarcliff Manor, NY: Author.

Hauerwas, Stanley. 1981. "Abortion: Why the Arguments Fail." In *A Community of Character: Toward a Constructive Christian Social Ethic.* Notre Dame, IN: University of Notre Dame Press.

Kittay, Eva Feder. 1999. *Love's Labor: Essays on Women, Equality, and Dependency.* New York: Routledge.

Kittay, Eva Feder, and Meyers, Diana T., eds. 1987. *Women and Moral Theory.* Totowa, NJ: Rowman and Littlefield.

Levine, Carol. 1999a. "The Loneliness of the Long-Term Caregiver." *New England Journal of Medicine* 340(20): 1587–1590.

Levine, Carol. 1999b. "Home Sweet Hospital: The Nature and Limits of Private Responsibilities for Home Health Care." *Journal of Aging and Health Care* 11(3): 341–359.

Levine, Carol, ed. 2000. *Always on Call: When Illness Turns Families into Caregivers.* New York: United Hospital Fund.

"Looking for a Family Resemblance: The Limits of the Functional Approach to the Legal Definition of Family." 1991. *Harvard Law Review* 104(7): 1640–1659.

Mahowald, Mary B. 1993. *Women and Children in Health Care: An Unequal Majority.* New York: Oxford University Press.

Mintz, Steven, and Kellogg, Susan. 1988. *Domestic Revolutions: A Social History of American Family Life.* New York: Free Press.

Murdoch, Iris. 1970. *The Sovereignty of Good.* London: Routledge and Kegan Paul.

Nelson, Hilde Lindemann, and Nelson, James Lindemann. 1989. "Cutting Motherhood in Two: Some Suspicions Concerning Surrogacy." *Hypatia* 4(3): 85–94.

Nelson, Hilde Lindemann, and Nelson, James Lindemann. 1992. "Frail Parents, Robust Duties." *Utah Law Review* 1992(3): 747–763.

Nelson, Hilde Lindemann, and Nelson, James Lindemann. 1995. *The Patient in the Family.* New York. Routledge.

Nelson, James Lindemann. 1990. "Partialism and Parenthood." *Journal of Social Philosophy* 21(1): 107–118.

Nelson, James Lindemann. 1992. "Taking Families Seriously." *Hastings Center Report* 22(4): 6–12.

Nelson, James Lindemann. 2003. "Just Expectations: Family Caregivers, Practical Identities, and Social Justice in the Provision of Health Care." In *Hippocrates' Maze: Ethical Explorations of the Medical Labyrinth.* Lanham, MD: Rowman and Littlefield.

Nussbaum, Martha C. 1990. *Love's Knowledge: Essays on Philosophy and Literature.* New York: Oxford University Press.

Okin, Susan Moller. 1989. *Justice, Gender, and the Family.* New York: Basic Books.

O' Neill, Onora, and Ruddick, William, eds. 1979. *Having Children: Philosophical and Legal Reflections on Parenthood.* New York: Oxford University Press.

Quinlan, In re. 70 N.J. 10–55, 355 A.2d 647–672, certiorari denied, 429 U.S. 922 (1976).

Rachels, James. 1989. "Morality, Parents and Children." In *Person to Person,* edited by George Graham and Hugh LaFollette. Philadelphia: Temple University Press.

Rawls, John. 1971. *A Theory of Justice.* Cambridge, MA: Harvard University Press.

Rhoden, Nancy K. 1988. "Litigating Life and Death." *Harvard Law Review* 102(2): 375–446.

Rothman, Barbara Katz. 1986. *The Tentative Pregnancy: Prenatal Diagnosis and the Future of Motherhood.* New York: Viking.

Ruddick, Sara. 1989. *Maternal Thinking: Toward a Politics of Peace.* Boston: Beacon Press.

Ruddick, William. 1988. "Are Fetuses Becoming Children?" In *Biomedical Ethics and Fetal Therapy,* ed. Carl Nimrod and Glenn Griener. Waterloo, ON: Wilfrid Laurier University Press.

Ruddick, William. 1989. "When Does Childhood Begin?" In *Children, Parents, and Politics,* ed. Geoffrey Scarre. Cambridge, Eng.: Cambridge University Press.

Sabatino, Charles. 2000. "What the States Are Doing." (Lecture, Conference on End of Life Decision-Making: What Have We Learned Since Cruzan? 2000 Annual Meeting). Boston, MA: American Society of Law, Medicine and Ethics.

Schneider, Carl E. 1992. "Bioethics and the Family: The Cautionary View from Family Law." *Utah Law Review* 1992(3): 819–847.

Schoeman, Ferdinand. 1980. "Rights of Children, Rights of Parents, and the Moral Basis of the Family." *Ethics* 91(1): 6–19.

Schoeman, Ferdinand. 1985. "Parental Discretion and Children's Rights: Background and Implications for Medical Decision-Making." *Journal of Medicine and Philosophy* 10(1): 45–61.

Teitelbaum, Lee. 1992. "Intergenerational Responsibility and Family Obligation: On Sharing." *Utah Law Review* 1992(3): 765–802.

U.S. President's Commission for the Study of Ethical Problems in Medicine and Biomedical and Behavioral Research. 1983. *Deciding to Forego Life-Sustaining Treatment: A Report on the Ethical, Medical, and Legal Issues in Treatment Decisions.* Washington, D.C.: U.S. Government Printing Office.

Walker, Margaret Urban. 1987. "Moral Particularity." *Metaphilosophy* 18(3–4): 171–185. Reprinted in *Moral Contexts.* 2002. Lanham, MD: Rowman and Littlefield.

Wallerstein, Judith S.; Lewis, Julia M.; and Blakeslee, Sandra. 2000. *The Unexpected Legacy of Divorce.* New York: Hyperion.

White, Patricia. 1992. "Appointing a Proxy Under the Best of Circumstances." *Utah Law Review* 1992(3): 849–860.

Williams, Bernard A. O. 1981. "Persons, Character, and Morality." In *Moral Luck: Philosophical Papers, 1973–1980.* Cambridge: Cambridge University Press.

FEMINISM

• • •

As a social and political movement with a long, intermittent history, feminism has repeatedly come into being, generated change, and subsided into oblivion. As an eclectic body of theory, feminism entered the academy in the early 1970s as a part of the women's studies movement, where its contribution to scholarship in the arts, social sciences, and humanities has perhaps been particularly significant. Despite the variety of its political positions, social commitments, and theoretical vantage points, feminism's common concern is with the social pattern, widespread across cultures and history, whereby power and entitlements are distributed asymmetrically to favor men over women. This asymmetry has been given many names, including the subjugation of women, sexism, male dominance, patriarchy, systemic misogyny, phallocracy, and the oppression of women. A number of feminist theorists simply call it gender, and that usage will be adopted here.

The concept of gender rests on the assumption that there are two sexes, male and female. The cultural meanings assigned to those sexes through complex social processes establish a power relation in which masculinity predominates over femininity, and the things associated with masculinity predominate over their feminine counterparts. The term *gender* refers to this power relation, which operates through society's institutions and practices by conferring the control of resources and the right to social goods on men while relegating women to subordinate positions in service of men's interests and concerns. But because gender always works in a complicated interconnection with other abusive power systems such as race, ethnicity, sexual orientation, class, age, and disability, some women enjoy more power than some men. By the same token, these other power systems produce greater amounts of privilege for some women than for others.

One of the characteristic features of gendered power relations is androcentrism: the (usually unstated) view that man is the point of reference for what is normal for humans. According to the logic of androcentrism, if man is the yardstick or measure for being human, then women, not being men, must be defective humans. Furthermore, because androcentrism presumes that men are the point around which everything else revolves, the feminist insistence that women too are full–fledged human beings is just as much about men as everything else is—it is a threat to masculinity, or an attempt to usurp men's rightful place in the natural order of things.

Racism and discrimination against gays and lesbians employ the same sort of logic: the white race and heterosexuality are the norm for human beings, so anything other than the norm must be defective—not just statistically but morally abnormal. From this it follows that the demand to de–center the dominant group (or, to use another spatial metaphor, to dismantle the hierarchy that puts the dominant group on top) must be seen as a threat to the group—a threat to "the Southern way of life" or to "the family as we know it." Looking at the demand in this way keeps the focus on the dominant group, so that it, rather than unjust treatment of the subgroup, remains the center of attention.

Criticism and Construction

As a political movement, feminism has sought to undermine or overthrow the social mechanisms through which gender operates to oppress women. Because gender identity cannot be understood or even perceived outside its complicated interaction with other abusive power systems, feminists resist those as well. A feminist politics is not only a politics of resistance, however. It is also a politics of construction. It seeks to build a more just society—one that is as good for all kinds of women as it is for all kinds of men. So, for example, "first-wave" U.S. feminists such as Elizabeth Cady Stanton, Sojourner Truth, and Lucretia Mott worked for the right of women to own property, not to be enslaved, and to vote.

As a field of scholarship, feminism likewise pursues two goals. The first is criticism. Feminists have uncovered and opposed gender bias in the humanities, social sciences, natural sciences, the arts, and professions such as law and medicine. Sandra Harding, for example, has criticized the view, widely shared by scientists themselves, that science is value–free. She argues that scientific knowledge is produced largely by men who command significant amounts of social prestige, and that the perspective of these men is necessarily colored by assumptions and values arising from the kinds of activities in which they engage. As science leaves this per-spective unexamined, it assumes an objectivity that it does not in fact possess.

What Donna Haraway has dubbed the "god trick"—the ideal of a perspectiveless and timeless view from nowhere that purports to secure objectivity—strikes many feminists as both politically suspect and impossible to achieve. Femi-nist epistemologists such as Lorraine Code and Helen Longino argue that greater objectivity is attained by taking careful and rigorous account of knowers' social locations than by ignoring the effects of power on what kinds of knowledge is legitimated, whose knowledge is considered authoritative, and which knowers are ignored or excluded as a result.

As well as questioning sexist understandings of objectiv-ity, feminists have criticized the gender bias that inheres in other key theoretical concepts and indeed in mainstream theories themselves. But like political feminism, academic feminism does more than criticize—it also constructs. Femi-nist economists, for example, have not rested content with condemning the masculine bias inherent in the individual-ism and competition of much economic theory; they have constructed economic models that begin from the fact of human dependency and connection. Feminist historians have not only pointed to the gender gaps created by their profession's focus on military campaigns and other male–dominated activity in the public sphere, but have used women's diaries, letters, and other writings to construct histories of women and of domestic life. Feminist construc-tions in philosophy include a shift from mainstream episte-mology's preoccupation with necessary and sufficient condi-tions for knowledge, to the theoretical importance of the social location of the knower. Equally significant has been the construction of feminist moral theory, particularly the ethics of care and feminist responsibility ethics.

Feminist Epistemology

While on its face there seems to be something paradoxical about feminist criticisms of reason, given that the forms of argumentation on which these criticisms depend are them-selves a part of what is under attack, the burgeoning literature on this topic may be understood, not as a repudia-tion of reason *tout court,* but as a dissatisfaction with a particular picture of reason. This picture, which underlies much of contemporary nonfeminist ethics as well as other areas of mainstream philosophy, is that of a pure, universal reason, abstracted from historical and social contexts, oper-ating dispassionately and objectively to produce true propo-sitions. Feminists fault this picture as much for what it excludes as for what it portrays.

For one thing, the picture excludes the emotions, rather than acknowledging that feelings such as empathy, resent-ment, or anger play a useful role in reasoning—especially moral reasoning. The picture in particular excludes what people care about, rather than acknowledging that what they care about can itself be a reason for thinking or acting the way they do. It excludes trust, rather than acknowledging that trust is what keeps one's reasoning from becoming paranoid. And it excludes narrative or figurative modes of reasoning, rather than acknowledging that people often use stories and images to make sense of the world.

One important strategy for feminist epistemologists, then, has been to identify the tension between the explicit content of philosophical arguments, which appears gender–neutral, and the models, metaphors, and imagery underlying these arguments, which covertly favor the experiences and preoccupations of privileged men. A second important strategy has been to question the tradition that divorces reason from other human attributes. Many feminists have emphasized the role of the emotions in rational reflection, while others have emphasized the point that human reasoners are embodied, and that the social constructions surrounding differences in embodiment count among the conditions that make knowledge possible. Still others have emphasized the essentially social nature of human existence, arguing that knowledge is not "in the head" of solitary reasoners, but rather is produced and imparted in communities of knowers, and that abusive power systems operate in these communi-ties to discredit unjustifiably certain kinds of reasoning while authorizing others.

Borrowing from Marxist analysis, in the 1980s feminist standpoint theorists such as Nancy Hartsock and Patricia Hill Collins drew an analogy between women in gendered societies and workers in capitalist societies. They contended that just as the false presuppositions that sustain the ideology of capitalism are most visible from the hard–won perspective of the worker who has participated in consciousness–raising and political engagement, so too the false presuppositions that sustain the ideology of gender are best seen from the standpoint of those who have had to acquire detailed, self–reflective knowledge of the gender system simply in order to be able to function within it. Feminist standpoint theorists are less interested in claiming a single, unified standpoint that is representative of all women, however, than in taking seriously the knowledge that informs women's practices—whether domestic, emotional, intellectual, or professional.

Ethics of Care

One such practice is that of giving care. In the United States, but also in many other societies, women do far more unpaid, hands–on caregiving than men—they change the diapers, wash the dishes, clean the bathrooms, take the dog to the vet, feed and dress the children, take care of sick or disabled family members, and provide long–term care for elderly relatives. Even when married women have full–time jobs, they still almost invariably do the vast majority of the housework, childcare, and elder care. Nearly 75 percent of unpaid elder care is done by women, and after a divorce or in cases where the parents never married, 75 percent of dependent children live with and are cared for by their mothers rather than their fathers—a figure that approaches 100 percent when the children are infants or toddlers. Paid caregivers are mostly women, as well. Almost 96 percent of professional nurses are women, and the percentage of women providing daycare for children is close to 99 percent. In Canada, women do 80 percent of all caregiving, both paid and unpaid.

The Harvard psychologist Carol Gilligan, taking seriously the idea that women's experience of caregiving produces its own kind of moral reasoning, questioned whether the scale of moral maturity developed by her colleague, Lawrence Kohlberg, was as universally applicable as he supposed. At the first stage of Kohlberg's scale, morality is conceived of as a system of punishment and obedience. At Stage Two, it is motivated by personal reward. At Stage Three, it is taken to be a matter of helping and pleasing other people. At Stage Four it is understood as a set of rules for maintaining the social order. Those who reach Stage Five can sum up those social rules in a principle such as "the greatest good for the greatest number," while those at Stage Six are able to think of morality in terms of self–chosen universal principles of justice. Not everyone, claimed Kohlberg, reaches the more advanced stages of moral maturity.

Gilligan, noting that men consistently scored higher on the Kohlberg scale than women, questioned the reliability of the scale rather than accept its implication that women tend to be less morally mature than men. She claimed that many of the girls and women in her own developmental studies simply reasoned about moral matters "in a different voice." Instead of talking about rights and rules, they were using the language of relationships and connection. Rather than reasoning abstractly, their thinking was contextual and concrete. She called this a "care" orientation toward morality, and opposed it to the "justice" orientation displayed at stages Four, Five, and Six on Kohlberg's scale. Gilligan was careful not to say that the "different voice" is the voice of all women across cultures and through time, any more than the voice of justice is the voice of all men. She did, however, argue that gender shapes the experience of men and women differently, and that gendered experience—particularly the experience of living in a society that expects girls and women to perform vast amounts of caring labor—produces "different modes of moral understanding."

Nel Noddings, Virginia Held, Sara Ruddick, Joan Tronto, and Eva Kittay are among the most prominent of the feminist theorists who have used Gilligan's moral psychology to construct an ethics of care. They have examined caregiving for the moral understandings internal to the practice, offering accounts of not only what it is to care well, but also of the social and political framework in which this practice takes place. While care theorists have by no means created a unified account, it is nevertheless possible to identify three characteristic features of the ethics on which most, but not all, care theorists agree:

1. a caring relationship;
2. engagement with another's will; and
3. particularism.

Caring well both requires and is an expression of a caring relationship. The caregiver must care about the person she cares for, not only to keep the caregiving from becoming impersonal, cold, or self–serving, but because caring is a value in itself. To care in this sense is to feel concern for one's charge (Kittay's term for the person receiving the care). But while caring engages the emotions, the word does not refer solely to a cluster of feelings. As Held points out, it is also a moral term. It is a good thing to care about others; a bad thing not to care. Because it is a moral term, it can be used to guide how and when to act on one's feelings, as well as to evaluate specific instances of caregiving.

On the view of a number of care ethicists, the caring relationship requires engagement with another's will—the caregiver must treat her charge not simply as an object of her care, but as someone with wants, intentions, and desires of his own. Noddings calls on caregivers to practice what she calls engrossment, which consists of such close attention to the feelings, needs, ideas, or wants of their charges that the caregivers' own will is displaced. Other care ethicists emphasize the importance of self–knowledge, lest the caregiver confuse her own will with the will of her charge.

Caring well also requires the caregiver to pay attention to the particulars of a caring relationship rather than being guided by abstractly formulated rules or principles. It is by being closely attentive to this particular person, who needs this particular kind of care, in these specific circumstances, rather than by reflecting on general moral precepts, that morally admirable care is given. This is not to say that caregivers ought never to engage in abstract thinking. But the point is to remain within the caring relationship, which requires attention to the person for whom one cares rather than attention to moral abstractions.

A number of feminist ethicists have argued (repeatedly) that each of the three central features of the ethics of care reinforces the stereotype of the self–effacing wife and mother, prescribing courses of action and ways of thinking that are bad for women. In particular, the critics have identified three dangers. First, if the caregiver cares about the person she cares for, her feelings will not permit her to leave her charge's needs unmet, which poses the danger of exploitation. Second, the caregiver might become so engrossed in the needs and wants of her charge that she gives up her own sense of right and wrong, thereby losing her integrity. And third, if the caregiver attends closely to the particular needs and circumstances of her charge, her field of vision cannot accommodate the broader concerns of social justice.

Kittay's solution to the problem of exploitation is to call for financial, economic, and logistical support for caregivers. She argues that if one begins from the fact of human dependency instead of from the assumption that "all men are created equal," then caring for those who need it can be seen as one of the requirements of justice—as can support for those who provide this care. Diemut Bubeck has a different solution. Her idea, modeled on military service, is that men and women alike could spend some period of their lives in a "caring service" whose mission would be to provide respite care for unpaid dependency workers.

As for the problem of integrity, one solution is to build self–care into the ethics of care so that it does not become an ethics of self–erasure. However, if the caregiver's only motive for taking care of herself is that she can then better care for her charge, she stands in danger of losing herself altogether. Cheshire Calhoun's 1995 account of integrity provides a different solution. She argues that integrity is not only the personal virtue of holding fast to the moral values

that are central to one's self–conception, but also a social virtue, exercised by reliably standing for one's own best moral judgments to other people. If integrity involves being the kind of person others can depend on, it cannot be threatened by caring well. Indeed, for the caregiver to do what she knows to be wrong would count as defective care, because it would mean that her charge could not rely on her.

In response to the claim that the ethics of care is too focused on the personal and the particular to attend to issues of social justice, Tronto proposes to redraw the boundary that political theorists and others have marked between morality and politics. As caregiving is a practice embedded in social life, she claims, it has to be understood in a political context and not just a moral one. A politics of care that complements the ethics of care would, in Tronto's view, recognize and support the caring labor on which every society depends. Such a politics would shift the goals of social policy from preserving autonomy to fostering interdependence; from promoting interests to meeting needs. It would value citizens even when they cannot fend for themselves.

Responsibility Ethics

The ethics of care is based on a morally crucial relationship between people that has too often been ignored or dismissed by nonfeminist ethicists, but relationships other than those involving care are also morally important, and they too give rise to responsibilities. Nor are relationships the only source of the moral demands made on people. For these reasons, several feminist ethicists have gone beyond care to develop an ethics of responsibility.

Margaret Urban Walker is less interested in the abstract questions that philosophers have traditionally raised about the conditions under which someone is morally responsible (Was he free to act otherwise? Did she form the proper intention?) than in examining how practices of responsibility operate within actual moral communities. People hold one another to their promises, excuse them, demand an explanation, give them a standing ovation, let them stew in their own juice, award them the Nobel Prize, and sentence them to death by lethal injection. In these and other ways responsibility is assigned, accepted, taken, deflected, redirected, and renegotiated.

How one is expected to participate in society's practices of responsibility depends just as much on one's gender, class, age, ethnicity, and race as it does on one's own achievements. Who gets to do what to whom is largely determined by the social power that is distributed according to these demographics, as is the matter of who must account to whom. And just as social position influences whether and to what extent one may take, assign, or avoid responsibility, so too it plays a role in determining who may set or change the rules that govern when, how, and by whom this may be done.

As Walker points out, however, the system is rigged. The social forces that allow some people to take responsibility for the things that are pleasant or rewarding, while imposing on other people the kinds of responsibility that keep them from attaining many of the good things in life, are the same forces that hide the fact that this is going on. Some of these forces naturalize the uneven distribution of responsibility, concealing the coercion that sustains the arrangement by representing it as natural—as when women are said to have a maternal instinct that qualifies them to care for children while men do not. Other forces normalize the unfairness, focusing so much attention on the norms or standards for fulfilling a particular responsibility that the question of why a particular kind of person must assume the responsibility is completely hidden from view. Incessantly barraging women with the norms for looking attractive, for example, is a wonderful way of concealing the unfairness of requiring them to take far more responsibility for their appearance than men.

Practices of responsibility look forward as well as backward. In *The Unnatural Lottery,* Claudia Card points out that people who have suffered from unfair distributions of responsibility can do more than make backward–looking assignments of blame for past wrongs. A woman who has been raped, for example, can adopt a forward–looking stance that allows her to take responsibility for what happened to her—not in the sense of blaming herself, but in the sense of refusing to be a victim. She can be responsible for rebuilding her life at the same time as she holds her attacker responsible for his deed.

Normally, adults are expected to know the moral rules and to be aware of the standards by which other people judge them. That is part of what it means to be a morally competent person. But in "Responsibility and Reproach," Calhoun observes that morally competent people can lose their competence in abnormal moral contexts, such as the one that feminists take themselves to inhabit. If, for instance, the normal moral context allows men to deflect responsibility for changing their babies' diapers, then even a well–meaning man is unlikely to see the sexism behind his assumption that when he does change a diaper, he is doing something nice rather than doing merely what he ought. As he is behaving irreproachably according to the standards of the moral context he inhabits, it hardly seems fair to blame him. One could, after all, excuse him for the same reason one excuses young children's wrongdoing—that he is not responsible for his attitude because he has not yet learned the

moral rules that govern the abnormal moral context feminists occupy. But Calhoun thinks he should be held responsible anyway. When feminists reproach people who engage in sexist behavior, she argues, they teach them that what they are doing is wrong, motivate them to change their behavior, and show them respect rather than treating them like children. This is one way in which feminists can take responsibility (in Card's sense) for sexism.

The ethics of care and responsibility ethics display some common themes. Both reject the idea that persons are essentially self–sufficient and unconnected, insisting instead that selves are always nested in webs of relationship. Both emphasize the differences among people rather than making abstract generalizations about human nature. Both use gender as a central category of analysis. Both use the language of responsibilities rather than rights or duties. And both begin from careful examinations of actual, real–time personal interactions. This on–the–ground quality is highly characteristic of feminist ethics—it is a way of avoiding the mistake of theorizing from too limited a set of examples.

Feminist Bioethics

In Canada and the United States, the bioethics movement and second–wave feminism both began in the late 1960s, but the two discourses had little to say to one another for the better part of two decades. It was not until 1989 that the U.S. journal of feminist philosophy, *Hypatia,* published two special issues devoted to feminism and medical ethics. The few essays by feminists published up to that time in the premier U.S. journal in bioethics, the *Hastings Center Report,* dealt solely with ethical issues surrounding women's reproductive systems.

All that has changed. The 1990s saw a steady stream of conferences, monographs, anthologies, and essays in learned journals that examine bioethical issues through a feminist lens. Susan Sherwin's *No Longer Patient: Feminist Ethics & Health Care* appeared in 1992, as did *Feminist Perspectives in Medical Ethics,* edited by Helen Bequaert Holmes and Laura M. Purdy. The International Network on Feminist Approaches to Bioethics, begun in 1993 by Holmes and Anne Donchin, has some 300 members worldwide and has sponsored several conferences on feminist bioethics, in conjunction with the International Association of Bioethics. In 1995, the prestigious Kennedy Institute of Ethics devoted its Advanced Bioethics Course to feminist perspectives on bioethics, and the plenary lectures of that course were then published in a special issue of the *Kennedy Institute of Ethics Journal.* In 1996, the *Journal of Clinical Ethics* published special sections in each of its four issues on feminism and bioethics. That same year saw the publication of an anthology edited by Susan M. Wolf, *Feminism and Bioethics: Beyond Reproduction.* In 1998, the *Journal of Medicine and Philosophy* devoted an entire issue to the feminist ethic of care. Anne Donchin and Laura M. Purdy's anthology, *Embodying Bioethics: Feminist Advances,* appeared in 1999. In 2001, the journal *Bioethics* published an issue devoted to feminist bioethics. Textbooks and readers in bioethics routinely include essays written by feminists.

Feminist bioethics largely consists of criticism directed at practices surrounding the care of women's bodies, and in particular, the parts of women's bodies that mark them as different from men. There has been an ongoing focus on women's reproductive practices, in the form of arguments in defense of abortion, debates about the wisdom of various methods of assisted reproduction, arguments against sustaining postmortem pregnancies, ethical analyses of various sorts of maternal–fetal conflicts, concern about HIV testing of newborns and pregnant women, pleas for better prenatal care for pregnant women, debates about the use and abuse of the birth control implant Norplant, arguments for and against amniocentesis and other genetic testing of fetuses, and discussions about hormone replacement therapy for postmenopausal women. And when feminist bioethicists have moved "beyond reproduction," as Susan M. Wolf puts it, they have tended to criticize practices of healthcare for women—weighing in, for example, on the debates over the medical management of breast cancer, arguing that tying healthcare insurance to employment disadvantages elderly women, or protesting the injustice of a healthcare delivery system that devotes a disproportionate amount of high–tech care, such as arterial angioplasty and organ transplantation, to men. While this criticism can be seen as a political and moral protest against the sexism that permeates the healthcare system, it has been argued that the preoccupation with women's bodies, and especially women's reproductive health, tends to reinforce the androcentric view that men are normal but women, being abnormal, require special accommodations both within healthcare and within bioethics.

Not all of feminist bioethical criticism focuses on women's (reproductive) health. Mary Mahowald has, for example, used standpoint theory to criticize healthcare providers who systematically discount their patients' knowledge about their illness and treatment. Virginia Warren has pointed out that medicine's preoccupation with crisis issues diverts attention from what may be called housekeeping issues, which are perceived as women's work and are on that account not valued. Susan M. Wolf has argued that gendered differences in medical treatment, suicidal behavior, healthcare insurance, and social expectations about self–sacrifice offer a reason to suppose that legalizing physician–assisted suicide would further oppress women. A number of feminists have criticized the cost–cutting measures resulting in shorter hospital stays that unfairly exploit the gendered division of labor within families, where, compared to men, women do vastly disproportionate amounts of caregiving, even if this means that they are restricted to part–time employment or give up their jobs altogether.

Feminist bioethicists' constructions have consisted mainly of reconceptualizing problems in areas of healthcare practice and policy ranging from postmenopausal motherhood to home healthcare, and then offering solutions based on those reconceptualizations. With the major exception of the work of some feminist bioethicists on the ethic of care, however, constructions in theory have been almost nonexistent. Much more could be done both to expand the ethic of care so that it furnishes conceptual tools for social and political analysis, and to use the practice of medicine itself to enrich ethical theory. That so little of this work has been done is not surprising, not only because feminist bioethics is a very young discourse but also because bioethics in general has failed to produce much distinctive theory, contenting itself with the pragmatic strategy of agreeing on middle–level ethical principles where it can, and scavenging from the standing political and moral theories when it must. Feminist bioethicists, however, do not have the luxury of that sort of pragmatism, because it is the business of feminism to be deeply suspicious of the standing political and moral theories, on the grounds that they are shot through with gender bias and so cannot be regarded as trustworthy. Many feminists argue that their task is to construct new theory rather than to refine theories that leave everything exactly as it was.

Why ought feminists theorize about ethical issues arising from biomedical practice? Why, that is, should there be a feminist bioethics at all? One answer is that medicine ought to be of particular concern to feminists because it is one of the hegemonic discourses of our time, commanding enormous amounts of social prestige and authority. Because it is so powerful that no other discourse except, possibly, that of international capitalism competes with it, it interacts with gender at many levels and in many different ways. Feminists continue to criticize that interaction, but they also wish to learn from it. By studying how power, in the guise of gender, circulates through the healthcare system, they contribute to the body of normative theory that might guide this socially valuable institution in the direction of greater justice.

HILDE LINDEMANN NELSON

SEE ALSO: *Abortion; Abuse, Interpersonal: Abuse between Domestic Partners; Adoption; Aging and the Aged: Old Age;*

Authority in Religious Traditions; Autonomy; Body: Cultural and Religious Perspectives; Care; Children: Rights of Children; Circumcision, Female Circumcision; Coercion; Compassionate Love; Embryo and Fetus; Environmental Ethics: Ecofeminism; Fertility Control; Gender Identity; Maternal-Fetal Relationship; Psychiatry, Abuses of; Reproductive Technologies; Research Policy: Subjects; Sexual Ethics; Sexism; Women as Health Professionals

BIBLIOGRAPHY

Alcoff, Linda, and Potter, Elizabeth, eds. 1993. *Feminist Epistemologies.* New York: Routledge.

Bubeck, Diemut. 1995. *Care, Gender, and Justice.* Oxford: Clarendon Press.

Card, Claudia. 1996. *The Unnatural Lottery: Character and Moral Luck.* Philadelphia: Temple University Press.

Calhoun, Cheshire. 1989. "Responsibility and Reproach." *Ethics* 99: 389–406.

Calhoun, Cheshire. 1995. "Standing for Something." *Journal of Philosophy* 85: 451–63.

Code, Lorraine. 1991. *What Can She Know?* Ithaca, NY: Cornell University Press.

Collins, Patricia Hill. 1990. *Black Feminist Thought.* New York: Routledge.

Donchin, Anne, and Diniz, Debora, guest eds. 2001. *Bioethics* 15(3).

Donchin, Anne, and Purdy, Laura M., eds. 1999. *Embodying Bioethics: Feminist Advances.* Lanham, MD: Rowman and Littlefield.

Frye, Marilyn. 1983. *The Politics of Reality: Essays in Feminist Theory.* Freedom, CA: Crossing Press.

Gilligan, Carol. 1982. *In a Different Voice: Psychological Theory and Woman's Development.* Cambridge, MA: Harvard University Press.

Haraway, Donna. 1991. *Simians, Cyborgs, and Women: The Reinvention of Nature.* New York: Routledge.

Harding, Sandra. 1986. *The Science Question in Feminism.* Ithaca, NY: Cornell University Press.

Hartsock, Nancy. 1983. "The Feminist Standpoint: Developing the Ground for a Specifically Feminist Historical Materialism." In *Discovering Reality,* ed. Sandra Harding and Merrill Hintikka. Dordrecht: Reidel.

Held, Virginia. 1993. *Feminist Morality: Transforming Culture, Society, and Politics.* Chicago: University of Chicago Press.

Holmes, Helen Becquaert, and Purdy, Laura M. 1989. "Special Issue: Ethics and Reproduction." *Hypatia* 4(3). Reprinted 1992, as *Feminist Perspectives in Medical Ethics.* Bloomington: Indiana University Press.

Holmes, Helen Becquaert, and Purdy, Laura M. 1989. "Special Issue: Feminist Ethics and Medicine." *Hypatia* 4(2).

Jaggar, Alison. 1991. "Feminist Ethics: Projects, Problems, Prospects." In *Feminist Ethics,* ed. Claudia Card. Lawrence: University Press of Kansas.

Jaggar, Alison, and Young, Iris Marion, eds. 1998. *A Companion to Feminist Philosophy.* Oxford: Blackwell.

Kittay, Eva Feder. 1999. *Love's Labor: Essays on Women, Equality, and Dependency.* New York: Routledge.

Little, Margaret Olivia. 1995. "Seeing and Caring: The Role of Affect in Feminist Moral Epistemology." *Hypatia* 10(3): 117–137.

Little, Margaret Olivia, ed. 1996. "Special Issue: Feminist Perspectives on Bioethics." *Kennedy Institute of Ethics Journal* 6(1).

Little, Margaret Olivia, and Veatch, Robert M., eds. 1998. "Special Issue: The Chaos of Care and Care Theory." *Journal of Medicine and Philosophy* 23(2).

Longino, Helen. 1993. "Subjects, Power and Knowledge: Description and Prescription in Feminist Philosophies of Science." In *Feminist Epistemologies,* ed. Linda Alcoff and Elizabeth Potter. New York: Routledge.

Mahowald, Mary Briody. 1992. "To Be or Not Be a Woman: Anorexia Nervosa, Normative Gender Roles, and Feminism." *Journal of Medicine and Philosophy* 17(2): 233–251.

Mahowald, Mary Briody. 1993. *Women and Children in Health Care: An Unequal Majority.* New York: Oxford University Press.

Mahowald, Mary Briody. 1996. "On Treatment of Myopia: Feminist Standpoint Theory and Bioethics." In *Feminism and Bioethics: Beyond Reproduction,* ed. Susan Wolf. New York: Oxford University Press.

Nelson, Hilde Lindemann. 2001. *Damaged Identities, Narrative Repair.* Ithaca, NY: Cornell University Press.

Nelson, Hilde Lindemann, and Nelson, James Lindemann. 1995. *The Patient in the Family: An Ethics of Medicine and Families.* New York: Routledge.

Noddings, Nel. 1984. *Caring: A Feminine Approach to Ethics and Moral Education.* Berkeley and Los Angeles: University of California Press.

Overall, Christine. 1987. *Ethics and Human Reproduction: A Feminist Analysis.* Boston: Allen & Unwin.

Overall, Christine. 1993. *Human Reproduction: Principles, Practices, Policies.* Toronto: Oxford University Press.

Petchesky, Rosalind Pollack. 1985. *Abortion and Woman's Choice: The State, Sexuality, and Reproductive Freedom.* Boston: Northeastern University Press.

Purdy, Laura M. 1996. *Reproducing Persons: Issues in Feminist Bioethics.* Ithaca, NY: Cornell University Press.

Roberts, Dorothy. 1997. *Killing the Black Body: Race, Reproduction, and the Meaning of Liberty.* New York: Vintage.

Rothman, Barbara Katz. 1989. *Recreating Motherhood: Ideology and Technology in a Patriarchal Society.* New York: Norton.

Ruddick, Sara. 1986. *Maternal Thinking: Toward a Politics of Peace.* Boston: Basic Books.

Scheman, Naomi. 1993. *Engenderings.* New York: Routledge.

Sherwin, Susan. 1992. *No Longer Patient: Feminist Ethics and Health Care.* Philadelphia: Temple University Press.

Tong, Rosemarie. 1997. *Feminist Approaches to Bioethics: Theoretical Reflections and Practical Applications.* Boulder, CO: Westview.

Tong, Rosemarie, ed. 1996. "Special Section: Feminist Approaches to Bioethics." *Journal of Clinical Ethics* 7(1, 2, 3, and 4).

Tronto, Joan C. 1993. *Moral Boundaries: A Political Argument for an Ethic of Care.* New York: Routledge.

Walker, Margaret Urban. 1998. *Moral Understandings: A Feminist Study in Ethics.* New York: Routledge.

Warren, Virginia. 1992. "Feminist Directions in Medical Ethics." *HEC Forum* 4(1): 19–35.

Wendell, Susan. 1996. *The Rejected Body: Feminist Philosophical Reflections on Disability.* New York: Routledge.

Wolf, Susan M., ed. 1996. *Feminism and Bioethics: Beyond Reproduction.* New York: Oxford.

INTERNET RESOURCE

International Network on Feminist Approaches to Bioethics. Available from <http://www.fabnet.org>.

FERTILITY CONTROL

• • •

I. MEDICAL ASPECTS

The ability of individuals to regulate their own childbearing represents one of the great medical advances of the twentieth century. As a result of demographic trends, which indicate an earlier onset of sexual activity and smaller family size, a woman may spend as long as thirty-five years purposefully avoiding pregnancy. An array of contraceptive methods is necessary to provide individuals with options that are most appropriate to their lifestyle, motivation, desire for effectiveness and convenience, and acceptance of medical risk. Two fundamental trends have affected contraceptive practice since 1960: the development of safe, continuous, and highly effective hormonal contraception, and more recently, an increased awareness of the role of barrier contraceptives for the dual purposes of pregnancy prevention and protection against sexually transmitted infections.

Currently available contraceptive methods include permanent methods that cause sterility—such as vasectomy in men and tubal occlusion in women—and reversible methods. Reversible methods include oral contraceptives (OCs); subdermal implants (Norplant®); progestin injections (depot-medroxyprogesterone acetate; DMPA; Depo-Provera®); intrauterine devices (IUDs); barrier methods (male and female condoms, diaphragm, cervical cap, and spermicidal products); and "natural" methods such as celibacy, periodic abstinence (natural family-planning and fertility-awareness methods), and withdrawal.

General Considerations

It is unreasonable to assume that there is an ideal contraceptive method for each couple; more commonly, couples alternate among various methods over time. A number of general considerations can help to guide an individual (or couple) in the selection of an appropriate contraceptive method.

FREQUENCY OF SEXUAL INTERCOURSE. Couples who have frequent intercourse (arbitrarily defined as more than two to three episodes of intercourse per week) should consider the more continuous, non-coitusrelated methods of contraception: OCs, IUDs, implants, injectables, or if childbearing is completed, permanent sterilization. For less sexually active couples (those who have intercourse less than once per week), an episodic method, such as a barrier contraceptive, would provide protection without exposure to method-related risks at other times.

NUMBER OF SEXUAL PARTNERS. Individuals who have multiple sexual partners, or whose partners have other partners, should be advised to consider one or more barrier methods, with the dual purposes of protection against sexually transmitted infections (STIs) and prevention of pregnancy. For couples who desire an optimal degree of pregnancy prevention, a combined approach of a barrier method plus a highly effective contraceptive will compensate for the relatively high pregnancy rate associated with barrier methods. Additionally, women in this category should not wear an IUD, as the risk of pelvic inflammatory disease (PID) and tubal infertility in IUD wearers is increased significantly in women with multiple sexual partners. For couples who are involved in a mutually monogamous relationship, no method of reversible contraception, including the IUD, increases the risk of PID or tubal infertility.

USER ACCEPTABILITY. Personal attitudes regarding the acceptability of certain methods may influence the success of use. These include religious beliefs, which may preclude the use of "mechanical" and hormonal contraceptives; tolerance of "nuisance" side effects, such as breast changes and vaginal bleeding; willingness to touch the genitals (of self or partner); and aesthetic concerns, such as tolerance of the "messiness" of spermicidal creams and jellies.

MOTIVATION AND SELF-DISCIPLINE. The degree of motivation to avoid pregnancy has a strong impact upon the successful use of contraceptives. Women who contracept to *delay* pregnancy have a higher failure rate than those who are intent on pregnancy prevention. Self-discipline also must be assessed, as women who are highly motivated may do well with intercourse-related (barrier) methods, while individuals who are poorly motivated should choose continuous non-intercourse-related methods such as OCs, IUDs, implantable or injectable methods, or sterilization.

ACCESS TO MEDICAL CARE. Because of the risk of medical complications, certain methods should be used only on the condition of reasonable access to medical care. This concern centers mainly on IUDs and to a lesser extent, hormonal methods. Users of barrier methods, natural methods, and those who have been successfully surgically sterilized have a negligible risk of life-threatening method-related complications.

EFFECTIVENESS. Desire for high effectiveness versus willingness to accept a degree of risk of failure is a primary concern for many contraceptors. Those who insist upon a high degree of efficacy are best advised to use a combination OC (discussed below), an IUD, an implantable or injectable method, or sterilization. Alternatively, for individuals who will accept a higher method failure rate, coupled with an understanding that such failures will result in a choice between delivery and abortion, less effective methods, including barriers and natural methods, may be used.

SAFETY. Medical safety is a major concern for most contraceptors, and concerns regarding health risks are a major reason for discontinuation of use. Paradoxically, adolescents are more likely to avoid or prematurely discontinue contraceptives for fear of adverse health effects, yet they comprise the age group least likely to experience them. The risks associated with contraceptive use are dependent on the following four variables, with an example of each:

1. Age. The risk of arterial complications (adverse effect on the heart and blood vessels, e.g., heart attack) of OCs is age-related; this risk is greatly compounded by cigarette smoking.

2. Underlying medical conditions. Women with underlying cardiovascular risk factors (e.g., hypertension, glucose intolerance, hyperlipidemia, cigarette use) are more likely to experience myocardial infarction (heart attack) while using OCs.

3. Sexual behaviors. A pattern of multiple sexual partners increases the risk of STIs. In particular, IUD wearers would have a greater risk of PID resulting in primary tubal infertility (fallopian tubes blocked by scar tissue).

4. Method-specific risk. Complications are intrinsic to the method, regardless of age, health, and sexual behaviors. Examples include the risk of hepatic adenomas (liver tumors that are noncancerous but that may hemorrhage) in OC users; and pelvic actinomycosis (infection) in long-term IUD users.

A key component of contraceptive efficacy and safety resides in the quality and clarity of instruction and counseling given to the user. Initial instruction should include a description of the methods of contraception currently available, their relative effectiveness, the advantages and disadvantages of each method, and, if appropriate, a comparison of short- and long-term costs. Once a method has been chosen, instruction should center on method-specific advice, such as information regarding method use and danger signals that should be reported to the provider. If the individual will be learning the use of a relatively complex method, or one with an increased likelihood of side effects, it is prudent to provide a simple backup contraceptive method, such as condoms, should the user decide to abandon the initial method. Method-specific counseling should be supplemented with a written fact sheet or other instructional material at a reading and comprehension level appropriate to the individual. Finally, the user should be encouraged to telephone or visit the office of the provider, as necessary, for further advice or modification of contraceptive use.

Oral Contraceptives

The oral contraceptive (OC) is the method of reversible contraception used most widely in the United States. Two types are available: combination OCs, which contain fixed (monophasic) or variable (multiphasic) doses of synthetic estrogen and progestin, and progestin-only pills (POPs, mini pills). OCs primarily prevent pregnancy by preventing ovulation (release of an egg from the ovary). The estrogen and progestin in the pill exert negative feedback on the hypothalamus (the part of the brain that controls hormone production by the pituitary gland) to suppress the release of the hormone GnRH, which in turn decreases secretion of the pituitary hormones LH and FSH, preventing ovulation.

OCs also thicken cervical mucus, which promotes an environment hostile to sperm and alters the endometrium (the lining of the uterus), so that implantation of an embryo is unlikely to occur even if an egg "breaks through" (is released) and is then fertilized. The failure rate of combined oral contraceptives when used correctly and consistently is 0.1 pregnancies per one hundred women per year. In typical use, the failure rate is three pregnancies per one hundred women per year.

Research continues on a male birth control pill. The initial study, announced in 1996, showed that the pill lowered sperm counts significantly with few, if any, side effects. This contraceptive is composed of a progestin and testosterone.

BENEFICIAL EFFECTS OF OCS. Prevention of pregnancy: When used correctly, OCs are highly effective in preventing pregnancy. This includes ectopic pregnancies (those that implant outside the uterus), thus preventing an important cause of maternal morbidity and mortality. There is no increase in the rate of spontaneous abortion or fetal anomalies in former users of OCs, and no long-term reduction in fertility has been demonstrated.

Prevention of acute salpingitis (also called pelvic inflammatory disease, or PID): Even when controlled for sexual behavior and for the coincident use of barrier contraceptives, studies have shown that OC users have a decreased risk of acute salpingitis. It also appears that cases of salpingitis are less severe in OC users overall when compared to controls. Paradoxically, OC users seem to have a higher rate of chlamydial endocervicitis (an STI, with inflammation of the cervix, which may or may not progress to PID).

Prevention of genital tract cancers: Data from the Centers for Disease Control and Prevention's (CDCP) Cancer and Steroid Hormone (CASH) study show a 50 percent reduction in risk for the development of both endometrial and ovarian cancer. Past use of OCs appears to bestow this protective effect for as long as fifteen years after the user has discontinued OC use. The relationship of OCs and cervical dysplasia (abnormal cells of the cervix that, if not monitored, sometimes progress to cancer) and carcinoma is somewhat more complex because of confounding biases, but overall, OC use neither causes nor protects against cervical neoplasia (abnormal tissue formation).

Relief of menstrual symptoms: OCs provide excellent therapy for primary dysmenorrhea ("normal" painful or difficult menstruation that is not related to a disease) because they suppress the endometrium (the lining of the uterus). Consequently, the endometrium does not produce as much prostaglandin, the substance that produces cramping of the uterus. There is a more variable effect on premenstrual syndrome, in that while many women have a decrease in symptoms, others have no change, and a small percentage have worsening symptoms. Because of shorter and lighter menses, the incidence of iron deficiency anemia is reduced by 65 percent. There is also a reduced risk of toxic shock syndrome.

Reduced risk of benign breast disease: OC users have a significant reduction in the incidence of benign (noncancerous) breast conditions, including fibroadenoma and fibrocystic change.

Prevention and treatment of functional ovarian cysts: As a result of the pharmacologic suppression of GnRH release and consequent blunting of pituitary gonadotrophin release, women who use OCs are less likely to develop functional ovarian cysts than women who do not use hormonal contraception. This effect appears to be dose-related, and users of low-dose OC products have less protection than those using stronger formulations. If OCs are given in an attempt to suppress an existing ovarian cyst, it is necessary to utilize a relatively strong product (e.g., Ovral) in order to achieve an effective degree of hypothalamic/pituitary suppression.

Other beneficial effects: For reasons that are unclear, OC users also have a lower incidence of rheumatoid arthritis and peptic ulcer disease.

ADVERSE EFFECTS OF OCS. The most common OC-related side effects are relatively minor. However, the patient may perceive them as major, and this may result in OC discontinuation and subsequent pregnancy. Effective management of minor or "nuisance" OC side effects consists mainly of patient education, and occasionally, medical intervention. Side effects include nausea, weight gain, spotting or breakthrough bleeding between menstrual periods, failure to have a menstrual period during the seven days off OCs, new onset or exacerbation of headaches, and chloasma (darkening of facial skin). Complications, while rare on low-dose combined oral contraceptives, can be serious.

Vascular complications: While initial studies indicated a direct relationship between estrogen dose and an increased risk of deep vein thrombosis (clotting) and pulmonary thromboembolism, more recent studies with low-estrogen-dose products have demonstrated only a minimally elevated attributable risk of these complications. For this reason, OC products containing thirty-five mcg of estrogen or less should be used routinely. In early studies of unselected women using relatively high-dose products, OC users also demonstrated an increased risk of myocardial infarction and stroke in comparison to controls. As a result of exclusion of women with major cardiovascular risk factors and a progressive trend toward the use of lower-dose products, OC users as a group no longer have an elevated attributable risk of OC-induced morbidity or mortality from arterial disease.

Hypertension: The estrogen and progestin components of OCs act in concert to occasionally cause the development of blood-pressure elevation in a small number of OC users. Hypertension is reversible with discontinuation of OCs.

Carbohydrate intolerance: The progestin component of OCs is known to cause peripheral glucose resistance and consequent elevation of insulin levels. In most cases, these effects are minor and are not clinically significant. If a diabetic woman is started on OCs, frequent blood glucose monitoring is necessary initially, as insulin requirements may change. OCs should not be given to diabetics who have clinically manifested vascular or kidney disease or to those with such cardiovascular risk factors as smoking, hypertension, hyperlipidemia (elevated fatty substances in the blood), or age over forty.

Breast cancer: The relationship between OC use and breast cancer has been studied extensively since the mid-1970s. In aggregate, the studies show that the relative risk of breast cancer in a present or former OC user is 1.0, implying neither protection nor increased risk. This relationship was present with a number of subgroups, including women who had initiated OCs at an early age, those who used OCs for longer than ten years, women with a history of benign breast disease, and those with a positive family history. However, a number of studies performed in the early 1980s demonstrated a possible association between OC use and breast cancer in other subgroups. The only thread of consistency in these studies was to show a small increase in the risk of breast cancer for recent OC users who developed breast cancer at an age younger than thirty-five. In that there seems to be a small reduction in breast cancers in past OC users older than thirty-five, it has been hypothesized that OCs, like pregnancy and exposure to other hormonal contraceptives, may be a weak breast cancer promoter, and that OCs may hasten the growth of a tumor already in existence.

DMPA

On October 29, 1992, the U.S. Food and Drug Administration (FDA) approved contraceptive labeling for depot-medroxyprogesterone (DMPA); commonly known by its trade name, Depo-Provera. This culminated a twenty-year effort to make a long-acting injectable contraceptive available to American women. Based upon the findings of extensive clinical research done outside the United States over a decade, the FDA determined that while some concerns remained, DMPA was considered to be as safe as other hormonal contraceptives already on the market.

DMPA's mechanism of action is quite similar to that of all other hormonal methods of contraception: inhibition of ovulation; thickening of cervical mucus, which makes sperm penetration through the cervical mucus more difficult; and induction of endometrial atrophy, which prevents implantation in the highly unlikely event of fertilization. The chemical structure of DMPA is much closer to that of natural progesterone than that of the 19-nortestosterone progestins used in oral contraceptives and Norplant. This may account for the fact that DMPA users have little, if any, change in a number of metabolic parameters over time. In particular, there is no change in clotting factors, globulin levels, or glucose metabolism in DMPA users when compared to pretreatment levels. The slight decrease in total cholesterol levels seen in DMPA users is the result of a minor drop in high-density lipoprotein, the "good" cholesterol, although neither change is clinically significant. Interestingly, DMPA positively affects the central nervous system, causing the seizure threshold to increase, thus making seizures less likely in women with seizure disorders (e.g., epilepsy). Estrogen levels in DMPA users remain at early follicular phase levels, and while other menopausal symptoms do not occur, there is a possibility that some DMPA users may lose a small amount of bone mass over time.

With DMPA there are 0.3 failures per one hundred women during the first year of typical use. This high efficacy is due both to DMPA's efficiency in inhibiting ovulation and the fact that it is a relatively "user friendly" method of contraception. The long interval between injections, a two-week grace period for injections given beyond twelve weeks, and the absence of need for any user or partner intervention at intercourse all contribute to DMPA's high effectiveness.

DMPA is given as a deep intramuscular injection into the deltoid (upper arm) or buttocks every twelve weeks. Since administration most optimally is provided with a 1 1/2 inch needle, most DMPA users, particularly thin women, will prefer the buttocks site. The initial injection of 150 mg of DMPA must be given within the first five days after the onset of menses, unless the woman has effectively been using the pill or has an IUD, in which case the first injection can be given any time during the month. Subsequent 150-mg injections are given at twelve-week intervals, although pregnancy is highly unlikely during the following two-week grace period. If fourteen weeks or more have elapsed since the last DMPA injection, a negative highly sensitive urine pregnancy test must be documented before the next injection is given.

The ideal candidate for DMPA is a woman who is seeking continuous contraception; wants long-term birth spacing; desires a method that is neither coitus-dependent nor requires daily motivation; or who cannot use, or chooses not to use, a barrier method, an IUD, or an estrogen-containing method. It may be particularly appropriate for women who cannot use OCs because of a history of thrombophlebitis, hypertension, heavy smoking, or other cardiovascular risk factors. Women with sickle-cell anemia or seizure disorders actually may experience an improvement in their medical condition. DMPA is an excellent method for postpartum and post-abortal women and can be initiated immediately after completion of the pregnancy. Postpartum women who are lactating (nursing) should not be given DMPA until lactation has been established, usually one to two weeks after delivery. Women who desire a high degree of confidentiality in contraceptive use are attracted to DMPA because it does not require the personal possession of medications or devices, nor does it leave marks of administration or current use.

DMPA has few contraindications: active thrombophlebitis; undiagnosed abnormal genital bleeding; known or suspected pregnancy; active liver disease; a history of benign or malignant liver tumors; known or suspected carcinoma of the breast; and sensitivity (allergy) to the medication. Special conditions requiring more detailed medical evaluation and follow-up include a history of heart attack or stroke; diabetes mellitus; current migraine headaches; a history of severe endogenous depression; and chronic hypertension.

Menstrual changes are universal in women using DMPA and include episodes of irregular bleeding and spotting (lasting seven days or more during the first months of use) and amenorrhea (no menses). Sixty percent of women using DMPA for one year report amenorrhea, and the percentage increases with progressively longer use. Menstrual changes are the most frequent cause for dissatisfaction and discontinuation among women using DMPA, and appropriate patient education and selection and supportive follow-up measures can markedly reduce patient discontent. Medical intervention for irregular or heavy bleeding rarely is necessary, and anemia is uncommon. While counseling and reassurance are initial measures, medical therapy consisting of low-dose oral estrogen for one to three weeks may give temporary respite from bleeding. Women persistently dissatisfied may be better served by discontinuing this method and seeking alternative types of contraception rather than by repetitive medical or surgical intervention. In cases of heavy vaginal bleeding, gynecologic evaluation to rule out such unrelated conditions as vaginitis, cervicitis, or cervical lesions should be performed.

Another group of side effects that occur fairly frequently among DMPA users are pregnancy symptoms such as nausea, breast tenderness, abdominal bloating, and tiredness. While these symptoms are prevalent in the first few months of DMPA use, persistence is uncommon and they rarely are cause for discontinuation.

Weight gain occurs in two-thirds of DMPA users owing to the drug's anabolic effect and its resultant impact on appetite. On average, DMPA users gain four pounds per year for each of the first two years of use. Women concerned or dissatisfied with weight gain should be counseled that it may be controlled with adequate exercise and moderate dietary restriction. Many women notice weight stabilization or improvement with time. If these measures fail and weight gain becomes problematic, DMPA discontinuation may become necessary.

Headache is a relatively common complaint in DMPA users, although not all headaches are necessarily related to the hormone in the drug. If the headaches are mild and without neurologic changes, treatment may be attempted with oral analgesics.

After a 150-mg injection of DMPA, the mean interval until return of ovulation is four to six months. Conception usually is delayed in former DMPA users when compared with women discontinuing oral contraceptives or IUDs. The median time to pregnancy following the last injection is nine to ten months, and studies have shown that almost 70 percent of former DMPA users conceive within the first twelve months following discontinuation, and over 90 percent conceive by twenty-four months, a rate comparable to that of oral contraceptive users. Nulliparous women (those who have never given birth to a child) and those using DMPA for many years experience the same return of fertility as other women studied.

Recent medical studies have addressed other safety issues regarding DMPA use. A large study conducted by the World Health Organization (WHO) showed that in aggregate, there is no overall increased risk of breast, cervical, or ovarian cancers in users of DMPA. DMPA users have a reduction in endometrial cancer for as long as ten years after discontinuation of the method. While there was evidence of a weak association between DMPA use and breast cancer in the subgroup of women under thirty-five who had used the drug within the previous four years, most experts feel that this represents a very weak promoter effect at a level similar to OC use. A single study showed a 7 percent reduction in bone density in premenopausal DMPA users compared to controls, but it is not clear whether this is a true biologic effect caused by low estrogen levels or due to selection bias.

Until more work is done in this area, some believe that it is prudent to screen potential DMPA users for osteoporosis risk factors and to provide additional counseling or evaluation for those with multiple risk factors.

Norplant

Norplant is a sustained-release contraceptive system that acts continuously for five years. It consists of six silicone rubber capsules, each the length and diameter of a matchstick, which are surgically implanted under the skin of the upper arm. The synthetic progestin Levonorgestrel, a hormone found in many oral contraceptives, is slowly released into the bloodstream, resulting in a constant hormone level. The contraceptive effect of Norplant is due primarily to inhibition of ovulation, although secondary mechanisms include thickening of cervical mucus, and formation of an atrophic endometrium. Although 20 percent of Norplant users ovulate in year one and up to 50 percent ovulate by year five of use, studies suggest that when ovulation does occur, it is defective and the ovum is not subject to fertilization. The cumulative pregnancy rate of Norplant users is 3.8 pregnancies per one hundred women over five years; the first-year failure rate is only 0.09 per hundred women per year. Ectopic (tubal) pregnancies are reduced by two-thirds in comparison to noncontracepting women, although should Norplant fail, there is a greater conditional probability (proportionate risk) that the pregnancy will be located in the fallopian tube rather than in the uterus.

Studies that have evaluated the metabolic effects of Norplant have found minimal impact. There is no effect on cholesterol or lipoprotein metabolism, glucose metabolism, or propensity to blood clotting. Norplant is an appropriate method of contraception for women who desire long-term contraception, who have completed childbearing but do not desire permanent sterilization and have had problems with other methods of contraception (including combined OCs), and for postpartum women, whether nursing or not.

The technique of insertion of Norplant involves anesthetizing the skin with local anesthetic and creation of a four-millimeter incision, followed by placement of a twelve-gauge trochar to insert the capsules in a fan-shaped pattern. The procedure takes less than ten minutes and is well tolerated by most women. The method should be inserted within five days of the onset of the menses and provides a contraceptive effect within twenty-four hours. More problematic is Norplant removal, which requires substantially more skill and takes between fifteen and forty minutes. The ease of removal is related to a number of factors, including the correctness of the initial Norplant insertion, the amount of fibrous tissue that has developed around the capsules, and the skill of the clinician.

The most prevalent adverse effect of Norplant is the unpredictability and irregularity of menstrual cycles, especially in the first year of use. Cycles may be shorter or longer than usual and associated with more or less bleeding; there may be bleeding between cycles, or no bleeding at all. Although there is no *cure* for irregular bleeding patterns, short-term palliation of the problem can be achieved by the use of low-dose oral estrogen therapy (e.g., ethinyl estradiol 20 mcg orally per day for two to three weeks). Other side effects include mild weight gain, headaches, hair loss, and new onset or exacerbation of depression.

Intrauterine Devices (IUDs)

Although the IUD is used by only 1 to 2 percent of contracepting women in the United States, it is one of the most widely used methods worldwide. A popular method in the United States in the 1970s, IUD use dropped precipitously as a result of the high rate of pelvic infection and consequent tubal infertility experienced by women who used the Dalkon Shield IUD, which was removed from the market for this reason. Mainly because of business concerns related to the risk of product liability suits, manufacturers of most other IUDs voluntarily withdrew their devices over the next decade. The two IUDs currently available in the United States include a progesterone-releasing T-shaped IUD (Progestasert®), which must be exchanged yearly, and a copper-bearing T-shaped device called the Cu-T-380-A (ParaGard®), which exerts its contraceptive effect for eight years.

The IUD's mechanism of action is still a matter of conjecture. In copper IUDs, it is likely that copper ions released by the device have a toxic effect on sperm, rendering them incapable of fertilizing an ovum. Progesterone-releasing IUDs probably exert their contraceptive effect by converting the endometrium to a chronically atrophic state, preventing implantation of the zygote (fertilized egg). IUDs are known to be a relatively effective contraceptive, with failure rates in the range of 0.6 to 2.0 pregnancies per one hundred women per year. While many clinicians assume that the IUD increases a woman's risk of experiencing an ectopic (tubal) pregnancy, studies clearly show that users of progesterone-bearing IUDs have no increased risk of ectopic pregnancy when compared to nonusers of contraception, while users of copper IUDs experience profound protection.

Women best suited for the use of an intrauterine device are those who desire continuous contraception; who want long-term birth spacing or have completed their families but do not want to be sterilized; who require very high contraceptive efficacy; who desire a method that neither is coitus-dependent nor requires daily motivation; and who cannot use or choose not to use a barrier method or a hormonal method of contraception. IUD insertion and removal are simple office procedures that may result in temporary uterine cramping, but rarely require the use of local anesthesia or analgesia.

IUD use may result in relatively minor side effects such as heavy menstrual periods or cramping (less so with the progesterone-releasing type) and increased vaginal discharge. The relationship between IUD use and pelvic infection and consequent infertility has been studied in great detail. Early studies demonstrated that the major risk associations were recent insertion (within twenty days) and the type of IUD used (the Dalkon Shield bestowing the greatest risk). More recent studies have suggested that an IUD wearer's sexual behavior is the single most relevant risk factor for pelvic infection; a woman in a mutually monogamous sexual relationship has no increased risk of pelvic infection or tubal infertility ("blocked" or scarred tubes from PID) compared to the sexually active woman who uses no method. Conversely, women who have multiple concurrent sexual partners, or those who themselves are monogamous, but whose male partner has other sexual partners, appear to be at increased risk of IUD-associated pelvic infection.

In light of these considerations, contraindications to IUD use include the following:

- pelvic inflammatory disease within the past twelve months or recurrent PID (more than one episode in the past two years);
- post-abortal or postpartum endometritis or septic abortion in the past three months;
- known or suspected untreated endocervical gonorrhea, chlamydia, or mucopurulent cervicitis;
- undiagnosed abnormal vaginal bleeding;
- pregnancy or suspicion of pregnancy;
- history of impaired fertility in a woman who desires future pregnancy;
- known or suspected uterine or cervical malignancy;
- small uterine cavity;
- history of pelvic actinomycosis infection (not asymptomatic presence of the organism);
- known or suspected allergy to copper or, for copper IUD only, a history of Wilson's Disease (an inability to metabolize copper).

While young age may be associated with certain risky sexual behaviors, young age alone is not an absolute contraindication to IUD use. Correspondingly, a history of previous childbearing should not be an absolute prerequisite for IUD use. If a young woman is involved in a long-term mutually monogamous relationship and has no other risk factors, she may be considered a candidate for an IUD.

Barrier Methods

Barrier methods include mechanical barriers such as male and female condoms, the female diaphragm and cervical cap, and chemical barriers such as spermicidal products. Nonprescription barrier contraceptives are an important contraceptive option because of their wide availability, relative ease of use, and acceptably high efficacy when used correctly and consistently. While the contraceptive efficacies of the various barrier methods when used alone are comparable to each other (typically about twenty pregnancies per one hundred women per year), their use in combination adds significantly to their effectiveness. In addition, male latex condoms and female vaginal sheaths, when used consistently and correctly, provide a high degree of protection against both the acquisition and the transmission of a number of sexually transmitted pathogens, including gonorrhea, chlamydia, syphilis, and some viral pathogens, including hepatitis B virus and HIV (human immunodeficiency virus), the virus that causes AIDS (acquired immunodeficiency syndrome). Spermicidal products, in addition to their contraceptive effect, have in vitro microbicidal properties and appear to provide some protection against gonorrhea and chlamydia. Nonprescription barrier contraceptives include male latex and animal membrane condoms; female polyurethane vaginal sheaths; the contraceptive sponge; and spermicidal films, foams, jellies, creams, and suppositories. Contraindications include allergy to latex rubber (in the case of male condoms, diaphragm, or cervical cap), a history of significant skin irritation with acute or chronic exposure to spermicides, and inability to understand instructions for use.

The contraceptive diaphragm is a dome-shaped latex device that serves as a mechanical barrier against the cervix and also holds a spermicidal preparation in place within the vagina. The diaphragm is one of the oldest barrier methods of the modern era, and has retained its popularity because of its nonhormonal nature, ease of use, and reasonable efficacy. It may be an appropriate method of contraception for women who prefer an intercourse-related nonhormonal method of contraception; desire a barrier method that can provide continuous protection over twenty-four hours; and feel that the diaphragm is less noticeable during intercourse than other barrier methods. The diaphragm should fit comfortably with the anterior (front) rim tucked behind the pubic bone in front and the posterior (back) rim seated deep in the vagina and behind the cervix, so that the cervix is covered by the dome of the diaphragm. The largest, most comfortable diaphragm that fits well should be chosen. Use of a backup method of contraception until the return visit, or until the patient is sure that the diaphragm is staying in place during intercourse, should be advised.

No attempt should be made to use the diaphragm if the woman cannot be fitted with the device due to physical characteristics of the vagina, cervix, or uterus that interfere with proper placement, or if the proper size diaphragm is not available. Other contraindications include a recent history of frequent lower urinary tract infections (e.g., cystitis), especially if associated with prior diaphragm use; less than three months since cervical surgery; less than two weeks since mid-trimester abortion or less than six weeks postpartum (after delivery of a child); allergy to rubber or to all spermicides; inability to understand instructions for use; and inability to insert, remove, and care for the device correctly.

The cervical cap is a thimble-shaped latex device that fits over the cervix and stays in place by mild suction. When used with a spermicide, it is a reliable barrier method of contraception that can be used continuously for up to forty-eight hours. In use in European countries since the 1930s, it was approved by the FDA for contraceptive use in the United States in 1988. The efficacy of the cervical cap in preventing pregnancy is similar to that of the diaphragm in nulliparous women, although the failure rate of the cap is greater in parous women.

The Prentif Cavity Rim Cervical Cap® is the only cap currently approved by the FDA. It is available in four sizes: 22-, 25-, 28-, and 31-mm internal diameter. Because cervix size may vary considerably, these sizes fit approximately 70–75 percent of women. The cap may be an appropriate choice for women who have experienced frequent urinary tract infections, especially if they occurred in association with the contraceptive diaphragm. Because there is less pressure on the urethra and bladder, the cap may be more comfortable than a diaphragm and less likely to predispose the user to a lower urinary tract infection.

Natural Methods

The most effective methods of fertility control are those in which sexual intercourse is avoided entirely. Abstinence is defined as a limited period of time in which intercourse is avoided, while celibacy refers to a lifestyle decision in which an individual chooses to avoid intercourse for a longer time interval, which may be lifelong in some cases.

Fertility awareness methods are those in which sexually active individuals avoid unprotected intercourse during the "fertile period," which is defined as the time in each cycle that ovulation is estimated to occur. Since the ovum survives for about 48 hours after ovulation and sperm can survive in the fallopian tubes for up to five days, the length of the fertile period is about seven days in most women. Couples who practice the fertility awareness method use a barrier method of contraception with intercourse during the fertile period and no method for the remainder of the cycle. In the "natural family planning" technique, a variant of fertility awareness, intercourse is avoided entirely during the fertile period and mechanical contraceptive methods are not used at any time in the cycle. The latter approach generally is endorsed by religious groups who object to the use of other birth-control methods, which they consider to be "artificial" in nature.

Four techniques, which can be used alone or in combination, are used to estimate the fertile period.

- The *calendar* method, in which previous menstrual cycling patterns are charted and from which future ovulatory patterns may be predicted. This method is comparatively inaccurate, as factors such as stress or illness can affect the time of ovulation and thereby shorten or lengthen a given cycle. In addition, many women have such variable cycle lengths that the estimated duration of the fertile period can be as long as two weeks.

- The *basal body charting* or *temperature* method, which is based upon the fact that a woman's basal temperature will increase by 0.5° to 1.0°F twelve to twenty-four hours after ovulation and will remain elevated until the next menstrual period. Women using this method are expected to check their temperature each morning upon arising until the temperature rise has been confirmed. Once two days have passed after the temperature rise, the fertile period is considered to be completed, and unprotected intercourse can resume until the next menstrual period.

- The *cervical mucus* method, also called the "Billings" or "ovulation" method, which relies upon the fact that a woman's cervical mucus becomes copious and watery in the few days before ovulation. The presence of characteristic mucus at the vaginal opening is a sign of impending ovulation and, hence, defines the existence of the fertile period.

- The *sympto-thermal* method uses a combination of two or more of the above techniques. The use of the cervical mucus to signal the beginning of the fertile period and the basal body temperature rise to predict its completion is the most accurate of the fertility awareness methods.

The effectiveness of the fertility awareness methods depends upon the couple's consistency of use and ability to avoid unprotected intercourse during the fertile period. When practiced correctly and consistently, the sympto-thermal method has a failure rate as low as two failures per one hundred women per year, while for the typical use failure rate for all methods of periodic abstinence is twenty pregnancies per one hundred women per year.

Sterilization

Voluntary surgical sterilization (VSS) is the most prevalent form of contraception in the United States; 60 percent of those surgically sterilized are women who have had tubal ligation, and 40 percent are men with vasectomies. Most couples who choose surgical sterilization have completed their families, although for some individuals this choice is prompted by an inability or unwillingness to use reversible methods of birth control. Criteria once used to determine the appropriateness of sterilization based on age and parity (number of children born) are no longer appropriate, and a woman's considered, informed decision should be respected by the provider, regardless of her age, parity, and social circumstances.

TUBAL LIGATION. The most important point to be made in counseling a woman regarding tubal ligation is that the procedure must be considered permanent and should be performed only when she is sure that she desires no further children. Alternative (reversible) methods of birth control should be discussed to ensure that these methods have not been rejected on the basis of misunderstanding or other biases. Other important aspects of counseling include a description of the surgical risks of tubal ligation, failure rates, and a comparison to the various methods of sterilization available, including vasectomy for the woman's partner. If consent cannot be obtained from a severely mentally disabled woman, a legal guardian may provide consent in some cases.

Both the federal government and individual states have regulations regarding minimum age requirements and waiting periods from the time of written consent until the date that the operation may be performed if federal or state funding is to be used. For this reason, women who plan to undergo postpartum tubal ligation should receive counseling and consent before thirty-four weeks gestation.

The surgical approach to tubal ligation is primarily dependent upon whether the procedure is performed in the postpartum period, or longer than six weeks after delivery, in which case it is considered to be an interval tubal ligation. In a postpartum tubal ligation, a minilaparotomy performed within four to twenty-four hours of delivery is the preferred approach subsequent to a vaginal delivery. After receiving a regional or general anesthetic, a three-centimeter curvilinear or vertical incision is made immediately under the umbilicus. Once the peritoneal cavity has been entered, either the operator's finger can be used to sweep each tube into the incision or each tube can be grasped under direct vision. In either case, positive identification of the tube can be made by visualizing the fringelike portion at the abdominal end of each tube and by demonstrating that the nearby round ligament is uninvolved. After completion of the tubal occlusion, each excised tubal fragment must be sent for histological confirmation. In a woman delivered by cesarean section, any of the three techniques described below can be performed after repair of the uterine incision has been completed.

A number of techniques are available when there is direct access to the fallopian tubes via minilaparotomy or cesarean section. They include the following methods:

- modified Pomeroy method, in which two ligatures (sutures, "ties") are placed in the mid-portion of each of the tubes and then the pieces of tube between the ligatures are removed. The closed ends retract, leaving a gap between the closed-off tubal segments.
- Irving method, whereby the tubal stump nearest the uterus is tucked into a tunnel made in the myometrium (muscular structure) of the large upper part of the uterus.
- Uchida method, which involves excision of a five-centimeter segment of tube, followed by burying the tubal stump farthest from the uterus within the mesosalpinx (the free margin of the upper part of the broad ligament).

While the failure rates of the Irving and Uchida techniques are exceedingly low (less than 1/1,000) in comparison to the Pomeroy method (1/250), the former take longer to perform and therefore are relegated to special cases.

Interval tubal ligation may be performed with a laparoscope (a narrow lighted tube) via a low minilaparotomy incision (a small horizontal incision, 2–5 cm long, just above the pubic hairline), the former being much more prevalent in the United States. Laparoscopic approaches ("band-aid" surgery) include either open or closed laparoscopy, and both one- and two-puncture instruments (laparoscopes) are available. While a large majority of laparoscopic tubal ligations are performed under general anesthesia, there is a growing trend to perform these procedures under local anesthesia, thereby reducing cost and avoiding the risk of general anesthetic complications, which is the most common cause of tubal ligation deaths. If local anesthesia is used, the tubes must be bathed in a long-acting local anesthetic, then banded or clipped, rather than electrocoagulated (coagulation or clotting of tissue using a high-frequency electric current).

Minilaparotomy for interval tubal ligation is performed via a three-centimeter low horizontal incision. Because of the difficulty entailed in working through a small incision, the procedure is facilitated by using a uterine elevator, an instrument placed in the vagina to lift the uterus. The procedure may be performed with general, regional, or local anesthesia. Minilaparotomy is contraindicated when the patient is obese, has an enlarged or immobile uterus, or when adnexal disease (in the areas adjacent to the uterus, e.g., ovaries and tubes) such as endometriosis is suspected. Nonetheless, minilaparotomy can be a safer, simpler, and less expensive procedure than laparoscopy, which requires more technical equipment and endoscopy experience.

If minilaparotomy is chosen, any of the occlusion techniques outlined above for postpartum tubal ligation may be used. In addition, spring-loaded tubal clips are available that can be easily applied through a minilaparotomy incision. With the laparoscopic approach, three methods of tubal occlusion are available:

- Electrocautery, with a coagulation or "blend" current, used at two or three sites along the mid-fallopian tube. Either unipolar or bipolar cautery may be used; while bipolar cautery is safer (since it is less prone to cause bowel burns), it takes longer and has a higher failure rate. Unipolar electrocautery is faster and more effective, but there is a risk of sparking between the electrode and the bowel, resulting in an unrecognized injury. Fallopian tubes occluded by electrocautery may be quite difficult to reanastomose (reconnect, in the event the woman changes her mind and wants to try to achieve pregnancy) because of extensive scarring.

- Silastic (silicone rubber) rings may be applied with a forceps-type applicator to a loop of mid-portion fallopian tube. This approach avoids the risk of electrical injury to the bowel and preserves much larger segments of healthy ends of the severed fallopian tube should later reversal be considered.

- Spring-loaded clips may be placed at a single site in the middle of the tube and can be used with double-puncture laparoscopy or at minilaparotomy.

The provider must explain that with tubal interruption alone, no organ is removed; tubal sterilization merely prevents conception. The operation is not "desexing" and will not reduce libido, vary the woman's menses, or alter her appearance. There is usually no adverse change in sexual function following tubal sterilization; on the contrary, many women who feared pregnancy before the operation report increased satisfaction in sexual intercourse and are pleased with the operative result. However, 2 to 5 percent report less frequent orgasm and a similar percentage have delayed regret that the procedure was performed.

Only hypophysectomy (excision of the pituitary gland), bilateral oophorectomy (removal of both ovaries), and ovarian damage by radiation are certain methods of sterilization. Abdominal and tubal pregnancies have occurred (rarely) even after total hysterectomy (removal of the uterus). Oophorectomy and sterilization by radiation are usually followed within four weeks by vasomotor reactions (symptoms associated with menopause such as "hot flashes") and a gradual diminution in libido or sexual satisfaction during the next six months.

VASECTOMY. Sterilization of the man by vasectomy is both less dangerous and less expensive than tubal ligation, as it is routinely performed as an office procedure under local anesthesia. Through one or two small incisions in the scrotum, the vas deferens (the tube or duct that carries sperm) is isolated and occluded and usually a small segment of each vas is removed. Neither physiologic impotence nor changes in libido result from the procedure. Sterility cannot be assumed until postoperative ejaculates are found to be completely free of sperm. Failure of the vasectomy, as manifested by pregnancy in a partner, occurs in 0.1 percent of patients. Medical risks of vasectomy include hematoma (blood clot or bruise) formation, epididymitis (congestion or inflammation of the epididymis, the coiled tubular structure where sperm cells mature), spontaneous recanalization of the vas (reconnection of the ends with restored patency) (incidence of less than 1%), and the development of a spermatocele (cystic nodule containing sperm). Atrophy of the testes very rarely results from ligation of excessive vasculature (blood supply). Vasectomy often is reversible—up to 90 percent in some reports—but requires expensive microsurgery and special skill with no guarantee of success. Pregnancy results in only about 60 percent of cases after reversal; factors that influence success include (but are not limited to) the surgeon's skill, the type of procedure used, and time interval since vasectomy.

MICHAEL S. POLICAR (1995)
REVISED

BIBLIOGRAPHY

Berman, S. M. 1991. "Fertility Control and HIV Infection." *Archives of AIDS Research 5*, 1(2): 25–28.

Chica, M. D., and Barranco, E. 1994. "Fertility Control by Natural Methods: Analysis of 218 Cycles." *Advances in Contraception 10*, 1: 33–36.

Hatcher, Robert A., ed. 1994. *Contraceptive Technology*. 16th rev. ed. New York: Irvington.

Judkins, David R. 1991. *National Survey of Family Growth: Design, Estimation, and Inference.* Hyattsville, MD: U.S. Department of Health and Human Services, Public Health Service, National Center for Health Statistics.

Kubba, Ali. 1991. "New Thinking in Contraception." *Practitioner* 235(1508): 878–882.

Robertson, William H. 1990. *An Illustrated History of Contraception: A Concise Account of the Quest for Fertility Control.* Park Ridge, NJ: Parthenon.

Slawson, David C., and Shaughnessy, Allen F. 1994. "Norplant vs. Oral Contraceptives." *Journal of Family Practice* 38(6): 631–632.

Stedman, Thomas Lathrop. 2000. *Stedman's Medical Dictionary,* 27th ed. Philadelphia: Lippincott, Williams, and Wilkins.

Webb, Anne. 1994. "Long-Term Contraception: Assessing the Alternatives—Norplant and IUDs." *British Journal of Sexual Medicine* 21(2): 12–14.

II. SOCIAL AND ETHICAL ISSUES

The status of contraception, sterilization and abortion services in the United States has always been linked to the various social and political movements that have been engaged with issues of women's role in society, reproduction and sexuality. Different groups have advocated for and against family planning for different reasons and with different levels of success. While issues pertaining to reproductive control have always caused some degree of social conflict, this has been especially true since the 1970s when the abortion debate intensified and spilled over to other reproductive health services. The emergence of HIV and rising rates of other sexually-transmitted diseases have also contributed to the controversy surrounding fertility control in the United States and abroad as the new millennium dawns.

This entry begins with a discussion of fertility control in a historical context. One must be aware of this history in order to understand the current ethical debate and controversies surrounding family planning and abortion. The article then continues with discussions of the social, political, religious and moral perspectives. Although the circumstances may change, the issues surrounding fertility control will always be with us and will remain among the most unresolved in bioethics.

Historical Context

It is often said that if we are unaware of our history, we are doomed to repeat the mistakes of the past. Mistakes and dilemmas regarding birth control are particularly apparent when looked at from the perspectives of the women involved, rather than as a success of technology developed by the great men of medicine.

Advocates for birth control generally intended it to be an option for all women, regardless of race or class. The reality, however, was often that poor, otherwise unempowered women, often from minority backgrounds, were most in need of such advocacy, education and access to contraception. Upper-class women had greater access to information and methods of contraception through their private physicians and other social contacts. They could also pay for whatever was available at the time. They voluntarily reduced the number of children they had. The well-intentioned, beneficent efforts on the part of advocates for women and for birth control to improve access for poor minority women and empower them often had the effect of targeting these women for efforts to reduce the numbers of children they had. The ability of a woman to choose the number of children she had and when she had them might allow her to control other aspects of her life and family and to improve the quality of life for herself and others. It could also come dangerously close, on a population basis, to achieving the desires of eugenicists to reduce the numbers of poor minority, or otherwise undesirable people, in the population. One example of this tension is that involving immigrant Irish and Eastern European women in the late nineteenth century. There was a real concern on the part of eugenicists that the immigrant population was growing and reproducing while educated, upper class American women were successfully reducing the size of their families. Eugenicists may have wanted to control the fertility of immigrant women in order to maintain population proportions, especially those of the "desirable" component of the population. On the other hand, early advocates for birth control might have wanted to improve access to birth control in order to empower these women to control their own destinies to a certain extent. Promoting the autonomy of women and acting beneficently on their behalf, in this case, comes dangerously close to the less ethically acceptable motivation of the eugenicists.

The history of the birth control movement in this country over the past 125 years provides clear examples of the tensions which have always existed between empowering women to control their fertility and promoting limitations on fertility for the disadvantaged. Several important developments in the history of the American birth control movement have been chosen to illustrate these tensions and provide a context within which to analyze contemporary social, ethical and political issues (Powderly).

CONTRACEPTION IN LATE NINETEENTH CENTURY AMER-ICA.

Victorian beliefs regarding sexuality accepted promiscuity as a fact of life for men who were either not expected to or were unable to control their sexual urges. Women, on the other hand, were expected to control or even deny their sexuality (Gordon, 1981). Prostitutes were a common and accepted solution to this dichotomy. Despite the view that female sexuality was viewed as inextricably linked to reproduction, contraception was widely practiced among all social classes. The methods of contraception varied by class, however, due to cost and availability. The upper classes were more likely to use relatively expensive methods of contraception such as condoms, spermicides, and douches. They might also have had access to diaphragms and cervical caps smuggled in from Europe at a high cost. Withdrawal and rhythm were often the only methods available to the poor. At a time when menstrual cycles were only partially understood, pregnancies often resulted. Abortion, often self-induced and always dangerous, was resorted to frequently. It is estimated that one out of every five to six pregnancies in America ended with an abortion by the 1850s (Chesler). Mortality from septic abortions was extremely high. In 1888, it was estimated as being fifteen times greater than maternal mortality (LaSorte, Powderly).

During this era, American feminists supported the concept of "voluntary motherhood" (Gordon, 1981). Far from empowering women and providing them with sexual freedom, however, voluntary motherhood sustained traditional family roles for women. Limitation of family size enhanced their ability to fulfill their societal roles as wives and mothers according to this view. These feminists were joined by moral reformers who were concerned about excessive breeding among the lower classes. Immigrants were particular targets of this concern. Focusing efforts toward reduction of fertility on the lower class and members of minority groups has strong historical roots in the late nineteenth century (Powderly).

Although contraception was widely practiced in private and abortion was accepted as a necessity when it failed, many were not willing to risk expressing support for them in public or admitting to their use. This Victorian reluctance influenced public policy. Abortion was declared illegal for the first time in the United States in 1830. A majority of states had declared it so by 1870 (LaSorte). A great legal blow was dealt to contraception in 1873 with the passage of the statute that came to be known as the Comstock law. This federal statute made it illegal to transport obscene materials through the mail. Contraceptive devices such as condoms and diaphragms as well as literature were confiscated under this law, which was in effect until 1936. It lost its power in a case in which Margaret Sanger established the right of doctors and other qualified professionals to use the mail for such distribution. Contraceptives themselves remained in the obscenity statutes until 1971 (Wardell, Powderly).

MARGARET SANGER AND THE AMERICAN BIRTH CONTROL MOVEMENT.

Perhaps no name is more associated with birth control, family planning, and reproductive freedom for women than Margaret Sanger's. Sanger was born in 1879, the middle child in an Irish immigrant family with eleven children. She was impressed at a young age with the effect of frequent pregnancies on her mother, who suffered from tuberculosis and died at the age of fifty. Her mother's frequent pregnancies and their ultimate role in her early death angered Sanger. She went on to play a strong role in the birth control movement in the United States and abroad until her death in 1966. While her decision to devote her life to the promotion of access to birth control for all women was influenced by many factors, her own family background and experience certainly played an important role.

Sanger was trained as a nurse, although she left her training program early to marry William Sanger. Because of prohibitions against married nursing students in this era, she could not remain in the program once she married. She would remain conflicted throughout her life between her obligations to her family and the demands of her passionate cause—access to birth control for all women. This is a conflict that remains for many working mothers today in an era where there is often no choice.

Margaret Sanger's experience as a visiting nurse and midwife on New York City's Lower East Side provided the stimulus for her crusade. She often cited the case of Sadie Sachs, a twenty-eight year old Jewish immigrant and mother of three who was married to a truck driver named Jake. Unable to deal with another pregnancy and an additional child, Mrs. Sachs nearly died from a self-induced abortion. Sanger nursed her for weeks and listened to her pleas for reliable contraception. It is likely that Sanger offered her personal experiences with condoms and coitus interruptus, the common methods readily available at the time. Mrs. Sachs knew another pregnancy would kill her. The only advice her physician could offer her was to "tell Jake to sleep on the roof." If only these immigrant men could control their sexuality, there wouldn't be so many problems! There was no better or more constructive advice available to her. Three months later, Mrs. Sachs died of septicemia after another self-induced abortion. Her husband was distraught and her children left motherless. Margaret Sanger called it "the dawn of a new day in my life … I knew I could not go back merely to keeping people alive...." (Chesler; Wardell; Sanger, 1931, 1938; Powderly).

Early in her crusade, Margaret Sanger used her connections to the Socialist Party to promote her cause. She published a column entitled: "What Every Girl Should Know" in *The Call,* a New York Socialist daily, in 1912 and 1913. The columns elicited a range of responses and were ultimately challenged by Anthony Comstock. Early in 1913, one of the columns was entitled "What Every Girl Should Know—Nothing; by order of the U.S. Post Office" and was followed by a blank space. Several weeks later the censored column appeared (Chesler; Sanger, 1938). Birth control was not to become a priority issue for the Socialists, however. It couldn't compete with suffrage and labor issues. Sanger was disillusioned and disappointed that birth control was not viewed by her comrades as a priority issue for women.

In 1914, Sanger abandoned her own failing marriage and devoted herself to the development of *The Woman Rebel,* a magazine for working women that would cover issues of sexuality and contraception. She was indicted under the Comstock laws for sending the first issue of this magazine through the mail. While awaiting trial, she wrote *Family Limitation,* a practical pamphlet on birth control methods. The world was about to go to war and Sanger's arrest and cause were not receiving as much publicity as she had hoped for. She decided to flee the country and her children and go to Europe until she could command more visibility. While she continued her research on contraceptive methods, her husband, still a supporter, went to jail for dispensing one of her pamphlets. Sanger returned to heightened publicity for her cause and the charges against her were ultimately dropped (Chesler; Powderly).

Sanger began a cross-country speaking tour to promote the importance of knowledge for women regarding sexuality and birth control. While she promoted access to birth control for all women, she focused primarily on the poor. Sanger believed that uncontrolled fertility and large families were inextricably linked to poverty. Her efforts to empower poor women, however, would be viewed by some as racist and by others as having eugenic propensities. While many eugenicists supported the ideas of limiting population growth, particularly among those they viewed as undesirable (e.g. the poor, immigrants, those with mental problems or disabilities), they were greatly troubled by the idea that the upper classes would use birth control and the lower classes would continue to breed.

Margaret Sanger brought birth control directly to the poor women of Brooklyn on October 16, 1916, when she opened a free-standing clinic in Brownsville. Immigrant women from many cultures lined up with their baby carriages to learn how to prevent future pregnancies. In the few weeks the clinic was open, 464 women were provided with sex education and contraceptive information (Chesler; Powderly). The clinic was raided by the New York City Vice Squad and Sanger and her sister, Ethel Byrne, the clinic's nurse, were jailed. The trial produced an important legal victory for birth control. The New York State Court of Appeals interpreted the law to allow for prescription of contraceptives by physicians not only to prevent or cure venereal disease—an interpretation largely applied to men— but also for any health reason. This opened the door for physicians to prescribe contraceptives for women. It also produced another dramatic effect, however. Birth control from that point on was a physician-dominated enterprise. While Margaret Sanger's Brownsville clinic brought contraception to the community level and to poor women, it did so at a price. Nurses, and to a large extent, women, were not to control the provision of contraceptives. This is a legacy that lingers today. In populations with limited access to physicians, it is a clear disadvantage (Chesler; Powderly).

The compromises struck with the medical community are evident in Margaret Sanger's interactions with Robert Latou Dickinson. Dr. Dickinson, a Brooklyn gynecologist, was a champion of studies of female sexuality, fertility and contraception. While he was not a strong supporter of contraception early in his career, he became one of its strongest supporters and was on the Board of Planned Parenthood at the time of his death in 1950 at the age of eighty-nine. Dickinson and Sanger fought for the right to contraceptives, but he viewed her techniques as propogandist. He sought initially to evaluate the effectiveness of contraceptive counseling and techniques, using more traditional scientific methods. Influential in his field, Dickinson used his platform as president of the American Gynecological Society to promote professional interest in birth control. He set up a committee on maternal health at the prestigious New York Academy of Medicine to promote contraceptive research. He found, however, that without Sanger's "propoganda" he had trouble recruiting patients. While he had access to the medical establishment, she had access to the women who would be the subjects of the research and the users of contraceptives. Dickinson also, ultimately, sought Sanger's assistance in securing diaphragms for his own patients. He had been unable to acquire enough diaphragms through legal channels. Sanger had been smuggling them into the country, sometimes in "Three-in-One oil boxes." She had married the millionaire head of the Three-in-One oil company and used his fortune and resources to promote her cause (Wardell; Powderly). Sanger and Dickinson often disagreed vehemently on strategy, but also cooperated to achieve their mutually desired goals. Dickinson ultimately joined Sanger's Birth Control Clinical Research Bureau's advisory board. Together, they assured that birth control would be available to American women. It was, however, to be a male-dominated enterprise constructed on the medical model (Powderly).

STERILIZATION. Tubal sterilization was first proposed in the early nineteenth century for effective long-term contraception in women undergoing operative deliveries (C-sections). The first reported tubal sterilization was performed in 1880 (Lungren; Siegler and Grunebaum). While technology had evolved enough to attempt these procedures, it is important to recognize that they were still quite risky. A paper delivered at the Brooklyn Gynecological Society in 1891 reviewed the sixty-eight sections that had been performed in the United States from 1882–1891. The Brooklyn maternal mortality rate of 33 1/3 percent compared favorably with the national mortality rate of 40 percent (Powderly). Surely, if a woman survived one section, avoidance of another would be an important consideration. Many of the early tubal ligations were recommended to protect the life or health of the woman.

In the early twentieth century, however, eugenics was a dominant reason for tubal sterilization, particularly involuntary sterilization. Compulsory sterilization began to be recommended for individuals with hereditary disease, the "feeble-minded" (i.e. the insane and demented) and the mentally retarded. There were also racial overtones, as undesirable characteristics were perceived to occur more often in Negroes, Orientals, and the foreign-born. In addition, there were some moves to sterilize habitual criminals—a move that some promote to this day for repeat sex offenders. While recommendations for habitual criminals dealt largely with men, efforts to control hereditary and mental illnesses were most often directed at women (Reilly; Powderly). Efforts to "train" female inhabitants of mental institutions gave way to a priority to keep them from reproducing. The view that deviance was hereditary was supported in large part by studies of two families—the Jukes and the Kallikaks.

Richard Dudgale, a social reformer, studied 709 people over five generations in a family he called the "Jukes." Although Dugdale believed both heredity and environment were to blame for the propensity of the Jukes for crime, intemperance and prostitution, he gave real credence to heredity (Dugdale). He estimated that their care had cost society well over a million dollars. In 1912, Henry Goddard added to the belief that deviance was hereditary with his publication of *The Kallikak Family.* Goddard had been studing feeble-mindedness when he discovered the family, which he traced back over six generations. The progenitor had produced both a legitimate and an illegitimate line. The legitimate line produced upstanding citizens, while the illegitimate line produced large families with a disproportionate number of feeble-minded individuals (Reilly; Powderly).

Already concerned with the effects of immigration on population demographics, eugenicists were given superb ammunition with these two studies. The eugenics movement also received financial support from some of the country's most prominent philanthropists. Even Theodore Roosevelt supported the movement, urging Americans to avoid "racial suicide"—the upper classes must not be outnumbered in their progeny by immigrants and the lower class.

The nation's first involuntary sterilization law was passed in 1907 and 14 states had laws allowing involuntary sterilization by 1914. The effect of the laws varied. From 1907 to 1921, there were 3233 documented sterilizations performed under state laws. These sterilizations were seen by many within the mental hygiene movement as beneficial to society and, at the very least, as not harmful to the individual (Reilly). While there was much popular and professional support, eugenic sterilization was still controversial. Some statutes were drafted with more concern regarding constitutional constraints and more care about guardians' consent. Ultimately, however, the Supreme Court provided a boost for involuntary sterilization with its decision in *Buck v. Bell* in 1927. Oliver Wendell Holmes wrote: "It is better for all the world, if instead of waiting to execute degenerative offspring for crime, or to let them starve for their imbecility, society can prevent those who are manifestly unfit from continuing their kind." Sterilization programs were active through the 1940s and 1950s and not influenced by reaction to the Nazi sterilization programs (Reilly; Powderly; Lombardo). Eugenic sterilization virtually disappeared, however, in the 1960s in an era of awareness of patients' rights and the need for society to protect the vulnerable.

BIRTH CONTROL AND THE MODERN ERA. The 1960s and 1970s saw great technological advances in birth control, albeit all dependent on women. The development and approval of oral contraceptives, after controversial research on women in the third world, finally provided a highly effective form of contraception that was not associated with individual sex acts. Intrauterine devices (IUDs) also became popular choices for women and couples who wanted to control their fertility. Although IUDs would later become less available because of legal challenges related to side effects of the Dalkon Shield, they remained a method of choice for many women. By the end of the twentieth century, contraceptive rings and patches and long-acting contraceptives like Norplant, in addition to safer doses of oral contraceptives, would provide many accessible and affordable options for fertility control. The reduction in the use of barrier contraceptives, however, would increase concern about transmission of sexually transmitted diseases, including HIV.

In addition to technological advances, there were legal and policy victories for birth control. A significant victory in this regard occurred in New York City in 1957 when Dr. Louis M. Hellman fitted a severely diabetic postpartum woman with a diaphragm in violation of the policies of the commissioner of hospitals. The media had been notified in advance and the resulting coverage precipitated a policy change that allowed women to receive contraceptive counseling and devices in municipal hospitals in New York City (Hellman). Dr. Hellman went on to serve as deputy assistant secretary for population affairs in the Department of Health, Education and Welfare under President Nixon. He oversaw the Title X family planning initiatives that provided family planning services to five million women who desired them but could not afford them (Powderly).

The Supreme Court declared contraception a constitutional right for married couples in 1965 in the case of *Griswold v. Connecticut.* The Comstock laws were finally repealed in 1971 and the Supreme Court guaranteed a woman's right to abortion in *Roe v. Wade* in 1973. Women were now entitled to access to contraceptives and abortion services. This, however, did not ensure that they would have access. Some women did not have access to Title X funded services and could not afford contraceptives. Barriers to health care in general often extended to family planning services. For others, partners or spouses prohibited the use of desired contraceptives. Cultural and religious beliefs and prohibitions may also prove problematic. In addition, the fight against legalized abortion rages on and has escalated to violent outbursts that threaten the providers and users of abortion services. Coercion and social pressure may also result in women who do not desire contraception being forced to use them (Powderly).

Social and Political Issues

Numerous social and political issues have influenced fertility control in the modern world.

INTEREST GROUPS AND FAMILY PLANNING. *Providers of Family Planning Services.* Family planning services in the United States are offered by both private and public agencies. Public providers of family planning services at the local level include public health clinics in hospitals or neighborhood health centers, school-based clinics, Medicaid managed-care organizations and hospital-based clinics. At the county, state, regional and national levels, various

arms of government are involved with the setting of policy for these publicly supported clinics and in devising formulas to disburse funding. The major conduit for public funding of family planning services is Title X of the Public Health Act of 1970. Title X has never allowed funding for abortion services, however.

In the private sector, abortion and family planning services are offered both by for-profit and not-for-profit clinics, managed care organizations and by private physicians. The not-for-profit Planned Parenthood Federation of America, Inc., with affiliates across the country, continues to be one of the most important providers of family planning services in the private sector.

In theory, the public and private components of the family planning delivery system share similar goals: the dissemination of contraceptive services and education under a public health model, which includes the prevention of HIV infection and other sexually transmitted diseases as well as services specifically rendered to control fertility. The relationship between the public and private components is quite complicated and intertwined, however. Family planning services, like other publicly provided social services in the United States, are typically delivered through a system that relies at least partly on private agencies, or "subcontractors," rather than directly by the government itself.

In addition, family planning became intensely politicized in the United States after the election of Ronald Reagan in 1980. Since then, the agendas of public and private providers of family planning services have often been at odds. Difficulties with Title X-funded programs illustrate these contradictions. A significant proportion of Title X-funded services in many communities across the country is provided by Planned Parenthood, which is also a prime target of those who are politically conservative because of the organization's visibility as an abortion provider. Political appointees within the Department of Health and Human Services, which oversees Title X and related services, have, at times, been aligned with political groups committed to the defunding of this program, because of some conservatives' opposition to family planning programs. The number of publicly funded family planning programs and clinics across the country has declined; this decline reflects the bitter ideological wrangling over the concept of publicly funded family planning (Ettinger, 1992; Scott).

In 2002, nearly five million women received health care services at family planning clinics funded by Title X. They were predominantly young, poor, uninsured, and had never had a child. Seventy-one percent of women using Title X-funded clinics are 20 years of age or older and 63 percent are white. Sixty-five percent have incomes at or below the federal poverty level. It is estimated that these clinics are the only source of family planning services for more than 80 percent of the women they serve (AGI, 2002a; Kaeser et al; Planned Parenthood).

The Women's Movement. Since the re-emergence of a visible women's movement in the United States in the late 1960s, various groups associated with the movement have been forceful advocates for family planning and abortion services. The new feminists have demonstrated a keen interest in issues of reproductive rights and sexuality (Joffe, 1986). The campaign to make abortion legal and accessible was a major focus of the feminist movement in the 1960s. During the 1980s, when a woman's right to a legal and safe abortion was threatened, women's organizations played a highly visible role in pro-choice activities, working closely with such organizations as Planned Parenthood and the National Abortion Rights Action League.

With respect to other reproductive issues, however, the relation of sectors of the women's movement to its abortion allies has been more complex. At times, the responses of some feminist health activists to prevailing contraceptive practices and new contraceptive innovations have conflicted with sometime allies, such as Planned Parenthood. These activists, for example, raised doubts early on about the safety of oral contraceptives, objected to testing new contraceptive technologies on women in developing nations and, more recently, voiced reservations about the likely social abuses of Norplant, a long-acting, implantable contraceptive device (Seaman; Gordon, 1976; Moskowitz and Jennings).

The Pro-Family Movement. Beginning in the 1970s, a movement of sexual conservatism—the "pro-family" movement—became a significant presence in family planning politics (Petchesky; McKeegan). This movement's main concern has been the breakdown of sexual morality in contemporary society, as evidenced by high rates of abortion, adolescent pregnancy, out-of-wedlock births, and sexually-transmitted diseases. For sexual conservatives, widely available family planning services—especially those supported by public funds—represent a temptation to break with traditional morality (Marshner). Though the pro-family movement is most visible in anti-abortion activity, its interests and interventions extend to a broad range of reproductive and sexual matters—contraceptive services, sex education, adolescent pregnancy prevention efforts, and HIV prevention (Joffe, 1986; Nathanson).

Family planning services for adolescents have been a major focal point of pro-family activity (Joffe, 1993). Conservative activists have persuaded legislators in a number of states to adopt parental notification and consent rules for teenagers seeking abortions, and have sought regulations that would include parental notification policies for federally funded clinics providing contraceptive services.

The "gag-rule" controversy, which has spanned the presidencies of Ronald Reagan through George W. Bush, is further illustration of the efforts of conservatives to link attacks on abortion to those on family planning. Originally written as an administrative guideline during the Reagan administration, the gag rule forbade employees in Title X-funded family planning clinics to provide counseling about abortion options, even when women asked for such information. For many within the healthcare community and the public at large, this ruling raised concerns about free speech for health professionals. In the space of several years, the gag rule was upheld by the Supreme Court, overturned by congressional legislation, and promptly vetoed by George H.W. Bush, under intense pressure from conservatives. In one of his first acts after taking office in 1993, Bill Clinton abolished the gag rule, under similar pressure from the pro-choice and family planning communities. On his first day in office, George W. Bush restored the Reagan–era gag rule for international family planning programs. This is a pattern that is likely to continue, illustrating the strong relationship between politics and women's health issues, especially those involving fertility control (Planned Parenthood; RowBoat).

Welfare Conservatives. In contrast to the pro-family movement, whose defining issue is the breakdown of sexual morality and traditional families, "welfare conservatives" are concerned about the rising welfare costs resulting from adolescent pregnancies, illegitimate births and failure of fathers to make child support payments. Welfare conservatives have made a number of policy proposals that either mandate use of contraception as a condition of receiving welfare or other financial incentives for such contraceptive use, that penalize recipients financially for having additional children and that forbid adolescent mothers from receiving welfare assistance directly, providing instead that the grant go to their parents or guardians (Nathanson; Peirce).

The contraceptive implant, Norplant, introduced in the United States in 1990, quickly became implicated in a number of policies advocated by welfare conservatives. Once inserted, the implant prevents pregnancy for up to five years. Both the insertion and the removal, however, must be done by a trained health professional. After the insertion, no further "user compliance" is required, making this a far more effective contraceptive device than other birth control methods. Within eighteen months of the introduction into the United States of this new method, virtually all states approved the public funding of Norplant insertion for welfare recipients. The potential for coercion is evident. There have been instances where judges have required Norplant use as a condition of probation or child custody for women convicted on drug-related charges or of child abuse (Forrest and Kaeser). Provision of access to Norplant for adolescents has also raised ethical concerns (Moskowitz and Jennings). In addition, lack of access to providers trained to remove the implant may restrict choice for some women.

SERVICES TO POTENTIALLY VULNERABLE POPULATIONS. *Minority Communities.* Minority communities in the United States have long had a wary relationship with family planning advocates and services. The previously cited historical links between the founders of the birth control movement, such as Margaret Sanger, and those in the eugenics movement with an avowedly racist ideology created a lasting sense of distrust in minority communities as to the intentions of some within the family planning movement (Chesler; Gordon, 1976). Such distrust reached a height in the late 1960s and early 1970s when many of the Title X clinics appeared to be targeted specifically at African-Americans, leading some African-American leaders to accuse family planners of "genocidal" intentions (Littlewood). More recently, some community leaders—most notably, black clergy—have joined forces with the pro-family movement, arguing against such measures as condom distribution in inner-city high schools and offering Norplant to adolescent mothers (Moskowitz and Jennings).

At the same time, the rates of premarital sexual activity, sexually-transmitted diseases, adolescent pregnancy and abortion have been disproportionately higher for minorities than for others. Thus, there is a need for culturally-sensitive family planning and abortion services, and many minority organizations argue forcefully for their retention and expansion.

Adolescents. In the early 1990s, adolescents were entitled to receive low-cost or free confidential contraceptive services at Title X sites. Adolescents, as a group, did not receive any public funds for abortion. The field of adolescent medicine recognizes the need to provide education and family planning services to sexually active adolescents (American Academy of Pediatrics, 1999). The rising rates of sexual activity among adolescents, particularly young adolescents, has increased concern within the family planning community about adolescent pregnancy and this group's vulnerability to HIV and other sexually-transmitted diseases (Alan Guttmacher Institute, 1991). In the 1980s, a major response to both these issues was the establishment of school-based clinics on the theory that while few teens would make their way to a free-standing clinic, clinics located within the school would reach a much larger public. Programs were also established for pregnant adolescents and those with children to try to keep them in school. Predictably, such school-based programs were controversial from the start, strongly opposed by conservatives and just as strongly advocated by health professionals and public health advocates (Kirby et al; Moskowitz and Jennings).

A number of school districts, particularly those in large urban areas, began distributing condoms to students in response to the HIV epidemic. There has been massive controversy here as well, with many parent and church groups opposing such efforts. Generally speaking, however, HIV-related interventions in schools seem to be more acceptable to the public and to educators than specific efforts for pregnancy prevention. A national study of sex education in U.S. schools in the late 1980s found far more attention paid to HIV and sexually-transmitted diseases than to family planning education (Forrest and Silverman). While most would advocate abstinence for adolescents, particularly young ones, the alarming rate of unprotected sexual activity in this age group warrants realistic education and confidential access to safe, appropriate family planning services.

In October of 1998, there was an attempt to pass legislation restricting minor's access to family planning services. The proposed amendment would have mandated that parents of dependent adolescents be notified before their children received contraceptives from Title X-funded clinics (Congressional Record). Supporters of parental consent feel that available, confidential family planning services encourage sexual activity in adolescents and undermine parental authority. However, research has demonstrated that confidentiality is crucial to teens' willingness to seek services related to sexuality (American Academy of Pediatrics, 1999; Reddy et al; Planned Parenthood). Moreover, Planned Parenthood states that the fact that the average teen does not visit a family planning clinic until 14 months after she has become sexually active provides clear evidence that clinics do not encourage sexual activity. Requiring parental consent may not deter adolescents from having sex, but it could keep them from seeking reproductive health care in a timely fashion or at all. This could contribute to an increased rate of pregnancies as well as sexually transmitted diseases (AGI, 2000; Planned Parenthood). While the 1998 amendment was not passed, there is an ongoing attempt by political conservatives to fight access to family planning services for adolescents and even punish them for having sex. In a recent NYC case, a group of eighth graders who skipped school to attend a party where they allegedly had sex were forced to submit to pregnancy and other gynecological testing and to provide the results before they could return to school. A suit has been filed on their behalf by the New York Civil Liberties Union (Williams).

Services to the Disabled. Case law in the United States generally recognizes that developmentally disabled individuals have the same fundamental rights regarding procreative choice as those who are not disabled. There are, however, difficulties in implementing family planning services for disabled persons. The issue of informed consent for mentally disabled individuals is particularly relevant and remains ethically problematic. Is the individual capable of giving informed consent, and if not, who is the appropriate surrogate empowered to make such decisions (Stavis).

In spite of legal decisions supporting provision of such services, relatively few disabled persons are served in Title X clinics (Moore and Lieber). Few clinic staffs have received the specialized training necessary to work effectively with this population. In addition, many caretakers, particularly parents, have difficulty dealing with sexuality in this population and are reluctant to ensure that these individuals receive such services. In addition, disabled individuals and caretakers are often not aware of the entitlement of the disabled to family planning services, which implies a need for more outreach to this population.

In light of the compulsory sterilization programs of the past, the major ethical conflict regarding sterilization today is balancing the rights of a mentally retarded or mentally disabled person to sexual freedom with a protection of their best interests regarding childbearing. Many writings deal with the sterilization of the mentally retarded who are somewhat incapacitated or even totally incapable of giving informed consent (Macklin and Gaylin). The Committee on Ethics of the American College of Obstetricians and Gynecologists has issued a statement on "Sterilization of Women Who Are Mentally Handicapped," which urges all possible attempts to communicate with the person involved on whatever level is possible. Even in cases where it is clear that the individual has no ability to comprehend a pregnancy and childbirth and may be harmed by the experience, it is difficult to obtain a court order for sterilization because of the history of abuses. Perhaps it is more beneficent to take the middle ground in these cases. While routine sterilization of a mentally impaired individual without her consent is clearly wrong, restricting the sexual expression of a profoundly impaired individual who cannot comprehend her sexuality, much less pregnancy or coitus-related conception, is also not justified. In carefully considered circumstances, advocates for the patient may conclude that sterilization is in the patient's best interest. The decision should be made by an appropriate surrogate or proxy, based on the best interests of the patient after considering alternative methods of dealing with the situation. The prominence of this issue in the Senate confirmation hearings of Dr. Henry Foster as Surgeon General in the Clinton administration illustrates the importance of this issue and the lack of societal consensus (Powderly, 1996).

Religious and Moral Issues

Most people today, along with philosophical ethicists, religious ethicists and organized religions, generally accept the morality of contraception within marriage, often appealing to the need for family planning. While recognizing a link between marital sexuality and procreation, many concede that marital sexuality also has other significant purposes such as expressing and enhancing the love union of the partners and thereby the good of the marriage. Unlimited procreation, or at times any procreation, could be harmful to one of the spouses, the marriage itself, the good of already existing children or the needs of the broader society. Judgments about the ethical use of contraception outside of marriage depends upon one's understanding of the morality of extramarital sexual activity. As a matter of fact, many unmarried people today are sexually active. Indeed, the majority of adolescents in the United States have had sexual intercourse by the time they are nineteen years old (Demetriou and Kaplan; American Academy of Pediatrics).

Many feminists emphasize reproductive rights, freedom, control of one's body and autonomy to support their stand that women have the right to make contraceptive decisions in all cases (Harrison). Although society at large in the United States no longer condemns all extramarital sexuality as immoral and irresponsible, the mainstream churches and religions still generally maintain the immorality of sexual relations outside marriage (Lebacqz). The use of condoms enters into the discussion of extramarital sexuality not only because of the desire to prevent procreation, but also because condoms can help to prevent the transmission of HIV and other sexually-transmitted diseases. If one believes that extramarital sexual relations are morally responsible, then the use of contraception to prevent unwanted procreation is morally acceptable.

No perfect contraception exists, but most ethical reasoning sees no significant moral differences among the various means, provided they are not harmful to the individuals who use them or others. One could justify contraception on the basis of an absolute autonomy, giving the individual control over her body and the right to make all decisions concerning it, but most justifications of family planning, which by definition concerns more than the individual, avoid such a radical individual autonomy. The official teaching of the Roman Catholic church constitutes the strongest and the primary contemporary moral opposition to the use of contraception.

The widespread moral acceptance of contraception has taken place well within the twentieth century. Individuals do not make moral judgments in the abstract. As indicated previously, a number of significant social factors have influenced the acceptance of contraceptive practices. These include the increased life expectancy of all human beings, the massive improvements in infant and child health resulting in more survival, the realities and pressures of an increasingly urban and industrialized society, the changing role and function of women in society, the wider and more accurate understanding of the physiology of human reproduction, the recognition of the population explosion and the need to limit population, and the development of accessible, effective methods of contraception.

The Christian religions have played a significant role in ethical views on contraception in the West. The ancient world of both East and West knew the reality of contraception either by avoiding insemination of the female or by using potions or magic. In the Greco-Roman world, some philosophers and physicians apparently accepted attempts at contraception. On the other hand, the Roman Empire tended to encourage childbearing. Some influential philosophers insisted that procreation constituted the only purpose of sexual intercourse and thus, logically condemned contraception. The Hebrew scriptures contain no law condemning contraception.

The Christian approach to contraception also developed in a context in which contraception was associated with prostitution and extramarital sexuality, which Christians strongly opposed. In addition, early potions used for contraception (and some modern methods such as IUDs) could not clearly be differentiated from abortifacients and abortion was even less tolerable than contraception. The Christian condemnation of contraception followed from its understanding of human sexuality and the belief that the purpose of sexuality was procreation. Some medieval theologians and their successors, however, including Thomas Aquinas, maintained that procreation was not the only lawful purpose for sexuality, at least within marriage. The church, for example, accepted the marital sexuality of the sterile and those no longer able to procreate. The procreation of offspring also included the responsibility for the well-being and education of the children—some would extend this to justify not having so many children that you could not care for the pre-existing ones. However, the condemnation of contraception remained, with emphasis on its violation of the order of nature calling for the depositing of the male seed in the vagina of the female. This nature-based rationale also served as the basis for the condemnation of sodomy, oral and anal sex, and masturbation. This view is closely related to the Hebrew prohibition on "spilling" seed.

Although some Protestant laypersons were involved in the Anglo-Saxon countries, the Christian churches remained firm in their condemnation of artificial contraception, as distinguished from abstinence, well into the twentieth century. The Church of England became the first Christian church to accept officially the morality of artificial contraception for spouses. In 1930, the Lambeth Conference, by a vote of 193 to 67, adopted a resolution recognizing a moral obligation to limit or avoid parenthood and proposing complete abstinence as the primary and most obvious way while also accepting other methods (Fagley).

The Committee on Marriage and Home of the U.S. Federal Council of Churches issued an influential statement in 1931 in which the majority of its members accepted the careful and restrained use of contraception by spouses. Subsequently, the major Protestant churches and the most significant Protestant theological ethicists accepted contraception as a way to ensure responsible parenthood. The proponents of change pointed to aspects in the Christian tradition supporting such a move. Christians had gradually come to recognize the loving or unitive aspect of marital sexuality in addition to the procreative aspect. The procreative aspect itself included not only the procreation but also the education of offspring. This called for the good health of the parents. Protestantism justified the use of contraception as a way for spouses to realize responsible parenthood (Fagley).

Roman Catholic official teachings continue to steadfastly oppose artificial contraception, even within marriage. Some Catholic theologians have advocated the use of the infertile period for sexual intercourse, or the rhythm method. In 1951, Pope Pius XII taught that serious medical, eugenic, economic and social indications justified the use of the sterile periods even on a permanent basis. Unfortunately, the rhythm method often proves to be a rather ineffective method of contraception. This can have devastating consequences, especially if there are serious medical contraindications to pregnancy. Pope John XXIII and Pope Paul VI established a commission to study the question. The majority of the commission favored changing the teaching to allow for artificial contraception, but Pope Paul VI and Pope John Paul II have reiterated an absolute condemnation of artificial contraception. In *Humanae Vitae,* Paul VI states that the natural law "teaches that each and every marriage act must remain open to the transmission of life" and refers to "the inseparable connection, willed by God and unable to be broken by man on his own initiative, between the two meanings of the conjugal act: the unitive and the procreative meaning" (Paul VI). In practice, the vast majority of Catholic couples use contraception (Curran). The Catholic Church's continued prohibition of any method of artificial contraception is especially problematic in poor, overpopulated developing countries with large Catholic populations. In such countries, uncurtailed childbearing can have dire consequences for women and children.

The Catholic Church also opposes voluntary sterilization for contraceptive purposes. As far as therapeutic sterilization is concerned, the principle of double effect is generally applied. Therapeutic sterilization is that done for the good or health of the individual and not primarily for contraceptive purposes. Direct sterilization is that which aims at making procreation impossible either as a means or as an end and is always considered wrong. Indirect sterilization aims directly at the health or good of the individual and the actual procreative effect is secondary. Thus, a cancerous uterus can be removed, but hysterectomy to prevent harm to the pregnant woman would be considered direct and morally wrong (Boyle).

The fact that there is little or no discussion of punitive sterilization in the more recent literature hints at a consensus against the practice. However, Francis Hurth, a conservative Roman Catholic theologian in the 1930s, proposed limited cases in which punitive sterilization might be justified. Pope Pius XI went out of his way not to directly condemn punitive sterilization. This is interesting in light of the absolute prohibition on sterilization for contraceptive purposes in women desperate to limit the size of their families. Proponents of punitive sterilization maintain that if the state can inflict capital punishment for certain crimes, it can also inflict the lesser punishment of sterilization in limited, appropriate cases. Critics reply that punitive sterilization does not achieve the purposes of punishment and does not even inhibit future sex crimes (McCarthy). Punitive sterilization is virtually unsupported (Mason).

Other religious bodies today generally support artificial contraception in the context of responsible parenthood. The Eastern Orthodox church accepts responsible contraception while condemning abortion and infanticide. The multiple purposes of marriage, the lack of any definitive statement against contraception by the church, a synergistic cooperation between God and humans, and the need for responsible parenthood serve as the basis for the responsible use of contraception within marriage (Harakas; Zaphiris).

Orthodox Judaism gives a limited acceptance to some forms of contraception. Jewish law puts the duty of procreation on the male, and this obligation militates against the use of condoms or coitus interruptus. In this view, the most acceptable contraception is that which interferes the least with the natural sex act (Rosner). Conservative and Reform Judaism fully accept and endorse contraception provided it is not harmful to the parties involved.

Islam accepts contraception if it does not entail the radical separation of procreation from marriage. All forms of contraception are acceptable provided they are not harmful and do not involve abortion. Justification for contraception in Islam rests on reports that the Prophet Muhammad did not forbid the contraceptive practices of some of his companions (Hathout).

Ancient Hindu medicine and Hindu tradition did not contemplate contraception, but did sanction means to enhance contraception. In time, medical texts began to address contraception by advising a few oral preparations to prevent conception. When India embarked on a national family planning program after its independence in 1947, the discussions accepted the morality of contraception, but the main focus was the relative population size of the higher and lower castes (Desai).

Contemporary popular morality—the behavior and values of ordinary people—as well as contemporary philosophy, theological ethics, and religious bodies (with the major exception of the Roman Catholicism), accept the morality of contraception for spouses in practicing responsible parenthood. General agreement exists that on the microlevel of the family, the decision about contraception should be made by the spouses themselves in the light of their own health, the good of their marriage, the education and formation of their children, and population and environmental needs, both local and global (Curran). In fact, with the exception of those who are politically conservative and/or pro-family, most accept the right to fertility control even for those who are unmarried.

International Population Control

The highly politicized nature of family planning in the United States has had major implications for the developing world. In response to pressures by conservatives, the emphasis of U.S. population programs abroad shifted heavily to programs promoting natural family planning rather than the more reliable methods of artificial contraception. Most notably, the "Mexico City policy" adopted by the Reagan administration in 1984 stipulated that no U.S. aid would go to any international organizations that supported abortion, even if the U.S. funds were separated and used only for nonabortion services. The Mexico City policy was overturned in the early days of the Clinton administration in 1993, thus renewing a commitment on the part of the United States to international family planning efforts after a period of marked decline. The policy again became an issue in the administration of George W. Bush who withheld $34 million in funding for birth control, maternal and child health care and HIV prevention from the United Nations Population Fund in 2002 (Rosenberg; Planned Parenthood; UNFPA Funding Act, 2003). The loss of U.S. funding has a grave impact on UNFPA programs and the people they serve. UNFPA estimated that the $34 million loss would lead to two million unwanted pregnancies, 800,000 induced abortions, 4,700 maternal deaths, and 77,000 infant and child deaths. Restoration of U.S. funding would also save lives through HIV prevention campaigns. The $34 million would provide one-third of the annual needs for mass HIV prevention information campaigns aimed at behavior change. It would also cover the cost of 13 per cent of the condoms needed worldwide to prevent sexually transmitted infections, including HIV. President Bush also reversed the U.S. position in support of the 1994 global agreement that affirmed the right of all couples and individuals to determine freely and responsibly the number and spacing of their children and to have the information and means to do so (United Nations; RowBoat). Walking a political tightrope, he then announced major programs to deal with HIV infection abroad.

Family planning issues are an increasingly high priority for many developing nations. Concerns about the ability to feed rapidly growing populations, the dramatic spread of HIV infection and AIDS in the Third World, especially in parts of Africa, Asia, and Eastern Europe, and the large number of deaths that occur each year from illegal abortions create constituencies for family planning services within these countries. There are, of course, also often significant religious and cultural objections.

The rise of indigenous women's movements in the developing world has also served as a particularly important stimulus for additional family planning services which must be provided in a culturally sensitive manner (Bruce; Dixon-Mueller). The International Women's Health Coalition has been one of the most successful international population groups in terms of its ability to work closely with local, grass roots women's organizations in the design and delivery of family planning programs.

Current and Future Controversies

The future of accessible family planning services in the United States and abroad is unclear. During the administration of Bill Clinton, the influence of political conservatives in public policy debates about family planning was greatly diminished. Clinton's appointments to key health policy positions of individuals strongly committed to family planning, especially in the area of adolescent pregnancy prevention, sharply reversed the trends of the Reagan-Bush era.

Ideological battles were temporarily muted, but they will never entirely disappear because of a change in presidential administration. At the state and local levels, many of the bitter struggles over the public provision of reproductive health services continued. Bill Clinton attempted to reform health care in general and largely failed. The election of George W. Bush signaled an immediate return to the ideologically conservative policies of his father.

The abortion issue remains among the most politically explosive and unresolved issues in bioethics. Provision of abortion services has endangered funding for other family planning services and endangered the lives of providers and consumers alike. Concerns of political conservatives and anti-abortion groups have affected policy debates as diverse as end of life decision-making in New York State and Federal regulation of embryonic stem cell research. In August of 2002, George Bush revealed his decision on stem cell research. Had it not been for the terrorist attacks that occurred shortly thereafter, stem cells might have been the defining issue of his presidency. Bush allowed future work with stem cell lines already produced, but his policy did not allow for the development of additional cell lines. By sitting on the fence, Bush did not satisfy either side in the debate. Anti-abortion forces were not happy that the existing cell lines, obtained from aborted fetuses, would still be used. Those in favor of stem cell research did not think that the existing cell lines would be adequate to study the possible benefits of stem cells for those with diseases such as Parkinson's Disease, Alzheimer's Disease, and diabetes.

The historical context is important for the current ethical and policy debates related to fertility control. Efforts to empower all women, including poor women of color, must be balanced with a keen sense of the abuses evident in the history of the birth control movement. Racism and eugenic concerns have been consistent issues in debates about controlling fertility, and our targeted educational programs and initiatives must be sensitive to community concerns. Empowering women to make their own reproductive choices is a praiseworthy goal, but it is not a desirable one for some.

KATHLEEN E. POWDERLY

SEE ALSO: *Abortion; AIDS: Public Health Issues; Autonomy; Coercion; Conscience, Rights of; Embryo and Fetus; Eugenics; Family and Family Medicine; Genetic Testing and Screening: Reproductive Genetic Screening; Infanticide; International Health; Law and Morality; Maternal-Fetal Relationship; Natural Law; Population Ethics: Religious Traditions; and other Fertility Control subentries*

BIBLIOGRAPHY

Alan Guttmacher Institute. 1991. *Facts in Brief: Teenage Sexual and Reproductive Behavior in the United States.* New York: Carole Joffe.

Alan Guttmacher Institute. 2000. *Fulfilling the Promise: Public Policy and U.S. Family Planning Clinics.* New York: Author.

Alan Guttmacher Institute. 2002a. *Family Planning Annual Report: 2001 Summary.* Submitted to the Office of Population Affairs, Department of Health and Human Services. New York: Author.

American Academy of Pediatrics. Committee on Adolescence. 1990. "Contraception and Adolescents." *Pediatrics* 86(1): 134–138.

American Academy of Pediatrics. Committee on Adolescence. 1999. "Contraception and Adolescents." *Pediatrics* 104(5): 1161–1166.

American College of Obstetricians and Gynecologists. Committee on Ethics. 1988. "Sterilization of Women Who Are Mentally Handicapped." Committee Opinion 63. Washington, D. C.: Author.

Boyle, John P. 1977. *The Sterilization Controversy: A New Crisis for the Catholic Hospital?* New York: Paulist Press.

Brodie, Janet F. 1994. *Contraception and Abortion in 19th Century America.* Ithaca: Cornell University Press.

Bruce, Judith. 1987. "Users' Perspectives on Contraceptive Technology and Delivery Systems: Highlighting Some Feminist Issues." *Technology and Society* 9(3–4): 359–383.

Chesler, Ellen. 1992. *Woman of Valor: Margaret Sanger and the Birth Control Movement in America.* New York: Simon and Schuster.

Congressional Record (Online). 1998. 105th Cong., 2d sess. (8 October 1998).

Curran, Charles E. 1979. *Transition and Tradition in Moral Theology.* Notre Dame: University of Notre Dame Press.

Demetriou, Efstratios, and Kaplan, David W. 1989. "Adolescent Contraceptive Use and Parental Notification." *American Journal of Diseases of Children* 143(10): 1166–1172.

Desai, Prakash N. 1991. "Hinduism and Bioethics in India: A Tradition in Transition." In *Theological Developments in Bioethics: 1988–1990,* pp. 41–60, ed. Baruch A. Brody, B. Andrew Lustig, H. Tristram Engelhardt, Jr., and Laurence McCullough. *Bioethics Yearbook,* vol. 1. Dordrecht, Netherlands: Kluwer.

Dixon-Mueller, Ruth. 1993. *Population Policy and Women's Rights: Transforming Reproductive Choice.* Westport, CT: Praeger.

Dugdale, R. L. 1877. *The Jukes: A Study in Crime, Pauperism, Disease and Heredity.* New York: G.P. Putnam & Sons.

Fagley, Richard M. 1960. *The Population Explosion and Christian Responsibility.* New York: Oxford University Press.

Forrest, Jacqueline D., and Kaeser, Lisa. 1993. "Questions of Balance: Issues Emerging from the Introduction of the Hormonal Implant." *Family Planning Perspectives* 25(3): 127–132.

Forrest, Jacqueline D., and Silverman, Jane. 1989. "What Public School Teachers Teach About Preventing Pregnancy, AIDS, and Sexually Transmitted Diseases." *Family Planning Perspectives* 21(2): 65–72.

Gordon, Linda. 1976. *Women's Body, Women's Right: A Social History of Birth Control in America.* New York: Grossman.

Gordon, Linda. 1981. *Woman's Body, Woman's Right: Birth Control in America.* New York: Penguin.

Griswold v. Connecticut, 381 U.S. 479 (1965).

Harakas, Stanley Samuel. 1991. "Eastern Orthodox Bioethics." In *Theological Developments in Bioethics, 1988–1990,* pp. 85–101, ed. Baruch A. Brody, B. Andrew Lustig, H. Tristram Engelhardt, Jr., and Laurence McCullough. *Bioethics Yearbook,* vol. 1. Dordrecht, Netherlands: Kluwer.

Harrison, Beverly Wildung. 1985. *Making the Connections: Essays in Feminist Social Ethics,* ed. Carol S. Robb. Boston: Beacon Press.

Hathout, Hassan. 1991. "Islamic Concepts and Bioethics." In *Theological Developments in Bioethics: 1988–1990,* pp. 103–117, ed. Baruch A. Brody, B. Andrew Lustig, H. Tristram Engelhardt, Jr., and Laurence McCullough. *Bioethics Yearbook,* vol. 1. Dordrecht, Netherlands: Kluwer.

Hellman, Louis M. 1971. "Family Planning Comes of Age." *American Journal of Obstetrics and Gynecology* 109(2): 214–224.

Joffe, Carole E. 1986. *The Regulation of Sexuality: Experiences of Family Planning Workers.* Philadelphia: Temple University Press.

Joffe, Carole E. 1993. "Sexual Politics and the Teenage Pregnancy Prevention Worker in the United States." In *The Politics of Pregnancy,* pp. 289–300, ed. Annette Lawson and Deborah L. Rhode. New Haven, CT: Yale University Press.

Kaeser, Lisa, et al. 1996. *Title X at 25: Balancing National Family Planning Needs with State Flexibility.* New York: Alan Guttmacher Institute.

Kirby, Douglas; Waszak, Cynthia; and Ziegler, Julie. 1991. "Six School-Based Clinics: Their Reproductive Health Services and Impact on Sexual Behavior." *Family Planning Perspectives* 23(1): 6–16.

La Sorte, M.A. 1976. "Nineteenth Century Family Planning Practices." *Journal of Psychohistory* (4): 163–183.

Lebacqz, Karen. 1978. "Sterilization: Ethical Aspects." In *Encylcopedia of Bioethics,* vol. 4, pp. 1609–1613, ed. Warren T. Reich. New York: Macmillan.

Littlewood, Thomas B. 1977. *The Politics of Population Control.* Notre Dame, IN: University of Notre Dame Press.

Lombardo, Paul. 2003. "Facing Carrie Buck." *Hastings Center Report* 33(2): 14–17.

Lungren, S. S. 1881. "A Case of Caesarean Section Twice Successfully Performed on the Same Patient." *American Journal of Obstetrics* (14): 78.

Macklin, Ruth, and Gaylin, Willard, eds. 1981. *Mental Retardation and Sterilization: A Problem of Competency and Paternalism.* New York: Plenum.

Malthus, Thomas R. 1993. *An Essay on the Principle of Population.* New York: Oxford University Press.

Marshner, Connaught C. 1982. *The New Traditional Woman.* Washington, D.C.: Free Congress Research and Education Foundation.

Mason, John Kenyon. 1990. *Medico-Legal Aspects of Reproduction and Parenthood.* Brookfield, VT: Dartmouth.

McCarthy, John. 1960. *The Commandments,* vol. 2 of *Problems in Theology.* Westminster, MD: Newman.

Mckeegan, Michele. 1992. *Abortion Politics: Mutiny in the Ranks of the Right.* New York: Free Press.

Moore, Melinda, and Lieber, Carolyn. 1988. *Assessing Reproductive Health-Care Services: An Assessment of Service Availability to Learning and Developmentally Disabled Individuals Through Title X-Funded Clinics.* Washington, D.C.: Polaris Research and Development.

Moskowitz, Ellen, and Jennings, Bruce, eds. 1996. *Coerced Contraception? Moral and Policy Challenges of Long-Acting Birth Control.* Washington, D.C.: Georgetown University Press.

Nathanson, Constance A. 1991. *Dangerous Passage: The Social Control of Sexuality in Women's Adolescence.* Philadelphia: Temple University Press.

Paul VI. 1968. "Humanae vitae." *Acta Apostolicae Sedis* 60: 481–503. Translated under the title "Humanae Vitae (Human Life)." *Catholic Mind* 66 (September 30, 1968): 35–48.

Peirce, Neal. 1992. "Cold Approaches to a Hot-Button Issue." *National Journal* 24(15): 890.

Petchesky, Rosalind P. 1990. *Abortion and Woman's Choice: The State, Sexuality, and Reproductive Freedom,* rev. edition. Boston: Northeastern University Press.

Powderly, Kathleen E. 1996. "Contraceptive Policy and Ethics: Lessons from American History." In *Coerced Contraception? Moral and Policy Challenges of Long-Acting Birth Control,* pp. 23–33, ed. Ellen Moskowitz and Bruce Jennings. Washington, D.C.: Georgetown University Press.

Reddy, Diane, et al. 2002. "Effect of Mandatory Parental Notification on Adolescent Girls' Use of Sexual Health Care Services." *Journal of the American Medical Association* 288(6): 710–714.

Reilly, Philip R. 1991. *The Surgical Solution.* Baltimore: The Johns Hopkins University Press.

Roe V. Wade, 410 U.S. 113 (1973).

Rosenberg, Debra. "Another Round in the Abortion Wars." *Newsweek,* January 22, 2002.

Rosner, Fred. 1979. "Contraception in Jewish Law." In *Jewish Bioethics,* pp. 86–96, ed. Fred Rosner and J. David Bleich. New York: Sanhedrin.

Sanger, Margaret. 1931. *My Fight for Birth Control.* New York: Farrar Rinehart.

Sanger, Margaret. 1938. *Margaret Sanger: An Autobiography.* New York: W.W. Norton.

Scott, Jenny. "Public Funding for Family Planning Drops." *Los Angeles Times,* September 27, 1991, p. A33.

Seaman, Barbara. 1969. *The Doctor's Case Against the Pill.* New York: Avon.

Sherwin, Susan. 1992. *No Longer Patient: Feminist Ethics and Health Care.* Philadelphia: Temple University Press.

Siegler, A.M., and Grunebaum, A. 1980. "The 100th Anniversary of Tubal Sterilization." *Fertility and Sterility* 34: 610.

Stavis, Paul F. 1991. "Harmonizing the Right to Sexual Expression and the Right to Protection from Harm for Persons with Mental Disability." *Sexuality and Disability* 9(2): 131–141.

United Nations. 1991. *The World's Women, 1970–1990: Trends and Statistics.* New York: Carole Joffe.

United Nations Population Fund (UNFPA) Funding Act of 2003. H.R., 108th Cong., 1st Sess.

Wardell, Dorothy. 1980. "Margaret Sanger: Birth Control's Successful Revolutionary." *American Journal of Public Health* 70(7): 736–742.

Williams, Joe. "Girls Penalized for Sex?: School Made 'em Squirm, Suit Says." *New York Daily News,* July 10, 2003.

Zaphiris, Chrysostom. 1974. "The Morality of Contraception: An Eastern Orthodox Opinion." *Journal of Ecumenical Studies* 11(4): 661–675.

INTERNET RESOURCES

Planned Parenthood. 2003. *America's Family Planning Program: Title X., The United Nations Population Fund.,* and *The Impact of the Global Gag Rule.* Available from <www.plannedparenthood.org>.

Row Boat. 2003. *George W. Bush's War on Women.* Available from <http://bopuc.levendis.com/RowBoat/archives/-2003/03/16>.

III. LEGAL AND REGULATORY ISSUES

The ability to control fertility depends on available technology, moral and religious acceptability, and legal permissibility or the threat of sanction. The major fertility-control mechanisms are contraception and sterilization and, when neither is used or the chosen method fails, abortion. The mechanical and physiological characteristics of each method determine the ease and comfort of individual use, the likelihood of success, and the potential for coercion.

In many cultures men view children as proof of virility and power. They see attempts by women to limit or terminate pregnancy as an attack on male authority and reproductive potential, which in many societies equals wealth. For many women a desire to limit pregnancy must often be pursued furtively, with fear of violence and retaliation. Biology and the threat to a woman's independence, health status, and well-being make the control of fertility primarily a woman's concern. A woman's ability to limit and control her fertility may be a necessary precondition for equality and personal economic status.

Because they affect relationships between the sexes, population growth, and a woman's status, contraception, sterilization, and abortion are and have been problematic for many societies. Secular societies committed to individual rights and liberties are less likely to intervene in reproductive decisions. But all societies to some degree attempt to influence individual reproductive choices.

History of Contraception Use and Control

GENERAL. Various societies have interceded for centuries in the free use of contraception, largely for moral and/or religious reasons. Classical Islam permitted the use of birth control and even early abortion (Fathalla et al.). Biblical Judaism, based on interpretations of the story of Onan in Genesis 38: 8–10, condemned *coitus interruptus* and the use of male condoms. Christianity gradually evolved a doctrine, based on biblical references, interpretations of natural law, and the writings of Saint Augustine (354–430), that prohibited use of all contraceptive devices (St. John-Stevas). Widespread, class-linked knowledge of contraceptive practices was effectively withheld from most of the population following the condemnation of birth control by philosopher and religious Thomas Aquinas (1224 [or 1225]–1274) in the mid-thirteenth century (Fathalla et al.). As religion formed part of the basis for modern secular law, control of fertility became a subject of legal attention and regulation.

Abortion, as a method of fertility control, has always been especially controversial. Despite its morally and legally complex past and its tendentious present, there is evidence today that abortion remains a favored method of birth control for many women, both as a preferred method of fertility control and as a backup to failed contraception. An estimated 46 million abortions are performed worldwide each year (Alan Guttmacher Institute). Unintended pregnancy is the leading cause of abortion. Approximately 150 million married women want to stop having children but are not using contraception (World Health Organization [WHO]). In the United States, where contraception is readily available, 49 percent of pregnancies are unintended (Henshaw). The United States Center for Disease Control (CDC) reported 884, 273 legal induced abortions in 1998, a ratio of 264 abortions per 1,000 live births.

While contraception and abortion address the prevention or termination of any specific pregnancy, sterilization terminates individual fecundity. With the development of modern, comparatively safe, and effective means of sterilization (vasectomy, or surgical excision of the duct carrying sperm from the testicles; and salpingectomy, or surgical removal of one or both fallopian tubes), individuals can choose, by means of one medical intervention, to detach

sexual intercourse from reproductive consequences. If chosen by individuals, these simple and almost always irreversible interventions extend autonomy; if imposed by the state, they can become instruments of repression.

Whether contraception, sterilization, and abortion should be permitted, prohibited, or coerced by government has generated intense controversy in countries as different as the United States, Romania, India, Ireland, and China. In each country, legislators, judges, individuals, and special-interest lobbies have struggled to affect how citizens will think about their options for controlling fertility, how the individual decision-making process will be informed and supervised, how access to contraception, abortion, and sterilization will be ensured or precluded, and whether coercion will be encouraged, permitted, or prohibited (Weston; Thomas).

Both female and male condoms have been available for centuries. Roman women attempted to use goat bladders (Fathalla et al.), and some African women hollowed out okra pods (Robertson). A picture of a penile sheath is recorded as early as 1350 B.C.E., although male condoms did not come into general use in Europe until 1671 and became reliable only with the vulcanization of rubber in 1843 (Robertson). Monitoring and prohibiting use of birth-control devices such as condoms are difficult because of the inherently private nature of their use. Manufacture, distribution, sale, and advertising are more easily regulated and prohibited.

Despite the long history and the private nature of fertility control, various legal and theological systems have attempted prohibition. The early Christian (Roman Catholic and Protestant) argument against contraception, influential as the model for legal regulation, holds that God's purpose for sex is conservation of the species, which is frustrated when people have intercourse for nonprocreative purposes (St. John-Stevas). The Catholic Church first proscribed contraception in canon law in 1140 (St. John-Stevas). While not all religions have been as resistant to the idea of contraception as the Catholic Church, contraceptive use has traditionally been considered an appropriate area for moral guidance and proscription and not until the beginning of the twentieth century did significant numbers of Protestant theologians provide moral approval (Larson).

Religious regulation has been selective. Some forms of birth control were interdicted, while others were and have remained relatively unnoticed. In addition prolonged lactation, postpartum abstinence, delayed marriage, celibacy, and to some extent infanticide, are all techniques of fertility management that have been and continue to be used.

U.S. HISTORY. Puritan theology dominated the early American colonists. The Puritans considered sex-related matters part of the devil's province, to be shunned and ignored, and they tolerated little open discussion (Robertson). In the 1830s some popular literature on contraception, such as Robert Dale Owen's *Moral Physiology,* began to be generally available (Robertson, Reed). Not until 1873 did law begin regulating distribution of contraceptives in the United States. The Comstock Act ("An Act for the Suppression of Trade in, and Circulation of, Obscene Literature and Articles of Immoral Use") equated contraception with obscenity and made it a federal offense to use the postal service for transporting obscene materials, defined to include contraceptive and abortion information and equipment. The act also banned importation and interstate transportation of such items (Sloan). After the act's passage, many states adopted their own regulations on the sale, advertising, and display of contraceptive devices.

Margaret Sanger, a nurse affected by her work in poor communities where morbidity (the incidence of disease) and mortality from abortion was high, was a vociferous advocate for birth control (Reed; *People v. Sanger,* 1918). She founded a monthly magazine, *The Woman Rebel,* for which she was arrested and indicted under the Comstock Act. She fled to Europe and returned in 1916 to establish the first American birth-control clinic in Brooklyn, a borough of New York City (Chessler). In 1918 she was convicted and sentenced to thirty days in the workhouse under New York State's Comstock law. Years later a physician in one of Margaret Sanger's clinics who had ordered a package of contraceptives through the mail was charged with violating the Tariff Act of 1930, a statute based on the Comstock Act that prohibited importation of "any article whatever for the prevention of conception or for causing unlawful abortion." On appeal the federal circuit court for the second circuit held that the act did not apply when the article imported was not intended for an immoral purpose. Judge Augustus Hand declared that the Tariff Act was part of a "continuous scheme to suppress immoral articles and obscene literature," and refused to find proper medical use of a contraceptive by a licensed physician to be immoral or obscene (*U.S. v. One Package ...,* p. 739). Though the court did not invalidate the statute, its interpretation limited the sweeping definition of morality and obscenity that had previously held sway.

Statutes modeled after the Comstock Act continued to exist, however, until 1965, when the U.S. Supreme Court in the case of *Griswold v. Connecticut* invalidated a Connecticut statute prohibiting the use of contraceptives. The Court held, citing prior cases that had created a zone of privacy protecting certain personal behaviors, that these penumbral rights of "privacy and repose," based on several fundamental constitutional guarantees, protected the use of contraceptives by married persons (*Griswold v. Connecticut,* p. 481).

Griswold was followed by *Eisenstadt v. Baird* (1972), extending this reasoning to nonmarried individuals. The statute that was invalidated in *Eisenstadt* prohibited single persons from obtaining contraceptives to prevent pregnancy, and permitted contraceptives only on a physician's prescription for the purpose of disease prevention. The statute was held to violate the equal protection clause of the Fourteenth Amendment:

> [W]hatever the rights of the individual to access to contraceptives may be, the rights must be the same for the unmarried and the married alike.... If the right of privacy means anything, it is the right of the individual, married or single, to be free from unwarranted governmental intrusion into matters so fundamentally affecting a person as the decision whether to bear or beget a child. (*Eisenstadt v. Baird,* p. 452–453)

Minors gradually attained access to contraceptive advice and devices. In 1977, in the case of *Carey v. Population Services International,* the U.S. Supreme Court invalidated a New York State statute that had banned the sale or distribution of contraceptives to persons below the age of sixteen and had prohibited the advertising or display of contraceptives by any person, including a pharmacist. In 1983 the Supreme Court struck down a federal statute prohibiting unsolicited advertisements of contraceptives (*Bolger v. Young Drug Products Corp.*). In addition, under Title X of the Public Health Services Act and Title XIX of the Social Security Act, receipt of federal funds prohibits a requirement of parental consent for services and requires confidentiality. Efforts to require parental notification under these acts have been held unconstitutional (*Jane Does 1 through 4 v. State of Utah Dept. of Health, Planned Parenthood Association of Utah v. Dandoy*), and federally funded clinics provide a full range of advice and service for fertility control for adults and minors.

New Contraceptive Technologies

A revolution in birth control techniques has created new possibilities for individual choice and new dangers of coercive action by legislatures, bureaucrats, and judges. Additional dangers arise from inadequate new-product testing and from lack of information or misinformation about risks and benefits of use. Female condoms, levonorgestrel (Norplant), and Depo-Provera are increasingly available to women for contraception.

The female condom or vaginal pouch was approved by the U.S. Food and Drug Administration (FDA) in 1993. The device, developed and marketed by Wisconsin Pharmaceuticals, consists of a polyurethane sheath secured inside the vagina by a small metal ring and outside by a large metal ring. It is the only barrier contraceptive that is under the control of a woman, an increasingly important factor for women seeking to protect themselves from sexually transmitted diseases and human immunodeficiency virus (HIV) infection when their partners refuse or neglect to use condoms. The device was approved by the FDA despite concerns that it was not proved as effective as the male condom for prevention of pregnancy or prevention of transmission of infection.

Norplant, approved by the FDA in 1990, is a long-term implantable contraceptive comprised of six capsules that gradually release progestin, thereby providing effective contraception for five years. A two-capsule version provides protection for three years. Norplant, like other contraceptive devices, is morally neutral; it may enhance the range of individual choice or, because of its long-acting nature, lend itself to coercive action by others. It permits a woman to protect herself without conscious attention to contraception but makes her dependent on medical intervention for removal, a dependency many women resent.

Norplant suppresses ovulation, and changes the female physiology to discourage pregnancy. For women who choose this contraceptive technique, it offers 100 percent compliance and effectiveness without the need to attend to individual acts of intercourse or to daily medications. There are some side effects and contraindications for use, including the possibilities of weight gain, headaches, and a general feeling of malaise. Implantation and removal remain expensive in the United States, costing between $500 and $750 (Planned Parenthood).

The only way to stop the contraceptive effect of the device is to have it surgically removed. Removal is more complicated than insertion and more than one session may be required to remove all the capsules; removal may also be painful. Norplant provides either long-acting contraception or time-limited sterilization (Mertus and Heller; Arthur).

Norplant presents an easy potential for coercive use by judges and legislatures. Problematic uses include requiring Norplant as a condition of parole following a conviction for child abuse, and paying women on welfare for consenting to initial and continued placement of the contraceptive. The first is clearly coercive. The second is potentially coercive depending on the context of a woman's poverty. Various state legislatures have considered statutes that would pay women receiving welfare to use Norplant or mandate its use by women convicted of child neglect and drug use, or both (Mertus and Heller; American Medical Association Board of Trustees [AMA]).

Judicial or legislative imposition of Norplant may violate a woman's constitutionally protected rights to choose how to manage reproduction and to choose whether or not to consent to or refuse medical care (*Cruzan v. Director, Missouri Department of Health*). Any long-acting male contraceptive would implicate these same rights. In addition, because long-acting contraception amounts to temporary sterilization, it raises the specter of eugenics—policies that are often directed at people of color, the poor, the retarded, the mentally ill, and other persons designated by those in power as undesirable. Norplant offers effective contraception when chosen voluntarily by a woman informed of the risks and benefits, and a potential for tyranny when imposed by judges or legislatures.

Regulation of Contraceptive Technologies

In addition to enhancing individual choice and restricting abuse, regulation of new technologies must ensure access and quality control. The development of new technologies is regulated formally by the approval process of the FDA, and informally by compensation awards under tort law for harm caused by defective products.

The FDA regulates the development of new drugs and contraceptive devices under the Federal Food, Drug and Cosmetic Act of 1938. Under this law, a company interested in marketing new contraceptive drugs or devices must submit data, including results from various tests for safety, effectiveness, and dosage, as part of an extensive approval process. In addition to approving new drugs and devices, the FDA reviews labeling and assesses data in a postmarketing surveillance program. The FDA approval process has been criticized as expensive, time consuming, and a barrier to new techniques. It has also been praised for protecting consumers from the harm of untested substances.

The FDA approval process is not the sole factor dictating whether a reproductive technology reaches U.S. consumers, however. The American tort system is designed to compensate those injured, deter the marketing of dangerous and defective products, and resolve disputes between the injured person and the manufacturer.

A person may recover damages for dangerous or defective products, including contraceptive devices, if either negligence or a strict liability is established. Negligence requires proof that the manufacturer was at fault. However, sometimes the fault of a large company is difficult to establish, and therefore the interests of justice dictate that a victim should be allowed to recover damages without proving specific fault. According to the strict products-liability principle, if a product is sold in a defective condition, and is unreasonably dangerous to the consumer, there is liability regardless of the care taken, that is, regardless of negligence in any individual case. Strict liability may make manufacturers apprehensive about putting new contraceptive products on the market.

This is the case especially since the litigation experience of the A. H. Robins Company, developer and marketer of the Dalkon Shield, an intrauterine contraceptive device. In a series of court cases in the early 1980s, this device was proved to cause pelvic inflammatory disease, infertility, birth defects, perforated uterus, and spontaneous abortion. In a series of jury verdicts throughout the United States, A. H. Robins was forced to pay compensatory damages and punitive damages because plaintiffs proved that the company had understood the dangers of the device, withheld this knowledge from prospective users, and misrepresented the nature and safety of the device (Mintz). Despite this experience, cases brought by women seeking recovery for harm from contraceptive devices have usually found the manufacturer liable only under theories of negligence—for example, negligent failure to comply with the duty of care, negligent failure to warn of risks, or fraudulent misrepresentation (*Hilliard v. A. H. Robins Co., Tetuan v. A. H. Robins Co.*). In fact, even those courts purporting to apply strict liability seem to be applying a theory of negligent failure to warn under the rhetoric of strict liability (Henderson and Twerski; Fox and Traynor).

How tort law is interpreted is in a state of flux. Some judges and juries appear to view manufacturers as *deep pockets* (Reilly) and to see tort law as a vehicle for providing social insurance for injury victims. Many critics of large jury awards argue that the size of jury awards often bears no relationship to actual economic loss or to pain and suffering, and that awards of punitive damages are arbitrary and unfair. Supporters of the present pattern of trial awards argue that claims of a law crisis in this area are exaggerated because of manufacturers's dislike for how the law determines their liability (Fox and Traynor). However as long as manufacturers fear they will have to pay large financial penalties to women who suffer the consequences of their new products, many may be reluctant to market new products, a trend that may limit women's access to new contraceptive technologies.

Postcontraception, the *morning-after* pill, is widely dispensed on college campuses after unprotected intercourse and in emergency rooms for rape victims; it promises to be another barrier to unwanted pregnancy. The process generally entails two treatments of oral contraceptives within seventy-two hours of intercourse and is thought to prevent pregnancy either by blocking fertilization or by blocking implantation of the fertilized egg. An antihormone (mifepristone)

product called RU-486, discussed in the following section, has also shown promise as a morning-after pill.

Abortion

This article will not survey the legal history and the current status of abortion law and regulation. This discussion will be limited to RU-486 which, while functioning as an abortion inducer, is thought of by many users as similar to oral contraceptives.

RU-486 is a steroid analogue that, when used with prostaglandin (PG), is able to induce menses within eight weeks of the last menstrual period. It has been called a *menstrual regulator* in an attempt to distinguish it from contraceptives and abortion inducers, although to theologians the physiological function is clearly that of an abortion inducer. It was approved for use in France in 1988. Limited trials in the United States began in 1994. Shortly after its introduction in France, the manufacturer, Roussel Uclaf, attempted to halt distribution for fear of anti-abortion protests. The French government, a one-third owner of the company, ordered continued manufacture and distribution (Banwell and Paxman).

Whether RU-486/PG will become readily available will depend on each nation's interpretation of relevant abortion laws and regulations. If abortion "is defined to include techniques that operate before implantation is complete, RU-486/PG will be regulated by abortion law. If not, RU-486/PG might be considered similar to a contraceptive and could be made more widely available. This distinction is particularly important because abortion legislation generally imposes criminal penalties" (Banwell and Paxman, p. 1400).

While France considers RU-486/PG an abortion inducer, Germany, New Zealand, and Liberia use a definition of pregnancy in their abortion statutes providing that pregnancy begins only after complete implantation. In these countries, RU-486/PG and any other menses-inducing technique is regulated as a form of contraception. In countries with strict abortion laws in which pregnancy is defined as beginning with fertilization, even early use of RU-486/PG might be barred (Banwell and Paxman).

Many countries in Latin America and Africa have restrictive abortion statutes that require proof of pregnancy. Statutes that require proof of pregnancy will be difficult to use as a barrier to RU-486/PG. Other national statutes criminalize the intent to abort whether or not the woman is pregnant. In these countries, many of which are former French colonies, the widespread use of RU-486/PG is effectively precluded. In societies governed by Islamic law, where pregnancy may be terminated until quickening—when fetal movement is felt—RU-486/PG would likely be acceptable (Banwell and Paxman).

Sterilization

Sterilization is a particularly useful technique for men and women who are certain that they have fulfilled their reproductive agenda. For these individuals sterilization provides an uncomplicated and generally certain method of limiting fertility. Whereas sterilization done competently is 100 percent effective, cases have claimed damages for children conceived as the result of incomplete sterilizations.

The key legal issues in sterilization involve the need to ensure that the choice is made by a competent adult who has chosen voluntarily; the need to decide for some persons, almost always women, who are clearly incapable of deciding for themselves; and the need to prevent notions of eugenics from dictating sterilization policy and practice. Sterilization, because it requires only one medical intervention, has been particularly susceptible to government abuse.

Women or men who choose sterilization must be counseled about the risks and benefits of the intervention itself and about the very slim chances for reversal if permanent infertility is no longer desired. Some localities have regulations requiring a waiting period between a request for sterilization and the actual procedure. Others preclude caregivers from soliciting consent for sterilization from women during the birthing process. Both restrictions offer protection against coercion, especially for low-income women and women of color who have been historically at risk for nonconsensual sterilization.

Sterilization has been used by physicians and by state and federal governments since the turn of the century (Mertus and Heller), in order to limit the reproduction of low-income women and women of color. It has also been used as a method of eugenics "to weed out traits or characteristics that are held to be undesirable. Further, sterilization was simultaneously discouraged among affluent white women" (Mertus and Heller, p. 377).

The history of involuntary sterilization of incompetent and developmentally disabled individuals in the first half of the twentieth century is a history of "wholesale violations of constitutional rights carried out with the approval of the highest judicial tribunals." Eugenic sterilization—the attempt to rid the collective gene pool of hereditary mental and physical defects—was the result of the "enthusiastic application of Mendelian genetics" to population policy (*In re Conservatorship of Valerie N.*, p. 148).

In the early-twentieth century, thousands of young women and men were sterilized as the result of decisions by the directors of mental institutions or prisons in which they were housed, or by decisions of their conservators or guardians. The impulse to control the reproductive capacity of these people was fueled by the dual fears that children would perpetuate their parents's mental or physical *deformity* and would be a drain on state coffers. But there is another basis, never articulated as such in legislation or by the courts, and that is a general revulsion at the concept of mentally *defective* persons acting sexually. Indeed a 1913 California statute granted authority to *asexualize* committed mental patients and developmentally disabled persons prior to their release from state institutions (*In re Conservatorship of Valerie N.*). Sexuality, as well as reproductive capacity, was at issue.

By the second decade of the twentieth century, twenty-two states had eugenic sterilization statutes. Between 1907 and 1921, 3,233 sterilizations were performed, of which California was responsible for 2,558. By 1927 California had performed over 5,000 sterilizations, four times as many as had been performed by any national government worldwide. By 1960 approximately 60,000 persons had been subjected to compulsory sterilization in the United States, with nearly 20,000 in California (Mertus and Heller).

In 1927 the U.S. Supreme Court upheld a Virginia statute permitting the sterilization of the *mental defectives* (*Buck v. Bell*). The Court based its decision on two lines of reasoning: that if rendered unable to procreate, the person might more easily become self-supporting; and that society can choose to protect itself from further dissemination of defective genes. Justice Oliver Wendell Holmes wrote, "The principle that sustains compulsory vaccination is broad enough to cover cutting the Fallopian tubes.... Three generations of imbeciles are enough" (*Buck v. Bell*, p. 207).

Buck v. Bell, though never overruled, has been severely limited by later decisions. In 1942 the U.S. Supreme Court invalidated the Oklahoma Habitual Criminal Sterilization Act, which ordered the sterilization of anyone convicted of three crimes involving *moral turpitude;* however, the contested law excepted certain white-collar crimes. In *Skinner v. Oklahoma* (1942), declaring the Sterilization Act unconstitutional on equal-protection grounds, the Court ruled that procreation is a basic civil right that can be abridged only by showing compelling state interest. The Court referred to the right to marriage and procreation as a basic liberty and as one of the basic civil rights. The Court's reluctance to approve the Oklahoma statute appears to reflect apprehension that sterilization could be used oppressively.

The second half of the twentieth century has witnessed a revulsion against nonconsensual sterilization, based on the revelations of Nazi abuses and the emergence of various rights movements in the United States—civil, women's, welfare, mentally ill, the disabled, and prisoners. Sociological and medical research regarding the nature of mental illness and developmental disability also enlightened the public regarding the ability of developmentally disabled and mentally ill persons to lead constructive, competent, loving lives as partners and parents.

Beginning in the 1950s, numerous states repealed legislation permitting eugenic sterilization for institutionalized persons or limited the powers of conservators and guardians to procure individual sterilization. Yet in many states these statutes are still law. This has led to the ironic position, in many states, that no one can consent for the incapable, thus denying them access to sterilization even when sterilization is the only or arguably the best contraceptive solution—and even when it is required to protect health or life itself.

Arguments regarding sterilization for incompetent persons pit advocates of reproductive choice for the disabled against those who argue that the right to *bear or beget* a child includes the right to choose reproduction, contraception, or sterilization. Federal (*Hathaway v. Worcester City Hospital, Ruby v. Massey*) and state courts (*In re Moe; In re Grady; In re A. W.*) have generally held that developmentally disabled persons have fundamental privacy and liberty interests in making decisions about procreation and that these interests require sterilization to be an option for fertility control. Some state courts, however, have refused to authorize sterilization of an incompetent person unless the state legislature has specifically authorized the decision and specified a process (*Hudson v. Hudson, In re Eberhardy*). The U.S. Supreme Court has yet to examine the issue, but prior cases would seem to support a right of access to sterilization for incompetent persons.

Cases claiming rights of protection from sterilization most often involve consent for severely disabled young women for whom menstruation and pregnancy would be painful, provoking, upsetting, or possibly life-threatening (for example, one woman for whom the sight of her own blood caused a pattern of severe self-mutilation [*In re P. S.*]). In most states, courts appoint an independent guardian to protect the interests of the person and then base their decision on the standard of *best interest* (*In re P.S., In re Hayes*) or substituted judgment (*In re Moe, In re Grady*).

The dangers of forced sterilizations are apparent outside the realm of prisoners, developmentally disabled, and incompetent individuals, largely where issues of race and class are present. The indigent, who are often persons of color, have been particularly subject to sterilization abuses by public officials and collaborating physicians. Numerous cases have been documented of coerced sterilization of Native Americans (Kelly), Latinos (particularly those who spoke little or no English), and African Americans (*Relf v. Weinberger,* 1977). In response to one egregious incident (*Relf v. Weinberger*), the district court examined the practice of physicians at federally funded clinics who were using sterilization to limit the reproduction of African-American teenagers. The court invalidated federal regulations that permitted involuntary, coerced sterilization, including sterilization of minors or persons incapable of providing consent. The court further held that such sterilizations could not be funded under the Social Security Act or the Public Health Service Act. The court found that minors and other incompetents had undergone federally funded sterilization and that an indefinite number of poor people had been improperly coerced into accepting sterilization operations under the threat that various federally supported welfare benefits would be withdrawn unless they submitted.

Local statutes and federal regulations have further limited the use of sterilization. In New York City, for example, statutes passed in 1985 require completion of a complicated informed-consent process and a thirty-day waiting period before sterilization is permitted (New York City Charter and Administrative Code §17–401 et seq.). Federal regulations also prescribe special informed consent procedures and waiting periods for federally funded sterilizations (Code of Federal Regulations 1993b, 1993c).

Much current law attempts to protect vulnerable women and limit potential abuse by emphasizing voluntary, informed consent and limiting sterilizations to which individual, capable consent is not given. Even where there is no specific legislation to that effect, compulsory sterilization has become rare; those states that have retained compulsory sterilization statutes on the books have, for the most part, let them slip into disuse (Haavik and Menninger).

Discussion of eugenics as appropriate public policy for the protection of future generations has largely been discredited because of the Nazis's horrendous abuse of the concept, because of scientific and societal disaffection with eugenic theories, and because of increasing respect for those with developmental and other disabilities. Nonetheless eugenics is not yet dead. Increasing knowledge about genetics and new reproductive technologies such as in vitro fertilization, artificial insemination, and surrogate motherhood, may allow people to selectively create babies of *higher quality,* and may renew the specter of eugenics, albeit in a new light (Neuhaus).

An ethical policy controlling reproduction must offer a range of contraceptive services to women and men and simultaneously protect adults with reproductive potential from state coercion. New technologies offer increased protection from unwanted pregnancy and increased potential for overriding individual preferences.

NANCY NEVELOFF DUBLER
AMANDA WHITE (1995)
REVISED BY NATHANIEL STEWART

SEE ALSO: *Abortion; AIDS: Public Health Issues; Autonomy; Coercion; Conscience, Rights of; Embryo and Fetus; Eugenics; Family and Family Medicine; Genetic Testing and Screening: Reproductive Genetic Screening; Infanticide; International Health; Law and Bioethics; Law and Morality; Maternal-Fetal Relationship; Natural Law; Population Ethics: Religious Traditions;* and other *Fertility Control* subentries

BIBLIOGRAPHY

Alan Guttmacher Institute. 1999. *Sharing Responsibility: Women, Society and Abortion Worldwide.* New York: Alan Guttmacher Institute.

American Medical Association Board of Trustees. 1992. "Requirements or Incentives by Government for the Use of Long-Acting Contraceptives." *Journal of the American Medical Association* 267(13): 1818–1821.

Arthur, Stacey L. 1992. "The Norplant Prescription: Birth Control, Woman Control, or Crime Control?" *UCLA Law Review* 40(1): 1–101.

A. W., In re, 637 P.2d 366 (Colo. 1981).

Banwell, Suzanna S., and Paxman, John M. 1992. "The Search for Meaning: RU 486 and the Law of Abortion." *American Journal of Public Health* 82(10): 1399–1406.

Bolger v. Young Drug Products Corp., 463 U.S. 60 (1983).

Buck v. Bell, 274 U.S. 200 (1927).

Carey v. Population Services International, 431 U.S. 678 (1977).

Chessler, Ellen. 1992. *Women of Valor: Margaret Sanger and the Birth Control Movement in America.* New York: Simon & Schuster.

Code of Federal Regulations. 1993a. "Birth Control, Pregnancy, Child Placement, and Abortion." 28 C.F.R. 551.23.

Code of Federal Regulations. 1993b. "Sterilization of Persons in Federally Assisted Programs of the Public Health Service." 42 C.F.R. 50.201 et seq.

Code of Federal Regulations. 1993c. "Sterilizations." 42 C.F.R. 441.250 et seq.

Conservatorship of Valerie N., In re, 707 P.2d 760 (Cal. 1985).

Cruzan v. Director, Missouri Department of Health, 497 U.S. 261 (1990).

Eberhardy, In re, 294 N.W.2d 540, 97 Wis.2d 654, (Wis.Ct.App. 1980).

Eisenstadt v. Baird, 405 U.S. 438 (1972).

Fathalla, Mahmoud; Rosenfield, Allan; and Indriso, Cynthia. 1990. "Family Planning." In *The FIGO Manual of Human Reproduction* vol. 2 *Family Planning,* ed. Mahmoud Fathalla and Allan Rosenfield. Park Ridge, NJ: Parthenon.

Federal Food, Drug, and Cosmetic Act. 1938. 21 U.S.C. §301 et seq.

Fox, Eleanor M., and Traynor, Michael. 1990. "Biotechnology and Products Liability." *ALI-ABA Continuing Course of Study: Biotechnology Law* November 8.

Francome, Colin. 1984. *Abortion Freedom: A Worldwide Movement.* Boston: Allen & Unwin.

Grady, In re, 85 N.J. 235, 426 A.2d 467 (1981).

Griswold v. Connecticut, 381 U.S. 479 (1965).

Haavik, Sarah F., and Menninger, Karl A. 1981. *Sexuality, Law, and the Developmentally Disabled Person: Legal and Clinical Aspects of Marriage, Parenthood, and Sterilization.* Baltimore: Paul H. Brookes.

Hathaway v. Worcester City Hospital, 475 F.2d 701 (1st Cir. 1973).

Hayes, In re, 93 Wash.2d 228, 608 P.2d 635 (1980).

Henderson, James A., Jr., and Twerski, Aaron D. 1990. "Doctrinal Collapse in Products Liability: The Empty Shell of Failure to Warn." *New York University Law Review* 65(2): 265–327.

Henshaw, Stanley K. 1998. "Unintended Pregnancy in the United States." *Family Planning Perspectives* 30(1): 24–29.

Hilliard v. A. H. Robins Co., 196 Cal.Rptr. 117, 148 Cal.App.3d 374 (2nd Dist. 1984).

Hudson v. Hudson, 373 So.2d 310 (Ala. 1979).

Jane Does 1 Through 4 v. State of Utah Department of Health, 776 F.2d 253 (10th Cir. 1985).

Kelly, Joan. 1977. "Sterilization and Civil Rights." *Rights* 23(5): 9–11.

Larson, David R. 1991. "Contraception and Coercion: Theological Reflections, Update." *Loma Linda University Center for Christian Bioethics* 7(2): 4–5.

Leebron, David W. 1990. "An Introduction to Products Liability: Origins, Issues and Trends." *Annual Survey of American Law 1990* 2: 395–458.

Mastroianni, Luigi; Donaldson, Peter J.; and Kane, Thomas T., eds. 1990. *Developing New Contraceptives: Obstacles and Opportunities.* Washington, D.C.: National Academy Press.

Means, Cyril C., Jr. 1971. "The Phoenix of Abortional Freedom: Is a Penumbral or Ninth-Amendment Right About to Arise from the Nineteenth-Century Legislative Ashes of a Fourteenth-Century Common-Law Liberty?" *New York Law Forum* 22(2): 335–410.

Mertus, Julie, and Heller, Simon. 1992. "Norplant Meets the New Eugenicists: The Impermissibility of Coerced Contraception." *Saint Louis University Public Law Review* 11(2): 359–383.

Mintz, Morton. 1985. *At Any Cost: Corporate Greed, Women and the Dalkon Shield.* New York: Pantheon.

Moe, In re, 432 N.E. 2d 712, 385 Mass. 555 (Sup.Ct. Mass. 1982).

Mohr, James C. 1978. *Abortion in America: The Origins and Evolutions of National Policy, 1800–1900.* New York: Oxford University Press.

Neuhaus, John. 1988. "The Return of Eugenics." *Commentary* 15: 26.

People v. Sanger, 222 N.E. 192, 118 N.E. 637 (1918); 251 U.S. 536 (1919).

Petchesky, Rosalind P. 1990. *Abortion and Women's Choice: The State, Sexuality, and Reproductive Freedom,* rev. edition. Boston: Northeastern University Press.

Planned Parenthood Association of Utah v. Dandoy, 810 F.2d 984 (10th Cir. 1987).

Planned Parenthood of Central Missouri v. Danforth, 428 U.S. 52 (1976).

Preston, Yvonne. 1992. "China's Shadow Population." *Straits Times,* June 21, p. 1.

P.S., In re, 452 N.E.2d 969 (Sup. Ct. Ind. 1983).

Reed, James. 1978. *From Private Vice to Public Virtue: The Birth Control Movement and American Society Since 1830.* New York: Basic Books.

Reilly, John P. 1989. "The Erosion of Comment K." *University of Dayton Law Review* 14(2): 255–278.

Relf v. Weinberger, 372 F.Supp. 1196 (Dist. D.C.); motion denied, sub nom. *Relf v. Matthews,* 403 F.Supp. 1235 (Dist. D.C. 1975): order vacated, *Relf v. Weinberger,* 565 F.2d 722, 184 U.S.App.D.C. 147 (1977).

Robertson, William. 1990. *An Illustrated History of Contraception: A Concise Account of the Quest for Fertility Control.* Park Ridge, NJ: Parthenon.

Roe v. Wade, 410 U.S. 113 (1973).

Ruby v. Massey, 452 R.Supp. 361 (Dist. Conn. 1978).

Skinner v. Oklahoma ex-rel. Williamson, 316 U.S. 535 (1942).

Sloan, Irving J. 1988. *The Law Governing Abortion, Contraception and Sterilization.* New York: Oceana.

Stephen, Chris. 1992. "Romania: Abortions Skyrocket, Contraception Yet to Take Hold." *International Press Service* August 19.

St. John-Stevas, Norman. 1971. *Agonizing Choice: Birth Control, Religion, and the Law.* Bloomington: Indiana University Press.

Tetuan v. A. H. Robins Co., 241 Kan. 441, 738 P.2d 1210 (1987).

Thomas, Christopher. 1990. "A Society Defeats Its Own Rules." *Times* (London), January 6.

United States Code Annotated. 1930 "Tariff Act." 19 U.S.C.A. §305(a).

U.S. v. One Package Containing 120, More or Less, Rubber Pessaries to Prevent Conception, 86 F.2d 737 (1936).

Weston, Mark. 1990. "Where the World's Major Religions Disagree." *Washington Post,* January 23, p. Z12.

World Health Organization. 1997. *Abortion: A Tabulation of Available Data on the Frequency and Mortality of Unsafe Abortion,* 3rd edition. Geneva: World Health Organization.

INTERNET RESOURCE

Planned Parenthood Association of America. 2003. "Birth Control: Norplant and You." Available from <http:\www.plannedparenthood.org>.

FETAL RESEARCH

• • •

All of the research discussed in this entry involves women and men, as well as human embryos and fetuses. When implantation is a necessary condition for the research, as in the case of most fetal research, the fetus is implanted in the uterus of a woman. For all of the research considered in the entry, the oocytes (eggs) of at least one woman are required; in cases involving in vitro fertilization (IVF), the oocyte retrieval process can be onerous for the woman involved. In addition, sperm from at least one man are required for fertilization. Finally when research is conducted on the developing fetus, interventions also directly impact and take place through the body of the pregnant woman. For reasons of brevity, this entry focuses primary attention on the developing human embryo and fetus. However recognition of the inextricable connection between the fetus or embryo and the woman and man who provide the gametes that give rise to it or to the woman in whom gestation occurs is critical to ethical discourse, and is explicitly discussed where possible.

Four major types of research will be analyzed in this entry:

1. research on preimplantation embryos;
2. research on unimplanted embryos and fetuses beyond the fourteenth day of development;
3. research on implanted embryos and fetuses; and
4. research on aborted, live embryos and fetuses.

The topic of research on living tissue derived from fetal remains is discussed in a separate entry.

Preimplantation Embryo Research

The human preimplantation embryo can be defined as the developing organism from the time of fertilization to approximately the fourteenth day after fertilization, assuming a normal rate of development. The major preimplantation stages in human and other mammalian embryos are usually distinguished by such names as zygote, morula, and blastocyst. By the end of fourteen days the early human embryo has, except in rare cases, lost the capacity to divide into two individuals; it has also begun to exhibit a longitudinal axis that forms the template for the spinal column, an axis called the primitive streak (McLaren; Dawson, 1990a).

Preimplantation embryo research generally requires the associated procedure of IVF (although it would in principle be possible to retrieve an early embryo by flushing it from the uterus of a woman following in vivo fertilization of an ovum). Thus the question of research on preimplantation embryos did not arise until IVF techniques had been developed and validated, first in laboratory animals, then in humans. In 1959 M. C. Chang of the Worcester Foundation in Massachusetts was the first scientist to demonstrate unambiguously the fertilization of nonhuman mammalian oocytes in vitro. Chang's success was followed in 1969 by the first confirmed report of IVF with human gametes by three British researchers (Edwards et al.). Only nine years later the first human birth after IVF—the infant's name was Louise Brown—was reported by members of the same British research team (Steptoe and Edwards).

Given that IVF is required for preimplantation embryo research, the risks to the woman of ovarian stimulation and oocyte retrieval are relevant to the discussion. Ovarian stimulation with injectable gonadotropins has been associated in some studies with an increased risk of ovarian tumors (Harris et al.), though the association is controversial. In addition gonadotropins are associated with a risk of ovarian hyperstimulation syndrome, which is associated with ovarian enlargement, massive fluid and electrolyte imbalances, renal insufficiency, and in rare cases thromoembolism and death.

There are two major contexts for research on preimplantation embryos. The first is one in which the transfer of the embryo into the uterus of a woman (or perhaps, in the future, into a device that can support full-term fetal development) is planned. In the second context, no embryo transfer is envisioned and, accordingly, the death of the embryo or later fetus at a stage before viability is intended. These two research contexts raise somewhat different ethical issues.

RESEARCH FOLLOWED BY EMBRYO TRANSFER. In the years preceding the birth of Louise Brown in 1978, researchers devoted substantial attention to improving the prospects for successful IVF and embryo transfer. This research focused on methods for maturing oocytes, facilitating fertilization, and culturing or cryopreserving early embryos (Biggers). During the 1990s, researchers continued this type of research. New methods for assisting fertilization have been devised, including the drilling of a small hole in the outer shell of an oocyte or the injection of a sperm directly into an oocyte, a process known as intracytoplasmic sperm injection (ICSI) (Van Steirteghem). Similarly researchers have developed methods for removing one or two cells from an eight- or sixteen-cell embryo in order to perform preimplantation diagnosis of genetic or chromosomal abnormalities (Edwards, 1993). These techniques are performed so that only embryos without genetic abnormalities are transferred to the uterus, while affected embryos are discarded. In the twenty-first century, one can anticipate research that attempts to prevent the later development of a genetic disease (for example, cystic fibrosis) by treating an individual at the embryonic stage of life. If successful this kind of disease prevention by means of gene modification would be likely to affect all of the cells of the person, including his or her reproductive cells (Wivel and Walters).

The ethical issues that arise with preimplantation embryo research when embryo transfer is planned are at least analogous to those that arise with fetal research in anticipation of birth, with research on infants, and with research on children. That is, one attempts to perform a careful analysis of the probable benefits and harms of the research to the individual and to others; one seeks an appropriate decision maker, usually a genetic parent or a guardian, who can represent the best interests of the potential research subject; and one looks for a disinterested mechanism for prior ethical review of the proposed research. This kind of embryo research, in which the research procedures are often designated *therapeutic* or *beneficial,* is generally approved by commentators on the ethics of such research, even if they diverge widely in their attitudes toward IVF, the moral status of preimplantation embryos, and abortion (see, e.g., Ramsey, 1970; Catholic Church; Singer et al.).

RESEARCH NOT FOLLOWED BY EMBRYO TRANSFER. Research in this context may be proposed for a variety of reasons. The goal of the research may be to assess the safety and efficacy of clinical practices, for example, IVF or the use of contraceptive vaccines. Alternatively the goal may be epidemiological, for example, to estimate the frequency of chromosomal abnormalities in early human embryos. Another goal that has gained significant national and international attention is the use of embryos for the creation of stem cells (Thompson et al.). Stem cells are a unique type of cell that have the potential to mature into cells of a particular type (e.g., heart, blood, muscle, or brain cells). This versatility has been thought to hold significant scientific and therapeutic promise for treatment of such diseases as Alzheimer's, heart disease or kidney failure; furthermore, these cells may be essential to understanding early stages of human development. Finally in other cases research on embryos may have little reference to clinical medicine or human pathology. That is, research with preimplantation embryos may be much more basic, seeking to compare early development in various species of mammals or to explore the limits of embryo fusion or hybrid creation among different species.

Two distinct ethical questions have received primary attention in the international bioethics debate about preimplantation embryo research without embryo transfer. The first question is: Is research on such embryos morally permissible if it is not intended to benefit the embryos themselves? If the answer to the first question is negative, the second question is irrelevant. However, if the answer to the first question is affirmative, there remains a second question: Is it morally permissible to fertilize human oocytes for the sole purpose of performing research on the resulting embryos and in the absence of any intention to transfer the embryos for further development?

In their responses to the first question, proponents of nonbeneficial (to the embryos) research procedures adduce several arguments. First the research may produce benefits, either for clinical practice or in terms of basic knowledge, that are not attainable by any other means (U.S. Department of Health, Education and Welfare [HEW]; Warnock; Ethics Committee of the American Fertility Society; Robertson; National Bioethics Advisory Committee [NBAC]). One variant of this argument asserts that it is morally irresponsible to introduce new techniques (for example, cryopreservation of embryos) into clinical practice without first performing extensive laboratory studies of the technique (International Society of Law and Technology [ISLAT] Working Group).

Second, proponents of preimplantation embryo research note that the biological individuality of the embryo is not firmly established until approximately fourteen (or perhaps twenty-one) days after fertilization. Before that time twinning can occur, or two embryos can fuse into a single new embryo called a chimera (Hellegers; Dawson, 1987; Grobstein). If developmental individuality does not occur until after the preimplantation stage, research proponents argue, the preimplantation embryo is not protectable as a unique human being.

Third, proponents of research cite the apparently high embryo loss rate that occurs in natural human reproduction. The most reliable estimates are that approximately 50 percent of the human eggs that are fertilized either fail to develop or die within two weeks after fertilization occurs (Chard). To this factual evidence is added the metaphysical assertion that entities with such a high rate of natural death within two weeks of coming into being cannot be morally significant at this early stage of their existence. Proponents of

embryo research may acknowledge that adult persons have some moral obligations toward early embryos, but these obligations are viewed as relatively weak and are thought to be outweighed by, for example, substantial clinical benefits to many future patients (NBAC).

Opponents of preimplantation embryo research have replies to these arguments and adduce other arguments of their own. In response to the first argument of proponents, the opponents assert that the end of desirable clinical consequences does not justify the means of performing research that seriously damages or destroys the embryo. To the consequential argument of proponents, conservatives may counterpose a consequential argument of their own, namely, that negative consequences will result from research on early embryos. For example researchers may become desensitized to the value of human life, or bizarre human-nonhuman hybrids may be produced in the laboratory (Catholic Church, Dawson, 1990b).

The second and third arguments of the proponents are viewed as mere descriptions of natural phenomena that carry no particular moral weight. Twinning, recombination, and embryo loss, if they occur naturally and are beyond human control, are in this view no more morally relevant than other natural evils like earthquakes or volcanic eruptions. For their part, opponents put forward two additional arguments. First, the genotype of a new individual is firmly established at the time when the pronuclei from the sperm cell and the ovum fuse. This fusion, sometimes called syngamy, occurs at the conclusion of fertilization. Thus from a genetic standpoint, a new individual exists from syngamy forward. Second, opponents of preimplantation embryo research often adduce the potentiality argument: that the early embryo contains within itself all of the genetic instructions necessary for the development of a fetus, an infant, and an adult, provided only that the embryo is placed in an environment that will nurture its further development. Therefore the person that the early embryo may one day become should be respected in an anticipatory way even at the early stages of development, when it lacks many of the characteristics of persons in the full sense.

Proponents of research do not deny that a new genotype is established at the time of fertilization. They simply point to other factual considerations that are in their view more relevant to moral judgments about the acceptability of embryo research. In response to the potentiality argument, research proponents note that a single sperm cell and a single oocyte have the potential to become an embryo, yet opponents of embryo research do not accord special moral status to reproductive cells. Further only a few cells of the preimplantation embryo develop into the embryo proper;

the rest become the placenta, the amniotic sac, and the chorionic villi (McLaren). Finally with the advent of cloning technology (the creation of an embryo from a single somatic cell), a single somatic (i.e., skin, breast, or other) cell theoretically has the potential to become an embryo, and it would be impossible to accord special moral status to every somatic cell in a human's body. In other words potentiality is a continuous notion, or a matter of degree, not an all-or-nothing concept (Singer and Dawson).

Among proponents of research on preimplantation embryos there is a division of opinion on the second question noted above—whether the creation of human embryos specifically for research purposes is morally permissible. Proponents of the conservative answer to this question argue that only embryos left over from the clinical practice of IVF and embryo transfer should be used in research (Steinbock). Such embryos might include those selected out when the number of embryos available for transfer exceeds a number that is considered safe for the woman (between two and five, depending on patient age and other prognostic factors (American Society for Reproductive Medicine [ASRM]). Leftover or surplus embryos might also become available in the context of cryopreservation, if a couple completes its desired family size or if both genetic parents die in an accident while some embryos remain in frozen storage.

The principal argument of conservatives on the deliberate-creation question is a Kantian argument against using early human embryos merely as means. In the opinion of conservatives, creating embryos with the prior intent of destroying them at an early stage of development is incompatible with the respect that should be accorded to human embryos. Conservatives can accept the use of leftover embryos for research because there was at least at one time an intention to transfer the preimplantation embryos to the uterus of a woman, where they could develop into viable fetuses. In their view the research use of such *spare* embryos is a morally acceptable alternative to donation or discard (Steinbock). The primary argument of those who do not object to creating embryos for research is a composite. Proponents of this view argue, first, that our moral obligations to early human embryos are relatively weak. Further proponents of the liberal view note that good research design may require either a larger number of embryos than the clinical context can provide or unselected embryos rather than those that have been rejected for embryo transfer, perhaps because they are malformed or slow in developing (Ethics Committee of the American Fertility Society). Indeed while estimates are that approximately 400,000 cryopreserved embryos are in storage, only 2.8 percent of these are available for research (Hoffman et al.).

PRACTICE VS. ETHICS. In the 1990s international practice and ethical opinion regarding human embryo research diverged sharply. One polar position in practice was that of the United Kingdom, where research on preimplantation embryos was conducted in numerous laboratories under the supervision of voluntary and (later) statutory licensing authorities (United Kingdom, 1992). At the other pole was Germany, which prohibited the fertilization of ova for the practice of research, as well as any research that was likely to destroy or damage the embryo. In the United States, embryo research was legal though practically limited due to a legislative prohibition of federal funding for: (1) any research involving the creation of a human embryo for research purposes; or (2) any research in which a human embryo is destroyed, discarded, or knowingly subjected to risk of injury or death. This prohibition has been implemented yearly through a provision included in Congressional appropriations for the Department of Health and Human Services (DHHS) since 1996 (P.L. 107–116 [2002]).

Ethics advisory bodies have been far from unanimous in their evaluations of research involving preimplantation embryos. The earliest report on this topic, produced by the Ethics Advisory Board in 1979 for HEW, judged embryo research to be ethically acceptable if it was designed primarily to "assess the safety and efficacy of embryo transfer" (p. 106). During the 1980s and early 1990s, there emerged three general positions among such advisory bodies. Several Australian committees rejected the idea of any human embryo research. A few Australian committees and most of the committees based in continental Europe approved embryo research but rejected the deliberate creation of embryos for research purposes. In the Netherlands, the United Kingdom, Canada, and the United States, advisory committees tended to approve both human embryo research and the creation of embryos for research (Walters; National Institutes of Health [NIH]).

In the late 1990s and early 2000s, reports of stem cell derivation from human embryos (Thompson et al.) prompted reexamination of ethics and policy regarding embryo research (Green). International practice and ethical positions remain polarized. In 1999 the NBAC issued a report and recommendations that federal agencies should fund research on embryos left over after IVF for derivation of stem cells but not research involving embryos created solely for research purposes. Despite this recommendation, in 2001 the Bush administration decided to allow federal funding only for research on existing cell lines. In contrast the Human Fertilisation and Embryology Authority (HFEA) in the United Kingdom has continued to permit and license human embryo research and the creation of embryos for research but with enhanced guidelines specific to the derivation and use of stem cells.

Research on Unimplanted Embryos and Fetuses Beyond the Fourteenth Day of Development

The developing human organism is technically called an embryo during the first eight weeks following fertilization. It is called a fetus for the remainder of its development. In this section, prolonged in vitro culture of embryos and fetuses will be evaluated.

Prolonged embryo culture has been undertaken in several species of nonhuman mammals, especially rats and mice. In the early years of research, embryos at various stages of development were removed (or *explanted*) from the uteri of pregnant females and sustained in various kinds of laboratory devices that delivered oxygen and nutrients (New). More recently unimplanted mouse and cattle embryos have been sustained in culture to developmental stages more complex than those attained by preimplantation human embryos (Chen and Hsu; Thomas and Seidel).

As of 2003 no researchers are proposing to perform studies of either of these types with human embryos. The explantation mode of research will probably not be undertaken in humans because of the risks to the pregnant woman and because the need is questionable. However sustained culture of human embryos after IVF would in principle be possible. It is not clear whether the current lack of proposals to culture embryos in vitro beyond fourteen days is based on technical, ethical, or financial (given the bans on funding for embryo research) considerations. The longest well-documented periods for human embryo culture are eight days and thirteen days (Fishel et al.). Possible rationales for extending embryo culture beyond fourteen days could include studying differentiation, the anatomy and physiology of the embryo, the implantation process, or the effect of drugs or radiation on the developing embryo (Karp; Edwards, 1989; Sass).

There has been relatively little ethical discussion of embryo research beyond fourteen days. Most advisory committees have simply accepted the fourteen-day limit without extensive discussion. In the case of the Warnock Committee report from the United Kingdom, this limit was said to be appropriate because it correlates with the appearance of the primitive streak in the embryo (Warnock, 1984). The primitive streak is the first indication of the embryo's body axis, the last opportunity for twinning to occur, and a point before sentience is attained. Several commentators have suggested that the justification for the fourteen-day limit is relatively weak and have proposed extending the limit for in vitro human embryo research to approximately twenty-eight days (Edwards, 1989; Kuhse and Singer).

If embryo culture methods improve sufficiently, it may one day be possible to sustain either a nonhuman or a human embryo and fetus in vitro for an extended period, or even through an entire gestation. The technological support system that sustains such development will probably be called an artificial placenta. If prolonged embryo culture is employed with human embryos and fetuses, decisions will be required about whether to sustain development to the point of viability. At some point a transition will undoubtedly be made from laboratory research designed to test the technical feasibility of long-term culture to an actual attempt to produce a human child by means of ectogenesis (extrauterine development) (Kass; Fletcher; Karp; Walters).

Research on Implanted Embryos and Fetuses

The ethical questions that surround research on implanted embryos and on implanted fetuses are virtually identical, except for the different stages of development involved. This continuity in biological development and similarity in ethical analysis is so striking that both the U.S. National Commission for the Protection of Human Subjects of Biomedical and Behavioral Research (U.S. Commission for the Protection of Human Subjects) and the British Polkinghorne Committee employed the term *fetus* to refer to the developing entity from the time of implantation through the whole of gestation. In the following discussion the word fetus and its derivatives will be employed to refer to the embryo or fetus from the time of implantation in the uterus of a woman through the point at which physical separation from the woman occurs.

As in the case of preimplantation embryo research, one can distinguish two major contexts for fetal research. The first is one in which further development and delivery of an infant are anticipated. The second context is one in which induced abortion is either planned or in progress.

FETAL RESEARCH IN ANTICIPATION OF BIRTH. Many of the ethical issues involved in fetal research conducted at any stage of gestation in anticipation of birth closely parallel the ethical issues in research on newborns. The main reason for the close parallel is that the further development of the fetus or newborn into an adult person is planned. No research procedure that is likely to threaten the life or damage the health of a future person would be either proposed or carried out by responsible scientists. For this reason research not intended to benefit a particular fetus (in anticipation of birth) or a particular newborn is generally constrained by the no-risk or minimal-risk rule (U. S. Commission for the Protection of Human Subjects, Polkinghorne). That is, the research must be judged to pose either no risk at all (as in certain observational studies) or only minimal risk to the potential subject. For research intended to benefit a particular fetus or newborn, a careful weighing and balancing of likely benefits and harms to the subject is required (Polkinghorne; 45 C.F.R. 46.204).

The major difference between neonatal research and fetal research in anticipation of birth is that the fetus is contained within the pregnant woman's body, and any research intervention will require physical contact with, or at least physical proximity to, the pregnant woman. Thus fetal research inevitably and simultaneously affects a pregnant woman. For this reason it requires a careful weighing and balancing of the risks to her, as well as her informed consent.

Just as fetal research inevitably affects a pregnant woman, research on pregnant women inevitably affects the fetus. In the 1990s some commentators noted that a tendency to focus on fetal well-being resulted in the exclusion of women from clinical trials and in a paucity of information about the impact of medications and interventions on pregnant women or fetuses (Institute of Medicine). Their recommendations included presumed eligibility of pregnant women for participation in clinical studies, whether or not direct fetal benefit is anticipated. In the United States the revised Code of Federal Regulations accounts for the connectedness of the woman and fetus and modifies the minimal risk standard in that it allows for greater than minimal risk research in which the risk to the fetus is caused solely by interventions or procedures that hold out the prospect of direct benefit for the woman *or* the fetus (45 C.F.R. 46.204).

Many clinical procedures that are now routinely employed in obstetrical practice were first tested on pregnant women and fetuses in anticipation of birth. One early therapy was the use of exchange transfusions to overcome Rh incompatibility between a pregnant woman and her fetus. The worldwide epidemic of HIV infection and AIDS provided the context for important research affecting fetuses in the 1990s. In one groundbreaking randomized clinical trial, the antiviral drug azidothymidine (AZT) was administered to HIV-infected pregnant women in an effort prevent the transmission of infection to their fetuses, and was found to reduce the risk of vertical transmission by 66 percent (Sperling et al.).

One of the problems associated with early HIV research was that the impact of interventions to prevent maternal to child transmission was only measured with respect to fetal well-being; outcomes affecting pregnant women were not measured (Faden et al.). In the late 1990s the tendency to focus on fetal outcomes while ignoring those of women gained greater attention as one of several ethical issues surrounding experimental techniques now known as maternal-fetal surgery.

While surgical therapies for prenatally diagnosed lethal conditions have been investigated since the early 1980s, this type of fetal research gained considerable attention in the late 1990s and early 2000s due to several ethical issues associated reports on the use of maternal-fetal surgery to correct fetal myelomeningocele (Lyerly et al.). Myelomeningocele is a condition involving incomplete closure of the spinal cord during fetal development and may be associated with bowel and bladder dysfunction, weakness or paralysis of the lower extremities, and cognitive difficulties. Investigators hypothesized that some of the neurologic damage associated with myelomeningocele occurred in utero due to exposure of the spinal cord to amniotic fluid, and thus that closure of the defect prior to birth would be associated with fewer adverse consequences in the neonate. Therefore, surgical closure of the spinal cord defect before birth, involving an operation on the pregnant woman and fetus, has been attempted and has raised many clinical and ethical issues.

One issue raised was whether it was appropriate to perform interventions associated with greater than minimal maternal and fetal risks in order to correct a non-lethal fetal anomaly. Previously the risks of maternal-fetal surgery had been justified in part because their aim was to correct otherwise lethal fetal anomalies, such as severe urinary tract obstruction, hydrocephalus, and congenital diaphragmatic hernia. Myelomeningocele, on the other hand, is an anomaly that is compatible with a normal life. A related concern was that willingness to perform this procedure reinforced discriminatory attitudes toward individuals with disabilities, like those with spina bifida (Myelomeningocele). Another concern raised was the failure to collect data on outcomes related to women, even though the techniques involved experimental surgery on both women and fetuses. Commentators emphasized that both the woman and fetus needed to be considered research subjects. Other concerns included the tendency to view these procedures as *innovative therapy* rather than *research,* and the adequacy of the informed consent process in pregnant women with a potentially sick fetus. As techniques to diagnose and potentially treat prenatally diagnosed conditions improve, the ethical issues surrounding maternal-fetal surgery for myelomeningocele will continue to be relevant to the conduct of fetal research in anticipation of birth.

FETAL RESEARCH IN ANTICIPATION OF OR DURING IN-
DUCED ABORTION. Fetal research conducted before or
during induced abortion could have various aims. One
possible goal would be to develop better techniques for
prenatal diagnosis, for example, by means of fetoscopy or
chorionic villi sampling. Another possible goal would be to
study whether drugs, viruses, vaccines, or radioisotopes cross
the placental barrier between pregnant woman and fetus. A
third aim of such studies could be to develop techniques for
induced abortion that are safer for pregnant women or more
humane in the termination of fetal life. Fourth, during
abortion by hysterotomy (a seldom-used procedure similar
to a cesarean section), fetal physiology can be studied after
the fetus has been removed from the uterus of the pregnant
woman and before the umbilical cord has been severed
(Walters, 1975).

Commentators on the ethics of fetal research in anticipation of induced abortion have always been aware that a
pregnant woman who intends to terminate her pregnancy
can change her decision about abortion even after a research
procedure has been performed. In addition in rare cases an
attempt at induced abortion results in a live birth. Thus
except in the case of research procedures performed during
the abortion procedure itself, the distinction between a
fetus-to-be-aborted and a fetus-to-be-born is statistical rather
than metaphysical. One study performed for the U.S. Commission for the Protection of Human Subjects in the 1970s
estimated the change-of-decision rate between a visit to an
abortion facility and the scheduled time of termination to be
in the range of 1–2 percent (Bracken).

The possibility that a pregnant woman may change her
decision to undergo induced abortion after a research intervention sets an outer limit on the types of interventions that
prudent researchers would be willing to perform. For example it would be useful to know at what stages of pregnancy
alcohol, drugs, or viral infections are most likely to produce
malformations in human fetuses; however, in the view of
most commentators on the ethics of fetal research, such
studies ought not to be performed in humans. In the words
of the Peel Committee report, "In our view it is unethical for
a medical practitioner to administer drugs or carry out any
procedures on the mother with the deliberate intent of
ascertaining the harm that these might do to the fetus,
notwithstanding that arrangements may have been made to
terminate the pregnancy and even if the mother is willing to
give her consent to such an experiment" (United Kingdom,
1972, p. 6).

Even if research likely to cause serious damage to the
fetus is ethically proscribed, there are at least two different
ethical standards that can be adopted with respect to fetal

research in anticipation of or during induced abortion. The
first standard asks for equal treatment of the fetus-to-be-
born and the fetus-to-be aborted. In brief this standard
requires either that one should perform research procedures
on fetuses-to-be-born concurrently with performing the
same procedures on fetuses-to-be-aborted, or at least that
one should be *willing* to perform the same procedure on
both groups of fetuses. In practice this standard would be
virtually equivalent to the no-risk or minimal-risk rule
discussed in connection with fetal research in anticipation
of birth (McCormick; Walters, 1975; Ramsey, 1975;
Polkinghorne).

An alternative standard would reject the equal-treatment
requirement. What is proposed instead is a kind of case-by-
case approach to fetal research (U.S. Commission for the
Protection of Human Subjects; Fletcher and Ryan). For
example if the primary risk of a research procedure like
chorionic villi sampling is that it will cause abortion in a
small percentage of pregnant women, then it can be argued
that research on this diagnostic procedure should be performed on women who plan to undergo induced abortion. If
the research procedure itself is unlikely to injure the fetus,
then the major remaining risk is that the abortion that the
pregnant woman planned to have induced in the future
would instead occur spontaneously. The major ethical questions remaining in a case of this kind have to do with the
timing of abortion: Is a later rather than an earlier induced
abortion less respectful of the developing fetus? Does a later
abortion entail greater risks to the physical and mental
health of the pregnant woman?

An important dimension of the fetal research discussion
is the possibility that research procedures will cause pain to
the fetus (Steinbock). One of the difficulties in coming to
terms with this issue is that the word *pain* probably has
different meanings at different developmental stages. The
anatomical basis for simple spinal reflexes seems to be
present in human embryos at about 7.5 weeks post fertilization. Between the ninth and twelfth weeks of development,
the fetal brain stem begins to function as a rudimentary
information processor. However only at twenty-two to
twenty-three weeks of gestation is the cerebral neocortex
connected to the other parts of the brain (Flower). Presumably the fetal capacity to perceive pain would differ at each of
these three steps, but it is difficult to know precisely to what
extent painful stimuli would be felt or remembered.

Research on Aborted, Live Embryos and Fetuses

There are major conceptual difficulties involved in describing a previously implanted entity that is expelled or removed

alive from a pregnant woman's body (or removed alive from attachment to an artificial placenta). One candidate term is *abortus;* another is *fetus ex utero* or *embryo or fetus outside the uterus.* Adjectives applied to such entities include *previable* or *nonviable* and *viable.* A *viable fetus outside the uterus* is in fact a newborn infant, albeit one that may be seriously premature. In addition the notion of viability is elastic, sometimes seeming to mean the gestational age, weight, or length at which the smallest known infant has survived, at other times seeming to mean the stage at which a stipulated percentage of infants survive, given the assistance of technological means of life support.

Three circumstances can be envisioned in which the question of research on formerly implanted, living embryos or fetuses could arise. First, the surgical removal of an ectopic pregnancy could provide a still-living embryo or fetus. Second, a spontaneous miscarriage could result in the delivery of a live embryo or fetus. Third, an already implanted embryo or fetus could be aborted by means that make it either possible or likely that an intact, living embryo or fetus will result from the abortion procedure.

There is no clear consensus on the ethical justifiability of research on living human embryos or fetuses outside the uterus. In the United Kingdom, two official reports reflect a clear trend in a more conservative direction. In 1972 the Peel Committee affirmed the scientific value of research on clearly previable fetuses outside the uterus and permitted many kinds of research on such fetuses (United Kingdom, 1972). However the Polkinghorne Committee report of 1989 expressly rejected the position of the Peel Committee, arguing that the only morally relevant distinction was between living and dead fetuses, not the distinction between previable and viable fetuses (Polkinghorne). In the United States the U.S. Commission for the Protection of Human Subjects allowed no significant procedural changes in the abortion procedure solely for research purposes and restricted what could be done with the live, delivered embryo or fetus to intrusions that would not alter the duration of its life. Recommendation 1100 by the Parliamentary Assembly of the Council of Europe (1989) also discussed "the use of human embryos and fetuses in scientific research." Its recommendation clearly reflected the ambivalence of ethical opinion on research involving live embryos or fetuses outside the uterus. After stating that "Experiments on living embryos or foetuses, whether viable or not, shall be prohibited," the recommendation continued as follows: "None the less, where a state authorises certain experiments on nonviable foetuses or embryos only, these experiments may be undertaken in accordance with the terms of this recommendation and subject to prior authorisation from the health or

scientific authorities or, where applicable, the national multidisciplinary body" (Council of Europe, p. 6).

Conclusion

Since 1978 the ethical discussion of research involving implanted fetuses and live, aborted fetuses has matured, but it has proceeded largely along the lines established in the 1970s. In contrast the success of clinical IVF has given new impetus to the ethical debate about research on preimplantation embryos. In the future it is at least possible that new methods for sustained embryo and fetal culture in vitro will give rise to additional ethical challenges.

LEROY WALTERS (1995)
REVISED BY ANNE DRAPKIN LYERLY

SEE ALSO: *Cloning: Reproductive; Embryo and Fetus: Embryo Research; Embryo and Fetus: Embryonic Stem Cell Research; Maternal-Fetal Relationship; Research Policy; Research, Unethical*

BIBLIOGRAPHY

American Society for Reproductive Medicine. 1999. *A Practice Committee Report: Guidelines on the Number of Embryos Transferred.* Birmingham, AL: Author.

Biggers, John D. 1979. "In Vitro Fertilization, Embryo Culture and Embryo Transfer in the Human," Appendix. In *HEW Support of Research Involving Human in Vitro Fertilization and Embryo Transfer.* Washington, D.C.: Author.

Bracken, Michael B. 1975. "The Stability of the Decision to Seek Induced Abortion." In *Research on the Fetus,* Appendix. Washington, D.C.: U.S. Department of Health, Education, and Welfare.

Catholic Church. Congregation for the Doctrine of the Faith. 1987. *Instruction on Respect for Human Life in Its Origin and on the Dignity of Procreation.* Vatican City: Author.

Chang, M. C. 1959. "Fertilization of Rabbit Ova in Vitro." *Nature* 184(4684): 466–467.

Chard, T. 1991. "Frequency of Implantation and Early Pregnancy Loss in Natural Cycles." *Baillière's Clinical Obstetrics and Gynaecology* 5(1): 179–189.

Chen, L. T., and Hsu, Y. C. 1982. "Development of Mouse Embryos in Vitro: Preimplantation to the Limb Bud Stage." *Science* 218(4567): 66–68.

Council of Europe. Parliamentary Assembly. 1989. *Recommendation 1100: On the Use of Human Embryos and Fetuses in Scientific Research.* Strasbourg: Author.

Dawson, Karen. 1990a. "Introduction: An Outline of Scientific Aspects of Human Embryo Research." In *Embryo Experimentation,* ed. Peter Singer; Helga Kuhse, Stephen Buckle, et al. New York: Cambridge University Press.

Dawson, Karen. 1990b. "A Scientific Examination of Some Speculations about Continuing Human Pre-Embryo Research." In *Embryo Experimentation,* ed. Peter Singer, Helga Kuhse, Stephen Buckle, et al. New York: Cambridge University Press.

Edwards, Robert G. 1989. *Life Before Birth: Reflections on the Embryo Debate.* New York: Basic Books.

Edwards, Robert G., ed. 1993. *Preconception and Preimplantation Diagnosis of Human Genetic Disease.* Cambridge, Eng.: Cambridge University Press.

Edwards, Robert G.; Bavister, Barry D.; and Steptoe, Patrick C. 1969. "Early Stages of Fertilization in Vitro of Human Oocytes Matured in Vitro." *Nature* 221(5181): 632–635.

Ethics Committee of the American Fertility Society. 1990. "Ethical Considerations of the New Reproductive Technologies." *Fertility and Sterility* 53(6)(Supplement 2): 1S–104S.

Faden, Ruth; Kass, Nancy; and McGraw, Deven. 1996. "Women as Vessels and Vectors: Lessons from the HIV Epidemic." In *Feminism and Bioethics: Beyond Reproduction,* ed. Susan Wolf. New York: Oxford.

Fishel, S. B.; Edwards, Robert G.; and Evans, C. J. 1980. "Human Chorionic Gonadotropin Secreted by Pre-Implantation Embryos Cultured in Vitro." *Science* 223(4638): 816–818.

Fletcher, John C., and Ryan, Kenneth J. 1987. "Federal Regulations for Fetal Research: A Case for Reform." *Law, Medicine and Health Care* 15(3): 126–138.

Fletcher, Joseph F. 1974. *The Ethics of Genetic Control: Ending Reproductive Roulette.* Garden City, NY: Anchor.

Flower, Michael J. 1985. "Neuromaturation of the Human Fetus." *Journal of Medicine and Philosophy* 10(7): 237–251.

Green, Ronald M. 2001. *The Human Embryo Research Debates: Bioethics in the Vortex of Controversy.* New York: Oxford.

Grobstein, Clifford. 1988. *Science and the Unborn: Choosing Human Futures.* New York: Basic Books.

Harris, R.; Whittemore A. S.; Itnyre J.; and the Collaborative Ovarian Cancer Group. 1992. "Characteristics Relating to Ovarian Cancer Risk: Collaborative Analysis of 12 U.S. Case-Control Studies. III. Epithelial Tumors of Low Malignant Potential in White Women." *American Journal of Epidemiology* 136: 1204–1211.

Hellegers, André E. 1970. "Fetal Development." *Theological Studies* 31(1): 3–9.

Hoffman, David I.; Zellman, Gail L.; Fair, Christine; et al. 2003. "Cryopreserved Embryos in the United States and Their Availability for Research." *Fertility and Sterility* 75(5): 1063–1069.

Institute of Medicine. Committee on the Ethical and Legal Issues Relating to the Inclusion of Women in Clinical Studies. 1994. *Women and Health Research.* Washington, D.C.: National Academy Press.

International Society of Law and Technology Working Group. 1998. "ART into Science: Regulation of Fertility Techniques." *Science* 281: 651–652.

Karp, Laurence E. 1976. *Genetic Engineering: Threat or Promise?* Chicago: Nelson-Hall.

Kass, Leon R. 1972. "Making Babies—The New Biology and the *Old* Morality." *Public Interest* 26: 18–56.

Kuhse, Helga, and Singer, Peter. 1990. "Individuals, Humans and Persons: The Issue of Moral Status." In *Embryo Experimentation,* ed. Peter Singer, Helga Kuhse, Stephen Buckle, et al. New York: Cambridge University Press.

Lyerly, Anne D.; Gates, Elena A.; Cefalo, Robert C.; and Sugarman, Jeremy S. 2001. "Toward the Ethical Evaluation and Use of Maternal-Fetal Surgery." *Obstetrics and Gynecology* 98: 689–697.

McCormick, Richard A. 1975. "Experimentation on the Fetus: Policy Proposals." In *Research on the Fetus,* Appendix. Washington, D.C.: U.S. Department of Health, Education and Welfare.

McLaren, Anne. 1986. "Prelude to Embryogenesis." In *Human Embryo Research: Yes or No?,* ed. Gregory Bock, and Maeve O'Connor. London: Tavistock.

National Bioethics Advisory Commission. 1999. *Ethical Issues in Human Stem Cell Research. Report and Recommendations of the National Bioethics Advisory Commission,* vol. I. Rockville, MD: Author.

National Institutes of Health. Human Embryo Research Panel. 1994. *Report of the Human Embryo Research Panel,* 2 vols. Bethesda, MD: Author.

New, D. A. T. 1973. "Studies on Mammalian Fetuses in Vitro During the Period of Organogenesis." In *The Mammalian Fetus in Vitro,* ed. C. R. Austin. London: Chapman & Hall.

Polkinghorne, J. C. 1989. *Review of the Guidance on the Research Use of Fetuses and Fetal Material.* London: Her Majesty's Stationery Office.

Ramsey, Paul. 1970. "Moral and Religious Implications of Genetic Control." In *Fabricated Man: The Ethics of Genetic Control,* ed. Paul Ramsey. New Haven, CT: Yale University Press.

Ramsey, Paul. 1975. *The Ethics of Fetal Research.* New Haven, CT: Yale University Press.

Robertson, John A. 1994. *Children of Choice: Freedom and the New Reproductive Technologies.* Princeton, NJ: Princeton University Press.

Sass, Hans-Martin. 1989. "Brain Life and Brain Death: A Proposal for a Normative Agreement." *Journal of Medicine and Philosophy* 14(1): 45–59.

Singer, Peter, and Dawson, Karen. 1988. "IVF Technology and the Argument from Potential." *Philosophy and Public Affairs* 17(2): 87–104.

Singer, Peter; Kuhse, Helga; Buckle, Stephen; et al., eds. 1990. *Embryo Experimentation.* New York: Cambridge University Press.

Sperling, R. S.; Shapiro, D. E.; Coombs, R. W.; et al. 1996. "Maternal Viral Load, Zidovudine Treatment, and the Risk of Transmission of Human Immunodeficiency Virus Type 1 from Mother to Infant." *New England Journal of Medicine* 335(22): 1621–1629.

Steinbock, Bonnie. 1992. *Life Before Birth: The Moral and Legal Status of Embryos and Fetuses.* New York: Oxford University Press.

Steptoe, Patrick C., and Edwards, Robert G. 1978. "Birth After the Reimplantation of a Human Embryo." *Lancet* 2(8085): 366.

Thomas, Wendell K., and Seidel, George E., Jr. 1993. "Effects of Cumulus Cells on Culture of Bovine Embryos Derived from Oocytes Matured and Fertilized in Vitro." *Journal of Animal Science* 71(9): 2506–2510.

Thompson, James; Itskovitz-Eldor, J.; Shapiro, S. S.; et al. 1998. "Embryonic Stem Cell Lines Derived from Human Blastocysts." *Science* 282: 1145–1147.

United Kingdom. Department of Health and Social Security Advisory Group. 1972. *The Use of Fetuses and Fetal Material for Research: Report.* London: Her Majesty's Stationery Office.

United Kingdom. Human Fertilisation and Embryology Authority. 1992. *Annual Report: 1992.* London: Author.

U.S. Department of Health, Education and Welfare. Ethics Advisory Board. 1979. *HEW Support of Research Involving in Vitro Fertilization and Embryo Transfer: Report and Conclusions.* Washington, D.C.: Author.

U.S. National Commission for the Protection of Human Subjects of Biomedical and Behavioral Research. 1975. *Research on the Fetus: Report and Recommendations.* Washington, D.C.: U.S. Department of Health, Education and Welfare.

Van Steirteghem, André C. 1993. "High Fertilization and Implantation Rates After Intracytoplasmic Sperm Injection." *Human Reproduction* 8(7): 1061–1066.

Walters, LeRoy. 1975. "Ethical and Public Policy Issues in Fetal Research." In *Research on the Fetus,* Appendix. Washington, D.C.: U.S. Department of Health, Education and Welfare.

Walters, LeRoy. 1979. "Ethical Issues in Human in Vitro Fertilization and Research Involving Early Human Embryos." In *HEW Support of Research Involving Human in Vitro Fertilization and Embryo Transfer,* Appendix.Washington, D.C.: U.S. Department of Health, Education and Welfare.

Walters, LeRoy. 1987. "Ethics and New Reproductive Technologies: An International Review of Committee Statements." *Hastings Center Report* 17(Special supplement June): 3–9.

Warnock, Henry. 1984. *Report of the Committee of Inquiry into Human Fertilisation and Embryology.* London: Her Majesty's Stationery Office.

Wivel, Nelson A., and Walters, LeRoy. 1993. "Germ-Line Gene Modification and Disease Prevention: Some Medical and Ethical Perspectives." *Science* 262(5133): 533–538.

INTERNET RESOURCES

Human Fertilization and Embryo Authority. 2002. *Eleventh Annual Report and Accounts.* Available from <http://www.hfea.gov.uk/Downloads/Annual_Report/AR_2002.pdf>.

U. S. Code of Federal Regulations, Protection of Human Subjects. 45 CFR 46. 2003. Available from <http://ohrp.osophs.dhhs.gov/humansubjects/guidance/45cfr46.htm/>.

FETUS

SEE *Embryo and Fetus*

FREEDOM AND FREE WILL

• • •

Freedom is widely regarded as a highly desirable component of human personalities, interpersonal relations, and social and governmental arrangements. Despite multiple meanings, the main types of freedom can be defined and distinguished.

Types of Freedom

Diverse freedoms contrast with different types of restrictions, limitations, or restraints that negate them. Some freedom-inhibiting conditions are internal to persons, some external, some negative, some positive. Joel Feinberg (1980) developed a useful four-way typology of constraints: external positive, external negative, internal positive, and internal negative. Examples of these, respectively, are lack of money, being handcuffed, fear, and weakness. In the free will controversy, freedom of action equates with external freedom, both positive and negative, while freedom of will is a variety of internal freedom.

POSITIVE EXTERNAL FREEDOM. Positive external freedom is having the external means to achieve our ends and fulfill our desires or interests. These means are positive conditions in our environment such as money to pay our way, schools open to all, or accessible medical resources and personnel. A pregnant woman who desires an abortion but lacks the money to pay for it has insufficient positive external freedom. Whether society should pay for contraception services and abortions for the poor, thereby enhancing their positive freedom, is highly controversial (Edwards, 1997). Patients in great pain who desire analgesic medication may or may not have compassionate doctors who will prescribe adequate means to pain relief; if denied such means by uncaring, inattentive, or intimidated doctors, these patients lack external freedom.

NEGATIVE EXTERNAL FREEDOM. Negative external freedom is the absence of external pressures, constraints, or restraints that inhibit or prevent us from doing what we want or choose to do. Many negative conditions interfere significantly with freedom of action. We are negatively free externally when unencumbered by such restraints as chains, shackles, walls, and jails, and/or by such constraints as laws, institutional prohibitions, threats, intimidations, and coercive or covert pressures from others. Absence of external encumbrances usually correlates very directly with increased options for choice and action.

Many types of positive external freedom are widely recognized and cherished. Some of the most important are political freedoms or rights guaranteed by government. The Bill of Rights to the U.S. Constitution identifies and affirms such varieties of external freedom of action as freedom of religion, freedom of speech, freedom of the press, freedom to assemble peaceably, and freedom to petition government for redress of grievances. Other amendments guarantee the freedom to participate in political processes on an equal basis. These constitutionally guaranteed forms of freedom of action declare that government, other institutions, and specific individuals may not interfere with a person's choice of religion, with people expressing their thoughts, or with people communicating their beliefs, knowledge, and ideas through the press and other media. All of these kinds of freedom of action are both permitted and limited by our laws; none is absolute without qualification. All are highly desirable whether or not humans have free will and would be so even in a totally deterministic universe.

Historically, many classes of individuals were externally unfree in a great variety of undesirable ways. The fullest enjoyment of external freedom in the United States was once limited to competent, landowning, white males, whereas severe restrictions were imposed on the freedom of action of females, slaves, nonwhites, minors, mentally disturbed persons, the landless, homosexuals, and other disfavored groups such as animals. Gradually, as prejudices waned, usually after prolonged and bitter struggles, both the scope and types of freedom were extended to victims of unjust discrimination; but the process has not yet come to an end.

External social and governmental restrictions on freedom of action are not always undesirable. We are not and should not be free to do many things that would be harmful to the person and/or property of others or, more controversially, even to ourselves. Some external legal, moral, and social restraints on freedom of action are perfectly legitimate. When freedom of action conflicts with more legitimate goals and values, it must yield to their superiority.

External freedom of action is extremely valuable, but it is not sufficient for freedom in its fullest sense. Other kinds of freedom internal to persons are also highly desirable.

POSITIVE INTERNAL FREEDOM. Positive internal freedom consists of the effective presence of internal factors that contribute to people fulfilling their goals, desires, and interests; being self-reliant and self-directed—their own masters; and being in control of their own lives and destinies. These are elements of personality such as knowing who we are, our circumstances, the alternatives among which we must select, and the norms and facts relevant for making informed decisions; the ability to think, deliberate, and reason about our ends or goals, to prioritize and harmonize them, and to recognize effective means to achieve them; conscience, a moral sense of right and wrong; feelings, emotions, motives, desires, purposes, interests, and affections; and the ability to make our own choices for ourselves and to identify with our own purposes and projects, and the inner resources for acting as we will to act.

Occasionally freedom is said to consist of valuing and actualizing certain inner processes and states above all others. Saint Augustine (354–430), the early Christian church father, identified true freedom with complete conformity to the will of God; and the Stoics and the seventeenth-century Dutch philosopher Benedict Spinoza identified it with being rational and controlling or suppressing one's emotions.

Positive internal freedom may include free will, but most of its components would be highly desirable even in the absence of free will. Being positively free is what most bioethicists mean by being autonomous, or rationally autonomous, though whether this includes free will is not always clear. Respecting the rational autonomy of patients is a matter of valuing their positive internal freedom and acting accordingly.

NEGATIVE INTERNAL FREEDOM. Negative internal freedom is the absence of internal psychological or physiological obstructions that inhibit the proper functioning of the constituents of positive internal freedom—the absence of factors that inhibit knowing, deliberating, feeling, preferring, valuing, discerning right from wrong, self-control, making our own choices for ourselves, and acting effectively. Exercise of positive freedom is inhibited by such internal conditions as being overwhelmed by unconscious processes or motives, or by psychoses, neuroses, compulsions, addictions, or other nonvoluntary character defects and disorders. Genetic and neuromuscular conditions involving pain, weakness, disability, or hyperactivity may also undermine negative internal freedom.

Many conditions that undermine negative internal freedom have external causes, some medical in nature, some not. Negative internal freedom is absent in individuals who are temporarily stupefied by alcohol or by recreational or poorly administered psychotropic drugs, and in those who are more permanently impaired by brain damage, retardation, or a degenerative disease. People may also lose or lack independence if their capacities and options are reduced by lobotomies, psychosurgery, hypnosis, behavior modification, brainwashing, indoctrination, or massive ignorance. When used skillfully with the informed voluntary consent of patients, psychotherapy can increase human freedom, not decrease it. The Austrian neurologist Sigmund Freud (1856–1939) thought that the major purpose of psychoanalysis is to increase the freedom of otherwise freedom-impaired patients.

All four types of freedom have significant worth for human beings with or without free will and may be classified as intrinsic goods, valuable for their own sakes; as indispensable extrinsic goods, valuable as essential means to other human ends; or as both at once; but we can make such judgments justifiably only if we are sufficiently enlightened, fair-minded, and free!

Because healthy bodies and selves are our most directly efficient instruments, and because so many conditions that interfere with freedom are medical in nature, physicians and other healthcare professionals are uniquely positioned by their knowledge and power to enhance human freedom.

Free Will, Obligation, Responsibility, and Related Concepts

The concept of free will is inextricably bound up with many related but elusive concepts such as duty or obligation, responsibility, blameworthiness, and praiseworthiness.

THE FREE WILL POSITION. Defenders of free will insist that freedom in the most inclusive and desirable sense is something more than mere external freedom of action; it is a fundamental type of positive internal freedom. Free will involves more than a mere internal capacity for making choices, for choices may be either free or unfree. Free choices are informed and intentional as well as creative, originative, or "contracausal." Choices are not free if they are completely determined by ignorance or by preexisting desires, habits, beliefs, or by other psychological, physiological, genetic, social, or environmental conditions. When choices are so determined, we lack the power to choose otherwise and are inevitably destined to make exactly the choices we make and do exactly the things that we do. Representative defenders of free will include the fourteenth-century English philosopher William of Ockham, the eighteenth-century Scottish philosopher Thomas Reid, and such contemporary figures as C. A. Campbell, Roderick Chisholm, Rem B. Edwards, and Robert Kane.

Defenders regard free will as essential to human worth and dignity, partly because of its inherent value and partly because it is interwoven inextricably with other indispensable moral and legal concepts and practices such as obligation, responsibility, blameworthiness, and praiseworthiness.

Being *obligated*—having duties, whether moral, prudential, or whatever—is possible only if we have free will, genuinely open alternatives, and the ability to choose and act otherwise, defenders claim. Obligation presupposes being able to choose freely and act dutifully. Ought implies can, and cannot implies not obligated. In a deterministic universe devoid of free will, those who choose to do their duty can and must do so; oddly, those who do not cannot, and thus never have or had any duties at all. Actually, because neither ever encounters open alternatives or could ever choose or act otherwise, no one ever has any duties of any kind, for all persons are rigidly determined to choose and act exactly as they do.

Similarly, being *responsible* for our choices and the actions that issue from them just means that we understand the genuinely open alternatives before us, that we desire or intend some of them, and that our final decisions originate with us, rather than being programmed into us by heredity, our physical or social environment, fate, God, or any kind of external causes, however near or remote. These things may influence us, but they cannot completely determine us if we are to be responsible for what we decide and do.

The free will position also insists that blame and punishment as well as praise and reward are inextricably linked to being responsible. When we do wrong and are *blameworthy,* we may be justly blamed or punished only if we are responsible for our decision to do wrong, and only if we do it knowingly and intentionally, it originates with us, and it could have been otherwise—that is, only if it is informed, intentional, and free. And when we do what is right and are *praiseworthy,* we may be justly praised and rewarded only if we responsibly, knowingly, intentionally, creatively, and freely decide to do so. Blameworthiness cannot be defined simply as susceptibility to blame or punishment; nor can praiseworthiness be defined simply as susceptibility to praise or reward. The susceptibility must be just or appropriate, free will advocates insist; and this condition is satisfied only when we choose responsibly, that is, originatively or freely, knowingly, and intentionally and have the power to choose otherwise from genuinely open alternatives. If our choices do not originate with us, if they are programmed into us and we are predetermined to make only and exactly the choices that we make, then our programmers, but not we ourselves, are responsible for our decisions, and we cannot justly be held responsible or subjected to blame, punishment, praise, or reward.

Free will champions usually affirm *indirect* as well as the *direct* responsibility. We are indirectly responsible for our choices and actions, even when they are completely determined by our present character and strongest inclinations, as long as that character and those inclinations were significantly shaped by choices and efforts that we made earlier in life. Advocates of free will and self-creative responsibility typically do not hold that all our responsible choices are directly free or originative. Determinists are right that most of our present choices are completely determined by our existing dispositions and interests; but if we actively participated in forming them by earlier self-creative choices and efforts of will, then we are indirectly responsible for the choices and actions that issue from our self-established character.

HARD AND SOFT DETERMINISM. In his influential 1884 article, "The Dilemma of Determinism," the American psychologist and philosopher William James (1842–1910) distinguished between hard and soft determinism. *Hard determinists* usually accept every feature of the free will position except causal indefiniteness. They agree that a free will would be an originative or self-creative will, and that being obligated and responsible just means knowingly, intentionally, and originatively making right or wrong choices that could have been otherwise. Social practices involving obligation, blame/punishment, and praise/reward are just and justified only if we are free and responsible. Nevertheless, determinism is true and all our choices are caused or determined by antecedent conditions; none could be otherwise. Because we are not free and responsible, we are never justified in holding anyone obligated or responsible for anything. We can never justly blame or punish wrongdoers or praise and reward those who do right. Representative hard determinists include Spinoza; the English clergyman and chemist Joseph Priestley; the young Benjamin Franklin; the eighteenth-century American statesman and philosopher, who later recanted this position; and Paul Edwards.

Some hard determinists acknowledge that our established practices of being morally obligated as well as blaming, punishing, praising, and rewarding are so valuable morally and socially, so indispensable for the very existence of a livable community, that the illusion of free will should be sustained in order to perpetuate them (Smilansky, 2000). Others insist that hard determinists may legitimately abandon blame and punishment but retain obligation, praise, and reward. Without deluding anyone, hard determinists can approve, commend, encourage, praise, and reward right actions, even if they are not strictly obligatory. Such activities become integral parts of causal processes calculated to bring about decent social orders (Wolf, 1980, 1990; Pereboom, 1995, 2001).

Soft determinists do not embrace these drastic conclusions. They hold that causal determinism is perfectly compatible with human obligation and responsibility and the moral and social practices normally associated with them. Representative soft determinists include the seventeenth-century English philosopher Thomas Hobbes, the eighteenth-century American clergyman and theologian Jonathan Edwards, the eighteenth-century Scottish philosopher and historian David Hume, the nineteenth-century English philosopher and economist John Stuart Mill, and more recent figures such as Harry G. Frankfurt, Daniel Dennett, and Kai Nielsen.

COMPATIBILISM. Soft determinists are compatibilists who attack almost every element of the free will position and reject the free will view that causal determinism is incompatible with human freedom, obligation, responsibility, and just susceptibility to blame/punishment or praise/reward.

Compatibilists hold that freedom of action combined with inner conditions that do not presuppose causal indeterminism are quite sufficient for human obligation and responsibility—that free will is not needed in the first place. If we are free to do what we knowingly and intentionally most want to do, then we are responsible for doing it, and we can have moral and other kinds of obligation. Compatibilists attack the free will meaning of the term *responsible* and redefine the concept.

For the free will position, being responsible for making choices and the actions that flow from them means:

(1) Recognizing and understanding the alternatives, which are genuinely open metaphysically.
(2) Intending to or being motivated or predisposed to choose one or more of these alternatives without their being completely predetermined by our desire(s), dispositions, or anything else.
(3) Deliberating about the alternatives.
(4) Knowing that some alternatives are good or right, some bad or wrong, and perhaps some indifferent.
(5) Originating the choices and efforts that we make.
(6) Having the power to choose otherwise.

Compatibilistic soft determinists omit the self-originative features of this definition. For them, being responsible just means:

(1) Recognizing and understanding the alternatives, which need not be metaphysically open.
(2) Intending or being more strongly motivated or predisposed to choose one alternative over the

others, especially when these belong to our deep rational selves.

(3) Deliberating about the alternatives.

(4) Knowing that some alternatives are good or right, some bad or wrong, and perhaps some indifferent.

Origination, open alternatives, and the ability to choose otherwise are irrelevant; so, free will is irrelevant. Determinism is compatible with holding people under obligation and regarding them as responsible for what they choose and do. But is this compatibilistic redefinition of the term responsible acceptable? Can we really escape the deep-rooted intuition that we are not responsible for any choices and efforts that are programmed into us from beyond?

Objections and Responses

Past and present debates incorporate many objections to free will with corresponding replies.

CHOICE AND CHANCE. Free will itself is not compatible with having duties and being responsible because free choices are by definition uncaused and indeterministic, which means that they are mere uncontrolled chance events or accidents.

But, say free willists, chance events do not satisfy many conditions that define responsible free choices. They do not involve deliberation, knowledge of alternatives or of right and wrong, desires, dispositions and intentions, or the subjective experience of selecting or trying. When free choices are made, these conditions bring about inclinations without necessitating a particular choice. These conditions are the very essence of self-control and self-causation, not of chance.

UBIQUITOUS CAUSATION. Because all events have causes, free choices and all effort-makings have causes. There are no exceptions to deterministic causation.

Free will defenders respond that the very concept of causation is ambiguous, not clear and distinct. Free originative choices can be uncaused or "contracausal" in one sense, yet caused in another. Free choices have *necessary causal conditions* such as knowledge, desires, and (if moral) a sense of right and wrong; in their absence, free choices cannot occur. But these are not *sufficient causal conditions* in whose presence only one outcome must occur. Only with respect to sufficient causal conditions are free choices uncaused. With respect to necessary conditions, they are caused. The philosophical options are more complex than simple *indeterminism,* which denies the relevance of all causal considerations to free choice, versus *determinism,* which affirms the rigid causal determination of all choices. Partisans of free will may adopt *libertarianism,* which affirms that existing causal conditions

limit but do not necessitate choices that cannot occur in their absence.

Some proponents of free will claim that self-creative choices are made by an enduring substantive self that is exempt from normal event-causation (Chisholm; O'Connor). Others hold that choices are made by events within that stream of consciousness that constitutes personal selfhood (Edwards, 1969; Kane, 1985, 1996, 2002). Still others claim that agency causation is not so radically different from event causation (Clarke).

CAUSATION BY STRONGEST MOTIVES. Experience shows that all our choices are determined by the strongest desires or sets of cooperating desires belonging to our settled character.

In response, free willists argue that experience actually shows that effort-making and self-creative choosing occur only when character, dispositions, and desires are in conflict and prevailing inclinations are not settled in advance—only when given motives are not sufficiently powerful to resolve motivational conflict. Free choices function to resolve conflicting motives when none are sufficiently powerful themselves to overcome their competitors. Sometimes choice boosts an inclination that is in conflict with others and makes it the strongest. Usually our choices are completely determined by our strongest inclinations, but even then we are indirectly responsible for them if our earlier choices and efforts helped to create them.

THE ABILITY TO CHOOSE OTHERWISE. Being able to choose otherwise is merely hypothetical, not categorical or absolute. Even on deterministic grounds, we can choose or could have chosen otherwise *if* our desires, dispositions, character, or other conditions are or were otherwise. This is quite sufficient for responsible choice.

On the contrary, free willists respond, hypothetical conditions are still incompatible with the deep and ineradicable intuition that we are responsible only if our choices and efforts originate with us; if they originate in heredity and/or environment, these, not we, are responsible for them and the actions that issue from them. Complete determination is incompatible with individual responsibility, blameworthiness, and praiseworthiness.

THE SCIENTIFIC WORLDVIEW. Free will is incompatible with what natural science tells us about the universe and about ourselves.

Free willists reply that Newtonian science had no place for free will because it regarded everything, including human choices, as completely determined and absolutely predictable, given existing facts and natural laws; but this worldview is now obsolete. Quantum physics recognizes indeterminateness and unpredictability within the depths of nature, including human brains. Random quantum events are themselves not within our control, admittedly, but they make room for creative self-control, just as Newtonian physics excluded it. On a more macroscopic level, modern brain scans reveal indeterminate, unresolved conflicts within and between different regions of the brain that are resolved when "executive control" is exercised (Posner and DiGirolamo).

Objections and replies to problems of free will are almost inexhaustible, and every response seems to generate another round of objections and responses. Free will and philosophical issues relating to it have been debated for over 2,000 years and will be, perhaps, for thousands more.

REM B. EDWARDS

SEE ALSO: *Autonomy; Authority in Religious Traditions; Behavior Control; Behaviorism; Behavior Modification Therapies; Coercion; Conscience; Conscience, Rights of; Human Dignity; Insanity and the Insanity Defense; Institutionalization and Deinstitutionalization; Mentally Disabled and Mentally Ill Persons; Neuroethics; Patients' Rights; Psychiatry, Abuses of*

BIBLIOGRAPHY

Campbell, C. A. 1957. *On Selfhood and Godhood.* London: George Allen and Unwin.

Chisholm, Roderick. 1964. "Human Freedom and the Self." Lawrence: University of Kansas, Department of Philosophy. Reprinted in *Free Will,* ed. by Derk Pereboom. Indianapolis, IN: Hackett, 1997; and in *Free Will,* ed. by Robert Kane. Oxford: Blackwell, 2001.

Clarke, Randolph. 1996. "Agent Causation and Event Causation in the Production of Free Action." *Philosophical Topics* 24(2): 19–48.

Dennett, Daniel. 1984. *Elbow Room: The Varieties of Free Will Worth Wanting.* Cambridge, MA: MIT Press.

Edwards, Jonathan. 1754 (reprint 1957). *Freedom of the Will.* New Haven, CT: Yale University Press.

Edwards, Paul. 1958. "Hard and Soft Determinism." In *Determinism and Freedom in the Age of Modern Science,* ed. Sidney Hook. New York: New York University Press.

Edwards, Rem B. 1969. *Freedom, Responsibility, and Obligation.* The Hague, Netherlands: Martinus Nijhoff.

Edwards, Rem B. 1997. "Public Funding of Abortions and Abortion Counseling for Poor Women." In *New Essays on Abortion and Bioethics,* ed. Rem B. Edwards. Greenwich, CT: JAI Press.

Feinberg, Joel. 1980. *Rights, Justice, and the Bounds of Liberty: Essays in Social Philosophy.* Princeton, NJ: Princeton University Press.

Frankfurt, Harry G. 1971. "Freedom of the Will and the Concept of a Person." *Journal of Philosophy* 68(1): 5–20.

Frankfurt, Harry G. 1988. *The Importance of What We Care About: Philosophical Essays.* New York: Cambridge University Press.

Franklin, Benjamin. 1725 (reprint 1930). *A Dissertation on Liberty and Necessity, Pleasure and Pain.* New York: Facsimile Text Society.

Hobbes, Thomas. 1841. *The Questions concerning Liberty, Necessity, and Chance.* In *The English Works of Thomas Hobbes,* vol. 5. London: John Bohn.

Hume, David. 1739–1740 (reprint 1958). *A Treatise of Human Nature.* Oxford: Clarendon Press.

James, William. 1884. "The Dilemma of Determinism." *Unitarian Review and Religious Magazine* 22(September).

Kane, Robert. 1985. *Free Will and Values.* Albany, NY: State University of New York Press.

Kane, Robert. 1996. *The Significance of Free Will.* New York: Oxford University Press.

Kane, Robert, ed. 2001. *Free Will.* Oxford: Blackwell.

Mill, John Stuart. 1867. *An Examination of Sir William Hamilton's Philosophy …,* 3rd edition. London: Longmans, Green, Reader, and Dyer.

Nielsen, Kai. 1971. *Reason and Practice.* New York: Harper and Row.

Ockham, William of. 1991. *Quodlibetal Questions,* 2 vols., tr. Alfred J. Freddoso and Francis E. Kelley. New Haven, CT: Yale University Press.

O'Connor, Timothy. 1998. "The Agent as Cause." In *Metaphysics: The Big Questions,* ed. Peter van Inwagen and Dean Zimmerman. Oxford: Blackwell.

Pereboom, Derk. 1995. "Determinism *al Dente.*" *Noûs* 29(1): 21–45.

Pereboom, Derk. 2001. *Living without Free Will.* Cambridge, Eng.: Cambridge University Press.

Pereboom, Derk, ed. 1997. *Free Will.* Indianapolis, IN: Hackett.

Posner, Michael I., and DiGirolamo, Gregory J. 2000. "Attention in Cognitive Neuroscience: An Overview." In *The New Cognitive Neurosciences,* 2nd edition, ed. Michael S. Gazzaniga et al. Cambridge, MA: MIT Press.

Priestley, Joseph. 1778 (reprint 1977). *A Free Discussion of the Doctrines of Materialism, and Philosophical Necessity....* Millwood, NY: Kraus.

Reid, Thomas. 1788 (reprint 1977). *Essays on the Active Powers of Man.* New York: Garland.

Smilansky, Saul. 2000. *Free Will and Illusion.* Oxford: Clarendon Press.

Spinoza, Benedict. 1951. *Ethics.* In *The Chief Works of Benedict de Spinoza,* vol. 2, tr. Robert Harvey Monro Elwes. New York: Dover.

van Inwagen, Peter. 1983. *An Essay on Free Will.* Oxford: Clarendon Press.

Wolf, Susan. 1980. "Asymmetrical Freedom." *Journal of Philosophy* 77(3): 151–166.

Wolf, Susan. 1990. *Freedom within Reason.* Oxford: Oxford University Press.

FUTURE GENERATIONS, REPRODUCTIVE TECHNOLOGIES AND OBLIGATIONS TO

• • •

Since the early 1960s, scholars have struggled to define the nature and content of our obligations, if any, to future persons. These discussions began in the fields of environmental ethics and population policy and have had their most robust recent expression in the debate over risky reproductive technologies. This entry reviews the issues as they arise in decisions about reproduction, especially decisions involving reproductive technology.

The threshold issue is whether living persons have any duty to consider the welfare of future people. If that question is answered in the affirmative, then the content of the duty needs to be defined. The fact that reproductive conduct is existence inducing, however, greatly complicates the effort to determine exactly when a risky reproductive decision threatens the welfare of future persons.

Duties to Future Persons

Duties not to harm persons seem to presuppose their existence (Narveson). Yet, the future children whose interests are threatened by today's decisions do not exist and may never exist. Because their existence is entirely contingent, skeptics question whether it is coherent to talk of a duty to these "potential" people.

Until the middle of the twentieth century, courts in the United States agreed. Since then, however, nearly all courts have abandoned that view, concluding as most bioethicists do, that duties can run to future people who are foreseeably endangered by our actions (Buchanan et al.).

Moral philosopher David Heyd, in his 1992 book, *Genethics,* argued that an exception must be made for people who control whether or not a future person exists. He contended that creators, such as parents making reproductive decisions or scientists deciding whether to clone a human, cannot have obligations to future persons whose very existence they control. Although he conceded that we ordinarily do owe duties to future persons, he contended that this duty does not extend to persons whose existence we determine. Thus, a baby food manufacturer has an obligation not to harm babies who are born after its pureed peas are canned, but parents or scientists cloning humans have no obligation to future persons whose very existence they control. "There are no moral constraints," he argued, "in genesis decisions" (Heyd, p. 16).

Heyd's argument has central implications for the law and ethics of reproductive behavior. Heyd seems to assume that the right to deny existence includes the freedom to create people without accountability. This would excuse parents and fertility clinics from any obligation to consider the welfare of the children whom they are trying to create.

Heyd's view, however, does not appear to be widely shared. For example, in her 1998 book, *Child versus Childmaker,* Melinda A. Roberts noted that Heyd's view "implies that my neighbor's future child, but not my own, has a claim to my good behavior" (p. 20). Using his analysis, a homeowner who breaks a glass bottle in the backyard may have a duty to the neighbor's future children to pick up the glass, but not to the homeowner's own future children. That conclusion is difficult to defend persuasively. Heyd's theory assumes that the power to create a person implies the absence of any obligation to use that power responsibly. In his view, childbearing is inherently a selfish choice. Yet, this assumption is certainly not self-evident and it conflicts with commonplace expectations of responsible parenting.

Perhaps the key issue in the debate over the duty to future persons is whether a duty can be owed to a "person" who does not yet exist and may never exist. So characterized, the duty appears to be owed to preconception phantoms. Advocates of the duty contend, however, that the obligation being asserted is better understood as a conditional obligation that ripens only if and when an actual person is harmed (Peters, 1999). Whereas it may not be sensible to talk of duties to people who may never exist ("potential people"), it is sensible to talk of a duty to the people who do come to exist in the future ("future people"). Thus, the baby food manufacturer's duty runs only to actual, living people who consume its baby food. At that moment, the potential harmfulness of the earlier negligence crystallizes.

Harm to Future Persons

Many different theories have been offered to identify the circumstances in which reproductive behavior can cause harm to future persons. Each theory identifies a different vantage point from which to understand the interests of future persons. Collectively, they provide a useful set of tools for evaluating the impact of a novel reproductive technology.

At the outset, the inquiry into harmfulness requires a definition of what it means to harm someone. Under conventional analysis, harmful conduct is conduct that makes a person worse off than he otherwise would have been (Fishkin). Lawyers call this a "but for" test because it asks whether the victim would have avoided injury but for the conduct in dispute. Although this test can sometimes be applied to reproductive behavior without any novel difficulties, its application is often complicated by the fact that the injuries believed to be harmful could not have been avoided except by preventing the child from being born at all. A child conceived by cloning, for example, owes his life to this technology. When a disputed act is existence inducing, the only alternative to life with the disability caused by the existence-inducing technology is no life at all. If the conventional test for harmfulness is used, then the disability-causing technology is not harmful unless life with the disability is worse than the alternative—never existing at all. This comparison does pose special problems.

The remainder of this entry begins by exploring the simplest cases—those in which the traditional test of harmfulness seems most apt. The entry then examines the application of this test to injuries that are inextricably associated with life itself and reviews some alternatives that have been suggested to the comparison between life and nonexistence. Finally, it examines the dilemma posed when parents or clinics have a choice between two alternative paths to reproduction, one of which is safer than another.

Ordinary Harm

The easiest cases to analyze do not require a comparison between life and nonexistence. This is true whenever the behavior that caused the injury was not essential to the birth of the child. Consider, for example, the negligent repair of a fertile woman's uterus. A child who is subsequently born prematurely because of this carelessness has suffered injuries that could have been prevented if more care had been taken. Measuring the extent of her harm, therefore, does not require a comparison between life with her injuries and never existing at all. Instead, it requires only a comparison between life with her injuries and life without them.

In the context of reproductive technology, this kind of harm can occur both in routine settings and in exotic ones. Injuries caused by a fertility clinic's failure to properly store its frozen embryos are a straightforward example of this kind of ordinary, avoidable harm. Ordinary harm, however, can also occur in settings typically assumed to trigger the nonexistence comparison, such as multiple cloning or multiple embryo transfer. In a 1996 article, Roberts pointed out that any emotional injuries associated with being one of many identical clones can be avoided by cloning only one person from each source. That single child will consequently be better off than he would have been if additional identical siblings had been cloned.

Injuries caused by germ-line genetic engineering can also be understood in this way. A child who suffers injuries from the genetic engineering of her embryo need not have suffered these injuries if the embryo had been implanted without first manipulating its genes. Of course, she also would not enjoy the benefits, if any, conferred by the manipulation. Thus, she has been harmed by the manipulation if, but only if, it did more harm than good. Answering this question does not require a comparison between life and nonexistence.

The most interesting interpretive debate regarding the applicability of ordinary harm analysis to reproductive behavior involves parents who say that they will not conceive at all if they are not able to use a risky reproductive technique. Consider the case of a fertile couple who could conceive naturally but choose instead to employ a surrogate because the genetic mother fears the risks of childbirth, as occurred in the notorious case of "Baby M" (*In the Matter of Baby M,* 1988). If the parents would not have conceived at all had they been prevented from employing a surrogate, then their child's only alternative to surrogacy was nonexistence. For this reason, scholars such as John A. Robertson believe that no harm is done to this child by use of a surrogate unless the child suffers harms so serious that its life is worse than not existing at all.

The same surprising conclusion arises in other reproductive settings. Assume, for example, that parents can honestly contend that they will not have any children at all if they are not permitted to use a risky reproductive technique such as germ-line genetic engineering. If their claim is correct, then their future child's only alternative to the risks associated with germ-line genetic manipulation is not existing at all.

Roberts rejects the conclusion that no harm has been done in these cases. She has persuasively argued that children such as these are harmed whenever people could have prevented their injuries and chose not to do so (Roberts, 1996, 1998). From her perspective, the fertile couple's choice is a harmful one if it exposes the child to extra unnecessary risks. That the parents preferred not to avoid those risks does not make the choice any less harmful to the child. That child could have been born without his injuries.

Roberts's analysis squares with our intuitions. Surprisingly, however, it is less consistent than Robertson's is with the but-for test of causation. What matters under this test is what *would* have happened had the technology been banned, not what *could* have happened. If surrogacy had been prohibited, for example, the child would not have been born. The test does not take into account the fact that the same embryo could have been implanted in the genetic mother.

Nevertheless, the but-for test is only a starting point for the analysis of causation. Both philosophers and courts have recognized its occasional deficiencies and have fashioned a number of exceptions to ensure that the attribution of causation comports with common sense. Roberts's case for yet another exception is quite credible. Taken to its logical conclusion, conventional harm analysis would excuse even the intentional infliction of harm on future children, as long as being able to inflict it was essential to the procreative intent of the would-be parents. Thus, deaf parents who genetically engineer their children to be deaf cause no harm if this is the only way in which they are willing to have children. This makes no sense. The very intention that makes their conduct culpable also insulates it from moral responsibility.

In ordinary settings, the plaintiff's inability to satisfy the but-for test implies that the plaintiff would have been no better off if the defendant had behaved more responsibly. In the special context of existence-inducing conduct, however, the failure to satisfy the traditional but-for test of causation does not have this meaning. Nonexistence was not the child's only alternative to life with her injuries. Instead, the defendant could have prevented the child's injuries. The mere fact that the parents preferred not to do so seems an insufficient basis for concluding that no harm has been done by their choice.

To recap, reproduction decision making sometimes threatens future children with ordinary harm. Analyzing the harmfulness of these decisions is straightforward except when parents claim that they would not have conceived at all if not permitted to reproduce in a dangerous manner. In such cases, one can either treat the choice as harmless unless the injuries are so serious that life itself is harmful (a threshold that is the subject of the next section) or else replace the inquiry into what would have happened with an inquiry into what could have happened.

Life as a Harm

Sometimes, the underlying objection to a risky form of reproductive conduct is not that safer alternatives were foregone, but that the conduct in question is simply too dangerous to use, even as a last resort. Imagine, for example, an infertile couple who have been unable to conceive despite undergoing several cycles of in vitro fertilization (IVF) in which three embryos were implanted each cycle. For this couple, implanting a higher number of embryos may be the only feasible way to conceive. Yet, doing so greatly increases the risk of a dangerous multiple pregnancy and, with it, the risk of serious injury. Not using the higher number of embryos would reduce this risk—not by allowing the children to be born without injury but by preventing their birth. If the only alternative to the use of a risky reproductive technology is not having children at all, then no harm is done to the children under the but-for test unless life with the anticipated disabilities is worse than never existing at all. Thus, no harm is done unless life is worse than nonexistence.

The idea that life itself can be harmful has been very controversial, even though the nonexistence comparison is actually just a special application of the but-for test. Indeed, most American courts have concluded that the notion of a harmful life offends public policy because it suggests that life with a disability is less valuable than life without it and because it is logically incoherent. For these reasons and others, most courts in the United States have refused to allow lawsuits claiming that a child was harmed by birth with a serious disability. Most scholars and a few courts, however, disagree. Although evaluating the harmfulness of life itself does involve some conceptual puzzles, these puzzles seem soluble.

Because "it is necessary to be in order to be better off," critics believe that it is logically incoherent to say that someone could "be" better off if they had never been born (Feinberg). A related objection is that humans know nothing about nonexistence and, thus, cannot compare it to life. One judge put his concerns this way: "Ultimately, the infant's complaint is that he would be better off not to have been born. Man, who knows nothing of death or nothingness, cannot possibly know whether that is so.... To recognize a right not to be born is to enter an area in which no one can find his way" (*Gleitman v. Cosgrove*). Many scholars, however, argue that reference to nonexistence is not necessary to determine whether life with a catastrophic disability is harmful. Instead, the benefits of life can be balanced against the burdens. A life in which the burdens exceed the benefits can reasonably be characterized as harmful. Fortunately, injuries this serious are rare. The birth defects most commonly offered as examples are Lesch-Nyhan syndrome and Tay-Sachs disease.

Critics also contend that treating life itself as harmful is a repudiation of the value of human life and a threat to the welfare of living people with disabilities (*Blake v. Cruz*). Others believe, however, that respect for future persons dictates that they be spared these terrible injuries (*Turpin v. Sortini*). They also note that preventing the birth of a person with a disability is not inconsistent with vigorously protecting the welfare of people who are born with disabilities. Finally, they note that our comfort with decisions to refuse death-prolonging care reflects our recognition that life is not always a blessing (Peters, 1989).

Courts commonly offer one additional reason for rejecting wrongful life cases. They doubt that any harm ascertained using the nonexistence comparison can be rationally translated into money damages. Whether or not this is correct, it is not a reason for refusing to apply the nonexistence comparison in settings where money damages are not an issue. The difficulty of calculating damages for the injuries suffered by a cloned child, for example, may be a plausible argument for denying the child a civil action for compensatory damages, but it is not an argument against prohibiting cloning until it is more safe to perform.

In fact, outside of the courts, the most common objection to the nonexistence comparison is not that it is unmanageable or too readily assumes that life is not worth living, but that it is underprotective, that is, it dictates restraint only when the risks are truly catastrophic. The critics can be loosely sorted into two groups. The first group contends that the nonexistence comparison sets the threshold too high. They prefer a more demanding threshold such as a minimally decent quality of life or a probability of harm no greater than the risks associated with natural conception. Critics in the second group believe that reproductive conduct is harmful to future children, regardless of the absolute severity of the injuries, whenever parents or providers choose a risky route when a safer one is available.

The debate over a more demanding threshold was led at one time by scholars who felt that it was unethical to expose future children to the unknown risks associated with a new reproductive technology (Ramsey). They contended that it was unethical to impose this risk without the child's consent. The consent objection has lost emphasis in recent years, perhaps because parents have the same moral authority to consent to these risks on behalf of their future children as they have to consent to risky new treatments for their living children.

Although the consent objection has largely disappeared, it is still common to see discussions of reproductive conduct that measure the safety of a new technology against the risks of natural conception (Green). Despite the intuitive appeal of the comparison to natural conception, however, this benchmark is vulnerable to several objections when it is applied to treatments of last resort. First, the current level of risk for natural conception is not *natural* at all, but the

product of modern medical technology. Thus, the current level of risk is merely a historical coincidence. Second, though matching this level of risk may be desirable, it is not obvious why parents who face greater risks, but who have no safer alternatives, are acting unethically. The only alternative for their children is not existing at all. Finally, using the average risks of natural conception as a baseline, which means treating a riskier than average procedure as immoral, even if the injuries associated with the procedure do not prevent the affected children from having fulfilling lives. This is counterintuitive. For these reasons, no consensus in support of routine comparisons to natural conception has emerged.

Another school of ethicists offers a very different threshold for deciding when reproduction violates our obligations to future persons. Starting at least with the nineteenth-century English philosopher and economist John Stuart Mill, philosophers have argued that we owe our children a minimally decent quality of life (Cohen, 1996, 1997; Steinbock and McClamrock). Support for this benchmark is found not only in the ethics literature but also in the daily decisions that prospective parents make to avoid the birth of children with serious birth defects, through either preventive sterilization or prenatal screening and abortion. Support of the idea of a minimal quality of life is also found in the regulatory stance of the U.S. Food and Drug Administration (FDA). Unquestionably, the FDA would deny approval for an effective fertility drug that caused significant birth defects, even if those injuries were not so catastrophic as to make life itself harmful.

Given its intuitive appeal, it is surprisingly difficult to explain why the goal of a minimally decent quality of life should be obligatory and not merely aspirational. Although it may be useful after birth as a measure of the support obligations that parents and society owe to their living children, this benchmark seems less apt as a determinant of reproductive obligations. Its advocates have yet to explain convincingly why it is wrong to create a child whose life—despite being considered to be below the quality of life threshold—will, on balance, be beneficial. Thus, some respected scholars reject it (Robertson; Roberts, 1998).

Nevertheless, the persistence of the minimally decent life standard and its relatively broad support suggest that it is driven by an important intuition. Thus far, the best attempts to identify the source of this intuition turn on the distinction between death and nonexistence (Cohen, 1996; Kamm; Peters, 1989). Because death is a fate faced by actual persons, it seems more tragic than never existing at all. And because we view life as precious, we are hesitant to conclude that a living person's suffering is so profound that death would be better. This skews our burden–benefit calculus in favor of life.

Decisions regarding whether or not to reproduce are materially different. Although a decision not to reproduce does mean that a potential future person will never come to exist, it does not lead to the death of a living person. As a result, we may feel comfortable imposing a more demanding test for preconception decisions than we would impose for the discontinuation of life support. Injuries that are not so catastrophic that death would be a blessing may, nonetheless, be so serious that it would be better never to have had the child at all. According to this view, one can rationally decide to treat disabled babies aggressively while simultaneously concluding that it would be better not to conceive more children who will suffer from these injuries. Using this distinction, the FDA's decisions make sense. If this insight is persuasive, then any application of the nonexistence comparison that overlooks this distinction threatens to underprotect future children.

To summarize, the mere fact that a reproductive technology is more risky than natural conception does not mean that its use violates our obligation to future children. However, technologies that cause injuries so serious that life is not worth having do cause harm and, thus, require justification. When policymakers ask whether the risks of a reproductive practice are so serious that nonexistence would be better, they need to remember that preconception decisions do not lead to the death of a living person and, therefore, a more demanding minimal threshold can be imposed than would be appropriate after birth.

Avoiding Injury by Substituting a Different Child

Even if the but-for test is applied in a way that recognizes that life itself is sometimes harmful, the test remains vulnerable to the criticism that it overlooks an important and quite different category of harmful conduct. This category is composed of decisions to engage in risky reproductive behavior when a safer alternative is available. In this category of cases, parents and clinics can minimize future suffering by taking the safer route. Thus, for example, sperm banks can materially improve the health of the babies that they help to create by screening their sperm donors for transmissible illnesses.

Yet, the but-for test of harm cannot explain why a choice not to screen sperm is harmful. That is because screening would result in the birth of different children. Whenever the choice between two reproductive alternatives would result in the birth of different children, the but-for test dictates that the harmfulness of the choice be determined by asking whether the child who is born would have been better off not existing at all. That is because choosing

the safer route would not have made this child better off. Instead, this child would not have existed, and a different child would have been born. As a result, the options for the injured child were life with a disability or no life at all. If the injuries suffered are serious, but not so serious that never existing would be better, then no harm has been done to children created by the sperm bank. Even a clinic's failure to screen for HIV infection may not meet this threshold (Robertson).

This conclusion defies common sense. Because it focuses exclusively on the magnitude of the injury to a specific child, rather than on the presence or absence of safer alternatives, conventional analysis overlooks the harm caused when injuries could be avoided by substituting one future child for another. The harmfulness of a decision not to avoid injury by substitution lies not in the absolute magnitude of the threatened harm, but in the decision to take a risky route when a safer one was available. The but-for test cannot explain the harmfulness of these choices because choices such as these do not make a specific child worse off than she otherwise would have been. Instead, they substitute a different child. Yet, conventional analysis overlooks the fact that substituting improves the collective welfare of the class of future children.

Proponents of a duty to choose the child who will suffer least concede that tort compensation for the injured children will not be appropriate unless the injuries meet the wrongful life threshold (Peters, 1999). That is because these children could not have been born without their injuries. Their only options were life as it is and nonexistence. As a consequence, only those whose lives are worse than nonexistence have been individually harmed. Yet, taking avoidable risks can harm the welfare of the class of future children, even though there are no individual victims. Cumulatively, responsible decisions improve the welfare of future children as a class by substituting healthier children and, thus, reduce the suffering experienced by these children.

Giving content to our obligations to future persons in this manner was first discussed at length by Derek Parfit in his 1984 book, *Reasons and Persons*. Since then, others have applied the idea to reproductive technology (Brock; Peters, 1989). Parfit offered the example of a woman who is advised by her doctor not to become pregnant until she recovers from a temporary illness that causes moderate birth defects. Under the but-for test, she does no harm by refusing to wait, because waiting would change the identity of the resulting children. Parfit called this counterintuitive result the "nonidentity problem." To cure this gap in our understanding of harmful conduct, Parfit proposed a principle that he called Q that obliged parents and providers to have the child who will suffer least.

A primary obligation to avoid unnecessary suffering is intuitively appealing. It also seems consistent with the moral reasoning of John Rawls, outlined in his 1971 book, *A Theory of Justice*. Presumably, people acting under a veil of ignorance about their own circumstances, as according to Rawls, would agree that parents should try to have the children who will suffer least. This principle is also consistent with the utilitarian emphasis on beneficence because it calls for decisions that will maximize the welfare of the resulting children. When we are able to avoid injuries by substituting one child for another, we should do so unless doing so will threaten even more important interests.

This principle has surprisingly broad application to reproductive decision making. Parents deciding which embryo to transplant as part of an IVF procedure are making a choice that would be governed by this principle. Infertile patients deciding whether to clone a genetically related child or use donated embryos are making a similar choice, as are couples deciding whether to use donated sperm or to accept the risks associated with intracytoplasmic sperm injection (ICSI). ICSI is a treatment for male infertility that involves injecting a woman's egg with her partner's sperm. It poses extra risk because it bypasses the natural process for willing defective sperm.

The duty to choose the safest route to conception also provides an alternative way of resolving the debate, described briefly above, between Robertson and Roberts over the significance of reproductive alternatives that parents have available to them but decline to use. If avoiding injuries by substitution is better than declining to do so, then the disinterest of prospective parents in the safer option is not relevant to the assessment of harmfulness.

Concerns

One consequence of offering a more robust understanding of the interests of future children, like the theory of avoidability by substitution, is to expand the number of cases in which the interests of future children conflict with the interests of prospective couples, both fertile and infertile. Prospective parents have a liberty interest in making their own decisions free from governmental restriction. Critics charge that a broad conception of our obligations to future children will impose upon prospective parents an unwanted duty to undergo prenatal screening and to abort if tests are positive (Robertson). The enriched conception of the interests of future children described here does have broad implications, which apply to both artificial and natural conception.

While it is true that a broad conception will increase the number of cases in which we will appreciate that the children's interests conflict with parental liberty, rejecting

that conception will not eliminate the conflicts—it will only reduce them. In either event, a model for reconciling these competing interests will need to be developed. The strength of the notion of avoidability by substitution is that it helps us to appreciate potential conflicts that are overlooked entirely by conventional analysis. The significance of this new methodology is not that it requires intervention in every case, but that it requires justification in cases overlooked by more conventional notions of harm.

A second concern expressed about avoidability by substitution is that it characterizes conduct as harmful in circumstances in which no specific person has been harmed. For some philosophers, this is a serious problem (Roberts, 1998). One critic called it merely a "norm against offending persons who are troubled by gratuitous suffering" (Robertson, 1997, p. 76). Advocates claim, however, that it is genuinely person-affecting insofar as it reduces unnecessary human suffering (Brock).

Finally, proponents of avoidability by substitution have struggled to find a method for handling "different number" cases. Different number cases arise when the use of a risky reproductive method (such as cloning or the use of fertility drugs at a dosage associated with multiple pregnancies) will result in a different number of children than would have been produced using a safer alternative (such as natural conception or lower doses of the fertility drug). Moral philosophers have discovered that startling paradoxes plague the effort to compare the welfare of groups of different sizes. A tentative solution has been offered that combines average utility and total utility into a combined index that can be used to compare the moral implications of different number reproductive choices (Hurka). This proposal, however, has not yet been thoroughly tested.

The debate over avoidability by substitution is far from resolved. While avoidability by substitution seems to provide a useful explanation consistent with our intuitions, it raises problems that make it unattractive to some ethicists. Even if it is persuasive, it must be supplemented by the nonexistence comparison in cases in which prospective parents want to engage in a risky reproductive practice for which no safer alternative exists, such as postmenopausal pregnancy.

Conclusion

Reproductive behavior can be harmful to future children in three ways. First, reproductive practices can sometimes cause ordinary harm. These are injuries that could have been avoided if more care had been used, such as injuries caused by failure to store frozen embryos properly. Second, reproductive technology can result in a harmful life when the child who is born has a life that is not worth having. Finally, the interests of future children are harmed when the birth of an injured child could have been avoided by changes in conduct resulting in the birth of a different, healthier child. This kind of harm is avoidable by substitution. Clinics performing artificial insemination, for example, can prevent needless suffering by screening out high-risk donors. Responsible efforts to protect future children from harm should aim at minimizing each of the three types of harm to the extent that is consistent with parental procreative liberty.

PHILIP J. PETERS, JR.

SEE ALSO: *Aging and the Aged: Anti-Aging Interventions; Children; Environmental Ethics; Environmental Health; Hazardous Wastes and Toxic Substances; Maternal-Fetal Relationship; Population Ethics; Sustainable Development; Technology*

BIBLIOGRAPHY

Baby M, In the Matter of 1988. 537 A.2d 1227.

Bayles, Michael D. 1976. "Introduction." In *Ethics and Population* ed. Michael D. Bayles. Cambridge, MA: Schenkman.

Bayles, Michael D. 1980. *Morality and Population Policy.* University: University of Alabama Press.

Bell, Nora K., and Loewer, Barry M.. 1985. "What Is Wrong with 'Wrongful Life' Cases." *Journal of Medicine and Philosophy* 10: 127.

Blake v. Cruz. 1984. 698 P.2d 315, 321 (Idaho).

Brock, Dan W. 1995. "The Non-Identity Problem and Genetic Harms: The Case of Wrongful Handicaps." *Bioethics* 9(3/4): 269–275.

Buchanan, Allen; Brock, Dan W.; Daniels, Norman; et al. 2000. *From Chance to Choice: Genetics and Justice.* Cambridge, Eng.: Cambridge University Press.

Cohen, Cynthia B. 1996. "Give Me Children or I Shall Die! New Reproductive Technologies and Harm to Children." *Hastings Center Report* 26(2): 19–27.

Cohen, Cynthia B. 1997. "The Morality of Knowingly Conceiving Children with Serious Conditions: An Expanded 'Wrongful Life' Standard." In *Contingent Future Persons: On the Ethics of Deciding Who Will Live, or Not, in the Future,* ed. Nick Fotion and Jan C. Heller. Dordrecht, Netherlands: Kluwer Academic.

Feinberg, Joel. 1986. "Wrongful Life and the Counterfactual Element in Harming." *Social Philosophy and Policy* 4(1): 145–178.

Fishkin, James S. 1982. "Justice between Generations: The Dilemma of Future Interests." In *Social Justice,* ed. Michael Bradie and David Baybrooke. Bowling Green, OH: Bowling Green State University.

Gleitman v. Cosgrove. 49 N.J. 22, 63, 227 A.2d 689, 711 (1967)(Weintraub, C. J., dissenting in part).

Green, Ronald M. 1997. "Parental Autonomy and the Obligation Not to Harm One's Child Genetically." *Journal of Law, Medicine, and Ethics* 25(1): 5–15.

Hanser, Mathew. 1990. "Harming Future People." *Philosophy and Public Affairs* 19(1): 47–70.

Heyd, David. 1992. *Genethics: Moral Issues in the Creation of People.* Berkeley: University of California Press.

Hurka, Thomas. 1983. "Value and Population Size." *Ethics* 93: 496–507.

Kamm, Frances M. 1993. *Morality, Mortality,* vol. 1: *Death and Whom to Save from It.* New York: Oxford University Press.

Narveson, Jan. 1976. "Moral Problems of Population." In *Ethics and Population,* ed. Michael D. Bayles. Cambridge, MA: Schenkman.

Parfit, Derek. 1984. *Reasons and Persons.* Oxford: Clarendon Press.

Peters, Philip G., Jr. 1989. "Protecting the Unconceived: Nonexistence, Avoidability, and Reproductive Technology." *Arizona Law Review* 31(3): 487–548.

Peters, Philip G., Jr. 1992. "Rethinking Wrongful Life: Bridging the Boundary between Tort and Family Law." *Tulane Law Review* 67(2): 397.

Peters, Philip G., Jr. 1999. "Harming Future Persons: Obligations to the Children of Reproductive Technology." *Southern California Interdisciplinary Law Journal* 8(2): 375–400.

Ramsey, Paul. 1978. *Ethics at the Edges of Life: Medical and Legal Intersections.* New Haven, CT: Yale University Press.

Rawls, John. 1971. *A Theory of Justice.* Cambridge, MA: Harvard University Press.

Roberts, Melinda A. 1995. "Present Duties and Future Persons: When Are Existence-Inducing Acts Wrong?" *Law and Philosophy* 14: 297–327.

Roberts, Melinda A. 1996. "Human Cloning: A Case of No Harm Done?" *Journal of Medicine and Philosophy* 21(5): 537–554.

Roberts, Melinda A. 1998. *Child versus Childmaker: Future Persons and Present Duties in Ethics and the Law.* Lanham, MD: Rowman and Littlefield.

Robertson, John A. 1994. *Children of Choice: Freedom and the New Reproductive Technologies.* Princeton, NJ: Princeton University Press.

Robertson, John A. 1997. "Wrongful Life, Federalism, and Procreative Liberty: A Critique of the NBAC Cloning Report." *Jurimetrics* 38(1): 69–82.

Steinbock, Bonnie, and McClamrock, Ron. 1994. "When Is Birth Unfair to the Child?" *Hastings Center Report* 24(6): 15–21.

Turpin v. Sortini. 31 Cal.3d 220, 182 Cal. Rptr. 337, 643 P.2d 954 (1982).

Woodward, James. 1986. "The Non-Identity Problem." *Ethics* 96(4): 804–831.

G

GENDER IDENTITY

• • •

The term *gender* has a long history, with Greek roots signifying "birth, race, and family" and Latin roots signifying "birth, race, and kind." The psychologist John Money was among the first to use the term to refer to a person's felt identity as male or female, as distinguished from that person's biological sex traits (Money). The term also is used to refer to a person's nature or identity as male or female and to social aspects of sex such as the cultural roles of men and women.

Various biological traits distinguish male from female, but males and females are not distinct in categorical ways and the boundary between male and female is fluid rather than fixed: Human beings can exhibit atypical traits or intersexed conditions (Fausto-Sterling). Rather than having an XX or XY sex chromosome complement, for example, some people have an XXY or XYY complement. In some cases an individual may be born with only a single X chromosome. Some humans have indeterminate genitalia or both testicular and ovarian tissue. In regard to social roles male and female traits can overlap as well.

Gender Assignment of Newborns and Children

The sex of a newborn child is of keen interest to the parents, but some children are born with ambiguous genitalia, having both testicular and ovarian tissue, or genetic syndromes that confound a simple designation as male or female. The term *gender assignment* refers to practices that are used to discern and impose a gender identity on a newborn child.

Suzanne J. Kessler has described how cultural ideals of sex influence the practice of gender assignment. She showed that some physicians have made decisions about gender assignment in accordance with the size and expected function of a child's genitalia rather than in accordance with more complex hormonal and genetic assessments (Kessler, 1990; 1998). If a male child was likely to have a very small penis, for example, some physicians and parents used surgery to assign a female identity to that child. Advocates of this kind of intervention argue that a secure gender identity depends on having appropriate sexual genitalia.

The gender assignment of John/Joan has received a great deal of attention (Colapinto, 1997). In 1966 a physician burned the penis of boy beyond repair during a circumcision that involved an electrocautery needle. Fearful of what the boy's life would be like, his parents took him Johns Hopkins University for evaluation. The psychologist John Money proposed gender reassignment from male to female on the assumption that the loss of the penis was so damaging that it would be better for the child to be raised as female; he also believed that gender identity can be shaped after birth. With the consent of the parents, in 1967 physicians removed the boy's testicles at the age of 22 months, repositioned the urethra, and induced a preliminary vaginal cleft. The parents selected a girl's name and began to treat and raise the child as female (Colapinto, 2000).

From 1972 on Money reported the child's gender assignment as successful. He said that the case showed that gender identity is plastic and can be shaped during early childhood. One's sense of self as male or female is not, he held, determined by anatomy, genetics, or prenatal history. Health practitioners translated that evidence into practice guidelines and encouraged gender interventions. One advocate said that the possibility of female sex assignment with genetic males "must be considered whenever the severity of the genital abnormality is such that it is likely to be extremely difficult or impossible to correct for normal adult functioning" (Baker, p. 266).

In fact, the gender reassignment of this child failed. The child consistently rejected female identification and exhibited male-typical interests and behaviors. Eventually the child refused further interventions, and at that point the family told the child the truth. The fourteen-year-old immediately reclaimed a male identity, adopted a male name, started male hormone treatments, underwent breast removal, and eventually was treated with phalloplasty, the construction of a penis. None of those events were reported in the professional literature until 1997. Thirty years passed between the beginning of this experiment and its publicly described failure (Diamond and Sigmundson).

Some commentators believe that that failure provides evidence that gender assignments do not work, but that conclusion is not fully supported by the evidence. Gender assignment in children has not been well studied, but even if this case failed spectacularly, other interventions might succeed. It also should be noted that the intervention made sense at the time of an unsettled debate about the extent to which gender identity can be influenced after birth. The unfortunate outcome has rightly forced broad reconsideration of gender assignment practices. Various commentators have noted that gender assignment can reinforce dubious notions such as the view that a person cannot be male unless he has a large and intact penis and that it is better for a child to grow up as a sterile female than as a male with a very small or damaged penis.

Some commentators have argued that gender assignment violates children's autonomy (Dreger, 1999). That argument is not convincing because newborns and very young children lack the cognitive powers that justify respect for people's choices. More convincing are worries that early gender interventions are not effective or work to the advantage of anxious parents, not to the benefit of the children. Concerns of this kind suggest that gender assignment in the case of ambiguous genitalia or intersex conditions at the very least should not be treated as inherently shameful or as a social emergency.

Physicians should propose gender interventions to parents only after a rigorous evaluation of the risks and benefits. Among other things, practitioners should advise parents that some individuals live happily with atypical genitalia or intersex conditions and that gender assignment can be carried out later on if that is desired by the child (Dreger, 1998). Parents need support as they think through decisions about gender interventions with their children, and this support should include nonpathologized images of intersex people. In the 1990s the Intersex Society of North America began its education and advocacy efforts to improve options for intersex people and their healthcare providers, and this group explicitly rejects a pathological view of intersexuality.

Gender Identity Disorders

Some people assert a gender identity that is at odds with their anatomy and genetic traits. The American Psychiatric Association (APA) treats some of those people as suffering from gender identity disorder (GID). GID sometimes is called gender dysphoria, and it occurs in children, adolescents, and adults. According to the APA, people with this disorder are characterized by a "strong and persistent cross-gender indentification" (American Psychiatric Association, 2000, p. 581).

This preoccupation is said to pass into the pathological when there is strong and persistent cross-gender identification and clinically significant distress or impairment in social, occupation, or other important areas of function. The diagnosis is not applied to persons with cross-gender identification who have intersex conditions. To some extent *gender identity disorder* replaces what previously has been treated as *transsexualism,* a term that came into use in the 1940s. Although some commentators still use that term, *transgenderism* and *cross-gendered identities* have come into common use.

The prevalence of cross-gender identities has been poorly studied. There have been no studies of prevalence in the United States, although there have been some studies in smaller countries. According to those studies, cross-gender identities occur in 1 in 30,000 adult males and 1 in 30,000 adult females (American Psychiatric Association, 2000). There are various theories about why some people come to have cross-gender identities, although no single theory is accepted as conclusive. Researchers have explored prenatal hormonal exposure, birth order, genetics, brain structure, and various psychological and social learning theories (Green and Blanchard; Devor). Whatever the origins of cross-gender identification are, there is a general pattern of development: People have a sense of dissatisfaction with their sex characteristics and assigned gender, conclude that that dissatisfaction would be alleviated by change and therefore pursue varying degrees of reassignment (Devor).

Adults with cross-gender identities differ in regard to expectations from medicine and how far they want to conform their bodies to a particular gender (McCloskey).

Not everyone wants to assume every male or female trait. Transgendered men may elect to have testosterone treatment, excision of the breasts and genitals, reduction in thyroid cartilage to minimize the Adam's apple, and the construction of a vagina. Transgendered women may elect to have estrogen treatment, electrolysis of unwanted hair, and the construction of male genitalia. However, some transgendered people continue to value aspects of their originally assigned sex and want to keep them even as they add other transfomations. Also, not all instances of cross-dressing or atypical gender expression represent cross-gender identities. Some men and women cross-dress for sexual reasons; this phenomenon is known in psychiatry as transvestism. In these instances there is no discordance between one's biological traits and one's desired gender identity. The issue here is gender expression rather than identity.

There are no specific clinical or psychological tests to diagnose cross-gendered identities; the diagnosis is made on the basis of the case presentation. Moreover, there are no pharmaceutical or surgical treatments for this condition. Generally, behavioral or psychosocial treatments are used to orient a person to a gender identity; no hormonal or pharmacological treatments are known. Some studies have shown that cross-gender identification can be reduced in children through a variety of psychological and social interventions (Green). Advocates of treatment with children focus their interventions on helping children become content with their birth sex. They counsel, for example, that "young children should be taught that sex is irreversible" (Green and Blanchard, p. 1658).

Some practitioners justify therapy for children to alleviate the distress associated with cross-gender identities and behaviors and prevent the emergence of a homosexual orientation in adolescence and adulthood (Rosen et al.). Critics have contested both of those goals. In 1996 the Human Rights Commission of the City and County of San Francisco condemned the use of the diagnosis of GID. According to that group, the diagnosis of GID in children is used to screen for homosexuality and stigmatize gender nonconformity. Others have defended the use of the diagnosis and therapy: "Whether or not someone else agrees, parents have the legal right to bring a child for therapy to modify behavior they disapprove of and with the goal of preventing a later behavior of which they disapprove" (Green and Blanchard, p. 1659). Those commentators compare this option to parents' rights with respect to their children's education, religion, and diet.

Parents have a prima facie right to choose on behalf of their children, but that right is tempered by the moral right of children to be protected from undue risk and useless treatments. For reasons of beneficence parents should not use therapies that bring more harm than good to their children. Medical ethics also recognizes that maturing adolescents deserve a degree of choice in regard to birth control practices, psychiatric treatment, and involvement in research even when those choices conflict with parental wishes. Gender therapies for maturing adolescents require much stronger justifications than do those undertaken with much younger children.

Harry Benjamin holds a central place in the scientific study of transsexualism or transgenderism. Benjamin was a German national who immigrated to the United States and published *The Transsexual Phenomenon* in 1966. In that book he offered the first comprehensive treatment guide for transsexuals. In late 1970s a group of healthcare professionals codified his approach in the Harry Benjamin Standards of Care. Among other things, those rules require that people who seek gender interventions:

1. obtain a diagnosis of gender disorder;
2. begin a relationship with a therapist;
3. receive hormone therapy;
4. live as cross-dressed for a sustained period; and
5. after therapists authorize it, receive desired surgical interventions (Harry Benjamin International Gender Dysphoria Association).

These standards are observed widely in professional relationships with transgendered people. However, some commentators believe that the standards are paternalistic in the sense that they represent a degree of control over medical interventions that is not required elsewhere, for example, in cosmetic surgeries.

Transgender therapy has important implications for a person's social and legal status. The physician and tennis player Renee Richards, formerly Richard, gained the right to play in women's professional tennis as a transgendered woman (Richards). Other transgendered men and women have not been as successful in finding accommodation in society and the law. Individuals who undergo transgender therapy often face legal difficulties insofar as they may violate laws regarding cross-dressing and the use of public washrooms. Those people are sometimes restricted in their right to marry and have children. Prison housing also raises special problems because transgendered persons are especially vulnerable to mistreatment and violence. Some jurisdictions have adopted laws that prohibit discrimination against people having or being perceived as having a self-image or identity not traditionally associated with one's biological sex. Most jurisdictions have no such laws.

The Ethics of Transgender Interventions

Insofar as male-to-female transgenderism is more common than its opposite, some critics have seen in transgender therapy the extension of male privilege. Janice Raymond has argued that male-to-female transgenderism trivializes women because it treats femaleness as a trait that men may adopt as they wish. She characterizes female-to-male transgenderism as an attempt to bypass constraints on female participation in a male-dominated society (Raymond). Raymond would not ban transgender therapy, but she believes that a greater social emancipation of women would eliminate the reasons for seeking it. By contrast, other commentators believe that the origins of cross-gendered identities are ultimately beside the point: Those commentators think that the proper focus of interest in these identities is not prevention and treatment but social accommodation so that people may live in whatever modes of sex or gender expression they find desirable (Devor).

Some commentators object to gender interventions for adults on the grounds that medical interventions violate the natural law principle of bodily integrity. However, other commentators working within the same tradition have defended medical interventions on the grounds that they protect psychic health (Springer). It is also possible to argue on utilitarian grounds that if psychiatry has no meaningful treatment for cross-gendered identities, gender interventions can help people achieve happiness. Even commentators who defend a pathological interpretation of cross-gender identities agree that "the most reliable conclusion is that the overwhelming majority of post-operative transsexuals are content with their decision to undergo sex reassignment" (Green and Blanchard, p. 1660). Utilitarian ethics not only advocates the greatest happiness for the greatest number of people, as in the philosopher John Stuart Mill's formulation, it also asserts the liberty principle, a principle of noninterference with individual pursuits insofar as they do not harm others. A case can be made that atypical gender choices do not intrude on the rights of others any more than atypical religious or political views do.

Defending atypical gender identities and expression in adults does not of course establish what priority gender interventions should have in a health-care system. Some critics argue that too little research has been done on ways to improve the surgical needs of transgendered people (Devor). Some people have found that private insurers and government health programs are unwilling to pay for interventions because the interventions are voluntary and do not cure an underlying disorder. Other commentators have argued that gender interventions meet an important psychic need, that they work, and that their limitations can be overcome through better selection standards (Gordon). Those commentators therefore argue that private insurers and the government should pay for gender therapies.

Gender, Identity, and Gender Expression

One of the striking aspects of recent medical history is the way in which affected parties have worked to mitigate injurious or harmful medical practices. For example, women's advocacy groups have helped reshape health-care practices that worked against the interests of women. Men and women with homosexual orientations have worked to change the medical perception of homosexuality as pathological (Bayer). People with AIDS have forced a reconsideration of problematic language and representations used to describe them (Treichler). In a similar way people with cross-gender identities and intersex conditions have challenged the assumptions behind diagnoses and treatments related to gender.

In 1993, participants at the International Conference on Transgender Law and Employment Policy issued the first version of the International Bill of Gender Rights. Among other things, that bill asserts the right of all people to self-definition in regard to gender and the right of free gender expression. It also asserts the right of people to control their bodies in regard to chemical, cosmetic, and surgical interventions as well as the right to receive competent and professional medical care. It also rejects the pathological interpretation of gender: "[I]ndividuals shall not be subject to psychiatric diagnosis or treatment as mentally disordered or diseased solely on the basis of a self-defined gender identity or the expression thereof" (International Conference). In the long run it is a goal of gender activists to move society away from the treatment and prevention of GID and toward acceptance of a much broader range of gender expression.

Gender activism generally rejects the idea that only people with a particular biological endowment may participate in masculinity or femininity. This approach is part of a larger critique of gender roles that are constructed from opposed conceptions of male and female (MacKenzie; Feinberg). A number of commentators point out that some societies have successfully incorporated more diffuse notions of gender identity and gender roles; Native American tribes are commonly cited examples (Williams; Jacobs, Thomas, and Lang).

This critique raises questions about whether gender assignment in children and the category of GID serve social rather than medical purposes. The APA has attempted to divest itself of responsibility for the enforcement of moral or political values: "Neither deviant behavior, e.g., political, religious, or sexual, nor conflicts that are primarily between the individual and society are mental disorders unless the deviance or conflicts is a symptom of a dysfunction in the person" that generates persistent stress, disability, or significant risk of suffering, death, pain, disability, or loss of freedom (American Psychiatric Association, 1987, p. xxii). Some commentators believe that the stress suffered by children, adolescents, and adults with cross-gender identities is primarily social in nature and thus is primarily a social problem, not an issue to be addressed through diagnosis and treatment.

Some commentators wonder whether medicine will continue to identify cross-gender identifications as pathological or whether another view will prevail. Certainly, attention to the views and counsel of the people under discussion and resistance to easy slippage between biology and culture will help medicine and ethics serve human beings as the people they are rather than as the people society would have them be.

TIMOTHY F. MURPHY (1995)
REVISED BY AUTHOR

SEE ALSO: *Body: Cultural and Religious Perspectives; Homosexuality; Life, Quality of; Paternalism; Psychiatry, Abuses of; Psychoanalysis and Dynamic Therapies*

BIBLIOGRAPHY

American Psychiatric Association. 1987. *Diagnostic and Statistical Manual of Mental Disorders,* 3rd edition, rev. Washington, D.C.: Author.

American Psychiatric Association. 2000. *Diagnostic and Statistical Manual—IV—TR.* Washington, D.C.: Author.

Baker, Susan W. 1981. "Psychological Management of Intersex Children." In *The Intersex Child,* pp. 261–269, ed. Nathalie Josse. Basel: S. Karger.

Bayer, Ronald. 1987. *Homosexuality and American Psychiatry.* Princeton, NJ: Princeton University Press.

Benjamin, Harry. 1966. *The Transsexual Phenomenon.* New York: Julian Press.

Colapinto, John. 1997. "The True Story of John/Joan." *Rolling Stone,* December 11, pp. 54–73, 92–97.

Colapinto, John. 2000. *As Nature Made Him: The Story of the Boy Who Was Raised as a Girl.* New York: HarperCollins.

Devor, Holly. 1997. *FTM: Female-to-Male Transsexuals in Society.* Bloomington: Indiana University Press.

Diamond, Milton, and Sigmundson, Keith. 1997. "Sex Reassignment at Birth: Long Term Review and Clinical Implications." *Archives of Pediatric and Adolescent Medicine* 151: 298–304.

Dreger, Alice Domurat. 1998. *Hermaphrodites and the Medical Invention of Sex.* Cambridge, MA: Harvard University Press.

Dreger, Alice Domurat, ed. 1999. *Intersex in the Age of Ethics.* Hagerstown, MD: University Publishing Group.

Fausto-Sterling, Anne. 2000. *Sexing the Body: Gender Politics and the Construction of Sexuality.* New York: Basic Books.

Feinberg, Leslie. 1999. *Trans Liberation: Beyond Pink or Blue.* Boston: Beacon.

Gordon, Eric B. 1991. "Transsexual Healing: Medicaid Funding of Sex Reassignment Surgery." *Archives of Sexual Behavior* 20(1): 61–74.

Green, Richard. 1987. *The "Sissy Boy Syndrome" and the Development of Homosexuality.* New Haven, CT: Yale University Press.

Green, Richard, and Blanchard, Ray. 2000. "Gender Identity Disorders." In *Kaplan and Sadock's Comprehensive Textbook of Psychiatry,* ed. Benjamin J. Sadock and Virginia A. Sadock. New York: Lippincott, Williams & Wilkins.

Jacobs, Sue Ellen; Thomas, Wesley; and Lang, Sabine. 1997. *Two Spirit People: Native American Gender Identity, Sexuality, and Spirituality.* Urbana: University of Illinois Press.

Kessler, Suzanne. 1990. "The Medical Construction of Gender: Case Management of Intersexed Infants." *Signs* 16(1): 3–26.

Kessler, Suzanne. 1998. *Lessons from the Intersexed.* New Brunswick, NJ: Rutgers University Press.

MacKenzie, Gordene Olga. 1994. *Transgender Nation.* Bowling Green, OH: Bowling Green State University Popular Press.

McCloskey, Deirdre N. 1999. *Crossing: A Memoir.* Chicago: University of Chicago Press.

Money, John. 1988. *Gay, Straight, and In-Between: The Sexology of Erotic Orientation.* New York: Oxford University Press.

Raymond, Janice. 1994. *Transsexual Empire: The Making of the She-Male.* New York: Teacher's College Press.

Richards, Renee. 1983. *Second Serve: The Renee Richards Story.* New York: Stein and Day.

Rosen, Alexander; Rekers, George A.; and Bentler, Peter M. 1978. "Ethical Issues in the Treatment of Children." *Journal of Social Issues* 34: 122–136.

Springer, Robert H. 1987. "Transsexual Surgery: Some Reflections on the Moral Issues Involved." In *Sexuality and Medicine,* vol. 2, ed. Earl E. Shelp. Dordrecht, Netherlands: D. Reidel.

Treichler, Paula. 1999. *How to Have Theory in an Epidemic: Cultural Chronicles of AIDS.* Durham: Duke University Press.

Williams, Walter L. 1992. *Spirit and the Flesh: Sexual Diversity in American Indian Culture.* Boston: Beacon Press.

INTERNET RESOURCES

Harry Benjamin International Gender Dysphoria Association. 2003. Available from <http://www.hbigda.org>.

International Conference on Transgender Law and Employment Policy. 2003. Available from <http://www.transgender.org. stlgf/gender.html>.

GENETIC COUNSELING, ETHICAL ISSUES IN

• • •

Genetic counseling is a complex communication process that takes place between a genetic counselor and one or more counselees, also called clients. It may involve a single encounter lasting thirty to sixty minutes or multiple encounters over months or years. The type and duration of the encounter is determined by the nature of the condition that led to the encounter. This includes whether the condition under discussion is genetic or nongenetic, the mode of inheritance, and the severity of the disorder, including its prognosis. Therapeutic and reproductive implications play a significant role as well as the counselor's evaluation of the effectiveness of the counseling encounter.

Effective and helpful genetic counseling should be guided by several ethical principles and human values judged by most workers in the field to be of vital importance (Wertz et al.). These include autonomy; beneficence and nonmaleficence; confidentiality; veracity and truth-telling; and informed consent. It is also crucial that varied cultural and ethnic factors be taken into account. The professional code of ethics for genetic counselors should also be considered (Palmer).

Since genetic counseling usually occurs in medical settings such as clinics, medical centers, or private offices, the ethical values that prevail in medical and nursing practice should also play a role in genetic counseling. These principles or values influence different aspects of the counseling process to different degrees. Their influence may also vary according to the cultural background, ethnicity, or religious beliefs of the counselees and their families. The latter factors should receive serious attention, since cultural, religious, or ethnic differences can profoundly influence the relative weight given to one value or principle over another. This is especially true when counseling involves individuals from other countries (Wertz et al.). Counselees from the so-called Third World may cherish religious tenets and ethical values drastically different from those of the Jewish and Christian faiths that inform so much of Western medical ethics (Fisher).

Autonomy and Nondirectiveness

A major facet of the counseling process, and one important goal of a successful counseling process, is a course of action (or inaction) that is determined according to the best available evidence. Genetic counselors generally agree that this decision should be made by the counselee, and that it should be made freely and without coercion (Fraser, 1974; Ad Hoc Committee on Genetic Counseling). Counselors want to avoid, to the extent possible, being accused of "playing god" and to resist any temptation to practice eugenics, the process of manipulating genes in order to "improve" genetic makeup. The manipulation is accomplished by directing the counselees about what reproductive decisions they should or should not make. This is inappropriate because respect for autonomy should be a predominant ethical value guiding the counseling process and its outcome. This is the clear consensus of genetic counselors from all over the world (U.S. President's Commission; Wertz and Fletcher).

If counselees are to make autonomous decisions, they must be fully informed about the disorder in question, free of coercion, aware of all the possible choices, and have access to any facilities and/or services to implement their decision. In its purest sense and with only rare exceptions, the nature of the decision is not an issue as long as the counselee has decided that such a decision is in her or his best interest. In this model of counseling the counselor makes every effort to be "nondirective," that is, to refrain as much as possible from providing any suggestion directly or indirectly to the counselee as to what decision she or he should make (Fraser, 1974, 1979; Hsia). No counselor can be totally unbiased and without any interest in the decision that is made. However, the aim in counseling is to create "an accepting psychologic climate" and thereby the possibility of a nondirective relationship (Antley).

An ethical dilemma may arise for the counselor if the counselee wants to make a decision that will have what the counselor strongly feels are mostly negative consequences. For example, a man and a woman are both affected by a serious homozygous recessive disorder (e.g., sickle-cell anemia) and are advised that all their children will be similarly affected. After being counseled, and with full knowledge of the genetic consequences, they decide to have their own biological children. This kind of decision is called dysgenic by some, because it has the potential of resulting in an increase in the number of deleterious genes in the next generation. This will be true if the couple has more than two children and they in turn live to reproduce in an environment where these genes have no selective advantage. Some counselors feel that the counselor may be justified in not honoring the principle of nondirectiveness because the net reproductive effect is likely to produce more harm than benefit (Yarborough et al.). It further results in a situation in which children who are destined to live a life of pain and suffering are knowingly brought into the world. Furthermore, there is the possibility of genetic harm to this population if this practice becomes more common. These harms must be balanced against the benefit to these parents of having their own biological children, even if these children are much more likely to suffer or to die an early death.

The counselor who feels that the principle of nondirectiveness ought not be violated under any circumstances should at least explore with the counselees the psychosocial and emotional reasons that led them to this decision. The counselor should assist them in a careful and deliberate examination of the benefits and harms that may effect them and their offspring (Kessler). Strong arguments have been advanced suggesting that by applying the principle of beneficence, the counselor is justified in attempting to persuade counselees to reconsider their decisions in certain cases without violating the rule of nondirectiveness (Yarborough et al.).

Beneficence/Nonmaleficence: Whose Needs Come First?

When the counselee is trying to balance the benefits and harms of a particular decision against one another, there may be a tendency to emphasize the benefits over the harms. In some cases, the benefit or beneficence for the counselee(s) may mean maleficence or harm for the child. If parents who know they will have a child with a serious genetically determined disease decide to go ahead because they believe they have a "right to bear children," they may benefit in having their own biological children. At the same time they might not be judged "responsible parents" because they may not have given serious enough consideration to the suffering and discomfort their offspring will suffer. Even if this factor has been considered, the parents may justify their decision on the religious grounds that they are merely following the dictates of a higher power, leaving it to God to determine whether or not they have children.

In some cases it may be difficult for counselor and counselee to agree on what constitutes a benefit and what a harm, since such determinations are often rather subjective, governed primarily by the counselee's values. For example, abortion of an affected fetus might be considered a benefit to some and harmful to others, depending on whose needs are considered primary. Providing information that there is a high probability that a counselee at risk to inherit a serious genetically determined disease of late onset has in fact

inherited it might seem a beneficent act by some who value knowledge of any sort, and a maleficent or harmful act by others who value information only when it leads to the prevention or correction of harm. In the tension between these contrasting ethical principles, medical ethical tradition suggests that nonmaleficence should be weighted more heavily than beneficence in cases where they are in conflict. This position is consistent with the maxim of *primum non nocere,* first do no harm (Beauchamp and Childress), since providing information without clear benefit has the potential for causing social and emotional harm.

Veracity and Truth-telling in Genetic Counseling

A major part of the genetic counseling process is the exchange of information about the medical and family history provided by the counselee and comprehensive genetic and medical information about the disease in question provided by the counselor (Fraser, 1974; Hsia). The counselee needs accurate information, including the correct diagnosis, in order to choose a beneficial course of action. Truth-telling is an essential ingredient of the relationship between genetic counselors and counselees. Part of the trust that exists between them is based on this virtue. As a consequence, the genetic counselor should provide truthful, accurate, and complete information to the counselee concerning the genetic disorder being considered.

On some occasions the genetic counselor might have very good reasons for violating this important trust. Failure to tell the truth will most often involve withholding information rather than lying. But the counselor bears the burden of justifying failure to tell the whole truth. This is the case even if the counselor is keeping back some information until a time when it may be more readily received, that is, when the counselee is judged to be better prepared to accept negative information and its attendant consequences. Some reasons that might be given for holding back information include:

1. The information, if transmitted, is likely to cause permanent damage to the self-image of the counselee or result in a serious or severe emotional reaction. This is the case when a female is found to have an XY sex chromosomal constitution rather than the normal XX sex chromosomes.
2. Refraining from transmitting the information will not have a significant effect on the options open to the counselee or her or his family nor will it compromise any therapy the counselee or the family should receive.

3. The counselee has a history of serious depression and the information, if fully given, has a good chance of exacerbating the depression with a significant risk of suicide.

4. The information reveals evidence that the putative father in a family is not the biological father of a particular child; if this information is provided, it is likely to lead to the breakup of the family and the child will no longer have a father.

5. A young man or woman has been found to be a presymptomatic carrier of a late-onset, autosomal (related to chromosomes that are common to both sexes), dominant condition and does not want a fiance to be told because it is feared she or he might break off the relationship.

The latter two cases, in which information is withheld from third parties, raise the question of the counselor's obligation or "duty to warn" others who might be affected by the presence of the genetic condition in a spouse or significant other. For some counselors, the "right to know" or the "duty to warn" provides strong justification for telling the whole truth at all times during the counseling process, regardless of the potential consequences. At the same time, a minority of counselees feel they have a right "not to know." These people would rather not be told about a serious genetic condition of late onset, especially if there is no effective therapy or other maneuver that will forestall its onset or significantly reduce its symptoms. If counselees do not wish to know about their incurable condition, the information may nevertheless have to be placed in the medical record so that future health-care givers will be alert to the counselee's status. The information can also be provided if counselees should change their minds. In general, genetic counselors will withhold information only where there is a strong likelihood for serious harm to the family or to the self-image or status of the individual (Wertz et al.).

Confidentiality and the Control of Genetic Information

Medical genetics is more concerned with the family than almost any other medical subspecialty. As part of the evaluation of a clinically significant genetic disorder, the genetic counselor is required to collect detailed family data and record it in the form of a *pedigree.* This enables the counselor and the medical geneticist to determine whether there is a pattern of occurrence in the family consistent with control by a single gene of major effect (often referred to as a "Mendelian" gene). The pedigree may also provide information that may indicate the presence of inherited chromosomal structural rearrangements called translocations. More often than not, the pedigree information is insufficient to make this determination. But when it does demonstrate the presence of an inherited defect, this knowledge can have serious, even grave, implications for the other genetically related members of the family. This is especially true when one is dealing with conditions that demonstrate autosomal or X-linked dominant or X-linked recessive modes of inheritance, because inheritance of a single mutant gene on an X or non-X chromosome can cause the full-blown clinical disorder.

Under the medical model that governs medical geneticists and genetic counseling, the counselee has the status of a patient. All information relative to his or her case is covered by the guarantee of privacy and confidentiality that is required of health professionals (Beauchamp and Childress). The medical geneticist or genetic counselor should get permission from the counselee to contact other family members to inform them that they are at risk for a serious genetically determined disorder. In general, this is not a problem; most counselees readily consent to having their relatives contacted or are willing to do this themselves. But in at least two instances the genetic counselor may face an ethical dilemma concerning the release of information to third parties.

1. The disorder is *not* treatable and can be diagnosed by prenatal diagnosis, so a couple at risk could theoretically avoid the birth of an affected child; or individuals at risk for this might wish to take special predictive tests and use the knowledge to get their affairs in order or in other ways to alter their life situation.

2. The disorder is treatable and can be cured or can have the symptoms and any complications significantly reduced by safe and readily available therapy; or the expression of the disorder can be prevented if it is detected before the symptoms have appeared.

The obligation to maintain confidentiality of patient records and genetic information obtained in a medical setting is not absolute and may be breached when there is adequate justification. The exceptions may be invoked only if there are extenuating or overriding personal or social circumstances. The State of Texas statute on confidentiality, for example, allows confidential information to be disclosed if there is the probability of imminent physical injury to the patient or others (Andrews). In the case of genetic disorders, the most compelling argument for breaching confidentiality besides those instances where it is required by law is the protection of third parties from harm (Andrews). In ethical terms this is sometimes cited as "the duty or obligation to warn" when there is a clear or imminent danger.

In the cases shown above, there would appear to be clear justification for breaching confidentiality in the second case but not in the first. In the first example, useful information might be provided to third parties, but there is no evidence of harm because the condition identified is not treatable. In the second example, the fact that there is a treatment or a method of preventing the condition means that failure to warn would result in harm to a third party. Since the burden of justification would be on the genetic counselor to show that the harm, however, conceived, is correctable or preventable, it makes sense not to breach confidentiality in instances where the potential harm is not clearly defined. The U.S. President's Commission for the Study of Ethical Problems in Medicine and Biomedical and Behavioral Research regarding confidentiality provided four conditions under which the requirements of confidentiality can be overridden and genetic information released to relatives or their physicians (1983).

Revealing genetic information, especially in cases of presymptomatic diagnosis, has other important implications for the counselee's eligibility for health insurance and possibly for life insurance. Depending on the condition involved, such information if revealed can also affect employability and opportunities for promotion. There is always a significant risk that sensitive information, if released, may find its way to individuals or agencies that might harm the counselee in the future.

Informed Consent in Genetic Counseling

Since a major component of genetic counseling is communication of information, and since the counselee is encouraged to make her or his own decision, problems or conflicts with informed consent are unusual. Informed consent is especially relevant in the counseling process when a procedure may result in potentially harmful or ambiguous outcomes, for example:

1. in connection with prenatal diagnosis, when the counselee or woman who is to undergo the test needs to understand its risks, benefits, errors, and limitations;

2. as a prelude to presymptomatic testing for a serious disorder without available treatment or methods of prevention, where a positive result can have profound implications for the individual's future life;

3. in connection with participation in a research protocol in which there may be questions about the future use of data or tissue or blood (especially DNA) in future studies or in the search for other genetic markers.

Ethnic and Cultural Influences

The population of the United States and many other industrialized nations is becoming more diverse. It is estimated that by the year 2010 nearly one-third of the population of the United States will be made up of minorities. Genetic counseling that promotes individual autonomy and is consistent with the ethical values discussed here will require that counselors be aware of and responsive to a wide and growing range of ethnic and cultural variations among those who are now and will be seeking genetic counseling (Fisher). Conflicts are almost certain to arise when the values and decisions of the ethnically and/or culturally different counselees conflict with those of the counselors and the Western values derived from Jewish and Christian sources that in general govern the decision-making process. The value systems that have been used traditionally in counseling will probably have to be applied in significantly different ways if the process and outcome of counseling is to be helpful and effective.

ROBERT F. MURRAY, JR. (1995)
BIBLIOGRAPHY REVISED

SEE ALSO: *Access to Healthcare; Autonomy; Beneficence; Confidentiality; Eugenics; Family and Family Medicine; Genetic Counseling, Practice of; Genetic Testing and Screening; Health Insurance; Professional-Patient Relationship; Responsibility*

BIBLIOGRAPHY

Ad Hoc Committee on Genetic Counseling. American Society of Human Genetics [Charles J. Epstein, Chairman]. 1975. "Genetic Counseling." *American Journal of Human Genetics* 27(2): 240–242.

Andrews, Lori B. 1987. *Medical Genetics: A Legal Frontier.* Chicago: American Bar Foundation.

Antley, Ray M. 1979. "The Genetic Counselor as Facilitator of the Counselee's Decision Process." In *Genetic Counseling: Facts, Values and Norms,* pp. 137–168, ed. Alexander M. Capron, Marc Lappé, Robert F. Murray, Jr., Tabitha M. Powledge, Sumner B. Twiss, and Daniel Bergsma. National Foundation-March of Dimes Birth Defects Original Article Series, 15(2). New York: Alan R. Liss.

Bartles, Dianne M.; Leroy, Bonnie S.; and Caplan, Arthur L., eds. 1993. *Prescribing Our Future: Ethical Challenges in Genetic Counseling.* Hawthorne, NY: Aldine de Gruyter.

Beauchamp, Tom L., and Childress, James F. 1989. *Principles of Biomedical Ethics,* 3rd edition. New York: Oxford University Press.

Bosk, Charles L. 1992. *All God's Mistakes: Genetic Counseling in a Pediatric Hospital.* Chicago: University of Chicago Press.

Clarke, Angus, ed. 1994. *Genetic Counseling: Practice and Principles (Professional Ethics)*. London: Routledge.

Fisher, Nancy L. 1992. "Ethnocultural Approaches to Genetics." *Pediatric Clinics of North America* 39(1): 55–64.

Fraser, F. Clarke. 1974. "Genetic Counseling." *American Journal of Human Genetics* 26(5): 636–659.

Fraser, F. Clarke. 1979. "Introduction: The Development of Genetic Counseling." In *Genetic Counseling: Facts, Values and Norms*, pp. 5–15, ed. Alexander M. Capron, Marc Lappé, Robert F. Murray, Jr., Tabitha M. Powledge, Sumner B. Twiss, and Daniel Bergsma. National Foundation-March of Dimes Birth Defects Original Article Series, 15(2). New York: Alan R. Liss.

Hildt, Elisabeth. 2002. "Autonomy and Freedom of Choice in Prenatal Genetic Diagnosis." *Medicine, Health Care, and Philosophy* 5(1): 65–71.

Hsia, Y. Edward. 1979. "The Genetic Counselor as Information Giver." In *Genetic Counseling: Facts, Values and Norms*, pp. 169–186, ed. Alexander M. Capron, Marc Lappé, Robert F. Murray, Jr., Tabitha M. Powledge, Sumner B. Twiss, and Daniel Bergsma. National Foundation-March of Dimes Birth Defects Original Article Series, 15(2). New York: Alan R. Liss.

Kessler, Seymour. 1979. "The Genetic Counselor as Psychotherapist." In *Genetic Counseling: Facts, Values and Norms*, pp. 187–200, ed. Alexander M. Capron, Marc Lappé, Robert F. Murray, Jr., Tabitha M. Powledge, Sumner B. Twiss, and Daniel Bergsma. National Foundation-March of Dimes Birth Defects Original Article Series, 15(2). New York: Alan R. Liss.

Oduncu, Fuat S. 2002. "The Role of Non-Directiveness in Genetic Counseling." *Medicine, Health Care and Philosophy* 5(1): 53–63.

Palmer, Shane. 1992. "Guiding Principles, Resolutions, Clarify Stance." *Perspectives in Genetic Counseling: Newsletter of the National Society of Genetic Counselors* 14(1): 1, 4–5.

Patenaude, Andrea Farkas; Guttmacher, Alan E.; and Collins, Francis S. 2002. "Genetic Testing and Psychology. New Roles, New Responsibilities." *American Psychologist* 57(4): 271–282.

Suter, Sonia M. 1998. "Value Neutrality and Nondirectiveness: Comments on Future Directions in Genetic Counseling." *Kennedy Institute of Ethics Journal* 8(2): 161–163.

U.S. President's Commission for the Study of Ethical Problems in Medicine and Biomedical and Behavioral Research. 1983. *Screening and Counseling for Genetic Conditions*. Washington, D.C.: Author.

Wertz, Dorothy C., and Fletcher, John C. 1988. "Attitudes of Genetic Counselors: A Multinational Study." *American Journal of Human Genetics* 42(4): 592–600.

Wertz, Dorothy C.; Fletcher, John C.; and Mulvihill, John J. 1990. "Medical Geneticists Confront Ethical Dilemmas: Cross-Cultural Comparisons Among Eighteen Nations." *American Journal of Human Genetics* 46(6): 1200–1213.

White, Mary Terrell. 1997. "'Respect for Autonomy' in Genetic Counseling: an Analysis and a Proposal." *Journal of Genetic Counseling* 6(3): 297–313.

White, Mary Terrell. 1999. "Making Responsible Decisions. An Interpretive Ethic for Genetic Decision-making." *Hastings Center Report* 29(1): 14–21.

Willer, Roger A., ed. 1998. *Genetic Testing and Screening: Critical Engagement at the Intersection of Faith and Science*. Minneapolis, MN: Kirk House Publishing.

Williams, Clare; Alderson, Priscilla; and Farsides Bobbie. 2002. "Is Non-directiveness Possible Within the Context of Antenatal Screening and Testing?" *Social Science and Medicine* 54(3): 339–347.

Yarborough, Mark; Scott, Joan A.; and Dixon, Linda K. 1989. "The Role of Beneficence in Clinical Genetics: Nondirective Counseling Reconsidered." *Theoretical Medicine* 10(2): 139–149.

GENETIC COUNSELING, PRACTICE OF

• • •

Genetic counseling is a relatively new medical counseling service that aims to help those affected by genetic conditions or who face increased genetic risk. Clients seek this service asking questions about why a condition occurred, the chances that it may occur again in the future, and how they may be helped to cope with the uncertainty, risk, or prognosis of a diagnosis. Genetic counseling is often provided by a team of genetics providers (medical geneticists, master's level genetic counselors, and genetic nurses) in a specialty clinic within a hospital, university medical center, or in a community outpatient setting. Attention is paid to the medical, informational, and emotional needs of clients and their family members related to genetic conditions or birth defects.

History

Genetic counseling began in the United States in the 1930s when the academic discipline of genetics emerged and Mendelian principles of single gene inheritance could be applied to human conditions. The first *practitioners* were academic geneticists who were approached by individuals with concerns about their own family history. In the 1940s the field of human genetics was established, followed by medical specialization in genetics that focused on the diagnosis and natural history of genetic conditions. Shortly thereafter in the 1970s, the profession of genetic counseling was established in the United States. Practitioners earn a master's degree and are trained in both human genetics and psychological counseling skills. As of 2002 there were estimated to be over 2,000 genetic counselors practicing in the United States and Canada. Genetic counselors are credentialed by the American Board of Genetic Counseling to uphold practice standards. These professionals work with medical geneticists and obstetricians to provide education and counseling related to risk or diagnosis of a genetic condition or congenital anomaly.

Definition

Genetic counseling makes genetic information available to clients and facilitates their use of that information. Genetic information is important to understanding the cause of conditions, making informed choices, and adapting to genetic risk. The range of information provided includes the medical diagnosis, the inheritance pattern, the risk of recurrence, medical management or surveillance, prognosis, schooling needs, support groups, financial issues, and reproductive options. Since clients often seek services around significant life events or crises, the information is often highly sensitive, such as predicting the health of future children, the likelihood of a late onset condition, or the loss of an affected child. Discussion of genetic conditions or risks may therefore elicit feelings of lowered self-esteem, guilt, shame, loss, and blame for parents of affected children. Overall addressing the cognitive, affective, and behavioral aspects of clients' responses to the information are central components to genetic counseling. A practice definition states that:

> Genetic counseling is a dynamic psychoeducational process centered on genetic information. Within a therapeutic relationship established between providers and clients, clients are helped to personalize technical and probabilistic genetic information, to promote self-determination, and to enhance their ability to adapt over time. The overarching goal is to facilitate clients' ability to use genetic information in a personally meaningful way that minimizes psychological distress and increases personal control. (Biesecker and Peters, p. 195)

Settings and Practice Goals

There are a variety of different settings for genetic counseling, including reproductive, pediatric/adult, and common disease clinics. Each one embodies a different set of aims. In the reproductive setting, the focus is primarily on decision making. Most often clients seen in a prenatal genetics clinic seek to understand their age-related risks for having a child with a chromosomal abnormality, such as Down syndrome. Increasingly they may also be seen in follow-up to an abnormal screening test that implicates higher chances for having a child with a birth defect or chromosomal disorder. These clients most often have no family history of the disorder(s) in question and are helped to understand what the conditions are, their likelihood for occurrence, and the options for managing or terminating the pregnancy. The goal is to promote client self-determination in exercising choice about the use of prenatal tests. Reproductive genetic counseling aims to deliver personalized genetic information to the client in a useful way; to explore the meaning of the information with the client in light of personal values and beliefs; to promote the clients' preferences for reproductive options with consideration of alternatives, consequences, and barriers; and to prepare the client for adapting to the outcomes of the choice(s) (Biesecker). When an abnormality is detected, there are few options for treating the condition and couples face painful decisions about whether or not to abort a desired pregnancy. Genetic counseling is particularly important when couples face such irreversible life-altering decisions.

In the pediatric and adult genetics setting, the goal is to facilitate client understanding and adaptation to a condition. In this setting clients often have a child or other relative who is affected with a genetic condition that they seek to better understand as part of their adaptation to (often unexpected) circumstances. Obtaining an accurate diagnosis of the condition by a medical geneticist is an essential component. Medical information provided to clients includes a description of the condition and its potential long-term consequences. The aims of genetic counseling in the pediatric or adult genetics setting are to discuss client understanding of cause as it relates to a scientific (genetic) explanation and the client's interpretation, to explore the role of personal beliefs in adaptation, and to promote feelings of personal control and mastery over the condition (Biesecker). Genetic counseling helps clients to cognitively integrate genetic information into their personal beliefs and frame of reference in a manner that is personally useful to them. Referrals are often made to support groups or to other parents with similarly affected children. School referrals for attention to special learning needs for the child may also be made. Parents often require a great deal of follow-up medical, educational, and support services for their child and themselves.

In the common disease setting, such as cancer genetics, cardiovascular genetics, or neurogenetics clinics, most often adults seek to understand their own risk for disease. The goal is to maintain the health of at-risk individuals. Specific aims are to increase accurate risk perception, to facilitate adaptation to genetic risk, to promote health-enhancing behaviors, and to prevent disease (Biesecker). Predictive genetic testing may be offered as part of the effort to refine risk more precisely and as a basis for making screening or prevention recommendations. Yet decisions about predictive testing are highly personal due to the lack of empirical evidence to guide practitioners in making medical recommendations based on test results. In many cases genetic testing offers risk estimates but little else. Clients' decisions about undergoing predictive testing often lie with the meaning the test result would have for adapting to living at risk. Increasingly such testing will also be used to manage risk by offering targeted interventions for those identified to be at increased genetic risk, but this is rarely the case.

Cancer genetics services have been established in response to the research and commercial availability of predictive testing for cancer risk. Tests have been developed for breast and ovarian cancer risk, colorectal cancer risk and for certain rare cancer syndromes. While medical recommendations are made for tested individuals found to be at increased risk, there remains a paucity of empirical evidence to support the majority of these recommendations. With time more precise risk estimations will be made using testing, targeted interventions will be known to be effective, and reduction in morbidity and mortality will be achieved. In the meantime, however, the imprecise nature of cancer genetics testing necessitates informed consent and emphasizes the importance of pre-test education and counseling in the common disease setting.

Non-Directiveness

Genetic counseling is often described as *non-directive,* meaning that clients are helped to make personal decisions without undue influence by the counselor. This practice principle emerged from reproductive genetic counseling where couples face decisions about having children or continuing an affected pregnancy. It remains an important ethical principle for guiding clients through their reproductive choices. Clients are helped to make personally relevant and informed choices for themselves. Nonetheless nondirectiveness is difficult to achieve since counselors have personal and professional biases and experiences that may be inadvertently expressed in how information is presented or emphasized in genetic counseling. While counselors may not intend to guide client decisions, it is reasonable to assume that genetic counseling influences them. Yet the majority of clients are capable of making their own decisions and can benefit from prenatal counseling by exploring their own beliefs, attitudes, and values related to their ability to parent a child affected with a particular condition. Genetic counseling that is client-centered focuses on meeting the needs of clients by working within the context of their sociocultural beliefs and lived experience. Even if a genetic counselor explicitly expresses her own beliefs during reproductive counseling, it is unlikely that a client will simply adopt them. However there are situations where conflicts in promoting personal reproductive choice do exist.

When a prenatal genetic counselor is employed by a commercial laboratory or prenatal testing center, there is more likely to be a potential conflict of interest. If the testing center promotes prenatal tests rather than promoting the choice of testing, then the counseling may emphasize the benefits of testing over the risks. There might be more frequent assumptions on behalf of the counselor that if the client was referred for prenatal testing, that the client is going to undergo testing rather than insuring that each client makes an informed and personal decision whether or not to undergo optional prenatal tests. Further, if the counselor's salary depends upon a certain number of tests being conducted, there is likely to be an even greater chance for persuasive prenatal genetic counseling.

In genetic counseling settings other than reproductive, non-directiveness has little relevance. In the common disease setting, for instance, making screening recommendations to promote health intends to be directive. Applying the notion of non-directiveness to genetic counseling in general has lead to a great deal of confusion in the literature (Kessler). In addition to directive health-related recommendations, communication in genetic counseling is often directive. Offering advice or making referrals may be also be construed as directive. The adoption of non-directiveness as a central tenet of genetic counseling has limited the use of (directive) therapeutic interventions that may be helpful to clients. Genetic counseling may be practiced in a more hesitant manner if counselors fear directing their clients' decisions when fully engaging with them may be more productive. Issues related to non-directiveness continue to be actively debated in the professional literature.

Client-Centered Practice

Interpretation and use of genetic information by clients depends somewhat on their personality traits and characteristics. Clients come from a variety of sociodemographic and ethnocultural backgrounds that shape their beliefs, values, and available resources. Clients also may belong to affected families who have experience with a condition under discussion. Others may not have had experience with it. These variables shape client needs, attitudes, and priorities. Genetic counseling necessitates assessment of these variables in order to tailor the information and counseling to meet client needs. A couple with two children affected with cystic fibrosis that faces a decision about prenatal testing with a subsequent pregnancy is expert on the disorder and its impact on the family. A couple who is found to be at increased risk for having a child with cystic fibrosis based on carrier screening with no family history of the condition may have little idea of what having an affected child may mean for the child or themselves. Genetic counseling would differ in meeting the needs of these clients, even though at face value, each involves a fetus at 25 percent risk for being affected with the same condition, cystic fibrosis.

Since genetic conditions affect families, there may also be differences in how relatives view or use genetic information. Genetic counselors working with various family members have obligations to protect the privacy of individual clients and to support different decisions made within the same family. The offer to undergo predictive genetic testing, for instance, may result in some individuals who are interested and others who are not. Yet test results for one relative may reveal the at-risk status of another. So protecting personal testing decisions within families can be challenging. Genetic counseling aims to help relatives anticipate such consequences prior to undergoing testing. Rarely family members may choose not to reveal risk of a genetic condition to relatives. In this circumstance, genetic counselors may be persuasive in encouraging clients to notify their relatives so that each at-risk person may be informed and equipped to make his or her own decision about whether or not to undergo genetic testing. There is debate about the duty of genetics providers to warn at-risk relatives in situations where family members choose otherwise.

As more genetic discoveries emerge and genetics medicine moves into an era in which diagnoses are refined by genetic information, more tests are developed, and treatments tailored, all healthcare providers will need to understand some aspects of medical genetics. Nurses, primary care physicians, and even social workers and psychologists will be faced with helping clients to make decisions about using new genetic technologies. This sea change suggests a significant need for professional genetics education to prepare a variety of healthcare providers to care for clients in the future. Genetic counselors are important providers for helping to train others. In the meantime, it is important that clients who encounter new genetic technologies have access to appropriately trained and certified genetics providers. As genetic testing is increasingly utilized as a tool for medical management and not merely as a means to obtain risk information, there is likely to be less psychological turmoil for clients in making decisions about undergoing testing. However carrier testing or pre-symptomatic testing for serious, late-onset disorders without medical treatment will continue to elicit strong thoughts and feelings from clients. Certain genetic testing will continue to need to be accompanied by psychoeducational genetic counseling provided by well-trained clinicians to facilitate personal decision making. As the number and background of professionals involved in genetic testing expands, there is a greater potential threat to well-informed decision making. The maintenance of a high training and practice standard for genetic counseling is a priority in anticipating some of the consequences of the diffusion and proliferation of genetic testing.

Genetic counseling has evolved rapidly in its short history from the reproductive arena to pediatric and adult genetics clinics and more recently into common disease clinics. With this expansion, its goals have become more diverse and specific to the setting. As genetics medicine further emerges and new genetic tests are introduced, promoting informed choice about use of genetic tests will continue to necessitate pre-test genetic education and counseling. Ethical controversies related to duty to warn relatives, risks to the confidentiality of genetic information, and conflicts of interest related to commercial incentives for testing will expand and policies and even legislative protections will emerge.

BARBARA BOWLES BIESECKER (1995)
REVISED BY AUTHOR

SEE ALSO: *Autonomy; Beneficence; Confidentiality; Eugenics; Family and Family Medicine; Genetic Counseling, Ethical Issues in; Genetic Discrimination; Genetic Testing and Screening; Professional-Patient Relationship*

BIBLIOGRAPHY

Andrews, Lori; Fullarton, Jane; Holtzman, Neil; et al., eds. 1994. *Assessing Genetic Risks: Implications for Health and Social Policy.* Washington, D.C.: National Academy Press.

Bartels, Dianne M.; LeRoy, Bonnie S.; and Caplan, Arthur L., eds. 1993. *Prescribing Our Future: Ethical Challenges in Genetic Counseling.* New York: Aldine de Gruyer.

Biesecker, Barbara B. 2001. "Mini Review: Goals of Genetic Counseling." *Clinical Genetics* 60: 323–330.

Biesecker Barbara B, and Marteau, Theresa M. 1999. "The Future of Genetic Counseling: An International Perspective." *Nature Genetics* 22(2): 133–137.

Biesecker Barbara B, and Peters, Kathryn. 2001. "Process Studies in Genetic Counseling: Peering into the Black Box." *American Journal of Medical Genetics* 106: 191–198.

Kessler, Seymour. 1997. "Psychological Aspects of Genetic Counseling. XI. Nondirectiveness Revisited." *American Journal of Medical Genetics* 72: 164–171.

Reed, Sheldon C. 1974. "A Short History of Genetic Counseling." *Social Biology* 21(4): 332–339.

GENETIC DISCRIMINATION

• • •

Genetic discrimination is the term commonly assigned to actions taken against or negative attitudes toward a person based on that person's possession of variations in the genome, or variations in the genome of his or her biological relatives. A component of stigmatization, genetic discrimination differentiates social treatment based on assumptions about the value of information suggested by a particular genetic configuration in predicting present and future health status (Condit, Parrott, and O'Grady). The details of one's genome are typically available through genetic tests (Burke). The nature of genetics is such that information derived from one person's genetic composition may implicate or be attributed to the biological siblings and/or descendants of that person. Genetic discrimination illustrates the danger of a misinterpretation—or oversimplification—of information suggested by some genes. Fear of genetic discrimination is often cited as a reason for avoidance of genetic testing services (Rothenberg and Terry).

Empirical evidence of genetic discrimination in contemporary society is somewhat slight (Nowlan). Early reports of genetic discrimination by adoption agencies have not been repeated (American Society of Human Genetics). Nevertheless, fears of genetic discrimination by employers and insurance companies continue to influence decisions regarding submission to genetic testing and participation in certain forms of genetic research. The result may negatively influence individuals' health (Rothenberg and Terry). Efforts to address genetic discrimination include legislation, industry self-restraint, and private action, each controversial for what it suggests about the ability to prevent forms of discrimination.

Genetic Information

Some variations in the genome have demonstrated value in predicting the health status of a person. Where a disease is monogenic, like Huntington's disease, its onset is foretold by the presence or absence of a mutation in a single gene (Guttmacher and Collins). The presence and location of single nucleotide polymorphisms (each commonly referred to as a "SNP," pronounced "snip"), may inform decisions in drug therapy by predicting an ability to metabolize a drug or a risk of toxicity (Guttmacher and Collins; Syvanen). In other instances, an enzyme or protein may yield similar information. Efforts to map the human genome with greater specificity, as well as efforts in pharmacogenomics, rely upon comparisons of the patterns of genetic variation in large numbers of people.

Media coverage and other efforts to relate complex concepts in genetics to a lay audience have revealed a tendency to oversimplify the relationship between one's genome and one's destiny. Specifically, the predictive value of genetic information is often overstated. Behavioral genetics, for example, remains in its infancy; few genetic mutations or polymorphisms are thought predictive of intelligence or cognitive ability. With the exception of monogenic diseases, which are relatively rare, the predictive relationship between the genome and disease is compromised by the relative lack of knowledge about the influence of environmental factors. The wide range of more common diseases is a function of interactions between the genome and such factors as diet, climate, and physical activity. Finally, a gap typically exists between knowledge of the discovery of a causal relationship attributable to a particular genetic variation and knowledge of a treatment for the condition at issue.

The result of this oversimplification is genetic determinism (Rothstein, 1999), alternatively termed "genetic reductionism" (Lee, Mountain, and Koenig) or "genetic essentialism" (Nelkin). The terms describe the phenomenon through which the importance of genetic factors is emphasized at the relative expense of environmental and social factors. Together, determinism and discrimination are elements of stigmatization (Condit, et al.). As explained by Celeste M. Condit, Roxanne L. Parrott, and Beth O'Grady in their 2000 article, discriminatory attitudes about genetics get much of their stigmatizing impact from excessively deterministic attitudes about genetics.

Insurance

Discrimination might manifest in several ways. The use of genetic information by insurers figures prominently in assessments of public attitudes and fears about genetic research and medicine. Theoretically, genetic tests obviate the need for the family medical history common in medical underwriting practices. Relatively few instances of discrimination by an insurance company have been reported, whether because discrimination is difficult to recognize or prove, or because the practice is not prevalent (Rothenberg and Terry).

Within the context of life insurance, the question is whether companies should either require genetic testing or have access to the results of genetic tests documented in medical records in deciding whether to underwrite a policy.

Insurance is characterized by a commercial transaction in which the company pays a benefit upon the death of the policyholder in exchange for a premium proportional to the mortality risk assumed by the insurance company (Cook; Nowlan). The fear is that a life insurer would decline to underwrite a policy for a person or family of persons who possess genetic variations that suggests early death. Insurance companies wish to avoid financial harm caused by adverse selection. Adverse selection results when persons who believe they are at a lower risk of illness or early death choose to purchase less insurance or leave the market, while persons who believe they are at higher risk purchase greater amounts of insurance. Ultimately, the money paid in premiums by persons of lower risk is no longer sufficient to cover the expense incurred by insuring persons of higher risk.

Medical underwriting is not as common in the context of medical or health insurance as compared to life insurance (Nowlan). Countries with a national health service extend resources to nearly all citizens without regard to health status; medical underwriting becomes relevant only in the small market for private health insurance. Nevertheless, fears are particularly pronounced in the United Kingdom, where—contrary to other countries, including the United States—life insurance is a requisite to the purchase of a home or other real estate (Cook).

The private health insurance market is much more prominent in the United States than in other countries, but is made available primarily through group plans subsidized by the employer in a voluntary arrangement (Rothstein, 2000). Medical underwriting is a greater possibility in the relatively small market of private individual policies, which can be very expensive.

Employment

Initial fears suggested that employers who had access to genetic information would refuse to hire persons with inherited characteristics that suggested greater use of health resources by either the employee or family members. Employers would try to control expenses on healthcare and perhaps absenteeism by pricing premiums in accordance with health status of the employee. Recent legislation in the United States prohibits employers from charging employees of higher risk a higher premium (*Health Insurance Portability and Accountability Act of 1996 (HIPAA)*). Cases of genetic discrimination primarily involve an employer's attempt to require genetic testing or access to the results of genetic tests already included as medical records as a prerequisite or condition of employment. While state and federal statutes regulate the employer's use of results from genetic testing, other statutes that impose upon the employer a duty to ensure worker safety partially restore access to such medical information (Rothstein).

Eugenics

The eugenics movement and other misguided attempts to translate science into government policy provide support for contemporary fears of stigmatization. Proponents of eugenics, a dominant scientific philosophy from the late nineteenth century through the mid-twentieth century, sought to improve the quality of the human race through social policy based on flawed theories about heritable characteristics (Galton and Galton). Agents of the government dissuaded persons perceived as mentally deficient or possessing an inherently criminal nature from reproducing, sometimes through laws mandating sterilization of groups of persons (Markel). Eugenic principles were consistent with social classification policies implemented in support of Nazi Germany, and contributed to the mass exterminations of persons.

With regard to the issue of *race,* many who cite concerns of genetic discrimination emphasize the dangers attendant to the racialization of disease or conflating social categories with genetic variations (Lee, et al.). Despite evidence that patterns of genetic variation are greater within racialized groups than between them, resistance to historical patterns of classifying persons by race is neither easy nor simple.

The association of disease with an identifiable human population is a dangerous and often unintended consequence of technology. In the later years of the twentieth century, efforts in the United States to implement policies to help persons afflicted with sickle-cell disease, a heritable disease, proved disastrous. A push for early diagnosis and treatment yielded several state laws that mandated screening African Americans for the disease. The years following the passage of these laws were marked by an increase in acts of discrimination by government, insurers, and employers against persons afflicted with the disease, as well as against persons who were merely carriers of the trait (Markel). The disease became associated with African-Americans in a way that illustrated the dangers and improvidence of conflating *race* with a particular genetic composition. The foregoing demonstrates the perils of premature and perhaps short-sighted policymaking.

At the beginning of the twenty-first century, there were reports of discord within the Jewish community regarding genetic testing (Schwartz, Rothenberg, Joseph, et al.). Following the identification of mutations in BRCA1 and BRCA2 that are associated with a higher risk of breast or ovarian cancer, many supported testing as critical to prevention and treatment of women who carry the mutation, while others discouraged participation based on fear of stigmatization (American College of Medical Genetics). This reaction against genetic testing was based in part on a controversial history of research on Tay-Sachs disease. The knowledge gap between the ability to predict a condition and the ability to treat it created uncertainty and the opportunity for misinterpretation of existing information.

Fear vs. Fact

Some have observed that the greatest danger with respect to genetic discrimination stems from unsubstantiated fears of discrimination. Several studies document the effect of anxiety about the possibility of genetic discrimination on participation in genetic testing or screening procedures (Geer, Ropka, Cohn, et al.). Exaggerating the size of the problem promotes genetic determinism and feeds fears that inhibit participation in research and therapy.

The literature identifying the factors motivating an individual to participate in tests that yield genetic information useful in determining susceptibility to disease or illness reveal several themes. The desire to help a relative is commonly cited as a motivating factor (Applebaum-Shapiro, Peters, O'Connell, et al.). The relative paucity of empirical data as to the prevalence of discrimination does not influence public attitudes regarding a willingness to participate or fears of discrimination or stigmatization (Hall and Rich).

An individual's wish to avoid negative treatment based on deterministic attitudes can manifest in several ways. An individual may refuse to be tested for a particular trait even if necessary for diagnostic purposes. Alternatively, the person may opt to test anonymously or to pay for the test without filing an insurance claim—even if the test is covered—in an attempt to keep such information from the employer or medical insurer. For example, in the first years after the significance of the BRCA1 and BRCA2 mutations was announced and a predictive test made available, there emerged anecdotes in which persons took steps to conceal information from becoming a part of their medical records (Schwartz, et al.).

Social Policy

The power of the fear of genetic discrimination to direct behavior is central to debates regarding the need for curbs on such discrimination through social policy (Greely). The degree of restriction is often related to the degree of harm threatening economic and other values. In the United Kingdom, the strong relationship between life insurance, home ownership, and the effect of perceptions of danger on the national economy prompted a national investigation (Cook). At least partially to avoid more restrictive measures, the British life insurance industry declared a voluntary, qualified moratorium on policies. Some have suggested that industry self-restraint is preferable to overreaching or imprecise legislation (Nowlan). Critics contend that industry self-restraint can not serve as a sufficient deterrent to actions that could otherwise yield economic benefit.

Legislation plays a relatively more prominent role in policies regulating genetic discrimination in the United States. Absent a single, uniform statute at the federal level, the laws of individual states address genetic discrimination. The actions of employers and other entities are also subject to provisions within federal statutes that regulate the workplace and the marketplace (Pagnattaro). Legislation passed in the 1990s regulates the dissemination of medical records that could contain the results of genetic tests (*HIPAA*). Such regulation reflects the heightened value afforded privacy and confidentiality, particularly within the United States, in an era of advanced medical and informational technology.

Several scholars have criticized the use of legislation prohibiting genetic discrimination as premature and unnecessary government interference in a free market system (Epstein). Citing flaws in the legislative approaches to discrimination in other contexts, these scholars question the fairness of protecting the concealment of information that may have legitimate value. Others emphasize the absence of evidence of genetic discrimination by health or life insurance companies (Nowlan). To enact legislation on the basis of a problem that exists primarily through anecdotes, critics argue, is to validate fears that are unsubstantiated (Nowlan).

Still others praise legislation prohibiting genetic discrimination as an effective means of allaying the fears of the public (Greely). Legislation is a vehicle for establishing a shared consensus on the values underlying the matter. The cost of "symbolic" legislation, however, remains a matter for debate (Hellman).

Conclusion

More important than the prohibition of the actual behavior is the need to allay the concerns of persons acting on the basis of such fears. This is the challenge facing those who would shape public policy on the use of genetic information. Deterministic attitudes underlie fears of discrimination, as well as the actual discriminating conduct. The ability to surmise from one person's genetic information details about another will influence traditional notions of autonomy and even self-determination. The idea that stigmatization might follow from participation in genetic testing or other research is an obstacle to the optimization of the benefits in health and resources that are increasingly available through advances in genetic technology.

PHYLLIS GRIFFIN EPPS

SEE ALSO: *Access to Healthcare; DNA Identification; Eugenics; Genetic Counseling, Ethical Issues in; Genetics and Human Self-Understanding; Human Dignity; Human Rights; Justice; Patients' Rights; Population Ethics; Race and Racism*

BIBLIOGRAPHY

American Society of Human Genetics, Social Issues Committee, and American College of Medical Genetics. 2000. "Genetic Testing in Adoption." *American Journal of Human Genetics* 66(3): 761–767.

Applebaum-Shapiro, S. E.; Peters, J. A.; O'Connell, J. A.; Aston, C. E.; et al. 2001. "Motivations and Concerns of Patients with Access to Genetic Testing for Hereditary Pancreatitis." *American Journal of Gastroenterology* 96: 1610–1617.

Burke, Wylie. 2002. "Genetic Testing." *New England Journal of Medicine* 347(23): 1867–1875.

Condit, Celeste M.; Parrott, Roxanne L.; and O'Grady, Beth. 2000. "Principles and Practices of Communication Processes for Genetics in Public Health." In *Genetics and Public Health in the 21st Century: Using Genetic Information to Improve Health and Prevent Disease,* ed. M. J. Khoury, W. Burke, and E. Thomson. New York: Oxford University Press.

Cook, E. David. 1999. "Genetics and British Insurance Industry." *Journal of Medical Ethics* 25: 157–162.

Epstein, Richard A. 1994. "The Legal Regulation of Genetic Discrimination: Old Responses to New Technology." *Boston University Law Review* 74: 1–23.

Galton, David J., and Galton, Clare J. 1998. "Francis Galton: And Eugenics Today." *Journal of Medical Ethics* 24: 99–105.

Geer, Katherine P.; Ropka, Mary E.; Cohn, Wendy F.; et al. 2001. "Factors Influencing Patients' Decisions to Decline Cancer Genetic Counseling Services." *Journal of Genetic Counseling* 10(1): 25–40.

Greely, Henry T. 2001. "Genotype Discrimination: The Complex Case for Some Legislative Protection." *University of Pennsylvania Law Review* 149: 1483–1505.

Guttmacher, Alan E., and Collins, Francis S. 2002. "Genomic Medicine—A Primer." *New England Journal of Medicine* 347(19): 1512–1520.

Hall, M. A., and Rich, S. S. 2000. "Genetic Privacy Laws and Patients' Fear of Discrimination by Health Insurers: The View from Genetic Counselors." *Journal of Law, Medicine and Ethics* 28: 245–247.

Health Insurance Portability and Accountability Act of 1996 (HIPAA), Pub. L. No. 104–191, 110 Stat. 1936. 1996.

Hellman, Deborah. 2003. "What Makes Genetic Discrimination Exceptional?" *American Journal of Law and Medicine* 29: 77–116.

Lee, Sandra Soo-Jin; Mountain, Joanna; and Koenig, Barbara A. 2001. "The Meanings of 'Race' in the New Genomics: Implications for Health Disparities Research." *Yale Journal of Health Policy, Law, and Ethics* 1: 33–68.

Markel, Howard. 1992. "The Stigma of Disease: Implications of Genetic Screening." *American Journal of Medicine* 93: 209–215.

Nelkin, Dorothy. 2002. "A Brief History of the Political Work of Genetics." *Jurimetrics Journal* 42: 121–132.

Nowlan, William. 2002. "A Rational View of Insurance and Genetic Discrimination." *Science* 297: 195–196.

Pagnattaro, Marisa Anne. 2001. "Genetic Discrimination and the Workplace: Employee's Right to Privacy v. Employer's Need to Know." *American Business Law Journal* 29: 139–185.

Rothenberg, Karen, and Terry, Sharon. 2002. "Before It's Too Late—Addressing Fear of Genetic Information." *Science* 297: 196–197.

Rothstein, Mark A. 1999. "Behavioral Genetic Determinism: Its Effects on Culture and Law." In *Behavioral Genetics: The Clash of Culture and Biology,* ed. R. A. Carson and M. A. Rothstein. Baltimore: Johns Hopkins University Press.

Rothstein, Mark A. 2000. "Genetics and the Work Force of the Next Hundred Years." *Columbia Business Law Review* 2000: 371–402.

Schwartz, Marc D.; Rothenberg, Karen; Joseph, Linda; et al. 2000. "Consent to the Use of Stored DNA for Genetics Research: A Survey of Attitudes in the Jewish Population." *American Journal of Medical Genetics* 98: 336–342.

Syvanen, Ann-Christine. 2001. "Accessing Genetic Variation: Genotyping Single Nucleotide Polymorphisms." *Nature Reviews Genetics* 2: 930–940.

INTERNET RESOURCE

American College of Medical Genetics. 1996. "Statement on Population Screening for BRCA–1 Mutation in Ashkenazi Jewish Women." Available from <http://www.faseb.org/genetics/acmg/pol-24.htm>.

GENETIC ENGINEERING, HUMAN

• • •

The development of recombinant DNA techniques in the 1970s enabled scientists to create genetically engineered organisms. In 1975 molecular biologists and geneticists held a conference in Asilomar, California, to discuss the biosafety issues relating to the new technology as well as policies for regulation and oversight. In 1978 fertility specialists used in vitro fertilization (IVF) techniques to assist a British couple in conceiving Louise Brown, the world's first "test tube" baby. In the early 1980s researchers began using embryo-splitting technologies to produce desirable livestock clones for agriculture. By the end of the decade universities and biotechnology companies were manufacturing and patenting transgenic mice for use in drug testing and medical research.

During the course of those events many people expressed concern that these discoveries and innovations eventually would lead to human genetic engineering (HGE). In early discussions of HGE (circa 1965–1980) scientists, journalists, and scholars conjured up the familiar allegories of Mary Shelly's *Frankenstein* and Aldous Huxley's *Brave New World* to question the wisdom of pursuing the new technologies (Gaylin; Boone). Science fiction novels such as *Mutant 59* and *The Boys from Brazil* depicted the disastrous effects of genetic engineering experiments gone awry. The biotechnology critic Jeremy Rifkin (1983) warned of the Faustian bargain of genetic engineering and the dangers of meddling with nature. Theologians such as Paul Ramsey (1970) and bioethicists such as Leon Kass (1972) spoke about the dangers of "playing God" and disrupting family relationships. However, scientists, such as Joshua Lederberg (1966) and James Watson (1971) and philosophers such as Jonathan Glover (1984) and Joseph Fletcher (1965) embraced the possibilities of using HGE to advance scientific and social goals.

Two Key Distinctions and Four Basic Categories

While the public debate continued, scientists, clinicians, and scholars began to envision potential medical uses of HGE as they developed a framework for justifying the application of gene transfer technologies to human beings. Two key distinctions defined this framework: the somatic versus germline distinction and the therapy versus enhancement distinction (Walters; Anderson, 1985, 1989). Those distinctions implied four types of HGE:

> Somatic gene therapy (SGT)
>
> Somatic genetic enhancement (SGE)
>
> Germline gene therapy (GLGT)
>
> Germline genetic enhancement (GLGE)

Anderson (1989) and others argued that SGT could be justified on the grounds that it was morally similar to other types of medical treatments, such as pharmaceutical therapy and surgery. The goal of SGT is to transfer genes into human somatic cells to enable those cells to produce functional proteins in the appropriate quantities at the appropriate time. In 1990 the first SGT clinical trial involved an attempt to transfer normal adenosine deaminase (ADA) genes into patients with ADA deficiency, a disease of the immune system caused by mutations that prevent the patient from producing sufficient quantities of ADA (Walters and Palmer). Because SGT targets somatic cells, it probably will not transmit genetic changes to future generations as a result of the fact that genetic inheritance in human beings occurs through germ cells. However, there is a slight chance that an SGT protocol will result in an accidental gene transfer to germ cells, and that chance increases as one performs the experiment earlier in human development. For example, SGT administered to a developing fetus entails a significant risk of accidental gene transfer to germ cells (Zanjani and Anderson).

The goal of GLGT, in contrast, is to transfer genes into human germ cells to prevent the development of a genetic disease in a child who has not yet been born. A GLGT protocol for ADA deficiency would attempt to transfer normal genes into the parents' gametes or a zygote so that the progeny would have the correct gene and therefore would not develop the disease. Because GLGT targets germ cells, it is likely to transmit genetic changes to future generations; therefore, it poses far greater risks than does SGT. According to many authors and organizations, SGT can be morally justified but GLGT cannot because it is too risky. Thus, many clinician-scientists who saw the promise of SGT attempted to draw a firm moral boundary between SGT and GLGT.

After the first SGT experiments began, many writers made the case for crossing the line between somatic therapy and germline therapy (Zimmerman; Berger and Gert; Munson and Davis). Those writers argued that some germline interventions are morally justifiable because they promote medical goals such as disease prevention and the relief of suffering. Most of the approximately 5,000 known genetic diseases cause disabilities, premature death, and suffering. Although couples often can use nongenetic methods such as prenatal genetic testing and preimplantation genetic testing to give birth to children without genetic diseases, for some diseases germline therapy offers the only hope of producing a healthy child who is genetically related to the couple. For example, if a male and a female are both homozygous for a recessive genetic disease such as cystic fibrosis (CF), the only way they can produce a healthy child is to use gene transfer techniques to create embryos with normal genes (Resnik and Langer).

Therapy versus Enhancement

Many of the writers, clinicians, and scientists who defended genetic therapy also had moral qualms about genetic enhancement. In genetic enhancement the goal of the intervention is not to treat or prevent a disease but to achieve another result, such as increased height, intelligence, disease resistance, or musical ability. Thus, according to many authors, there is a moral distinction between genetic therapy, which is morally acceptable, and genetic enhancement, which is morally unacceptable or questionable (Suzuki and Knudtson; Anderson, 1989; Berger and Gert). Until society achieves a moral consensus on genetic enhancement, HGE protocols should not attempt to enhance human beings genetically.

By making these two fundamental distinctions, SGT proponents were able to obtain public approval of and funding for SGT experiments and dispel some of the fears associated with HGE. Under this twofold classification, SGT experiments were ethical and should be conducted but others types of HGE experiments were unethical or at least ethically questionable and should not be conducted.

Whereas the somatic versus germline distinction has stood the test of time, the therapy versus enhancement distinction has been criticized (Juengst, 1997; Stock and Campbell; Parens; Resnik, 2000a). Some critics of the second distinction argue that many genetic *enhancements* would be morally acceptable. For example, some day it may be possible to transfer disease-resistance genes to human beings. If childhood immunizations, which enhance the human immune system in order to prevent disease, are morally acceptable, what is wrong with *genetic immunizations?* It also may be possible some day to manipulate genes that affect the aging process. If nongenetic means of prolonging life such as organ transplants are morally acceptable, what is wrong with genetic means of prolonging life?

Other critics question the cogency of the distinction because it is founded on the concepts of health and disease (Parens). Therapy is an intervention designed to treat or prevent disease; enhancement is an intervention that serves another purpose. However, how should one define health and disease? Several decades of reflection on these concepts have not solved the problem (Caplan). According to an influential approach, disease is an objective concept that is defined as a deviation from normal human functioning that causes suffering and places limitations on a person's range of opportunities (Boorse; Buchanan et al.).

For example, CF is a disease because patients with CF do not breath normally. As a result, they have a variety of symptoms, such as shortness of breath and a persistent cough, which cause suffering and interfere with physical activity. CF patients also usually die many years before the normal human life span of seventy-plus years. Thus, a genetic intervention designed to treat or prevent CF is therapeutic.

However, this approach has some well-known problems and limitations. First, social and cultural factors play an important role in delineating the normal range of values that define disease. For example, dyslexia is recognized as a disease in developed nations because it interferes with reading, but it does not cause that problem in a nonliterate society. An adult in the United States who is shorter than four feet tall is regarded as having a disease—dwarfism—but the same adult living in an African pygmy tribe would be regarded as normal. Modern psychiatrists recognize depression as a mental illness, but it was regarded as a lifestyle or bad mood a hundred years ago.

Second, social and political values affect the range of opportunities in society and therefore have an impact on diseases; societies choose who will be disabled (Buchanan et al. 2000). For example, if a person has an allergy to cigarette smoke, he or she would have a difficult time breathing in a society in which smoking is permitted in public places. That person may become disabled, and his or her condition therefore would be a disease. However, that person would not have those difficulties is a society that bans smoking in public. The allergy would not prevent that person from working or participating in public activities. He or she therefore would not be disabled and would not have a disease.

Third, health usually is not defined as merely the opposite of disease. According to an influential definition of health, "Health is a state of complete physical, mental, and social well-being and not merely the absence of disease or infirmity" (World Health Organization [WHO]). This definition implies that some enhancements of human functioning are necessary to promote health because health is understood not only as the absence of disease but as an ideal state of functioning and flourishing. Thus, immunizations that enhance the immune system promote health, as do exercise regimens that enhance human musculature and endurance.

As a result of these and other problems with the therapy versus enhancement distinction, several authors have argued that it does not mark any absolute moral or metaphysical boundaries. One cannot equate *therapy* with *morally acceptable* or *morally required,* and one cannot equate *enhancement* with *morally unacceptable* or *morally forbidden.* To determine the moral justifiability of a genetic intervention in a particular case, one must assess that intervention in light of the relevant facts as well as moral values and principles such as autonomy, beneficence, and justice (Resnik and Langer). Some writers who criticize the distinction nevertheless maintain that it may be useful in setting an agenda for policy discussions or for raising moral warning flags (Buchanan et al.).

Inheritable Genetic Modifications

In the early debates about germline interventions most writers viewed GLGT and GLGE as methods for transferring genes to human germs cells such as sperm, ova, and zygotes or to human germ tissues such as the testes and ovaries. A human germline intervention would be similar to a genetic engineering experiment in a mammal in that it would attempt to transfer a gene into the DNA in the chromosomes in the cell nucleus. Writers on both sides of the GLGT debate agreed that random gene insertion would be an extremely risky procedure and that targeted gene replacement (TGR) would pose the fewest risks to progeny (Resnik, Steinkraus, and Langer).

Several important scientific and technical developments in the 1990s challenged this way of thinking about genetic interventions in the germline. In 1997 the experiment that produced Dolly, the world's first cloned sheep, demonstrated that nuclear transfer (NT) techniques could be applied to human beings (Pence). In this procedure one removes the nucleus from a zygote and transfers a nucleus from another egg or a somatic cell to the enucleated egg. The resulting embryo has a donor nucleus combined with the cytoplasm of the recipient. An NT procedure, like a GLGT procedure, produces inheritable genetic changes. However, an NT procedure does not attempt to modify human chromosomes. Since the early 1990s scientists and scholars around the world have had a vigorous debate about the ethical and social issues of human cloning (Kristol and Cohen). Several European countries, including Germany and France, have outlawed all human cloning. At the time of this writing the United States was considering a ban on human cloning, although no bill has been signed into law.

While the world was debating the ethics of NT, researchers conducted a more modest form of genetic manipulation in human beings: ooplasm transfer (OT). OT already has resulted in over thirty live births (Barritt et al.). In OT one infuses ooplasm (the cytoplasm from an egg) into a zygote. The resulting embryo has its original nucleus and a modified ooplasm containing ooplasm from the donor egg. OT also produces inheritable genetic changes because it modifies DNA that resides in the mitochondria: mitochondrial DNA (mtDNA). Because the mitochondria facilitate many important metabolic processes in cells, mtDNA plays an important role in cellular metabolism. Some metabolic disorders are caused by mutations in mtDNA. Less than 1 percent of human DNA consists of mtDNA; the majority of human DNA, nuclear DNA (nDNA), resides in the nucleus.

Although OT experiments and NT experiments do not appear to be as risky as experiments that manipulate human chromosomes, they are not risk-free because they can result in a mismatch between nDNA and mtDNA known as hetereoplasmy, which can affect the expression of both nDNA and mtDNA (Resnik and Langer; Templeton).

Artificial chromosomes pose an additional challenge to the earlier paradigm because they would not modify the chromosomes but would carry genes on a separate structure that would be segregated from the chromosomes (Stock and Campbell). One reason for developing artificial chromosomes is to avoid tampering with existing chromosomes. However, because an artificial chromosome could carry dozens of genes, it would transmit genetic changes to future generations.

As these developments unfolded, scholars discussed ethical and policy issues related to NT, OT, and artificial chromosomes (McGee; Bonnickson; Pence; Robertson, 1998; Stock and Campbell; Parens and Juengst; Davis). Some writers suggested that it would be useful to develop a typology for different interventions in the human germline to allow a distinction between various techniques, procedures, and methods (Richter and Baccheta; Resnik and Langer). For example, some techniques, such as TGR, attempt to modify the nDNA in human chromosomes. Other procedures, such as OT, attempt to change the composition of mtDNA. One could classify these procedures according to the degree of risk they entail, with OT being *low-risk* and TGR being *high-risk* (Resnik and Langer).

In light of the scientific, technical, and philosophical developments that occurred after the early discussions of germline interventions, in 2001 a working group convened by the American Association for the Advancement of Science proposed that people use the term *inheritable genetic modification* (IGM) instead of GLGT or GLGE because it provides a more accurate description of the techniques and methods that have been the subject of so much debate. According to the working group, IGM refers to "the technologies, techniques, and interventions that are capable of modifying the set of genes that a subject has available to transmit to his or her offspring" (Frankel and Chapman, p. 12). Under that definition, TGR, OT, NT, and the use of artificial chromosomes all would be classified as types of IGM. IGM could include methods that are used to treat or prevent diseases as well as methods intended to enhance human traits.

Arguments for and against IGM

There is not sufficient space in this entry for an in-depth discussion of the arguments for and against applying IGM procedures to human beings, and so the entry will provide only a quick summary of those arguments (for further discussion, see Resnik, Steinkraus, and Langer; Walters and Palmer; President's Commission; Holtug).

ARGUMENTS FOR IGM. The following arguments have been made in favor of IGM.

1. IGM can benefit patients by preventing genetic diseases as well as the disability, pain, and suffering associated with those diseases (Zimmerman; Berger and Gert; Munson and Davis). IGM also can benefit patients who will enjoy the effects of enhancements of health, longevity, intelligence, and so on (Stock and Campbell; Glover; Silver).

2. IGM can benefit parents by enabling them to have healthy children who are genetically related to the parents (Zimmerman; Robertson, 1994).

3. IGM can benefit society by reducing the social and economic burdens of genetic disease. Society also can benefit from IGM if enhancements of human traits increase human knowledge, productivity, performance, aesthetic experience, and other social goals (Harris; Silver).

4. IGM can benefit the human gene pool by enabling society to promote "good" genes and weed out "bad" genes. For a critique of this argument, see Suzuki and Knudtson (1989).

5. Parents have a right to use IGM to prevent genetic diseases and promote the overall health and well-being of their children (Robertson, 1994).

ARGUMENTS AGAINST IGM. The following arguments have been made against IGM.

1. IGM can cause biological harms to patients that result from genetic defects caused by IGM procedures, such as underproduction or overproduction of important proteins, the production of a protein at the wrong time, and the production of nonfunctional proteins. Although some procedures, such as OT, are safer than other procedures, such as TGR, IGM entails many risks that scientists do not understand fully (Resnik and Langer). IGM also could cause psychological harms to patients, who may view themselves as products of their parents' desires or as mere commodities (Kass, 1985; Andrews).

2. IGM could cause harm to a mother who carries a genetically modified child. For example, IGM might carry an increased risk of preeclampsia or complications during labor and delivery.

3. IGM could harm future generations. Because some genetic defects may not manifest themselves until the second or third generation, it may be difficult to estimate the potential harm to future generations (Suzuki and Knudson).

4. IGM could harm the gene pool by reducing genetic diversity, which is important for the survival of the human species (Suzuki and Knudston). For a critique, see Resnik (2000b).

5. IGM could cause harms to society, such as the increased social and economic burden of caring for patients with genetic defects caused by IGM, increased discrimination and bias against racial and ethnic groups and people with disabilities, the breakdown of the traditional family and traditional methods of reproduction, the loss of respect for the value of human life as a result of treating children as commodities, and the loss of human diversity (Kass, 1985; Kitcher; Kimbrell; Parens and Asch; Andrews, 2000).

6. IGM could waste health-care resources that could be better spent elsewhere (Juengst, 1991).

7. IGM could violate the rights of children, including the right not to be harmed, the right to an open future, and the right not be the subject of an experiment (Kimbrell; Andrews, 2000; Davis; McGee; Kass, 1985; Resnik, Steinkraus, and Langer).

8. IGM subverts natural reproduction and the natural human form (Rifkin; Kass, 1985). See Resnik, Steinkraus, and Langer (1999) for a discussion of this argument.

9. IGM is a form of "playing God" because people do not have the wisdom or the authority to design themselves (Rifkin; Kimbrell; Ramsey). See Peters (1997) for a critique of this view.

10. IGM is the vain pursuit of human perfection (Kass, 1985). See McGee (1997) for a critique of this view.

11. IGM is nothing more than a modern version of the eugenics movement (Kevles). It will repeat all the errors of the Social Darwinists and the Nazis (Kass, 1985). See Buchanan et al. (2000) and Kitcher (1997) for a discussion of this view.

12. IGM will cause social injustice by increasing the gap between the genetic "haves" and the genetic "have-nots." See Buchanan et al. (2000) and Mehlman and Botkin (1998) for further discussion of this argument.

Policy History

Many governments, regulatory agencies, and international bodies have taken a dim view of IGM. In the United States the National Institutes of Health (NIH) formed the

Recombinant DNA Advisory Committee (RAC) in 1975 to regulate and oversee recombinant DNA experiments supported by NIH funds. The RAC has the authority to regulate NIH-sponsored human gene therapy experiments, including IGM experiments. The RAC will not consider proposals for germline alterations because those procedures do not involve attempts to treat individual patients but instead involve attempts to change the genes passed on to future generations (Recombinant DNA Advisory Committee 1995).

The U.S. Food and Drug Administration (FDA) has the authority to regulate human experiments supported by private funds in the United States. The FDA sets ethical standards for human experimentation related to the development of new drugs, biologics, and medical devices. If a company wants to obtain approval of and market an item governed by the FDA, that company must submit data to the FDA that conform to its ethical guidelines. The FDA has stated that it has the authority to regulate human gene therapy as well as human cloning (U.S. Food and Drug Administration 2002a, 2002b). Although the FDA has not published a statement about its authority to regulate IGM, it would appear to have the authority to regulate any IGM procedures that involve new biologics, which could include human embryos. However, an important loophole in the FDA's regulatory authority is the fact that the agency does not have the authority to regulate assisted reproduction per se; it can only regulate drugs, biologics, and medical devices used in assisted reproduction. There are no federal laws and few state laws pertaining to assisted reproduction (Annas). It is possible that fertility clinics could perform IGM procedures such as OT or even cloning without any government regulation or oversight unless new legislation is enacted (Frankel and Chapman).

Outside the United States the Council for the Organization of Medical Sciences (CIOMS), the World Health Organization (WHO), and the United Nations Educational, Scientific, and Cultural Organization (UNESCO) have stated that the safety and efficacy of germline therapy must be evaluated thoroughly before any procedure takes place (CIOMS, WHO, and UNESCO). The International Bioethics Committee (IBC), sponsored by UNESCO, issued a report on human gene therapy that opposed germline manipulation at present as well as all forms of genetic enhancement (International Bioethics Committee). A group of advisers to the European Commission issued a report in 1993 that concluded that germline gene therapy is not ethically acceptable at the present time (Group of Advisors). Several countries, including Denmark and Germany, have banned germline gene therapy (National Bioethics Advisory Committee).

In the United Kingdom the Human Fertilization and Embryology Authority (HFEA) regulates and oversees IVF and infertility clinics. In 1998 the Human Genetics Advisory Commission (HGAC) and HFEA released a consultation paper opposing germline manipulation as well as cloning for reproductive purposes (Human Genetics Advisory Commission/Human Fertilization and Embryology Authority).

Professional societies also have not embraced IGM. The Council for Responsible Genetics (CRG), a genetics watchdog group, has opposed human germline engineering since the 1990s (Council for Responsible Genetics). The American Medical Association (AMA) does not oppose germline gene therapy, but it holds that genetic interventions should be limited to SGT for the present time. The AMA endorses genetic therapy but opposes genetic enhancement (American Medical Association). The American Society for Reproduction Medicine (ASRM) has not taken an official position on IGM but has called for a moratorium on NT until ethical and safety issues can be resolved (American Society for Reproduction Medicine).

Conclusion

It is likely that societies will debate the ethical and legal aspects of IGM for many years. The field of biotechnology is advancing so rapidly that interventions that were merely conceivable at the end of the twentieth century are fast becoming a practical reality. It is to be hoped that people will develop effective and well-balanced laws and policies pertaining to IGM before the first genetically engineered baby is born.

DAVID B. RESNIK

SEE ALSO: *Aging and the Aged: Anti-Aging Interventions; Enhancement Uses of Medical Technology; Genetics and Human Behavior; Health and Disease: History of the Concepts; Human Nature; Medicine, Philosophy of; Neuroethics; Transhumanism and Posthumanism*

BIBLIOGRAPHY

American Medical Association, Council on Ethical and Judicial Affairs. 1998. *Code of Medical Ethics, Current Opinions with Annotations.* Chicago: American Medical Association.

American Society for Reproduction Medicine. 2000. "Human Somatic Nuclear Transfer." *Fertility and Sterility* 74: 873–876.

Anderson, French. 1985. "Human Gene Therapy: Scientific and Ethical Considerations." *Journal of Medicine and Philosophy* 10: 275–291.

Anderson, French. 1989. "Why Draw a Line?" *Journal of Medicine and Philosophy* 14: 681–693.

Andrews, Lori. 2000. *The Clone Age: Adventures in the New World of Reproductive Technology.* New York: Henry Holt.

Annas, George. 1998. "The Shadowlands—Secrets, Lies, and Assisted Reproduction." *New England Journal of Medicine* 339: 935–937.

Barritt, John; Willadsen, Stephen; Brenner, Carl; and Cohen, Jonathan. 2001. "Cytoplasmic Transfers in Assisted Reproduction." *Human Reproduction Update* 7: 428–435.

Berger, Edward, and Gert, Bernie. 1991. "Genetic Disorders and the Ethical Status of Germline Therapy." *Journal of Medicine and Philosophy* 16: 667–683.

Bonnickson, Andrea. 1998. "Transplanting Nuclei between Human Eggs: Implications for Germ-Line Genetics." *Politics and the Life Sciences* 17: 3–10.

Boone, Charles. 1988. "Bad Axioms in Genetic Engineering." *Hastings Center Report* 18(4): 9–13.

Boorse, Christopher. 1977. "Health as a Theoretical Concept." *Philosophy of Science* 44: 542–577.

Buchanan, Alan; Brock, Dan; Daniels, Norman; and Wikler, Dan. 2000. *From Chance to Choice: Genetic and Justice.* Cambridge, MA: Cambridge University Press.

Caplan, Arthur. 1997. "The Concepts of Health, Disease, and Illness." In *Medical Ethics,* 2nd edition, ed. Robert Veatch. Sudbury, MA: Jones and Bartlett.

Council for Responsible Genetics. 1993. "Position Paper on Human Germ Line Manipulation." *Human Gene Therapy* 4: 35–37.

Council for the Organization of Medical Sciences, World Health Organization, and United Nations Educational, Scientific, and Cultural Organization. 1990. "Declaration of Inuyama and Reports of the Working Groups." *Human Gene Therapy* 2: 123–129.

Davis, Dena. 2001. *Genetic Dilemmas.* New York: Routledge.

Fletcher, Joseph. 1965. *Morals and Medicine.* New York: Beacon Press.

Frankel, Mark, and Chapman, Audrey, eds. 2000. *Human Inheritable Genetic Modifications: Assessing Scientific, Religious, and Policy Issues.* Washington, D.C.: American Association for the Advancement of Science.

Gaylin, Willard. 1977. "The Frankenstein Factor." *New England Journal of Medicine* 297: 665–666.

Glover, Jonathan. 1984. *What Sort of People Should There Be?* New York: Penguin Books.

Group of Advisors on the Ethical Implications of Biotechnology of the European Commission. 1993. *The Ethical Implications of Gene Therapy.* Brussels: European Commission.

Harris, John. 1992. *Wonderwoman and Superman: The Ethics of Human Biotechnology.* New York: Oxford University Press.

Holtug, Nils. 1997. "Altering Humans—The Case for and against Human Gene Therapy." *Cambridge Quarterly of Healthcare Ethics* 6: 157–174.

Juengst, Eric. 1991. "Germ-Line Gene Therapy: Back to Basics." *Journal of Medicine and Philosophy* 16: 587–592.

Juengst, Eric. 1997. "Can Enhancement be Distinguished from Therapy in Genetic Medicine?" *Journal of Medicine and Philosophy* 22: 125–142.

Kass, Leon. 1972. "Making Babies—The New Biology and the 'Old' Morality." *The Public Interest* 26: 18–56.

Kass, Leon. 1985. *Toward a More Natural Science.* New York: Free Press.

Kevles, Daniel. 1985. *In the Name of Eugenics.* Cambridge, MA: Harvard University Press.

Kimbrell, Andrew. 1997. *The Human Body Shop.* Washington, D.C.: Regnery.

Kitcher, Philip. 1997. *The Lives to Come.* New York: Simon & Schuster.

Kristol, William, and Cohen, Eric. 2001. *The Future Is Now: America Confronts the New Genetics.* New York: Routledge.

Lederberg, Joshua. 1966. "Experimental Genetics and Human Evolution." *The American Naturalist* 100(915): 519–531.

McGee, Glenn. 1997. *The Perfect Baby.* Lanham, MD: Rowman and Littlefield.

Mehlman, Maxwell, and Botkin, Jeffrey. 1998. *Access to the Genome.* Washington, D.C.: Georgetown University Press.

Munson, Ron, and Davis, Larry. 1992. "Germline Gene Therapy and the Medical Imperative." *Kennedy Institute of Ethics Journal* 2: 137–158.

National Bioethics Advisory Commission. 1997. *Report on Cloning Human Beings.* Washington, D.C.: Author.

Parens, Erik, and Asch, Adrienne, eds. 2000. *Prenatal Testing and Disability Rights.* Washington, D.C.: Georgetown University Press.

Parens, Erik, and Juengst, Eric. 2001. "Inadvertently Crossing the Germline." *Science* 292: 397.

Parens, Erik, ed. 1999. *Enhancing Human Traits.* Washington, D.C.: Georgetown University Press.

Pence, Greg. 1998. *Who's Afraid of Human Cloning?* New York: Routledge.

Peters, Ted. 1997. *Playing God?: Genetic Determinism and Human Freedom.* New York: Routledge.

President's Commission for the Study of Ethical Problems in Medicine and Biomedical and Behavioral Research. 1982. *Splicing Life: The Social and Ethical Issues of Genetic Engineering with Human Beings.* Washington, D.C.: President's Commission.

Ramsey, Paul. 1970. *Fabricated Man: The Ethics of Genetic Control.* New Haven, CT: Yale University Press.

Recombinant DNA Advisory Committee. 1995. "Recombinant DNA Research: Actions under the Guidelines." *Federal Register* 60 (810: 20731–20737, April 27).

Resnik, David. 2000a. "The Moral Significance of the Therapy/Enhancement Distinction in Human Genetics." *Cambridge Quarterly of Healthcare Ethics* 9: 365–377.

Resnik, David. 2000b. "Of Maize and Men: Reproductive Control and the Threat to Genetic Diversity." *Journal of Medicine and Philosophy* 25: 451–467.

Resnik, David, and Langer, Pamela. 2001. "Human Germline Therapy Reconsidered." *Human Gene Therapy* 12: 1449–1458.

Resnik, David; Steinkraus, Holly; and Langer, Pamela. 1999. *Human Germline Gene Therapy: Scientific, Moral and Political Issues.* Austin, TX: R.G. Landes.

Richter, Gerd, and Baccheta, Matthew. 1998. "Interventions in the Human Genome: Some Moral and Ethical Considerations." *Journal of Medicine and Philosophy* 23: 303–317.

Rifkin, Jeremy. 1983. *Algeny.* New York: Viking Press.

Robertson, John. 1994. *Children of Choice.* Princeton, NJ: Princeton University Press.

Robertson, John. 1998. "Oocyte Cytoplasm Transfers and the Ethics of Germ-Line Intervention." *Journal of Law, Medicine, and Ethics* 26(3): 211–220.

Silver, Lee. 1998. *Remaking Eden: How Genetic Engineering and Cloning Will Transform the American Family.* New York: Avon.

Stock, Gregory, and Campbell, John. 2000. *Engineering the Human Germline.* New York: Oxford University Press.

Suzuki, David, and Knudtson, Peter. 1989. *Genethics.* Cambridge, MA: Harvard University Press.

Templeton, Allan. 2002. "Ooplasmic Transfer—Proceed with Care." *New England Journal of Medicine* 346: 773–775.

Walters, Le Roy. 1986. "The Ethics of Human Gene Therapy." *Nature* 320: 225–227.

Walters, Le Roy, and Palmer, Julie. 1997. *The Ethics of Human Gene Therapy.* New York: Oxford University Press.

Watson, James. 1971. "Moving Toward Clonal Man." *Atlantic Monthly* 227(5): 50–53.

Zanjani, Esmail, and Anderson, French. 1999. "Prospects for in Utero Human Gene Therapy." *Science* 285: 2084–2088.

Zimmerman, Burke. 1991. "Human Germline Therapy: The Case for Its Development and Use." *Journal of Medicine and Philosophy* 16: 593–612.

INTERNET RESOURCES

Human Genetic Advisory Commission/Human Fertilization and Embryology Authority. 1998. "Cloning Issues in Reproduction, Science and Medicine." Available from <http://www.dgwsoft.co.uk/homepages/cloning/>.

International Bioethics Committee. 1994. "Report on Human Gene Therapy." Available from <http://www.unesco.org/ibc/en/>.

U.S. Food and Drug Administration. 2002a. *Human Gene Therapy and the Role of the Food and Drug Administration.* Available from <http://www.fda.gov/cber/>.

U.S. Food and Drug Adminstration. 2002b. *Use of Cloning Technology to Clone a Human Being.* Available from <http://www.fda.gov/cber/genetherapy/clone.htm>.

World Health Organization. "Definition of Health." Available from <http://www.who.int/aboutwho/en/>.

GENETICS AND ENVIRONMENT IN HUMAN HEALTH

• • •

All living things interact with multiple environments, both physical and biological. With regard to the flourishing of plants and animals, environmental features such as temperature, humidity, sunlight, and altitude often set boundaries crucial to development. Biological interactions between living things frequently are another major factor in growth and survival, for example, where parasites and predators cause illness or injure plants and animals. So it is with human health and flourishing as well, where environmental hazards and infectious diseases account for the vast majority of illnesses resulting in death.

The publication of Rachel Carson's *Silent Spring* (1962) and the subsequent emergence of a worldwide environmental movement has raised social awareness of the dangers to human health posed by industrial chemicals. Of the several million chemicals listed by the American Chemical Society, about 75,000 are used as pesticides, cosmetics, pharmaceuticals, food additives, or industrial agents. Most new chemicals must be tested for potential toxicity to humans and other living things before they can be approved for sale. In the United States, the Food and Drug Administration (FDA) requires extensive animal and clinical testing of new drugs, vaccines, and approved drugs proposed for new uses, as well as animal testing for food additives and cosmetics. Under various pesticide laws, including the Toxic Substances Control Act of 1976, the U.S. Environmental Protection Agency (EPA) also requires toxicity testing of new chemicals before they are brought to market. In addition, the Occupational Safety and Health Administration, Consumer Product Safety Commission, Department of Agriculture, Department of Transportation, and their state and local counterparts, each have additional responsibilities regarding the control of chemical agents.

These regulatory policies have done much to improve environmental quality and protect humans from industrial hazards. Nonetheless, individuals do not bear the burdens of environmental risk equally and vary remarkably in their responses to chemical exposures and pharmaceuticals. Such variation may reflect differences in sex, age, nutrition, lifestyle decisions to smoke cigarettes or drink alcoholic beverages, recreational exposures to similar chemicals, concurrent occupational exposures, and use of protective gear or medicines. In addition, variation in individual response may reflect inherited differences in a person's ability to metabolize specific chemicals, thus affecting individual risks of disease and other adverse effects.

The products of the Human Genome Project are allowing new investigations of these inherited differences that appear to make some individuals more vulnerable to specific environmental exposures or more susceptible to environmentally-induced diseases. The study of these inherited differences and their potential influence on individual response to environmental agents is the subject of the field of ecogenetics.

Ecogenetics: Individual Variation in Susceptibility to Environmental and Chemical Agents

Ecogenetics examines how genes and environmental factors interact with each other to affect human health and disease. Genes are sequences of DNA in humans' twenty-three pairs of chromosomes in each nucleated cell. Genes specify the sequence of proteins, which are the main effector molecules of cells, serving as enzymes (catalysts), structural molecules (like collagen), antibodies to fight off infections, and binders of oxygen or xenobiotics (including pharmaceuticals or chemicals in the environment). Environmental factors include social and familial environment, intrauterine environment, cigarette smoking, alcohol, other substance abuse, stress, and exposures to chemical, physical, and biological agents. Some environmental exposures such as ultraviolet light, X rays, and certain industrial chemicals cause damage to DNA (genetic mutations), which alter gene function as well as the structure and function of the protein specified by that gene. Although many such mutations appear to be of little consequence, some may lead to disease.

There are many examples of gene-environment interactions combining to affect human health. Body weight and obesity, for example, appear to be the result of food intake, energy expenditure, and various genetic determinants. For infectious diseases such as malaria and tuberculosis, genetic features appear to affect both individual susceptibility and the severity of the illness. Another example is response to pharmaceutical products, where some drugs with limited side effects (at usual doses in most individuals) may cause severe problems for persons with genes associated with decreased capacity to metabolize the drug. Without exposure to the drug, however, these genetic variants may be innocuous. For example, cytochrome P450 enzymes form a family of dozens of related enzymes with distinct and overlapping characteristics. One specific P450 enzyme,

debrisoquine 4-hydroxylase, has been associated with marked variation in the metabolism of more than thirty drugs.

Biochemical and molecular techniques are being used to develop new genetic markers of host susceptibility to environmental and chemical agents. To cause poor health, many chemicals must be activated by enzymes to intermediates that attack DNA (as appears to be the case in many environmentally-induced cancers and birth defects). Other enzyme systems detoxify potentially toxic compounds, and variation in the genes that specify the sequence of enzymes involved in these biotransformation steps can result in people with similar exposures having very different disease risks.

An example of this type of gene-environment interaction affecting health outcomes is deficiency in the enzyme glutathione S-transferase (GST), which is believed to be an important predisposing factor in the development of some environmentally-induced cancers. About 45 percent of persons of European ancestry lack detectable activity of a particular form of GST. Several studies examining GST levels in lung tissue suggest that GST-deficient smokers are at higher risk of developing lung cancer, presumably because this enzyme detoxifies carcinogenic chemicals. Thus, GST-normal smokers are partially protected against lung cancer. In addition, high GST activity is an important protective factor against liver cancer resulting from exposure to aflatoxin (a toxin from fungi that grow on peanuts and corn).

An additional example of this type of ecogenetic phenomenon is provided by variation in the liver enzyme N-acetyl transferase (NAT), which has been associated with marked differences in blood levels of several drugs, including the anti-tuberculosis drug isoniazid (at standard doses). Roughly 50 percent of individuals of European or African ancestry have the slow acetylator phenotype (the form of the gene and enzyme with lower metabolic activity) associated with higher levels of still-active drug and a propensity to adverse effects. The same detoxification mechanism metabolizes several other chemicals, including the human bladder carcinogens beta-naphthylamine, benzidine, and 4-amino-biphenyl—all former mainstays of the dyestuff industry worldwide. People who are slow acetylators are at higher risk for bladder cancer, as expected from the hypothesis that they would be less able to detoxify these potent carcinogens by acetylation to inactive products. DNA probes are available to assay this kind of genetic variation in peripheral blood cells, rather than having to administer a test drug and measure metabolites in urine.

Gene-environment interactions also can be seen in many other kinds of diseases, not just cancers. For example, the common organophosphorus pesticide, parathion, is converted to its toxic intermediate, paraoxon, by the P450 system and then inactivated by a circulating plasma enzyme, paraoxonase. About half of individuals of European descent have low paraoxonase activity. For similar exposures, people with lower activity of this enzyme are likely to be at higher risk for neurologic toxicity and take longer to recover. High blood cholesterol levels are related both to diet and to inherited variation in several genes affecting the proteins that carry fat (lipoproteins) and their cell receptors. Cholesterol- and fat-reducing diets and drugs can reduce coronary heart disease deaths and heart attacks; however, responses to diet and drugs appear to differ among people with different genetic causes of high levels of fat components in the blood. Chronic anemias due to iron deficiency are a major health problem throughout the world. Although iron can be supplied inexpensively by fortification of flour, a small percentage of individuals carry genes (for types of anemia called thalassemias or for an iron metabolism disorder known as hemochromatosis) that cause these individuals to absorb iron excessively. These people might be injured by additional dietary intake of iron.

Integrating Genetic and Environmental Information in Clinical Research

The risks posed by exposure to chemical and environmental agents are related to the level of exposure, the intrinsic potency of the agent, and the susceptibility of the person exposed. In general, the highest exposures are in patients receiving potent drugs or radiation as medical treatments and in workers manufacturing or cleaning up chemicals in various operations. Therefore, it is logical and efficient to investigate potential risks to human health in patients and in workers with known exposures to specific agents. Studies of risks to the general population from contamination of groundwater or from air pollution, consumer products, or hazardous waste sites are far more difficult to conduct because the levels of exposure are typically much lower and thus the likelihood of identifying adverse effects is significantly reduced. In addition, although chemical exposures may cause immediate toxicity to the skin, eyes, lungs, heart, liver, nervous system, reproductive organs, or other target sites in the body, some effects may be unrecognized at first, including mutations in specific genes that may eventually lead to cancer or birth defects. Repeated exposures at relatively low doses also may have cumulative toxic effects that are difficult to identify. The challenge of establishing that impairment of brain function can result from lead exposure, for example, illustrates the difficulty of assessing the role of chronic, low-level environmental exposures in disease.

These considerations highlight the importance of ecogenetic research combining careful exposure-assessment studies with investigations of genetic influences on disease. Such a multidisciplinary approach is being explored in a coordinated manner through the Environmental Genome Project (EGP), a research initiative supported by the National Institute of Environmental Health Sciences, a component of the National Institutes of Health. The goals of the EGP are to: (1) identify some of the more common genetic differences between individuals that appear to affect response to environmental hazards; (2) conduct epidemiological studies investigating the role of gene-environment interactions in the development of common diseases like asthma, cancer, and heart disease; and (3) promote the use of information regarding gene-environment interactions in public health initiatives.

The EGP will develop in several stages. In the first phase of the project, experts will identify a set of approximately 500 genes that appear to play a role in the development of environmentally-induced diseases. These will include xenobiotic metabolism and detoxification genes, DNA repair genes, signal transduction genes, and genes involved in oxidative processes. Having identified a set of genes that appear to be involved in environmental response, the second phase of the project will catalogue common genetic differences in these genes—differences that may affect the functioning of the associated enzymes. Finally, in the third phase of the EGP, researchers will study the biological implications of these genetic differences using functional assays and population-based studies of gene-environment interactions. Organizers of the project expect that the first two phases of the EGP will be completed in late 2004. The third phase of the project will require significantly more time to complete, however, and will involve numerous epidemiological studies conducted over the next ten to twenty years.

Since many of the genes believed to play an important role in how humans respond to environmental hazards appear to affect health only in the presence of specific environmental exposures, deciphering the relationships that exist between genetic variants and individual response has the potential to improve public health significantly. Identifying those persons most at risk, for example, and encouraging them to avoid those environmental hazards to which they are most susceptible, may help prevent or delay disease onset in large segments of the population without pharmacological interventions. In addition, projects like the EGP might eventually lead to:

1. more accurate estimates of disease risks;
2. targeted disease-prevention strategies or medical-monitoring programs to detect disease earlier;

3. pharmaceutical products with fewer adverse effects; and

4. a better understanding of biological mechanisms of disease.

A great deal of work will need to be done to elucidate specific genetic risk profiles for environmentally-induced diseases as we move into the era of genetic medicine. In the meantime, both the population-wide approach that emphasizes environmental measures and the genetic approach that aims to identify individuals at increased risk are likely to be advocated. It is certainly prudent, for example, that everyone follow a diet that avoids excess fat, cholesterol, and salt. At the same time, genetic tests may soon be able to identify those persons at highest risk of developing coronary heart disease and high blood pressure. Taken together, these two strategies may provide a powerful approach to encouraging individuals to change their diets and lifestyles in ways that promote good health.

Ethical Issues in Ecogenetics

Although ecogenetics is still in its infancy as a scientific field, a number of important ethical considerations can be anticipated and should be addressed before genetic tests are used to screen individuals or populations for inherited susceptibilities to chemical or environmental agents. For example, long before the development of molecular genetics, J.B.S. Haldane suggested in *Heredity and Politics* (1938) that it might be reasonable to exclude persons who are susceptible to potter's bronchitis (a common problem among British potters at the time) from work in that occupation. Since workplace exclusion, stigmatization, and discrimination can result from knowledge of genetic risk factors for disease, studies of gene-environment interactions raise a number of ethical and social issues of great importance.

How one defines the extent of an individual's risk, for example, is an issue deserving of attention. Susceptibility to one kind of chemical may not predict susceptibility to chemicals with unrelated metabolism or structure. Thus, no one should be branded as "hypersusceptible" to chemical exposures on the basis of being identified as vulnerable to a specific environmental hazard or chemical. Since much confusion often surrounds the interpretation of genetic information, with laypersons frequently overstating the predictive value of a test, educational programs that aim to improve public understanding of ecogenetic tests will be critical to the long-term success of this new field.

Another issue that will be important to clarify for the general public is that, even after a genetic risk factor has been identified and is well characterized, the cause of disease in a specific individual often will be unclear. The well-recognized interaction of cigarette smoking with workplace asbestos exposure in causing lung cancer reveals some of the scientific uncertainties and ethical problems associated with assignments of disease causation in individual cases. The mere fact that a person has a gene that predisposes him or her to a specific disease—and then goes on to develop that disease—does not establish that the genetic susceptibility was the cause of the disease. Other genetic or environmental factors, for example, may have contributed substantially to the outcome.

Another ethical consideration is that since genetic differences sometimes occur with markedly different frequencies across racial or ethnic groups, targeted genetic testing programs could place disproportional burdens on members of some racial or ethnic groups. Related to this is the problem of group stigmatization, where social disadvantage results from the general association of a susceptibility gene with a particular racial or ethnic group.

Although tests for genetic predispositions to chemical and environmental agents could lead to targeted preventive approaches and improved assessments of individual risk, it is important that the future availability of such techniques does not diminish the commitment to eliminate hazardous environmental exposures. For example, the ability to identify genetic sensitivities to toxins in the workplace may inadvertently shift the focus of risk-management efforts away from the improvement of unhealthy environmental conditions if employers find it less costly to dismiss genetically sensitive workers than to eliminate workplace hazards.

In addition, the potential *geneticization* of environmental disease may inappropriately place unreasonable expectations on those persons with known genetic sensitivities. Individuals known to be particularly susceptible to the harmful effects of a particular chemical agent, for example, may face social pressures to remove themselves from those environments in which that chemical is found (e.g., to move to a different neighborhood or change jobs). Ironically, if we are successful in reducing environmental exposures to levels sufficient to protect most of the population, genetic differences between individuals will account for a larger proportion of the remaining risk among those exposed. This possibility could foster more deterministic attitudes regarding the significance of genetic information, for example, resulting in research funding being diverted from traditional preventive strategies for improving public health to approaches stressing genetic causes of disease.

Lastly, while genetic markers of susceptibility are being developed for use in healthcare settings, it is important to be mindful of the possibility that information about gene-environment interactions may be used in other contexts before those associations are well validated. In this regard, a recent Equal Employment Opportunity Commission (EEOC) claim brought forth against the Burlington Northern Santa Fe Railroad Company illustrates the potential for not-yet-validated associations to be used inappropriately. The EEOC dispute in question involved the railroad company testing workers for an alleged genetic predisposition to carpel tunnel syndrome. Although the extent to which the gene in question may be a predisposing factor in the development of carpel tunnel syndrome is largely unknown, that did not prevent the company from attempting to use this information in their efforts to avoid responsibility for workers' compensation claims. Whether other employers will adopt similar practices based on new ecogenetic information is a matter to watch carefully in the coming years.

GILBERT S. OMENN
ARNO G. MOTULSKY (1995)
REVISED BY RICHARD R. SHARP

SEE ALSO: *Genetic Counseling, Ethical Issues in; Genetic Counseling, Practice of; Genetic Discrimination; Genetics and Human Self-Understanding; Genetic Testing and Screening; Health and Disease; Health Insurance*

BIBLIOGRAPHY

Andrews, Lori B.; Fullarton, J. E.; Holtzman, N. A.; and Motulsky, A. G. 1994. *Assessing Genetic Risks: Implications for Health and Social Policy.* Washington, D.C.: National Academy Press.

Carson, Rachel. 1962. *Silent Spring.* Boston: Houghton Mifflin.

Draper, Elaine. 1991. *Risky Business: Genetic Testing and Exclusionary Practices in the Hazardous Workplace.* New York: Cambridge University Press.

Eaton D. L., and Bammler, T. K. 1999. "Concise Review of the Glutathione S-Transferases and Their Significance to Toxicology." *Toxicological Science* 49: 156–164.

Grandjean, Philippe. 1991. *Ecogenetics: Genetic Predisposition to the Toxic Effects of Chemicals.* New York: Routledge, Chapman, and Hall/World Health Organization.

Guttmacher, A. E., and Collins, F. S. 2002. "Genomic Medicine—A Primer." *New England Journal of Medicine* 347: 1512–1520.

Haldane, John Burdon Sanderson. 1938. *Heredity and Politics.* New York: Norton.

Holtzman, Neil A. 1989. *Proceed with Caution: Predicting Genetic Risks in the Recombinant DNA Era.* Baltimore: John Hopkins University Press.

International Agency for Research on Cancer, IARC Working Group on the Evaluation of Carcinogenic Risks to Humans.

1987. *Overall Evaluation of Carcinogenicity: An Updating of IARC Monographs on the Evaluation of Carcinogenic Risks to Humans,* vols. 1–42, suppl. 7. Lyons, France: Author.

Khoury, M. J.; Adam, M. J.; and Flanders, W. D. 1988. "An Epidemiologic Approach to Ecogenetics." *American Journal of Human Genetics* 42: 89–95.

Motulsky, Arno G. 1978. "Bioethical Problems in Pharmacogenetics and Ecogenetics." *Human Genetics* Supplement 1: 185–192.

Nebert, D. W., and Russell, D. W. 2002. "Clinical Importance of the Cytochromes P450." *Lancet* 360: 1155–1162.

Olden, Kenneth, and Wilson, Samuel. 2000. "Environmental Health and Genomics: Visions and Implications." *Nature Reviews Genetics* 1: 149–153.

Omenn, Gilbert S. 2000. "Public Health Genetics: An Emerging Interdisciplinary Field for the Post-Genomic Era." *Annual Review of Public Health* 21: 1–13.

Omenn, Gilbert S., and Motulsky, Arno G. 1978. "'Eco-genetics': Genetic Variation in Susceptibility to Environmental Agents." In *Genetic Issues in Public Health and Medicine,* ed. Bernice H. Cohen, Abraham M. Lilienfeld, and Pien-Chien Huang. Springfield, IL: Charles C. Thomas.

Sharp, Richard R. 2001. "The Evolution of Predictive Genetic Testing: Deciphering Gene-Environment Interactions." *Jurimetrics* 41: 145–163.

Sharp, Richard R., and Barrett, J. Carl. 1999. "The Environmental Genome Project and Bioethics." *Kennedy Institute of Ethics Journal* 9: 175–188.

U.S. Congress, Office of Technology Assessment. 1983. *The Role of Genetic Testing in the Prevention of Occupational Disease.* Washington, D.C.: U.S. Government Printing Office.

U.S. Congress, Office of Technology Assessment. 1991. *Medical Monitoring and Screening in the Workplace.* Washington, D.C.: U.S. Government Printing Office.

Weber, Wendell W. 1997. *Pharmacogenetics.* New York: Oxford University Press.

GENETICS AND HUMAN BEHAVIOR

• • •

I. SCIENTIFIC AND RESEARCH ISSUES

Interest in the possible effects of genetic inheritance on human behavior is a perennial one, with its modern roots dating back the writings of Sir Francis Galton in the late nineteenth century. The issue is often framed as a debate over "nature versus nurture." After the "rediscovery" of the work of Gregor Mendel (1822–1884) in the twentieth century, the issue came to be couched in terms of genes versus environments and their respective influences on the organism, while more recently the talk has been of DNA and its role in relation to other causal factors. Themes revolving around genetics and environment are especially contentious when behavioral and mental traits (and disorders) are brought into the picture. This has been the case for views about the self and responsibility, as well as in society in general, where the specter of eugenics is quickly raised. According to the Nobel Laureate Thorsten Wiesel, "Perhaps most disturbing to our sense of being free individuals, capable to a large degree of shaping our character and our minds, is the idea that our behavior, mental abilities, and mental health can be determined or destroyed by a segment of DNA." The inflammatory appearance in 1994 of *The Bell Curve* by social scientists Richard Herrnstein and Charles Murray, which argued IQ is substantially inherited and may differ among races for genetic reasons, represents a major example of this social contentiousness. Another highly fractious example revolved around the University of Maryland's project on genetics and criminal behavior, and especially the September 1995 conference. The conference was strongly criticized by groups opposed to any inquiries into genetics and crime, and some of these groups' representatives invaded the conference and had to be escorted away by the authorities (Wasserman and Wachbroit).

The academic discipline that studies the effect of genetics on human behavior is termed *behavior genetics* or *behavioral genetics*. In addition to studying humans, this discipline has a long history of examining the behaviors of simpler organisms, including the round worm (*C. elegans*), the fruit fly, (*Drosophila*), and the common mouse (*Mus*), as well as dogs, primates, and many other organisms. The organized discipline began to coalesce from a wide variety of disciplines in the 1960s with the appearance of the first textbook in the subject, *Human Genetics* by John Fuller and Robert Thompson. The disciplines contributing to behavioral (and psychiatric) genetics included biology (including genetics), psychology, statistics, zoology, medicine, and psychiatry. Especially significant was the psychology of *individual differences,* which perhaps provided the main themes of the new subject (see psychiatric geneticist Irving Gottesman's 2003 article for a brief but excellent historical introduction and references).

In the realm of behavioral disorders and genetics, the years since 1970 have seen a shift from the view of psychiatric disorders being primarily environmental (due to poor parenting, for example) to the contemporary view that amalgamates both genetic and what are called *nonshared* environmental influences as major causal determinants of mental disorders. This has not been a shift without controversy, and it reflects broader shifts in psychosocial studies of the contributions of nature and nurture (Reiss and Neiderhiser). Further, though psychology has paid increasing attention to behavioral genetics, cultural anthropology and sociology have been strongly resistant to any genetic approaches (Rowe and Jacobson).

Major Methods of Studying Genetic Influences

Traditional genetics, of the type investigated by Mendel and his followers, was able to identify genes that had large effects and often displayed typical patterns, such as those involving dominant, recessive, or sex-linked traits. Genes that affect human behaviors and exhibit such patterns are well-known, including Huntington's disease (caused by an autosomal dominant mutation) and phenylketonuria, or PKU (a recessive mutation). Symptoms of Huntington's disease's include degeneration of the nervous system, usually beginning in middle age and resulting in death. In this devastating disease, there is usually a gradual loss of intellectual ability and emotional control. The genetic pattern is that of a condition caused by a rare, single, dominant gene. Since affected people have one copy of the dominant disease gene and one copy of a recessive gene (for a "normal" nervous system), half of their offspring develop the disease. Huntington's never skips a generation. Since the gene is dominant, the person who inherits it will manifest the disease (if he or she lives long enough). If one full sibling has the condition, there is a fifty-fifty chance that any other sibling will also get the disease.

In contrast to dominant conditions, recessive conditions show a very different pattern of occurrence. *Recessive* means that both copies of the gene must be of the same form (the same allele) in order to show the condition. Two parents, neither of whom shows a trait, can have a child affected by a recessive trait (this happens if both parents are carriers of one copy of the recessive allele—the child thus has two copies, one from each parent, and manifests the condition). Recessive traits can skip generations because parents and their offspring can carry one copy of the recessive gene and not display the associated trait. In the population there are many recessive genes that cause various abnormal conditions. Each particular recessive allele may be rare, but since there are many of them, their combined impact on a population can be substantial.

Among humans, a classic example of recessive inheritance is the condition of phenylketonuria (PKU). Individuals with PKU usually are severely mentally impaired. Most never learn to talk; many have seizures and display temper tantrums. PKU is a form of severe mental retardation that is both genetic and treatable. It is genetic in that it is caused by a recessive genetic allele. Without two copies of that particular allele, a person will not develop the set of symptoms, including mental impairment, that is characteristic of PKU. However, scientific knowledge has led to a treatment. It was discovered that the recessive PKU gene prevents the normal metabolism of a substance that is common in food, making many normal foods toxic to the individual with two PKU alleles. A special diet that is low in the offending substance can prevent or minimize the nervous system damage that leads to the profound intellectual disabilities of untreated PKU individuals.

The example of PKU demonstrates that inherited (genetic) conditions can be treated—that knowledge of specific causation can result in effective treatment. This is an extremely important point both ethically and philosophically, because it is often misunderstood and misinterpreted.

Well over one hundred different genes are known for which relatively rare recessive alleles cause conditions that include severe mental impairment among their symptoms. The rapidly developing knowledge of basic genetic chemistry, from molecular genetics to biotechnology and the Human Genome Project, which produced a mapping of some 30,000 human genes early in the twenty-first century on April 15, 2003, holds out the hope that many more of these devastating genetic conditions may soon be treatable. As part of the Human Genome Project, genes for Huntington's disease and PKU have been identified and sequenced, though as yet no new therapies have been developed for these disorders.

In spite of these clear scientific successes related to Mendelian genetic-pattern disorders, many human traits—including normal traits, as well as somatic, behavioral, and psychiatric disorders—have *not* exhibited clear Mendelian patterns of inheritance. For those traits, an extension of Mendel's work to quantitative traits that was first developed by Sir Ronald Fisher, has been used extensively. Beginning in the 1990s, an additional, more molecular, set of techniques was developed to examine possible influences of genetics on human behavior. These two broad approaches to studying the influences of nature and nurture in psychiatry are termed *quantitative* (or *epidemiological*) and *molecular*. A brief summary of the two approaches is presented here, including some examples of their results and their problems (an overview of them can be found in Neiderhiser and in Schaffner [2001], and a systematic analysis is presented in *Behavioral Genetics* by Plomin et al.).

QUANTITATIVE METHODS. Quantitative, or epidemiological, methods are utilized to distinguish genetic and environmental contributions to quantitative traits or features of an organism, as well as to assess correlations and interactions between genetic and environmental factors that account for differences between individuals. These methods do not examine individual genes, but report on proportions of differences in traits due to heredity or environment, or to their interactions, broadly conceived. The methods include family, twin, and adoption studies. Adoption studies examine genetically related individuals in different familial environments, and thus can *prima facie* disentangle contributions of nature and nurture. Twin studies compare identical and fraternal twins, both within the same familial environment and (in adoption studies) in different familial circumstances.

Twin studies have been used extensively in psychiatry to indicate whether a disorder is genetic or environmentally influenced, and to what extent. Twin studies make several assumptions to analyze gathered data, including that the familial environment is the same for twins raised together but different for twins raised apart, an assumption called the *equal environments assumption.* Though critics of genetic influence often question this assumption empirical studies have confirmed it (Kendler et al.). The example of schizophrenia may help make some twin results clearer. Employing what are termed *concordance studies* of twins, Gottesman and his associates have reported over many years that the risk of developing schizophrenia if a twin or sibling has been diagnosed with the condition is about 45 percent for monozygotic (MZ) twins, 17 percent for dizygotic (DZ) twins, and 9 percent for siblings (Gottesman and Erlenmeyer-Kimling). This concordance pattern supports what is called a non-Mendelian polygenic (many genes) quantitative trait etiology for schizophrenia with a major environmental effect (> 50%), i.e., more than half of the differences in liability to schizophrenia among individuals is due to environmental factors. Twin studies can also be used to estimate the heritability of a trait or a disorder, which for schizophrenia is about 80 percent. *Heritability* is a technical term, one that is often confusing even to experts, and one which only loosely points toward the existence of underlying genetic factors influencing a trait. Investigators note that "it does *not* describe the quantitative contribution of genes to … any … phenotype of interest; it describes the quantitative contribution of genes to *interindividual differences* in a phenotype studied in a particular population" (Benjamin et al., p. 334). If there are no interindividual differences in a trait, then the heritability of that trait is zero—leading to the paradoxical result that the heritability of a human having a brain is virtually zero. Heritability is also conditional on the environment in which the population is studied, and the heritability value can significantly change if the environment changes.

Keeping these caveats in mind, heritability estimates for many major psychiatric disorders appear to be in the 70 to 80 percent range, and personality studies indicate heritabilities of about 30 to 60 percent for traits such as emotional stability and extraversion, suggesting that these differences among humans are importantly genetically influenced. But even with a heritability of schizophrenia of about 80 percent, it is also wise to keep in mind that approximately 63 percent of all persons suffering from schizophrenia will have *neither first- nor second-degree* relatives diagnosed with schizophrenia, reinforcing the complex genetic-environmental patterns found in this disorder.

Twin studies were also the basis of a distinction between *shared* and *nonshared* environments. The meaning of environment in quantitative genetics is extremely broad, denoting everything that is not genetic (thus environment would include *in utero* effects). The shared environment comprises all the nongenetic factors that cause family members to be similar, and the nonshared environment is what makes family members different. Remarkably, quantitative genetics studies of normal personality factors, as well as of mental disorders, indicate that of all environmental factors, it is the *nonshared* ones that have the major effect. A meta-analysis of forty-three studies undertaken by psychologists Eric Turkheimer and Mary Waldron in 2000 indicated that though the nonshared environment is responsible for 50 percent of the total variation of behavioral outcomes, *identified and measured nonshared environmental factors* accounted for only 2 percent of the total variance. Turkheimer infers that these nonshared differences are nonsystematic and largely accidental, and thus have been, and will continue to be, very difficult to study (Turkheimer, 2000). This possibility had been considered in 1987 by Robert Plomin and Denise Daniels but dismissed as a "gloomy prospect"— though it looks more plausible.

Epidemiological investigations have also identified two important features of how genetic and environmental contributions work together. The first, genotype-environment *correlation* (GℰE), represents possible effects of an individual's genetics on the environment (e.g., via that individual's evoking different responses or selecting environments). Such effects were found for both normal and pathological traits in the large Nonshared Environmental Adolescent Development (NEAD) study, described in detail in the 2000 book *The Relationship Code,* written by David Reiss

and colleagues. Secondly, different genotypes have different sensitivities to environments, collectively called genotype×environmental *interaction* (G×E). Differential sensitivity is important in many genetic disorders, including the neurodevelopmental models of schizophrenia genetics and in a recent study on the cycle of violence in maltreated children (discussed later).

MOLECULAR METHODS. Classical quantitative or epidemiological studies can indicate the genetic contributions to psychiatric disorders at the population level, but they do not identify any specific genes or how genes might contribute (patho)physiologically to behavioral outcomes. According to psychiatric geneticist Peter McGuffin and his colleagues, "quantitative approaches can no longer be seen as ends in themselves," and the field must move to the study of specific genes, assisted by the completed draft versions of the human genome sequence (McGuffin et al., p. 1232). In point of fact, a review of the recent literature indicates that most research in behavioral genetics, and especially in psychiatric genetics, has taken a "molecular turn."

It is widely acknowledged that most genes playing etiological and/or pathophysiological roles in human behaviors, as well as in psychiatric disorders, will *not* be single locus genes of large effect following Mendelian patterns of the Huntington's and PKU type discussed earlier. The neurogeneticist Steven Hyman notes that mental disorders will typically be heterogeneous and have multiple contributing genes, and likely have different sets of overlapping genes affecting them. Mental disorders will thus be what are called *complex traits,* technically defined as conforming to *non-*Mendelian inheritance patterns.

There are two general methods that are widely used by molecular behavioral and molecular psychiatric geneticists in their search for genes related to mental disorders: (1) linkage analysis, and (2) alleleic association. Linkage analysis is the traditional approach to gene identification, but it only works well when genes have reasonably large effects, which does not appear to be the case in normal human behavior or in psychiatry. Allelic association studies are more sensitive, but they require "candidate genes" to examine familial data. An influential 1996 paper by statisticians Neil Risch and Kethleen Merikangas urged this strategy.

Studies in schizophrenia are again illustrative of these approaches, as are the Alzheimer's disease genetic studies reviewed later. Though there was an erroneous 1988 report of an autosomal dominant gene for schizophrenia on chromosome 5 that is seen as a false positive, evidence has been accumulating for genes or gene regions of small effect related to schizophrenia on many chromosomes, including 1q, 2, 3p, 5q, 6p, 8p, 11q, 13q, 20p, and 22q (Harrison and

Owen). Replication difficulties with these results in different populations of schizophrenics and their families have been a recurring problem, however.

Environmental Research and the Envirome

It is clear from epidemiological studies that more than half the variance of typical behavioral traits, as well as half of the liability for psychiatric disorders (including schizophrenia), is environmental. This has fueled major searches for various environmental causes. In schizophrenia, this work has been reviewed by Ming Tsuang and his colleagues, who note that the major environmental risk factors in schizophrenia are due to the nonshared environment. These include problems in pregnancy (e.g., pre-eclampsia) and obstetric complications, urban birth, winter birth, and maternal communicational deviance. Thus far, *identified* predisposing environmental factors have small values in comparison with genetic risk factors. Using a term coined in 1995 by James C. Anthony, Tsuang et al. have proposed that the entire *envirome* needs to be searched for extragenetic causes of disorders, including schizophrenia. These factors are believed to affect susceptible genotypes, involving G×E interactions.

Though evidence for susceptibility genes for major mental disorders continues to accumulate, there has been no strongly replicated result that might be used in diagnosis or in early detection and prevention interventions. Of all the *psychiatric* disorders that have been investigated to date by genetic strategies, only Alzheimer's disease (AD) provides both a classical Mendelian etiological picture and complex trait patterns, and thus can function as a concrete prototype for psychiatric genetics and for research on genetic influences on human behavior in general. There are three Mendelian forms of early-onset AD, due to dominant mutations in genes APP, PS1, and PS2. The strongly replicated APOE4 locus associated with late-onset Alzheimer's disease (LOAD), in contrast, is a *susceptibility gene,* neither necessary nor sufficient for the disease. The APOE4 and APOE2/3 alleleic forms also interact with other genes and with the environment. APOE alleles 2 and 3 appear to protect individuals with the APP mutation (Roses). Other susceptibility genes for LOAD continue to be investigated. a possible locus on chromosome 12 has been identified, and one was reported in 2000 on chromosome 9 (Pericak-Vance et al.; Roses).

Cognitive Abilities and Intelligence

Though there are more data about the inheritance of intelligence than about any other complex behavioral characteristic of humans, the word *intelligence* is viewed even by the proponents of IQ testing as misleading because it has too many different meanings. IQ researchers seem to prefer to use the expression "general cognitive ability," represented by the letter g (Jensen; Plomin, DeFries, et al., 2001). The notion of substantial genetic influences on individual variation in g or "intelligence" remains controversial even after almost a century of investigation.

Most investigators in behavioral genetics view the level of intellectual functioning (abstract reasoning, ability to perform complex cognitive tasks, score on tests of general intelligence, IQ) as a strongly heritable trait. In 1963, psychologists Nikki Erlenmeyer-Kimling and Lissy Jarvik summarized the literature dealing with correlations between the measured intelligence of various relatives. After eliminating studies based on specialized samples or employing unusual tests or statistics, they reviewed eighty-one investigations. Included were data from eight countries on four continents spanning more than two generations and containing over 30,000 correlational pairings. The overview that emerged from that mass of data was unequivocal. Intelligence appeared to be a quantitative polygenic trait; that is, a trait influenced by many genes, as are such physical characteristics as height and weight.

The results did not suggest that environmental factors were unimportant, but that genetic variation was quite important. The less sensitive trait of height (or weight) can be used to illustrate this distinction. It is well known that an individual's height can be influenced by nutrition, and inadequate diets during development can result in reduced height. The average height of whole populations has changed along with changes in public health and nutrition. Yet at the same time, individual differences in height (or weight) among the members of a population are strongly influenced by heredity. In general, taller people tend to have taller children across the population as a whole, and the relative height of different people is strongly influenced by their genes. This also appears to be the case with intelligence. The Erlenmeyer-Kimling and Jarvik survey data suggest that about 70 percent of the variation among individuals in measured intelligence is due to genetic differences. The remaining 30 percent of the variation is due to unspecified (and still unknown) environmental effects.

Two decades later, in 1981, Thomas Bouchard and Matt McGue at the University of Minnesota also compiled a summary of the world literature on intelligence correlations between relatives. They summarized 111 studies, 59 of which had been reported during the seventeen years since the Erlenmeyer-Kimling and Jarvik review. Bouchard and McGue summarized 526 familial correlations from 113,942 pairings. The general picture remained the same, with roughly 70 percent of normal-range variation attributable to genetic differences and about 30 percent due to environmental effects.

However, researchers examining the behavioral genetics of cognitive ability estimate the heritability of g (or IQ) as substantially lower, about 30 to 35 percent. Statisticians Bernie Devlin, Michael Daniels, and Kathryn Roeder argue that the much of the difference between the high and low heritabilities can be accounted for by a substantial maternal environmental component. As in the height and weight example above, there is also a substantial general environmental component that increased IQ scores by about 30 points between 1950 and 2000. This is known as the Flynn effect (see Flynn).

Robert Plomin and colleagues have attempted to identify specific genes or gene regions, also known as quantitative trait loci (QTLs), that influence IQ. Though there has been one publication reporting an IQ-related gene (see Plomin, Hill, et al.), replication has not yet been forthcoming.

Much is known about the genetics of mental retardation and learning disabilities. The most common single causes of severe general learning disabilities are chromosomal anomalies (having too many or too few copies of one of the many genes that occur together on a chromosome). These genes may reside on additional chromosomes, for example trisomy 21 (an extra chromosome 21, or three instead of the normal two) is the cause of Down's syndrome, and the "fragile X" condition may by itself account for most, if not all, of the excess of males among people with severe learning disabilities (Plomin, DeFries, et al., 2001). A large number of rare single-gene mutations, many of them recessive, induce metabolic abnormalities that severely affect nervous system function and thus lead to mental retardation. Because the specific alleles involved are individually rare and recessive, such metabolic abnormalities can cause learning-disabled individuals to appear sporadically in otherwise unaffected families. The new field of molecular genetic technology holds a promise of future therapeutic regimens for many learning disabilities.

Personality Studies

Dimensions of personality tend to be familial (Benjamin et al.). Modern studies of twins and adoptees suggest that for adults, some major dimensions are influenced by differences in family environments, while some are not. For the dimension of extroversion, which encompasses such tendencies as sociability and impulsivity, genetic factors account for about 30 to 60 percent of the variation among adults, with about 50 percent of the variation being environmental in origin.

But, surprisingly, none of the variation among adults appears to be related to environmental differences within families.

For neuroticism, which taps such traits as anxiousness (a characteristic state of anxiety), emotional instability, and anxious arousability (a tendency to react with anxiety to events), about 40 percent of the adult variation appears to be caused by genetic differences, and again none of the variation is from environmental differences that are shared by members of the same family. In contrast, social desirability, which measures a tendency to answer questions in socially approved ways and to want to appear accepted by and acceptable to society, does not show evidence of genetic causation. Essentially all of the measurable variation in social desirability appears to be environmental, with about 20 percent due to family environment.

Some authors, including Robert Plomin and colleagues, the authors of *Behavioral Genetics* (2001), suggest that because extroversion and neuroticism are general factors involved in many other personality scales or dimensions, most of the others also show moderate genetic variation. For example, a twin study involving eleven personality scales found genetic influence of various degrees for them all (Tellegen et al.). On average, across the eleven personality scales, 54 percent of the variation was attributable to genetic differences among the people, and 46 percent to environmental differences.

Tendencies toward affective (mood) disorders, including psychotic depression and bipolar disorder type I (manic depression), also are clearly influenced by genetics. A lack of familial co-occurrence has established the separateness of schizophrenia from the affective psychoses. Unipolar depression and bipolar affective disorder do co-occur, and there may be a genetically influenced major depressive syndrome distinct from manic depression. The affective disorders probably include a diversity of genetic conditions.

Other Traits

Although data are sparse for many traits, modern studies are revealing genetic involvement in many conditions of importance to society. Plomin and colleagues point out that, for males, the best single predictor of alcoholism is alcoholism in a first-degree biological relative. Alcoholism clearly runs in biological families. Severe alcoholism affects about 5 percent of males in the general population, but among male relatives of alcoholics the incidence is about 25 percent. The incidence remains about the same for adopted-away sons of male alcoholics. However, biological children of nonalcoholics are not at increased risk for alcoholism when raised by alcoholic adoptive parents.

Behavioral and psychiatric geneticists have studied genetic influence on antisocial behavior and adult criminality. Studies tend to report that shared environment is more important as a cause in juveniles and that genetics plays more of a role in adults (Lyons et al.). These studies have been extremely contentious, however (Wasserman and Wachbroit). Since the early 1990s several molecular studies of genetics and violence have also emerged, two of which are cited here. In 1993 Hans Brünner and his group reported on a Dutch family with a missing gene on the X chromosome which governed the monoamine oxidase A (MAOA) enzyme, an enzyme that metabolizes some key neurotransmitters (Brünner et al.). The Dutch families' males exhibited an unusual number of antisocial behaviors of varied sorts (assaults, rape, arson, etc.). Males, lacking a second X chromosome, were more vulnerable to the effects of this mutation. The mutation was subsequently determined to be extremely rare, and behavioral geneticists largely lost interest in the MAOA gene. In August 2002, however, a major study involving about 1000 New Zealand families found that a less severe MAOA gene mutation had a significant effect on males' display of antisocial behaviors, including their being convicted for violent offenses (Caspi et al.). But the antisocial behaviors only appeared in those subjects (in as much as 85% of them) who had experienced abuse during childhood, indicating an important G × E interaction effect of gene with environment. This carefully designed study is yet to be replicated, but it has received widespread attention.

Both twin and adoption studies that indicate obesity is highly heritable, probably about 70 percent (Grilo and Pogue-Geile). In addition, a large adoption study of obesity among adults found that family environment by itself had no apparent effect—in adulthood, the body mass index of the adoptees showed a strong relationship to that of their biological parents, but there was no relationship between weight classification of adoptive parents and the adoptees. The relation between biological parent and adoptee weight extended across the spectrum, from very thin to very obese. Once again, cumulative effects of the rearing home environment were not important determinants of individual differences among adults (Stunkard et al.).

Philosophical and Theoretical Perspectives

Biologists, psychologists, and philosophers have engaged in high-level theorizing about the effects of genes on traits in general and on human behavior in particular. Perhaps the most vigorous and ongoing discussion has been generated by a variety of papers and books that can be loosely characterized as a "developmentalist challenge" to the separability of genetic and environmental contributions to an organism's features (Schaffner, 1998). Over the years, the biologist Richard Lewontin's views have been particularly influential in this regard. Similar views critical of an overemphasis of genetic influence on traits have been articulated by several other scholars (see *Cycles of Contingency* [2001], by Susan Oyama, Paul Griffiths, and Russell Gray, which presents a number of contributions to "developmental systems theory" [DST]). Thus far, DST has largely been directed at critiquing DNA priority in molecular developmental and evolutionary claims, and at recommending more epigenetic-driven research. It is conceivable that as DST develops further, it will be applied more specifically to the relation of nature and nurture in a number of psychiatric disorders.

Integrated Approaches

Some recent articles suggest that research integrating quantitative and molecular approaches with neuroscientific strategies will be the most fruitful way to provide a framework for genetic and environmental effects on organisms. Reiss and Neiderhiser recommend an "integrated" approach. In their 1991 book *Schizophrenia Genesis*, Irving Gottesman and Dorothea Wolfgram envision the future promise of neuroscience programs to assist progress in schizophrenia. The increasingly important neurodevelopmental perspective approach to schizophrenia has been championed by Tsuang and colleagues and implemented in recent papers from the Pittsburgh group (Mirnics et al.). In addition, a series of ethical issues have arisen in neuroscience that mirror many of those first generated by behavioral genetics, including issues of reduction, determinism, and responsibility. A new term, *neuroethics,* has been coined to describe these issues (Marcus).

The completion of the draft mapping of the human genome has led to a realization that the next stage of inquiry into examining human behavioral traits, and both somatic and mental disorders, will need to be very complex, involving functional genomics, proteomics (the study of proteins and their effects) (Pandey and Mann), and enviromics (Anthony). These will be difficult and complex projects that will also need to attend carefully to developmental issues, since most human diseases, including psychiatric disorders, probably represent the culmination of "lifelong interactions between our genome and the environment" (Peltonen and McKusick, p. 1228). Animal models will be helpful here, as will new technologies using DNA genetic chips, also known as *microarrays.*

Conclusion

There are diverse methodological approaches to studying the effects of genetics on human behavior and in relation to psychiatric disorders. The working out of the partitioning of genetic and environmental causes and their interactions at multiple levels of aggregation in complex systems, as humans are, will require many research programs extending over many years, hopefully producing a number of useful interim results such as those discussed above. These results, however, will not silence the continuing debates over the roles that genes and environments play in the complex choreography of organism development and behaviors.

GLAYDE WHITNEY (1995)
REVISED BY KENNETH F. SCHAFFNER

SEE ALSO: *Genetic Counseling, Ethical Issues in; Genetic Counseling, Practice of; Genetic Engineering, Human; Genetics and Environment in Human Health; Genetics and Human Self-Understanding; Genetics and Racial Minorities; Genetics and the Law; Human Dignity; Human Nature; Privacy and Confidentiality in Research;* and other *Genetics and Human Behavior* subentries

BIBLIOGRAPHY

Anthony, James C. 2001. "The Promise of Psychiatric Enviromics." *British Journal of Psychiatry* 40 (suppl.): 8–11.

Benjamin, Jonathan; Ebstein, Richard P.; and Belmaker, Robert H. 2002. *Molecular Genetics and the Human Personality.* Washington, D.C.: American Psychiatric Publications.

Bouchard, Thomas J., Jr., and McGue, Matt. 1981. "Familial Studies of Intelligence: A Review." *Science* 212(4498): 1055–1059.

Brunner, H. G.; Nelen, M.; Breakefield, X. O.; et al. 1993. "Abnormal Behavior Associated with a Point Mutation in the Structural Gene for Monoamine Oxidase A." *Science* 262(5133): 578–580.

Caspi, Avshalom; McClay, Joseph; Moffitt, Terrie E.; et al. 2002. "Role of Genotype in the Cycle of Violence in Maltreated Children." *Science* 297(5582): 851–854.

Devlin, Bernie; Daniels, Michjael; and Roeder, Kathryn. 1997. "The Heritability of IQ." *Nature* 388(6641): 468–471.

Flynn, J. R. 1999. "Searching for Justice: The Discovery of IQ Gains over Time." *American Psychologist* 54: 5–20.

Fuller, John L., and Thompson, William Robert. 1960. *Behavioral Genetics.* New York: Wiley.

Gottesman, Irving. I. 2003. "A Behavioral Genetics Perspective." In *Behavioral Genetics in the Postgenomic Era,* ed. R. Plomin, J. DeFries, I. Craig, P. McGuffin, et al. Washington, D.C.: American Psychological Association.

Gottesman, Irving I., and Erlenmeyer-Kimling, L. 2001. "Family and Twin Strategies As a Head Start in Defining Prodromes and Endophenotypes for Hypothetical Early-Interventions in Schizophrenia." *Schizophrenia Research* 51(1): 93–102.

Gottesman, Irving I., and Wolfgram, Dorothea L. 1991. *Schizophrenia Genesis: The Origins of Madness.* New York: Freeman.

Grilo, C. M., and Pogue-Geile, M. F. 1991. "The Nature of Environmental Influences on Weight and Obesity: A Behavior Genetic Analysis." *Psychology Bulletin* 110(3): 520–537.

Harrison, P. J., and Owen, M. J. 2003. "Genes for Schizophrenia? Recent Findings and Their Pathophysiological Implications." *Lancet* 361(9355): 417–419.

Herrnstein, Richard J., and Murray, Charles A. 1994. *The Bell Curve: Intelligence and Class Structure in American Life.* New York: Free Press.

Hyman, Steven E. 2000. "The Genetics of Mental Illness: Implications for Practice." *Bulletin of the World Health Organization* 78(4): 455–463.

Jensen, Arthur R. 1998. *The g Factor: The Science of Mental Ability.* Westport, CT: Praeger.

Kendler, K. S.; Neale, M. C.; Kessler, R. C.; et al. 1993. "A Test of the Equal-Environment Assumption in Twin Studies of Psychiatric Illness." *Behavioral Genetics* 23(1): 21–27.

Lewontin, Richard C.; Rose, Steven P. R.; and Kamin, Leon J. 1984. *Not in Our Genes: Biology, Ideology, and Human Nature.* New York: Pantheon.

Lyons, M. J.; True, W. R.; Eisen, S. A.; et al. 1995. "Differential Heritability of Adult and Juvenile Antisocial Traits." *Archives of General Psychiatry* 52(11): 906–915.

Marcus, Steven, ed. 2002. *Neuroethics: Mapping the Field: Conference Proceedings.* New York: Dana Foundation.

McGuffin, Peter; Riley, Brien; and Plomin, Robert. 2001. "Genomics and Behavior. Toward Behavioral Genomics." *Science* 291(5507): 1232–1249.

Mirnics, K.; Middleton, F.; Marquez, A. A.; et al. 2000. "Molecular Characterization of Schizophrenia Viewed by Microarray Analysis of Gene Expression in Prefrontal Cortex." *Neuron* 28(1): 53–67.

Neiderhiser, Jenae M. 2001. "Understanding the Roles of Genome and Envirome: Methods in Genetic Epidemiology." *British Journal of Psychiatry* 40 (suppl.): 12–17.

Oyama, Susan; Griffiths, Paul E.; and Gray, Russell D. 2001. *Cycles of Contingency: Developmental Systems and Evolution.* Cambridge, MA: MIT Press.

Pandey, A., and Mann, M. 2000. "Proteomics to Study Genes and Genomes." *Nature* 405(6788): 837–846.

Peltonen, Leena, and McKusick, Victor A. 2001. "Genomics and Medicine. Dissecting Human Disease in the Postgenomic Era." *Science* 291(5507): 1224–1229.

Pericak-Vance, M. A.; Grubber, J.; Bailey, L. R.; et al. 2000. "Identification of Novel Genes in Late-Onset Alzheimer's Disease." *Experimental Gerontology* 35(9–10): 1343–1352.

Plomin, Robert, and Daniels, D. 1987. "Why Are Children in the Same Family So Different from One Another?" *Behavioral and Brain Sciences* 10: 1–60.

Plomin, Robert; DeFries, John C.; McClearn, Gerald E.; et al. 2001. *Behavioral Genetics.* New York: Worth.

Plomin, Robert; Hill, L.; Craig, I. W.; et al. 2001. "A Genome-Wide Scan of 1842 DNA Markers for Allelic Associations with General Cognitive Ability: A Five-Stage Design Using DNA Pooling and Extreme Selected Groups." *Behavioral Genetics* 31(6): 497–509.

Reiss, David, and Neiderhiser, Jenae M. 2000. "The Interplay of Genetic Influences and Social Processes in Developmental Theory: Specific Mechanisms Are Coming into View." *Developmental Psychopathology* 12(3): 357–374.

Reiss, David; Neiderhiser, Jenae M.; Hetherington, E. Mavis; et al. 2000. *The Relationship Code: Deciphering Genetic and Social Influences on Adolescent Development.* Cambridge, MA: Harvard University Press.

Risch, Neil, and Merikangas, Kathleen. 1996. "The Future of Genetic Studies of Complex Human Diseases." *Science* 273(5281): 1516–1517.

Roses, Allen D. 2000. "Pharmacogenetics and the Practice of Medicine." *Nature* 405(6788): 857–865.

Rowe, David C., and Jacobson, Kristin C. 1999. "In the Mainstream: Research in Behavioral Genetics." In *Behavioral Genetics: The Clash of Culture and Biology,* ed. Ronald A. Carson and Mark A. Rothstein. Baltimore: Johns Hopkins University Press.

Schaffner, Kenneth F. 1998. "Genes, Behavior, and Developmental Emergentism: One Process, Indivisible?" *Philosophy of Science* 65(June): 209–252.

Schaffner, Kenneth F. 2001. "Nature and Nurture." *Current Opinion in Psychiatry* 14(Sept): 486–490.

Stunkard, A. J.; Foch, T. T.; and Hrubec, Z. 1986. "A Twin Study of Human Obesity." *Journal of the American Medical Association* 256(1): 51–54.

Tellegen, A.; Lykken, D. T.; Bouchard, T. J., Jr.; et al. 1988. "Personality Similarity in Twins Reared Apart and Together." *Journal of Personality and Social Psychology* 54(6): 1031–1039.

Tsuang, Ming. 2000. "Schizophrenia: Genes and Environment." *Biological Psychiatry* 47(3): 210–220.

Turkheimer, Eric. 2000. "Three Laws of Behavior Genetics and What They Mean." *Current Directions in Psychological Science* 9: 160–161.

Turkheimer, Eric, and Waldron, Mary. 2000. "Nonshared Environment: A Theoretical, Methodological, and Quantitative Review." *Psychology Bulletin* 126(1): 78–108.

Wasserman, David T., and Wachbroit, Robert S. 2001. *Genetics and Criminal Behavior.* Cambridge, Eng.: Cambridge University Press.

Wiesel, T. 1994. "Genetics and Behavior." *Science* 264: 1647.

II. PHILOSOPHICAL AND ETHICAL ISSUES

Behavioral genetics has been a focus of intense controversy both within and outside the field almost from its inception.

Much of the controversy within the field involves conceptual and methodological issues such as the question: Do twin studies yield the most scientifically reliable conclusions about the degree to which genes shape behavior? Rather than address those issues, this entry examines some of the social and ethical issues that may arise as a result of what researchers in behavioral genetics claim to know regarding the role of genes in shaping human behavior. Special attention is given to what may be referred to as the promise or the threat of eugenics, depending on one's philosophic perspective, as that relates to developments in the field.

Historical Background

Eugenics is characterized by the devising of interventions aimed at improving the quality of the human genome. Those interventions can be either social behavioral or molecular. In *The Republic* Plato recommended using the power of the state to arrange marriages of the best with the best. A practical problem with that approach is that it is a very crude and haphazard way to improve the human genome. Philosophical and scientific thinking for roughly the next 2,000 years was locked into Platonic and Aristotelian premises, specifically the belief that the *nature* or *essence* of each living thing is eternal and immutable. However, the emergence of evolutionary theory from the work of Charles Darwin radically undermined that premise.

The *immutable* natures of all plants and animals in fact have been changing constantly (or perishing) in response to environmental forces over millions of years. In the nineteenth century emerging agricultural sciences showed was that such change need not be left to slow and chaotic natural forces; instead, the tools of science could be used to effect deliberately changes that suited various human needs. Darwin's cousin Sir Francis Galton took the next logical step and suggested that deliberate reproductive control could be applied to human beings as well. In 1883 he started using the term *eugenics* to describe those efforts.

In the early part of the twentieth century the eugenics movement was endorsed by many prominent scientists, intellectuals, and political leaders (Kevles), including Charles Eliot, the president of Harvard University. Still, the tools available for eugenic purposes remained crude and ethically problematic. It is one thing, morally speaking, to create social practices that would encourage the marriage of the best with the best; it is quite another to use the coercive powers of the state to sterilize individuals who are judged unfit to reproduce "their kind."

In the early twentieth century enthusiasm for eugenics might be said to have reached a peak in 1927 with the U.S.

Supreme Court decision *Buck v. Bell*. Oliver Wendell Holmes there upheld the constitutionality of state sterilization laws with the ringing words "Three generations of imbeciles is enough!" The rise of Nazism and the appropriation by the Nazis of the rhetoric of eugenics to justify their atrocities resulted in a tarnishing of the eugenics movement in the middle part of the century. To this day those unsavory connotations remain attached to the term *eugenics*.

The second half of the twentieth century saw the discovery of the DNA molecule by Francis Crick and James Watson, followed by the very rapid development of genetics as a science and the dissemination of genetic insights and techniques into other areas of science, such as behavioral genetics in psychology. That effort culminated in the mapping of the entire human genome, beginning in the 1990s to April 2003. One consequence of those scientific successes is that eugenics has regained a considerable degree of scientific and moral legitimacy.

A primary reason for the renewed legitimacy is the fact that molecular biology offers the promise of tools that can achieve with great precision whatever eugenic goals *we* might embrace. Furthermore, the emphasis by advocates of the *new eugenics* is on the voluntary use of those tools by individuals as opposed to their forcible imposition by the state. In addition, the emphasis of advocates for eugenics is not on improving the quality of *the* human genome. Instead, that emphasis is individually therapeutic, as in traditional medicine. The dominant goal is to improve the lifetime welfare of future possible children who otherwise would be faced with genetic deficiencies that would compromise the length and quality of their lives. However, there are critics of all forms of eugenics, whether new or old, whether aimed at eliminating debilitating medical conditions or enhancing desirable human traits such as intelligence (Rifkin; Kass).

Eugenics: Some Broad Moral and Political Issues

Who should be the *we* that would have the moral authority to determine eugenic goals? Should this be part of the authority and responsibility of the state, or should such decisions be left to autonomous individuals? If people chose to invest that authority in a liberal democratic state, would careful adherence to legitimate democratic processes be sufficient to guarantee the moral legitimacy of the eugenic policies that emerged from those processes? If conscientious adherence to such democratic processes were insufficient, what extrapolitical norms could justifiably be invoked for purposes of assessing those processes and policies critically? What would be the source of the moral authority of those norms?

Alternatively, if the coercive powers of the state were judged to be problematic, especially with regard to intimate and personal matters such as the genetic endowment of children, eugenic goals could be left to the choices of individuals and the private organizations that would provide the means necessary for achieving those goals, such as genetic testing and alternative means of reproduction. This would be what Philip Kitcher refers to critically as "laissez faire eugenics." If such eugenic outcomes were both privatized and uncoerced, would that guarantee the moral and political legitimacy of those outcomes? Troy Duster thinks not. Or would a state be correctly judged to be irresponsible for allowing any and all voluntary eugenic decisions to happen in an entirely unregulated fashion primarily because the best interests of future children would be at risk?

These questions are raised in the context of a liberal, pluralistic, secular, tolerant democratic state that seeks to maximize the scope of individual liberty as long as that liberty is not used to threaten the equally valuable rights and liberties of others or undermine important public interests. This type of state recognizes that there are many reasonable visions of what it means to live a good life and that consequently a state must refrain from using its coercive powers to impose a preferred vision of a good life on those who would not choose it for themselves (Rawls). It is a state that will not allow sectarian religious preferences to shape public policy, especially if a policy is needed to guide intimate life decisions. Thus, critical religious appeals to the language of "playing God" will have little legitimacy as rational support for public policies that might be aimed at outlawing "private eugenic efforts" by parents to shape the genetic endowment of their children (Peters; Evans).

Eugenics: Some Policy Issues

A state that did nothing to regulate any of the medical technologies that might be used to shape or choose the genetic endowment of future children might be regarded as irresponsible. After all, one version of the argument might go, how can a compassionate and responsible society allow children to be born with serious medical disorders, such as cystic fibrosis or Tay-Sachs disease, that would very adversely affect the length and quality of their lives when that society has the technology to prevent such harm? Alternatively, how can a compassionate and responsible society allow genetic and medical researchers to experiment with alterations in the genetic endowments of embryos if there is any risk of significant harm to the children who eventually would be born?

Both of these questions suggest a necessary and legitimate role for the state in regulating the development and use of technologies that have a eugenic purpose. However, that leaves unspecified the norms that justifiably could be invoked in a liberal pluralistic society for purposes of shaping both the content and the purpose of those policies. For example, should a compassionate and responsible society use tax monies to underwrite basic research aimed at providing the capacity to shape the genetic endowment of future children? This society already spends billions of public dollars each year through the National Institutes of Health to address an enormous range of human health problems, many of which have genetic roots. Alternatively, the genetic research that people imagine necessarily would involve the destruction of numerous embryos that were only a few days old. That would violate the deep moral convictions of many people in the society who are concerned about protecting all human life from the moment of conception. Are their concerns sufficient to take such public funding off the table?

If the destruction of embryos is a legitimate societal concern, less offensive policy options are available for achieving eugenic goals. There could be public funding for eugenic education. This could take many forms, but the general idea is that future parents would know what options were available to them for shaping naturally or technologically the genetic endowment of their children. A society could encourage widespread and complex genetic testing long before marriage by underwriting the cost of that testing so that individuals would be motivated to refrain from having children altogether, refrain from having children with partners who were genetic mismatches, or refrain from reproducing except through the use of an alternative reproductive technology.

Utopian Eugenics

The policy options cited above would come under the rubric of *utopian eugenics,* a phrase introduced by Philip Kitcher. That phrase is intended to suggest the desirability of a society pursuing a range of eugenic goals within the constraints of a liberal pluralistic political framework. Broad public genetic education and public support for access to genetic testing would increase the capacity of individuals to make autonomous eugenic choices regarding their own children in the light of their deepest values. Such public support also would demonstrate responsible but noncoercive regard for the well-being of future children who otherwise would be vulnerable to the profoundly harmful vagaries of the genetic lottery.

The word *harm* merits special emphasis in understanding the thrust of utopian eugenics. Kitcher and others are morally and politically comfortable with eugenic policies aimed at giving parents tools for preventing substantial genetic harm to their future children. However, many

people (Parens) are less comfortable with eugenic interventions aimed at enhancing the genetic endowment of future children. This raises two questions, one moral and the other conceptual: Is there a significant moral difference between genetic interventions aimed at minimizing genetic harm and genetic interventions aimed at enhancing traits? Can a sharp conceptual distinction be drawn between what are called genetic harms and what are called genetic enhancements? These questions are discussed and analyzed thoroughly, along with their practical implications, by Allen Buchanan and coauthors.

Behavioral Genetics and Eugenics: Distinctive Moral Concerns

The questions raised above might be characterized as generic questions about eugenics. The examples used have all been about physical diseases with strong genetic links. However, the actual history of the eugenics movement has largely involved what today would be labeled behavioral genetics. That is, what those advocates wanted eliminated from the human gene pool were genes associated with being feeble-minded, lazy, alcoholic, violent, inclined to criminality, and so on. This raises a host of other moral and political and philosophic issues that are much more perplexing than the issues listed above.

If an individual has a gene variant that will result in affliction with cystic fibrosis or Huntington's disease or an early-onset form of Alzheimer's disease, such disease processes are seen to be accidental afflictions of that individual's body. Those diseases do not alter people's fundamental nature as persons, as rational moral agents. However, if an individual is feeble-minded (or a genius), alcoholic, or inclined to criminality as a result of his or her genetic endowment, this seems to be integral to his or her nature as a person, as a choice-making creature. It also raises the troubling question of whether individuals with such genetic endowments can be held accountable for the behaviors that seem to flow from those endowments. The argument, stated very crudely, would be that people do not hold individuals responsible for having cystic fibrosis; consequently, those individuals should not be held responsible for their criminal behavior if that behavior is just another product of their genetic endowment.

Other troubling social consequences may be associated with behavioral genetics. Genes seem to "travel" in clusters: Family resemblances are a common social phenomenon. Those resemblances also show up among members of ethnic and racial groups. None of these observations are intrinsically troubling. However, if a particular racial or ethnic group is perceived socially to have many members who are less intelligent, more violent, more prone to engage in criminal activity, and so on, and if those undesirable traits are believed to be genetically rooted, those social groups as a whole will be vulnerable to serious social stigmatization.

The practical argument is obvious: If members of *that group* cannot benefit from social investments in education, why waste resources on *them*. In this way the worst social prejudices can be given scientific and political legitimacy as well as insulation from moral criticism. That is, if individuals in the disfavored group are denied various social opportunities, those denials can be justified morally on the grounds that those individuals are genetically incapable of taking advantage of those opportunities. This issue has been the focus of a political firestorm that initially was generated by Arthur Jensen and then reignited by Charles Murray and Richard Herrnstein.

Behavioral Genetics: Key Elements of the Science

Moral judgments about personal responsibility for behavior or social discrimination must take into account relevant well-established scientific facts. Thus, it would be morally wrong to hold an individual who is completely in the grip of psychotic delusions responsible for his or her behavior in the same way one does with a person with normal rational capacities and moral sensibilities. At least two popular beliefs associated with genetics represent a gross distortion of the actual science and an equally gross distortion of related moral judgments.

The first belief is that people's fate is in their genes, that the genetic endowment of an individual is a *future diary* of that individual. In other words, people's behavior is at least very strongly determined by their genes. The second belief is that for any biological fact about people there is a *gene for* that biological fact. Thus, if scientists look hard enough, they eventually will find a *gene for* depression, a high IQ, aggression, criminality, being gay, and so on. A headline from *Time* magazine (Lemonick) is illustrative: "The Search for a Murder Gene."

What is referred to colloquially as *the* Huntington's gene would reinforce both of these popular misconceptions. That is, if an individual has inherited this gene, it is almost 100 percent certain that that person will have the disease (although there is considerable variation in the age at onset and the intensity of the disorder). That person is fated in a very strong sense. No personal behavior and no environmental variables can alter that fate. However, this picture of genetic determinism seems to have an extremely limited range of application. No human behavior of even minimal complexity seems to be genetically controlled in that simple

a fashion (Ehrlich and Feldman; Beckwith and Alper; Ridley; Schaffner).

This entry does not address the philosophic issues and arguments associated with the free will–determinism debate or the debates in the philosophy of mind about whether mental events are nothing more than mechanistic brain states. However, a review of core scientific propositions that would be endorsed by a wide range of behavioral geneticists and a linking of those propositions with core scientific propositions in the neurocognitive sciences probably would provide a better basis for identifying and addressing related moral and political issues such as the question of the possibility of moral responsibility.

The Nature of Human Nature

Steven Pinker is the author of a provocative book titled *The Blank Slate: The Modern Denial of Human Nature*. There are three "myths" he intended to undermine in that book: (1) the belief that human beings are born as blank slates (from the philosopher John Locke) that are shaped completely by experience, (2) the belief in the ghost in the machine (from the philosopher Renée Descartes), which holds that the mind is a nonphysical entity that is connected mysteriously to people's physical bodies, and (3) the belief (from the philosopher Jean-Jacques Rousseau) that human beings are born as "noble savages," that they are born morally innocent and corrupted later by social institutions. Pinker contends that none of these beliefs can be supported by contemporary science.

Pinker argues that human beings have a nature at birth, that what is referred to as the mind is really the human brain, that the architecture of the brain is the product of eons of evolutionary development, that very complex interactions among many genes (as well as complex environmental factors) are ultimately responsible for that brain architecture, and that the detailed architecture of the brain varies from one individual to another as a result of the genetic variation and environmental influences that distinguish individuals. This genetic variation among individuals includes both cognitive and emotional differences.

Pinker is comfortable with the idea that from birth some individuals are more shy or more outgoing than others, more happy or more depressed, more inclined to be socially conformist or to engage in antisocial behavior, more inclined to be forgiving or to erupt in anger, and so on. For Pinker the same thing is true with respect to the display of intellectual abilities. He sees all these behavioral predispositions as ultimately being rooted in the genetic endowment of each individual; this is why he rejects the notion that humans at birth are noble savages or blank slates.

Some people consider the picture Pinker has painted excessively deterministic and mechanistic, both eviscerating any basis for moral responsibility for human behavior and reinforcing deep social prejudices against certain racial and ethnic groups. However, that conclusion is not warranted. What Pinker writes (p. 48) and what generally would be endorsed by behavioral geneticists is the following: "Most psychological traits are the product of many genes with small effects that are modulated by the presence of other genes, rather than the product of a single gene with a large effect that shows up come what may." He goes on to note that the effects of most genes are probabilistic and that the environment often modulates the effects of particular genes in complex ways. This is why identical twins do not live identical lives.

Behavioral Genetics and Eugenics: Contemporary Ethical Concerns

In 2002 in Great Britain the Nuffield Council on Bioethics addressed these issues and reached essentially the same conclusions. That is, the council sees no reason why research in behavioral genetics necessarily yields a fatalistic picture of human life in general or an undermining of the human capacity for moral judgment and moral responsibility. The genetic endowment of individuals establishes a range of behavioral options and predispositions related to personality, but the precise way in which those predispositions manifest themselves in a particular individual is a complex product of environmental chance and the deliberative capacities of that individual.

Those deliberative capacities can be influenced for better or worse by the formal and informal social learning opportunities offered in particular social contexts. For example, an individual may have a genetic endowment that predisposes him or her to react depressively to a range of disappointments and frustrations. However, an individual who is reflectively aware of those behavioral predispositions as a result of diligent parenting, sensitive friends, or personal reading may adopt a range of psychological and behavioral strategies that minimize the potentially damaging results of those depressive feelings. Alternatively, that reflective awareness might suggest taking medications aimed at altering the brain chemistry that sustains those feelings of depression. In either case what is illustrated is a responsible reaction to what might be described as innate features of one's personality. Kay Jamison's struggle with depression, as recounted in *An Unquiet Mind* (1995), is illustrative of these points.

If the picture sketched here is roughly correct and if the work of behavioral geneticists does not undermine people's capacity to be responsible moral agents, are any other moral issues raised by this research? The work of the Nuffield Council (2002) is helpful in responding to this question. The council points to two large concerns that potentially raise moral issues: medicalization and eugenics.

The term *medicalization* typically is used to express a specific criticism: that what once was regarded as a normal behavior or bodily state now is regarded as abnormal because there are medical interventions that give people control over that behavior or state. Some people are *just shy*. This is a fact about some individuals that is accepted routinely. However, if antidepressants such as Paxil can alleviate such behavioral dispositions and allow individuals to be more sociable (per social expectations), such individuals may no longer be accepted as shy persons. Instead, they may be *diagnosed* as shy and advised (expected) to seek appropriate medical help.

There is no simple response to this issue. One legitimate fear is that the range of social tolerance for personality types and traits will be narrowed excessively to the detriment of such individuals. That is, those individuals may be subjected to excessive social scrutiny and social pressure to conform to a narrow range of socially acceptable behavior. This seems contrary to the core values of a liberal society. However, in other cases medicalization of behavior that once was regarded as normal may be beneficial to both individual and social welfare. Attention deficit hyperactivity disorder (ADHD) illustrates this point. Children who are identified as having ADHD benefit greatly from drugs such as Ritalin. The practical moral problem is that the behavioral and diagnostic boundaries of this disorder are fuzzy and controversial, and this can lead to morally troubling problems of overdiagnosis and underdiagnosis.

The other concern raised by the Nuffield Council is the eugenics issue. Dean Hamer and coworkers announced in 1993 the discovery of "the gay gene." Hamer later retracted that claim, recognizing that the basis for the sexual orientation of individuals is much more complex than the workings of a single gene. However, his original claim helped establish in the public mind that there soon may be a genetic test for "being gay" that would allow potential parents in the future to use preimplantation genetic diagnosis (PGD) to weed out gay embryos. Similar beliefs suggest that in the future it will be possible to pick out or create through germline genetic engineering smarter or happier or nonviolent or nonalcoholic embryos. This refers back to the eugenics issues that were raised earlier in this entry.

Those issues may be addressed more thoughtfully by recalling a key scientific claim about behavioral genetics. These types of behavioral phenomena are only indirectly the product of very complex interactions among many genes as well as environmental factors, all of which are very poorly understood. Nobody knows which genes, in what way, to what degree, and at what point in development yield the neural capacities that establish a range of intellectual abilities. This is true whether one's concerns are with happiness, aggressiveness, schizophrenia, or addiction (Hamer; Beckwith and Alper). Furthermore, if society's legitimate social goals include shaping human behavior in various ways, there also are available as tools a very large range of social practices and medical interventions.

Behavioral Genetics and Eugenics: Some Ethical Guidelines

The Nuffield Council on Bioethics) has suggested several criteria for assessing from a moral point of view eugenic interventions aimed at improving behavioral outcomes: effectiveness, safety, reversibility, and choice.

If researchers discover genes associated with intelligence, it is likely that any one of those genes will have only very small and uncertain effects on the intellectual potential of an embryo. Consequently, embryonic genetic intervention to improve intelligence appears to be an ineffective approach. IQ scores as measured by standardized tests increased twenty to thirty points during the twentieth century. Clearly, that improvement did not result from radical genetic changes.

Safety must be a critical moral consideration, especially if the individuals whose behavior is to be affected do not have the capacity to give consent, as would be true for children and embryos. Giving Paxil to a moderately shy child may be morally objectionable when researchers are not certain of the long-term effects of that drug and the behavior to be altered is only moderately dysfunctional. Gene therapy would be problematic on this criterion for children or adults because there has been little success and some serious bad outcomes. The risks of gene therapy may be reasonable if individuals are faced with a life-threatening disorder, but that is not the case when the goal is behavioral alteration.

Reversibility is the third criterion the Nuffield Council emphasizes. It is difficult to imagine that anyone would want to be less intelligent, less happy, vulnerable to addiction, or more prone to violence. However, if researchers engage in behaviorally oriented genetic alterations, they may overshoot the mark: An individual could end up experiencing feelings of happiness in socially inappropriate situations.

The Nuffield Council notes that physicians are very reluctant to do genetic testing of children for medical disorders to which a child might be vulnerable as an adult and for which there is no medical intervention. The council recommends similar reticence if genetic tests related to what might be described as presymptomatic personality disorders were developed.

For example, a child might seem as happy as any other child in the neighborhood, but parental concerns about a family history of depression might motivate them to pursue genetic testing of that child for depression. That testing would yield no obvious good for the child but could put the child at risk for stigmatization or a maladaptive response from the parents. In addition, such nonsymptomatic nontherapeutic genetic testing represents a violation of the privacy rights and autonomy rights of that child. Also, assuming that the test identified a genetic pattern associated with depression in the child's family, everything known today would suggest that this represented no more than increased susceptibility for that disorder, not certainty that it would express itself or that its expression would be severe.

There are considerations of justice and the protection of fair equality of opportunity that are relevant to this discussion. Some writers (Silver) fear that differences in wealth will permit the rich to purchase a superior genetic endowment, especially with regard to valued behavioral traits, for their children, establishing permanently superior genetic castes. However, this is a plausible concern only extremely far into the future, if ever.

Still, there are relevant considerations of justice in the present that are related to improving the genetic endowment of future children (Fleck). Genetic testing in vitro of eight-cell embryos, or preimplantation genetic diagnosis, permits the selection of embryos that are free of certain serious genetic defects. However, this intervention costs about $40,000 per successful pregnancy. It seems reasonable to ask whether such interventions should be publicly funded as a matter of social justice and perhaps as a matter of genetic social responsibility as well.

Conclusions

Relative to scientific understanding and technical capacities in the field of behavioral genetics, fears of behavioral eugenics are exaggerated. People have very little capacity, using the tools of molecular biology, to alter with confidence the genetic endowments of future children.

No emerging knowledge in the fields of behavioral genetics and developmental biology or the neurosciences would justify concluding in a global fashion that human beings can no longer be held morally responsible for their behavior because their behavior has been determined in a mechanistic fashion by their genes (Wasserman).

However, as knowledge of the behavioral sciences becomes more refined and certain, society will be forced to make increasingly nuanced judgments about the capacity for responsible moral action by individuals whose genetic endowment includes significant susceptibility to aggression or depression or other socially or medically deviant behaviors. That is, society will have no right to advance global assertions of moral responsibility by all individuals in all circumstances. In some circumstances moral or legal responsibility for specific actions will be diminished or eviscerated as a result of biological facts beyond the control of the individual.

A liberal society should accord substantial respect for the procreative liberty of potential parents, including their right to determine the genetic endowments of their future children. However, a responsible liberal society will take seriously its obligations to protect those children from embryonic behavioral genetic experimentation that would threaten their future capacities for autonomy or the future interests generally valued by all human beings. No simple moral algorithm can indicate how such balances should be struck in making public policy.

RICHARD A. SHWEDER (1995)
REVISED BY LEONARD M. FLECK

SEE ALSO: *Autonomy; Freedom and Free Will; Genetic Counseling, Ethical Issues in; Genetic Counseling, Practice of; Genetic Engineering, Human; Genetics and Environment in Human Health; Genetics and Human Self-Understanding; Genetics and Racial Minorities; Genetics and the Law; Human Dignity; Human Nature; Privacy and Confidentiality in Research;* and other *Genetics and Human Behavior* subentries

BIBLIOGRAPHY

Beckwith, Jon, and Alper, Joseph. 2002. "Genetics of Human Personality: Social and Ethical Implications." In *Molecular Genetics and Human Personality,* ed. Jonathan Benjamin, Richard Ebstein, and Robert Belmaker. Washington, D.C.: American Psychiatric Publishing.

Buchanan, Allen; Brock, Dan; Daniels, Norman; and Wikler, Dan. 2000. *From Chance to Choice: Genetics and Justice.* New York: Cambridge University Press.

Duster, Troy. 1990. *Backdoor to Eugenics.* New York: Routledge.

Ehrlich, Paul, and Feldman, Marcus. 2003. "Genes and Cultures: What Creates Our Behavioral Phenome?" *Current Anthropology* 44: 87–95.

Evans, John H. 2002. *Playing God: Human Genetic Engineering and the Rationalization of Public Bioethical Debate.* Chicago: University of Chicago Press.

Fleck, Leonard. 2002. "Just Caring: Do Future Possible Children Have a Just Claim to a Sufficiently Healthy Genome?" In *Medicine and Social Justice: Essays on the Distribution of Health Care,* ed. Rosamond Rhodes, Margaret Battin, and Anita Silvers. New York: Oxford University Press.

Hamer, Dean. 2002. "Rethinking Behavior Genetics." *Science* 298: 71–72.

Hamer, Dean; Hu, S.; Magnusun, V.; and Pattatucci, A. 1993. "A Linkage between DNA Markers on the X Chromosome and Male Sexual Orientation." *Science* 261(5119): 321–327.

Jamison, Kay Redfield. 1995. *An Unquiet Mind: A Memoir of Moods and Madness.* New York: Vintage Books.

Jensen, Arthur. 1969. "How Much Can We Boost IQ and Scholastic Achievement?" *Harvard Educational Review* 39(1): 1–123.

Kass, Leon. 2002. *Life, Liberty, and the Defense of Dignity: The Challenge for Bioethics.* San Francisco: Encounter Books.

Kevles, Daniel. 1985. *In the Name of Eugenics: Genetics and the Uses of Human Heredity.* Berkeley: University of California Press.

Kitcher, Philip. 1996. *The Lives to Come: The Genetic Revolution and Human Possibilities.* New York: Simon & Schuster.

Lemonick, Michael. 2003. "The Search for a Murder Gene." *Time,* January 20, p. 100.

Murray, Charles, and Herrnstein, Richard. 1994. *The Bell Curve.* New York: Free Press.

Nuffield Council on Bioethics. 2002. *Genetics and Human Behavior: The Ethical Context.* London: Nuffield Council on Bioethics.

Parens, Eric, ed. 1998. *Enhancing Human Traits: Ethical and Social Implications.* Washington, D.C.: Georgetown University Press.

Peters, Ted. 1997. *Playing God: Genetic Determinism and Human Freedom.* New York: Routledge.

Pinker, Steven. 2002. *The Blank Slate: The Modern Denial of Human Nature.* New York: Viking.

Rawls, John. 1993. *Political Liberalism.* New York: Columbia University Press.

Ridley, Matt. 1999. *Genome: The Autobiography of the Species in 23 Chapters.* New York: HarperCollins.

Rifkin, Jeremy. 1984. *Algeny.* New York: Penguin Books.

Schaffner, Kenneth. 1999. "Complexity and Research Strategies in Behavioral Genetics." In *Behavioral Genetics: The Clash of Culture and Biology,* ed. Ronald Carson and Mark Rothstein. Baltimore: Johns Hopkins University Press.

Silver, Lee. 1997. *Remaking Eden: Cloning and Beyond in a Brave New World.* New York: Avon Books.

Wasserman, David. 2001. "Genetic Predispositions to Violent and Antisocial Behavior: Responsibility, Character, and Identity." In *Genetics and Criminal Behavior,* ed. David Wasserman and Robert Wachbroit. Cambridge, Eng., and New York: Cambridge University Press.

GENETICS AND HUMAN SELF-UNDERSTANDING

• • •

Genetics on the simplest level is the name of a class of problems of organic chemistry: how to name and describe the structure and function of the DNA that forms the core structure within the nucleus of all living cells. The particles of the molecule are arranged in a structure called the double helix, and this doubled form traces the function of the molecule and the transmission of data between generations of organisms as each is copied for replication. Scientists have come to understand and believe that genes, the smallest unit within that molecular system, direct chemical reactions that create larger proteins that drive the processes necessary for cell growth and cell death. Much remains to be discovered about *how* this occurs, but *that* it occurs—that proteins direct biological processes, and that they in turn are directed by genetic or epigenetic activity—is largely a settled question.

Why then, does the idea of genetics excite such controversy? The problem lies in what one makes of this genetic narrative, and how the epistemic task of genetics implies fundamental ontological and moral assumptions. Hence, the meaning of *genetics* is only partially addressed as a problem of scientific definitions. It also queries some of the most profound of issues in philosophy (such as the meaning of identity), social theory (such as the meaning of justice), and theology (such as the balance between imaginative human actions and proper human duties).

Genetics as Science and as Ontology: A Simultaneous Debate in Bioethics

Bioethics as a field grew contemporaneously and concordantly with genetics; bioethics began with speculation about the meaning of gene research (Jonson). Nothing has concerned the field of bioethics, a field largely marked by concern for the unknowable and speculative future implications of activities in the biological sciences and medicine, more profoundly than genetics. Genetics is a metaphor and a medical hope. It is at once a final cure for diseases, a prophecy for illness and for abilities, and perhaps a harbinger of troubling

injustice when used as definitive of moral status. Genetic knowledge in the late twentieth century became the central way to make meaning of the single most contentious and heavily freighted problem in human self understanding, that of origins and kinship and the way that birth circumstance was or was not determinate of fate. As philosophy and theology has much to say about kinship, fate, and family, bioethics has much to say about genetic knowledge of the same issues.

There is long history of moral advice directed toward genetic science, stressing the profound dangers attendant upon the kind of knowledge that genetics presents. Genetic knowledge represents a powerful and new understanding of how basic biological processes can be expected to unfold relative to older systems of human understanding as presented in religious or moral traditions, and genetic knowledge can be destabilizing to these systems. Since the relationship between present states of being and the unknown future had, up until the late nineteenth century, been in the purview of magic, philosophy, or religion, the unease surrounding genetic knowledge is understandable—fate, behavior, and character are powerful grounds of contention in any case. Yet by the first years of the twenty-first century, the relationship between the science of genetics and the critique of this science began to be shaped by its own dynamics as well. Genetic knowledge itself began to stand in for modern scientific knowledge, for scientism, and for instrumentality. Bioethicists found a belief in genetic causation vexing, perhaps reductionist; this critique became a stable feature of the literature of bioethics. It was a hallmark of the debate: Researchers would describe new discoveries in genetic science, and bioethicists would describe the attendant dangers. This can be illustrated well in the first (1995) edition of the *Encyclopedia of Bioethics,* in which researchers (Whitney, Anderson and Friedman) delineate, with clear enthusiasm, the emerging science of the mapping of the human genome—at that point just begun as a project, and philosophers, (Flew, Shweder, Juengst and Walters) raise the specter of Nazis, insurance company misuse of information, "playing God," and making "designer babies."

Nearly a decade has passed since that edition, five decades from the first discoveries that lead to modern DNA research (Watson, Crick, 1953, Franklin) and three decades from the Asilomar conference on recombinant genetic methodology, in which ethical issues took center stage in genetic research (Soll and Singer, 1973.).

Despite dramatic changes in the scientific knowledge base over the last several decades of the twentieth century, and despite an emerging praxis of medical and agricultural genetics, many of the identical concerns about hubris and post-human futures are persistently raised in bioethical discussions of genetics, and little of the original choreography of the debate has altered. Why this might be the case, and why bioethicists might find genetic knowledge to be fraught with a particular sort of meaning, is the subject of this article.

Knowing and Meaning to Know

Genetic knowing long has implied a moral sense, a way in which we could come to know, utterly, and with certainty, our human selves. Thus genetic testing becomes the first issue of concern, and remains one of the most troubling ones. Genetic testing is where the process of differentiation begins, and is the most direct and immediate way that genetic knowledge inserts into the particular and individual lives of most members of society. Genetic testing leads to application as soon as it leaves the realm of the laboratory, and its rationale is only evident in application. If humans are constituted in particular and tangible physical ways, and if one comes to understand particular facts as expressing the very truth of one's being (things like gender, or size, or impulse regulation), then knowing more precisely or more clearly who one is implies that one might know more precisely what to do. One might, through knowing who one is more exactly, know the scope of possible actions. This could produce knowledge about how to live morally, how to construct the artifice of social order with compassion, wisdom, and insight. Further, the self might well be altered as humans alter other species. If humans can alter our species in the way that we can alter other parts of the natural world once thought immutable, the question emerges: how can we do so in a just and thoughtful manner?

One can argue at this juncture that it has always been the case that all science involves this sort of venture of self generation, and many have noted that genetic knowledge is a matter of more facts amassed, as opposed to a greater interpretive power (Jonson). In this argument, genetic knowledge is not unlike the new understanding of gametes that took place in the middle of the 1800s, a form of understanding of human reproduction that implicated theology as well as science. The shift from Aristotelian notions of the beginning of life to theories first developed when lenses could be ground and microscopes constructed allowed a democracy of meanings to be attached to reproduction. Large shifts in understanding occurred throughout the seventeenth, eighteenth, and nineteenth centuries. Darwinian explanations marked ontological revolutions as well as epistemic ones, disrupting and destabilizing fixed philosophical, social, and theological ways of understanding nature and moral location.

Maynard Olson argues that the understanding and interpretation of the double helix is another such leap in self understanding, and a prelude to even more potentially destabilizing—or potentially liberating—ways of organizing human societies. If humans' sense of ourselves as both free and freely choosing rests on a detachment from our bodily selves, it will be likely come to be seen as mistaken. We are, in this genomic age, as much shaped by this understanding of ourselves as genetically capacitated as we are by the understanding of ourselves as having souls and psyches.

Assembling Knowledge

Genetics suggests a set of ideas about the nature, goal, and purpose of human life. It suggests, then, a definition of the self relative to the human location in the phenomenological universe. Like all science, genetic science suggests a method—not only a set of facts, but a way of ordering, framing, and using the facts. Genetics—with the goal of understanding a large and complex phenomena, organism, or mechanism—seems to demand understanding, defining, and naming all the parts of the thing, knowing the smallest discreet part of the whole, and knowing how the activities of each part connect. Hence, the task is to define the parts list and the function of each part, as a way of describing the activities of the phenomena. What genetic science threatens are not only the ideal forms, but the relationships and activities of phenomena in the actual, moving, and existing world.

The search for atoms and wave particles in physics parallels the search for genes and chromosomes in biology. Genetics functions on the basic idea that pieces of the whole need to be fully understood, and that a reconstruction of both the structure and functional pathways of each event within the whole is critical to the organizing principle itself: Parts determine the whole. Further, like all knowledge, the fulcrum of genetics lies against the notion that naming and defining creates being and allows for possession: Names determine relationships. To name a thing is to define its identity, and hence to identify it as a thing that can be owned, exchanged, used, bought, and sold.

Finally, like all knowledge, genetics is also about power and control (of the unknowable future, of the unknowable body, and of the unknowable other). Genetics understands itself by disassembly, through the knowing and naming activity, done primarily by mapping in the lab and testing in the clinic. It is a critical Hellenistic notion that making is knowing and in the creation of a "working parts list" and a "manual," one can know the essence of the thing (Peters, 2002). The idea that having a parts list then assumes assembly is both what is intriguing and troubling about the meaning of genetics (Fleishacker). At the beginning of the twenty-first century, the hopes for the next logical stage—reassembly—were merely theoretical, yet the prospect of manufacture seems inevitable and troubling to many critics.

The result of such reassembly—a commodity without human connection, named as a clone or as a designer baby—haunts the field, and this specter transforms the debates about genetic testing into something far larger. It becomes a debate in which knowing *which one am I?* becomes a kind of knowing *who could I be?* In this scenario, if one creates an object rather than a human person, one could have an unjust power over the production. Hence, genetic knowledge, testing, and even basic research stands in for the clinical results of the research at its farthest reach. Meaning and mythos overcome actual science, as ethicists and society look at the next stage. The sense of the power behind the discourse has driven both the enthusiasts of genetic science and the catastrophists.

The concerns about the meaning of genetic knowledge center around five topical areas: issues of identity; issues of relationships and kinship; issues of health/illness, ability/disability; and issues of justice. Identity is at the core of reflections on human meaning. Of all the answers to this question of identity, it is perhaps the emerging research and applications of genetic information that offer a definitive response. After the human genome has been fully charted, it will be possible to answer the identity question with a set of mathematical coordinates, an identity bar code that would be distinctly individual. Genetics is, among many other things, a way to name and to describe the processes that make one distinctive and particular. An understanding of how DNA shapes the self unfolds within older contextual ideas about identity. In the words of many that describe the genetic mapping projects, knowing and naming can help us "crack the code of Life," or "tell us who we are and why we behave the way we do," or "explain our traits." The genetic explanation—not the reductionist causality of one gene making one behavior—allows an understanding that genes, proteins, and the environment complexly and intricately signal one another and hence "write" the narrative of human action. If genes and proteins and signals allow for differing levels of biological products in our bodies, and if we react with pleasure, anxiety, or disease to these products, then the horizon of possibilities against which all action is taken is in part suggested by the limits of our creaturely, molecular selves.

The idea that inheritable characteristics determine family ties is an old notion, but the idea that membership in a class of people is similarly determined is an idea that gained ground only in the eighteenth century, when colonial expansion raised the problem of inclusion of others into categories of science. Membership, and hence moral status and social privilege, became linked not to narratives of place, dress, or speech, but rather to something more tangible: the phenotype of persons. This physicality of how one knew what was valid, the linking of truth with the observation of physical facticity, transformed both the science and the polity of modernity.

Identity is paradoxical for Americans. It is a country premised on the idea that who you were did not matter; who your parents were was not the determinant factor in this new land. For many, the radical change in heritage would be the interruption of centuries of closed familial possibilities, and the possibilities of shifting identity that urban and industrial concentrations required. Yet the mutable, spontaneous and creative re-imagining of the self has collided with another narrative, that of a deeply pre-organized and highly structured internal code, a code which, for better or for worse, is passed between generations. Hence, Americans hold two things in tension—that we are free of all previous and unchosen commitments, and that we are increasingly to be understood as having our fate scripted into our very cells.

The Remembrance of History

Paradoxically, what grounds concerns about the speculative future of science is the past—what is called "the shadow of history" (Juengst). Given the emergence of bioethics directly after the trials of the Nazi doctors at Nuremberg, it is not surprising that there is hardly any account of modern genetics that does not begin with a detailed account of the classic tragic and paradigmatic slippery slope of bioethics—the passage of Germany's most imminent scientists from physiologic metrics, to behavioral genetics, to eugenics, mass murder, and torture based on Aryan racial science. The death camps of the Shoah were particularly horrific in their painstaking record on the "science experiments" on the imprisoned Jewish, gypsy, and homosexual subjects, conducted under the rubric of exploring the question of human difference understood as racialized genetic difference.

In the United States, most intellectuals of the Progressive Era held the assumption that breeding was linked to human behavior in the straightforward way that it was linked to animal behavior. Few doubted Francis Galton's extrapolation of Darwin's understanding of hereditary traits, and the widespread acceptance of physical and mental characteristics as hereditary—and thus subject to social engineering—was a feature of arguments from sources as disparate as American socialists and industrialist Henry Ford (Kevles and Hood). The measuring and mapping of the human body was driven by a need to account for conditions of vast social difference, emerging class distinctions made newly apparent by the industrial revolution and colonialism, and to justify such social inequalities with seemingly natural and logical categories (Duster; Gilman). Marking the physical differences between individuals and groups implied a ranking of worth and of deviance; it further implied that danger could be logically eliminated from a world cleansed and purified.

Genetics understood as eugenics could be used as the justifying modern ideology both to encourage "good" (i.e., healthy, large, white, socially obedient, Aryan) births, and to eliminate "sickly" or "weak" (mentally or physically disabled) births and people. While it is clear that the ideas of inheritance, family resemblance, and hereditary have ancient textual and historical power, this marriage of science and tradition clearly amplified the ideology. Hence, fears of the widespread misuse of genetics and its linkage to a "science out of control" were largely formulated in the period 1845 to 1945. This period, and the eugenic sterilizations that peaked in the 1920s and 1930s in the American context (finally ending only in 1973 with *Valerie N. v. State of California*), delineates the concern: since genetics was code for the worst excesses of state discrimination, is not the past inevitable prologue?

Issues of Justice

The idea of difference implies hierarchy. Genetic testing is conducted to find and define the metric of difference from an agreed-upon norm. Critics of genetic testing raise two problems: first, that the idea of testing can be used unfairly as a basis for allocation of scarce goods, such as admission to competitive institutions or privileged social locations (jobs, professional schools, university); second, the very idea of a norm is an invalid one, and one that creates and reifies social hierarchies that destabilize democracy.

One new bioethical argument has been raised by disability advocates. They argue that genetic tests are an imperfect way of understanding humanity. Genetic testing, which notes allelic variation, can point to difference but is not sensitive to how the differences will express in any one human body, nor any one human circumstance or exposure. Further, genetic testing can alert one to differences but cannot alter the genome of the person tested. Used in the context of a prenatal test, each parent must decide if the pregnancy should proceed or if the different genetic code and its attendant disease will create a child with a disability so profound that such a child would be better off having never lived. Then, argue advocates for the disabled, if such a child's life is considered too burdensome, will such a judgment be fatally linked to disabled persons already born? Since at this point only the person and not the genetic

disease can be eliminated, will this have implications for the moral status of the disabled community?

A second troubling aspect of a widening use of genetic knowledge lies at the other end of the possible curve of genetic endowment and the notion of the normal. If researchers could intervene to alter disease-causing genes, might science not go further to enhance traits labeled as desirable? Justice issues arise not only in the classic distributive sense—wealthy individuals and classes of individuals will have a unique access to the first uses of enhancements—but also in the deeper sense that genetic science might disrupt the social compact by introducing such different abilities.

The final issue of justice asks a different genre of question: Will increased genetic knowledge and use of genetic information and interpretation allow for healthcare that is more or less just? There are at least two possible responses. First, as noted above, enhancement or differential access to genetics could deepen differences, particularly if such changes are heritable, allowing a persistent benefit across multiple generations. But the very quality of genetics that allows for wide applicability may well mean that genetic methods could be both widely available and less beholden. Chronic conditions that could be cured would mean that certain types of drug therapies would not be needed. Justice, argue Alan Buchanan, Daniel Brock, and Norman Daniels (2000), becomes a matter of making just choices rather than adjudicating and adjusting the unfairness of a genetic lottery. Many critical aspects of the problem of justice are not different in meaning from other types of sophisticated, highly technological medical interventions such as organ transplants, chemotherapy, or implantable cardioversion devices, which allow for similarly vast differences between persons, countries, and healthcare system membership. Genetic medicine can seem to be paradoxically more unjust precisely because it has the potential to become far more widespread in application, and because of its heritable character.

Issues of Relationships and Kinship

Linked to the issue of identity are the issues of family, kinship, and citizenship. Increasingly, genetic identity is used as a way of describing these sorts of relationships. Families in earlier historical periods defined the boundaries of love and relationship. With each new genetic advance from in vitro fertilization to cloning, the question is raised about whether bonds of love and family would be severed, and in some extreme accounts, the question of whether both genders would be needed at all, as genetic materials that carry identity could be disaggregated and reassembled at will, without regard to family bonds.

Genetic science made significant progress in the years around the turn of the twenty-first century. The Human Genome Project, which provoked concern in many bioethicists, had been largely completed by 2003, and many more genetic tests are available and even commonplace in prediagnostic use. Further, the field of population genetics has emerged as a new force in medicine, anthropology, and popular culture via genealogy. Genes and genetic testing have become a feature not only of the clinical world, but of the world in which families search for roots to their past history. The search for roots has long been a part of establishing authenticity, and in the twentieth century this search for roots became a popular staple of fiction and culture, with genetic testing kits to find ancestry available through the Internet. For many groups, searches for genealogy were linked to the larger project in which cultures that had been destroyed or threatened were remembered and preserved. Such endeavors are not without scientific grounding: genetic science has noted for years that predictable mutation rates allow for dating when populations reached bottlenecks, encountered plagues, etc. The Y chromosome is slow to change, and single nucleotide polymorphisms (SNPs) can be noted and interpreted and used as markers in human populations. Since each male inherits one Y chromosome from his father, the Y SNP model haplotypes can be and have been used to trace genetic origins.

Specific populations that have attempted to confirm their narratives of origin with genetic testing include the Melungians and the Lemba.

The Melungians are a group of related families in loosely-linked communities in the mountains of Appalachia, called a *tri-racial isolate* by social scientists of the 1930s who wrote the first ethnographic studies to describe them. The Melungians, though, have embraced an origin story that they are really lost Turkish sailors; they have enlisted the resources of the University of Virginia's genetics department to further these claims, and are supported by the Turkish government.

The South African tribe of Bantus called the Lemba, like other tribes in Africa, has claimed ownership of a narrative of Jewish heritage. The Lemba observe a practice curiously distinct from surrounding Muslim or African native traditions: they observe Sabbath, they have menstrual rituals, and they have a particular priestly caste—the Bubas—that hold significantly more leadership. In the case of the Lemba, DNA mapping tests have been preformed, and the distinctive Cohen haplotype occurs in the same frequency as

it does in Ashkenazi Jewish populations; this is very suggestive of a valid claim of Jewish origin.

The question raised by these cases involves the idea of identity: After the genetic tests are completed, will the facts of genetics trump the narratives of inclusion? Will the genetic information disrupt the story and weaken the claim of inclusion, or will it strengthen it?

Identity and Authenticity

This new use of genetic testing has raised a series of intriguing questions. If genetics is what makes one a "real" Native American or a "real" Jew, then is the DNA self the authentic self? Increasingly, DNA testing does establish criminal identity, parentage, and paternity. At stake in this discourse is how one defines and creates identity. In reflecting on this problem, the work of Charles Taylor is useful. Taylor notes that modernity threatens an authentic sense of identity in several ways.

For Taylor, the sense of self is diminished by "three malaises." First is an increasing individualism, the idea that the conscience and the consciousness of the self is shaped by our attachment to freedom understood as autonomy from hierarchy, order, and authority. The self is understood less as a person within a social structure but far more narrowly, and this may well "flatten and narrow our lives, making them poorer in meaning, and less concerned with others or society." Genetic knowledge, in this view, portends an ever greater threat in this direction—it is not just the individual person but her *genes* that seem to direct the will. Taylor's second malaise is the cluster of fears about the use of instrumental reason, technology, and efficiency as both explanatory and justifying. For Taylor, who understands the usefulness and libratory possibility of technology, the critique is still important; he argues that devices, technological solutions, and a cost-benefit strategy will also "flatten" the moral self. Taylor's final concern is that a focus on the value of an atomized self, in a technological world driven primarily by instrumental reason, produces a world with less active citizenship and a diminished moral sense. If one understands that the condition of the world is such that it stands in need of healing and repair, and that medical genetics might well play a critical role in understanding and addressing many disease states, then one can turn to Taylor: "We are embodied agents, living in dialogical conditions, inhabiting time in a specially human way, that is making sense of our lives as a story that connects the past from which we have come to our future projects. That means if we are to properly treat a human being, we have to respect this embodied, dialogical, temporal nature" (p. 106).

For Taylor, the struggle to find the meaning of the authentic self is never fully completed or realized. He is not thinking here primarily of the problem of phenome to genome, but his model allows reflection on a similar set of issues.

Genetic identity is vexed by a concern that science is leading toward a post-evolutionary state, understood by bioinformatics professor Pierre Baldi as the result of an evolution and relationality that could be entirely planned on our collective behalf. If genetic codes and hence knowledge of the gene-protein-phenotype relationship is finite, it all potentially can be known. "[S]ooner rather than later we will know all the letters and genes in the human genomes, all the protein families, as well as their structures and functions … in many ways we are reaching the end of our evolutionary odyssey … All the things that have been created and molded by evolution stand a chance of being seriously challenged" (Baldi, 2003). Baldi's thoughtful optimism may be premature, as others have argued for a more iterative ethics, one that worries step-by-step about the actual thing one can do in science, rather than the problems created by a speculative future scenario (Olsen). Yet meaning is made through one's sense of journey and direction as much as by one's attention to the drama. One understands and makes meaning of genetic knowledge through attention to the past, and to the future, as well as to the present.

Philosopher Bernard Williams considers the novel by Nigel Dennis called *Cards of Identity,* in which "an organization, called the 'Identity Club' engages in making people over, giving them a new past and a new character—a new identity." Williams notes that the key feature in the process was the choice of a new name. For Williams, what matters for identity is the relationship between the many, or the type, and the one, or the particular. Existence can be discontinuous, and identity is not to be confused with role. One's role or social identity is constructed, always shared: "[I]ndeed it is particularly important that it is shared and an insistence on such an identity, (say, Native American) is an insistence on the way that it is shared, by 'social processes'." Williams argues that such an identity, if embraced, is "an aid to living." Here, Williams notes that social identity is understood to be causative: "thought to explain or underlie a lot of the individual's activities, emotions, reactions and in general, life. And such an identity, particularly, if chosen is a search for a sort of a homecoming." Williams argues:

> It is also typical of such identities that they are not just analogous to the classifications of nature, but closely related to nature … they seek to affirm and *origin.…* it is typical in such cases that they have some sense that they are not just opting for one group among others, but … finding something

that was there; or coming home—one kind of obedience to Nietzsche's splendid instruction "become what you are." In such a case, what I have come to lies outside my will, something that is given, although I must choose to take it up. (p. 10)

Identity is political, and it is, for Williams, linked to the project of the Enlightenment itself—a project of understanding and discovery of what was there all the time.

Life in the Imagined Future

Can one, with the human genome mapped, the "parts list" on ready file—not only for humans, but for an increasing range of our favorite or feared animals, plants, and viruses—go beyond the familiar critiques? What does genetic knowledge mean for us now, that we in fact have lived through the calamitous times so feared by critics in the 1990s? What does it mean to think genetically? Is it different than how a philosopher would think in 1955, 1925, 1825, or 1155? What part of this is knowing that human genes make a series of proteins that control pathways of more protein-protein chemical reactions, allowing this author to create and the reader to read these words and allowing them to be seen and stored by other proteins in the neurons? Does it become merely another metaphor, akin to, for example, the culturally ubiquitous metaphor of the body that is formed of clay by a Master Potter's hand? Or does, it, as was predicted in 1995, "make us rethink many of our moral concepts and theories."

In part, moral concepts and theories have been revised with the acquisition of genetic knowledge. Parents and physicians are willing to understand and act on behalf of an embryo on the basis of genetic information alone: they terminate, complete, or choose a particular pregnancy based on prenatal genetic diagnosis. Courts and police find completely credible the notion that samples of DNA at a crime scene can prove that a particular suspect was there and use this to arrest and convict one person, or to free others.

But remarkably, given the level of concern, moral concepts appear to be remarkably resilient. While it is true that new reproductive techniques did change the variety of ways that pregnancies could be begun, the years around the turn of the twenty-first century also saw significant increases in adoption, including interracial and international adoptions, and the evidence that genetic material mattered more than other familial bonds was conflicted. Some of the advanced reproductive technology stressed genetic ties, but others (as in the use of surrogate eggs from young women implanted in older women, or the use of sperm banks) stressed gestational or non-genetic bonds as increasingly important. The last half of the twentieth century was notable both for a deepening sense of ourselves as driven by genetic coding, and for a deepening sense of fundamentalist religious fervor, spirituality, and attention to alternative medicine—quite an unexpected paradox. Genetic rhetoric in the period just after the mapping of the human genome, rather than accentuating perceived racialized divisions, steadily and officially proclaimed our unity as a remarkably coherent human species with highly conserved genetic similarities to other organisms. It has became commonplace to understand that genetic codes matter a great deal, at the same time that it has become commonplace to add that the complexities of environment and epigenetic factors, chaos theory, and randomness also play significant roles.

Conclusion

History, even very recent history, can be held to up to the prognostic ability of bioethicists who reflect on the future and predict its course. How has bioethics as a field done, in this way, against the unfolding of the knowledge only speculated about in the 1990s? To be sure, few if any of the predicted catastrophic or euphoric scenarios have occurred in any empirical way.

Is it prudent to have concerns about the potential consequences of genetic knowledge? To be sure. It has been fears and not faith that have driven the thoughtful design of many of bioethical regulations. Fearsome events may well await us, but the trends have not been in that direction, as a review of the world since the 1990s teaches. To the contrary, the importance of families has not waned, nor have kindred and kind been neglected. Children, as families have chosen to have fewer children overall, remain highly valued, and the bond between generations seems entirely unaffected at least by genetic testing, although there has been increased vigilance in all matters genetic. A deeper sense of faith in the ethical and moral integrity of research and in the core duties of medical science may well be in order.

By 2003, there were new laws, and far more robust ones, that protect privacy and insurance misuse; there also existed national oversight bodies in most industrialized countries, and bodies at the international, national, state, and non-governmental organization (NGO) levels, to regulate or at least publicly examine genetic policies and techniques. Bioethics centers and ethics debate in general flourished at the beginning of the twenty-first century, despite new and pivotal research in genetics taking center stage in many science policy debates. The President of the United States, George W. Bush, made human embryonic stem cells the subject of his first public address, and the U.S. Congress debated the science and ethics of genetic policies, especially cloning and genetic modification. The ethical discourse

about meaning and agency moved from the academic margins to the center of the debate. Decades after James Watson, Francis Crick, Rosalind Franklin, and Linus Pauling moved the chemistry that enabled the basic theory of genetics towards the modern intellectual project of genetic sequencing, and decades after computational and structural biology coalesced this sequence into a credible account of how human persons develop, few would claim a victory for an unreflective position in the debates about the influence of nature versus nurture.

The human genome, our *nature,* is clearly understood as responsive and interactive with the environment, adaptive yet constrained. Few can credibly deny the reality of the genetic-protein explanation of the physical world. It is, for now, the best account of the phenomenological terrain, and it is the text and tool that facilitates the exploration of the details and the variable of our human selves. Will we reach unbreachable ethical boundaries in this terrain? Will the "moral harm" that might exist become too dangerous to contemplate, and will the existence of moral harms outweigh moral duties to simply know and name as much about the world as we can? Are there horizons beyond which we cannot venture, and entities we ought not to know, mysteries that allow humanity to exist? Or have we a human duty to our human curiosity? Can one argue for a duty to heal and in the pursuit of the goal of healing, allow for all knowledge, and all pursuit, no matter where it might lead? Such worrisome questions remain, despite both increased regulatory efforts and a series of gravely sobering and stochastic human events. An article such as this can only hope to highlight competing moral appeals as they emerge in the literature of bioethics and in the literature of science—it cannot hope to solve the quandaries, and humility in prognostication about our genetic future, for good or for ill, would be a wise and prudent path. Genetic knowledge places us in a position of unprecedented choices—not yet about our final telos, but in a very real way, in a position to understand both the gravity and the temptations of the road we travel there.

LAURIE ZOLOTH

BIBLIOGRAPHY

Buchanan, Allen; Brock, Dan; Daniels, Norman; and Wikler Daniel. 2002. *From Chance to Choice: Genetics and Justice.* Cambridge, Eng.: Cambridge University Press.

Cohen, Cynthia B., ed. 1999. *New Ways of Making Babies: The Case of Egg Donation.* Bloomington: Indiana University Press.

Dennis, Carina; Gallagher, Richard; and Watson, James. 2002. *The Human Genome.* Hampshire, Eng.: Palgrave Macmillan.

Duster, Troy. 2003. *Backdoor to Eugenics.* New York and London: Routledge.

Fleischacker, Samuel. 2003. Speech to the Northern Illinois Ethics Consortium.

Gilman, Sander. 2003. *Jewish Frontiers: Essays on Bodies, Histories, and Identities.* New York: Palgrave Macmillan.

Jonsen, Albert R. 2003. *The Birth of Bioethics.* New York: Oxford University Press.

Juengst, Eric T. 1990. "The NIH 'Points to Consider' and the Limits of Human Gene Therapy." *Human Gene Therapy* 1(4): 425–433.

Kevles, Daniel J., and Hood, Leroy; eds. 1992. *Code of Codes: Scientific and Social Issues in the Human Genome Project.* Cambridge, MA: Harvard University Press.

Lauritzen, Paul, ed. 2001. *Cloning and the Future of Human Embryo Research.* New York: Oxford University Press.

Nigel, Dennis. 2002. *Cards of Identity.* Normal, IL: Dalkey Archive Press.

Olson, Maynard. 2003. Speech for the Fred Hutchinson Cancer Research Center in Seattle, WA.

Peters, Ted. 2003. *Playing God?: Genetic Determinism & Human Freedom,* 2nd edition, Forward by Francis Collins. New York and London: Routledge.

Taylor, Charles. 1992. *The Ethics of Authenticity.* Cambridge, MA: Harvard University Press.

Wasserman, David, and Wachbroit, Robert, eds. 2001. *Genetics and Criminal Behavior.* Cambridge, Eng.: Cambridge University Press.

Williams, Bernard. 2002. *Truth and Truthfulness: An Essay in Genealogy.* Princeton, NJ: Princeton University Press.

GENETICS AND RACIAL MINORITIES

• • •

Advances in genetic research such as the completion of the Human Genome Project (HGP) have significant implications for the health of members of racial minority groups. Research on human genetic variation is anticipated to increase biomedical understanding of disease etiology and affect social and cultural meanings of race. In this entry the ethical implications of genetic research for the health of members of racial minorities are discussed. Racial minorities are defined as groups that historically have been identified by race and as a result have limited access to resources and opportunities. This entry discusses the implications of advances in human genetics for the understanding of race and ethnicity and the impact of racial categories on research into human genetic variation. It addresses the effect of these implications on the national priority to decrease health disparities among racial groups in the United States. Discussion topics include genetic determinism and reification of race, the protection of research participants and informed consent, and the distribution of benefits from human genetic research and its implication for justice in regard to the health and well-being of members of racial minorities.

Human Migration, Genetic Diversity, and Race

Since its genesis in the sixteenth century, the concept of *race* as a biological *kind* has been a focal point of debate (Boxill). Controversy over the use of the term has emerged in regard to the values that have been attached to groups identified by race and the characteristics that have been attributed to them. Throughout the twentieth century scholars consistently challenged the validity of biological differences between populations that were linked to race. Scientific research consistently has revealed that more genetic variation exists within than between populations (Lewontin). Despite this finding, race has become increasingly salient in understanding disparities in the health status of population groups and continues to be an important factor in both biomedical research and clinical medicine.

Central to arguments over race is a lack of agreement on its definition. In a manner that often is implicit, biomedical researchers and clinicians use a potpourri of surrogate concepts, including skin color, hair type, national origin, and citizenship, to identify race. This situation is complicated by the common practice of relying on self-reports, which often are based on factors that have little to do with biology. In addition, racial categories change over time and tend to be context-dependent, as is illustrated by the history of U.S. Census racial and ethnic categories (Lee et al.). Since the insertion of the term *race* into scientific discourse, the definition of race has been a moving target, and this has contributed to confusion about its meaning and implications for biomedical research and clinical care.

In 1996 the American Association of Physical Anthropologists issued a statement that included the following assertion: "Pure races, in the sense of genetically homogenous populations, do not exist in the human species today, nor is there any evidence that they have ever existed in the past." Although it acknowledges that differences between individuals exist, the statement emphasizes that those differences are the result of hereditary factors and the effects of natural and social environments. Genetic differences between populations result from the effect of the history of human migration and reproduction and consist of a gradient of varying frequencies of all inherited traits, including those that are environmentally malleable.

Critical to comprehending human genetic variation is an understanding of the meaning of population genetic structure, which is best understood as the pattern of genetic differences among genomes, the full sets of human genes found in the nucleus of each cell. These genes are arranged linearly on chromosomes and consist of strings of chemical units called nucleotides (Weiss). The genome interacts with the environment to produce phenotypes, or all observable traits of individual appearance and behavior. Patterns within the genome vary across a species, depending on the history of mating within that species. The patterns or genetic frequencies of human populations have been affected by mutation, migration, natural selection, and random genetic drift to varying extents. These forces have resulted in the genetic variation that exists among human populations. Genetic differences between global populations do not map neatly onto the racial categories that have emerged through sociohistorical processes. Instead, race, defined by discrete group boundaries, serves as a poor proxy for the continuum of human genetic variation.

Racial Categorization in Human Genetic Variation Research

The completion of the HGP has resulted in new and well-funded themes of scientific inquiry in medicine. A central goal of human genetic research is identifying the genetic and environmental causes of human disease. Recent advances such as high-throughput genomic sequencing technology have increased the efficiency of large-scale rapid genotyping and ushered in a new era of genetic epidemiological research. This research has focused on the identification of single-nucleotide polymorphisms (SNPs). As was discussed briefly above, the genome is specified by the four nucleotide "letters" A (adenine), C (cytosine), T (thymine), and G (guanine) that form patterns. SNP variation occurs when a single nucleotide, such as an A, replaces one of the other three nucleotide letters: C, G, or T. SNPs are believed to be associated with individual differences in susceptibility to disease; environmental insults such as bacteria, viruses, toxins, and chemicals; and drugs and other therapies.

The search for these genetic clues has led to efforts to map SNPs and use that information to identify the multiple genes associated with complex diseases such as cancer, diabetes, vascular disease, and some forms of mental illness. For most SNPs, all populations have all the possible genotypes for a SNP, but populations may differ in regard to the frequencies of individuals with each of the different genotypes.

Although the location of SNPs is believed to hold the key to identifying the genetic basis for the onset of disease and influencing responses to drug therapeutics, it has been posited that SNPs do not travel independently. Instead, SNPs are located in what has been identified as blocks of alleles that are inherited as units. The patterns of the SNP alleles in those blocks are called haplotypes. Studies show that most SNPs are in haplotype blocks that have been transmitted for many generations without recombination. Because each block has only a few common haplotypes, identifying haplotypes eliminates much of the tedious work of attempting to find single SNPs that are correlated meaningfully with disease. In effect, the task of locating frequently elusive needles in the enormous haystack of the human genome has been mitigated by the knowledge that these needles, or SNPs, tend to be located in groups. It is expected that the 10 million common SNPs will be reduced to 200,00 to 300,000 tag SNPs that will signal the location of regions that affect disease more readily through genome scans.

To create a genetic test that will screen for a disease in which the disease-causing gene already has been identified, scientists collect blood samples from a group of individuals affected by the disease and analyze their DNA for SNP patterns. Next, researchers compare those patterns to patterns obtained by analyzing the DNA from a group of individuals not affected by the disease. This type of comparison, which is called a disease gene association study, can detect differences between the SNP patterns of the two groups, indicating which pattern most likely is associated with the disease-causing gene. Eventually, SNP profiles that are characteristic of a variety of diseases will be established. As part of that effort an increasing amount of research has called for the DNA sampling of individuals identified with specific racial minority populations. The collection of DNA samples has resulted in the racial categorization of genetic material stored in governmental and commercial genetic databases.

Scientific Racism and Eugenics: Cautionary Tales

In considering the ethical implications of race in human genetics research, it is prudent to review the lessons learned from the history of scientific racism in medicine. In the United States and abroad scientific racism has resulted in the exploitation of racially identified populations in the name of scientific and medical progress. Although science often has been portrayed as *value-free,* scientific theories have been used to support beliefs in the inferiority of racialized populations. Historically, race began as a biological taxonomy by which humans were categorized according to phenotypic differences such as skin color and facial features and by supposed personality traits. Despite general rejection of such definitions, scientific research is at times compromised by a priori assumptions that build on notions of race as biology.

The term *eugenics,* which was coined by Francis Galton early in the twentieth century, has been incorporated into various state-sponsored programs around the world (Galton). The most notorious of those programs was guided by the German program of *Rassenhygiene,* or "racial hygiene," that led ultimately to the Holocaust. In the early 1900s the eugenics program was promoted through scientific organizations such as the Society for Racial Hygiene and the Kaiser Wilhelm Institute for Anthropology, Human Genetics and Eugenics. Later, when incorporated into Nazi ideology after the rise of Adolph Hitler, the racial hygiene program led to a broad spectrum of egregious scientific experimentation and the eventual extermination of millions of Jews, Gypsies, homosexuals, and other individuals deemed undesirable by the Third Reich (Weigmann).

During that period of state-sponsored racism, other nations, such as Great Britain, Norway, and France, were adopting their own brands of eugenics policies. Eugenics gave scientific authority to social fears and lent respectability to racial doctrines. Powered by the prestige of science, it was coupled with modernizing national projects that promoted claims of social order as objective statements grounded in the laws of nature (Dikotter). Unfortunately, history provides several examples of how the marriage of scientific racism and national political agendas has led to the unfair treatment of socially and politically vulnerable racial minorities. In South America, for example, eugenic policies have been the key to a national revival in which indigenous concerns over racially diverse and socially disparate societies have led to race-based initiatives to regulate human reproduction. Brazil and Argentina have experienced the use of science in the name of forging "superior and cosmic national races" (Stepans).

Perhaps the longest single study involving the exploitation of human subjects in medical research was the Tuskegee Syphilis Study conducted by the U.S. Public Health Service. The study, which was called the Tuskegee Study of Untreated Syphilis in the Negro Male, began in 1932 and did not end until 1972. The study involved the recruitment of over 300 black men with syphilis who were told by researchers that they were being treated for "bad blood," a local term used to describe several ailments, including syphilis, anemia, and fatigue (Jones). Those men did not receive proper treatment even after penicillin became available as an effective therapy in 1943. In exchange for taking part in the study, the men received free medical examinations, free meals, and burial insurance. The Tuskegee Study caused a public outcry that led the assistant secretary for health and scientific affairs to appoint an Ad Hoc Advisory Panel that concluded that the Tuskegee Study was "ethically unjustified" (Brandt). It is a "powerful metaphor that has come to symbolize racism in medicine" (Gamble) and a cautionary tale about the vulnerability of racial minorities in biomedical research.

Ethical Issues of Identifying Race in Genetics

The development of genomic research technologies has the potential for a dramatic enhancement of biomedical prevention and treatment of disease. Efforts to identify genetic mutations associated with disease may yield significant findings that uncover important clues to the onset of common diseases. Critical to these endeavors is a growing need to understand human genetic variation. In the absence of cost-effective ubiquitous genotyping technology, researchers have tended to favor population-based sampling. Strategies of using racially identified populations in the mapping of genetic markers, however, should be viewed with due consideration of the potential ethical implications of such research. Of particular concern are the potential for stigmatization and discrimination, informed consent, and distributive justice.

REIFICATION OF RACE: STIGMATIZATION AND DISCRIMINATION. Historically, race, genetics, and disease have been linked inextricably, producing a calculus of risk. Sometimes these associations are accurate, and sometimes they reflect underlying social prejudice. One risk in medical research is that any racial or ethnic identifiers used in human genetic variation research will come to be reified as biological constructs, fostering a genetic essentialism. This essentialism could obscure the fluid nature of the *boundaries* between groups and the common genetic variation within all groups.

An example is sickle-cell anemia, an autosomal recessive disease that is caused by a point mutation in the hemoglobin beta gene (HBB). It is a condition that has been racialized as a "black disease" in the United States. However, closer scrutiny reveals that the incidence of sickle-cell anemia is associated with zones of high malaria incidence, because carriers of that gene have some degree of protection against malaria. The condition is the result of human migration and the interaction of genes with the environment. Its emergence as a racial disease is an artifact of U.S. history. If the source of slaves to the Americas had been Mediterranean regions, where the incidence of the disease is also appreciably high, rather than from Africa, sickle-cell disease might have become known as a southern European disease. The reification of race results in such conflations.

Stigma and discrimination are potentially harmful consequences that are associated with the reification of race and genetic essentialism, particularly if curative measures are not available. Insurance companies and managed-care organizations in particular have an economic stake in controlling the potential costs of "high-risk" clients (Knoppers). In addition, social prejudice could arise in the identification of correlations between genes and disease. Race may be treated as an independent variable in the calculus of risk and result in real social harms for individuals in regard to the anticipation that they will fall ill.

INFORMED CONSENT: PROTECTING POPULATIONS. Harm from race-based genetic research may extend beyond the individuals at risk for a particular disease if targeted genetic testing implicates socially identifiable groups. Increasing attention to the ethical implications of research on human genetic variation has resulted in a shift of emphasis from individuals to "groups." The question of who should "consent" to genomic research demands a discussion of who are the potential victims of research-related harms (Kass and Sugarman). Although the informed consent process focuses on individual participants in scientific studies, risks stemming from population-based research may affect those who are not direct participants but are implicated by their identification with particular groups (Wilcox et al.; Faden and Beauchamp).

Acknowledgment of such harms has fueled a growing debate over whether individuals alone are sufficient to consent to research participation or whether others who subscribe to or are ascribed membership in a racial group also should participate in this process as potential victims of research (Greely). Several scholars and policy makers have advocated "community consultation," arguing that internal review boards (IRBs) should implement new mechanisms that supplement individual consent with group permission (Weijer; Foster and Sharp; Clayton). Others have countered that giving groups the moral authority to bestow informed consent is conceptually flawed and logistically confusing (Juengst). In dispute are the assumptions that (1) there is a singular, self-evident social body that represents a particular individual human subject, (2) that social body has the moral authority to *speak* for all the members of a particular group, and (3) consultation with that social body absolves researchers of responsibility for prospective harms.

Population-based DNA sampling and the identification of racial minorities in research on human genetic variation have broadened the debate over informed consent. At issue are the responsibilities of researchers and clinicians for preventing future harms associated with knowledge that links race, disease, and genes and the need for the participation of research populations in the scientific process.

DISTRIBUTIVE JUSTICE: THE PROMISE OF PERSONALIZED MEDICINE. The decision to identify race in human genetic research may have important ramifications for the establishment of research priorities that could have implications for helping exacerbate or ameliorate health disparities between groups. An example of such research is the field of pharmacogenomics. It is well recognized that most drug therapies exhibit wide variability among individuals in terms of efficacy and toxicity. It has been estimated that over 100,000 patients die and 2.2 million are injured annually by adverse drug reactions (Lazarou et al.). For many medications differences in reactions are due in part to SNPs in gene-coding drug-metabolizing enzymes, drug transporters, and/or drug targets. The ultimate goal of such research is to develop "individualized" drug therapy that will reduce adverse side effects and provide cost-effective medicines (March et al.)

The adoption of pharmcogenomics has serious implications for the practice of clinical medicine. The population-based approach to the marketing of healthcare products raises the possibility that drug development will build on and strengthen notions of racial difference. Furthermore, *racial thinking* may have ramifications for the perceived beneficiaries of pharmacogenomics research in that racially identified consumer groups may unduly dictate the scientific development of therapeutics. This may lead to a racial segmentation of the market in which drugs are directed at groups in a way that will increase the economic health of the companies investing in therapeutics.

In the unlikely event that genotyping becomes so common that patients are able to identify themselves in terms of the multitude of SNPs involved in disease gene associations and drug metabolism, human genetic variation research will continue to use racially identified populations. Genetic research offers the potential for significant progress toward the mitigation of health disparities between populations in the United States. However, history serves as an important reminder that every leap in scientific advancement must be tempered by careful consideration of its ethical implications.

SANDRA SOO-JIN LEE

SEE ALSO: *Bioethics, African-American Perspectives; Eugenics; Genetic Counseling, Ethical Issues in; Genetic Counseling, Practice of; Genetic Engineering, Human; Genetics and Environment in Human Health; Genetics and Human Self-Understanding; Genetics and Racial Minorities; Genetics and the Law; Harm; Health Insurance; Holocaust; Human*

Dignity; Human Nature; Minorities and Research Subjects; Privacy and Confidentiality in Research; Race and Racism

BIBLIOGRAPHY

American Association of Physical Anthropologists. 1996. "Statement of Biological Aspects of Race." *American Journal of Physical Anthropology* 101: 569–570.

Boxill, Bernard. 2001. "Race and Philosophical Meaning." In *Race and Racism,* ed. Bernard Boxill. Oxford: Oxford University Press.

Brandt, Allan. 1985. "Racism and Research: The Case of the Tuskegee Syphilis Study." In *Sickness and Health in America: Readings in the History of Medicine and Public Health,* ed. Judith Walzer Leavitt and Ronald L. Numbers. Madison: University of Wisconsin Press. Originally published in *Hastings Center Report* 8(6): 21–29.

Clayton, Ellen Wright. 1995. "Why the Use of Anonymous Samples for Research Matters." *Journal of Law, Medicine, and Ethics* 23: 375–377.

Dikotter, Frank. 1998. "Race Culture: Recent Perspectives on the History of Eugenics." *American Historical Review* 103(2): 467–478.

Faden, Ruth, and Beauchamp, Tom. 1986. *A History and Theory of Informed Consent.* New York: Oxford University Press.

Foster, Morris, and Sharp, Richard. 2000. "Genetic Research and Cultural Specific Risks—One Size Does Not Fit All." *Trends in Genetics* 16(2): 93–95.

Galton, Francis. 1897 "Eugenics: Its Definition, Scope, and Aims." *American Journal of Sociology* 10(1): 1–25.

Gamble, Vanessa. 1997. "Under the Shadow of Tuskegee: African Americans and Health Care." *American Journal of Public Health* 87: 1773–1778.

Greely, Henry. 2001. "Human Genomics Research: New Challenges for Research Ethics." *Perspectives in Biology and Medicine* 44(2): 221–229.

Jones, James H. 1981. *Bad Blood: The Tuskegee Syphilis Experiment.* Collier Macmillan.

Juengst, Eric. 1998. "Groups as Gatekeepers to Genetic Research: Conceptually Confusing, Morally Hazardous and Practically Useless." *Kennedy Institute of Ethics Journal* 8(2): 183–200.

Kass, Nancy, and Sugarman, Jeremy. 1996. "Are Research Subjects Adequately Protected?" *Kennedy Institute of Ethics Journal* 6(3): 271–282.

Knoppers, Bertha. 2000. "Population Genetics and Benefit Sharing." *Community Genetics* 3(4): 212–214.

Lazarou, Jason; Pomerantz, Bruce H.; and Corey, Paul N. 1998. "Incidence of Adverse Drug Reactions in Hospitalized Patients." *Journal of the American Medical Association* 279(15): 1200–1206.

Lee, Sandra Soo-Jin; Mountain, Joanna; and Koenig, Barbara. 2001. "The Meaning of 'Race' in the New Genomics: Implications for Health Disparities Research." *Yale Journal of Health Policy, Law, and Ethics* 1: 33–75.

Lewontin, Richard. 1972. "The Apportionment of Human Diversity." In *Evolutionary Biology,* ed. Theodor Dozhansky.

March, Ruth; Cheeseman, Kevin; and Doherty, Michael, et al. 2001. "Pharmacogenetics—Legal, Ethical, and Regulatory Considerations." *Pharmacogenetics* 2(4): 317–327.

Stepans, Nancy Leys. 1996. *The Hour of Eugenics: Race, Gender, and Nation in Latin America.* Ithaca, NY: Cornell University Press.

Weigmann, Katrin. 2001. "In the Name of Science." *EMBO Reports* 21(101): 871–875.

Weijer, Charles. 1999. "Protecting Communities in Research: Philosophical and Pragmatic Challenges." *Cambridge Quarterly Journal of Health Care Ethics* 8: 501–513.

Weiss, Kenneth. 1995. *Genetic Variation and Human Disease.* Cambridge, Eng.: Cambridge University Press.

Wilcox, Allen J.; Taylor, Jack A.; Sharp, Richard R. 1999. "Genetic Determinism and the Overprotection of Human Subjects." *Nature Genetics* 21(4): 362.

INTERNET RESOURCE

National Center for Biotechnology Information. Available from <http://www.ncbi.nlm.nih.gov/About/primer/snps.html>.

GENETIC TESTING AND SCREENING

• • •

I. REPRODUCTIVE GENETIC TESTING

Reproductive genetic testing comprises a set of techniques for sample collection and analysis, the aims of which are to detect fetal anomaly. This article will describe the most important of these techniques and consider their bioethical aspects. This will include both those reproductive genetic technologies that are used in established pregnancies and preimplantation genetic diagnosis, performed before the establishment of a uterine pregnancy.

Methods for Obtaining Samples for Prenatal Diagnosis

Amniocentesis is frequently used synonymously with the term *prenatal testing*. Amniocentesis is in fact merely a technique for removal, via a needle puncture of the uterus, of amniotic fluid from the sac which surrounds the fetus during pregnancy. This fluid contains fetal cells on which analyses can be performed. The usefulness of amniocentesis is tightly linked to expanding knowledge about genetics, the development of techniques of fetal analysis, and changing legal and social norms.

In 1955, it was first demonstrated that fluid could be removed from the amniotic sac, that fetal cells could then be cultured, and that the total number of chromosomes—including the sex chromosomes—could be ascertained—a process called karyotyping. The first use of karyotyping was to identify male fetuses of women who carried serious genetic conditions on their X chromosome. However, this was initially of limited usefulness as no information other than fetal sex was obtainable, the safety of the procedure needed further investigation, and pregnancy termination for fetal anomaly was not legal.

The later finding that a karyotype showing three rather than two copies of a chromosome (trisomy 21) was indicative of Down syndrome presented the possibility of much broader use for amniocentesis. Not only was Down syndrome an important cause of mental retardation, it was also predicted by a pregnant woman's increasing age rather than by her genetic history. When, in the mid-1970s, a large study demonstrated the safety of amniocentesis (NICHD National Registry for Amniocentesis Study Group) at approximately the same time that the Supreme Court decision in *Roe v. Wade* made abortion legal in the United States, the way was opened to the population-based use of this technique for women of advanced maternal age.

Serious maternal complications from amniocentesis are rare; the primary medical risk of amniocentesis is fetal loss from the procedure. For this reason, the age, at which amniocentesis is routinely offered, is driven by an equation that looks for equipoise between the risk of procedure-related miscarriage and the age-related risk of Down syndrome. It is worth noting that one can infer from this equation an equivalence between the negative outcome of a fetal death and birth of a child with a disability, an equivalence which, as discussed below, would be contested from various positions critical of prenatal testing. Nevertheless, as rates of procedure-related miscarriage have decreased—due primarily to the use of real-time ultrasound to guide the needle—the age at which women are routinely offered amniocentesis has also decreased. At the beginning of the twenty-first century, it is standard of care to offer amniocentesis to women over age thirty-five.

Although amniocentesis is most closely associated with trisomy 21, any chromosomal abnormality can be detected through karyotyping, and the sample of fluid obtained can be used to diagnose any fetal anomaly for which a cytogenetic, biochemical, or DNA test has been developed (e.g., Tay-Sachs, sickle cell anemia, Huntington's disease).

EARLY AMNIOCENTESIS AND CHORIONIC VILLUS SAMPLING. Amniocentesis is performed in the middle of the second trimester of pregnancy. By this time, pregnant women have often experienced *quickening* (perceived fetal movement) and the fetus is nearing the age of viability. These factors have led to a search for earlier modes of fetal sample collection, including first trimester ("early") amniocentesis and chorionic villus sampling (CVS).

Although there was initial enthusiasm for early amniocentesis performed in the eleventh through thirteenth weeks of pregnancy, recent data suggest that this procedure may pose significantly greater fetal risks than traditional amniocentesis, including high rates of pregnancy loss and risk of fetal malformations (e.g., club foot) (Bianchi, 2000). In addition, early amniocentesis is more technically difficult and thus more often will fail to obtain a fluid sample adequate for cell culture. Enthusiasm for the procedure has waned, although it is possible that future solutions to these problems will revitalize interest.

Rather, it is CVS that appears likely to become the procedure of choice for earlier fetal sample collection. The chorionic villi are precursors of the placenta and have proved a good source of fetal tissue. CVS can be performed safely as early as the tenth week of pregnancy, either transabdominally or transvaginally; the risks have been found to compare well with second trimester amniocentesis (Bianchi, 2000). In addition, the waiting period for results following CVS is shorter than in amniocentesis—three to eight rather than ten to fourteen days. Since there is considerable documented anxiety for parents waiting for prenatal test results, this represents a significant advantage.

MATERNAL SERUM FETAL CELL RECOVERY. Both CVS and amniocentesis are invasive techniques. They share disadvantages of potential fetal harm and are relatively costly to perform. Thus, there continues to be interest in finding a non-invasive, less expensive technique that could be used to gather a fetal sample early in pregnancy. There is only one such technique on the horizon in 2003—maternal serum fetal cell recovery.

It is known that a small number of fetal cells are sloughed off and cross into maternal blood circulation. After isolation from a maternal blood draw, these cells can then be used for any desired fetal analysis. However, fetal cells are numerically rare in maternal blood and their identification and isolation is difficult. In addition, the type of cell most amenable to detection and isolation is not ideal for chromosomal analysis (Holzgreve and Hahn). Nevertheless, work on this technique progresses and a prospective multi-center trial of this technique as a screen for chromosomal anomalies began in the mid-1990s (Bianchi, 2002). Early results were promising for chromosome analysis, but the future goal of fetal cell recovery remains broader than this: To be able to perform not only analysis of chromosomal abnormalities, but to capture the larger number of fetal cells needed for DNA techniques. This goal holds the promise of genetic analysis for any disorder of interest.

Screening Tests and Diagnostic Tests

The above techniques are used for diagnosis in high-risk women. But almost all pregnant women are offered a variety of other prenatal screening tests.

Although the distinction quickly becomes complicated, in its simplest form, screening tests are offered to a population of apparently healthy persons in order to find those few at increased risk. Ideally, screening tests are easy and inexpensive to perform and interpret, and do not entail risk for the person screened. Screening tests have high rates of initial positive results and thus a large percentage of people who have positive screening tests will prove not to have the screened-for problem on follow-up diagnostic testing.

In contrast, diagnostic tests are offered to individuals known to be at increased risk of a condition in order to answer the question, "Does this person have this disease?" Diagnostic tests are generally more complicated and expensive to perform and interpret, and may entail risk. They are expected to have higher standards of sensitivity and specificity: to do a much better job at identifying all and only cases of the disorder.

The screening and diagnostic testing regimens typically offered to pregnant woman and couples at the beginning of the twenty-first century are presented in Table 1. Each begins by asking a question that assigns the woman to a risk level. It is important to realize that each screening test has its own percentage of initial positive results; thus, each additional screen raises the risk for any individual woman of getting an initial positive result at some time during pregnancy. In addition, these tests are not all done at the same time in pregnancy. For example, an African-American woman,

less than thirty-five years old, would be offered carrier testing for sickle cell disease in her first trimester and would also be offered multiple marker screening in her second trimester.

MSAFP and Multiple Marker Screening

While amniocentesis for Down syndrome is perhaps better known, the test which truly revolutionized prenatal diagnosis was maternal serum alpha fetoprotein (MSAFP) screening, which became the first screening test offered to all pregnant women solely for the purpose of discovering risk for a fetal anomaly.

MSAFP screening was developed to detect neural tube defects (NTDs) in the fetus. NTDs comprise a set of defects involving the development of the brain and spine and leading to varying degrees of physical and cognitive impairment, some of which are incompatible with life; they are among the most common of serious birth defects. Finding fetal NTDs is complicated by the fact that over 90 percent occur to women at no known risk, making it necessary to offer testing to the entire population of pregnant women to detect any reasonable percentage of fetal NTDs.

Alpha fetoprotein is a substance produced by the developing fetus and present in maternal blood during pregnancy. In the early 1970's, it was found that higher than normal levels of MSAFP correlated with increased risk of fetal NTDs. This suggested the possibility of an inexpensive, minimally invasive, screening modality for NTDs (Brock, Bolton, and Monaghan).

In the 1980's, researchers linked lower than normal levels of MSAFP to Down syndrome and other chromosomal abnormalities, thus expanding the utility of the test (Merkatz, Nitowsky, Macri, et al.). Early pilot projects demonstrating the feasibility of MSAFP testing increased enthusiasm for it as a prenatal screening test, and the screening became firmly established as standard of care in the United States when an American College of Obstetrics and Gynecology "Legal Alert" warned obstetrical providers that failure to offer the test might leave them open to liability in the case of a baby born with a detectable anomaly (ACOG, 1985).

However, one concern about using MSAFP to detect Down syndrome was that it had much lower sensitivity and specificity for chromosomal abnormalities that it did for NTDs. When it was found that the addition of other biochemical markers improved the ability of the screen to predict Down syndrome, these quickly became added to the analysis. Most providers perform multiple marker screening, with a *triple marker* screen including human chorionic gonadotrophin and unconjugated estriol being the most common. Since all these analytes are gathered from the same

TABLE 1

Current Screening Practices

Screening question	Answer	Next Step	Next Step	Next Step
What is your age?	>35	Referral for amniocentesis/CVS		
Is there any genetic disorder in your family?	Yes	Referral for carrirer testing **or** amniocentesis/CVS *(Depending on characteristics of the disorder and the mode of genetic transmission)*		
What is the race/ ethnicity/country of origin of woman (and partner)?	African-American	Offered sickle cell carrier testing	If both partners are carriers, referral for amniocentesis/CVS	
	Ashkenazi-Jewish	Offered Tay-Sachs (and possibly an Ashkenazi-Jewish panel, including, e.g. Canavan disease) carrier testing	If both partners are carriers, referral for amniocentesis/CVS	
	Southeast Asian, Greek Southern Italian	Standard blood work-up looking for anemia may be used to suggest need for a next step	Offered alpha or beta thalassemia carrier testing	If both partners are carriers, referral for amniocentesis/CVS
	European-American	Offered cystic fibrosis carrier testing; some places may make this offer to ALL pregnant women	If both partners are carriers, referral for amniocentesis/CVS	
Are you beginning prenatal care <16 weeks of pregnancy	Yes	Offered multiple marker screening	If result is positive HIGH, referred for ultrasound If result is positive LOW, referred for amniocentesis	If result is inconclusive, referred for amniocentesis
Suggested one-age screening protocol				
Are you beginning prenatal care in the first trimester?	Yes	Offered PAPP-A screening, adjusted by maternal age, and ultrasound to assess fetal nuchal translucency	If joint results are positive, referred for amniocentesis	

SOURCE: Author.

blood sample, the test has not changed from the point of view of the pregnant woman.

One important aspect of multiple marker screening is that it cannot be done until the fifteenth week of pregnancy, and most women are screened at sixteen weeks and above. This means that diagnostic work-up for a positive test is done toward the end of the second trimester, and a woman who wanted to terminate a pregnancy based on the results of a diagnostic test would be facing a late second trimester termination.

Suggestions for a One-Age Screening Protocol

Since the 1970s, maternal age has been used as a screen for offering amniocentesis to pregnant women, with biochemical screening offered to younger women since the late 1980s.

However, there is debate about these guidelines (see, for example, Rosen, Kedar, Amiel, et al.; Haddow, Palomaki, Knight, et al.; Pauker and Pauker; Egan, Benn, Borgida, et al.; Dommergues, Audibert, Benattar, et al.). This controversy seems to be based largely on the trend toward women bearing children at later ages (from 1974 to 1997, the United States has seen a 2.7-fold increase in live births among women ages 35–49) (Egan, et al.). This age increase means a dramatic increase in the number of amniocenteses performed, with concomitant procedure-related losses and economic costs.

The most radical suggestion for changing the routine is to screen women of all ages in an identical manner (see last row of Table 1). The most promising of such approaches include ultrasound measurement of the thickness of subcutaneous edema in the neck of the fetus (fetal nuchal translucency) combined with new types of serum marker screening (e.g., PAPP-A). When these techniques are performed in the first trimester of pregnancy, and the results are combined with the risk based on maternal age alone, this regimen is believed to have an 80 to 90 percent detection rate for trisomy 21 and other chromosomal abnormalities (Nicolaides, Heath, and Liao). Although fetal nuchal translucency screening has not been accepted as standard of care, the American College of Obstetrics and Gynecologists stated at the end of the twentieth century that it shows promise (1999).

The advantages of a single screening modality for women of all ages are that it would decrease the number of amniocenteses in older women and, with these more sensitive screening modalities, also increase the detection rate in younger women. (In terms of raw numbers, younger women have the greatest number of affected pregnancies.) Several sets of modeling data suggest that with this approach the overall detection rate would improve and the fetal loss rates would decrease (Rosen, Kedar, Amiel, et al.; Haddow, Palomaki, Knight, et al.; Dommergues, Audibert, Benattar, et al.). The disadvantage, however, would be that, since amniocentesis has a virtual 100 percent sensitivity, some fetuses with Down syndrome that would have been detected through universal screening of women over thirty-five would be missed, and some women over thirty-five would bear a child with Down syndrome who would not otherwise have done so. The ethical, and political, debates concern the fact that a medical service that was accepted as a right for pregnant women of a certain age would be withheld from those same women unless they had demonstrated risk. This may well appear to be an unacceptable form of sudden healthcare rationing to older pregnant women.

It is also worth noting that none of these one-age screening models refer to the detection of neural tube defects, but rather appear to exist in a separate universe of consideration and calculation. Thus, they would not solve the problem of multiple screenings and multiple chances for initial positive results and concomitant anxiety.

Prenatal Screening and the Experience of Pregnancy

The advent of MSAFP screening transformed the experience of pregnancy for the *low risk* woman—that is, the great majority of pregnancies. As is clear from Table 1, it is possible for a woman to go through a period of waiting for results of one test only to then begin all over again with testing for another condition. For example, a thirty-year old Southeast Asian woman might have a standard blood work-up that revealed anemia, be offered thalassemia carrier testing along with her partner, and, when both proved to be carriers, be offered CVS; she might have a negative result and then, some weeks later, be offered multiple marker screening and receive a positive result; she might then choose to undergo amniocentesis. All of this could produce a healthy baby and a disastrously upsetting and expensive pregnancy. There appear to be no empirical data on the frequency of such experiences. However, variations on this theme are frequently reported by obstetric providers.

General Ethical Issues in Prenatal Diagnosis

In addition to the issues involved in one mode of screening or another, there are overarching ethical issues that concern the entire project of prenatal diagnosis. These involve contestations over the meaning, experience, and implications of these tests. Specifically, there is a lack of clarity about the centrality of pregnancy termination to an offer of prenatal testing; whether testing resolves or creates maternal anxiety; and the relationship of individual reproductive choices to societal effect. This latter includes the effects of prenatal testing on those with disability and, more broadly, the relationship between prenatal screening programs and eugenics. Related to the latter is a question about the effectiveness of individual autonomous choice as a safeguard against eugenic abuses related to prenatal testing. All these issues affect and are affected by the lack of a mechanism for rational deliberative decision-making in the United States about why and which prenatal tests are developed and offered.

PRENATAL TESTING AND ABORTION DECISION MAKING. The performance of any medical test is predicated on a hypothesis of benefit which defines the way in which the results of the test will lead to actions that help prevent disease or ameliorate its burden. Implicitly, the person whose disease burden is being ameliorated is the person being tested. Although it is everyone's hope that identification of a fetus with a particular condition will lead to prevention or cure of that disease, this is very rarely true today and the only way to prevent the fetus being born with the condition is through termination of the pregnancy.

Religious objections. From the viewpoint of conservative religious positions that object to abortion under all circumstances, the link of prenatal testing and abortion is clear, and offering women this choice is deeply objectionable.

Cost benefit literature. There is another body of literature in which the centrality of abortion decision making to prenatal testing is quite clear—literature that assesses the effectiveness of testing programs by comparing the economic costs of prenatal testing to economic savings. The costs include such items as sample collection, analysis, and results communication; savings include monies not spent on medical care for children who would have been born with disability but instead are not born. One of the major variables in the equation is the minimum number of women who need to choose termination in order for the screening program to be cost-effective, assuming that not all women who test positive will go on to end the pregnancy. Thus, the calculation both acknowledges the autonomous choice involved in prenatal screening programs in the United States and the need for those autonomous choices to lean, in sum, in the direction of pregnancy termination.

However, most literature that discusses the benefits of prenatal testing talks about the reassurance provided about the health of the fetus for the large majority of women—those who test negative—and the chance for women or couples who choose not to terminate to prepare emotionally for the birth of child with a disability. Generally stated last is the enhancement of *reproductive choice* in the case of a positive test result.

REASSURANCE AND ANXIETY. The issue of reassurance and, conversely, anxiety in relation to prenatal testing has received considerable attention. Women themselves often cite *reassurance* as a benefit of testing. Much empirical research has focused on the issue of anxiety for that group of women who receive an initial positive result. These data suggest that women's anxiety is raised following a positive result but that, in general, this anxiety is relieved by a negative result. Data suggest that for some women, however, the anxiety persists, along with difficulty believing their fetus is healthy.

Some feminist critics also suggest an irony in which the reassurance provided by testing may be necessary, in great part, due to anxiety raised by the testing itself. In general, these critics claim that the expansion of prenatal testing has radically changed the experience of pregnancy and that while the number of fetal anomalies has, of course, not increased, the perception of risk among pregnant women has increased greatly.

INFORMATION PROVISION. Another aspect of prenatal testing, sometimes cited by theoretical literature and pregnant women as an advantage for those unwilling to terminate a pregnancy, is the opportunity to have time to prepare emotionally for the birth of a child with a disability. However, there are no empirical data demonstrating that advance preparation actually has an effect on adjustment to the birth of a child with a disability. In addition, the majority of women who receive positive results do terminate their pregnancies. Data suggest that close to 90 percent of women terminate following a diagnosis of a chromosomal

disorder such as trisomy 21; the rate of termination for NTDs is more variable, reflecting the greater variation in the severity of the detected anomaly (Cragan, Roberts, Edmonds, et al.).

Thus, the most obvious advantage of prenatal testing must remain the ability to terminate a pregnancy which would result in a child with a disability. This suggests that the bifurcated conversation in the United States about prenatal testing—in which cost effectiveness calculations make assumptions which are omitted or contradicted in the clinical literature and most patient education materials—may make it difficult to have a societal conversation about the larger effects of prenatal testing on society.

The Effects of Individual Reproductive Choices on Society

In addition to advantageous or deleterious effects on individual women and couples, concerns exist about the effects of prenatal testing on society.

THE DISABILITY CRITIQUE. The most forceful critique of prenatal testing is that made by disability theorists (Parens and Asch). Their most straightforward claim is that prenatal testing represents "search and destroy" missions against those who would be born with disability and is, simply, a eugenic program. A more subtle disability critique states that the choice to abort an otherwise desired fetus on the basis of one trait or characteristic sends the message that the lives of those with disability are not valuable and that the disability makes the child unacceptable (Asch and Geller); this has been termed the *expressivist argument.* Objections to the expressivist argument share a skepticism about the ability of individual acts to constitute a message. Objections to the disability critique in general often point to the increasing societal protections of individuals with disability that have co-occurred with the growth of prenatal testing.

THE LIMITS OF AUTONOMY. The argument that prenatal testing is not eugenic and not disvaluing of living individuals with disability rests largely on the way that testing programs protect the autonomy of women's or couple's decisions in regard to the use of testing and test results. A central ethical issue, therefore, concerns the actuality and the limits of such autonomy. Specifically: Are women or couples making autonomous decisions in regard to prenatal testing? Can the aggregate effect of autonomous choices be eugenic? And, if they can, how problematic is this?

Are prenatal testing decisions truly autonomous? Individual autonomy is a foundational principle in Western bioethics, and there is virtually universal agreement that women and/or couples should make informed decisions about the use of testing and should not be coerced into pregnancy terminations following a positive prenatal test. The disagreement that exists, therefore, is about the possibility and actuality of such autonomy.

On a narrow level, there is concern that women do not understand the implications of an offer of prenatal testing; this has led to attempts to improve the informed consent process. Yet empirical research suggests that such attempts are only partly successful in the prenatal testing arena, as is true of informed consent in general. Empirical data suggest that, especially *low risk* women who are offered prenatal testing in a context of routine prenatal care, are likely to conflate prenatal testing for fetal anomalies with tests which can directly benefit themselves and their fetus (Press and Browner). It is possible that this misunderstanding is enabled by healthcare providers who are likely to find greater liability risk in the woman who refuses testing and has a baby born with a disability than one who does not fully understand the implications of prenatal screening and participates regardless; it may also reflect a reluctance on the part of both providers and pregnant women to discuss pregnancy termination. Some critics suggest, however, that some women would not have started down the prenatal testing path if they had truly understood the implications in terms of pregnancy termination; they argue that this may represent a compromise of their autonomy.

A broader concern is that the very existence of large-scale prenatal testing compromises the possibility of individual autonomous decision making. Feminist critics, among others, point out that prenatal screening has become routinized, with an offer of some sort of prenatal screening standard of care for all pregnant women. These critics assert that in this setting, not being screened, while a possible choice, becomes a marked one that requires justification to one's healthcare providers and one's peers. Concern has also been expressed that mothers who decide to forgo testing and give birth to a child with a disability will be blamed by society and even, perhaps, denied healthcare insurance for the child. There is little empirical support at this time for these latter claims.

Can the aggregate impact of autonomous choices be eugenic? Even if each choice to use prenatal testing and terminate a pregnancy is informed and autonomous, the net effect might be considered eugenic. And, in fact, there are those who do not consider this to be problematic. Thus, for example, some public health statements clearly cite the measure of success of screening for neural tube defects as the lowering of the number of children born with these defects. Some bioethicists also suggest that eugenics, premised on individual, autonomous choices, is not necessarily bad.

How Are Decisions About Prenatal Test Offers Made?

These positions would seem to require a clear social consensus of what changes in the gene pool would be *eu*-genic. Yet, at the turn of the twenty-first century there exists no body in the United States, as there is in other countries, that decides on the available panel of prenatal tests. Nor is there a forum for public discussion of this issue. Some tests stumble into becoming standard of care due to medico-legal concerns (e.g., MSAFP testing). At other times, decisions are made on an ad hoc bases. Thus, a strongly perceived need by obstetric providers for guidance about cystic fibrosis (CF) screening led to the convening of an National Institutes of Health (NIH) Consensus Development Conference. This group recommended the routine offer of CF carrier screening in pregnancy, but concerns that physicians were not prepared for this change in practice led to the creation of an ad hoc panel charged with creating recommended protocols for implementation (National Institutes of Health Consensus Development Conference). The existence of the panel has not calmed concerns that physicians are not ready to meet the challenge of offering a new population-based test.

As genes for Mendelian disorders and those that confer susceptibility to more common disorders are found in increasing numbers, the lack of any orderly process from gene discovery to test development and then to making that test available to the public becomes increasingly problematic. At this point, healthcare providers are the de facto gatekeepers, relying on recommendations from professional organizations, actions of insurance payers, patient demand, and their own consciences in making decisions about what tests to offer. As genetic knowledge increases, this will become an ever more pressing societal problem.

Preimplantation Genetic Diagnosis

If prenatal testing is about which children will not be born, preimplantation genetic diagnosis (PGD) can be said to be about which children will be born.

PGD began as an alternative to prenatal testing for fertile couples known to be at high risk of genetic disease. It comprises a series of highly technical steps. The scenario involves inducing superovulation in the woman to increase the number of eggs in one reproductive cycle, the harvesting of those eggs, and the creation of six to eight embryos by in-vitro fertilization (IVF). In the most common protocol, the resulting embryos are allowed to develop until they reach the eight- to twelve-cell stage, and then one or two cells are removed from each embryo for genetic analysis. Those embryos that carry the genetic defect are discarded. Depending on the number of unaffected embryos, some or all are implanted. Which embryos are chosen and what happens to those that remain are issues of ethical contention.

Many issues raised by PGD are outside the scope of this article. However, two issues raised by PGD are also directly related to dilemmas discussed in the context of prenatal diagnosis: First, what is abortion? Second, how does one decide which babies will be born, and with what traits and/or diseases?

WHAT IS ABORTION? One of the advantages commonly cited for PGD is that it avoids the problem of abortion. This assumes a definition of abortion as the interruption of an established pregnancy. However, abortion can also be defined as "the arrested development of an embryo at a more or less early stage" (from the *Random House Dictionary of the English Language*), a definition which would include the discarding of embryos, affected or unaffected, within PGD. It would also appear that those individuals (and points of view) most uncomfortable with abortion in the prenatal setting would be most likely to endorse this broader definition of abortion and thus be unlikely to see PGD as a solution to the abortion issue.

WHICH BABIES WILL BE BORN? PGD involves an issue not raised by prenatal diagnosis—more embryos are produced by PGD than can be used. The existence of these "excess embryos" demands that criteria be found on which to predicate decisions about which children should be born. Although, in practical terms, these decisions are often made on the basis of simply finding sufficient unaffected embryos for implantation, the possibility of deciding which embryos to implant has provoked considerable discussion. For example, is it appropriate to base a decision about which of two unaffected embryos to implant based on the preference of the parents for a child of one sex rather than the other?

Some of the discussion of how to choose embryos for implantation has a proscriptive edge, such as the view that to bring to birth a child with any impairment, however slight, if it could have been avoided, is to harm the child; more categorical is the view that procreative beneficence demands the selection of the "best" children. The logical extreme of this latter position is suggested by the view that "the question is not which individuals have worthwhile lives, but which of two possible worlds would be better: a world where disabled individuals are brought to birth or a world where non-disabled individuals are brought to birth" (Bennett, p. 468).

Much of this sort of discussion belies a belief in the ability of genetic analysis to do things that are neither currently possible nor likely to be so in the future—for example, to isolate the embryo that will become the most intelligent child. Nevertheless, these openly eugenic views,

which are not found in the literature on prenatal testing, would appear to be premised on the belief that abortion is not involved in PGD and that the choice involves a more acceptable *selection for* rather than *selection against*. However, such an assumption would likely not satisfy those who have the most concerns about abortion. And for those critics (see, for example, the feminist and disability critiques) whose concerns do not involve abortion, this discussion around PGD lays bare the eugenic thrust they see in all prenatal testing.

Conclusion

Discussions of both prenatal testing and preimplantation genetic diagnosis appear to assume that the continuing march of reproductive technology is inevitable. It is possible that the overriding issue in all of reproductive genetics is whether society will see the development and use of these techniques as matter for democratic deliberation and decision, or whether the implementation of new technologies will continue in the established piecemeal fashion, and ethical discussion will continue to be reactive.

NANCY PRESS

KILEY ARIAIL

SEE ALSO: *Abortion; Cloning: Reproductive; Disability; Embryo and Fetus; Eugenics; Eugenics and Religious Law; Genetic Counseling, Ethical Issues in; Genetic Counseling, Practice of; Genetic Discrimination; Maternal-Fetal Relationship; Mistakes, Medical; Moral Status; Reproductive Technologies; Value and Valuation;* and other *Genetic Testing and Screening* subentries

BIBLIOGRAPHY

American College of Obstetrics and Gynecology (ACOG). 1985. "Professional Liability Implications of AFP Tests." DPL Alert. Washington, D.C.: Author.

American College of Obstetrics and Gynecology (ACOG). 1999. "First-trimester Screening for Fetal Anomalies with Nuchal Translucency: ACOG Committee Opinion." Washington, D.C.: Author.

Asch, Adrienne, and Geller, Gail. 1996. "Feminism, Bioethics, and Genetics." In *Feminism and Bioethics: Beyond Reproduction*, ed. Susan M. Wolf. New York: Oxford University Press.

Bennett, R. 2001. "Antenatal Genetic Testing and the Right to Remain in Ignorance." *Theoretical Medicine and Bioethics* 22(5): 461–471.

Bianchi, Diana W.; Crombleholme, Timothy M.; and D'Alton, Mary E. 2000. *Fetology: Diagnosis & Management of the Fetal Patient.* New York: McGraw-Hill Medical Publishing Division.

Bianchi, Diana W.; Simpson, Joe Leigh; Jackson, L.G.; et al. 2002. "Fetal Gender and Aneuploidy Detection Using Fetal Cells in Maternal Blood: Analysis of NIFTY I Data. National Institute of Child Health and Development Fetal Cell Isolation Study." *Prenatal Diagnosis* 22(7): 609–615.

Brock, D. J. H.; Bolton, A. E.; and Monaghan, J. M. 1973. "Prenatal Diagnosis of Anencephaly through Maternal Serum-alphafetoprotein Measurement." *The Lancet* 2(7835): 923–924.

Cragan, Janet D.; Roberts, Helen E.; Edmonds, Larry D.; et al. 1995. "Surveillance for Anencephaly and Spina Bifida and the Impact of Prenatal Diagnosis—United States, 1985–1994." *Morbidity and Mortality Weekly Report, Centers for Disease Control Surveillance Summary* 44(SS–4): 1–13.

Dommergues, Marc; Audibert, Francois; Benattar, Clarisse; et al. 2001. "Is Routine Amniocentesis for Advanced Maternal Age Still Indicated?" *Fetal Diagnosis and Therapy* 16: 372–377.

Egan, James F. X.; Benn, Peter; Borgida, Adam F.; et al. 2000. "Efficacy of Screening for Fetal Down Syndrome in the United States from 1974 to 1997." *Obstetrics and Gynecology* 96(6): 979–85.

Haddow, James E.; Palomaki, Glenn E.; Knight, George J.; et al. 1994. "Reducing the Need for Amniocentesis in Women 35 Years of Age or Older with Serum Markers for Screening." *New England Journal of Medicine* 330(16): 1114–1118.

Holzgreve, Wolfgang, and Hahn, Sinuhe. 2001. "Prenatal Diagnosis Using Fetal Cells and Free Fetal DNA in Maternal Blood." *Clinical Perinatology* 28(2): 353–65, ix.

Merkatz, Irwin R.; Nitowsky, Harold M.; Macri, James N.; et al. 1984. "An Association between Low Maternal Serum A-fetoprotein and Fetal Chromosomal Abnormalities." *American Journal of Obstetrics and Gynecology* 148(7): 886–894.

National Institutes of Health Consensus Development Conference Statement on Genetic Testing for Cystic Fibrosis. 1999. "Genetic Testing for Cystic Fibrosis." *Archives of Internal Medicine* 159(14): 1529–39.

NICHD National Registry for Amniocentesis Study Group. 1976. "Midtrimester Amniocentesis for Prenatal Diagnosis." *Journal of the American Medical Association* 236: 1471–1476.

Nicolaides, Kypros H.; Heath, Victoria; and Liao, Adolfo W. 2000. "The 11–14 Week Scan." *Ballieres Best Practice & Research* 14(4): 581–594.

Parens, Eric, and Asch, Adrienne, eds. 2000. *Prenatal Testing and Disability Rights (Hastings Center Studies in Ethics).* Washington, D.C.: Georgetown University Press.

Pauker, S.D., and Pauker, S.E. 1994. "Prenatal Diagnosis—Why 35 is a Magic Number." *New England Journal of Medicine* 330(16): 1151–1152.

Press, Nancy, and Browner, C.H. 1997. "Why Women Say Yes to Prenatal Diagnosis." *Social Science and Medicine* 45(7): 979–989.

Rosen, D. J. D.; Kedar, I.; Amiel, A.; et al. 2002. "A Negative Second Trimester Triple Test and Absence of Specific Ultrasonographic Markers May Decrease the Need for Genetic Amniocentesis in Advanced Maternal Age by 60%." *Prenatal Diagnosis* 22(1): 59–63.

II. NEWBORN GENETIC SCREENING

Throughout the United States, and in many other countries around the world, newborns are tested within the first few days to weeks of life for a varying array of metabolic disorders. Until recently, newborns were typically screened for only a handful of disorders, but recent technological advances and new knowledge about genetics have led to pressure for greatly expanded screening. At first glance, newborn screening might seem unremarkable. Much of medical practice is devoted to the early detection of disease to allow the delivery of effective interventions, and new developments are often received enthusiastically. But newborn screening programs have several features that individually and collectively pose particular ethical challenges.

All U.S. states require that newborns be screened, either prior to discharge or, if delivered outside a healthcare facility, within the first two to three days of life (AAP). Maryland, Wyoming, and, for some but not all tests, Georgia and Massachusetts require that parents give their permission for screening, though many states do permit parents to refuse screening (generally for religious reasons). This option may be difficult to exercise in practice, however, since few states require that parents even be told that screening is occurring, much less that they have a right to refuse. Thus, one of more remarkable aspects of newborn screening is that parents are not even nominally part of the decision-making process for their new infants (AAP; Paul; Clayton).

Those who argue against either notifying parents or seeking their permission reason that all children should be screened, and it would thus be a waste of money and effort to talk with parents (Cunningham). Proponents of mandatory screening argue that most parents would agree to screening, but that they might be unduly worried if they knew about the test (Cunningham). They assert further that parents who refuse would be harming their own children. These arguments raise two separate issues: (1) the justifiability of excluding parents, and (2) the characteristics of newborn screening programs (and the disorders they seek).

The Role of Parents

The role of parents in making healthcare decisions for their infants is addressed elsewhere in this encyclopedia. In general, parents are presumed to have a role to play in such decisions, which can be overridden only to avert serious harm. But clinicians cannot decide not to talk with parents simply because they think it would take too much time, would make parents worry, or that it would be a waste of effort because parents usually agree to the clinician's recommendations anyway.

These principles suggest to the advocates of seeking parental permission that parents cannot justifiably be denied the opportunity to be informed about and participate in decisions about newborn screening. Most parents agree to screening, and informed parents are more likely to ensure that screening is performed, as well as to obtain any follow-up that may be required (Andrews). Even if parents refuse screening, it is unlikely that their children will come to harm, for the disorders sought in these programs are very rare.

Newborn Screening Programs

Universal newborn screening was first adopted for phenylketonuria (PKU), an inherited metabolic disorder that causes severe mental retardation unless treatment is started in the first few weeks of life (NAS). Children with this disease have few symptoms early on, but the metabolic abnormality can be detected in the first few days of life by testing either the urine or the blood. Thus, several factors converged to support the idea of early detection:

- The disease has a devastating outcome
- Treatment is highly effective in averting this outcome, but only if it is started early
- Affected children cannot be detected on the basis of symptoms in time to start effective treatment
- Screening reliably detects most affected children (NAS)

When clinicians were slow to adopt these tests in their clinical practice, in part because they were uncertain about the efficacy of treatment, advocates went to their legislators to get them to enact laws requiring PKU screening (AAP; Clayton; NAS).

In the two decades that followed the enactment of these initial laws, the diseases that were added to the testing panels generally had similar characteristics. Congenital hypothyroidism requires early treatment to prevent severe retardation, and it frequently is not detected clinically during the newborn period. The risk of overwhelming bacterial infection faced by young children with sickle-cell disease can be greatly reduced by giving prophylactic penicillin. Children with galactosemia are often critically ill by the time the condition is detected on the basis of their symptoms, an outcome that can be averted by using a formula that does not contain lactose (milk sugar). Typically, programs were expanded to these and other disorders in response to a combination of mounting medical evidence and political pressure by families and clinicians.

Pressure to expand the number of disorders being screened for expanded dramatically during the 1990s, largely as a result of the development of tandem mass spectrometry ("MS/MS") (AAP). This technology permits the detection of a large number of metabolic abnormalities on a single specimen of blood. Unfortunately, no treatment exists for many of the disorders detectable by MS/MS, which raises issues of whether to test for these abnormalities, and of what to tell families whose children may have one of the untreatable diseases.

Until recently, most state statutes focused on identifying affected children. Most state programs tried to ensure that these children were directed to appropriate sources of care, but few actually ensured the availability of needed medications and diets. Since children do not have universal access to healthcare, some children received no treatment, and some parents suffered job lock. Increasingly, states, practitioners, and clinicians have begun to work together to develop systems to ensure the delivery of care for these children (AAP), a laudable goal which is threatened by the increasing pressure to privatize newborn screening.

The Problem of False Positives

Screening tests are assessed according to their sensitivity (the percentage of affected individuals detected) and their specificity (the percentage of unaffected individuals who are correctly excluded from further testing). The actual number of people who receive inaccurate initial screening results depends in large part on the frequency of the disease in the population. The more common the disease, the more likely it is that a person who receives a positive (abnormal) test result will actually be affected. (The rhetoric of screening and testing is confusing in that "positive" test results almost always mean that something is wrong.) As the disease becomes less frequent, the proportion of initial results that turn out to be "false positives" increases. Suppose a disease has an incidence of 1 in 10,000 and a population of 100,000 people is tested with a screening test that has a sensitivity of 90 percent (so that 9 out of 10 affected people will test positive) and a specificity of 99 percent (so that 99 out of 100 unaffected people will test negative). The results overall would be as follows:

	Test positive	Test negative
Affected	9 "true positive"	1 "false negative"
Unaffected	999 "false positive"	98,991 "true negative"

Put another way, for every person who was truly affected (and tested positive), 100 people who did not have the disease would also (falsely) test positive. In addition, nine people who did have the disease would test negative. While most people who get false positive test results are ultimately reassured by further testing, some may continue to be worried. Affected children who are missed in these programs may face substantial delays in diagnosis if clinicians reason that the child could not have the disorder because it would have been identified in the newborn period.

The disorders sought in newborn screening programs typically are quite rare, usually having frequencies in the 1-in-5,000 to 1-in-15,000 range. Some of the diseases that are being added being to newborn screening panels are as rare as 1 in 100,000. Without denying the benefits that can come to affected children who are detected in these programs, it is important to acknowledge the possible harms that may befall the many children who inevitably receive falsely abnormal results. The newborn period is a particularly vulnerable time. Parents are just beginning to know and bond with their infants. Bad news, even if incorrect, can interfere with the formation of this central relationship and lead parents to view their new infants as medically fragile. One study revealed that almost 10 percent of parents whose infants received initial false-positive screening results for cystic fibrosis were still worried a year later that their children were affected or otherwise sickly.

Thus, the trend has been to increase the disorders for which newborns are screened, including some for which the benefits of early invention are unclear or may be absent, all the while causing a growing number of infants to receive false-positive test results, which will cause some of them harm.

The Implications of These Disorders

Most of the disorders sought by newborn screening are inherited, usually as autosomal recessive disorders. If parents have a child with one of these diseases, they have a one in four chance in each subsequent pregnancy of having another affected child. Children with such a disease can have affected children themselves if they have children with partners who have one or two copies of the same mutated gene. Some screening protocols, such as those for sickle-cell disease and cystic fibrosis, also detect carriers (children who have a single copy of a mutated gene). While these children do not have the disease, the presence of a mutated gene signals an increased risk of having a truly affected child, both for them and for their parents. From an ethical perspective, it seems obvious that parents should be told about all of these implications, but this sort of communication often does not occur.

One of the more difficult ethical questions is whether parents should be encouraged to alter their future reproductive plans in order to decrease the costs of disease to society.

The general consensus is that decisions about having children are to be made by the prospective parents according to their own values, and that genetic counseling is to be nondirective (Andrews, Fullerton, Holtzman, et al.).

Another complex issue is whether decreasing the number of affected children born, whether as a result of state intervention or even of independent decisions by prospective parents, should be seen as an additional goal or benefit of newborn screening. Some governmental officials have made this argument, even calculating the decreased healthcare expenditures that follow from the birth of fewer affected children in their efforts to calculate the cost efficacy of newborn screening (Cunningham). Others, including advocates of disability rights and opponents of prenatal diagnosis, find these arguments distasteful and potentially coercive (Asch).

Unintended Consequences

Untreated women with PKU are profoundly retarded and rarely have children. As a result of the successful implementation of newborn screening and treatment for PKU, however, many affected females are now in their reproductive years, have intelligence in the normal range, and can and do become pregnant. Unless these women adhere to the highly restrictive and burdensome PKU diet prior to conception and throughout their pregnancy, their children will be born with severe brain injury.

These children typically do not have PKU themselves because their fathers are not likely to be carriers since those mutations are not common. The injuries they suffer during pregnancy result instead from the high levels of phenylalanine that exist in their mothers' blood when they eat a normal diet, levels which are particularly toxic to the developing brain. The irony then is that improving the lives of women with PKU creates a high level of risk to the children they may bear. Clearly, these women need to be educated about the importance of adhering to the proper diet prior to and during pregnancy. The ethical dilemma is whether it is ever appropriate, and if so, how, to bring pressure to bear to lead these women to either follow this onerous diet or avoid childbearing altogether (Robertson and Schulman).

Newborn Screening Samples as DNA Databanks

Birth is the only time of life when the government collects blood from virtually everyone. Some states discard these samples within a few months after birth, while others retain them indefinitely. In the past it was not possible to extract much information from these samples because most metabolites deteriorate quickly, but recent advances, particularly in DNA testing, have created new possibilities. Newborn samples can be used for DNA identification, for further investigation when a child subsequently becomes sick, or for research, for which they may be particularly attractive as a true population sample. However, all these uses are secondary to the purpose for which they were initially collected—to detect children with diseases that urgently require treatment.

The appropriateness of using these samples for these other purposes raises many of the questions that attend any use of stored tissue samples for research, including: (1) whether it is necessary to ask the donor (or in this case the parent) for permission; (2) when, if ever, it is appropriate to inform individuals of their personal results; and (3) what sort of review needs to occur before these samples can be used. The fact that these samples are typically obtained without parental knowledge or permission makes these issues that much more urgent, particularly in a society that is so deeply concerned about issues of genetic privacy. It would be rather ironic if a system of universal DNA identification were developed as a by-product of newborn screening rather than as a result of an explicit policy decision.

Conclusion

The particular ethical issues posed by newborn screening arise because these programs are required and run by the government, typically do not involve parents in decision making, often implicate reproductive decision making, and can provide samples for a growing number of secondary uses. These unique factors suggest that parents should have a greater role to play in these programs, and that these programs should remain narrowly focused on detecting diseases for which treatment is urgently needed to avert serious sequelae.

ELLEN WRIGHT CLAYTON

SEE ALSO: *Cloning: Reproductive; Disability; Embryo and Fetus; Eugenics; Eugenics and Religious Law; Genetic Counseling, Ethical Issues in; Genetic Counseling, Practice of; Genetic Discrimination; Genetics and Human Self-Understanding; Infants; Informed Consent; Maternal-Fetal Relationship; Mistakes, Medical; Moral Status; Reproductive Technologies; Value and Valuation;* and other *Genetic Testing and Screening* subentries

BIBLIOGRAPHY

American Academy of Pediatrics (AAP), Newborn Screening Task Force. 2000. "Serving the Family From Birth to the Medical Home, Newborn Screening: A Blueprint for the Future, A Call for a National Agenda on State Newborn Screening Programs." *Pediatrics* 106 (suppl.): 383–427.

Andrews, Lori B. 1985. "New Legal Approaches to Newborn Screening and the Rationale behind the Recommendations for Quality Assurance in Newborn Screening." In *Legal Liability and Quality Assurance in Newborn Screening,* ed. Lori B. Andrews. Chicago: American Bar Foundation.

Andrews Lori B.; Fullerton, Jane E.; Hotlzman, Neil A., et al., eds. 1994. *Assessing Genetic Risks: Implications for Health and Science Policy.* Washington, D.C.: National Academy Press.

Asch, A. 1989. "Reproductive Technology and Disability." In *Reproductive Laws for the 1990s,* ed. S. Cohen and N. Taub. Clifton, NJ: Humana Press.

Clayton, Ellen W. 1992. "Screening and Treatment of Newborns." *Houston Law Review* 29(1): 85–148.

Cunningham, George. 1990. "Balancing the Individual's Rights to Privacy against the Need for Information to Protect and Advance Public Health." In *Genetic Screening: From Newborns to DNA Typing,* ed. Bartha M. Knoppers and Claude M. Laberge. Amsterdam: Excerpta Medica.

Faden, Ruth; Chwalow, A. J.; Holtzman, Neil A.; et al. 1982. "A Survey to Evaluate Parental Consent as Public Policy for Neonatal Screening." *American Journal of Public Health* 72: 1347–52.

Hannon, W. Harry, and Grosse, Scott D. 2001. "Using Tandem Mass Spectrometry for Metabolic Disease Screening Among Newborns." *Morbidity and Mortality Weekly Report* 50(RR03): 1–22.

National Research Council, Committee for the Study of Inborn Errors of Metabolism. 1975. *Genetic Screening: Programs, Principles, and Research.* Washington, D.C.: National Academy Press.

"Newborn Screening for Sickle Cell Disease and Other Hemoglobinopathies." 1989. *Pediatrics* 83(5/2): 813–914

Paul, D. 1999. "Contesting Consent: The Challenge to Compulsory Neonatal Screening for PKU." *Perspectives in Biology and Medicine* 42: 207–219.

Robertson, J. A., and Schulman, J. D. 1987. "Pregnancy and Prenatal Harm to Offspring: The Case of Mothers with PKU." *Hastings Center Report* 17(4): 23–33.

Tluczek A.; Mischler, E. H.; Farrell, P. M.; et al. (1992). "Parents' Knowledge of Neonatal Screening and Response to False-Positive Cystic Fibrosis Testing." *Journal of Developmental Behavioral Pediatrics.* 13(3): 181–186.

Waisbren S.E., Hanley, W; and Levy, H. L.; et al. 2000. "Outcome at Age 4 Years in Offspring of Women with Maternal Phenylketonuria: the Maternal PKU Collaborative Study." *Journal of the American Medical Association* 283(6): 756–762.

III. POPULATION SCREENING

One of the sequelae of the Human Genome Project has been a resurgence of interest in using clinical genetic testing tools at the population level to promote public health goals (Khoury, 1996; Coughlin). This resurgence raises a number of bioethical issues for public health policy-makers and the health professionals involved in delivering genetic services: questions about the limits of public health authority in this domain, the justice of population-based genetic interventions, the social costs of such screening, and the ethical allegiances of the clinicians involved. In this entry, these issues will be reviewed through the lens of one problem that seems to animate all the rest: the problem of defining *prevention* for the purposes of a *public health genetics.*

Background

Mass genetic screening programs have a relatively long history amongst modern genetic services, starting with the screening of newborns for prophylactic therapy against metabolic disorders in the 1960s and continuing into adult carrier testing programs for recessive genetic diseases such as Tay-Sachs (Kaback; Blitzer and McDowell), sickle cell disease (Bowman; Duster), and the thalassemias (Angastiniotis, Kyriakidou, Hadjiminas) in specific at-risk populations in the 1970s. The early adult screening programs shared two features that warranted, and garnered, significant attention within bioethics and health policy (National Academy of Sciences; President's Commission). First, they targeted specific socially-defined populations, which raised issues of group-specific stigmatization and discrimination (Kenan and Schmidt; Markel). Second, the information about carrier status the screens provided was primarily useful for reproductive rather than therapeutic decision-making, raising issues of parental autonomy, paternalism and procreative choice (Juengst, 1988; Thompson et. al).

The 1980s witnessed a second wave of adult genetic screening programs, aimed at detecting pregnant women at risk for delivering children with genetic birth defects and chromosomal abnormalities (Cunningham and Kizer; Haddow, Palomaki, Knight). These programs are intended to have universal application within populations, and have been routinized into the obstetrical care of pregnant women in many countries, raising issues of voluntariness and informed consent (Press and Browner; Marteau). They have also provoked an outspoken reaction from the community of people with disabilities, who argue that such programs work against attempts to reform social attitudes about disability (Parens and Asch).

Today, these three *traditional* forms of population genetic screening—newborn screening, risk-group carrier testing, and pregnancy screening—continue to make up the vast bulk of population genetic screening activities that are funded and evaluated as state public health initiatives. At the same time, the disease targets of these screening efforts have changed, as public health programs see rationales for shifting specific tests from one form of testing to another. Thus, many states have added sickle cell testing to their universal newborn screening panels (Olney), and calls have been made for universal screening of pregnant women for maternal PKU (Kaye, et. al) and fetal hemoglobinopathies (Cuckle). Moreover, genetic tests originally reserved for clinical use in families at risk for diseases such as cystic fibrosis or fragile-X syndrome have also begun to be used as population screens, both as part of newborn screening panels and prenatal testing programs (Caskey; Cuckle). In all such shifts, the tests have moved in the direction of earlier and more universal screening.

The new wave of interest in *public health genetics* generated by advances in genomic science focuses on tests that would have universal application within multi-ethnic populations, like pregnancy testing, but, like newborn screening, would measure the tested individuals' personal risk for disease, with an eye toward prophylactic action. Moreover, in addition to screening for signs of rare *genetic diseases,* like all the traditional forms of screening, the emphasis is on the detection of molecular markers that confer statistically increased risks for more complex, and more common, chronic diseases of adulthood, like coronary artery disease, cancer, or diabetes (Khoury, Burke, Thompson).

The discussion of using these new tests as public health tools has been dominated by questions of feasibility and utility (Omenn, Holtzman). As one review concludes:

> Several issues must be addressed, however, before such tests can be recommended for population-based prevention programs. These issues include the adequacy of the scientific evidence, the balance of risks and benefits, the need for counseling and informed consent, and the costs and resources required. Ongoing assessment of the screening program and quality assurance of laboratory testing are also needed. (Burke et al., p. 201)

These concerns mirror those expressed in the literature on using predictive genetic risk assessments as a part of medical care in clinical settings (Geller, et. al.). The use of these same tests as population screening tools would place them in the larger context of the existing population genetic screening programs, however, and it is in that context that they become most bioethically challenging. As these tests become integrated into the shifting mix of existing *population-based prevention programs,* they expose fundamental questions about the goals of the enterprise that have not been so apparent in the past. What should population-based genetic screening strive to accomplish, and by what criteria should one measure success?

Phenotypic and Genotypic Prevention

The ubiquitous answer to these questions in the literature of public health genetics is *the prevention of disease,* a classic public health goal. This goal is operationalized as the reduction over time in measures of the morbidity and mortality caused by the target disease within the screened population. To flesh out the kinds of interventions that should be counted in those measures, most authors appeal to the public health field's traditional lexically-ordered scheme of primary, secondary and tertiary *levels of prevention,* and attempt to categorize population genetic screening tests accordingly. Thus, for example, one public health guidance document states:

> Primary prevention genetic services are services intended to prevent a birth defect, genetic disorder, or disease before it occurs. Genetic counseling is a form of primary prevention. Genetic counseling provides couples with information about their pregnancy, and reproductive risks and pregnancy options. Secondary prevention genetic services are services intended to prevent the unfavorable sequelae of an existing disorder or genotype. Newborn screening is a classic example of secondary prevention. Tertiary prevention genetic services are services aimed at ameliorating the unfavorable consequences of existing disorders, through enabling services such as parent-to-parent support and empowerment. (Kaye et al.)

Using this scheme provides a logic for shifting tests into the newborn, prenatal and preconception stages, because traditionally "primary prevention" has been considered the ultimate goal of public health interventions.

Unfortunately, this scheme also introduces an important equivocation into public health discourse between two different ways in which genetic screening might be thought to be *preventive*: genetic screening as a technique for preventing the expression of a genetic disease in an individual and genetic screening as a technique for preventing the intergenerational transmission of disease genes. For convenience, the first kind of prevention may be called *phenotypic prevention,* since its goal is to prevent the manifestation of a particular clinical phenotype. Similarly, the second sort of prevention may be called *genotypic prevention,* (or *geno-prevention*) because its goal is to prevent the birth of people with particular genotypes. Equivocating between these two senses of prevention in discussions of population screening

results in the attribution of genotypic preventive goals to public health genetics. That, in turn, generates the deeper questions of public authority, social justice, and professional allegiance that animate bioethical concern in this area.

Phenotypic Prevention

The dominant rhetoric of contemporary public health genetics stresses phenotypic forms of prevention as the primary goal of population genetic screening (Coughlin). This is not surprising. Phenotypic prevention is a straightforward medical pursuit that few would criticize: it is designed to further the health interests of individual patients by allowing them to avoid foreseeable medical problems. Almost all public health efforts outside of population genetic screening employ this concept of prevention, and even within public health genetics there are typical phenotypic prevention efforts at each of the three *levels of prevention* (Holtzman).

The concept of phenotypic prevention rests on several assumptions, however, which are worth unpacking. First, phenotypic prevention assumes that there are people who survive the intervention to benefit from having their foreseeable health problems forestalled. Thus, for example, proposals to *prevent* occupational disease by firing all susceptible employees instead of cleaning up the workplace seem inherently wrong-headed. Second, it assumes that diseases are best defined at the level of the actual health problems that they occasion for individual people, rather than in terms of their preclinical etiology. Otherwise, preclinical interventions like dietary changes would be directly curative, not prophylactic. Third, it assumes that diseases are distinct from the people they burden, so that it becomes appropriate to use metaphors of external defense to describe the beneficiaries, as *vulnerable* to *attack* by disease without the *protection* of prevention.

Along with these assumptions, the concept of phenotypic prevention enjoys a high degree of moral authority as an imperative for medicine and society. In fact, the promise of phenotypic preventive measures to "protect the helpless from harm" has been compelling enough in our society to allow both primary and secondary forms of phenotypic prevention to become established in effectively mandatory programs as a matter of public policy (President's Commission).

Of course, if primary prevention is the prevention of the onset of a genetic disease in an at-risk patient, then most of the preconception, preimplantation, and prenatal genetic screening interventions usually classified as *primary prevention strategies* cannot, in fact, qualify for that status. Neither pre-implantation embryo screening nor selective termination can serve to prevent the onset of a heritable disease in affected patients. At most, they are capable of preventing cases of a disease within a family (or a population), by allowing parents (or a society) to avoid the birth of at-risk individuals.

This conceptual confusion does lead to some cognitive dissonance in the literature. The Centers for Disease Control and Prevention, for example, illustrates the concept of *primary prevention* in genetics by listing "medical and community-based interventions focused on carrier detection and premarital counseling as ell as on prenatal diagnosis and pregnancy termination," but then adds the confusing parenthetical remark that "(This last may not be considered primary prevention)" (Khoury et al., 1997, p. 1718). It is also telling that one can find carrier screening, intrauterine diagnosis and selective termination classified in the literature as an example of primary prevention (Kaye, et. al.), secondary prevention (Wertz, Fletcher, and Berg), and even tertiary prevention (Porter)! Clearer thinkers: Holtzman (1989) sets carrier screening, amniocentesis and selective termination outside of preventive medicine's traditional trichotomy, by labeling them as a form of genetic disease *avoidance*. Similarly, the editor of the journal Community Genetics declares that:

> Calling termination of pregnancy after prenatal diagnosis "prevention" is a perversion of terminology. I suggest that we should use the term "reproductive choice." By analogy with prevention, one might define different levels of reproductive choice. Primary reproductive choice would then consist of actions to avoid conception of affected offspring, while secondary reproductive choice would bar implantation or birth of affected embryos and fetuses. (ten Kate, p. 87)

In fact, when they incorporate reproductive genetic screening programs into their menu of preventive interventions, public health geneticists have been forced to slip between two very different senses of *prevention*. They have conflated screening to prevent the phenotypic expression of a genotype in a particular patient (*phenotypic prevention*) with screening to prevent the birth of individuals with a particular genotype (*genotypic prevention*). These two visions of screening reflect quite distinct concepts of disease prevention, with different histories within healthcare, different philosophical assumptions, and different degrees of moral authority.

Genotypic Prevention

Genotypic prevention is a pursuit that is much more controversial than phenotypic prevention. That is understandable, for several reasons:

First, it is often hard to know what ends genotypic preventive measures are intended to serve. Genotypic preventive measures are usually described as a way of furthering the procreative interests of prospective parents, by allowing them to avoid the birth of individuals with foreseeable health problems (like AID following adult carrier testing for cystic fibrosis mutations, or selective termination following intrauterine diagnosis of Down's syndrome).

At the same time, these same interventions are often evaluated in terms of the economic and public health interests of society, according to their ability to reduce the incidence of genetic disease in a population. Thus, the famous "success stories" of genetic screening (like the Mediterranean carrier screening programs for beta-thalassemia, or Tay-Sachs screening in the Ashkenazi-American population) most often counted as successful in terms of these societal criteria (Rao, et. al.; Blitzer and McDowell). In those stories, in fact, the commitment to channeling screening efforts through the individual's voluntary reproductive choices is itself portrayed as simply a savvy strategy for achieving the profession's underlying goal of reducing society's healthcare costs (Caskey; Palomaki; Chappele, et. al.).

Secondly, whether geno-prevention is pursued in the cause of family planning or the public health (or both), it must make two sets of related assumptions. First, it assumes that the diseases it prevents are best understood at the level of the genotype, rather than through the pathophysiology of their expression, just as AIDS is understood in terms of its causal HIV infection rather than the infection's clinical sequelae. Understanding genetic disease through the lens of the germ theory in this way means that the language of "molecular disease," and "DNA-based diagnosis" seems apt, and it makes sense to contrast preventing the vertical transmission of pathogenic disease genes with palliative or symptomatic interventions like low phenylalanine diets.

Second, proponents of geno-preventive efforts must assume important personal (or social) value judgments about the burden of the cases of disease being prevented. Genes are not, like germs, external infectious agents that can be kept (or cleaned) out of a living person's body. Instead, genotypic prevention has to involve avoiding the birth of individuals conceived with the pathological genotype. The beneficiaries of such an intervention cannot be the individuals whose births are avoided: if the genotypic transmission has been successfully prevented, there can be no such individuals.

That means that to justify geno-prevention someone (parents or society) must make the judgment that the burden of coping with cases of a disease outweighs any other value that individuals with a given genotype might bring to a family or community, and warrants action to exclude individuals with those mutations from the lives of the wild type.

Finally, genotypic prevention already has a bad track record as a social and professional goal. Genotypic prevention has been accepted before as a societal imperative, on the coat-tails of the public health movement's successes with the primary prevention of infectious disease (Allen). The "Eugenics Movement" of the first half of the twentieth century is remembered primarily for the discriminatory immigration restrictions and coercive sterilization laws it produced (Reilly), and the ease with which it was appropriated to support genocide (Muller-Hill). The horrific consequences of ranking genotypic preventive goals over individual interests still effectively undermine any claims to moral authority it might make.

Unfortunately, as its controversial features already suggest, to the extent that population genetic screening becomes associated with a professional allegiance to genotypic prevention, it inherits all the history, assumptions and moral liability of that concept, and the prospects for a well-reasoned public assessment of its merits dim considerably.

Against this background, the professional confusion over the true goals of contemporary genotypic prevention services and the fact that all geno-preventive services require the judgment that some genotypes are predictably burdensome enough to others to outweigh any other potential their bearers might have, makes it easy for critics of new approaches to genotypic prevention to remind the public of the excesses of the historical eugenics movement, and label any new efforts accordingly, with powerful political effect (Hubbard).

Moreover, inviting external political challenges is not the only trouble that endorsing genotypic prevention would create for public health genetics. it would also create substantive philosophical tensions within the field which could threaten the ethical integrity of the field. Since genotypic prevention is also unnecessary as a rationale genetic screening and counseling services, some argue that it is time for public health authorities to explicitly eschew this old eugenic legacy as a professional goal.

Ethical and Social Implications

As a professional ethical matter, accepting genotypic prevention as a proper goal of public health genetics has chilling implications. Expanding the geneticist's preventive goals of genetic medicine to include reducing the incidence of pathological genotypes broadens their responsibilities beyond their presenting patients to the next generation's aggregate population. Since the latter will always be a bigger

group, its preventive health needs will always be greater by at least some scores (e.g., disease care costs), and therefore, for some, more compelling. This makes it very easy for genetic medicine to elevate what began as a serendipitous "by-product" of its services—the reduction of disease burden and cost to society—to a central position within its mission, without even noticing when it does so.

Again, such criteria do have a long history in applied human genetics, as basic ingredients in the various programs of "negative eugenics" this century has witnessed. They even continue to be explicitly used by some genetic services programs seeking to justify their public support in economic terms (Chappele, et al; Cuckle). As a result, there is no need to guess at the internal dangers that adopting such ideals would pose for the professional ethics of genetic medicine: the experiment has already been conducted. Experience shows that there are at least four important hazards for the profession:

1. First, the field would have to decide where within the spectrum of human genetic variation to define the pathological genotypes it would seek to prevent (Juengst, 1988). Most of the proponents of preventive genetic screening programs skirt this problem by stipulating that they are only talking about "severe congenital abnormalities" that produce "serious handicaps." (Cuckle). These caveats address this line-drawing problem in a time-honored way, by appealing to common sense notions of severity. In doing so, the proponents of geno-preventive germ-line intervention are following the footsteps of authors like Dr. Nathan Fasten, when he wrote in 1935 that:

> Here one must pause to comment that it is difficult to define clearly the standards of desirability or the standards of perfection in the human family. Even so, most normal persons would agree that the hopeless cases of physical and mental defectives, those that are incapable of care for themselves, particularly where it is certain that such defects are the results of hereditary factors, are no asset to society and should be eliminated as quickly as possible. (p. 354)

So far, Dr. Fasten appears to be anticipating the modern argument. However, Dr. Fasten's own list of what "most normal persons" should include in the class of "hopeless cases" is telling:

> Here are included the feeble-minded, the insane, the paupers, the confirmed criminals, and the grave sex offenders. This group, in general, is a tremendous burden on society. Genetic evidence has been accumulating to reveal that most of these defects are due to heredity. Social workers also

have discovered that from this stock the largest percentage of the dependent individuals originate. Geneticists and social workers, therefore, believe that nothing but good can come from efforts in the direction of the rapid elimination of this branch of society. (p. 355)

Of course, it would be unfair and anachronistic to insinuate that the contemporary advocates of genetic screening subscribe to eugenic ideologies like Fasten's: they clearly do not. The point in resurrecting him is simply to illustrate that it is often hard to know, in the thick of things, how much one's professional assessments of pathology are influenced by larger cultural ideologies and social values.

If genetic medicine is to prevent its practitioners from being lured away into other social agendas, it still must address the challenge of defining its domain. As the intensity of the debates over the prenatal sex selection as a professional practice already demonstrates (Warren), drawing these boundaries will involve just as difficult a set of value judgments as attempts to use genetic technologies to *enhance* specific human traits. As Dr. Fasten reminds us, without more operational definitions, rhetorical appeals to "severity" and the intuitions of the "reasonable person" will not help brighten any of the lines that will need to be drawn across the spectrum of human traits as genetic medicine's power matures.

2. Moreover, it is increasingly clear that preventing the birth of a particular "pathological" genotype will not always mean preventing a clinical health problem. The more we learn about human genetics at the molecular level, the more complicated the story becomes. One increasingly prominent feature of that story over the last few years has been the deterioration of the theory of specific causation within genetics (Strohman). Not only are most health problems "polygenic" to some degree, but even the traditional "single gene disorders" are turning out to be molecularly heterogeneous (Holtzman). As the number and variety of different specific mutations that can all cause the same disease increases, so does the challenge of detecting and correcting them all in a patient. Worse yet, the causal complexity works in both ways: even the paradigmatic examples of clean Mendelian "singe gene" disorders, like "recessive" cystic fibrosis and "dominant" Huntington's disease are turning out to be multifactoral enough that carrying one of their (multiple) pathognomic genotypes no longer guarantees that one will experience a problematic clinical syndrome (cf. Tsui; Benjamin).

In other words, genotypes are not turning out to function very well as germs. The complexity of their expression as health problems undermines the confidence with which a clinician can predict the occurrence of severe health problems from a DNA diagnosis. Since genotypic prevention is conceptually committed to a deterministic etiology of specific causation, geno-preventive measures risk making (and acting on) both false negative and false positive prognoses. This means that they also risk intervening unnecessarily in cases that the environmental forces of expression and penetrance would have naturally mitigated.

3. Thirdly, as a consequence of its deterministic assumptions, genotypic prevention cannot help stigmatizing genotypes, and (since they are inseparable) the people whom they mark, as undesirable or pathological in themselves (Markel, Parens, and Asch). This kind of reductionism, reducing personal identities to disvalued health problems and disvalued health problems to one stigmatizing sign, is at the root of much of the social discrimination that people with disabilities must already overcome (Fine and Asch). To have public health authorities endorse genotypic prevention as a goal can only exacerbate these challenges, because it provides a medical sanction for exclusionary attitudes.(Saxton; Kaplan; Faden). The concern is that, if a given genotype carries such a disvalue for health professionals, it would not seem unreasonable for the public to chastise those who avoid screening as "irresponsible reproducers" and hold them accountable for their recklessness by denying them opportunities or services, like medical care for affected offspring (Thompson, et. al).

4. Finally, the ways in which genotypic preventive goals tend to overshadow individual interests also endangers the therapeutic relationship within genetic medicine. To the extent that genetic services programs are evaluated in terms of their success to reducing the incidence of particular genotypes, genetic service providers will inevitably have an stake in seeing that their clients make the "right" reproductive decisions: i.e., decisions not to bear children at risk for genetic disease. This is a pressure that is already creating tension within medical genetics, as the field attempts to accommodate itself to healthcare delivery systems that are managed with societal healthcare costs in mind. For example, there has been a lively debate in the British medical literature about how genetic services should interpret the societal expectation that they will "pay their own way" within the national health budget (Chappelle; Clarke). Genotypic prevention, in other words, imports a professional goal that encourages practitioners to influence the reproductive decisions their clients make, despite their professed respect for the reproductive autonomy of those they serve.

Fortunately, all of these professional ethical risks—the subordination of professional integrity to social ideology, the inappropriate reliance on simplistic science, the professional disvaluing of human minorities, and the willingness to invade the sphere of reproductive privacy on behalf of society's economic interests—are dangers which human geneticists have succumbed to and overcome before (Kevles; Allen). Moreover, they are also the dangers in response to which the contemporary *client-centered* professional ethic of medical genetics has largely been shaped. In contemplating the future of germ-line gene therapy, it may be helpful to recall how this existing moral tradition handles the question of genotypic prevention, and consider its relevance for public health genetics. Doing so shows that genotypic prevention is not only a dangerous goal for genetic medicine to espouse, it is also completely unnecessary.

The Existing Tradition

One of the reasons it is easy to slip between the phenotypic and genotypic senses of *prevention* in discussing genetic medicine's goals is that the desire to bear children free from specific genetic diseases can and often does provide a rationale for prospective parents' interest in the specialty's services. But that does not pose a professional ethical problem for clinical geneticists: whether the intervention is genetic counseling, adult carrier screening, intrauterine diagnosis, preimplantation screening, providers of genetic services can help parents achieve their geno-preventive goal in good conscience, because it falls within the sphere of reproductive choices which parents are free to make in a tolerant society. Even the sharpest critics of genotypic prevention as a professional and public policy will agree that individual decisions about these interventions are inseparable enough from core personal values and beliefs to warrant the same respect we give to other fundamental freedoms (of religion, for example)(Saxton; Fine and Asch).

However, it is not necessary to conflate the *patients'* goals with the *professional* goals of genetic medicine in order to display respect for reproductive autonomy. In doing so, advocates of increased screening blur a distinction that clinical geneticists providing more traditional genetic service have worked hard to clarify: the distinction between the profession's mission in providing its services and the personal interests of their clients (Botkin).

Clinical geneticists argue that their professional goals in offering reproductive genetic testing and counseling services have little to do with the content of the autonomous reproductive choices that their clients make. Their mission is to treat a special class of reproductive health problems their clients face as prospective parents: *the reproductive planning problems posed by their risk of having a child with a genetic disease* (NSGC; Bartels). The advocates of this ethos assert that "the fundamental value of genetic screening and counseling is their ability to enhance the opportunities for individuals to obtain information about their personal health and child-bearing risks and to make autonomous and noncoerced choices based on that information," not the elimination of genetic disease (President's Commission). From this perspective, the geneticists' goals are not so much "preventive" as directly therapeutic: the reproductive planning problems they address are already fulminant when their clients engage their services, and their treatment consists of giving them the information, counseling, and options they need to address their problems in terms of their own values and beliefs (Kessler).

This approach to defining the mission of reproductive clinical genetics has several important features for our purposes. The first is its emphasis on the practitioner's primary professional obligations to his or her presenting clients—usually prospective parents—rather than with the next generation. Thus, practitioners are warned that:

> Counselors may find themselves pulled by an allegiance to the unborn child—whose well-being is, after all, the ultimate object of their concern as well as the motivating interest of the parents. As understandable as this concern may be, in the end it must give way to the duty owed to the counselee— the parents (Capron, p. 334).

Secondly, since in practice *reproductive health* largely boils down to the ability to fulfill one's procreative ambitions, the geneticists' treatment goals can only really be accomplished within the context of their patients' own life plans and beliefs. Because the content and consequences of the reproductive decisions that the geneticist helps facilitate reflect personal moral judgments made within the sphere of the patients' procreative liberty, they are understood to be beyond the geneticists' professional domain of concern. As a consequence, geneticists are expected to be strictly *nondirective* in the counseling they provide, and to help their clients to make their own value judgments about the relative burden of the disease their children may inherit. The practical result of this orientation is a strongly client-centered ethos that, historically, anticipated the rise of *patient autonomy* in the ethics of other medical specialties by twenty years.

In part, this tradition has historical roots in the reaction of postwar medical geneticists to the excesses of their eugenic predecessors. However, it also reflects an important strategy for dealing with the predictive and moral uncertainties of the reproductive decisions that geneticists' help their clients make (Juengst, 1989). The tradition is often inaccurately accused of prescribing "value-neutrality" and criticized accordingly (Caplan), but it would be more accurate to label it as "value-sensitive," since it instructs clinical geneticists to discern and work with their clients' values, rather than be blind to them.

The consequence of this client-centered, non-directive ethos is that genetic medicine has no need to adopt geno-preventive goals in order to explain or justify the interventions it performs on behalf of its clients. In fact, it is free to repudiate "public policy intended to change the genetic makeup of the populations" (Council of Regional Genetics Networks), and thereby to distance itself from the liabilities that the geno-preventive concept brings to the profession. One recent statement of this ethos is worth citing at length, because of the ways it clearly displays its roots in the field's concern with the hazards of espousing geno-preventive goals for their services:

> Reproductive genetic services must ultimately serve personal—not public—interests, in improving the overall reproductive lives of women. Whatever societal gains might be realized through the eugenic use of reproductive genetic services should be heavily outweighed by the personal needs of women and their families. The ideals of self-determination in family matters and respect for individual differences, ideal that lie behind the client-centered view of reproductive genetic services, are jeopardized whenever the primary goal of these services becomes the prevention of the birth of individuals with a disorder or a disability. To the extent that voluntary reproductive genetic services are evaluated even indirectly in eugenic terms, societal pressures have the potential to threaten the important interests of individual women and their families. (Thomson et al., p. 1161)

Of course, there are still plenty of ethical tensions within this model of genetic medicine (e.g. cf. Bartels). For example, as more can be done to address the phenotypic problems associated with fetal genotypes identified through genetic testing, it becomes harder to interpret prenatal testing as solely aimed at addressing a parental reproductive health problem. In these cases, the fetus emerges as a *presenting patient* for the medical geneticist, with its own claims to professional allegiance. Similarly, to the extent to which the profession fails to distinquish between their commitment to a non-directive counseling style and their professional obligation to establish the limits of their services, concerns about a laissez faire, commercialized, "consumer eugenics" will remain. Genetic medicine also has to grapple with the fact that, unless the profession is willing to use genotypic preventive measures of success, it may find its reproductive testing

and counseling services excluded from cost-conscious healthcare coverage plans as relative luxuries.

Moreover, despite its prominence in the rhetoric of the field, it is also true that this client-centered ethos does not command universal allegiance amongst human geneticists: in fact, 59% of geneticists surveyed do still endorse the "reduction in the number of carriers of genetic disorders" as a professional goal for their field (Wertz and Fletcher). Nevertheless, on the whole, rejecting genotypic prevention in favor of focusing on the interests of the presenting patient serves its advocates well in clinical genetics. By keeping the specialty's loyalties with the particular patients at hand, and its professional prescriptions within the context of those patients' own values and goals, it inoculates the field against infection by the dangerous agendas of negative eugenics.

The bad news for proponents of population genetic screening, of course, is that returning to the client-centered ethos of medical genetics does mean that they will have to forego their appeals to genotypic prevention in making their case. Whether or not genetic screening has any promise for "purifying the human gene pool" should remain totally irrelevant to its acceptance as a public health tool. Given the political, professional and social dangers of going down the eugenic road, any short-term benefits of doing so could carry a very heavy price for all concerned.

Conclusion

Genetic medicine is quickly leaving the stage in its history when it only has information and solace to provide its patients. As it becomes increasingly incorporated into public health, it will be important not to forget the moral tradition that sustains it. Affirming the traditional commitment of geneticists to the physical health and reproductive autonomy of their clients and patients means relinquishing genotypic prevention as a formal goal for the profession. In contemporary political argot, public health genetics should continue to be an empowering, not an exclusionary science: it should continue to be about helping living people address their individual health problems, and not about protecting the *gene pool* or society from those people, as some form of expensive pollution. Speaking clearly about the place of *prevention* in public health genetics is one way the pioneers of the new era can reaffirm this fundamental conviction.

ERIC T. JUENGST

SEE ALSO: *Coercion; Eugenics; Eugenics and Religious Law; Genetic Counseling, Ethical Issues in; Genetic Counseling, Practice of; Genetic Discrimination; Genetics and Human Self-Understanding; Informed Consent; Justice; Public Health*

Law; Value and Valuation; and other *Genetic Testing and Screening* subentries

BIBLIOGRAPHY

Allen, G. E. 1989. *Eugenics and American Social History, 1880–1950. Genome* 31: 885–889.

Angastiniotis, Michael; Kyriadou, Sophia; Hadjiminas, Minas. 1986. "How Thalassemia Was Controlled in Cyprus" *World Health Forum* 7: 291–297.

Bartels, D, et al., eds. 1993. *Prescribing Our Future: Ethical Challenges in Genetic Counseling.* Hawthorne, NY: deGruyter.

Benjamin, C. M., et al. 1994. "Proceed with Care: Direct Predictive Testing for Huntington's Disease." *American Journal of Human Genetics* 55: 606–617.

Blitzer, M.G., and McDowell, G. A. 1992. "Tay-Sachs Disease as a Model for Screening In-born Errors." *Clinical Laboratory Medicine* 12: 463–480.

Botkin, Jeffrey. 1990. "Prenatal Screening: Professional Standards and the Limits of Parental Choice." *Obstetrics and Gynecology* 75: 875–880.

Bowman, James. 1977. "Genetic Screening Programs and Public Policy." *Phylon* 38: 117–142.

Burke, Wylie; Coughlin, Steven; Lee, Nancy; et al. 2001. "Application of Population Screening Principles to Genetic Screening for Adult-Onset Conditions" *Genetic Testing* 5: 201–211.

Cao, A.; Rosatelli, M. C.; Galanello, R. 1991. "Population-based Genetic Screening." *Curr Opin Genet Dev* 1: 48–53.

Capron, A. 1979. "Autonomy, Confidentiality and Quality Care in Genetic Counseling." In *Genetic Counseling: Facts, Values and Norms,* p. 334, ed. A. Capron, et al. New York: Alan R. Liss.

Caskey, Thomas. 1993. "Presymptomatic Diagnosis: A First Step Toward Genetic Health Care," *Science* 262: 48–49.

Chappele J. C.; Dale, R.; Evans, B.G. 1987. "The New Genetics: Will It Pay Its Way?" *Lancet* 1: 1189–1192.

Clarke, A. 1990. "Genetics, Ethics and Audit." *Lancet* 335: 1145–1147.

Coughlin, Steven. 1999. "The Intersection of Genetics, Public Health and Preventive Medicine." *American Journal of Preventive Medicine* 16: 89–91.

Council of Regional Networks for Genetic Services. 1994. *Code of Ethical Principles for Genetics Professionals.* Cornell, NY: Cornell University Medical College.

Cunningham, George, and Kizer, K.W. 1990. "Maternal Serum Alpha-feto Protein Activities of State Health Agencies: A Survey." *American Journal of Human Genetics* 47: 899–903.

Cuckle, Howard. 2001. "Extending Antenatal Screening in the UK to Include Common Mongenic Disorders" *Community Genetics* 4: 84–86.

Duster, Troy. 1989. *Backdoor to Eugenics.* NY: Routledge.

Faden, R. 1994. "Reproductive Genetic Testing, Prevention and the Ethics of Mothering." In *Women and Prenatal Testing: Facing the Challenges of Genetic Technology,* pp. 88–98, ed. E. Thomson and K. Rothenberg. Columbus: Ohio State University Press.

Fine, M., and Asch, A., eds. 1988. *Women with Disabilities: Essays in Psychology, Culture and Politics.* Philadelphia: Temple University Press.

Geller, Gail; Botkin, Jeff; Green, Michael; et al. 1997. "Genetic Testing for Susceptibility to Adult-Onset Cancer." *Journal of the American Medical Association* 277: 1467–1474.

Haddow, J. E.; Palomaki, Glenn; Knight, G. J. 1992. "Prenatal Screening for Down Syndrome with Use of Maternal Serum Markers" *New England Journal of Medicine* 321: 588–593.

Holtzman, N. A. 1989. *Proceed with Caution: Predicting Genetic Risks in the Recombinant DNA Era.* Baltimore: The Johns Hopkins University Press.

Hubbard, R. 1986. "Eugenics and Prenatal Testing." *Intl. J. Health Services* 16: 227–242.

Juengst, E. 1988. "Prenatal Diagnosis and the Ethics of Uncertainty." In *Medical Ethics: A Guide for Health Professionals,* pp. 12–25, ed. J. Monagle and D. Thomasma. Rockville, MD: Aspen.

Juengst, E. 1989. "Patterns of Reasoning in Medical Genetics." *Theoretical Medicine* 10: 101–105.

Kaback, Michael; Lim-Steele, D.; Dabholkar, D.; et al. 1993. "Tay-Sachs Disease Carrier Screening, Prenatal Diagnosis and the Molecular Era: An International Perspective, 1970–1993." *Journal of the American Medical Association* 270: 2307–2315.

Kaplan, Deborah. 1994. "Prenatal Screening and Diagnosis: The Impact on Persons with Disabilities." In *Woman and Prenatal Testing: Facing the Challenges of Genetic Technology,* pp. 49–67, ed. K. Rothenberg and E. Thomson. Columbus, OH: Ohio State University Press.

Kaye, Celia; Laxova, Roberta; Livingston, Judith, et al. 2001. "Integrating Genetic Services into Public Health: Guidance for State and Territorial Programs." *Community Genetics* 1(4): 175–196.

Kenan, Regina, and Schmidt, Robert. 1987. "Social Implications of Screening Programs for Carrier Status: Genetic Diseases in the 1970's and AIDS in the 1980's." In *Dominant Issues in Medical Sociology,* 2nd edition, ed. H. Schwartz. New York: Random House.

Kessler, S. 1980. "The Psychological Paradigm Shift in Genetic Counseling." *Social Biology* 27(1): 67–85.

Kevles, D. 1985. *In the Name of Eugenics: Genetics and the Uses of Human Heredity.* New York: Knopf.

Khoury, Muin, and the Genetics Working Group. 1996. "From Genes to Public Health: The Applications of Genetic Technology in Disease Prevention," *American Journal of Public Health* 86: 1717–1721.

Khoury, Muin; Burke, Wylie; and Thompson, Elizabeth, eds. 2000. *Genetics and Public Health in the 21st Century.* NY: Oxford University Press.

Markel, H. 1992. "The Stigma of Disease: Implications for Carrier Screening." *American Journal of Medicine* 93: 209–215.

Marteau, Therese. 1995. "Towards Informed Decisions about Prenatal Testing: A Review" *Prenatal Diagnosis* 15: 1215–1226.

Muller-Hill, B. 1988. *Murderous Science: Elimination by Scientific Selection of Jews, Gypsies, and Others, Germany 1933–1945.* New York: Oxford University Press.

National Academy of Sciences. 1975. *Genetic Screening: Programs, Principles and Research* Washington, D.C.: National Academy Press.

National Society of Genetic Counselors. 1992. "Code of Ethics." *Journal of Genetic Counseling* 1: 41–42.

Olney, Richard. 1999. "Preventing Morbidity and Mortality from Sickle Cell Disease: A Public Health Perspective" *American Journal of Preventive Medicine* 16(2): 116–122.

Omenn, Gilbert. 1996. "Genetics and Public Health." *American Journal of Public Health* 86: 1701–1703.

Palomaki, G. E. 1994. "Population Based Prenatal Screening for the Fragile X Syndrome." *Journal of Medical Screening* 1: 65–72.

Parens, Erik, and Asch, Adrienne, eds. 2000. *Prenatal Testing and Disability Rights.* Washington, D.C.: Georgetown University Press.

Paul, D. 1984. "Eugenics and the Left." *Journal of the History of Ideas* 45: 567–590.

Porter, I. 1982. "The Control of Hereditary Disorders." *Annual Review of Public Health* 3: 277–319.

President's Commission for the Study of Ethical Problems in Medicine and Biomedical and Behavioral Research. 1983. *Screening and Counseling for Genetic Conditions.* Washington, D.C.: U.S. Government Printing Office.

Press, Nancy, and Browner, Carole. 1995. "Risk, Autonomy and Responsibility: Informed Consent for Prenatal Testing." *Hastings Center Report* 25(3): S9–S12.

Reilly, P. 1991. *The Surgical Solution: A History of Involuntary Sterilization in the U.S..* Baltimore: The Johns Hopkins University Press.

Shohat, M.; Legum, C.; Romen, Y.; et al. 1995. "Down's Syndrome Prevention Program in a Population with an Older Maternal Age" *Obstetrics and Gynecology* 85: 368–373.

Snyder, L. H., and David, P. R. 1965. "Genetics and Preventive Medicine." In *Preventive Medicine: An Epidemiological Approach,* pp. 321–345, 3rd edition, ed. H. R. Leavell and E. C. Clark. New York: McGraw-Hill.

Sorenson, J. 1974. "Biomedical Innovation, Uncertainty and Doctor-patient Interaction." *Journal of Health and Social Behavior* 15: 366–374.

Strohman, Richard. 1993. "Ancient Genomes, Wise Bodies, Unhealthy People: Limits of a Genetic Paradigm in Biology and Medicine." *Perspectives in Biology and Medicine* 37: 112–145.

ten Kate, Leo P. 2000. "Editorial." *Community Genetics* 5(2): 87.

Thomson, Elizabeth, et al. 1993. "National Institutes of Health Workshop Statement on Reproductive Genetic Testing: Impact on Women." *American Journal of Human Genetics* 51: 1161–1163.

Tsui, L. 1992. "The Spectrum of Cystic Fibrosis Mutations." *Trends in Genetics* 8: 392–398.

Warren, Mary Ann. 1985. *Gendercide: The Implications of Sex Selection.* Totowa, NJ: Rowan and Allanheld.

Wertz, D., and Fletcher, J. 1989. *Ethics and Human Genetics: A Cross-Cultural Perspective.* Berlin: Springer-Verlag.

Wertz, D.; Fletcher, J.; and Berg, K. 1995. *Summary Statement on Ethical Issues in Medical Genetics: Report of WHO Temporary Advisers.* WHO Document WHO/HDP/CONS/95. Geneva, Switzerland: World Health Organization.

IV. PUBLIC HEALTH CONTEXT

Genetic testing and screening programs have long been part of public health programs in the United States. For decades public health authorities have recommended the screening of newborns for specific genetic (and nongenetic) conditions through genetic tests that use blood samples from infants. Neonatal genetic testing and screening increasingly are becoming part of public health practice in the modern genetic revolution. Genetic testing and screening in the delivery of health services and for occupational purposes (Shulte and DeBord) are becoming more common despite legal impediments.

The proliferation of genetic testing and screening in the interests of protecting public health may help improve health outcomes on a population basis, but it simultaneously raises significant legal, social, and ethical concerns. When should genetic tests be allowed without informed consent? Should genetic screening be allowed for every condition for which a reliable and accurate test is available? When should genetic screening programs be mandatory (required) or voluntary (optional)? How can public health authorities or others acquire, use, or disclose sensitive genetic test results? These and other ethical issues are discussed in this entry in the context of the classic debate between individual rights and the goal of protecting the public's health.

Genetic Testing and Screening: Similarities and Distinctions

Though often used interchangeably, genetic testing and screening are different concepts. *Genetic testing* refers to medical procedures that determine the presence or absence of a genetic disease, condition, or marker in individual patients (Gostin). Genetic tests involve an examination of chromosomes, DNA molecules, or gene products (such as proteins) to find evidence of certain mutated sequences.

Genetic tests can (1) confirm a diagnosis for a symptomatic individual, (2) assist with presymptomatic diagnosis (e.g., Huntington's disease) or assessment of the risk of development of adult-onset disorders (e.g., Alzheimer's disease), (3) identify carriers of one copy of a gene for a disease in which two copies are needed for the disease to be expressed, and (4) aid in prenatal diagnosis and newborn screening. Hundreds of genetic tests are available to predict diseases in individuals and the population (Secretary's Advisory Committee on Genetic Testing [SAGCT]). Many others are being developed.

Despite their great potential, technical limitations to genetic tests can inhibit the prediction of disease in individuals. A genetic test may not be able to identify every mutation of a gene (which can have mutations in several places along its base pairs) and thus may not indicate an abnormality. Different mutations in a gene have different effects. The cystic fibrosis gene, for instance, has 800 potential mutations with varied effects on health (SACGT). In addition, genetic tests do not measure the complex interactions between genes and environment that contribute to the onset of almost all diseases. As a result, a genetic test is limited in its ability to gauge an individual's susceptibility to causes of mortality such as heart disease accurately.

Screening entails the systematic application of a test to a defined population (Gostin). *Genetic screening* refers to programs designed to identify persons in a subpopulation whose genotypes suggest that they or their offspring are at higher risk for a genetic disease or condition. In many cases this requires the administration of genetic tests, as defined above. Thus, whereas genetic tests are used to reveal specific propensities among individuals, genetic screening programs help identify rates of genetic diseases or conditions among subpopulations and sometimes can uncover previously unknown or unrecognized conditions. The nature and scope of genetic screening programs vary. Some screening programs are mandatory: Persons must participate in a screening program unless they opt out (where allowed) for religious, philosophical, or other reasons. Most screening programs, however, are voluntary. Persons may choose to participate (opt in) but do not have to.

There are many examples of genetic screening for public health purposes. Women may be screened for genetically related breast cancers. Persons may participate in prenatal genetic screening programs to determine genetic disorders in embryos before implantation. Obstetricians may advise pregnant women in higher-risk groups about specific genetic tests. Fetal karyotyping, for example, can suggest an increased likelihood of carrying a fetus with Down's syndrome among older women. Screenings for conditions such as Tay-Sachs disease and cystic fibrosis are available. Perhaps the most prominent example of genetic screening among a subpopulation is the long-standing public health practice of screening newborns for genetic conditions. Most states require the screening of infants for treatable genetic disorders, particularly phenylketonuria (PKU), subject to refusal on religious or philosophical grounds (New York State Task Force on Life and the Law). Some statutes deem newborn screening voluntary, although in practice it almost always is done in the interest of protecting an infant's health.

Genetics and Public Health

Genetic testing and screening further public health goals of preventing and treating diseases in the population in many ways. Because many diseases and conditions result from interaction among genes, behavior, and environment, understanding the role genes play in contributing to diseases clarifies the ways in which environmental and behavioral influences may lead to the onset of diseases. With this knowledge public health professionals can shape their assessment, policy development, and assurance techniques more effectively. Public health professionals can promote the use of genetic tests and services when inexpensive and effective treatments are available to advance the collective health of the population. An example mentioned involves newborn screening programs, which are expanding in scope as new genetic causes and treatments of disorders are discovered.

Genetic testing and screening for multifactoral conditions such as cancer may allow susceptible persons to change their behaviors and environment, thus improving public health. Public health officials may be best equipped to conduct population research to evaluate the clinical validity and utility of genetic testing and screening. Also, those officials can play a substantial role in the dissemination of information to medical professionals and the public about the role of genetics in health (Gostin, Hodge, and Calvo).

The use of genetic tests and screening for public health purposes, however, can be problematic. Genetic tests that have high rates of inaccuracy can lead to low predictive values when they are incorporated into a genetic screening program. Significant numbers of tests results that are false positive (healthy persons are wrongly determined to be affected by a genetic disease or condition) and false negative (persons who are affected go undetected) can follow. Experience with genetic screening for sickle-cell anemia among African-Americans in the 1970s demonstrated the potential discrimination that may follow a public health screening program (New York State Task Force on Life and the Law). Beyond obvious individual harms, genetic screening programs that are not scientifically sound or justifiable on societal grounds have little utility in public health. With limited resources for preventive public health measures, genetic screening programs that produce small yields (the number of newly recognized cases derived from the screening) as a result of inaccurate testing or other failures can compromise public health goals. Stated simply, poorly administered or poorly designed genetic screening programs that use inaccurate tests or insufficiently target at-risk populations negatively affect individuals and result in minimal or no improvement in public health.

Ethical Concerns

Ethical issues pervade any public health strategy involving genetic tests or screening. This section examines some of the key ethical issues concerning individual informed consent, the design and application of genetic screening and testing, and privacy and discrimination. These and other issues are explored in the context of the sometimes divergent views of public health and individual ethical theories discussed below.

BIOETHICS AND PUBLIC HEALTH ETHICS. Ethical questions arising from genetic testing and screening in the context of public health require an understanding of the differing perspectives of individual and public health ethics. Principles of bioethics largely have an individualistic focus. Persons as individuals are entitled to autonomy, are owed fair and equitable treatment, and must not be harmed intentionally. These rights inhere in each person and, consequently, are owed to each person. Principles of public health ethics do not abandon this individualistic approach. Protection of individual rights is critical in public health practice that increasingly stresses an ethic of voluntarism.

In contrast, public health is focused on the health of communities. Protecting the health of communities sometimes may require individuals to act or contribute to the larger community goals. For example, screening infants for genetic diseases requires parents to allow their children's blood to be tested. The resulting infringement on individual autonomy and decision making under this scenario may be minimal, but the impact on public health can be extraordinary. Public health authorities suggest that this infringement is completely justifiable under a public health ethical framework that envisions individuals as members of society with certain communal goals.

Many bioethicists often perceive a conflict between individual ethical rights and duties and public health ethics. Public health programs and efforts seemingly interfere with individual decision making, bodily integrity, and other protected interests. Ideally, public health programs incorporate the ethical rights of individuals to promote individual participation, which is essential to accomplishing many communal health goals. Sometimes it is not possible to respect the ethical interests of individuals and accomplish legitimate public health goals. For example, it is problematic to allow persons to deny public health authorities access to their diagnoses of genetic disease, which the authorities need to conduct effective surveillance. The individual's claim of a breach of privacy rights under principles of autonomy could trump the community's goal of monitoring disease among the population. Public health ethics suggests that persons participate in public health measures even when some infringement of their individual rights may follow. This analysis provides an appropriate framework for considering the ethical issues discussed below.

INDIVIDUAL INFORMED CONSENT. Principles of autonomy strongly support the individual's right to informed consent before genetic testing or screening. Many law and policy makers, particularly at the state level, have passed legislation or created administrative regulations in the last decade that require specific, written informed consent (sometimes including genetic counseling). Before the administration of a test patients are entitled to explanations of the nature and scope of the information to be gathered, the meaning of positive test results, the underlying disease or condition, and any risks involved in the testing or activities that follow a positive result. Through advance informed consent it is hoped that patients can weigh the benefits of genetic testing against the risks. However, problems in understanding the complexities of genetic science and uncertainties in the meaning of positive test results can limit the value of informed consent (Press and Clayton).

Should genetic tests ever be allowed without informed consent? Public health officials may justify mandatory newborn screening programs without parental consent by reference to utilitarianism and corresponding legal principles that authorize the state to protect children. However, at least in regard to autonomous individuals, there is little justification to mandate genetic testing or screening without informed consent.

WHEN SHOULD GENETIC SCREENING BE PERFORMED? Although genetic screening may be enhanced through the use of accurate tests, there are other key considerations, including determining (1) the at-risk population to be targeted for screening, (2) the method or methods of screening, whether mandatory (required) or voluntary (optional), (3) the persons who have access to the screening program (Lin-Fu and Lloyd-Puryear), (4) whether there is an effective and affordable treatment for the condition being screened, (5) the corresponding benefits to individuals of screening in cases in which treatment is lacking, and (6) whether the screening program is well tailored to accomplish the underlying public health goals.

Each of these criteria underlying the implementation of a genetic screening program is critical. If the screening program targets too large a group and is thus over-inclusive, persons may unjustifiably be asked or required to participate without any individual or public health benefit. If the screening is mandatory, individual autonomy can be breached unfairly. In cases in which persons lack access to testing services, they are unfairly left out of a public health program designed to improve communal health. If there is no effective treatment for a genetic condition, is there a valid reason to screen anyone for it? Many public health officials would suggest that there is not.

PRIVACY AND DISCRIMINATION. Many persons view their genetic information as highly sensitive and take affirmative measures to protect the privacy of that information. According to Georgetown University's Health Privacy Project (2001), over 15 percent of people engage in privacy-protective behaviors (e.g., withholding information, providing inaccurate information, doctor hopping, or avoiding care) to shield themselves from misuse of their health information. Individuals are concerned about the privacy of their genetic data because breaches can lead to invidious discrimination against an individual or group (Hodge and Harris) by insurers, employers, government agencies, and other societal members. Health, life, and disability insurers may attempt to use genetic test results to limit or deny coverage. Employers may reject applicants for positions or advancement on the basis of their genetic flaws (Gostin, Hodge, and Calvo).

Complicating the privacy claims of individuals, however, are the legitimate claims of others who have a right to know about another person's genetic profile. Spouses, offspring, and close family members may claim a right to obtain knowledge of an individual's genetic test results. State courts in Florida and New Jersey have suggested that healthcare workers may be obligated to share the results of genetic tests with blood relatives of their patients in certain circumstances. Right-to-know claims may further principles of beneficence but can impinge on the privacy rights of individuals participating in public health genetic screening programs.

GENETIC EXCEPTIONALISM. Individual privacy and antidiscrimination concerns relating to genetic testing have led many states to adopt genetic-specific privacy and antidiscrimination laws that are intended to protect persons from wrongful acquisition, use, or disclosure of individually

identifiable genetic data. These laws treat genetic information differently from other medical or personally identifiable information and typically establish heightened protections (Gostin and Hodge). Within the context of public health uses of genetic testing or screening programs the trend toward genetic exceptionalism presents its own ethical and practical concerns.

Genetic exceptionalism suggests that genetic information is unique. Many people believe that genetic information is different from other health data for several reasons. Foremost among those reasons is its predictive nature. Unlike most other medical records, which describe an individual's past or current health condition, genetic tests can identify (with varying degrees of confidence) the increased risk of future disease in otherwise healthy individuals. Other qualities add to the perception that genetic information is different. It remains largely stable throughout life. Genetic footprints are remarkably identifiable. Genetic conditions are inherited, and this means that genetic information necessarily reveals information about an individual's current family members and future offspring. Finally, although genetic tests are limited in their capabilities, genetic information can transcend health status to reveal predispositions and personal characteristics (Gostin, Hodge, and Calvo).

There are drawbacks to treating genetic information differently. Strict protection of autonomy, privacy, and equal treatment of people with genetic conditions may threaten the accomplishment of communal goods, including public health surveillance. As scientists discover more medical conditions that are gene-based, it will become increasingly difficult to distinguish genetic data from other medical data. Genetic information is part of the continuum of an individual's medical record and cannot be separated from those data easily. Some privacy advocates argue that genetic information is more sensitive than other health information because it can provide significantly more personal information about an individual's existing and future medical conditions. However, *nongenetic* electronic health records also may provide many personal details. Electronic health records include private demographic, financial, and family history information as well as a patient's social, behavioral, and environmental factors (Gostin and Hodge).

Genetic-specific statutes may be considered unfair because they treat people who are facing the same social risks differently on the basis of the biological cause of their otherwise identical health conditions. Why, for example, should medical information about a woman who has developed breast cancer of genetic origin (e.g., BRACA 1 or 2) be given greater protection than information about a woman who has developed breast cancer because of environmental or behavioral factors such as smoking (Rothstein)?

On a practical level, treating genetic diseases as distinct from other medical diseases or conditions may enhance the stigma of genetic testing and screening programs even as lawmakers attempt to remove their stigmatizing effects. This can create public fears and misapprehension about genetics that may discourage individuals from seeking testing or participating in screening programs and may thwart future scientific progress.

Conclusion

The public health benefits of genetic testing and screening support their existing and future uses in the population, yet the underlying risks to individuals and populations require caution and awareness. Ethical issues related to the administration of testing and screening with informed consent, the privacy rights of individuals, and concerns about discrimination cannot be resolved easily. Balancing individual rights with the community's interests in promoting public health requires an understanding of the sometimes divergent positions of bioethics and public health ethics. Exceptionalizing protection of individual rights that are based on distinctions of genetic tests or information from other health data is difficult. Ultimately, choices about the use of genetic tests and the administration of genetic screening in the population must be made collectively in the interests of promoting improvements in public health.

JAMES G. HODGE, JR.

SEE ALSO: *AIDS; Autonomy; Confidentiality; Genetic Counseling, Ethical Issues in; Genetic Counseling, Practice of; Holocaust; Informed Consent; Public Health; Public Health Law; Public Policy and Bioethics; Race and Racism; Utilitarianism;* and other *Genetic Testing and Screening* subentries

BIBLIOGRAPHY

Gostin, Lawrence O. 2000. *Public Health Law: Power, Duty, Restraint.* Berkeley: University of California Press.

Gostin, Lawrence O., and Hodge, James G. 1999. "Genetic Privacy and the Law: An End to Genetics Exceptionalism." *Jurimetrics: The Journal of Law, Science, and Technology* 40: 21–58.

Gostin, Lawrence O.; Hodge, James G.; and Calvo, Cheye M. 2001. *Genetics Law and Policy: A Review.* Denver, CO: National Conference of State Legislatures.

Hodge, James G., and Harris, Mark E. 2001. "International Genetics Research and Issues of Group Privacy." *Journal of BioLaw and Business* Special Supplement: Global Genomics: 15–21.

Lin-Fu, Jane S., and Lloyd-Puryear, Michele. 2000. "Access to Genetic Services in the United States: A Challenge to Genetics

in Public Health." In *Genetics and Public Health in the 21st Century: Using Genetic Information to Improve Health and Prevent Disease,* ed. Muin J. Khoury, Wylie Burke, and Elizabeth J. Thomson. New York: Oxford University Press.

New York State Task Force on Life and the Law. 2000. *Genetic Testing and Screening in the Age of Genomic Medicine.* New York: Author.

Press, Nancy, and Clayton, Ellen Wright. 2000. "Genetics and Public Health: Informed Consent beyond the Clinical Encounter." In *Genetics and Public Health in the 21st Century: Using Genetic Information to Improve Health and Prevent Disease,* ed. Muin J. Khoury, Wylie Burke, and Elizabeth J. Thomson. New York: Oxford University Press.

Rothstein, Mark R. 1998. "Genetic Privacy and Confidentiality: Why They Are So Hard to Protect." *Journal of Law, Medicine and Ethics* 26: 198.

Secretary's Advisory Committee on Genetic Testing. 2000. *Enhancing the Oversight of Genetic Tests: Recommendations of the SAGCT.* Bethesda, MD: Author.

Shulte, Paul A., and DeBord, D. Gayle. 2000. "Public Health Assessment of Genetic Information in the Occupational Setting." In *Genetics and Public Health in the 21st Century: Using Genetic Information to Improve Health and Prevent Disease,* ed. Muin J. Khoury, Wylie Burke, and Elizabeth J. Thomson. New York: Oxford University Press.

INTERNET RESOURCES

Centers for Disease Control and Prevention Office of Genetics and Disease Prevention. 2003. Available from <http://www.cdc.gov/genomics/default.htm>.

Georgetown University Health Privacy Project. 2001. *Landmark Health Privacy Law Issued by Clinton Administration.* Available from <http//www.healthprivacy.org>.

V. PREDICTIVE GENETIC TESTING

In June 2000 international leaders of the Human Genome Project (HGP) confirmed that the rough draft of the human genome had been completed a year ahead of schedule. In February 2001 special issues of *Science* and *Nature* published the working draft sequence and analysis. A complete, high-quality DNA reference sequence was announced in April 2003, two years earlier than the originally projected completion date. Although a major goal of the HGP is to provide tools to treat, cure, and ultimately prevent genetic disease, the immediate outcome has been a surge in the number of genetic tests that can be used to determine an individual's risk for developing an ever-increasing number of genetic diseases.

The ability to provide currently healthy individuals with DNA-based risk assessments for diseases that will manifest in the future, especially in the absence of effective treatment for those diseases, presents challenges for those at risk, health professionals, and society. This entry explores some of those challenges, concentrating on tests that can detect mutations associated with adult-onset disorders.

Available Tests

The beginning of the era of genetic prediction can be dated to 1983, when Huntington's disease (HD) became the first disease to be mapped to a previously unknown genetic location through the use of restriction enzymes that cleave deoxyribonucleic acid (DNA) at sequence-specific sites (Gusella et al.). Huntington's disease is a late-onset autosomal dominant neuropsychiatric disorder. The child of an affected parent has a 50 percent chance of inheriting the genetic mutation that causes HD. Disease onset usually occurs in the fourth decade of life and is marked by a movement disorder, alterations in mood, and cognitive decline. There is no treatment or cure.

Inherited variations of these DNA sequences, which also are known as restriction fragment length polymorphisms (RFLPs), can be used as genetic markers to map diseases on chromosomes and to trace the inheritance of diseases in families. The discovery of these markers represented a significant advance in HD research. Not only did the markers provide a possible clue for finding the HD gene and understanding the mechanism by which the gene causes brain cells to die, this discovery meant that predictive testing for some individuals at risk for HD was possible through the use of a technique called linkage. Linkage testing requires the collection and analysis of blood samples from affected and elderly unaffected relatives of the at-risk individual who asks for testing to trace the pattern of inheritance of the HD gene in a specific family. Linkage testing is labor-intensive and expensive and can result in erroneous conclusions caused by incorrectly attributed paternity, misdiagnosis, and the distance between the gene and the markers used for testing. The discovery of the HD gene in 1993 (Huntington's Disease Collaborative Research Group) made testing more accurate, less expensive, faster, and possible for every person at risk for HD.

Since that time new discoveries in molecular genetics have shifted the focus from relatively rare single-gene disorders such as HD to common adult-onset disorders that cause substantial morbidity and mortality. Examples include the identification of mutations in the BRCA1 and BRCA2 genes as causes of susceptibility to breast and ovarian cancers (Miki et al.; Wooster et al.), the discovery of multiple genetic mutations associated with the risk of colorectal cancer (Laken et al.; Lynch and Lynch), the reported association between the APOE e4 allele and late-onset Alzheimer disease (Strittmatter et al.), associations between factor V Leiden

and thromboembolic disease (Hille et al.; Ridker et al.; Simioni et al.), and the identification of the HFE gene for hereditary hemochromatosis (Beutler et al.; Edwards et al.). In the second decade of the twenty-first century it has been predicted that genetic tests will be available for diabetes, asthma, dyslexia, attention deficit hyperactivity disorder, obesity, and schizophrenia. These discoveries point to the potential use of genetic tests for population screening in adult populations and an increasing role in public health for genetic testing.

Evaluating New Tests

The National Institutes of Health–Department of Education–Department of Energy (NIH–DOE) Task Force on Genetic Testing stated in 1998 that any proposed initiation of population-based genetic screening requires careful attention to the parameters of both analytical and clinical validity. For DNA-based tests analytical validity requires establishing that a test will be positive when a particular sequence is present (analytical sensitivity) and establishing the probability that that test will be negative when the sequence is absent (analytical specificity). Clinical validity involves establishing measures of clinical performance, including the probability that the test will be positive in people with the disease (clinical sensitivity), the probability that the test will be negative in people without the disease (clinical specificity), and the positive and negative predictive value (PV) of the test. The positive PV is the probability that people with a positive test eventually will get the disease. The negative PV is the probability that people with negative test results will not get the disease.

Two features of most of the genetic diseases discussed as candidates for population-wide screening also affect the clinical validity of any test designed to screen for those diseases. The first is heterogeneity, or the fact that the same genetic disease may result from the presence of any of several different variants of the same gene (an example would be cystic fibrosis, with over 900 mutations found in the CF gene) or of different genes (such as the genes for breast cancer BRCA1 and BRCA2). The second is penetrance, the probability that disease will appear when the disease-related genotype is present. Both heterogeneity and penetrance may differ in different populations, causing difficulties in the interpretation of test results. The final Report of the Task Force on Genetic Testing stated that "clinical use of a genetic test must be based on evidence that the gene being examined is associated with the disease in question, that the test itself has analytical and clinical validity, and that the test results will be useful to the people being tested" (Task Force on Genetic Testing).

From a public health perspective the value of implementing these tests on a population-wide basis will depend to a large extent on whether early treatment of diseases discovered through screening improves the prognosis (Burke et al.). That can be determined only through randomized clinical trials, an expensive process for the array of tests likely to be developed in the near future. However, experience with hormone replacement therapy (HRT) for healthy postmenopausal women in which HRT was found to cause more health problems than a placebo (Writing Group for the Women's Health Initiative Investigators) and a widely used knee surgery technique for osteoarthritis that was found to be ineffective (Moseley et al.) suggests that such trials may be a necessary component of any proposed large-scale screening effort.

Critics of this approach say that the prospective studies necessary to gather this type of information can take years. If widespread use of a test is withheld until the positive predictive value is determined fully and the risks and benefits of testing are known clearly, manufacturers and laboratories could be inhibited from developing tests, and consequently, people will be denied the benefits of being tested. Even without an effective treatment these benefits might include a reduction in uncertainty, the ability to avoid the conception or birth of a child carrying the disease-causing mutation, escape from frequent monitoring for signs of disease or prophylactic surgery, and freedom from concerns about employment or insurance discrimination.

In the absence of a consensus on the public health benefits of widespread screening, tests continue to be developed and in some cases marketed directly to physicians and consumers. For example, in June 2002 Myriad Genetics, based in Salt Lake City, Utah, announced that it would market genetic tests for familial cancers to the general public despite the fact that those tests were appropriate only for a very small percentage of the population. This practice has been the subject of some controversy (Holtzman and Watson), especially in cases in which predictive tests have become available without adequate assessment of their positive predictive value or benefits and risks. Without this information it is difficult for providers or consumers to make thoughtful and fully informed decisions about whether to offer or to use the tests. In another case a test based on the association of the APOE e4 allele with late-onset Alzheimer's disease was marketed directly to physicians just months after the first paper about that association was published. The genetics community decried this development, asserting that the actual interpretation of those associational data for any single individual could not be determined and that any test result based on it would be misleading if not worthless.

The public outcry was so great that the test was withdrawn from the market in a matter of months.

The Testing Process

Requests for testing can arise from a variety of circumstances and for a number of reasons. For example, although genetic test results can be used to guide individual healthcare and reproductive decisions, genetic testing often is sought to fulfill familial, domestic, or vocational responsibilities (Burgess and d'Agincourt-Canning). For this reason healthcare professionals must be adept at presenting and discussing the potential ramifications of testing in light of the at-risk individual's reason for requesting testing. Genetics practice also calls for pretest and posttest counseling and formal informed consent procedures to ensure that people deciding whether to undergo genetic testing are informed about the risks and potential harms, benefits, and limitations of the test, as well as alternatives and treatment options (National Advisory Council for Human Genome Research; Holtzman and Watson).

At the beginning of the twenty-first century, the volume of genetic testing was not great and the vast majority of testing occurred in genetic centers or in consultation with highly trained geneticists and genetics counselors. As the number of tests increases, the demand for testing may outstrip the capacity of genetics-trained individuals to respond. This scenario suggests that it is likely that more and more testing decisions will be made by physicians with little formal training or experience in genetics. Some question the ability of physicians to perform this function and continue to recommend referrals to health professionals with specific training in genetics to ensure proper counseling, informed consent, and correct interpretation of test results (Giardello et al.).

A related issue is the fear that physicians will be more likely to take a directive approach to decisions about testing. This approach is antithetical to the concept of the value-neutral nondirective counseling that is a main tenet of all genetic counseling. Historically, this commitment to nondirective counseling can be understood as a moral stance designed to disassociate modern genetics from the eugenics movements of the first half of the twentieth century, which often advocated forced sterilization for individuals deemed to be genetically abnormal (Paul).

Philosophically, nondirective counseling also reflects the centrality of respect for autonomy (the right to self-determination or self-governance) in modern bioethics. Because decisions about genetic testing often involve reproduction and/or an individual's most personal desires and fears, the genetics community has adopted the view that the role of the genetics professional is to help an individual make a decision about testing that is consistent with that person's most strongly held values. Genetic counselors in training are taught specifically not to let their own opinions and attitudes influence the information that is given to people or recommendations for a course of action.

The Decision to Be Tested

The process of genetic testing can challenge traditional concepts of autonomy and privacy. The desire to be tested on the part of one individual can place pressure on other family members if their cooperation is required for the test to be done. In testing for familial cancers, for example, it is often necessary for a family member who is already affected to be tested first to identify the specific disease-associated mutation in the family. If the affected family member refuses to cooperate, that refusal can frustrate the desire of other family members to learn about their risk. This need to identify an index case also makes it difficult for an individual who wishes to be tested to keep that decision private.

Some authors have advanced the concept of *relational responsibility* as playing a key role in decisions regarding testing (Burgess and d'Agincourt-Canning). This ethical concept emphasizes that decisions about genetic testing occur within complex social relationships that are embedded in and shaped by notions of responsibility to specific others. Thus, although testing guidelines often emphasize that the decision whether to undergo genetic testing should be solely that of the individual for his or her own purposes and free from coercion by a spouse or another family member, research suggests that in reality people often make decisions about testing on the basis of the wishes and desires of others, primarily close family members, about whom they care deeply. Rosamund Rhodes has taken the notion of relational responsibility further, arguing that individuals have a moral duty to pursue genetic information about themselves, especially in cases in which that information has ramifications for others, such as spouses or children (Rhodes).

Ordering Tests

Once the decision has been made to pursue testing, tests for relatively common disorders usually are obtained from commercial laboratories (GeneTest). Blood is drawn and mailed to the laboratory, and the test results are conveyed back to the healthcare professional who ordered the test. That person then has the responsibility of conveying the results, usually in person, to the individual who has been tested. Genetic tests for rare disorders sometimes are available only from laboratories in academic medical centers that

have a particular interest in the disease in question. Those laboratories may not have satisfied the ongoing quality and proficiency assessments required of commercial laboratories, thus raising questions about the reliability of testing obtained from this source.

Sharing Genetic Information

When a test has been performed and a result has been obtained, other considerations come into play. Perhaps the most vexing is whether and when a person has a moral duty to share genetic information. Genetic test results for a specific individual also reveal information about that person's relatives. Parents and children share half their genes, as do siblings. If a woman learns that she carries a gene associated with breast cancer, does she have a responsibility to share that information with her sister? Many writers agree that that responsibility exists, with Dorothy Wertz and colleagues suggesting that at the level of the person genetic information, although individual, should "be shared among family members" as a form of shared familial property (Wertz et al.). Indeed, most people, once they are aware of the implications of genetic information for other family members, willingly share the information with those for whom it is especially relevant.

However, what if a woman with a breast cancer mutation does not wish to share that information? May her physician breach her confidentiality and warn her sister? Several groups have addressed this issue in depth (President's Commission for the Study of Ethical Problems in Medicine and Biomedical and Behavioral Research; Andrews et al.). Guidelines published by the American Society of Human Genetics Social Issues Subcommittee on Familial Disclosure in 1998 state that the legal and ethical norm of patient confidentiality should be respected, with breaches of confidentiality permitted only in exceptional cases. Those exceptions are (1) when attempts to encourage disclosure by the patient have failed, when the harm is highly likely to occur and is serious and foreseeable, when the at-risk relative or relatives are identifiable, and when the disease is preventable/treatable or medically accepted standards indicate that early monitoring will reduce the genetic risk and (2) when the harm that may result from failure to disclose outweighs the harm that may result from disclosure (Knoppers et al.). At least one author has argued that knowledge about the risk for conceiving a child with a deleterious gene does not pose the type of serious, imminent harm that generally would require disclosure (Andrews).

In regard to the issue of disclosure Ruth Macklin suggests the institution of a patient "Miranda" warning so that before genetic testing occurs, a patient would be warned about the circumstances that would result in the disclosure of genetic information to other family members regardless of the patient's intentions to disclose (Macklin).

Two court decisions appear to indicate an increasing trend toward disclosure. In *Pate v. Threkel*, Florida, 1995, a physician was held to a duty to warn patients of the familial implications of a genetic disease. In *Safer v. Estate of Pack*, New Jersey, 1996, the court held that a physician has a duty to warn relatives known to be at risk for a genetic disorder regardless of potential conflicts between the duty to warn and the obligations of confidentiality. The courts have not yet addressed a physician's obligation to disclose information concerning individuals whose occupations may place the lives of others in danger, such as pilots and air traffic controllers.

The completion of the Human Genome Project will result in a proliferation of genetic tests for a wide variety of disorders. Some public health advocates argue for a broader role for population-based testing, whereas critics believe that further work needs to be done to understand the value of testing on a widespread basis. Concerns exist about the ability of consumers and physicians to make informed decisions about whether to use genetic tests and are exacerbated by a growing trend on the part of commercial laboratories to market the tests directly to consumers. Once a test has been ordered and the results have been obtained, questions remain about the duties of both individuals and healthcare professionals regarding disclosure of test results.

KIMBERLY A. QUAID

SEE ALSO: *Autonomy; Cancer, Ethical Issues Related to Diagnosis and Treatment; Children: Mental Health Issues; Dementia; Genetic Counseling, Ethical Issues in; Genetic Counseling, Practice of; Genetic Discrimination; Genetics and Human Self-Understanding; Health Insurance; Informed Consent;* and other *Genetic Testing and Screening* subentries

BIBLIOGRAPHY

Andrews, Lori. 1997. "The Genetic Information Superhighway: Rules of the Road for Contacting Relatives and Recontacting Former Patients." In *Human DNA: Law and Policy: International and Comparative Perspectives,* ed. Bartha M. Knoppers and Claude Laberge. The Hague: Kluwer Law International.

Andrews, Lori; Fullerton, Jane; Holtman, Neil, et al. 1994. *Assessing Genetic Risks: Implications for Health and Social Policy.* Washington, D.C.: Institute of Medicine.

Beutler, Ernest; Felitti, Vincent; Gelbart, Terri, et al. 2000. "The Effect of HFE Genotypes on Measurements of Iron Overload in Patients Attending a Health Appraisal Clinic." *Annals of Internal Medicine* 133: 328–337.

Burgess, Michael M., and d'Agincourt-Canning, Lori. 2001. "Genetic Testing for Hereditary Disease: Attending to Relational Responsibility." *Journal of Clinical Ethics* 12: 361–372.

Burke, Wylie; Coughlin, Steven; Lee, Nancy, et al. 2001. "Application of Population Screening Principles to Genetic Screening for Adult-Onset Conditions." *Genetic Testing* 5: 201–211.

Edwards, Corwin Q.; Griffen, Linda M.; Ajioka, Richard S., et al. 1998. "Screening for Hemochromatosis: Phenotypes versus Genotypes." *Hematology* 35: 72–76.

Giardello, Francis M.; Brensinger, Jill D.; Petersen, Gloria M., et al. 1997. "The Use and Interpretation of Commercial APC Gene Testing for Familial Adenomatous Polyposis." *New England Journal of Medicine* 336(12): 823–827.

Gusella, James F.; Wexler, Nancy S.; Conneally, P. Michael, et al. 1983. "A Polymorphic DNA Marker Genetically Linked to Huntington Disease." *Nature* 306: 234–238.

Hille, Elysee T., Westendorp, Rudi G.; Vandenbroucke, Jan P., et al. 1997. "Mortality and the Causes of Death in a Family with Factor V Leiden Mutation (Resistance to Activated Protein C)." *Blood* 89: 1963–1967.

Holtzman, Neil A., and Watson, Michael S., eds. 1998. *Promoting Safe and Effective Genetic Testing in the United States: Final Report of the Task Force on Genetic Testing, National Human Genome Research Institute.* Baltimore: Johns Hopkins University Press.

Huntington's Disease Collaborative Research Group. 1993. "A Novel Gene Containing a Trinucleotide Repeat That Is Expanded and Unstable on Huntington's Disease Chromosomes." *Cell* 72: 971–983.

Knoppers, Bartha M.; Strom, Charles; Clayton, Ellen Wright, et al., for the American Society of Human Genetics Social Issues Subcommittee on Familial Disclosure. 1998. "Professional Disclosure of Familial Genetic Information." *American Journal of Human Genetics* 62(2): 474–483.

Laken, Steven J.; Petersen, Gloria M.; Gruber, Stephen B., et al. 1997. "Familial Colorectal Cancer in Ashkenazim Due to a Hypermutable Tract in APC." *Nature Genetics* 17(1): 79–83.

Lynch, Henry T., and Lynch, Jane F. 1998. "Genetics of Colonic Cancer." *Digestion* 59: 481–492.

Macklin, Ruth. 1992. "Privacy Control of Genetic Information." In *Gene Mapping: Using Law and Ethics as Guides,* ed. George Annas and Sherman Elias. New York: Oxford University Press.

Miki, Yoshio; Swensen, Jeff; Shattuck-Eidens, Donna, et al. 1994. "A Strong Candidate for the Breast and Ovarian Cancer Susceptibility Gene BRCA1." *Science* 266: 66–71.

Moseley, J. Bruce; O'Malley, Kimberly; Petersen, Nancy J., et al. 2002. "A Controlled Trial of Arthroscopic Surgery for Osteoarthritis of the Knee." *New England Journal of Medicine* 27(2): 81–88.

National Advisory Council for Human Genome Research. 1994. "Statement on the Use of DNA Testing for Presymptomatic Identification of Cancer Risk." *Journal of the American Medical Association* 271: 785.

Paul, Diane. 1995. *Controlling Human Heredity, 1865—Present.* Atlantic Highlands, NJ: Humanities Press.

President's Commission for the Study of Ethical Problems in Medicine and Biomedical and Behavioral Research. 1983. *Screening and Counseling for Genetic Conditions: A Report on the Ethical, Social and Legal Implications of Genetic Screening, Counseling and Education Program.* Washington, D.C.: U.S. Government Printing Office.

Rhodes, Rosamond. 1998. "Genetic Links, Family Ties, and Social Bonds: Rights and Responsibilities in the Face of Genetic Knowledge." *Journal of Medicine and Philosophy* 23(1): 10–30.

Ridker, Paul M.; Glynn, Robert J.; Miletich, Joseph P., et al. 1997. "Age-Specific Incidence Rates of Venous Thromboembolism among Heterozygous Carriers of Factor V Leiden Mutation." *Annals of Internal Medicine* 126: 528–531.

Simioni, Paolo; Prandoni, Paolo; Lensing, Anthonie W., et al. 1997. "The Risk of Recurrent Venous Thromboembolism in Patients with an ARG^{506}→Gln Mutation in the Gene for Factor V (Factor V Leiden)." *New England Journal of Medicine* 336: 399–403.

Strittmatter, Warren J.; Saunders, Ann M.; Schmechel, Donald E., et al. 1993. "Apolipoprotein E: High-Avidity Binding to B-Amyloid and Increased Frequency of Type 4 Allele in Late-Onset Familial Alzheimer's Disease." *Proceedings of the National Academy of Science of the United States of America* 90: 1977–1981.

Wertz, Dorothy; Fletcher, John; and Berg, Kare. 1995. *Guidelines on Ethical Issues in Medical Genetics and the Provision of Genetic Services.* Geneva: World Health Organization.

Wooster, Richard; Neuhausen, Susan L.; Mangion, Jonathan, et al. 1994. "Localization of a Breast Cancer Susceptibility Gene, BRCA2, to Chromosome 13q12–13." *Science* 265: 2088–2090.

Writing Group for the Women's Health Initiative Investigators. 2002. "Risks and Benefits of Estrogen Plus Progestin in Healthy Postmenopausal Women: Principal Results from the Women's Health Initiative Randomized Controlled Trial." *Journal of the American Medical Association* 288(3): 321–333.

INTERNET RESOURCES

GeneTests. 2003. Available from <http://www.genetests.org>.

Task Force on Genetic Testing. 1998. Available from <http://www.hopkinsmedicine.org/tfgtelsi/>.

VI. PEDIATRIC GENETIC TESTING

DNA-based clinical testing is available for over 900 genetic diseases, and research-based testing is offered for hundreds of others. Such testing can aid in making diagnoses, assessing recurrence risks, and providing accurate prognoses. Often genetic testing is initiated prior to the onset of symptoms. This type of testing is known as pre-symptomatic or predictive genetic testing, and is typically offered for adult-onset diseases such as Huntington's chorea or certain types of cancer. Huntington's chorea, or Huntington's disease, is a progressive, fatal, neurological condition that affects movements and memory. Individuals who carry the gene for Huntington's disease usually begin showing symptoms around age 40, though this can vary dramatically between individuals and families. The types of cancer that can be associated with inherited DNA mutations include breast cancer, ovarian cancer, and certain types of colon cancer.

Though DNA-based clinical testing has become a part of routine management for numerous diseases, it presents a unique set of circumstances that separate it from other types of testing. Since a number of genetic mutations are inherited from parents, testing either children or parents will often reveal increased risk for other family members. In the cases of autosomal dominant conditions such as Huntington's disease or Hereditary Breast and Ovarian Cancer syndrome, an affected parent has a 50 percent chance of passing on the defective gene to his or her child.

There are a number of ethical issues associated with the use of pre-symptomatic testing for adult-onset disorders. One important area of discussion focuses on whether genetic testing for these diseases should be initiated in children. Several professional organizations, including the American Academy of Pediatrics and the American Society for Human Genetics, have formal positions stating that children under the age of eighteen years should not undergo genetic testing for adult-onset disorders. The American Society for Human Genetics states: "if medical or psychological benefits of a genetic test will not accrue until adulthood, as in the case of … adult-onset diseases, genetic testing generally should be deferred" (American College of Medical Genetics, pp. 1233–1241), and the World Federation of Neurology Research Group on Huntington's Chorea explicitly recommends not testing any minors.

These policies are driven by the argument that since these are adult-onset disorders for which there is no treatment or medical intervention during childhood, there is no medical benefit to testing. Additionally, children are unable to understand the complexities involved in the testing and therefore cannot provide informed consent. Testing these children, then, potentially could be seen as harmful, as it takes away their right not to know their genetic status.

Proponents of genetic testing in children argue that there are situations when the benefits of testing, either medical or emotional, outweigh the potential harms. This article will explore these arguments in detail, and present a proposal for appropriate use for predictive tests in children.

Pre-symptomatic genetic testing for adult-onset disorders typically involves a detailed informed consent process. This process can include discussions of the natural course of the disease, prognosis, risks to other family members, and treatment options. Some informed consent processes, such as the one outlined by the Huntington's Disease Society of

America, require a psychiatric assessment to determine how test results will be viewed, and what potential reactions might occur. This process can be lengthy and challenging for an adult, and would not be possible for a child. The question, then, is raised as to whether parents can consent for the pre-symptomatic genetic testing for children.

Medical decision making for adults is largely guided by respect for persons and autonomy, whereas in pediatrics it is guided by beneficence. With regards to adult medicine, medical decisions made by competent adults who have undergone an appropriate informed consent process are typically respected. In a pediatric setting, the parents traditionally have had the responsibility of medical decision making, where a competent adult is challenged to make decisions not for his or her own care, but for the child's. This is based on the assumptions that parents are typically interested in maintaining their children's best interests and safety; parents are in a position to know what those best interests are by virtue of knowing their children better than anyone else; parents usually must deal with the financial, emotional, and practical aspects of such decisions; and Western society typically has strived to maintain privacy and parental control within a family unit whenever possible. In other words, the autonomy of parents traditionally is respected as long as it supports the benefit of the child; the challenge then becomes balancing the rights of the children with the rights of parents.

Can Predictive Genetic Testing be Harmful?

There are some situations where the desires of the parent, regardless of how well meaning, may not be in the best interest of the child. In the case of pre-symptomatic genetic testing, a parent often has a need to know what the genetic status of a child is, but that information may or may not be beneficial to the child, and even could be harmful. The purpose of an informed consent process for pre-symptomatic testing is to enable individuals to make decisions about whether they want this information, and to consider how it might affect how they live their lives. A child who has undergone genetic testing will never have the option not to know the results of that information. A positive test result in a child may result in potentially serious psychosocial affects on relationships, family, school performance, and self-concept. This is particularly true if the child has watched a great deal of suffering on the part of the parent. A negative test result can lead to survivor guilt or feelings of being ostracized from affected family members. Many adults choose not to undergo testing due to the psychological burden of incorporating a test result into their lives and futures, and opponents of predictive genetic testing in children feel that children should be offered that same freedom from knowledge.

Personal experience can also interfere with a child's ability to understand the complexities of a positive result, or the reassurance of a negative result. For example, a positive DNA test for the genes associated with Breast and Ovarian Cancer syndrome confers a lifetime risk of developing breast or ovarian cancer of approximately 50 to 80 percent, not 100 percent. Conversely, a negative test result for this child reveals that her risk of breast cancer is not zero, but rather that of the general population, which is approximately 10 percent. A child who has watched her mother die from breast cancer may view this positive result as a prediction of her future and a death sentence, instead of indicating an increased risk. This is a heavy burden to place on a child who is already struggling with the loss of a parent.

The nature of genetic material presents an additional challenge to testing individuals of any age, but these issues can be magnified when dealing with children. By definition, genetic testing often reveals information about other family members, and healthcare providers should consider prior to testing how that information will be addressed. Specifically, genetic testing can reveal cases of non-paternity that can have an adverse affect on the relationship between parent and child.

Can Predictive Genetic Testing be Beneficial?

There are potential benefits to pre-symptomatic genetic testing in children. From a parental standpoint, knowing the genetic status can help parents plan financially and emotionally for their child's future. A positive result may mean long-term care issues that can be offset by advanced financial planning. A parent who is afflicted with a genetic disease may seek comfort in knowing that he or she did not pass on the defective gene to a child, even if symptoms of that disease are years away. In the cases of Huntington's disease and certain types of cancer, an affected parent may not survive long enough for their child to reach adulthood, meaning the parent may die not knowing if their child will suffer a similar fate.

The child herself may be comforted by a negative result. There is a strong argument for the emotional benefit of being able to tell a child who is afraid of the disease of a parent that he or she is unlikely to develop the same disease. This is particularly true in an adolescent, who may have been able to identify his or her own risk through research, even if this information was never discussed at home or with a medical practitioner.

In addition, there are potential medical benefits to be considered. In the case of familial adenomatous polyposis (FAP), a familial colon cancer syndrome, colon cancer has been reported in children as young as ten years of age. Approximately 75 percent of those individuals carrying a DNA mutation associated with FAP will develop pre-cancerous polyps before age twenty. In families where this disease has been identified, children of affected parents have a 50 percent chance of having inherited the mutation. For these children, a positive test result would mean a much more rigorous medical course, involving annual colonoscopies to monitor the development of polyps, and most likely a prophylactic colectomy in the future, both measures that could save lives. A negative test result would spare these children from such invasive screening, and reveal their lifetime risk of colon cancer to be that of the general population.

Though it is generally understood that children do not possess the competence to make medical decisions, the situation is less clear for adolescents. Obviously there is no perfect age that competence can be assumed, nor is there a minimum age at which it can be specified as absent. There are adolescents who are capable of engaging in the informed consent process and making medical decisions for themselves. One would hope that, when possible, the decisions of the parent would encompass conversation with the child or adolescent and involve the minor to whatever degree is appropriate for maturity, interest, and responsibility.

The Rule of Earliest Onset

One proposal for determining the appropriate use of predictive tests is the "rule of earliest onset." Simply put, the rule states that "genetic testing should be permitted no earlier than the age of first possible onset of disease" (Kodish, p. 391). This guideline allows for the possibility that medical benefit may outweigh potential harms. Employing this basic rule provides several advantages. First, predictive testing is limited to those children for whom there is a potential medical benefit. Though this does not eliminate the possibility that decisions to test will be fueled by additional motivations, it ensures that benefit to the child will be present. Secondly, by delaying testing until an age when symptoms may occur, one maximizes the likelihood that the now older child can participate in the decision-making process. Finally, it is a family-specific guideline for testing that accounts for variation in the age of onset. For example, even though the majority of Huntington's disease occurs in adults, approximately 10 percent of cases are juvenile. In these families, the disease is typically transmitted through a father whose own disease had an earlier than expected presentation. If predictive testing for a child is being considered, and the history reveals that in this particular family the father is the affected individual and his symptoms developed in his twenties, then the rule of earliest onset for this family would suggest testing an adolescent.

Conclusions

Predictive genetic testing in a pediatric setting is complicated by the complexity of the information, the fact that testing decisions are being made by someone other than the person being tested, and the potential impact of the test results. Traditionally it has been thought that predictive genetic testing should not be offered to children under the age of eighteen, and many professional policies have been developed in support of this.

These policies are based on the assumption that "medical or psychological benefits of a genetic test will not accrue until adulthood." This article has discussed situations where there is arguably either a medical or emotional benefit to the child that would warrant testing, and presented a proposal for the use of predictive genetic testing in pediatrics.

REBECCA MARSICK
ERIC D. KODISH

SEE ALSO: *Disability; Eugenics; Eugenics and Religious Law; Genetic Counseling, Ethical Issues in; Genetic Counseling, Practice of; Genetic Discrimination; Genetics and Human Self-Understanding; Infanticide; Infants; Pediatrics;* and other *Genetic Testing and Screening* subentries

BIBLIOGRAPHY

Codori, A. M.; Petersen, G. M.; Boyd, P. A.; et al. 1996. "Genetic Testing for Cancer in Children. Short-term Psychological Effect." *Archives of Pediatrics & Adolescent Medicine* 150: 1131–1138.

Elger, B. S., and Harding, T. W. 2000. "Testing Adolescents for a Hereditary Breast Cancer Gene (BRCA1): Respecting their Autonomy is in their Best Interest." *Archives of Pediatrics & Adolescent Medicine* 154: 113–119.

Hanson, J. W., and Thomson, E. J. 2000. "Genetic Testing in Children: Ethical and Social Points to Consider." *Pediatric Annals* 29: 285–291.

Kodish, E. D. 1999. "Testing Children for Cancer Genes: The Rule of Earliest Onset." *Journal of Pediatrics* 135: 390–395.

Maat-Kievit, A.; Vegter-Van Der Vlis, M.; Zoeteweij, M.; et al. 1999. "Predictive Testing of 25 Percent At-risk Individuals for Huntington Disease (1987–1997)." *American Journal of Medical Genetics* 88: 662–668.

Meiser, B., and Dunn, S. 2000. "Psychological Impact of Genetic Testing for Huntington's Disease: An Update of the Literature." *Journal of Neurology, Neurosurgery, and Psychiatry* 69: 574–578.

Meiser, B.; Gleeson, M. A.; and Tucker, K. M. 2000. "Psychological Impact of Genetic Testing for Adult-onset Disorders. An Update for Clinicians." *Medical Journal of Australia* 172: 126–129.

Nelson, R. M.; Botkjin, J. R.; Kodish, E. D.; et al. 2001. "Ethical Issues with Genetic Testing in Pediatrics." *Pediatrics* 107: 1451–1455.

Ross, L. F., and Moon, M. R. 2000. "Ethical Issues in Genetic Testing of Children." *Archives of Pediatrics & Adolescent Medicine* 154: 873–879.

Seashore, M. R. 2000. "Genetic Screening and the Pediatrician." *Pediatric Annals* 29: 272–276.

INTERNET RESOURCES

American Academy of Pediatrics. 2001. "Ethical Issues with Genetic Testing in Pediatrics (RE9924)." Available from <http://www.aap.org>.

American College of Medical Genetics. 1995. "Points to Consider: Ethical, Legal and Psychological Implications of Genetic Testing in Children and Adolescents," pp. 1233–1241. Available from <http://www.acmg.net>.

American Medical Association. 1995. "Genetic Testing of Children." Available from <http://www.ama-assn.org>.

GRIEF AND BEREAVEMENT

• • •

The term *grief* can be defined as a type of stress reaction, a highly personal and subjective response that an individual makes to a real, perceived, or anticipated loss. Grief reactions may occur in any loss situation, whether the loss is physical or tangible, such as a death, significant injury, or loss of property; or symbolic and intangible such as the loss of a dream. The intensity of grief will vary, depending on many variables such as the meaning of a loss to the individual experiencing it. It should be recognized that loss does not inevitably create grief. Some individuals may be so disassociated from the loss object that they experience little or no grief, or their response may be characterized by intense denial.

This definition of acute grief distinguishes it from other terms such as *bereavement* or *mourning*. Bereavement refers to an objective state of loss. If one experiences a loss, one is bereaved. Bereavement refers to the fact of loss, whereas grief is the subjective response to that state of loss. Mourning has had two interrelated meanings within the field. On one hand, it has been used to describe the intrapsychic process through which a grieving individual gradually adapts to the loss, a process that has also been referred to as "grieving" or "grief work." The term has also been used to refer to the social aspect of grief, the norms and patterned behaviors and rituals through which an individual is recognized as bereaved and socially expresses grief. For example, in the United States, wearing black, sending flowers, and attending funerals are common illustrations of appropriate mourning behaviors.

Paradigms of Grief

Grief was first empirically described in 1944 by Eric Lindemann, a psychiatrist who studied survivors of the Coconut Grove Fire, a 1942 Boston fire that swept through a nightclub, killing many. Lindemann described grief as a syndrome that was "remarkably uniform" and included a common range of physical symptoms, such as tightness of throat, shortness of breath, and other pain, as well as emotional and other responses. It should be recognized that Lindemann's research was based on a sample of primarily young survivors of sudden and traumatic loss.

This medical model of grief was continued most clearly in the work of George Engel (1961). Engel believed that grief could be described as a disease, one having a clear onset in a circumstance of loss; a predictable course that includes an initial state of shock; a developing awareness of loss characterized by physical, affective, cognitive, psychological, and behavioral symptoms; and a prolonged period of gradual recovery, with the possibility that this recovery may be complicated by other variables. He noted that other disease processes also are influenced by psychological and social variables. Even the fact that grief is universal and rarely requires treatment, Engel argued, is not unlike other diseases. Engel also noted that whether or not a disease requires medical treatment or is even recognized as a disease is a social convention. Epilepsy, alcoholism, and many forms of mental illness are recognized as diseases but were not at other times in human history or in other cultures.

Another paradigm that attempts to offer insight into the nature of acute grief is the psychological trauma model. This model, based on the work of the Austrian neurologist Sigmund Freud (1917), views grief as a response to the psychological trauma brought on by the loss of a love object. Acute grief is a normal defense against the trauma of loss. To Freud, grief is a crisis, but one that will likely improve over time and that generally does not require psychiatric intervention.

Perhaps one of the more influential models to account for acute grief is the attachment model developed by John Bowlby (1980). This approach emphasizes that attachment, or bonding, is a functional survival mechanism, an instinct found in many of the higher animals. Given the prolonged periods of infancy and dependency, attachment is necessary for the survival of the species. When the object of that attachment is missing, certain behaviors arise that are instinctual responses to that loss. These behaviors, including crying, searching, and clinging, were seen by Bowlby as biologically based responses that seek to restore the lost bond and maintain the attachment. When these bonds are permanently severed, as in death, these behaviors continue until the bond is divested of emotional meaning and significance. These behaviors also serve a secondary purpose. By expressing distress, they engage the care, support, and protection of the larger social unit. This psychobiological model sees grief as a natural, instinctual response to a loss, a response that continues until the bond is restored or the grieving person detaches and divests of the bond.

These early approaches continue to influence understandings of grief, though more contemporary models emphasize that grief is a natural response to major transitions in life and that bonds between the grieving individual and the lost object continue, albeit in different forms, after the loss (Klass, Silverman, and Nickman). In addition, more recent approaches emphasize that a significant loss may shatter assumptions, causing grieving individuals to reconstruct their sense of self, their spirituality, and their relationship to others and the world at large. While this may be a painful process, it also may be a catalyst for growth.

Manifestations of Grief

Individuals can experience acute grief in varied ways. Physical reactions are common. These includes a range of physical responses such as headaches, other aches and pains, tightness, dizziness, exhaustion, menstrual irregularities, sexual impotency, breathlessness, tremors and shakes, and oversensitivity to noise.

Bereaved individuals, particularly widows, do have a higher rate of mortality in the first year of loss (Osterweis, Solomon, and Green). There may be many reasons for this—the stress of bereavement, the change in lifestyle that accompanies a loss, and the fact that many chronic diseases have lifestyle factors that can be shared by both partners. It is important that a physician monitor any physical responses to loss.

There are affective manifestations of grief as well. Individuals may experience a range of emotions such as anger, guilt, helplessness, sadness, shock, numbing, yearning, jealousy, and self-blame. Some bereaved persons experience a sense of relief or even a feeling of emancipation. This, however, can be followed by a sense of guilt. As in any emotional crisis, even contradictory feelings, such as sadness and relief, can be experienced simultaneously.

There can be cognitive manifestations of grief. Included here is a sense of depersonalization in which nothing seems real. There can be a sense of disbelief and confusion, an inability to concentrate or focus. Bereaved individuals can be preoccupied with images or memories of the loss. These cognitive manifestations can affect functioning at work, school, or home. Many persons also report experiences in which they dream of the deceased or have a sense of the person's presence, even sense-based experiences of the other.

Grief has spiritual manifestations. Individuals may struggle to find meaning and to reestablish a sense of identity and order in their world. They may be angry at God or struggle with their faith.

Behavioral manifestations of grief can also vary. These behavioral manifestations can include crying, withdrawal, avoiding or seeking reminders of the loss, searching behaviors, over activity, and changes in relationships with others.

The reactions of persons to loss are highly individual and influenced by a number of factors. These include the unique meaning of the loss, the strength and nature of the attachment, the circumstances surrounding the loss such as the presence of other crises, reactions and experiences of earlier loss, the temperament and adaptive abilities of the individual, the presence and support of family and other informal and formal support systems, cultural and spiritual beliefs and practices, and general health and lifestyle practices of the grieving individuals.

The Course of Grief

There have been a number of approaches to understanding the process or course of acute grief. Earlier approaches tended to see grief as proceeding in stages or phases. Colin Murray Parkes (1972), for example, described four stages of grief: shock, angry pining, depression and despair, and detachment. Recent approaches have emphasized that grief does not follow a predictable and linear course, stressing instead that it often proceeds in a roller-coaster-like pattern, full of ups and downs, times when the grief reactions are more or less intense. Some of these more intense periods are predictable—holidays, anniversaries, or other significant days—but other times may have no recognizable trigger.

More recent approaches have emphasized that grief involves a series of tasks or processes. J. William Worden

(1992) described four tasks to grief: recognizing the reality of the loss, dealing with expressed and latent feelings, living in a world without the deceased, and relocating the deceased in one's life. Therese A. Rando (1993) suggested that grieving individuals need to complete six "R" processes: recognize the loss, react to the separation, recollect and reexperience the deceased and the relationship, relinquish the old attachments to the deceased and the old assumptive world, readjust to the new world without forgetting the old, and reinvest. (While the language of both Worden and Rando is specific to death-related loss, their models can be adapted to other losses as well.) These and other similar models reaffirm the very individual nature of grief, acknowledging that these tasks or processes are not necessarily linear and that any given individual may have difficulty with one or more processes or tasks.

The critical point to remember is that the course of grief is not linear. Nor is there any inherent timetable to grief. Grief reactions can persist for considerable time, gradually losing intensity after the first few years. Recent research as well emphasizes that one does not "get over the loss." Rather, over time, the pain lessens, and the grief becomes less disabling as individuals function at levels comparable to (and sometimes better than) preloss levels. Bonds and attachments to the lost object continue, however, and periods of intense grief can occur years after the loss (Klass, Silverman, and Nickman). For example, the birth of a grandchild can trigger an experience of grief in a widow who wished to share this event with her deceased spouse.

Help and Grief

Persons experiencing acute grief can help themselves in a number of ways. Because grief is a form of stress, lifestyle management including adequate sleep and diet, as well as other techniques for stress reduction, can be helpful. Bibliotherapy or the use of self-help books can often validate or normalize grief reactions, suggest ways of adaptation, and offer hope. Self-help and support groups can offer similar assistance as well as social support from others who have experienced loss. Others may benefit from counselors, particularly if their health suffers or their grief becomes highly disabling, impairing functioning at work, school, or home, or if they harbor destructive thoughts toward self or others. Parkes (1980) particularly stressed the value of grief counseling when other support is not forthcoming.

Pharmacological interventions also may be helpful particularly when the grief is disabling, that is, severely compromising the individual's health or ability to function. Such interventions should be focused on particular conditions, such as anxiety or depression, that are precipitated or exacerbated by the bereavement. Pharmacological interventions should be accompanied by psychotherapy.

Most individuals seem to ameliorate grief in that, over time, they can remember the loss without the intense reactions experienced earlier. Nevertheless, anywhere from 20 to 33 percent seem to experience more complicated grief reactions (Rando).

Complicated Grief

While models of complicated grief vary (Rando; Worden), complicated grief reactions generally involve intensifications and exaggerations of the earlier described responses to grief that effectively impair the individual's ability to function. Complicated grief can also be evident in masked reactions—that is, the grief is masked by another problem such as substance abuse.

One factor that can complicate grief is disenfranchisement. The term *disenfranchised grief* refers to a grief that results when a loss is not socially sanctioned, publicly acknowledged, or openly mourned. Grief may be disenfranchised because a loss is not recognized (e.g., the loss of an animal companion), a relationship is not recognized (e.g., a friend or therapist), the griever is not acknowledged (e.g., a very young child or a person with developmental disabilities), the death evokes shame or censure (e.g., an execution), or the way the person expresses grief is considered inappropriate or unacceptable. In such cases, the person has experienced a loss, but has "no right to grieve," no expectation of public acknowledgement or support (Doka, 1989, 2002).

Ethical Issues in Grief

Ethical issues in grief may emerge from three sources. First are general issues for counselors. Grieving persons can be highly vulnerable. Counselors have to have personal integrity and follow the ethical standards of their profession, including maintaining confidentiality, preventing harm to the client or others, assuring competence, and upholding standards of professional behavior. Counselors should familiarize themselves with their respective codes of ethics. They may wish to review as well the Code of Ethics of the Association for Death Education and Counseling.

In addition to the normal standards of professional conduct, counselors should be aware of two other ethic-related issues that might arise in grief counseling. Ethical issues within the course of the medical treatment of the deceased person may affect responses to grief. For example, a person who decided to terminate treatment may struggle with that issue within the grief process. In similar ways, ethical decisions made after the death—such as the disposition of the remains or inheritance—may also be reviewed in the grieving process. For example, the deceased may make requests regarding the disposition of remains or property that families may be reluctant to follow. Such situations can exacerbate grief—intensifying guilt or anger and causing conflicts that lessen mutual support and add concurrent stresses.

KENNETH J. DOKA

SEE ALSO: *Care; Death; Dementia; Healing; Health and Disease; Medicine, Anthropology of; Mental Health, Meaning of Mental Health; Mental Health Therapies; Pain and Suffering; Palliative Care and Hospice*

BIBLIOGRAPHY

Bowlby, John. 1980. *Attachment and Loss: Loss, Sadness, and Depression.* New York: Basic.

Doka, Kenneth J. 1989. *Disenfranchised Grief: Recognizing Hidden Sorrow.* Lexington, MA: Lexington Books.

Doka, Kenneth J., ed. 2002. *Disenfranchised Grief: New Directions, Challenges, and Strategies for Practice.* Champaign, IL: Research Press.

Engel, George. 1961. "Is Grief a Disease? A Challenge for Medical Research." *Psychosomatic Medicine* 23: 18–22.

Freud, Sigmund. 1917 (reprint 1957). "Mourning and Melancholia." In *The Standard Edition of the Complete Psychological Works of Sigmund Freud,* vol. 14, ed. James Strachey. London: Hogarth Press.

Klass, Dennis; Silverman, Phyllis; and Nickman, Steven. 1996. *Continuing Bonds: New Understandings of Grief.* Bristol, PA: Taylor and Francis.

Lindemann, Eric. 1944. "Symptomatology and Management of Acute Grief." *American Journal of Psychiatry* 101: 141–148.

Osterweis, Marion; Solomon, Fredric; and Green, Morris. 1984. *Bereavement: Reactions, Consequences, and Care.* Washington, D.C.: National Academy Press.

Parkes, Colin Murray. 1972. *Bereavement: Studies of Grief in Adult Life.* New York: International Universities Press.

Parkes, Colin Murray. 1980. "Bereavement Counselling: Does It Work?" *British Medical Journal* 281: 3–6.

Rando, Therese A. 1993. *The Treatment of Complicated Mourning.* Champaign, IL: Research Press.

Worden, J. William. 1992. *Grief Counseling and Grief Therapy: A Handbook for the Mental Health Practitioner,* 2nd edition. New York: Springer.

HARM

· · ·

Harm is a central concept both in the practice of medicine and in ethics. Hence, it is no surprise that in bioethics harm plays a prominent role. The proper goal of medicine is to prevent, alleviate, or eliminate harm to patients that result from disease or injury. Moreover, some medical interventions themselves have a serious potential to cause additional (iatrogenic) harm—for instance, pharmacological side effects or even death from surgery.

General prohibitions against inflicting harm on others supposedly belong to the principles of any moral code, and an attitude of non-malevolence (taking care that others do not suffer harm) is widely regarded as a core virtue and as a decisive source of moral motivation. Beyond this, bioethics is concerned with harm-related judgments, obligations, prohibitions, and problems. The harm at stake is most often harm to patients. Such debates as those about professional duties toward patients, about matters of resource allocation, or about the limits of patient self-determination all deal in part with actual or potential suffering, dysfunction, pain, or death of patients. Some problems, however, relate to potential harm to third parties. For example, HIV-positive patients risk infecting uninformed sexual partners and pregnant women who consume drugs risk harm to their unborn children. Other ethical questions deal with harm to health professionals themselves—when, for instance, a physician faces treating a contagious patient under substantial personal risk. And finally, various arguments in bioethics address the possibility of long-term social harm resulting from certain permissive practices (the so-called slippery slope argument). For example, critics of prenatal selection against severe genetic diseases predict shrinking social solidarity with the handicapped and with their justified claims to social support.

While its central role in bioethics thus cannot be disputed, *harm* remains a vague and contested concept that in and of itself does not provide much moral guidance. What counts as harm varies greatly, as do the scope and relative importance of the prescriptions not to inflict, to prevent, or to remove harm.

Conceptual Questions

An instance of harm may be assessed with reference to kind, degree, and duration. Risk assessment, not considered here, also includes the probability of harm's occurrence. According to the *Oxford English Dictionary,* harm is "evil (physical or otherwise) as done to or suffered by some person or thing; hurt, injury, damage, mischief." As far as harm is relevant to moral deliberation, however, this broad concept must be restricted.

First, harm should be understood as person- (or animal-) regarding, that is, as consisting of events or states of affairs that are negative for someone—as expressed in Joel Feinberg's definition of harms as "setbacks to interest" (p. 31). As long as the sticky question of what counts as interests remains open, this concept of harm is still neutral to various ethical positions. Problems start with determining who counts as a bearer of interests; for instance, do embryos (as potential persons), the deceased or permanently unconscious (as former persons), or animals bear interests? These issues, although obviously important for evaluating abortion, transplantation, decisions to end treatment, or animal protection, will not be pursued here.

Secondly, ethics in general ethics and bioethics in particular have to restrict their focus on those instances of harm that are in some way or other linked to human action. It would not make sense to morally deliberate about ineluctable evils, deplorable though they may be. Rather, harm is ethically relevant only if it occurs or persists in consequence to human agency, be it by action or omission, from intention or negligence, but not from unavoidable ignorance. Thus, what counts as harm with relevance to bioethics is context-relative: harm is contingent upon professional knowledge and medico-technical progress.

Thirdly, bioethics, reflecting both ordinary moral and non-moral language usage, commonly differentiates between harm on the one hand and mere loss or lack of benefit on the other. Harm is not simply conceptually complementary to benefit (interest satisfaction), but it also represents a significant disservice to its *victim*. Along the scale of interest satisfaction, there are numerous positions of submaximal satisfaction (disbenefits) that it seems inappropriate to call *harms*. There is thus an asymmetry between harm and benefit in the sense that harm pertains exclusively to the basics of well-being. It may be wrong to prevent someone from obtaining a luxury good, but nevertheless, its consequence does not qualify as harm. Another argument elucidating this asymmetry emphasizes that harm has or leads to distinct phenomenal qualities of bodily or psychological painfulness and suffering, which is by no means true for all instances of lacking benefit (e.g., Noddings). Moreover, pity for someone's experience of harm is a motivation distinct from other forms of benevolence (e.g., Sidgwick).

Not to inflict, to prevent, or to remove harm usually takes moral precedence over providing those benefits the lack of which does not count as harm. Such asymmetry between harm and benefit has been traditionally acknowledged (e.g., by John Stuart Mill), but a more systematic focus on harm is a rather recent development of applied ethics, with its eye to more concrete moral rules (a notable exception being Jeremy Bentham's 1789 taxonomy of "pains" by sources, kinds, and circumstances). The improvement of people's well-being being a more or less central goal of any moral code, concrete efforts must first focus on the most important obstacles to well-being, that is, on existing or potential harm.

Understanding harm as a significant setback to someone's interests already implies that usually it ought to be avoided. In this sense harm is a weak normative concept, carrying a presumption of evaluative negativity. However, not every infliction or non-prevention of harm to another person is, all things considered, necessarily wrong, and in just this sense harm is not a strong normative concept. For instance, not to treat a particular patient in a tragic triage situation may be a deplorable but ethically-justified decision. Likewise, foregoing life-saving surgery on a competent patient because he autonomously decided against it, by no means "wrongs" him, in the sense of violating legitimate moral claims (Feinberg). Where harming thus does not necessarily mean wronging, the same is, of course, also true the other way round. One ought not conflate people's legitimate claims to justice or self-determination with those of not being harmed. Less clear cut is the distinction between harms and *offenses*, where the latter cause unpleasant, though not harmful, mental states. In the context of medicine, patients might be frustrated, shocked or irritated by inefficient hospital structures or by physicians who behave rudely. Whether such states of offendedness turn into proper harm seems to be but a matter of degree and duration.

Harm and Harm-Referring Duties in Bioethics

Assessing harm and distinguishing it from offenses, minor hurts, or non-harmful instances of lacking benefit requires an analysis of harm's nature and of how to determine its significance. Particularly in the context of healthcare, many instances of harm and potential harm to patients are widely uncontested, namely: severe lack of functioning resulting from bodily or mental disease, enduring pain, substantial suffering, gross disfigurement, or premature death. Another, easily neglected category of possible harm in the context of medical practice is of a psychosocial nature: for example, patients may experience absorbing anxiety, mistrust, alienation, helplessness, loss of self-control, loneliness, or annoyance due to structural and human deficits. In particular, the work of feminist ethicists (e.g., Noddings; Warren) and physician-ethicists (e.g., Cassell; Pellegrino and Thomasma) has created a new awareness of widely neglected kinds of harm to patients that occur in daily medical practice and that can largely be reduced or avoided when caregivers are humane and sympathetic. Even beyond the individual patient-caregiver relationship, general loss of trust in contemporary biomedical institutions and practices, in researchers and clinicians seems to be a prevalent and deeply troubling problem (O'Neill).

Finally, harm may occur as a setback to patients' higher-level "critical interests" in living a life they consider good (Dworkin). Notably, decisions about one's time and manner of dying are likely to relate to such highly personal, critical interests. Focusing on these issues would involve yet another conceptual enlargement of (modern) medical harm.

All of these states or events are setbacks to individuals' interests in basic well-being, and thus univocally considered harmful. In principle, they can be relevant to bioethics whenever they potentially occur or persist as a consequence of intentional behavior, where behavior must be understood in a broad sense. Hence, ethically-relevant harm can result from both omission and commission, from individual or collective acts, from a patient's own decision or from someone else's.

Harm can be intended, merely foreseen, or accepted as a lesser evil when compared to the consequences of all available alternatives, and it can be intended with regard to an identified or to a statistical addressee. Take a patient's premature death, to illustrate the broad variance of agents and victims and of causal and intentional modes under which ethically relevant-harm can occur in medicine. This premature death could, for instance, be the consequence of: a physician's decision to stop life-saving treatment, a negligently wrong treatment, an unfortunate research intervention, the patient's own decision against further treatment, a rationing policy, or a negligent infection from undisclosed sexually transmittable disease.

To emphasize it once more: it seems hard to find even one bioethical problem that does not somehow involve aspects of harm to patients or, less frequently, to health professionals or third parties. In all these matters, however, dissent arises when it comes to the comparative evaluation of a particular harm's negativity; in setting standards for professional, social, or personal responsibilities for people's health, and corresponding duties; and in the assessment of distinguishing harm from mere lack of benefit in healthcare.

With regard to duties, some scholars in ethics formulate a distinct duty of nonmaleficence, expressing a prohibition on actions with foreseeable harmful effects. Others, however, include this prohibition as part of a duty of beneficence. This, and whether such obligation is construed as a prohibition on causing net harm to someone (such that, say, shooting a murderer to save the lives of his three victims would not count as maleficent), or on harming itself (the shooting would be maleficent, though perhaps justified), is a question of terminological and classificatory preference. The duty of nonmaleficence is still indeterminate under any of these descriptions, not only because they reintroduce the problems of harm assessment but also because they are silent about permissible limits and trade-offs.

Recognizing a distinct principle of nonmaleficence is fairly common in medical (in contrast to general) ethics. It is meant to guide actions by caregivers in those situations that are most likely to produce harm. However, depending on both formal tailoring of concepts and on normative perspectives, there exist formal and substantial differences among bioethical perspectives in what is understood as nonmaleficence. Tom Beauchamp and James Childress, for

instance, turn to the four duties of beneficence originally distinguished by William Frankena in 1973. Frankena's classification of duties is based on a distinction between harm and benefit and on the action's causal mode:

1. not to inflict harm;
2. to prevent harm;
3. to remove harm; and
4. to promote good.

Beauchamp and Childress modify Frankena by subsuming the first duty under nonmaleficence and leaving the last three duties under beneficence. Their distinction between the two duties of nonmaleficence and beneficence thus corresponds to the difference between negative and positive duties (i.e., duties of omission versus duties of commission), again depending on aspects of causality. Beauchamp and Childress do not, however, take this classification as such to be normatively decisive; rather, they intend to capture ordinary language usage, mirroring the empirical fact that noninfliction of harm often is achievable at lower cost to the agent than is obeying positive duties. It is in this generalized sense that the obligation of nonmaleficence frequently has priority over beneficence.

Along these lines, Allen Buchanan and Dan Brock have suggested that appeals to nonmaleficence in medicine be understood as specific reminders: in Hippocratic times, not to forget that some treatments were only burdensome and not beneficial; in contemporary times, to correct "for professional biases toward over-treatment of non-communicating patients in conditions of great risk or profound uncertainty" (Buchanan and Brock, p. 256). These reminders pay attention to medicine's increasing potential not only to benefit patients but also to inflict iatrogenic harm upon them (Sharpe and Faden).

The duty of nonmaleficence may conflict with the autonomy of patients who request treatment that physicians consider harmful (e.g., unjustified surgery, futile chemotherapy, or drugs). With an eye to precisely this conflict, H. Tristram Engelhardt, Jr., understands the duty of nonmaleficence as a justification to limit patients' self-determination.

Problems with Harm in Medicine

As to the more precise nature of harm and to the scope of harm-related duties, bioethics inherits some of the controversies of general ethical theory. A crucial question is to what extent there are objective criteria for identifying and evaluating harm. If such criteria could be found, this might, for example, justify a physician's overriding a patient's own "harmful" preferences. Or, such criteria could be adduced in surrogate decision making for noncommunicating patients, as well as in matters of allocative justice (where it becomes crucial to evaluate medical interventions in terms of their comparative tendencies to avoid or alleviate net harm).

The issue of determining criteria is linked to the objectivity/subjectivity debate concerning people's well-being and ability to live a good life (see Griffin), and the setbacks to these. With most experts agreeing that there is an irreducible plurality of harms, the subjectivist view takes harm to be a significant setback only to actual wants or desires, possibly after procedural safeguards have been met. Here, for instance, a patient's death due to intentional non-resuscitation would be harmful only if the patient, when informed and asked, would opt for treatment. In the objectivist view, harm is a significant setback also to interests that are want-independent, but related to ideals of a good life. Here, death due to non-resuscitation could be harmful to a patient, regardless of whether he or she wants it.

The fundamental distinction between "want regard" and "ideal regard" (as a difference between subjective versus objective concepts of interest) was introduced by Brian Barry in political philosophy. In that area, lack of autonomy in forming one's wants is less obviously a danger than it is in medicine, where patients can so easily be ill informed, manipulated, or otherwise incompetent when forming their preferences. Therefore, at least certain procedural safeguards—such as standards of informed consent—are not inconsistent with "want regard" in medicine. Other safeguards, like elevating standards for patient competence to a level commensurate with the expected harm that would result from acting in accordance with patient choice (e.g., Buchanan and Brock), arguably cross over into "ideal regard." In any case, there is room for hybrid positions between the extremes of pure want regard and ideal regard. Consider forcing a Jehovah's Witness to be transfused with blood. Justifying this by reference to the patient's presumed objective interest in the preservation of his life falls under ideal regard. Arguing that the patient would want the transfusion if she were not bound to her irrational belief system puts harm assessment by want regard under some ideal-regarding constraint.

A common argument in favor of taking harm as an objective concept stresses the broad consensus in what "rational persons desire to avoid for themselves" (Culver and Gert, p. 70). Reference to the obvious consensus about the desirability of avoiding disease, disability, pain, premature death, and suffering, presupposed in daily medical work, is familiar from the debate over concepts of disease (Culver

and Gert). To concur on this point does not imply acknowledging universal standards for all sorts of harm. Rather, pain, disability, and premature death are seen as universal harms simply in being setbacks to very basic interests, the satisfaction of which is instrumental to practically all conceptions of a good life. It would, of course, not come as a surprise to find this true for many kinds of harm, in contrast to mere lack of benefits.

Even more serious problems with defining medical harm hinge on the need to compare two instances of harm, such as those from alternative treatment courses or from alternative resource distributions. Such ranking judgments are needed on kinds of harm (for example, pain versus addiction; premature death versus disfigurement; disease versus a restricted lifestyle) and on how much, when, and for how long harm is to be accepted, and for what purpose. At least implicit comparative evaluations of risks of harm and benefit are involved in virtually any treatment decision or medical indication (Veatch). Here, more fundamental disagreement starts: Some authors emphasize the great variability in comparative harm assessment, pointing to its relatedness to the context of each patient's irreducibly personal or parochial conception of a good life (e.g., Engelhardt; Veatch). This position has nurtured so-called autonomy-centered bioethics, which considers the assessment of harms and benefits to be the patients' business only. In contrast to this position, other scholars want to keep at least some objective ground for evaluations: medical interventions should, according to them, be determined futile not by patients, but by professional standards whenever they appear to be disproportionately harmful and thus "not reasonable" (Brody); or these scholars see interpersonal variability in ranking harm—though it exists—as not predominant and therefore not ruling out a beneficence-centered bioethics.

Other fundamental problems relate to the legitimate scope and relative importance of the obligations to prevent or to remove harm. First, some such actions, although morally laudable, are not required of the agent because they pose undue burdens or risks for him. For example, a therapist need not risk his own death in treating a violent patient. But how far do these agent prerogatives go? And how are they determined and justified? Secondly, harm preventing or removing actions sometimes ought to give way to other overriding duties (e.g., the duty to remove still greater harm from another or to respect patient self-determination). However, there are many different views as to what counts as overriding duty. Between the two extremes—understanding nonmaleficence as the trivially indeterminate principle "avoid harm (whatever that is) unless it is outweighed" or having as many specified duties as there are different normative theories—attempts have been made to give a more specific meaning to nonmaleficence without leaving the middle ground of broader consensus.

How to Handle Pluralist Harm Assessment

Undeniably, different people have very different notions of what *medical harm* would be for themselves or for others. Autonomy-centered bioethics has seen its task as spelling out procedures to foster a "morality of mutual respect" (Engelhardt) and patients' self-determination. This approach leads to particular concern for informed consent, policies for advance directives, substituted judgment, and so on. A contrasting approach urges that instead of inviting radical individualism in assessing medical harm, we redetermine medicine's substantive goals. Daniel Callahan, for example, argues that such individualism results in net harm to all by consuming too many resources for marginal benefits and setting wrong priorities in our lives. Stressing the importance of expectations and cultural presumptions in determining what individuals view as harm, Callahan hopes to find arguments acceptable to the whole of society—in favor, for instance, of decreasing individual expectations for life-prolonging treatment in old age.

Other authors concur that individualistic harm assessment is the wrong paradigm for medicine: "Moral atomism" is viewed as impoverishing medical practice socially and morally, that is, as giving up grounds on which a sense of community and good decision making should develop (Pellegrino and Thomasma). Others see "moral atomism" as leading to a waste of physicians' power to assist patients in pursuing their goals (Brody, p. 50), or as leading to paralysis in crucial policy questions, such as how to determine the best treatment interests of incompetent patients (Emanuel). Ezekiel Emanuel opts for communitarian healthcare settings, where groups of patients and physicians shape medicine according to their shared assessment of harms and benefits; others are confident that the consensus on harm in the context of medicine is substantial (Pellegrino and Thomasma; Cassell; Brody). They see the main problem in "the view that the physician respects autonomy by taking a negative, hands-off stance" (Brody, p. 50), which they argue ought to be given up in favor of assisting patients, in a critical and trustworthy manner, to assess harms and benefits.

Prominent Controversies on Medical Harm

A prohibition on killing is often taken to be the most important negative duty of nonmaleficence, death being a major harm for most people. Generally, the same is true for the medical context, with the contested exception of assistance in dying. Proponents of active voluntary euthanasia for terminally-ill patients are not only prepared to give priority to patient self-determination in these situations, but would not even consider the resulting death a harm and its intentional provision maleficent—rather to the contrary. Controversies over these issues across many cultures result from different views on the allegedly harmful or benefiting nature of a patient's death from assistance—be it by active killing, by withholding or withdrawing life support, assisted suicide, or indirect euthanasia. Those who insist on normative differences between these various forms of assistance often give normative weight to the involved causal or intentional differences. A prominent instance of such an argumentation is the controversial Roman Catholic doctrine of double effect, according to which, for example, indirect euthanasia can be justified in spite of the death that may result, since the latter is not intended but merely foreseen as a by-product of beneficent painkilling. Other opponents of aid in dying argue with the social harm than could be expected from one or several of these practices once, established as legitimate option for the terminally ill (the slippery slope argument).

Yet another debate centering on the concept of harm-concerns cases of sexually-active patients who carry a sexually-transmittable virus (e.g., HIV) and refuse to inform their partners. Legal prescriptions aside, bioethicists are divided as to whether the treating physician, who cannot convince his patient to the contrary, has a duty to inform those at risk. Obviously the obligation to prevent harm to others conflicts with the professional obligation to confidentiality; violating confidentiality might also lessen the general trust in physicians' patient advocacy.

The heated controversies on prenatal diagnosis, gene therapy, and wrongful birth and wrongful life issues focus on possible harm to future children or their parents, but also on those who are living with genetic handicaps. Once again, bioethicists dissent on what to identify as harm, how to evaluate its negativity, and how to balance related duties against other ethical obligations.

In summary, there is a remarkable tension between harm's undisputed importance in bioethics and the numerous different ways in which it comes to be conceptualized and evaluated, thus mirroring the plurality of existing ethical approaches.

BETTINA SCHOENE-SEIFERT (1995)
REVISED BY AUTHOR

SEE ALSO: *Animal Welfare; Bioterrorism; Buddhism, Bioethics in; Circumcision; Competence; Death; Death, Definition and Determination of; Double Effect, Principle or Doctrine of; Environmental Ethics; Ethics; Harmful Substances, Legal*

Control of; Holocaust; Homicide; Human Rights; Infanticide; Injury and Injury Control; International Health; Law and Morality; Malpractice; Mistakes, Medical; Moral Status; Pain and Suffering; Paternalism; Psychiatry, Abuses of; Research, Unethical; Smoking; Utilitarianism and Bioethics; Warfare

BIBLIOGRAPHY

Barry, Brian. 1965 (reprint 1990). *Political Argument: A Reissue with a New Introduction.* Berkeley: University of California Press.

Beauchamp, Tom L., and Childress, James F. 2001. *Principles of Biomedical Ethics,* 5th edition. New York: Oxford University Press.

Bentham, Jeremy. 1789 (reprint 1963). *An Introduction to the Principles of Morals and Legislation.* New York: Hafner.

Brody, Howard. 1992. *The Healer's Power.* New Haven, CT: Yale University Press.

Buchanan, Allen E., and Brock, Dan W. 1989. *Deciding for Others: The Ethics of Surrogate Decisionmaking.* New York: Cambridge University Press.

Callahan, Daniel. 1991. *What Kind of Life: The Limits of Medical Progress.* New York: Simon & Schuster.

Cassell, Eric J. 1991. *The Nature of Suffering: And the Goals of Medicine.* New York: Oxford University Press.

Culver, Charles M., and Gert, Bernard. 1982. *Philosophy in Medicine: Conceptual and Ethical Issues in Medicine and Psychiatry.* New York: Oxford University Press.

Dworkin, Ronald. 1993. *Life's Dominion: An Argument about Abortion, Euthanasia, and Individual Freedom.* New York: Knopf.

Emanuel, Ezekiel J. 1991. *The Ends of Human Life: Medical Ethics in a Liberal Polity.* Cambridge, MA: Harvard University Press.

Engelhardt, H. Tristram, Jr. 1996. *The Foundations of Bioethics,* 2nd edition. New York: Oxford University Press.

Feinberg, Joel. 1984. *Harm to Others.* New York: Oxford University Press.

Frankena, William K. 1973. *Ethics,* 2nd edition. Englewood Cliffs, NJ: Prentice-Hall.

Griffin, James. 1986. *Well-Being: Its Meaning, Measurement and Moral Importance.* Oxford: Clarendon.

Mill, John Stuart. 1863 (reprint 1979). *Utilitarianism.* Indianapolis, IN: Hackett.

Noddings, Nel. 1989. *Women and Evil.* Berkeley: University of California Press.

O'Neill, Onora. 2002. *Autonomy and Trust in Bioethics.* New York: Cambridge University Press.

Pellegrino, Edmund D., and Thomasma, David C. 1988. *For the Patient's Good: The Restoration of Beneficence in Health Care.* New York: Oxford University Press.

Sharpe, Virginia A., and Faden, Alan I. 1998. *Medical Harm: Historical, Conceptual, and Ethical Dimensions of Iatrogenic Illness.* New York: Cambridge University Press.

Sidgwick, Henry. 1966. *The Methods of Ethics,* 7th edition. New York: Dover.

Veatch, Robert M. 1991. *The Patient-Physician Relation: The Patient as Partner, Part 2.* Bloomington: Indiana University Press.

Warren, Virginia L. 1992. "Feminist Directions in Medical Ethics." In *Feminist Perspectives in Medical Ethics,* ed. Helen Bequaert Holmes and Laura M. Purdy. Bloomington: Indiana University Press.

HARMFUL SUBSTANCES, LEGAL CONTROL OF

• • •

At the beginning of the twenty-first century, opium, its constituent morphine, and the derivative heroin were viewed with fear and suspicion. As both popular and professional attitudes in the United States turned against drug use in the United States around 1980, physicians began to fear prescribing potentially addictive analgesics, and likewise, patients began to fear taking them. This attitude contrasts sharply with that of one of the leading American physicians in the mid-nineteenth century, George Wood, of the University of Pennsylvania, who wrote in 1868 that opium produces "an exaltation of our better mental qualities, a warmer glow of benevolence, a disposition to do great things, but nobly and beneficently, a higher devotional spirit, and withal a stronger self-reliance, and consciousness of power" (Vol. 1, p. 712).

Clearly, the ethical position a person takes regarding the availability of a drug is affected profoundly by whether that person believes that the drug is risky in any amount or that reasonable doses of the drug are a boon to humankind. These two positions have alternately influenced experts and the public since at least the eighteenth century in English-speaking countries. In times when one of these attitudes has held sway, the opposite ethical position has been dismissed as wrongheaded and refuted both morally and scientifically.

Attitudes toward Alcohol

Alcohol, a drug with a long history of easy availability and widespread consumption in the West, provides instructive examples of these dramatic shifts of opinion and their impact on ethical positions. The history of fermented beverages such as beer and wine goes back millennia, and distilled spirits began to be produced by about 1300 in Europe. For centuries afterward, nearly pure alcohol was produced in small amounts, and extraordinary characteristics were attributed to it. *Aqua vitae,* as certain distilled alcohol products were termed, was said to prolong life. In its qualities it approached the quintessence, or fifth element (along with earth, air, fire, and water). The "spirit" derived from distillation, according to John French, a seventeenth-century English physician, had wonderful "vertues … for there is no disease, whether inward or outward, that can withstand it" (p. 132).

In England, new scientific data challenged the old beliefs during the "gin epidemic" of the eighteenth century. For the first half of the century a battle raged between the populace—especially in London, where gin was cheaper than an equal volume of beer —and some religious and secular leaders who were appalled by the spiraling number of public drunks, "weak, feeble, and distempered children" (Plant, p. 9), and deaths attributed to the massive and cheap consumption of distilled spirits. Hogarth's print *Gin Lane* of 1751 captures the social destruction resulting from a substance that once had been thought of as an unadulterated good.

The new view of distilled spirits was incorporated into voluntaristic plans for self-improvement, most notably the religious movement led by John Wesley. In his attempt to revitalize the Church of England and establish a strict morality of behavior, Wesley argued for a distinction between fermented spirits and distilled spirits. He described distilled spirits as "a certain, tho' a slow poison," although he conceded that they might have medicinal uses (Wesley, p. xix). Eventually Wesley's Methodism moved, especially in the United States under the guidance of Wesley's chosen missionary, Francis Asbury, to a rejection of alcohol in any form.

In addition to moral objections, in the United States criticism of alcohol was based upon social and medical observations. Benjamin Rush, perhaps the most distinguished American physician of his time, launched an attack on alcohol that was based on his experiences as a physician in the War of Independence. Rush countered the popular notion that distilled spirits were a healthy means of invigorating soldiers and field workers, and a stimulant to intellectual activity. However, like Wesley, he focused on spirits, not on all forms of alcohol. His pamphlet *An Inquiry into the Effects of Ardent Spirits upon the Human Body and Mind,* written in the 1780s (reprinted in Musto, 2002a, p. 27), was distributed by the thousands throughout the nation and was still being reprinted and distributed four decades later.

TEMPERANCE MOVEMENTS. Later reformers, most notably Lyman Beecher in his monumental *Six Sermons on Intemperance* (reprinted in Musto, 2002a, p. 44), which first appeared in 1826 (reprinted 1828), adopted a more extreme attitude, condemning not only distilled spirits but all alcoholic beverages. Moderation was no longer recommended as an ideal; instead, it was presented as a dangerous delusion that would draw many people into alcohol abuse. Alcohol itself, Beecher argued, not the amount or type consumed, was an evil.

Thus, the United States experienced a positive attitude toward alcohol consumption in the eighteenth century, followed by a reversal dominated by the image of alcohol as a fundamentally evil substance that led to widespread prohibition in the 1850s. That first peak of prohibition faded under the resentment of the public, the difficulty of enforcement, and the monumental distraction of the Civil War. Later in the nineteenth century, opposition to alcohol revived, centering on the burgeoning urban saloon, a center of political and moral corruption, and a symbol of the rising fear of recent immigrants crowding into the cities. This anti-alcohol campaign was even more successful than the previous crusade, achieving by 1920 a total legal prohibition of alcohol except for sacramental, industrial, and medicinal uses.

AFTER PROHIBITION. After 1933, the year of the repeal of the Eighteenth Amendment, the backlash against Prohibition made advocacy of alcohol control an object of ridicule until about 1980; then another change in attitude toward alcohol—perhaps the beginning of a third temperance movement— once again put the issue of the damaging social consequences of alcohol in the forefront of public concern. In 1984 the federal government established a national drinking age of twenty-one, and since 1989, all containers for beverage alcohol manufactured for sale in the United States have been required by federal law to bear a government label warning against the dangers of alcohol. Since the 1980s state drunk-driving laws have been made much more punitive. Per capita consumption of alcohol, which hit a third historical peak in 1980, has been in a gradual decline since that time.

Attitudes toward Other Drugs

The image of alcohol did not wax and wane in isolation from the public's perception of drugs such as morphine, heroin, and cocaine, although the peaks of their favorable and unfavorable public images did not coincide precisely with those of alcohol. The use of cocaine rose rapidly after its introduction into the United States in the mid-1880s. Not until the Harrison Act of 1914 did the federal government prohibit the sale of cocaine without a prescription. A similar restriction on alcohol, National Prohibition, was enacted five years later, and by the mid-1920s the federal government had moved to eliminate heroin completely as a legally obtainable substance (Musto, 2002b).

When one reviews the history of drugs and alcohol in the United States, it is apparent that the ethical debate and extent of control have been related to the healthy or poisonous image of those powerful substances. Interestingly, neither extreme was buried by the victory of the contrary position. The ascendancy of one point of view seems to have created the conditions for the gradual emergence of the opposite attitude. A further point worth noting is that in the campaign against drugs and alcohol, the American practice has been to condemn them as being without any but the most limited value as medicine, and to hedge any exemption with tight restrictions. The periods of favorable and unfavorable attitudes are rather lengthy compared with the human life span, and so each tends to be seen as the settled opinion of science and society, and the presence or absence of controls seems to be based on what appear to be established premises.

The Control of Drugs and Alcohol

The control of drugs and alcohol involves both practical and philosophical considerations. Practically, a nation or locality has a limited array of controls, and those controls usually depend on the compliance of the public.

EFFECT OF LICENSING AND TAXATION. During the English gin epidemic, Parliament was limited to using a variety of license fees and taxes, which were not always easily enforced, to curb the production of gin. Success in the campaign did not begin to be acknowledged by observers until after 1750, by which time, presumably, the baleful effects of gin and the prolonged campaign against it by reformers had changed public attitudes toward that form of alcohol.

Control of opiates and cocaine initially took a different turn because, by the late nineteenth century, the licensing of physicians and pharmacists had become widespread in the United States. As a result, the first form of control over those drugs, after a period of free access, consisted of making them available by prescription only, although commonly a small amount would be permitted in an over-the-counter remedy.

To alert the public, the Pure Food and Drug Act of 1906 required that the amount of drugs in a remedy be included on the label.

During the Progressive Era (approximately 1890–1920), reformers worked to give the central government more power, so that the benefit of uniform national laws could be applied to problems such as tainted meat, adulterated medicines, the destruction of forests, and drug abuse. With regard to drug abuse, the knotty constitutional problem was addressed by basing the Harrison Act of 1914, which was meant to regulate the distribution of opiates and cocaine, on the federal power to tax. Each transaction, from importation to retail purchase, had to be recorded, and a small tax had to be paid. Evasion of that law would be punished as a violation of the tax statutes. The restriction on maintenance doses of opiates for addicts was effected through Treasury Department regulations that were promulgated to carry out the Harrison Act. That part of the regulation was overturned by the U.S. Supreme Court in 1916 as a violation of states' rights, but it was effectively reinstated on another basis by the Court in 1919 during a peak of concern over drug addiction and in the face of the impending prohibition of alcohol.

The impact of alcohol prohibition on the severity of other drug laws illustrates a common factor in the control of drugs that might be called the *hydraulic model*, which implies that repression of one drug shifts use to another substance. This analysis encourages a blanket control of drugs and is especially popular at times when it is believed that abuse of a particular drug is a sign of an "addictive personality" (as in the late twentieth century) or the affliction of "inebriety" (late nineteenth century). These diagnoses suggest that the afflicted individual is pressured to use alcohol and drugs, and that if one substance is not available, he or she will switch to another.

EFFECTIVENESS OF DRUG CONTROL MEASURES. The question of "availability" raises the controversial issue of the effectiveness of control measures. Do laws against drugs accomplish much more than raising the price of drugs? Can prescription controls or international interdiction reduce the supply of drugs? Can prohibition reduce the supply of alcohol? The answers to these questions are elusive, but one can say that in general the reduction in drug and alcohol use that accompanied the restrictions in the United States beginning with World War I (and ending with the start of a second drug epidemic in the 1960s) occurred during a period of extraordinary antagonism toward drugs. Drugs came under progressively more severe laws, with the exception of alcohol, whose prohibition was repealed in 1933.

Confidence in legal control was reinforced by the obvious decline in drug use, and alcohol consumption fell from 1.7 U.S. gallons per capita in 1910, to about 0.6 gallons between 1920 and 1930, and did not return to the 1910 level until the mid-1960s (Rorabaugh, p. 232). Anti-drug legislation became increasingly severe, even after Prohibition was repealed in 1933, including mandatory minimum sentences and, in 1956, federal enactment of the death penalty as an option in some cases of drug trafficking.

To understand the doubts concerning legal sanctions in the late-twentieth-century drug "epidemic," it is necessary to compare the two drug epidemics. During the first wave of drug use, laws did not exist until the public's fear demanded them. The more recent wave of drug use found the most severe drug laws in effect at a time when a favorable attitude toward drug use was spreading across many sectors of American life. The apparent weakness in the enforcement of these laws, their clash with a new attitude among experts and the public, and the failure to recall the earlier experience with drugs led to ridicule and comfortable evasion of the law. A renewed harmony between anti-drug attitudes and anti-drug laws followed in the 1980s and later.

In the 1930s, at the end of the epidemic that peaked at about the time of World War I, the United States, after requiring general anti-drug and anti-alcohol education through state laws, adopted a policy of silence regarding drugs. When silence was not possible, exaggeration was instituted to complement the increasing severity of the drug laws. That policy may account for the loss of public memory of that early "epidemic"; the style of calling any drug use fraught with extreme danger (for the purpose of discouraging experimentation) contributed to the lack of balanced knowledge about drugs that characterized both adults and youth in the 1960s. The ultimate effect of the policy was to undercut the credibility of official statements on drug use.

In addition to the issue of changes in attitudes toward drugs and the practical problem of what control mechanisms exist, there is the broader question of control philosophy. Should drugs be controlled at all? Should the state try to protect citizens from their own desire to use drugs? Is drug control a law-enforcement problem, a public-health task, or a moral or religious issue? For Beecher (1828), alcohol had to be controlled because, whereas drunkenness ruined health and family life, it also impaired the individual's ability to hear and respond to God's message of salvation. Alcohol produced temporal death and eternal damnation.

Beecher's British contemporary John Stuart Mill rejected American prohibition laws and similar restrictions on the buyers of alcohol as an unjustified interference with liberty. Mill was particularly harsh on actions designed to protect individuals from themselves. To questions of policy he applied this prime principal: "Over himself, over his own body and mind, the individual is sovereign" (p. 11).

The debate between law-enforcement and public-health approaches to drug and alcohol abuse is particularly sensitive to public attitudes toward the nature of the drugs themselves. In an era of drug toleration, public-health methods and medical treatment in general are advocated and practiced. The concern is not so much with a drug itself as with the bad effects that it may have on an unwise or excessive user. As the attitude turns against the use of drugs in any amount, frustration and anger support police action, arrests, and punishments for violations of a strict rejection of drug use that leaves no room for *recreational* drug use.

The War against Drugs

The nature of the American drug experience changed quickly in the mid-1960s. The use of illegal drugs, which had existed at the fringes of society for more than three decades, moved to the center of youth culture. The drugs of choice were cannabis and other psychedelics, such as LSD. Advocates claimed that using those substances gave a person an experience of ultimate reality, a kind of insight that saints had achieved only after lengthy meditation and asceticism. Aldous Huxley gave an early cachet to psychedelic use with two accounts, *The Doors of Perception* (1954) and *Heaven and Hell* (1956), based on his use of mescaline. Huxley believed, however, that such experiences were best confined to an intellectual elite. In the 1960s Timothy Leary expanded that concept in the 1960s to include everyone. "Turn on, tune in, and drop out" was his advice to America. A striking example of faith in the drug revolution was Charles Reich's *The Greening of America* (1970), which saw marijuana as the "truth serum" that would create a new consciousness and a new society.

Passage of the Drug Control Amendments of 1965—an early response to the use of psychedelics, stimulants such as amphetamine, and sleeping medications such as barbiturates—was intended to restrict licit pharmaceutical production. Legal production of amphetamines was reduced from 100,000 pounds annually to less than 1,000 pounds by 1990. By 2002 the amount had risen to 20,000 pounds, largely as a result of the use of amphetamines in treating hyperactive children. The basis of anti-drug laws beginning in 1965 was shifted from the taxing power of the federal government to the Interstate Commerce Clause, a precedent that would be followed in the future.

Another significant element in the 1965 law was the creation, within the U.S. Food and Drug Administration, of the Bureau of Drug Abuse Control (BDAC), which would have as its targets all dangerous drugs except the opiates, cocaine, and marijuana; those traditional substances continued to be the province of the U.S. Treasury's Bureau of Narcotics. Then, because separating out the turfs of the two control agencies proved difficult, they were merged in 1968 as the Bureau of Narcotics and Dangerous Drugs (BNDD) and moved from the U.S. Treasury Department and the U.S. Department of Health, Education, and Welfare Department to the U.S. Department of Justice.

The Nixon administration (1969–1974) confronted growing public alarm over rising drug use among youth and, in response, created the basic element of the war on drugs that continues to the present (Musto and Korsmeyer). One of the Nixon administration's major goals was to reduce crime. Persuaded by the successful record of methadone treatment in the District of Columbia that indicated adopting such treatment could lower crime rates, Nixon gradually came to favor the use of methadone as a substitute for the illegal opiates used by addicts. The fact that Nixon, who was known to have a visceral antagonism to drug use, would initiate a national policy of substituting a legal addiction for an illegal one surprised many people.

Out of the Nixon era came the first "drug czar"; the first federal strategy (1972) that attempted to coordinate all federal anti-drug efforts; the creation of the Drug Enforcement Administration (DEA), the successor to the BNDD and the Office of Drug Abuse Law Enforcement (a temporary effort by the federal government to affect local drug dealers); and the National Institute on Drug Abuse (NIDA).

Under Nixon the budget to fight drugs rose to heights never before attained in the federal government; thousands of additional BNDD and DEA agents were trained and were placed internationally as well as nationally. Nevertheless, throughout the Nixon era the American people grew more tolerant of the use of drugs, particularly cannabis. Public opinion did not turn against drugs until about 1980, at the end of Jimmy Carter's presidency. The 1970 Drug Abuse Prevention and Control Act reflected a liberalization of the drug laws through the elimination of mandatory minimum sentences and a provision for clearing the record of an individual convicted of personal possession of cannabis. Although Nixon would seek a resumption of mandatory minimum sentences in 1974, as his administration was collapsing, that punishment was not resurrected until the Anti- Drug Abuse Acts of 1986 and 1988.

Perhaps the most alarming change in drug use habits in the 1970s and 1980s was the use of "crack" cocaine, a method that allows the user to inhale cocaine fumes and results in an intense brain response. The deaths of prominent sports figures from cocaine use crystallized public opinion against drugs and led Congress and a series of presidents to wage a war on drugs that was unprecedented in American history. Drug law convictions crowded prisons and caused a backlash to the anti-drug campaign.

Decriminalization

In the era of increased drug use that started about 1965, an attack on prohibitory laws began with criticism of the extraordinarily long sentences meted out to persons who possessed small amounts of marijuana. By 1970 the federal law had been softened and advocates of legalizing marijuana were organized. With the rise in cocaine and heroin use, many people called for legalizing or "decriminalizing" those drugs on the grounds that their dangers had been exaggerated. In 1972 the term *decriminalization* was proposed in the first report of the U.S. Commission on Marihuana and Drug Abuse as a compromise between arresting persons with small amounts of marijuana for personal use, and allowing a free market in marijuana. Decriminalization would allow use while still permitting a national policy warning against the drug and maintaining legal sanctions against those who produced and distributed large amounts of the plant.

Libertarians, such as the economist Milton Friedman, added a philosophy of freedom from state interference in private acts, such as drug use, to the debate over controls. Although the public has been increasingly opposed to drug use (reflected also in reduced consumption of tobacco and alcohol) and in favor of strict anti-drug laws since about 1980, analyses questioning the campaign against drugs have continued (Friedman).

Opposition to the "war against drugs" has centered on two themes: interdiction of drugs from foreign nations and domestic enforcement of stricter anti-drug laws. Critics have argued that interdiction has not affected the availability of drugs, especially cocaine, the chief target of the U.S. Coast Guard and the other "uniformed" services as well as the U.S. Drug Enforcement Administration. With regard to domestic policy, application of harsh criminal penalties to drug offenders is condemned as a source of prison crowding that does little or nothing to reduce crime or hard-core drug use.

A recent suggestion offered by those opposed to overreliance on the criminal justice approach is "harm reduction," a phrase that attempts to describe Dutch drug policy. The Netherlands is noted for allowing personal use of drugs, providing sterile needles to drug injectors, and generally tolerating drug availability. The expectation is that in the long run this policy will allow more users to survive and experience a life less dominated by, or free from, drug use.

Criticism of any policy that would appear to encourage or facilitate drug use has been severe. Arguments against legalization include the observation that laws pressure users into treatment, the symbolic importance of an anti-drug policy, and the fear that drug use would increase if drugs were easily available and inexpensive.

Conclusion

The history of drug and alcohol control illustrates the slowly shifting assumptions societies make regarding those powerful substances. At the extreme of each attitude the good or evil nature of drugs seems so obvious that contrary notions are rejected with dispatch. Consequently, the ethical debate is deeply influenced by these alterations in attitude. These contrary positions also make an indefinitely sustainable drug policy difficult to frame.

DAVID F. MUSTO (1995)
REVISED BY AUTHOR

SEE ALSO: *Addiction and Dependence; Alcohol and Other Drugs in a Public Health Context; Alcoholism; Bioterrorism; Environmental Ethics; Hazardous Wastes and Toxic Substances; Smoking*

BIBLIOGRAPHY

Aaron, Paul, and Musto, David F. 1981. "Temperance and Prohibition in America: A Historical Overview." In *Alcohol and Public Policy: Beyond the Shadow of Prohibition,* eds. Mark H. Moore and Dean R. Gerstein. Washington, D.C.: National Academy Press.

Acker, Caroline Jean. 2002. *Creating the American Junkie: Addiction Research in the Classic Era of Narcotic Control.* Baltimore: Johns Hopkins University Press.

Beecher, Lyman. 1828. *Six Sermons on Intemperance,* 4th edition. Boston: T. R. Marvin. Reprinted in Musto, ed., *Drugs in America,* 2002a.

Campbell, Nancy D. 2000. *Using Women: Gender, Drug Policy, and Social Justice.* New York: Routledge.

French, John. 1667. *The Art of Distillation; or, A Treatise of the Choicest Spagyrical Preparations, Experiments, and Curiosities Performed by Way of Distillation.* London: E. Coles for T. Williams.

Friedman, Milton. 1991. "The War We Are Losing." In *Searching for Alternatives: Drug-Control Policy in the United States,* eds. Melvyn B. Krauss and Edward P. Lazear. Stanford, CA: Hoover Institution.

Kleiman, Mark. 1992. *Against Excess: Drug Policy for Results.* New York: Basic Books.

Lender, Mark E., and Martin, James K. 1982. *Drinking in America: A History.* New York: Free Press.

MacCoun, Robert J., and Reuter, Peter. 2001. *Drug War Heresies: Learning from Other Vices, Times, and Places.* New York: Cambridge University Press.

Mill, John Stuart. 1975 (1859). *On Liberty,* ed. David Spitz. New York: W. W. Norton.

Musto, David F. 1999. *The American Disease: Origins of Narcotic Control,* 3rd edition. New York: Oxford University Press.

Musto, David F., ed. 2002a. *Drugs in America: A Documentary History.* New York: New York University Press.

Musto, David F., ed. 2002b. *One Hundred Years of Heroin.* Westport, CT: Auburn House.

Musto, David F., and Korsmeyer, Pamela. 2002. *The Quest for Drug Control: Politics and Federal Policy in a Period of Increasing Substance Abuse, 1963–1981.* New Haven, CT: Yale University Press.

Nadelmann, Ethan A. 1991. "Thinking Seriously about Alternatives to Drug Prohibition." *Daedalus* 121(3): 85–132.

Plant, Moira. 1985. *Women, Drinking, and Pregnancy.* New York: Tavistock Methuen.

Rorabaugh, William J. 1979. *The Alcoholic Republic.* New York: Oxford University Press.

Rush, Benjamin. (n.d.). *An Inquiry into the Effects of Ardent Spirits upon the Human Body and Mind.* Philadelphia: Thomas Bradford. Reprinted in Musto, ed., *Drugs in America* (2002a).

U.S. National Commission on Marihuana and Drug Abuse. 1972. *Marihuana: A Signal of Misunderstanding.* Washington, D.C.: U.S. Government Printing Office.

U.S. Office of National Drug Control Policy. 2002. *National Drug Control Strategy.* Washington, D.C.: U.S. Government Printing Office.

Wesley, John. 1747. *Primitive Physick; or, An Easy and Natural Method of Curing Most Diseases.* London: Thomas Trye.

Wilson, James Q. 1990. "Against the Legalization of Drugs." *Commentary* 88(2): 21–28.

Wood, George B. 1868. *A Treatise on Therapeutics, and Pharmacology, or Materia Medica,* 3rd edition, 2 vols. Philadelphia: J. B. Lippincott.

HAZARDOUS WASTES AND TOXIC SUBSTANCES

• • •

Developed nations such as the United States annually use more than 60,000 hazardous chemicals in their agricultural and manufacturing processes. Because at least 10,000 are introduced each year, often we know very little about their effects. When we began massive use of such chemicals, we did not know that by the 1970s human breast milk would become more contaminated with toxins than any allowable manufactured foods. We did not realize that measurable amounts of DDT would appear in the polar ice caps. We did not suspect that by 2000 Silicon Valley would have more Superfund sites, twenty-nine, than any other single U.S. location—all because of toxic wastes from manufacturing high-tech products such as disk drives and semiconductors. We did not realize that, because of their long lifetimes, many hazardous chemicals would be able to migrate from their present waste sites and would threaten persons living thousands of years in the future. On the whole, we have assumed that dangerous chemicals are *innocent until proved guilty.* Because we do very little sophisticated epidemiological testing and rarely take account of food-chain and synergistic effects, thousands of chemicals have become both important to our agricultural and manufacturing processes and ubiquitous in our environment. Hence, it is often difficult to prove that any one chemical is responsible for specific harms, even when we know that it is theoretically able to cause many *statistical casualties.*

Hazardous wastes, byproducts of manufacturing, scientific, medical, and agricultural processes, have at least one of four characteristics: ignitability, corrosivity, reactivity, or toxicity (Wagner). Hazardous substances become wastes only when they have outlived their economic life. They include solvents, electroplating substances, pesticides such as dioxin, and radioactive wastes. Toxic substances, a subset of hazardous substances, have the characteristic of toxicity: the ability to cause serious injury, illness, or death.

Many persons became aware of the threat of hazardous wastes and toxic substances when American scientist Rachel Carson (1907–1964) wrote *Silent Spring* (1962), one of the earliest warnings of the dangers of pesticides, or when Michael Brown wrote his spellbinding account of hundreds of cancers, genetic damage, and birth defects near Love Canal, New York, and other waste sites in 1980. Indeed, hazardous-waste management has become one of the most serious environmental problems facing the world. In the United States alone, more than 5 billion pounds of toxic chemicals are released each year into air, water, and land. Approximately 80 percent of hazardous waste has been dumped into thousands of landfills, ponds, and pits throughout the world, from Love Canal in New York, to Mellery in Belgium, to North-Rhine in Germany. It has polluted air, wells, surface water, and groundwater. It has destroyed species, habitats, and ecosystems. It also has caused fires,

explosions, direct-contact poisoning, and numerous cases of cancer, genetic harms, neurological disorders, and birth defects.

Surprisingly, one-quarter of the mercury and nearly one-half of all dioxin released into the American environment is from the healthcare industry. The mercury comes from blood temperature gauges and batteries, for example, while the dioxin comes from burning chlorinated plastics, like the PVC tubing used in kidney dialysis. Both mercury and dioxin are emitted by hospital incineration, and each patient-day is responsible for 9 kilograms of solid waste. Much of the dioxin emitted is from biochemical waste, 60 percent of which is not handled adequately.

In part to protect workers and the public from the dangers associated with hazardous substances, the U.S. Congress passed laws such as the 1954 Atomic Energy Act; the 1975 Hazardous Materials Transportation Act; the 1976 Resource Conservation and Recovery Act (RCRA); the 1976 Toxic Substances Control Act (TSCA); the 1977 Clean Water Act; the 1977 Clean Air Act; and the 1980 Comprehensive Environmental Response, Compensation, and Liability Act known as CERCLA or Superfund (Dominguez and Bartlett). These laws include provisions that require monitoring pollutants, reporting spills, preparing manifests describing particular wastes, and special packaging for transporting specific types of hazardous materials. The Clean Air Act regulates smelter emissions, for instance, and the Clean Water Act regulates mining-caused water pollution (Young). RCRA was passed to fill a statutory void left by the Clean Air Act and the Clean Water Act, which require removal of hazardous materials from air and water but leave the question of the ultimate deposition of hazardous waste unanswered. Although RCRA addresses the handling of such waste at current and future facilities, it does not deal with closed or abandoned sites. CERCLA focuses on hazardous-waste contamination when sites or spills have been abandoned; through penalties and taxes on hazardous substances, CERCLA provides for cleaning up abandoned sites.

Despite laws that govern dangerous substances, and despite the fact that 50,000 environmental assessments are prepared annually in the U.S., many to evaluate waste sites under the 1969 National Environmental Policy Act, hazardous wastes remain a major problem. One reason is that well-financed industrial waste polluters can dominate underfunded government regulators. Another reason is that the North American Free Trade Agreement (NAFTA) has allowed more U.S. waste to go to countries such as Mexico. The U.S.-to-Mexico waste flow doubled, for example, from 1994 to 1999, and yet Mexico has only one licensed hazardous waste facility. A third factor is that the use of toxic substances and the management of hazardous wastes raise ethical issues that have not been adequately addressed by existing regulations. These issues include siting, rights of future generations, workers's rights, free and informed consent, compensation, due process, appropriate ethical behavior under conditions of uncertainty, where to place the burden of proof regarding alleged waste harms, and workers's and the public's right to know.

Equity Issues

Those who can afford to avoid hazardous wastes and toxic substances typically do so. Those who cannot are usually poor or otherwise disadvantaged. For this reason, public and workplace exposure to such hazards raises questions of intergenerational, geographical, and occupational equity. Intergenerational-equity problems deal with imposing risks and costs of hazardous wastes and toxic substances on future persons. Geographical-equity issues have to do with where and how to site waste dumps or facilities using toxic substances. Occupational-equity problems focus on whether to maximize the safety of the public or of the people who work with hazardous materials because we often cannot protect both groups at once. For example, effective decontamination and safety assurance at waste sites typically require more worker exposure to toxins but reduce public risk. Using mechanical or nonhuman decontamination and safety procedures, however, is safer for workers but usually increases public risk because such procedures are less effective than those controlled closely by people (see Kasperson).

Intergenerational equity requires us to ask whether we ought to mortgage the future by imposing our debts of buried (or stored) hazardous wastes on subsequent generations. Current plans for future U.S. government storage of high-level radioactive waste, for example, require the steel canisters to resist corrosion for as little as 300 years. Nevertheless, the U.S. Department of Energy admits that the waste will remain dangerous for longer than 10,000 years. Government experts agree that, at best, they can merely limit the radioactivity that reaches the environment, and that there is no doubt that the repository will leak over the course of the next 10,000 years (Shrader-Frechette, 1993). To saddle our descendants with the medical and financial debts of such waste, much of which is extremely long-lived, is questionable at best: We have received most of the benefits from the use of industrial and agricultural processes that create hazardous wastes, whereas future persons will bear most of the risks and costs. This risk/cost-benefit asymmetry suggests that, without good reasons or compensating benefits, future generations ought not be saddled with debts of

their ancestors. Moreover, any alleged economies associated with storage of hazardous waste are, in large part, questionable because of the practice of discounting future costs (such as deaths) at some rate of x percent per year. For example, at a discount rate of 10 percent, effects on people's welfare twenty years from now count only for one-tenth of what effects on people's welfare count for now. Or, more graphically, with a discount rate of 5 percent, 1 billion deaths in 400 years count the same as one death next year. A number of moral philosophers, such as Derek Parfit, have argued that use of a discount rate is unethical, because the moral importance of future events, like the death of a person, does not decline at some x percent per year.

Another issue related to intergenerational equity is what sort of criteria might justify irreversible damage to the environment, such as that caused by deep-well storage of high-level nuclear waste. On the one hand, irreversible management schemes for nuclear waste, because they are premised on the nonretrievability of the waste, theoretically impose fewer management burdens on later generations, but they also preempt future choices about how to deal with the hazards. On the other hand, schemes that are reversible allow for wider choices for future generations, but they also impose greater management burdens. If we cannot do both, is it ethically desirable to maximize future freedom or to minimize future burdens? The technical problems associated with storing long-lived hazardous waste for centuries are forcing us to take a great gamble that our descendants will not breach the waste repositories through war, terrorism, or drilling for minerals; that groundwater will not leach out and transport toxins; and that subsequent ice sheets, faulting, seismic activity, and geological folding will not uncover the wastes.

Using and storing toxins also raises questions of environmental justice, that is, spatial or geographical equity in the risk distributiuon (Shrader-Frechette, 2002). One such issue is whether it is fair to impose a higher risk (of being harmed by seepage from a hazardous-waste dump, for example) on persons just because they live in a certain spot. Or, is it ethical for people in one area to receive the benefits of products created by using toxic substances, while people in another area bear the health risks associated a hazardous-waste dump? How does one site hazardous facilities equitably, and how does one transport toxic substances safely (see English)?

Questions about the equity of risk distribution are central to the issue of managing toxic substances because thousands of persons—such as the 1984 victims of the Union Carbide toxic leak in Bhopal, India—have already died as a consequence of exposure to hazardous substances.

Current trade agreements also allow much hazardous waste of developed nations to be shipped to developing ones. Economic comparisons of alternative chemical technologies and different waste sites typically ignore the externalities (or social costs) such as the inequitable distribution of health hazards benefits associated with them. Geographical and intergenerational inequities are typically *external* to the benefit-cost schemes used as the basis for public policy. Consequently, decision makers almost always ignore them (Shrader-Frechette, 2002).

The most serious problems of geographical equity in the distribution of risks associated with dangerous substances arise because developed nations often ship their toxic chemicals and hazardous wastes to developing countries. One-third of U.S. pesticide exports, for example, are products that are banned for use in the United States. These exports are annually responsible for 40,000 pesticide-related deaths, mainly in developing nations (Shrader-Frechette, 1991). Likewise, the United Nations estimates that as much as 20 percent of the hazardous waste produced in developed nations is sent to other countries where health and safety standards are virtually nonexistent. The Organization of African Unity has pleaded with member states to stop such traffic, but corruption and crime have kept the waste transport going (Moyers). Indeed, exporting toxic substances and hazardous wastes may be the current version of the infant-formula problem. During the last three decades of the twentieth century, U.S. and multinational corporations have profited by exporting infant formula to developing nations and by encouraging young mothers not to nurse their children. They have been able to do so only by extremely coercive sales tactics and by misleading persons in developing countries about the relative merits and dangers of the exports.

Some of the greatest risks associated with toxic substances and hazardous wastes, whether in developed or developing nations, are borne by workers. One of the main questions of occupational equity is whether it is just to impose higher health burdens on workers in exchange for wages. Is it fair to allow persons to trade their health and safety for money? This question is particularly troublesome in the United States, because many other countries—such as the Scandinavian nations, Germany, and the former Soviet Union—have standards for occupational exposure to risks from toxins that are just as stringent as standards for public exposure. The United States, however, follows the alleged *compensating wage differential* (CWD) of Scot economist Adam Smith (1723–1790), presupposing that wages compensate workers for increased occupational exposures to toxic substances. As a consequence, U.S. regulators argue that, in exchange for facing higher risks than the public faces

from toxic substances, workers receive higher wages that compensate them for their burden. Other countries do not accept the economic theory underlying the CWD and argue for equal health standards, for making public and worker exposure norms the same (Shrader-Frechette, 1991).

Consent and Right to Know

One reason critics question the theory underlying the CWD is its presupposition that, by virtue of accepting certain jobs, workers exposed to serious hazards give free, informed consent to the risks. Yet, from an ethical point of view, those most able to give free, informed consent—those who are well educated and who have many job opportunities—are usually unwilling to do so. Those least able to give genuine consent to a risky workplace or neighborhood—because of their lack of education or information and their financial constraints—are often willing to give allegedly informed consent.

The 1986 U.S. Right-to-Know Act requires owners or operators of sites using hazardous materials to notify the Emergency Response Commission in their state that toxins are present at a facility. However, at least three factors suggest that this law may fail to ensure full conditions for the free, informed consent of persons likely to be harmed by some hazardous substance. First, owners or operators (rather than a neutral third party) provide the information about the hazard. Often those responsible for toxic substances and hazardous wastes do not inform workers and the public of the risks they face, even after company physicians have documented serious health problems. Employers in the chemical industry, for example, frequently spend money on genetic screening to exclude susceptible persons from the workplace rather than to monitor their health on the job (Draper). Second, the existence, location, and operational procedures of dangerous facilities are likely things to which citizens and workers have not given free, informed consent in the first place. Third, mining is not included among the industries required to report their toxic emissions to state and federal regulators. For example, Utah's Bingham Canyon Copper Mine, owned by Kennecott Copper, ranks fourth in the nation in total toxic releases, yet it and other mining companies do not report their releases (Young).

Sociological data reveal that, as education and income rise, people are less willing to accept either work in hazardous facilities or risky jobs; those who do so tend to be poorly educated or financially strapped. The data also show that the alleged CWD does not operate for poor, unskilled, minority, or nonunionized workers. Yet these are precisely the people most likely to have risky jobs, such as handling nuclear wastes. In other words, the very persons *least* able to give free, informed consent to occupational risks are precisely those who *most* often work in risky jobs (Shrader-Frechette, 1993).

At the international level, a similar situation occurs. The persons and nations least able to give free informed consent to the location of facilities for using or storing toxic substances are typically those who most often bear such risks. Hazardous wastes shipped abroad, for example, are usually sent to countries that will take them at the cheapest rate, and these tend to be developing nations that are often ill informed about the risks involved. In 1989, the United Nations passed a resolution requiring any country receiving hazardous waste to give consent before it is sent. Because socioeconomic conditions and corruption often militate against the exercise of free informed consent, however, it is questionable whether the U.N. resolution will have much effect (Shrader-Frechette, 1991).

Industrial offers of financial benefits—for storing hazardous waste in a developing nation or in an economically depressed community—create a coercive context in which requirements for free informed consent are unlikely to be met. Likewise, high wages for desperate workers who agree to take risky jobs may jeopardize their legitimate consent. In such contexts, we must admit either that our classical ethical theory of free informed consent is wrong or that our laws and regulations fail to provide an ethical framework in which those most affected by hazardous substances can give free informed consent to the risk.

Given the many consent-related problems relevant to risk from hazardous substances, a crucial issue is: Who should give consent? Liberty and grass-roots self-determination require local control of whether a hazardous facility is sited in a particular area. Yet, equality of consideration for people in all regions and minimizing overall risk often require federal control. Should a particular community be able to veto the location of a hazardous facility, even though that site may be the best in the country and may provide the most equal protection of all people? Or should the national government have the right to impose such risks on a local community, even against the wishes of that group?

On the one hand, federal jurisdiction is more likely to protect the environment, to avoid the tragedy of the commons, to gain national economies of scale, and to avoid regional favoritism. Federal jurisdiction is also more likely to provide compensation for victims of spillovers from another locale and to facilitate the politics of sacrifice by imposing equal burdens on all. On the other hand, local jurisdiction is more likely to promote diversity, to offer a more flexible vehicle for experimenting with waste regulations, and to enhance citizen autonomy and liberty. Local jurisdiction also is likely to encourage cooperation through participation in decision making, to discourage some kinds of inequitable federal policies, and to help avoid many violations of rights.

Compensation

Current U.S. laws do not typically provide for full exercise of due-process rights by those who may have been harmed by toxins or hazardous wastes. Many of the companies that handle dangerous substances do not have either full insurance for their pollution risk or adequate funds to cover their liability themselves. RCRA and CERCLA, however, require such companies both to show that they are capable of paying at least some of the damages resulting from their activities and to clean up their sites. Because enforcement of liability and coverage provisions of these laws is difficult, many hazardous-waste industries often operate outside the law. Furthermore, most insurers have withdrawn from the pollution market, claiming that providing such coverage carries the risk of payments for claims that would bankrupt them.

Just as insurers fear potentially large liability claims in cases involving hazardous-waste substances, so do members of the public. For example, in 1987 when the U.S. Congress chose Yucca Mountain, Nevada, as the likely site for the world's first permanent facility for high-level nuclear waste, local residents and the state asked for unlimited, strict-liability coverage for any nuclear-waste accident or incident. The U.S. Department of Energy's response to the citizens, based on the 1957 Price-Anderson Act, was that the government would allow the waste facility to bear only limited liability. Consequently, the U.S. nuclear program, including radioactive-waste management, has operated under a government-imposed limit for liability coverage. This limit, designed to protect the nuclear-waste industry from bankruptcy caused by accidents, is less than 3 percent of the government-calculated costs of the April 1986 Chernobyl nuclear catastrophe, and Chernobyl was not a worst-case accident (see Shrader-Frechette, 1993).

Limits on government or industry liability for hazardous-waste and toxic-substance incidents are problematic for several reasons. First, liability is a well-known incentive for appropriate, safe behavior. Second, refusal to accept full and strict liability suggests that hazardous- and radioactive-waste sites are not as safe as the government maintains they are. Third, if government officials may legally limit due-process right then, in the case of an accident at a hazardous-waste facility, the main financial burdens will be borne inequitably by accident victims rather than by the perpetrators of the hazard. Fourth, because much less is known about the dangers from hazardous wastes and toxic substances than about more ordinary risks, full liability seems a reasonable requirement. And finally, the safety record of hazardous facilities, in the past, has not been good. Every state and every nation in the world have extensive, long-term pollution from toxins. Even in the United States, the government has been one of the worst offenders. A congressional report has argued that cleaning up the hazardous and radioactive wastes at government weapons facilities would cost more than $300 billion (U.S. Congress; Shrader-Frechette, 1993). Such problems argue for citizens's rights to full liability.

Uncertainty, Human Error, and the Burden of Proof

Inadequate compensation for victims of toxins, inequitable distribution of the risks associated with hazardous wastes, and the uncertainties and potential harm associated with such substances provide powerful arguments for reducing or eliminating exposure to them. To decrease exposures and to move *beyond dumping*, however, we must have market incentives for reducing the volume of toxic substances and hazardous wastes (Piasecki; Higgins). To reduce the volume of these threats, we must know exactly what effects they cause, and we must make risk imposers accountable for their behavior. Ensuring accountability is not easy. Adequate tests for medical responses to low-level chemical exposures require samples of thousands of persons, because so many toxic substances produce health effects synergistically, because there are many uncertainties about actual exposure to hazardous substances, because the effects of such exposure often are unknown (Ashford and Miller), and because phenotypical characteristics among individuals often vary by a factor of 200. All four variables cause extreme differences in humans's responses to toxins.

Uncertainties about exposure and about the consequences of exposure to hazardous substances are compounded by the fact that the industries that produce toxic substances and hazardous wastes—and that profit from them—usually perform the required tests to determine toxicity and health effects. Pesticide-registration decisions (about allowing use of the chemicals) in the West, for example, are tied to a risk-benefit standard that combines scientific and economic evidence. Because industry does most or all of the testing, and because environmental and health groups are forced to show that the dangers outweigh the economic benefits of a particular pesticide, there is much uncertainty about the real hazards actually faced by workers and consumers. As a consequence, virtually no groups want toxic substances or hazardous wastes used or stored near them. Hence the protest: *Not in my backyard*—NIMBY.

NIMBY responses also arise as a consequence of public mistrust of human institutions for controlling hazardous wastes and toxic chemicals. All dangerous technologies are unavoidably dependent upon fragile, sometimes short-lived, human institutions and human capabilities. Faulty technology, after all, did not cause the injuries and deaths at Three Mile Island, Bhopal, Love Canal, or Chernobyl. Human error did. Human error and misconduct also may be the insoluble problem with using toxic substances and managing hazardous wastes. According to risk assessors, 60 percent to 80 percent of industrial accidents are due to human mismanagement or corruption (Shrader-Frechette, 1993). For example, at the nation's largest incinerator for hazardous wastes, run by Chemical Waste Management, Inc., in Chicago, a 1992 grand jury found evidence of criminal conduct, including deliberate mislabeling of many barrels of hazardous waste. They also discovered deliberate disconnection of pollution-monitoring devices. More generally, corruption in the waste-disposal industry has been rampant in the United States ever since the 1940s, when the Mafia won control of the carting business through Local 813 of the International Brotherhood of Teamsters. In the mid-1990s, three Mafia families still dominated hazardous-waste disposal and illegal dumping: the Gambino, Lucchese, and Genovese/Tiere crime groups (see Szasz). Given the potential for human error and corruption, citizens are frequently skeptical regarding whether hazardous and toxic substances will be handled safely, with little threat to workers or to the public.

Because of scientific unknowns and uncertainties about human behavior and corruption, several moral philosophers have argued that potentially catastrophic situations—involving hazardous wastes and toxic substances—require ethically conservative behavior (Cranor; Shrader-Frechette, 1991; Ashford and Miller). Such situations often require one to choose a *maximin* decision rule to avoid situations with the greatest potential for harm, as John Rawls (1971) has argued. Ethical conservatism, in a situation of uncertainty, also may require society to place the burden of proof—regarding risk or harm—on the manufacturers, users, and disposers of hazardous substances, rather than on their potential victims. This, in turn, may mean that we will need to reform our laws governing so-called *toxic torts* (Cranor).

Given the longevity and the catastrophic potential of many toxic substances and hazardous wastes, we may need to reevaluate the human and environmental price we have paid for our economic progress. Although our society may not be able to avoid use of certain toxic substances and disposal of some hazardous waste, it is clear that we need to maximize the equity with which we distribute the risks associated with such threats. We also need to guarantee, so far as possible, that potential victims of toxins are informed about the risks they face and that they freely consent to avoidable risk impositions. Finally, we ought to ensure that those put at risk from toxic substances and hazardous wastes are compensated, so far as possible, for harm done to them. Because of numerous uncertainties about their effects, and because of the catastrophic potential and the longevity of many hazardous materials, our behavior regarding them ought to be ethically conservative.

KRISTIN SHRADER-FRECHETTE (1995)
REVISED BY AUTHOR

SEE ALSO: *Environmental Ethics; Environmental Health; Environmental Policy and Law; Future Generations, Reproductive Technologies and Obligations to; Technology*

BIBLIOGRAPHY

Ashford, Nicholas A., and Miller, Claudia. 1991. *Chemical Exposures: Low Levels and High Stakes.* New York: Van Nostrand Reinhold.

Beder, Sharon. 2002. *Global Spin.* Devon, Eng.: Green Books.

Brown, Michael H. 1979. *Laying Waste: The Poisoning of America by Toxic Chemicals.* New York: Pantheon.

Carson, Rachel. 1962. *Silent Spring.* Boston: Houghton Mifflin.

Colborn, Theodora; D. Dumonoski; and J. P. Meyers. 1996. *Our Stolen Future.* New York: Dutton.

Cranor, Carl F. 1993. *Regulating Toxic Substances: Philosophy of Science and the Law.* New York: Oxford University Press.

Davis, Devra. 2002. *When Smoke Ran Like Water.* New York: Basic Books.

Dominguez, George S., and Bartlett, Kenneth G., eds. 1986. *Hazardous Waste Management.* Boca Raton, FL: CRC Press.

Draper, Elaine. 1991. *Risky Business: Genetic Testing and Exclusionary Practices in the Hazardous Workplace.* Cambridge, Eng.: Cambridge University Press.

Ebenreck, Sarah. 1983. "A Partnership Farmland Ethic." *Environmental Ethics* 5(1): 33–45.

English, Mary R. 1992. *Siting Low-Level Radioactive Waste Disposal Facilities: The Public Policy Dilemma.* New York: Greenwood.

Greenberg, Michael R., and Anderson, Richard F. 1984. *Hazardous Waste Sites: The Credibility Gap.* New Brunswick, NJ: Center for Urban Research.

Higgins, Thomas E. 1989. *Hazardous Waste Minimization Handbook.* Chelsea, MI: Lewis.

Kasperson, Roger, ed. 1983. *Equity Issues in Radioactive Waste Management.* Cambridge, MA: Oelgelschlager, Gunn, and Hain.

La Dou, Joseph. 1992. "First World Exports to the Third World: Capital, Technology, Hazardous Waste, and Working Conditions: Who Wins?" *The Western Journal of Medicine* 156(5): 553–554.

Moyers, Bill D. 1990. *Global Dumping Ground: The International Traffic in Hazardous Waste.* Washington, D.C.: Seven Locks Press.

Needleman, Herbert. 1998. "Childhood Lead Poisoning." *The American Journal of Public Health* 88: 1871–1877.

Nordquist, Joan. 1988. *Toxic Waste: Regulatory, Health, International Concerns.* Santa Cruz, CA: Reference and Research Services.

Parfit, Derek. 1985. *Reasons and Persons.* New York: Oxford University Press.

Piasecki, Bruce, and Davis, Gary A. 1987. *America's Future in Toxic-Waste Management: Lessons from Europe.* Westport, CT: Quorum.

Piasecki, Bruce, ed. 1984. *Beyond Dumping: New Strategies for Controlling Toxic Contamination.* Westport, CT: Quorum.

Postel, Sandra. 1987. *Defusing the Toxics Threat: Controlling Pesticides and Industrial Waste.* Washington, D.C.: Worldwatch Institute.

Rawls, John. 1971. *A Theory of Justice.* Cambridge, MA: Harvard University Press.

Samuels, Sheldon W. 1986. *The Environment of the Workplace and Human Values.* New York: Liss.

Shrader-Frechette, Kristin. 1991. *Risk and Rationality: Philosophical Foundations for Populist Reforms.* Berkeley: University of California Press.

Shrader-Frechette, Kristin. 1993. *Burying Uncertainty: Risk and the Case Against Geological Disposal of Nuclear Waste.* Berkeley: University of California Press.

Shrader-Frechette, Kristin. 2002. *Environmental Justice: Creating Equality, Reclaiming Democracy.* New York: Oxford University Press.

Szasz, Andrew. 1986. "Corporations, Organized Crime, and the Disposal of Hazardous Waste: An Examination of the Making of a Criminogenic Regulatory Structure." *Criminology* 24(1): 1–27.

U.S. Congress. 1983. *Hazardous Waste Disposal: Hearings Before the Subcommittee on Investigations and Oversight of the Committee on Science and Technology, U.S. House of Representatives, Ninety-Eighth Congress, First Session, March 30–May 4.* Washington, D.C.: U. S. Government Printing Office.

Wagner, Travis P. 1990. *Hazardous Waste Identification and Classification Manual: The Identification of Hazardous Waste Under RCRA and the Classification of Hazardous Waste Under HMTA.* New York: Van Nostrand Reinhold.

Waertenberg, Daniel; Reyner, D.; and Scott, C. S. 2000. "Trichloroethylene and Cancer." *Environmental Health Perspectives* 108: 161–176.

Wargo, John. 1998. *Our Children's Toxic Legacy.* New Haven: Yale University Press.

Wynne, Brian, ed. 1987. *Risk Management and Hazardous Waste: Implementation and the Dialectics of Credibility.* New York: Springer-Verlag.

Young, John. 1992. *Mining the Earth.* Washington, D.C.: Worldwatch Institute.

INTERNET RESOURCE

U.S. Department of Health and Human Services, Public Health Service. 2001. "Ninth Report on Carcinogens" Available from <http://niehs.nih.bov/roc/ninth/known3>.

HEALING

. . .

Health and Wholeness

Healing is an action whose goal is the restoration of health. The English word *health* literally means *wholeness* and *to heal* means *to make whole.* Ancient Greek had two words generally translated as "health": *hygieia,* meaning "a well way of living," and *euexia,* meaning "good habit of body." Leon Kass (1985) notes that the English and both Greek words for health are totally unrelated to all the words for disease, illness, and sickness. This is also true for German, Latin, and Hebrew. In addition, the Greek terms for health, unlike the English, are unrelated to all the verbs for healing. Health for the ancient Greeks was a state or condition unrelated to, and prior to, both illness and healers. The English emphasis on wholeness, Kass also notes, is comparatively static and structural, implying a whole distinct from all else and complete in itself and connoting self-sufficiency and independence. The Greek terms, in contrast, stress the functioning of the whole, and not only its working but its working well. Kass sums up this Greek understanding of health by defining it as a natural as opposed to a moral norm that reveals itself in activity as a standard of bodily excellence or fitness. It is the well-working of the organism as a whole, an activity of the living body in accordance with its specific excellences.

The work of healing in Western culture is the proper activity of the profession of medicine. Howard Brody (1987) calls medicine a craft in which scientific knowledge is applied to particular patients for the purpose of "a right and good healing action," employing the now-classic phrase of Edmund Pellegrino (1982). Unlike the Greek, the English language sets up a relationship between medicine, whose business is healing, and health that is problematic. Kass states the problem this way: Health and only health is the doctor's proper business; but health, understood as wellworking wholeness, is not the business only of doctors.

HEALTH AS EQUILIBRIUM. A less formal starting point than Kass's from which to examine the relationship between health and medicine is Pellegrino's definition of health as a state of accommodation, defined in different terms by each person. We feel healthy, he says, when we have found an equilibrium between our already-experienced shortcomings and our aspirations and have adjusted our goals to the gap between them. This means that health cannot be understood apart from a person's life history, or to use José Ortega y Gasset's phrase, one's "personal project" (p. 45). Healing, according to this definition of health, occurs when a new equilibrium is found between one's hopes and one's failures that can be incorporated into one's personal project. As such, healing must be based on an authentic perception of the experience of illness in the particular person.

THE CONTEXT OF HEALING. It follows that for an action of someone who professes to heal to be a right and good healing action, it must be situated in the context of a personal history so as to restore the direction of a personal project. This requires that a dialogue be established between healer and patient whose goal is the creation of a common ground of meaning shared by the healer and the patient. How extensive that common ground must be to constitute a right and good healing action is open to question. In taking a medical history, physicians have traditionally tended to restrict the province of illness to the *facts of diseases,* leaving unexplored the *fact of illness*—that is, the physical, psychological, and moral vulnerability the patient suffers in the attack on his or her very being that Pellegrino calls "the ontological assault of illness" (1982). However, this concentration on facts and diseases does not result from simple, unreflective traditionalism. Rather, it has enabled the profession of medicine to set very definite limits to the boundaries of healing and thereby to maintain control over the responsibilities that physicians take upon themselves as healers.

THE BOUNDARIES OF HEALING. The attempt by physicians such as Pellegrino to enlarge the boundaries of what counts as healing has often produced frustration and anger. For example, Franz J. Ingelfinger, in a classic editorial in the *New England Journal of Medicine,* rebukes those who would expand medical treatment to include families, not just individuals: "The curious idea is abroad that the doctor should be a factotum of health. By some singularity of reasoning, his role as healer is disparaged, and the words 'care, not cure' are becoming as tiresome as 'death with dignity'" (p. 565). He continues by lamenting that if the doctor is insensitive to the "multiple environmental conditions that threaten our mental and physical selves, he is regarded as failing the holistic image that many—both lay and medical—wish to impose on the physician" (p. 565). Ingelfinger concludes by asserting that the physician's primary concern, in spite of utopian claims to the contrary, should be sickness, not overall health; medicine should concentrate on "scientifically accurate diagnosis and treatment."

THE NATURE OF HEALING. The resistance of physicians such as Ingelfinger to what they regard as an unwarranted expansion of their role in society signals a fundamental disagreement within Western society about the nature of healing. Holistic approaches to medicine challenge traditional assumptions about who can be called a healer, what the goal of healing should be, and, most important, who can say what constitutes a right and good healing action: the healer or the one to be healed. Those who take positions like Ingelfinger's insist that only those who engage in "scientifically accurate diagnosis and treatment" deserve to be called healers, that healing aims at the cure of disease, and that the healer's profession alone can determine what constitutes a right and good healing action.

Those who disagree with these assumptions often attack their opponents as simply *uncaring*. Victor Kestenbaum, however, argues that the point of departure and method, not the lack of feeling, is the real issue. By distinguishing between caring and curing and limiting medicine to the latter, Ingelfinger and his colleagues take as normative the physician's perception of illness, shaped by the method of science, and then seek to derive global professional obligations from it. Thus they cut the phenomenon of illness to fit a prior conception of role and discourse. Pellegrino, Kestenbaum notes by way of contrast, starts with illness as experienced by the patient and derives professional obligations from the distinctly human dimensions of being ill and in distress. The responsibilities of the healer follow from the complexity and scope of the phenomenon of illness, not from the self-declared duties of the profession.

The Healing Profession

In the 1950s Pedro Laín Entralgo observed that "the curative activity of the physician is always determined by the reality of the human being towards which it is directed, that is, by the 'personal' conditions of the disease and of the patient" (p. xv). Pellegrino believes that this accommodation to the reality of the patient follows from the promise that the medical profession, in the person of the physician, makes to the patient: "The promise of help that shapes the nature of every healing act and defines the requirements for successful healing—even when cure is not possible" (p. 160). But,

Pellegrino notes, considerable confusion exists between doctor and patient about what healing means. Physicians, he says, often fail to comprehend what the patient understands by the promise of healing; patients often fail to understand what the physician thinks he or she is promising. Physicians, in response, are moving toward a restricted sense of promise, emphasizing technical competence, whereas patients expect not only competence but compassionate help as well. The wider the gap between professional promises and lay expectations, the more difficult becomes the collaboration between physician and patient to discover the equilibrium that constitutes genuine healing. As the gap increases, Pellegrino also notes, patients will be more tempted to seek alternatives to the "medical model" and lose the benefits of scientific competence.

COMPETENCE AND COMPASSION. Healing requires, Pellegrino insists, both competence (in scientifically accurate diagnosis and treatment) and compassion (the capacity to enter into the experience of illness with the patient). Competence is a necessary but not sufficient condition of healing. Healing "must be shaped at every step by the purposes of the healing acts—by the good of the person who is ill—his bodily good, of course, but also his concept of health, his value system, and his sense of the kind and quality of life he thinks is worthwhile" (p. 161). Pellegrino sums this up by declaring that the physician therefore has the obligation to protect the moral agency of the patient, to enhance it even in the face of the special vulnerabilities of being ill.

This protection of the moral agency of the patient lies at the heart of compassion; it is essential to the performance of a right and good healing action. Healing thus requires that the conversation between physician and patient encompass more than what can be accommodated by scientifically accurate medical language. As Jay Katz has observed, despite the quantity of words overflowing patients' medical charts, the world shared by doctor and patient is often one of profound silence, offering not the humaneness of shared understanding but the humaneness of services silently rendered (Katz).

The Silent World of Medicine

Yet modern scientific medicine owes its success to silence of a sort, a disbelief in words that Laín Entralgo traces to two tenets of the Hippocratic school of medicine. First, the latter rejected the use of words as a therapeutic tool; medicinal remedies were preferred to exorcism, which relied on the curative power of "fine words used in the manner of charms" (Laín Entralgo, p. 47). In addition, Hippocratic physicians trusted the patient's symptoms to reveal the causes of disease and dismissed the patient's own words about the source of his or her condition as unreliable opinion.

THE CLINICAL GAZE. Michel Foucault (1973), in his discussion of the antecedents of modern medicine, discovers a similar kind of silence in the "clinical gaze," a reorganization of medical perception that took place in the eighteenth century. Disease ceased to be perceived as an alien force inserted into the body and subject to the words of exorcism; instead, disease was the body itself, become diseased. Healing became the task of deciphering corporal space, a work of seeing instead of speaking. The model physician is Hippocrates, who applied himself only to observation, despising all preconceived systems that might bias the observer. This clinical gaze flourishes only in the relative silence of theories, imaginings, and whatever serves as an obstacle to the sensible immediate. In addition, when physicians question the patient, they question only what they can see—the body become diseased—and only in the language proposed by the body. All other languages, including that spoken by the patient, must fall silent before the absolute silence of observation. Within this double silence, Foucault says, things seen can be heard at last, and heard solely by the virtue of the fact that they are seen. It is in this sense that "the clinical gaze has the paradoxical ability to hear a language as soon as it perceives a spectacle" (p. 108).

The conversation that emerges from this double silence is an interior dialogue that the observer has with him- or herself, not a dialogue with the object of gaze. In the context of the physician-patient encounter, the language describing what the physician has seen gives structure to the encounter, not any language the patient might speak. The profundity of this silence derives from its absoluteness: Not only must the patient keep quiet about theories and imaginings that might relate to his or her illness, absolutely nothing the patient says can have any significance for the physician because no language can exist that has priority over the language of observation. This muting of the patient's own voice gives rise to what Foucault calls "the great myth of a pure Gaze that would be pure Language: a speaking eye" (p. 114). What it sees, it gathers and organizes; and as it sees, and sees more clearly, it speaks and teaches. The speaking eye becomes "the servant of things and the master of truth" (p. 115).

THE LANGUAGE OF CURING. Secretiveness, or what Foucault terms "esotericism," arises from this model for the physician-patient relationship because, as Foucault observes, one sees the visible (the true) only because one knows the language.

Unlike Molière's physicians, who spoke Latin merely in order not to be understood, Foucault's clinicians speak openly about that which anyone can see but only they can understand, because through the language of clinical description they have the means to see and hear at the same time, having access to a language that masters the visible. At this point, the earlier epistemological silence (Foucault's "double silence") that results from a constriction of perception changes into the silence of which Jay Katz speaks, a silence made even more baffling and profound by having as its vehicle a multitude of words that make every pretense of being understandable.

In effect, this model of medical perception insists that healing cannot be spoken or even thought of apart from the language of curing, that is, scientifically accurate diagnosis and treatment. This clinical perception and its promise of truth tend to overshadow all other claims to truth, reducing the promise to help those who suffer illness to the promise to be scientifically competent. Attempting to expand that visual horizon—particularly in the direction of the perspective of the patient—risks introducing an unacceptable noise into the silence of the medical clinic, an unwelcome and meaningless distraction from the work of curing.

Healing and Cultural Reality

Healing, of course, is a much broader cultural phenomenon than that encompassed by Western scientific medicine. Admittedly, the success of Western medicine at curing has helped justify its claim to be the model for healing in the world today. Yet, as Eric Cassell notes, "the success of medicine has created a strain: the doctor sees his role as the curer of disease and 'forgets' his role as healer of the sick, and patients wander disabled but without a culturally acceptable mantle of disease with which to clothe the nakedness of their pain" (Cassell, 1976, p. 51). This strain also appears in the way patients perceive their physicians. Western culture has conferred upon doctors the role of the care of the sick; but although doctors' role as the curers of disease is clear, their role as healers remains obscure. The latter role, Cassell adds, depends less on their ability to provide a scientifically accurate explanation of their patient's illness than to provide an explanation consistent with the culture of the patient. The reality that counts is cultural reality, and the system used by the healer or doctor need be accurate only in terms of the culture in which it is being used, for it serves to explain illness. The importance of the healer's explanation, Cassell insists, cannot be overemphasized.

THE HEALING RELATIONSHIP. As Cassell sees it, the healer's knowledge, imparted to the patient, helps move the world of illness from the unknown to the rational world. This knowledge allows the patient to "work on" the illness and to make an essential link between conscious process and body process that, Cassell says, marks the "educated" patient. Such healing is not cognitive alone. In addition to educating the patient, healers also play an active physical part in providing a link between symbolic reason and the body: They use their hands. Cassell calls this the "tenderness phenomenon," as important as education in the process of healing. He associates this phenomenon with parenting, and, in this sense, healers serve as parents. In addition to other aspects of the parental role, we transfer to them the right to lay hands on us, to be tender to us, and to pass through our territorial defenses.

The connectedness that underlies the tenderness phenomenon works in both directions. Healer and sufferer become exquisitely sensitive to one another; each can sense the feelings of the other. If healers can accept that the feelings they have can come from the patient, they can use their own feelings in the presence of the patient to provide a vital link with the patient's interior emotional state that is otherwise closed to the clinical observer. Cassell emphasizes that the ability of healers to establish this connectedness with the patient is not an exception to the role of healer but is rather an integral part of the healing function. It shatters the silence of which Katz writes, and substitutes for clinical detachment the "constant will of one trying to recognize" (Brody, 1992, p. 263).

Establishing this connectedness does not make of the healer a great person but does place both healer and patient in the presence of a deep human mystery that is greater than both of them. It is to be present at a creation that Elaine Scarry likens to the rediscovery of language: "Physical pain is not only itself resistant to language but also actively destroys language, deconstructing it into the pre-language of cries and groans. To hear those cries is to witness the shattering of language. Conversely, to be present when the person in pain rediscovers speech and so regains his powers of self-objectification is almost to be present at the birth, or rebirth, of language" (p. 172).

Explanation, education, and connectedness form the core of Cassell's understanding of the healing relationship. The problem with the scientific explanation of illness is not that it is incorrect, since, as Cassell notes, "we know that it need not be correct, since for most of the history of medicine it has not been correct" (1976, p. 128). Put differently, the virtue of scientifically accurate diagnosis and treatment does not lie in its correctness. The fact that it seems correct does not entitle it to stand as the only and sufficient explanation of illness. Although science has been empowered by Western

culture to dictate diagnosis and disease categories, Cassell notes that it has little or nothing to say about sick persons, their behavior, patient-healer communication, and so on. "If the whole point of the clinical encounter is to decide what is the right and the good thing to do for a specific patient, then traditional medical theory is sorely lacking" (1991, p. 6).

The Power of the Healer

Although he recognizes the limitations of traditional medical theory, Cassell does not intend to belittle or dismiss the role that the scientific explanation of disease has in Western culture or the promise it holds for the world. He wishes, in fact, to acknowledge its power: "The therapeutic power of the doctor-patient relationship grows in importance as the technology of cure becomes more powerful" (1991, p. 69). Yet, unfortunately, even as the importance of the relationship between doctor and patient grows under the stimulus of technology, so does the isolation of the patient, who becomes lost in a maze of tests, procedures, and treatment teams. To disregard this relationship only adds insult to the injury inflicted by isolation. "It has been one of the most basic errors of the modern era in medicine to believe that patients cured of their diseases—cancer removed, coronary arteries opened, infection resolved, walking again, talking again, or back home again—are also healed; are whole again" (1991, p. 69). What has been forgotten, he says, is that technology itself has no power—humans acquire power by employing the technology.

The importance of power in the therapeutic relationship has been explored at length by Howard Brody (1992). He analyzes the healer's power in three components: Aesculapian, charismatic, and social. The healer acquires Aesculapian power by virtue of training in the craft of healing. The power is impersonal, transferable to any other healer of comparable skill and experience. Charismatic power is founded on the healer's personal qualities and character and cannot be readily transferred. It is independent of the disciplinary knowledge and skill belonging to Aesculapian power. Social power arises from the social status of the healer within a particular society. It derives its authority in part from the implied contract between the healing profession and society that empowers the profession to determine truth in regard to illness.

The power to heal involves a complex interplay among all three kinds of power; it is a mistake, Brody notes, to limit the power of healing to Aesculapian power alone. Any discussion of what constitutes a right and good healing action must entail an exploration of the proper use of the other forms of power that the healer possesses. These forms of power risk what Brody calls "the dark side of the force."

This is "a lust, half childish, half sadistic, to use whatever power we might have to victimize others less powerful, and to enjoy it—to glory in the fact that they and not we are the victims, and to escape for a moment into the fantasy that since we can avoid their victimhood through our power, we are invulnerable and need never again feel fear" (Brody, 1992, p. 21).

THE VIRTUE OF COMPASSION. Healers can find the antidote to the dark side of the force by acknowledging the feelings of vulnerability and weakness that arise in them as they face the patient. They can do this only if they are open to the experience of being ill and in distress. To do this effectively, Brody says, healers need more than to be told they have an obligation to be open; they need to develop the virtue of compassion, an internalized habit of character that becomes an instinctive attitude of openness and vulnerability.

A major irony in the healer-patient relationship emerges here. To be compassionate in response to the suffering of the patient is itself a powerful act of healing. In showing compassion, the healer empowers the patient in a way that merely curing disease cannot. Curing disease eliminates a threat to bodily function and integrity; alleviating suffering, without which healing is a mere charade, restores the sufferer's connections with humanity and the ability to make sense of his or her own life. Yet, Brody says, this act of empowerment is possible only to the extent that the healer is willing to adopt a position of relative powerlessness, to acknowledge that the patient's suffering has incredible power over her or him and that it is impossible to remain unchanged in the face of it.

SHARED POWER. Western medical training urges compassion as a duty of the profession but at the same time warns, "Don't get too involved." Brody interprets this warning as a form of false reassurance that the power to heal does not entail the felt powerlessness of compassion. This denial of the power that the patient's suffering has over the physician is a rejection of the concept of shared power, which Brody states is the essential element in the ethical use of power. This denial also betrays a fundamental misperception of power as a zero sum game, that is, the belief that anything that increases the power of the patient within the healing relationship must necessarily decrease the healing power of the physician.

This *competitive* notion of power conforms to the type of moral reasoning that Carol Gilligan discovered among non-minority males in North American culture. The dominant male culture emphasizes the importance of finding the rules that govern a relationship and then selecting courses of action in keeping with the rules, even if such devotion to

rules means sacrificing someone's interests to the considerations of abstract justice (Gilligan). She counters with a type of moral reasoning common to the women she studied: They tend to focus on the nuances of personal relationships and seek solutions that protect the interests of all affected parties and that avoid bringing harm to anyone.

RESTRUCTURING THE POWER OF HEALING. Following the lead of Gilligan, other voices have appealed to an understanding of moral relationships from the perspective of women, such as Nel Noddings (1984), whose work on caring has influenced nursing ethics (Bishop and Scudder); and Virginia Warren (1989), who applies a feminist point of view to the conduct of medical ethics itself. Although these critics represent a wide range of opinion on the means to be used and even on the foundational reasons for doing so, most of them would agree with Susan Sherwin that there is a need to develop conceptual models for restructuring the power associated with healing and to clarify how "excessive dependence can be reduced, how caring can be offered without paternalism, and how health services can be obtained within a context worthy of trust" (p. 93). Sherwin notes with approval that, for many mainstream medical ethicists, compassion is frequently claimed to be more compelling than justice, a tendency she finds especially common in the contribution of physicians to medical ethics.

If this need for compassion is admitted, the significant question then becomes, What can allow a physician to experience the powerful suffering of a patient in a way that encourages the physician to share power and therefore to become not only a curer but also a healer? What is needed is a way for healers, and physicians in particular, to experience the felt reality of shared power without seeing it as a betrayal of their Aesculapian power, no matter how evident in this process its limitations may appear to become.

THE LIMITS OF AESCULAPIAN POWER. The strategy employed by many patient advocacy groups of leaving physicians' Aesculapian power undisturbed while severely restricting their social and charismatic power avoids the issue by ceding to physicians their chosen territory. Such an approach abandons the project of power sharing and attempts to render the healer-patient relationship "doctor-proof" by segregating Aesculapian power from the other forms of power. This strategy errs because it assumes that "we can wring morally acceptable actions out of any physician no matter how good or bad his motives if only we have the right rules for him to follow" (Brody, 1992, p. 55). As feminist critics have noted, this strategy endorses the *masculine* assumption that solving moral problems means discovering the right rules while leaving intact the existing power relationships. It cannot succeed because, as Brody points out, it mistakenly presumes that the healer's power comes in two neatly differentiated categories: power that helps fight illness, and power that can be used to violate patient's rights. But no such easy distinction is possible because the same powers can be easily redirected for good or ill.

The realization of shared power can take place only if those who profess to heal acknowledge responsibility for all the forms of power they possess. They must be reassured that owning up to their charismatic and social power does not imply that their Aesculapian power is fraudulent, although it may require them to admit that something like the placebo effect is present in almost every healing encounter (1992). For physicians to profess to heal requires the realization that their Aesculapian power, despite the warrant of its scientific accomplishments, is limited in both its scope and effectiveness. Curing does not ensure healing, and healing is possible even if there cannot be cure; nor is every human ill subject to cure. Such an admission, however, does not exempt those who profess to heal from attending to the needs of the poor, the oppressed, or those victimized by war, prejudice, and despotism. It only reminds them that their social and charismatic powers alone have authority in these difficult areas.

AESTHETIC DISTANCE. Compassion, lest it degenerate into codependency, does need to maintain a certain strength and thus a certain distance from the plight of the sufferer. Brody characterizes this distance as aesthetic rather than emotional; it resembles the reader's approach to a work of fiction (1992). To regard the suffering patient as a text, attended to at an aesthetic distance, still permits and even encourages intense emotional involvement. In reading the text presented by the sufferer, the healer must maintain in his or her imagination that separate vantage point from which the experience of the sufferer can be reinterpreted and reconnected to the broader context of culture and society.

Healing and Community

Healing reconnects the sufferer both to the self and to the world. The final and perhaps least appreciated aspect of healing is the need for this reconnection to take place in the context of a community, a need as real for the healer as it is for the sufferer. Healing requires from the healer a commitment over time to become a person capable of compassion and therefore of healing, who has the deep knowledge of how to fuse power and powerlessness, strength and vulnerability. This openness to vulnerability required of healers is more than a simple disposition to the notion of vulnerability. As Brody notes, there is a difference between being

"disposed" to something and striving over time to become something. It is the latter that is the mark of virtue.

In cultivating compassion as a professional virtue, healers must be willing to be formed by a compassionate community, "confident that they will receive empathic compassion and support from each other as they attend to the sufferings of their patients" (Brody, 1992, p. 267). In this arena, Brody ruefully notes, implicit issues of power have most stood in the way of the profession's reform. The self-imposed image of the physician as a powerful, scientific, objective individual, he says, works against the development of any effective peer support system. But it also cripples the physician's ability to be present to those in pain, which, as Stanley Hauerwas notes (1985), should be the goal of medical training.

For Hauerwas, "the physician's basic pledge is not to cure, but to share through being present to the one in pain" (p. 220). This pledge is difficult to carry out on a day-to-day basis. No individual has the resources to see so much pain without that pain hardening him or her. Pain, as Scarry notes, is destructive of human community; hence the prime directive of the healer to be present to those in pain carries with it an embodied threat to the ability to continue to be a healer. She or he must not only be formed as a healer by a compassionate community, but must also be continually sustained and nurtured by such a community—the kind of community, Hauerwas notes, that the Christian church claims to be.

There is a rich and varied tradition of healing not only within the Christian church but also in virtually every religious tradition. In fact, the role of healer in early societies encompassed not only the people's health but their entire welfare, including their spiritual welfare. The specialization that has accompanied modern civilization, however, makes discussion of the relationship between healing and religious belief problematic in that it is no longer clear who is priest, who is healer, and whose authority should predominate. The relation of medicine to particular religious traditions (Numbers and Amundsen) and the relevance of theological ideas, particularly that of covenant, to medical ethics (May) have opened up areas of fruitful exploration for both medicine and religion. But it may be well to concentrate, as Hauerwas does, not on these theoretical relationships but on the practical relation between communities, between those who practice religion and those who practice healing.

It is in this sense, Hauerwas says, that those who profess to heal need religion—not to provide miracles when there is a failure to cure, not even to supply a foundation for their moral commitments, but rather as a source of the habits and practices necessary to sustain them over the long haul as they care for those in pain. There needs to be a body of people who have learned the skills of presence to keep the world of the ill from becoming a separate world, both for the sake of the ill and for those who care for them. "Only a community that is pledged not to fear the stranger (and illness always makes us a stranger to ourselves and others) can welcome the continued presence of the ill in our midst" (Hauerwas, p. 223).

In the final analysis, healing is a communal action whose goal is the restoration not only of physical and mental wholeness to those who suffer illness but also of their integrity as persons, that is, as beings-in-relation to themselves and to other persons. It is a communal action in two senses: It reaches out to those isolated by illness to reconnect them to the human family; and it is sustainable only within a community that practices compassion as a virtue. The future of the healing professions everywhere depends as much on this nurture as on technical competence and the wise use of material resources. Those who profess to heal must know that no one is fully healed until all are healed.

J. PAT BROWDER
RICHARD VANCE (1995)
BIBLIOGRAPHY REVISED

SEE ALSO: *African Religions; Alternative Therapies; Body: Cultural and Religious Perspectives; Care; Christianity, Bioethics in; Compassionate Love; Daoism, Bioethics in; Disability; Grief and Bereavement; Health and Disease; Hinduism, Bioethics in; Human Dignity; Life, Quality of; Medicine, Art of; Narrative; Native American Religions, Bioethics in; Professional-Patient Relationship; Teams, Healthcare; Trust; Virtue and Character*

BIBLIOGRAPHY

Bishop, Anne H., and Scudder, John R., Jr. 1991. *Nursing: The Practice of Caring.* New York: National League for Nursing Press.

Bolton, Jonathan. 2000. "Trust and the Healing Encounter: An Examination of an Unorthodox Healing Performance." *Theoretical Medicine and Bioethics* 21(4): 305–319.

Brody, Howard. 1987. *Stories of Sickness.* New Haven, CT: Yale University Press.

Brody, Howard. 1992. *The Healer's Power.* New Haven, CT: Yale University Press.

Cassell, Eric J. 1976. *The Healer's Art: A New Approach to the Doctor-Patient Relationship.* New York: Penguin Books.

Cassell, Eric J. 1991. *The Nature of Suffering and the Goals of Medicine.* New York: Oxford University Press.

Cohen, Michael Howard. 2001. *Future Medicine: Ethical Dilemmas, Regulatory Challenges, and Therapeutic Pathways to Healthcare and Healing in Human Transformation.* Ann Arbor: University of Michigan Press.

Foucault, Michel. 1973. *The Birth of the Clinic: An Archaeology of Medical Perception,* tr. Alan M. Sheridan Smith. New York: Pantheon.

Gilligan, Carol. 1982. *In a Different Voice: Psychological Theory and Women's Development.* Cambridge, MA: Harvard University Press.

Grady, Christine. 1998. "Science in the Service of Healing." *Hastings Center Report* 28(6): 34–38.

Hauerwas, Stanley. 1985. "Salvation and Health: Why Medicine Needs the Church." In *Theology and Bioethics: Exploring the Foundations and Frontiers,* pp. 205–224, ed. Earl E. Shelp. Dordrecht, Netherlands: D. Reidel.

Ingelfinger, Franz J. 1976. "The Physician's Contribution to the Health System." *New England Journal of Medicine* 295(10): 565–566.

Kass, Leon R. 1985. *Toward a More Natural Science: Biology and Human Affairs.* New York: Free Press.

Katz, Jay. 1984. *The Silent World of Doctor and Patient.* New York: Free Press.

Kestenbaum, Victor. 1982. "Introduction: The Experience of Illness." In *The Humanity of the Ill: Phenomenological Perspectives,* pp. 3–38, ed. Victor Kestenbaum. Knoxville: University of Tennessee Press.

Laín Entralgo, Pedro. 1956. *Mind and Body: Psychosomatic Pathology: A Short History of the Evolution of Medical Thought,* tr. Aurelio M. Espinosa, Jr. New York: P. J. Kenedy & Sons.

May, William F. 1983. *The Physician's Covenant: Images of the Healer in Medical Ethics.* Philadelphia: Westminster.

May, William F. 2000. *The Physician's Covenant: Images of the Healer in Medical Ethics,* 2nd edition. Montville, NJ: Westminster Publishing House.

Moravcsik, Julius M. 2000. "Health, Healing, and Plato's Ethics." *Journal of Value Inquiry* 34(1): 7–26.

Noddings, Nel. 1984. *Caring: A Feminine Approach to Ethics and Moral Education.* Berkeley: University of California Press.

Numbers, Ronald L., and Amundsen, Darrell W., eds. 1986. *Caring and Curing: Health and Medicine in the Western Religious Traditions.* New York: Macmillan.

Ortega y Gasset, José. 1963. *Meditations on Quixote,* notes and intro. Julian Marais, tr. Evelyn Rugg and Diego Marin. New York: Norton.

Pellegrino, Edmund D. 1982. "Being Ill and Being Healed: Some Reflections on the Grounding of Medical Morality." In *The Humanity of the Ill: Phenomenological Perspectives,* pp. 157–166, ed. Victor Kestenbaum. Knoxville: University of Tennessee Press.

Pellegrino, Edmund D. 2001. "The Internal Morality of Clinical Medicine: A Paradigm for the Ethics of the Helping and Healing Professions." *Journal of Medicine and Philosophy* 26(6): 559–579.

Pellegrino, Edmund D., and Thomasma, David C. 1997. *Helping and Healing: Religious Commitment in Health Care.* Washington, D.C.: Georgetown University Press.

Pellegrino, Edmund D., and Thomasma, David C. 1997. *A Philosophical Basis of Medical Practice: Toward a Philosophy and Ethic of the Healing Professions.* New York: Oxford University Press.

Scarry, Elaine. 1985. *The Body in Pain: The Making and Unmaking of the World.* New York: Oxford University Press.

Sherwin, Susan. 1992. *No Longer Patient: Feminist Ethics and Health Care.* Philadelphia: Temple University Press.

Warren, Virginia L. 1989. "Feminist Directions in Medical Ethics." *Hypatia* 4(2): 73–89.

HEALTH AND DISEASE

• • •

I. History of the Concepts

II. Sociological Perspectives

III. Anthropological Perspectives

IV. Philosophical Perspectives

V. The Experience of Health and Illness

I. HISTORY OF THE CONCEPTS

Health and disease are among the fundamental experiences of human life. The concepts that people in various cultures have used in an attempt to understand and respond to those experiences have to do with the way humans relate to nature and culture. The concepts of health and disease have far-reaching consequences for diagnosis and therapy, the attitude and behavior of physicians, how patients deal with disease, social attitudes and structures, the shape of moral choices, and the cultural significance of sickness and wellness behaviors.

Health and disease are not merely medical terms; they are also vital themes in art, philosophy, theology, sociology, and psychology. In fact, these very disciplines remind medicine again and again of its distinctly *anthropological* character, in the sense that medicine deals with the nature and destiny of humans. Neither medicine nor the concepts of health and disease with which it deals can be properly understood by using the starkly contrasting categories of natural sciences and human sciences as a framework. Just as medicine cannot be reduced to either of the two, so it is also necessary to connect nature and culture in order to understand health and disease.

A universally valid definition of health has been as hard to formulate as a universally valid definition of disease.

Health and disease are physical, social, psychological, and spiritual phenomena that can be represented in concepts that are both descriptive and normative (the latter meaning based on norms), although these two sorts of concepts have not always been clearly distinguished in the historical development of these ideas. Humans not only determine what will be regarded as health and disease; at the same time they also interpret these experiences and decide how to respond to them.

Concepts of disease and health are especially important because they influence the manner and goal of medical treatment. Thus a mechanical or technologically structured understanding of disease (which views the human as a defective machine) requires a mechanical or technologically structured therapy (regarded as repair) and therapeutic relationship (a relationship of technician to defective machine). More personal or holistic concepts urge corresponding types of therapy and healer–patient relationships.

Contemporary medicine increasingly faces the task not only of overcoming sickness but also of preserving health. Prevention and rehabilitation play increasingly important roles alongside curative therapies. Treatment is understood to include attentive caring and support. Chronic suffering and death place different demands on the doctor–patient relationship than do acute illnesses. In light of such developments, concepts of health and disease require new definitions. A historical retrospective may assist in arriving at those definitions.

This entry does not attempt to offer a thorough cross-cultural analysis of concepts of health and disease; rather, it presents essential dimensions and changes in these concepts in the general course of history, their relationships with sociocultural backgrounds, and their practical and ethical consequences (Diepgen, Gruber, and Schadewaldt; Riese; Rothschuh; Schipperges, Seidler, and Unschuld; Temkin). A consideration of these historical developments can stimulate new reflections and initiatives, but history differs from any theoretical system. History has its own rules and logic. A progressionist explanation of the gradual development of notions of health and disease is inadequate. There are continuities and discontinuities, progress and regress, even within a single event or movement. This complex nature of history in general characterizes the history of medicine and specifically the history of the concepts of health and disease.

Health and disease suggest a variety of meanings from psychological, social, and spiritual perspectives. The word *illness* in the English language refers to the subjective or personal side of disease, whereas *disease* refers to the medical conception of pathological abnormality. It is possible for a person to feel ill without having a disease, and conversely, to have a disease without feeling ill. The term *sickness* transcends both of these concepts by focusing on social consequences. The concept of the *sick role* corresponds to the social nature of disease. The way in which societies vary in their interpretations of physical and mental disorders and in their treatment of and symbolic reactions to them reflects the cultural dimension of disease.

Nonetheless, some basic categories will be useful in the following discussion. One category is the explanation of disease, illness, and sickness. From a physical perspective, the different approaches of the past attribute disease to either liquid or solid components of the body or to the relationship between the body and the soul. Other distinctions refer to whether diseases should be regarded as existing entities (the ontological notion of disease) or as phenomena affecting individual persons in a variety of ways (the symptomatic notion of disease); and whether and to what extent the constitution and disposition of the individual (endogenous factors) and/or external (exogenous) factors play a significant role in determining health and disease.

A second category concerns response to disease, illness, and sickness. These responses have frequently been shaped by the explanation of disease, illness, and sickness. These two categories evolved into the science and clinical practice of medicine.

Primitive Peoples

There is no life without disease and pain; their ubiquitous nature is demonstrated by history. The skeletons of the first humans (500,000 B.C.E.) display bone disturbances and fractures. It is difficult to offer accurate descriptions of the health and disease of historically primitive peoples, because claims must depend on limited and problematic archaeological, paleopathological, and written sources (Clements).

At the dawn of human history, medicine had a magicomystical, demonic-religious character. Exogenous factors such as spirits, spells, and gods were considered responsible for disease. Personified living entities, spirits, took over a healthy body and made off with the soul of the person or allowed foreign elements to invade the body. Spirits, dead or living, could exercise fateful effects, acting out of revenge for breaches of taboos. Disease, directly related to sin and wrongdoing, represented not only an individual but also a social destiny. What befell one person befell the whole family, group, or tribe.

The diagnostic and healing powers of the healer or priest-doctor were supernatural. The healer had to be able to recognize which forces were at work in any given case. He did this by reading the stars or by drawing meaning from minerals, plants, and animals. Amulets and magic spells, oracles, atonement and confession, exorcism, bloodletting, and ceremonies of purification functioned as both preventive measures and cures. The whole community took part in the healing process; even pets were brought into it. Primitive peoples exhibited great cleanliness for the sake of prevention and strictly observed their cultural taboos.

There are remnants of these primitive notions of disease in today's lay language. For example, in English slang menstruation is sometimes called "the curse"; the German word for lumbago, *Hexenschuss,* means witch's wound. To what extent one can observe these assumptions about sickness and health, and the social structures that correspond to them, among the primitive peoples of today is hard to say. Modern civilization and medicine have left their impact in every part of the world. Primitive peoples, too, change over time.

Ancient Cultures

Precursors to medical systems and theories of disease were found in the ancient cultures of Mesopotamia and Egypt between the fourth millennium B.C.E. and the first, which established connections between concepts of nature and religion, on the one hand, and views of sickness and health on the other. Parallels between Chinese, Tibetan, Indian, and Greek perceptions of sickness and health indicate that these cultures may have derived these ideas from the same sources. Ancient American cultures also shared similar perceptions.

For these cultures health and disease were physical as well as religious phenomena. Sickness was still associated with sin, even as empirical interpretation of health and disease began to spread. Egyptian papyri (2000–1500 B.C.E.), for example, describe the courses of various diseases and categorize them according to regions of the body. The papyri list causes, symptoms, and prognoses, as well as empirical interventions. Putrefaction within the body in the form of spoiled material (*materia peccans*) caused sickness; these substances had to be removed if the patient were to be cured. The Greek historian Herodotus (fifth century B.C.E.) describes monthly purifications in Egypt.

Dietetic, medicinal, and surgical interventions were used, and much attention was given to public health. The medicine of ancient cultures combined religious ritual with empirical treatment. The Babylonian code of Hammurabi (d. 1750 B.C.E.) contained the first list of surgical fees and penalties in the case of failure; each varied according to the social status of the patient.

The explanatory dimensions of medicine, such as symptomology, nosology (the classification of diseases), diagnosis, and etiology (the study of the causes of diseases), as well as clinical dimensions such as prognosis, therapy, and prevention, began to establish themselves in these centuries. The traditional healer became the professional doctor; specialization developed. In this era, empirical observation, causal explanation, magic, and faith coexisted in medical theory and practice.

Greece and Rome

More extensive and reliable historical sources exist for ancient Greece and Rome. The ancient Greeks (500 B.C.E.) explained health and disease cosmologically and anthropologically, that is, in close relation to nature in general and to human nature in particular. Medicine sought not only to cure disease but also to maintain health. The pre-Socratic philosophers, who were the physicians of this time, developed a universal model of health, whose outlines can be found in the medical texts of Hippocrates (c. 460–c. 377 B.C.E.) and other physicians of the Corpus Hippocraticum (400 B.C.E.–200 C.E.). These pre-Socratic physicians must be distinguished from magicoreligious healers, who still existed at that time (Kudlien).

The great physician Galen (129–c. 199 C.E.) elaborated a model of health and disease as a structure of elements, qualities, humors, organs, temperaments, times of day, and times of year (Schöner). Health was understood in this perspective to be a condition of harmony or balance (*isonomia*) among these basic components that make up both nature in general and the individual body. Disease, on the other hand, was regarded as discordance, or the inappropriate dominance (*monarchia*) of one of the basic components. Disease in the perspective of humoral (pathology determined by bodily fluids) was interpreted as the disproportion (*dyscrasia*) of bodily fluids or humors: phlegm, blood, and yellow and black bile. Solidistic pathology traced disease to disturbances among the solid components of the body (shape, consistency, distance, etc.). The pneumapathological (spirit) approach attributed disease to a failed relationship between body and soul. Health (*eucrasia*) was characterized by equilibrium in the body.

Dietetics was considered of primary importance to the therapeutic process, followed by medication and lastly by surgery, a hierarchy exactly opposite to the prevailing Western approach of today. In the ancient perspective, dietetics involved much more than a health-conscious regulation of food and drink. Rather, it entailed a broad concept of how one should live a healthy life. Dietetics was concerned with six aspects of life that, although natural, did not regulate themselves, as did such physiological functions as respiration and digestion. Because they required human manipulation, these six aspects of life were called "non-natural" (*sex res non naturales*). These areas included how humans deal with:

1. air and light;
2. food and drink;
3. sleep;
4. motion and rest;
5. secretions; and
6. passions of the mind (Rather).

According to Galen, and in contrast to contemporary views, health and sickness were not the only states of existence. Rather, there was a third condition, an intermediate state of *neutrality* that existed between health and sickness: Medicine was therefore conceived as the science of health, sickness, and neutrality. In this notion of medicine, the overcoming of sickness was secondary to the preservation of good health or to aiding patients in living with impediments and handicaps. Galen said that because health precedes illness both in time and in esteem, one should try first to preserve health and only second to cure the illness as far as possible.

Philosophy and medicine mutually influenced one another in antiquity, although Hippocrates is said to have separated medicine from philosophy. Health and disease are not only empirical descriptions. They always have philosophical implications and practical effects. The Greek philosopher Plato (c. 428–c. 348 B.C.E.) defined medicine as the theory of health, and in the perspective of his ethical concept of health, he legitimized the active euthanasia of the physically handicapped and the mentally ill. Plato and his student Aristotle (384–322 B.C.E.) developed a typology of three physicians with corresponding types of relationships with the patient. The *slave doctor* commands, and the patient has to obey. The *doctor for freemen* explains the treatment to the patient and the patient's family. Doctors understood to be *medically educated laymen* signified individuals who take responsibility for their own health, sickness, and death.

While abortion and active euthanasia were forbidden as therapeutic acts for the Hippocratic physician, the Stoics justified these practices in situations in which the patient had lost or was in danger of losing moral autonomy and rational awareness. Harmony of the mind was placed above health and disease, above wealth and poverty. For the Stoic philosopher Seneca (c. 4 B.C.E.–65 C.E.), disease meant physical pain (*dolor corporis*), the suspension of joy (*intermissio voluptatum*), and the fear of death (*metus mortis*)—implying that disease combines physical, psychological, social, and mental dimensions. While being persecuted by the Roman emperor Nero, Seneca ended his own life through active euthanasia with the help of his friend and doctor Statius Annaeus.

The Middle Ages

The Christian Middle Ages (500–1300) interpreted health and sickness in a theological perspective. Cosmological (or natural) and anthropological (or human) approaches were subordinated to, without being supplanted by, the supernatural notion of transcendence. Christian beliefs and natural causes for health and disease were not mutually exclusive. Sicknesses could be described simultaneously as physical entities and as acts of God's intervention. The Christian, Arabic, and Jewish traditions all viewed health or *quality of life* as the outcome of a good relationship with God.

Medicine consisted of theory and practice, each of which was further divided. Medical practice consisted of dietetics, medicaments (therapeutic substances), and surgery. Galen's humoral pathology prevailed throughout the Middle Ages, and dietetics in antiquity's broad sense of the term continued to function as the most important form of treatment. The emphasis on spirituality did not run counter to medical aid and health education. As the vessel of the soul, the body warranted careful attention.

During the Middle Ages, a variety of specific health rules (*Regimina sanitatis*) were developed for people of various ages, occupations, and classes, as well as for both sexes. One famous example, the *Regimen Sanitatis Salernitanum* from the thirteenth century, has survived in various medical customs and was published in all major European languages.

According to the medieval Christian viewpoint, the figure of Christ as healer (*Christus medicus*) stood behind every doctor, and behind every patient was the figure of the suffering Christ. Health, disease, and healing gained their meaning from this perspective. These concepts were related intimately to the idea of salvation history (eschatology), seen as a progression of the world starting with its establishment in paradise (*constitutio*), through its earthly existence (*destitutio*), and finally to resurrection (*restitutio*).

These concepts also had their practical consequences, manifested in biographies and other documents of arts and literature. Each transition from health to sickness and from sickness to health represented this eschatological process on an individual level. Even though sickness, suffering, and death had salvific significance or were essential traits of human life, they were fought with dietetics and medical therapy. But they were also to be accepted, because earthly life is different from paradise. In this regard, Saint Augustine (354–430) remarked that people have to say "yes" to some forms of pain but are not forced to love them.

The Greco-Roman link between health, beauty, and morality was abandoned during the Middle Ages. Every sick, suffering, or handicapped individual had the right to receive medical treatment. Hospitals, first founded during the Middle Ages, were open to all suffering and helpless people, based on Jesus' words: "I was sick, and you cared for me" (Matthew 25: 26). At the same time, however, the Bible was used to justify excluding lepers from society.

The classical and Christian concept of the seven cardinal virtues (prudence, temperance, fortitude, justice, faith, hope, and love) applied to healthy people as well as to the sick, doctors, and the community. Suicide and euthanasia were regarded as sins because they were deliberate attempts to shorten life. Therefore the ancient Hippocratic oath was continuously accepted in this epoch. The art of dying (*ars moriendi*) was considered a central part of the art of living (*ars vivendi*). Sickness could be traced to inherited sin, personal guilt, demonic possession, or a test from God. Job of the Old Testament represented a classic example of the latter.

In contrast to present-day attitudes, health was also viewed as negative in the moral and religious sense ("corrupting health": *sanitas perniciosa*) and sickness as positive ("a healing sickness": *infirmitas salubris*). Coping with illness was believed to manifest a person's fortitude; furthermore, a life without physical or psychical damage or pain was thought to produce a false image of earthly life and the human condition. A contemporary biographer, writing about the constant illness of the saintly German abbess Hildegard of Bingen (1098–1179), who was also a prominent naturalist and physician, said that her whole life could be compared to a "precious dying."

The Modern Era

With the coming of the modern era at the time of the Renaissance, which began in the fourteenth century, an emphasis on this world, nature, and the individual replaced the medieval focus on the hereafter. The secularization of paradise—or the hope of realizing beauty, youth, and health in an earthly life—has influenced human thought and action and the course of medicine up to the present. Empirical observation, causal explanation, and rational therapy became the ideals of education, research, and practice in medicine. Nevertheless, magic, astrology, and alchemy continued to play a role in medicine for quite some time.

At the transition from the Middle Ages to the modern era, the German physician and philosopher Paracelsus

(1493–1541) designed an all-encompassing system of medicine. Along with philosophy, astronomy, and alchemy, ethics acquired a fundamental role. Paracelsus replaced the ancient humoral pathology with three rudiments from alchemy: salt, mercury, and sulfur. Dominance of one of these biochemical components over the others led to different types of diseases. Disturbances in the spiritual principle also led to disease. According to Paracelsus, the general factors that contributed to disease belonged to nature as well as culture: (1) cosmic influences (*ens astorum*); (2) material influences (*ens veneni*); and (3) individual constitution (*ens naturale*), spirit (*ens spirituale*), and God (*ens Dei*). Paracelsus's concept of disease is ontological or essentialistic: Disease is a "thing," which he compared with a parasite, a separate organism. This notion contrasts with the Hippocratic concept, which explained sickness as an individual, symptomatic phenomenon.

The utopian writings of the English statesman Thomas More (1478–1535), the English philosopher Francis Bacon (1561–1626), and the Italian philosopher Tommaso Campanella (1568–1639) include basic categories for determining health and disease as well as guiding principles for eugenic public health policies. Their concepts justified suicide and euthanasia—but only under the condition that it be done freely (at the decision of the individual). During the Renaissance the different types of euthanasia, still relevant in the discussions of the subject today, were already established. Not everyone supported active euthanasia as a social reaction to sickness. The German theologian Johann Valentin Andreae (1586–1654), unlike More and Bacon, expressly rejected euthanasia in his 1619 work *Christianopolis.* He stated that "reason commands that human society should be more gently disposed toward those who have been less kindly treated by nature" (p. 274).

The philosophy of the French mathematician René Descartes (1596–1650), with its mechanical model of health and disease, became highly important for the concepts of disease and therapy. According to Descartes, the body is a perfect clockwork mechanism set in motion by God to function mechanically. The soul, also divinely created, acts independently from the body. This dualistic system of body (*res extensa*) and soul (*res cogitans*) was widely accepted in medicine and produced a mechanistic view of physiology, still accepted in the present, that also existed in lay interpretations of health and disease. Scientific explanation concerned the discovery of the fixed rules of mechanistic structures and their processes. Clinical medicine concerned the detection of damaged structure, malfunction, and departure from these rules, and the restoration of proper anatomic structures and physiology.

During the Enlightenment (eighteenth century), the real beginnings of a public health movement began to take shape. The German philosopher Gottfried Wilhelm Leibniz (1646–1716) made numerous recommendations for public health. The American statesman and philosopher Benjamin Franklin (1706–1790) formulated a characteristic phrase of the time: "Health is wealth." The German physician Johann Peter Frank (1745–1821) and the French philosopher Jean-Jacques Rousseau (1712–1778) represented the opposition between state policies and individual agendas. According to Rousseau, civilization and the state had ruined human health in its natural state. Frank, in contrast, believed that social reforms lead to progress. Several books were published primarily on prevention and rehabilitation. The German physician Christoph Wilhelm Hufeland (1762–1836), author of the widely distributed *Makrobiotik* (1797), manifested again the relationship between concepts of health, disease and therapy —especially as normative categories— with the social attitudes and reactions. He believed that physicians should not be allowed to engage in active euthanasia, pointing out that physicians who start to decide which sick persons are worthy of living become "the most dangerous people in the state."

The concepts of health and disease vacillate between anatomy and physiology. The definitions of disease and health of the Scottish physician John Brown (1735–1788) received great recognition in the medicine, philosophy, and literature of his time. His 1780 work *Elementa Medicinae* defined health and disease in terms of the relationship of opposing forces within a person: of organic excitability and external and internal stimuli, resulting in an excited or irritated condition of the organism. According to Brown, disease is the result of overstimulation (*sthenie*) or insufficient stimulation (*asthenie*). Health, on the other hand, is characterized by equilibrium between the capacity to be stimulated and internal and external stimuli. Treatment, therefore, functioned either to strengthen or subdue stimuli. Bloodletting and diet calmed a condition of overstimulation, whereas ether, camphor, and opium had the opposite effect. Equally important for the further progress of medicine was the anatomical foundation of pathology by the Italian physician Giovanni Battista Morgagni (1682–1771) with his fundamental work *De sedibus et causis morborum* (On the seats and causes of disease), published in 1761.

Romanticism and idealism, around 1800, introduced interpretations of health, disease, and death that are of general importance and transcend substantially the limits of medicine (Leibbrand). These three states were regarded as dialectically connected with one another and interpreted as the main stages of the genesis of Spirit out of nature, a

Hegelian theme (von Engelhardt). According to the German poet Friedrich von Hardenberg (1772–1801), who wrote under the pseudonym Novalis, there is always disease in health and health in disease; illness or sickness is given a central value: "Medicine should be an elementary science of every cultivated person" (Novalis, p. 474). Illness can be an experience or medium of personal growth. The personhood of the patient becomes a central claim: "Human being = person; that is the point of unity," (Heinroth, p. 158) categorically announced the german physician Johann Heinroth (1773–1843). The German philosopher Joseph Schelling (1775–1854) held that health is the harmonious relationship of the basic organic functions of sensibility, irritability, and reproduction. The German philosopher Georg Hegel (1770–1831) argued that life would be impossible without disease, that each organism contains the "germ of death" from birth, and that all therapy presupposes that disease is not a total loss of health but rather a conflict within physical or psychical forces. Only through disease and death of the individual does the universal and eternal world of the spirit come into being. "Above this death of Nature, from this dead husk, proceeds a more beautiful Nature, proceeds Spirit" (Hegel, p. 443).

MEDICINE AND THE NATURAL SCIENCES. Medicine in the remainder of the nineteenth century followed the model of the natural sciences and not that of natural philosophy and philosophical anthropology of the romantic-idealistic era. This increasingly self-conscious scientific medicine concentrated on curing disease and neglected the maintenance of good health. It also neglected the contributions of the arts, literature, and theology. The patient became more and more an object. The patient's subjectivity or personality was disregarded, and the history of the patient was reduced to the history of the disease. Anatomy and physiology were connected; the cell replaced tissue as the center of attention. Experimentation, statistics, and causal thinking became the basis for medical research. A Cartesian concern for mechanistic structure and function according to discernible rules became paramount.

The German pathologist Rudolf Virchow's (1821–1902) definition of disease was widely accepted: "Disease begins at that moment when the regulatory system of the body is not sufficient to overcome a disturbance. It is not life under abnormal circumstances, nor the disturbance as such which produces a disease, rather the disease begins with the insufficiency of regulatory mechanism" (p. 193). According to Virchow, the body's regulatory ability varied from person to person. The healthy body is capable of bringing an abnormal situation back into equilibrium. Disease was an observable phenomenon in the living body, caused by internal and external factors. The cell became the basis of disease, and—using a political metaphor—it deserves recognition, along with blood and nerves, as the "third estate." The infection of cells, and thus the body, by external infectious agents became the dominant explanation of disease. The clinical response was to eradicate the infection.

In the nineteenth century, dietetics lost its broader or anthropological meaning and came to refer simply to the intake of food and drink. Thus a 2,000-year-old tradition, already limited in the eighteenth century, reached its end. Nevertheless, the tradition of dietetics survived longer in the area of hygiene than in pathology. Scientific medicine in its modern form considered heredity, psychical, and social factors relatively unimportant to the etiology of disease. Infection was the decisive explanatory factor; therapeutic results from the period substantiated this theory. Thus, the development of concepts of health and disease and of clinical responses to them was synergistic, a historical process that continues into the present.

At the beginning of the twentieth century, constitutional pathology and anthropological medicine began to counteract the one-sided approach of infectious disease modules of medicine. Medicine recovered the importance of the individual and social circumstances in health and disease—constitutional pathology on the physical level, anthropological medicine on the psychical or mental level. Human beings were conceived as participating in nature as well as in culture. The German physician Viktor von Weizsäcker (1886–1957) reintroduced in his anthropological medicine "the person as subject," in regard to the patient, the doctor, and science.

In medicine as well as in biology, the concept of finality (*causa finalis*) regained attention; diseases not only have a physical cause (*causa efficiens*) but also manifest a sense of meaning. The controversy between monocausal thinking (*causalism*) and multifactorial thinking (*conditionalism*) influenced medicine during those decades around 1900 and is still lively: Can disease be deduced from one cause, or is it necessary to take different causes of different areas of reality into consideration? The concept of cause not only has consequences for the theory of disease origin and disease process but also affects medical therapy, prevention, and rehabilitation, all of which in turn shape the individual and social situation of the sick person.

Philosophers and theologians, as well as writers and artists, hoping to give people assistance that the natural sciences and medicine were unable to provide, continued to produce valuable interpretations of health and disease that took the spiritual or cultural nature of human experience into account, calling into question the established normative equation of health as positive and disease as negative. The French writer Marcel Proust (1871–1922) stated that humankind owes its major cultural accomplishments to sick and suffering people: "They alone founded religions and created masterpieces" (p. 405). Increasingly, arts and literature have been acknowledged as being helpful in coping with disease, pain, and death.

The German philosopher Martin Heidegger (1889–1976) claimed that he wrote his analysis of death in *Being and Time* (1927) especially for doctors; in this work, Heidegger emphasized that only the human beings have the consciousness of death and of their own death. The German physician and philosopher Karl Jaspers (1883–1969) defined disease and health in the perspective of his philosophical position. Neurosis being "a failure in the marginal situations (*Grenzsituationen*) of life," he visualized the goal of its therapy "as a self-realisation or as a self-transformation of the individual through the marginal situation, in which he is revealed to himself and affirms himself in the world as it is" (p. 275). Jaspers contended that psychiatry shared two major methodologies: that of "explanation," which characterizes the natural sciences (disease), and that of "understanding," which is typical of the human sciences (illness). The ethical and practical consequence of his concept of disease in the objective, subjective, and cultural sense is outlined in his concept of the existential communication between the physician and the patient. Existential communication combines the subjective and cultural dimensions in an ethical perspective.

In the twentieth century, psychology and sociology expanded the scientific understanding of health and disease, emphasizing the difference between *disease* as objective and physical, and *illness* and *sickness* as subjective and social. According to this general perspective, contemporary people associate disease with the following interpretations: challenge, enemy, punishment, weakness, relief, strategy, loss or damage, and value (Lipowski). Medicine concentrates on weakness, loss, and damage, that is, the physical components of this model.

In the sociological perspective the role of the sick person is characterized by:

1. freedom from daily duties,
2. freedom from the responsibility for the sick condition,
3. the obligation to want to become well again, and
4. the obligation to seek medical help (Parsons; Schaefer).

Descriptive and normative aspects permeate this sociological definition of the role of the sick person. Disease is not only described in its social causes and consequences; demands and expectations are formulated. Subsequent studies have revealed further processes of different levels (age, sex, socioeconomic state, type of disease, etc.) of defining a person as sick. Also important are the differentiation between "bad" and "ill," or criminal behavior and sickness, and the negative or stigmatizing consequences of diagnostic acts.

The 1947 World Health Organization (WHO) definition of health—"a state of complete physical, mental, and social wellbeing and not merely the absence of disease or infirmity"—has to be interpreted in its social and political context and purposes. These included attempts to justify international involvement in the internal affairs of countries. It is another matter whether medicine can offer explanations and therapies to achieve *complete,* multifunctional wellbeing, the definition of which includes social and spiritual as well as medical aspects. The WHO definition was used as the starting point for intense bioethical debates on the moral and political responsibilities of the international community in regard to healthcare—especially for corresponding projects in developing countries. But this definition, taken generally, is limited in its sharp contrast between health and disease and its exaggerated estimation of health. With good reason, health can also be regarded as the ability to bear injury, handicaps, and the anticipation of death, and to successfully integrate these abilities into one's life. Integration is the capacity to cope with death; death is a part of life and not only its contrary or end.

Conclusion

The history of concepts of health and disease is the history of concepts that explain and direct response to disease, illness, sickness, and health. These concepts are deeply rooted in physical and psychical experiences and have medical and social consequences. The importance of scientific explanations, with their roots in Cartesian medicine and developments in the nineteenth century, is obvious. Of equal importance, perhaps, are attempts to counterbalance an excessive emphasis on scientific medicine with anthropologic, social, ethical, and political dimensions of the concepts of health and disease. After all, for much of its history medicine has not been confined solely to disease but also took responsibility for health. Therapy in the past meant more than just curing; it also meant prevention or preservation of health and assistance in chronic disease and in dying. Disease was interpreted as a disturbance of the organism, the sick person, and his or her social situation. Furthermore, medicine did not have sole domain over health and disease; a multitude of important interpretations originated from the arts, theology, and philosophy. In this holistic perspective, people of the present also expect medical and social aid.

Sickness and health, in their natural and cultural breadth, remind medicine of its fundamentally scientific and humanistic nature. Health and disease are concerned with life and death and are closely connected to the physical, social, psychic, and spiritual nature of humans.

Today, disease and health are conceived as more closely connected (Canguilhem; Engel). The transitions and parallels are seen more strongly, and the interplay of the body, soul, spirit, and environment is more carefully observed. Attention is shifting from infectious diseases to chronic illness and death, though the experience of acquired immunodeficiency syndrome (AIDS) and other diseases prove the continuity of those events. The emergence of molecular medicine, with its reliance on genetic concepts of health and disease, may lead to a reintegration of the scientific and humanistic dimensions of the concepts of health and disease. The global scientific and economic limitations of medicine have made the concepts of health and disease a central topic in theory as well as in practice, for science as well as for everyday life.

Developing countries have special problems to overcome that stem from their own cultural changes and from their reception of Western medicine. The Western world must be critical of its own normative position in regard to these developing countries as in regard to its own concept of life. Disease should not be understood merely as a limitation or a loss, but also as a challenge. Coping with illness can manifest courage and compassion; meeting this challenge strengthens self-confidence, causes social reform, and enriches the world of culture.

DIETRICH VON ENGELHARDT (1995)
REVISED BY AUTHOR

SEE ALSO: *Addiction and Dependence; Aging and the Aged: Anti-Aging Interventions, Ethical and Social Issues; Alcoholism; Anthropology and Bioethics; Biology, Philosophy of; Consensus, Role and Authority of; Dementia; Emotions; Feminism; Genetics and Human Self-Understanding; Homosexuality; Insanity and Insanity Defense; Mental Illness; Metaphor and Analogy; Transhumanism and Posthumanism;* and other *Health and Disease* subentries

BIBLIOGRAPHY

Andreae, Johann Valentin. 1916. *Christianopolis,* ed. and tr. Felix Emil Held. New York: Oxford University Press.

Antonovsky, Aaron. 1987. *Unraveling the Mystery of Health.* San Francisco: Jossey-Bass.

Canguilhem, Georges. 1984. *Le normal et le pathologique,* 5th edition. Paris: Presses Universitaires de France.

Clements, Forest Edward. 1932. "Primitive Concepts of Disease." *American Archeology and Ethnology* 32(2): 185–243.

Diepgen, Paul; Gruber, George B.; and Schadewaldt, Hans. 1969. "Der Krankheitsbegriff, seine Geschichte und Problematik." In *Handbuch der Allgemeinen Pathologie,* vol. 1, ed. Franz Büchner. Berlin: Springer-Verlag.

Engel, George L. 1960. "A Unified Concept of Health and Disease." *Perspectives in Biology and Medicine* 3(4): 459–485.

Engelhardt, Dietrich von. 1984. "Der metaphysische Krankheitsbegriff des Deutschen Idealismus: Schellings und Hegels naturphilosophische Grundlegung." In *Medizinische Anthropologie,* ed. Eduard Seidler. Berlin: Springer-Verlag.

Hegel, Georg Wilhelm Friedrich. 1970. *Hegel's Philosophy of Nature,* tr. Arnold Vincent Miller. Oxford: Clarendon Press.

Heinroth, Johann Christian August. 1844. "An Heinrich Damerow, 1842." *Allgemeine Zeitschrift f'r Psychiatrie* 1:158.

Jaspers, Karl. 1973. "Die Begriffe Gesundheit und Krankheit." In *Allgemeine Psychopathologie,* 9th edition. Berlin: Springer-Verlag.

Kudlien, Fridolf. 1968. "Early Greek Primitive Medicine." *Clio Medica* 3(4): 305–336.

Leibbrand, Werner. 1956. *Die spekulative Medizin der Romantik.* Hamburg: Classen.

Lipowski, Zbigniew Jerzy. 1970. "Physical Illness, the Individual, and the Coping Processes." *Psychiatry in Medicine* 1(2): 91–102.

Novalis [Friedrich von Hardenberg]. 1981. *Schriften,* vol. 3. Darmstadt, Germany: Wissenschaftliche Buchgesellschaft.

Parsons, Talcott. 1973. "Definition von Gesundheit und Krankheit im Lichte der Wertbegriffe und der sozialen Struktur Amerikas." In *Der Kranke in der modernen Gesellschaft,* 4th edition, ed. Alexander Mitscherlich, Tobias Brocher, Otto von Merin, and Klaus Horn. Cologne: Kiepenheuer and Witsch.

Proust, Marcel. 1975. *Auf der Suche nach der verlorenen Zeit.* Frankfurt: Suhrkamp.

Rather, Lelland J. 1968. "The 'Six Things Non-Natural': A Note on the Origins and Fate of a Doctrine and Phrase." *Clio Medica* 3(4): 337–347.

Riese, Walther. 1953. *The Conception of Disease: Its History, Its Versions, and Its Nature.* New York: Philosophical Library.

Rotberg, Robert I., ed. 2000. *Health and Disease in Human History.* Cambridge: MIT Press.

Rothschuh, Karl Eduard, ed. 1975. *Was ist Krankheit? Erscheinung, Erklärung, Sinngebung.* Darmstadt, Germany: Wissenschaftliche Buchgesellschaft.

Schaefer, Hans. 1976. "Der Krankheitsbegriff." In *Handbuch der Sozialmedizin,* ed. Maria Blohmke, Christian von Ferber, Karl Peter Kisker, and Hans Schaefer. Stuttgart, Germany: Erike.

Schipperges, Heinrich; Seidler, Eduard; and Unschuld, U. Paul, eds. 1978. *Krankheit, Heilkunst, Heilung.* Freiburg, Germany: Alber.

Schöner, Erich. 1964. *Das Viererschema der antiken Humoral-pathologie.* Wiesbaden, Germany: Steiner.

Stempsey, William E., 1999. *Disease and Diagnosis.* Dordrecht: Kluwer.

Temkin, Owsei. 1973. "Health and Disease." In *Dictionary of the History of Ideas,* vol. 2, ed. Philip P. Wiener. New York: Scribners.

Virchow, Rudolf. 1869. "Über die heutige Stellung der Pathologie." *Tageblatt der 43. Versammlung deutscher Naturforscher und Ärzte,* 185–195.

Weizsäcker, Viktor von. 1951. *Der kranke Mensch: Einführung in die medizinische Anthropologie.* Stuttgart, Germany: Koehler.

II. SOCIOLOGICAL PERSPECTIVES

The sociology of health and disease has two distinct traditions, each with somewhat different implications for the field of bioethics. The first tradition is socioepidemiologic in nature, which is to say it focuses on understanding how the distribution of death and illness is influenced by such factors as age, gender, race, and social class. The second tradition is oriented to the doctor-patient relationship and is concerned with the meanings of illness for patients and practitioners, and with how these meanings reflect the nature of power and authority in society.

The Social Epidemiology of Illness

ORIGINS. Sociological perspectives on health and disease can be traced to the French sociologist Emile Durkheim's classic treatise, *Suicide* (1951). In this work, Durkheim examined the impact on the suicide rate of such variables as residence (urban or rural), marital status, and religious affiliation. Durkheim's basic assumption was that if suicide were purely an individual phenomenon, these variables would have no impact on group rates. Using public health statistics, Durkheim determined that the suicide rate was higher among urban dwellers than among those who lived in rural areas, that the rate of the unmarried exceeded that of the married, and that of Protestants exceeded that of Catholics. He theorized that social ties linking individuals to society inhibit suicidal impulses, while the absence of such ties does not. Much subsequent socioepidemiology of illness echoes Durkheim's findings that those with a greater stake in society fare better than those with a lesser stake.

Since Durkheim published this work, sociologists have dedicated themselves to showing that who becomes ill is not just a matter of individual constitutions, but is heavily influenced by the standard variables of sociological explanation; namely gender, race, and class. While the proposition that one's social position predicts one's health status is generally accepted, attention is also now being paid to the pathways that explain this phenomenon. Bruce Link and Jo Phelan, for example, argue that individually based risk factors need to be contextualized in order to consider what puts people at risk, and that social factors, such as socioeconomic status, are fundamental causes of disease because their association with disease remains constant even when intervening factors change.

GENDER. Despite their greater life expectancies, women report more morbidity and utilize health services more frequently than do men (Verbrugge). Explanations advanced for the higher rates of illness among women include less satisfying social and economic roles; greater stress; more cultural permission for reporting discomfort; and biological differences.

CLASS. The relationship between class and mortality and morbidity is well documented. At all age levels in the United States, there is an inverse relationship between morbidity and social class (Syme and Berkman). This means that as class standing increases, the prevalence of illness decreases, and vice versa. Similar relationships have been demonstrated for other countries in the industrialized West. There is also evidence that the association between socioeconomic status (SES) and health exists at all levels of the SES hierarchy (Adler, et al.). It has been argued that socioeconomic status is a key factor in the creation of disparities in health, and that the reduction of health disparities will rely on addressing the components of SES, particularly income, education, and occupation (Adler and Newman).

Although the link between social class and the prevalence of illness is not disputed, the reasons for it are. A number of explanations have been advanced to account for this relationship, including lack of access to healthcare resources; lifestyle (there is an inverse relationship between obesity, as well as tobacco and alcohol consumption, and social class); and increased exposure to economic and social stress. Work has been indicted as a causal factor in the relationship between social class and heart disease (Siegrist, et al.; Marmot and Theorell). Lower-class jobs provide less autonomy, more constraint, and less opportunity for expression than middle-class occupations. In addition, the causal direction of the link between class and illness has been questioned, with some analysts suggesting that since the less well are unable to compete in the economic system, they have their class standing lowered as a result. This is known as the *downward drift hypothesis.* There is some evidence to suggest that inequality itself, independent of income, is detrimental to health, and not only to those who have fewer resources but also to those with higher SES (Kawachi and Kennedy).

RACE. Race is another variable that affects mortality and morbidity. Vincente Navarro argues that once class is taken into account, differentials between whites and blacks disappear. This may be so, but at a pragmatic level there is a very real association of health status with urban poverty and race. This association accounts for morbidity and mortality associated with violence, infant mortality, and HIV infection associated with intravenous drug use and prostitution. The problems of the urban poor in gaining access to healthcare services have also been well documented. Compliance with treatment regimens is also an issue for inner-city populations, with the most common explanation being the cultural distance between providers and patients.

STRESS AND DISADVANTAGE. Stress has been used as a variable to explain relationships among gender, social class, race, and illness. While the "fundamental cause" concept (Link and Phelan) attempts to expand the causal pathways studied between SES and health, the "stress theory" specifies one particular aspect of the relationship between social position and health. Persons of lower SES experience more stressful environments, such as economic strain and insecure employment (Brunner), and these stressors influence susceptibility to disease by impacting (among other things) the nervous and immune systems. Stress seems to better account for variations in rates of mental, rather than physical, illness (Lin and Ensel). Despite the widespread agreement on how to measure it, there is confusion about what *stress* is. There is also widespread agreement that social supports and networks buffer stress, but there is some confusion about how (Kessler, et al.). Moreover, stress does not have an equal impact on men and women. Marriage, for example, buffers stress better for men than for women.

ELIMINATING HEALTH DISPARITIES. Having demonstrated that health disparities often follow the contours of social disadvantage, a great deal of work has been focused on how to specify the causal pathways of this disadvantage, with the goal of eliminating disparities in health. This has led to disagreement about what the causal pathways to health differentials are, and about the ways in which efforts to reduce disparities can reach the intended beneficiaries without widening the very gap they are intended to close. Medical innovations and public-policy interventions to reduce disparities are often introduced and carried out in a context of inequality (Mechanic), and it has been argued that targeting facets of socioeconomic status, such as a living wage, may go furthest in reducing health disparities (Link and Phelan; Adler and Newman).

Social Epidemiology and Bioethics

The social epidemiology of illness demonstrates that sickness does not fall equally upon rich and poor, men and women, or upon black and white. Distributional inequities are more than simple political and economic problems—they have an ethical dimension as well.

Bioethicists need to pay greater attention to issues of justice and equity at a political level; that is, to the ethical dimensions of political decisions. As the allocation of scarce resources becomes a public issue of greater salience, the underserved will need advocates. The championing of individual patient rights that marked bedside bioethics in its formative years needs to be extended to the class of uninsured and underinsured patients as healthcare grows in importance on the national political agenda.

As its scope of inquiry expands, bioethics may have the opportunity to play a greater role in policy making. However, there is a danger here as well. So long as bioethics is focused on the bedside, both the subject matter and the texts appropriate to it are limited. Once the links between class, race, gender, and illness are illuminated, the boundaries of bioethics become murky. The doctor-patient relationship may be fraught with moral complexity, but it is a rather neatly defined, bounded whole. This is not so for the entire distributive system of society.

The Social Construction of Illness

The second tradition in the sociology of illness is less concerned with the distribution of illness by race, class, and gender, and more concerned with the social meanings attached to illness. It is more concerned with the roles of provider and patient, and with what these roles say about the distribution of power and authority in society. The social epidemiological tradition is involved in the analysis of large data sets (such as national samples) to determine statistical correlations between health status and social traits such as gender, class, and race. The social-constructionist approach is more likely to involve firsthand observation of behavior in a limited number of settings. These observations of behavior provide a basis for drawing conclusions about the nature of healthcare more generally. Favored themes in the social-constructionist approach include the management of uncertainty, the difficulties of lay-professional communication, and the use and misuse of professional authority.

THE SICK ROLE. Sociological speculation about the nature of the doctor-patient relationship begins with Talcott Parsons's discussion of the "sick role" (1951). Although Parsons's unique insight is so commonplace today that we do not appreciate its originality, he was among the first to focus on the doctor-patient dyad as a role relationship with a set of reciprocal rights, duties, and obligations.

Parsons begins with a discussion of the basic social situation in which patients and physicians find themselves. Patients are: (1) not to blame for their condition, (2) powerless, and (3) technically incompetent. Physicians' existential position is one beset with uncertainty about what ails the patient and how best to treat it. In addition, they are unable to cure many of the ills of patients, and there are difficulties with access to both patients' bodies and the intimate details of their lives.

Each role consists of four interlocking imperatives that grow out of the social assumptions made about each actor. The sick patient is granted a temporary exemption from normal social responsibilities. In exchange for this exemption, the patient must seek technically competent help, must be motivated to get well, and must comply with treatment regimens. The passivity of the patient stems from what has been called the "power asymmetry," which Parsons says characterizes the relation of doctor and patient. The only positive action Parsons ascribes to the patient is to seek help. By making this a role obligation, Parsons ignores the complexities of help-seeking behaviors. Such complexities include the recognition of a condition as *illness,* of the cultural and economic barriers to access, and of the nature of lay networks. In addition, with his stricture on technically competent help, Parsons invalidates any and all alternatives to allopathic medicine.

Physicians, according to Parsons, occupy roles whose demands are dictated by their existential situation. First, physicians achieve their roles by mastering basic areas of knowledge. Some physicians are smarter than others, and some know more, but all have completed the same core medical curriculum. Parsons calls this "universal achievement." Second, physicians limit their ministrations to areas of competence. They are expert in areas of health and illness, and their advice is limited to these areas. Parsons identifies this as "functional specificity." The limits of functional specificity have widened as the links between lifestyle, stress, and illness have been documented. Nonetheless, there are limits. Physicians maintain an attitude of affective neutrality. Renee Fox and Harold Lief identify this as "detached concern." Physicians are involved with the problems of their patients, but not so involved as to interfere with rational decision-making. Finally, physicians act from a stance that

Parsons identifies as "collective neutrality." The physician is not guided by self-interest or the profit motive. Rather, physicians' actions are guided by altruism, by what will restore health, whatever the sacrifice or cost to the physician, patient, or collectivity.

Parsons's analysis describes normative patterns rather than empirical occurrences. His physicians live in a world in which they share values with patients and always act in the best interests of the patient. They also act as agents of social control. The physician provides legitimate excuses from work, directs treatment, and controls access to healing resources. Tension may arise because the interests of the social system and of the patient may not coincide.

THE SOCIAL CONSTRUCTION OF ILLNESS. Parsons's "sick role" is the first sociological theory to recognize that the experience of illness is determined by social factors. Many sociologists accept Parsons's basic insights but differ with him on how the experience of illness is shaped by values and beliefs that are implicit, tacit, unexamined, and variable across cultural groupings. Conflict theorists, for example, emphasize that society is made up of competing groups with different values, rather than, as Parsons argued, cooperating groups with shared values (Freidson). For these sociologists, the physician's role as a fiduciary whose actions express the interests of patients is disputed; the physician is seen instead as a *moral entrepreneur* who cloaks self-interest or the interests of his or her social class in a neutral scientific language.

Conflict, or *labeling,* theorists share with Parsons the understanding that physicians act as agents of social control but they differ about who benefits from these gatekeeping activities and what the consequences of these activities are. For Parsons, the physician's actions certifying illness serve the entire society by promoting an environment in which the individual designated as *sick* can later return to productive social and economic roles. There are no long-term consequences to the labeling of individuals.

Labeling theorists contend that labeling is used by the dominant classes to protect their interests, suppress the less fortunate, and reinforce established hierarchies (Becker; Freidson). Casting an individual in the sick role stigmatizes him or her and spoils life chances (Goffman; Scheff). Susan Sontag has argued that the vocabulary of illness leads those who are sick to blame themselves. Those who are vulnerable to labeling engage in a variety of social strategies to avoid it. Peter Conrad and Joseph Schneider have described how those with epilepsy, for example, attempt to stay "in the closet" with their condition rather than suffer the discrimination that attends candor.

Much of the work of labeling theorists depends on the contention that the locus of social control in the modern state has shifted. Conrad and Schneider observe that explanations of deviance now rely on "madness" instead of "badness." The dominant agents of social control are no longer clergy, but physicians. Social problems become medicalized, and the targets of therapeutic activity are more likely than not to be the socially disadvantaged. Jane Mercer, for example, found that the label *mentally retarded* was significantly more likely to be applied to members of minority populations.

In labeling theory a key variable of interest is social power. Labels are used to depress the social chances of the disadvantaged are also manipulated to aid the powerful. New categories of pathology emerge that create opportunities for healthcare professionals who use newly discovered syndromes to expand their power, while the social and structural conditions that generate problems remain, or become, invisible. For example, Stephen Pfohl views the discovery of the "battered-child syndrome" as a boon to pediatric radiologists and other pediatric professionals. The beating of children is not new, however, but its treatment as a medical problem is novel. Entire diagnostic classification systems may be viewed this way. Joel Kovel has criticized the American Psychiatric Association's *Diagnostic and Statistical Manual of Mental Disorders* (DSM-III; now replaced by the DSM-IV), the official diagnostic system of mental health professionals, for hiding social and political meanings in apparently neutral language. The purpose of the DSM, in this view, is to enable the psychiatric profession to control the institutions of mental health.

Individuals may actively seek some labels and avoid others. Tsunetsugu Munkata points out that in Japan the label *neurasthenia* is widely adopted to avoid the stigmatizing term *schizophrenia,* while Peter Conrad has shown how both parents and school professionals embrace the label of *hyperkinesis* to describe unruly children. Parents accepted the label because it absolved them of blame for their children's conditions; school officials accepted the term because it offered an individual-level explanation for restive behavior, allowing them to overlook deficiencies in school organization. Many illness designations signify entities whose precise, objective markers of disease are unclear. Sufferers, however, seek the legitimation of the disease label. Suffering is a powerful determinant of self-labeling, as the proper label serves to excuse and explain behavior that would otherwise be unacceptable. The early labeling theorists concentrated on labeling as a top-down phenomenon, stressing the repressive features of labels while ignoring the benefits some labels conferred.

The fact that the powerful resist—as well as discover, create, or construct—disease classification should also not be overlooked. Phil Brown and Edward Mikkelsen describe how the inherently conservative bias of epidemiological methods that depend on population-based measures retarded the identification of an environmentally generated cancer cluster in Woburn, Massachusetts. In another case, scientific medicine and organized mining interests retarded the recognition of "black lung" as an occupational disease (Smith). Both cases illustrate how the alliance of organized science with corporate interests can burden and delay successful efforts to discover or construct disease or the cause of disease.

Social Construction and Bioethics

Two key points of contention distinguish Parsons's theory of the sick role from labeling theory. The first is whether physicians have patients' interests reliably at heart. Parsons, in claiming that physicians have a "collectivity orientation," signals his confidence that they do. For labeling theorists, however, claims of altruism are utilized to cloak self-interest. This difference in attitude is very apparent in the writing from each orientation on the role uncertainty plays in medicine. From a Parsonian orientation, uncertainty is a problem to be overcome and a psychological burden to physicians (Fox, 1959). From a labeling orientation, uncertainty is a ploy that physicians magnify in order to control patients (Davis).

The second key difference between Parsons and the labeling theorists concerns patient autonomy. For Parsons, the only autonomous decision made by the patient is the one to seek care. After that, patients simply, and appropriately, follow the doctor's orders. Since the physician has the patient's best interest in mind, there is no reason for the patient to balk or to question. For labeling theorists, there is no reason for the patient to follow medical regimes without question, since there is no guarantee that the physician has the patient's best interest in mind.

Informed consent is based on the principles of autonomy and self-determination. Sociological description of the doctor-patient relationship, whether from Parsons or from the labeling theorists, illuminates the absence of autonomy and self-determination. Sociologists differ on the necessity and value of such principles.

The earliest sociological studies of death and dying (those of Barney Glaser and Anselm Strauss, published in 1965) described the extent to which autonomy and self-determination were missing in the doctor-patient relationship. Physicians operated in what Glaser and Strauss called a "closed awareness context." Physicians knew of fatal conditions but routinely did not pass this information on to patients, and they often colluded with family members to keep this information from patients. These practices were rationalized as kinder than being candid.

Because of informed consent, a veritable revolution occurred in the doctor-patient relationship. Candor replaced evasion. With informed consent, patients are more than ever the masters of their own treatment. The paternalism that marked Parsons's description of the doctor-patient relationship has given way to a more egalitarian, more formally contractual, relationship. While there is much to celebrate in these changes, something may have been lost. There are costs involved with a fuller patient autonomy. Under the banner of autonomy, physicians may hide behind their role as technical experts and leave weighty matters to patients. There are also new possibilities for the psychological abandonment of patients.

CHARLES L. BOSK (1995)
REVISED BY CHARLES L. BOSK
JACQUELINE HART

SEE ALSO: *Alternative Therapies; Anthropology and Bioethics; Bioethics, African-American Perspectives; Body; Eugenics: Historical Aspects; Feminism; Insanity and the Insanity Defense; Lifestyles and Public Health; Medicine, Sociology of; Mental Illness; Race and Racism; Sexual Identity; Women, Historical and Cross-Cultural Perspectives;* and other *Health and Disease* subentries

BIBLIOGRAPHY

Adler, Nancy E.; Boyce, Thomas; Chesney, Margaret A.; et al. 1994. "Socioeconomic Status and Health: The Challenge of the Gradient." *American Psychologist* 49(1): 15–24.

Adler, Nancy E., and Newman, Katherine. 2002. "Socioeconomic Disparities in Health: Pathways and Policies." *Health Affairs* 21(March/April): 60–76.

Bartley, Mel; Blane, David; and Davey, George, eds. 1998. *The Sociology of Health Inequalities.* Sociology of Health and Illness Monograph Series. Oxford: Blackwell.

Becker, Howard S. 1963. *Outsiders: Studies in the Sociology of Deviance.* New York: Free Press.

Brown, Phil, and Mikkelsen, Edward. 1990. *No Safe Place: Toxic Waste, Leukemia, and Community Action.* Berkeley: University of California Press.

Brunner, E. 1997. "Stress and the Biology of Inequality." *British Medical Journal* May 17: 1472–1476.

Conrad, Peter J. 1975. "The Discovery of Hyperkinesis: Notes on the Medicalization of Deviant Behavior." *Social Problems* 23(1): 12–21.

Conrad, Peter J., and Schneider, Joseph W. 1980. *Deviance and Medicalization: From Badness to Sickness.* St. Louis, MO: Mosby.

Cooper, Cary L., and Marshall, Judi. 1979. "Occupational Sources of Stress: A Review of the Literature Relating to Coronary Heart Disease and Mental Ill Health." *Journal of Occupational Psychology* 49(1): 11–28.

Davis, Fred. 1960. "Uncertainty in Medical Prognosis: Clinical and Functional." *American Journal of Sociology* 66(1): 41–47.

Durkheim, Emile. 1951 (1897). *Suicide: A Study in Sociology.* New York: Free Press.

Fox, Renée C. 1959. *Experiment Perilous: Physicians and Patients Facing the Unknown.* Glencoe, IL: Free Press.

Fox, Renée C., and Lief, Harold I. 1963. "Training for Detached Concern in Medical Students." In *The Psychological Basis of Medical Practice,* ed. Harold I. Lief, Victor Lief, and Nina Lief. New York: Harper & Row.

Freidson, Eliot. 1970. *The Profession of Medicine: A Study in the Sociology of Applied Knowledge.* New York: Harper & Row.

Glaser, Barney G., and Strauss, Anselm L. 1965. *Awareness of Dying.* Chicago: Aldine.

Goffman, Erving. 1963. *Stigma: Notes on the Management of Spoiled Identity.* Englewood Cliffs, NJ: Prentice Hall.

Kawachi, Ichiro, and Kennedy, Bruce P. 2002. *The Health of Nations: Why Inequality is Harmful to Your Health.* New York: New Press.

Kessler, Ronald C.; Price, Richard H.; and Wortman, Camille B. 1985. "Social Factors in Psychopathology: Stress, Social Support, and Coping Processes." *Annual Review of Psychology* 36: 531–572.

Kovel, Joel. 1988. "A Critique of the DSM-III." *Research in Law, Deviance, and Social Control* 9: 127–146.

Lin, Nan, and Ensel, Walter M. 1989. "Life Stress and Health: Stressors and Resources." *American Sociological Review* 54(3): 382–399.

Link, Bruce, and Phelan, Jo. 1995. "Social Conditions as Fundamental Causes of Disease." *Journal of Health and Social Behavior* 37(special issue): 1–26.

Link, Bruce G.; Northridge, Mary E.; Phelan, Jo C.; and Ganz, Michael L. 1998. "Social Epidemiology and the Fundamental Cause Concept: On the Structuring of Effective Cancer Screens by Socioeconomic Status." *Milbank Quarterly,* Special Issue: *Socioeconomic Differences in Health* 76(3): 375–402.

Marmot, Michael, and Theorell, Tores. 1988. "Social Class and Cardiovascular Disease: The Contribution of Work." *International Journal of Health Services* 18(4): 659–674.

Mechanic, David. 2002. "Disadvantage, Inequality, and Social Policy." *Health Affairs* 21 (March/April): 48–59.

Mercer, Jane R. 1973. *Labeling the Mentally Retarded: Clinical and Social System Perspectives on Mental Retardation.* Berkeley: University of California Press.

Munkata, Tsunetsugu. 1989. "The Socio-Cultural Significance of the Diagnostic Label 'Neurasthenia' in Japan's Mental

Health Care System." *Culture, Medicine, and Psychiatry* 13(2): 203–213.

Navarro, Vincente. 1991. "Race or Class or Race and Class: Growing Mortality Differentials in the United States." *International Journal of Health Services* 21(2): 229–235.

Parsons, Talcott. 1951. *The Social System.* New York: Free Press.

Pfohl, Stephen J. 1977. "The 'Discovery' of Child Abuse." *Social Problems* 24(3): 310–323.

Ross, Catherine E., and Mirowsky, John. 2000. "Does Medical Insurance Contribute to Socioeconomic Differentials in Health?" *Milbank Quarterly* 78(2): 291–321.

Rothman, David J. 1991. *Strangers at the Bedside: A History of How Law and Bioethics Transformed Medical Decision Making.* New York: Basic Books.

Scheff, Thomas J. 1966. *Being Mentally Ill: A Sociological Theory.* Chicago: Aldine.

Schneider, Joseph W., and Conrad, Peter J. 1980. "In the Closet with Illness: Epilepsy, Stigma Potential, and Information Control." *Social Problems* 28(1): 32–44.

Siegrist, Johannes; Siegrist, Karin; and Weber, Ingbert. 1986. "Sociological Concepts in the Etiology of Chronic Disease: The Case of Ischemic Heart Disease." *Social Science and Medicine* 22(2): 247–253.

Smith, Barbara. 1981. "Black Lung: The Social Production of Disease." *International Journal of Health Services* 11(3): 343–359.

"Socioeconomic Differences in Health." 1998. *Milbank Quarterly* (special issue) 76(3).

Sontag, Susan. 1978. *Illness as Metaphor.* New York: Farrar, Straus & Giroux.

Syme, S. Leonard, and Berkman, Lisa F. 1976. "Social Class, Susceptibility and Sickness." *American Journal of Epidemiology* 104(1): 1–8.

Thoits, Peggy A. 1985. "Self-Labeling Processes in Mental Illness: The Role of Emotional Deviance." *American Journal of Sociology* 91(2): 221–242.

Verbrugge, Lois M. 1989. "The Twain Meet: Empirical Explanations of Sex Differences in Health and Mortality." *Journal of Health and Social Behavior* 30(3): 282–304.

III. ANTHROPOLOGICAL PERSPECTIVES

Medical anthropologists focus on people's life worlds (the subjective experience or phenomenology of sickness and healing), their cultural systems of meaning (e.g., ideas about what causes disease and how it is diagnosed), and the material conditions in which experiences and beliefs are situated (e.g., local disease ecology). Medical anthropologists attempt to understand and describe the medical beliefs and practices of people whose cultures and life worlds are often very different from their own. They routinely are confronted with the problem of translating unfamiliar meanings and experiences into familiar (Western) terms and concepts without taking them out of context or subordinating them to Western assumptions about sickness, health, efficacy, autonomy, and the like (Lock and Gordon; Kleinman, 1988; Gaines).

The anthropological perspective makes it possible to examine and clarify bioethical issues from multiple cultural points of view. The current debate over the bioethics of organ harvesting—the surgical removal of transplantable body parts such as the heart, liver, and kidneys—illustrates why it is important to have a clear understanding of cultural points of view. For transplantation to succeed, organs must be removed either (1) from a living donor in cases in which the organ is not vital to the donor's survival (e.g., a single kidney) or (2) immediately after a donor's death, before the organs have begun to decompose.

In most Western societies the line between life and death in the context of organ harvesting is identified with brain death, the irreversible loss of higher brain functions. The decision to identify death with brain death is consistent with Western cultural notions: Selfhood is identified with the mind, and the mind is by convention situated in the brain. This arrangement has the practical advantage of leaving a working heart in a harvestable body, facilitating the collection of transplantable organs. Japanese culture, in contrast, recognizes a different relationship between selfhood and the body: The self is not identified with a single body region. From this perspective a brain-dead body with a functioning heart has not crossed the line from life to death and is not yet a harvestable resource (Lock, 2002). Clearly, cultural definitions of selfhood and personhood have a profound impact on people's responses to bioethical issues.

Orientations to the Body

The history of medical anthropology is to a large extent a history of scrutinizing and challenging Western assumptions about sickness, beginning with the distinction between biomedicine and traditional medicine. (Most medical anthropologists prefer the term *biomedicine* to the alternative terminology: *scientific, modern,* and *Western* medicine. For an explanation see Leslie.) At first glance the distinction appears to be a commonsense way to classify different kinds of medical systems; in practice it rests on a set of problematic assumptions.

First, it implies that *traditional* medical systems have something fundamental in common, whereas in reality so-called traditional systems are highly diverse in both their medical theories and their practices and share little as a category other than being different from biomedicine (Leslie and Young). Second, juxtaposing traditional medical systems with biomedicine implies that biomedicine is a monolithic system, beyond the reach of culture. However, social scientists have demonstrated significant variation in biomedical notions, technologies, and clinical practices both within communities and across cultures (Brodwin, 2000; Hahn and Gaines; Lindenbaum and Lock; Lock, 1993; Lock, Young, and Cambrosio). Third, comparing biomedicine to other medical systems also sets biomedicine as the standard of medical care because it is based on scientific principles; this conveys the idea that other medical systems are not as *real* or therapeutically effective.

A more useful way to compare medical systems across cultures is to start with the question, How do the beliefs and practices of a medical system orient healers and patients to their bodies? An answer from the Western perspective might be that because the body is the site of the pain and suffering associated with sickness, the body must be the focus of attention for patients and healers everywhere. In reality, medical systems are not equally interested in the body. Rather, those systems and their perspectives are distributed along a continuum that includes the biomedical perspective among many others.

At one end of the continuum are systems whose orientation to the body can be called externalizing in that their diagnostic and therapeutic ideas and techniques direct people's attention away from the sufferer's body. In those systems the medical gaze looks outward, scanning networks of people and beings (e.g., ancestral spirits, possession spirits, demons) for morally significant encounters and events involving the sick person or that person's close relatives. The diagnostic goal is to construct a useful etiology, that is, a string of circumstances and events that lead to the onset of suffering and distress and identify the ultimate source of the sickness. The therapist's goal in those systems is to insert himself or herself into the patient's sickness narrative and, once there, persuade or coerce the pathogenic agents to stop afflicting the patient. The classic account of diagnosis and treatment in an externalizing system is E. E. Evans-Pritchard's *Witchcraft, Oracles, and Magic among the Azande* (1937).

A sick person's body is a site of discomfort and distress, and in this sense sickness is the same all along the continuum. At the externalizing end, however, the patient's bodily experiences and transformations are mute. Typically, the body is a black box in that although people may have names for certain body parts and organs, they can posit no functions or systemic connections for them. Pain, suffering, and the visible transformations that accompany sickness and disease signify only themselves; they reveal nothing about processes and events that biomedicine recognizes are taking place inside. Although practitioners may give patients medicaments to take, those medicines are characteristically anodynes or substances that are intended to make the patient more comfortable while the actual cure is being pursued elsewhere. In short, in externalizing systems medical meanings and experiences are created and connected by discrete socio-logics rather than by a universal bio-logic (Lock and Gordon).

Anthropologists describe three broad types of therapeutic strategies that operate in externalizing medical belief systems: agonistic strategies, in which the goal is to eliminate or neutralize pathogenic agents; initiatory strategies, in which the goal is to bring the patient and the pathogenic agent into a permanent and manageable relationship (Boddy); and strategies of persuasion, in which the goal is to persuade the pathogenic agent through offerings or appeals to cease afflicting the patient (Lewis). Beyond these generalizations, externalizing systems are highly heterogeneous.

Biomedicine is at the opposite end of the continuum, among the internalizing systems, in which diagnosis and therapy orient patients and healers toward the body. Here sickness coincides with the limits of the body, and the goal of diagnosis and therapy is to get inside the body, to take control of its internal parts and processes. Circumstances and events outside the body are interesting only to the degree to which they lead to inferences about pathological processes taking place inside. It is in these systems that one finds theories of pathophysiology, the grammars that enable people to read bodily changes symptomatically.

Medical Efficacy

Common sense inclines people to suppose that because internalizing systems are able to read embodied symptoms, they are more empirical and realistic than externalizing systems are. Ethnographic research, however, indicates that all medical systems, externalizing as well as internalizing, are generally empirical and realistic. That is, they are capable of routinely producing self-vindicating outcomes, evidence that demonstrates their efficacy.

Medical efficacy can be demonstrated by two different kinds of results. First, efficacy is sometimes a capacity for producing hoped-for results, such as the amelioration of pain or the remission of symptoms. In practice it is not difficult for externalizing and internalizing systems to produce hoped-for results in light of the fact that the majority of medical problems consist of either (1) transient or recurrent symptoms that are perceived as being discrete disorders or (2) self-limiting diseases, episodes that end in either spontaneous remissions or death. In these circumstances medical practices acquire a reputation for hoped-for efficacy when three conditions are met: An intervention routine occurs between onset and outcome, remissions predominate over deaths and other unwanted outcomes, and superior alternative interventions are absent or inaccessible.

Second, efficacy can take the form of producing expected results. This occurs when practices and procedures are able to produce evidence that affirms the line of reasoning and the underlying assumptions that persuade patients and practitioners to select particular interventions. Expected results can be produced without also producing hoped-for results. Thus there is the grim joke that the operation succeeded but the patient died: The patient's body, once opened up, reveals a pathology that affirms the correctness of the assumptions and choices that have led from diagnosis to surgery, but the intervention is unsuccessful because of circumstances beyond the clinician's control. All medical systems, whether internalizing or externalizing, appear capable of distinguishing between hoped-for results and expected results.

In addition, serious sickness is a source of distressing feelings that are only incidentally connected to the pain and suffering of a sick person. Medical practices may have the effect of reducing such distress by connecting sickness events to local systems of moral and cosmological meaning. This power to give meaning to and impose moral order on chaotic and threatening events may be sufficient to perpetuate certain medical practices even when those practices have no great reputation for producing cures. Those practices sometimes are called healing rituals by anthropologists.

The Mind-Body Problem

One of the current debates in biomedicine surrounds the mind-body problem, which has arisen from the observation that sickness is simultaneously an objective phenomenon and a subjective phenomenon. In the language of the social sciences the objective (or bodily) component is called *disease,* and refers to abnormalities and dysfunctions in organs and organ systems. The subjective component is called *illness,* and refers to the patient's unique and holistic experience of either disease-related distress or certain other socially disvalued states, such as psychogenic mental disorders, that conventionally are bracketed together with diseases. Disease can occur in the absence of illness, as in the case of undiagnosed and asymptomatic hypertension, and illness can occur without disease, as in adjustment disorder and somatization disorder.

Anthropologists have critiqued the mind-body distinction in two ways. The first critique calls for a reconceptualization of the relationship between mind and body. The argument is that people need to free themselves from the

objective-subjective comparison and take account of the continuous interaction between mind and body: the capacity of the mind to affect bodily states positively and negatively, the mind's predilection for using bodily states as idioms of distress, and so on (see Csordas).

The second and more radical critique refers back to anthropology's task of translating unfamiliar meanings and experiences into intelligible concepts without subordinating them to Western assumptions about sickness, healing, and agency. Both Western culture and biomedicine assume the existence of a mind situated in the brain. In practice, the mind is one of the Western ways of talking about the self: the body's seat of consciousness, the subject of its experiences, the initiator of the body's purposeful actions, the repository of its memories, and the locus of moral agency. To anthropologists the Western mind/self is a cultural artifact; it exists because people have practices that make it exist in the same way that possession spirits exist in the Sudanese *zar* cult. Indeed, there are many cultures and systems of medicine that are *mindless* in the sense that they have no corresponding network of mental and moral meanings, and they constitute people and experiences in fundamentally different ways. Thus, the mind-body distinction has been criticized not because there is a need for more effective concepts for connecting psyche (mind) to soma (body) but because the notion of mind itself and the practices through which that notion emerges subordinate non-Western cultures and realities to a distinctively Western ontology (Good and Kleinman; Kleinman, 1988).

Patterns of Resort

The idea that in any community an individual's medical behavior is congruent with a unitary set of meanings concerning sickness and its causes, diagnosis, and treatment is an obstacle to translating medical realities between cultures. Anthropologists make a series of distinctions between medical traditions, sectors, and systems so that they compare cultural norms of medical behavior:

1. A medical tradition is a set of practices and technologies organized around historically situated ideas about etiology, symptomatology, and treatment. Biomedicine, Ayurvedic medicine, and the zar cult are examples of medical traditions. Traditions are simultaneously vocabularies for interpreting the world and plans of action and technologies for producing facts that confirm their interpretations of the world.

2. The actual forms a tradition takes in a specific community make up its medical sector. A particular medical tradition can be put into action in various ways. It can be used to justify a range of practices,

technologies, and routines, and it can be adapted to a variety of institutional settings. For example, in many less developed countries the biomedical tradition is practiced in four sectors: licensed professionals (physicians, nurses, etc.), fee-for-service injectionists (who inject clients with substances from the biomedical pharmacopeia), pharmacists (who can diagnose symptoms as well as prescribe treatments), and domestic settings (where the biomedical tradition is employed mainly to diagnose problems). Although the four sectors share a single tradition, they include different sets of options. In the first sector clinicians monopolize diagnosis and treatment choices and decide which etiologies will be tested and confirmed and which sets of cultural meanings and socioeconomic implications will be realized through these practices. Injectionists and pharmacists represent patron-dominated sectors of biomedicine in the sense that patients or members of their families make their diagnoses before consulting the practitioner. Practitioners may be asked for alternative diagnoses, but the ultimate decision is the patient's.

3. A medical system is equivalent to the collection of traditions and sectors that are available to the people in a particular community. Medical beliefs and practices are useful to patients and their families because those people know how to incorporate them into patterns of resort. These are the paths that people create in the course of actual sickness episodes as they navigate their way from one medical sector to another, picking and choosing from among their options.

The ethnographic literature suggests two main patterns of resort. In the first the patient or a surrogate simultaneously consults alternative traditions. People have various motives for following this strategy. In some cases patients believe that the effects of multiple interventions are cumulative; in other cases they are unsure which, if any, of the available traditions will provide an effective cure. In some communities, notably in southern Asia, the simultaneous pattern of resort reflects a therapeutic division of labor. Biomedicine is prized for its quick effects against causal agents such as microbes and its ability to treat symptoms such as high fevers. The Ayurvedic tradition is valued for its ability to counter the perceived side effects of biomedicines, especially antibiotics, and its ability to restore an equilibrium among the body's organs and humors, that is, the state synonymous with health. The alternative strategy consists of a sequential pattern of resort in which the individual exhausts the resources of a tradition or sector before moving on to an alternative tradition in the medical system (Young, 1983).

The paths that individuals follow through their medical systems are determined by a variety of factors. For example, patients who want to avoid stigmatizing etiologies (ones that would contaminate or spoil an individual's social identity) or diagnoses with a poor prognosis are likely to compare the range of diagnoses and etiologies that belong to the various traditions in their medical system and then start off with the tradition that offers the most favorable outcomes. The choice may be influenced by cost-benefit calculations. That is, a practitioner's or sector's economic and geographic accessibility are weighed against the perceived seriousness of the patient's sickness and the value of the patient to his or her family (Nichter).

Implications for Bioethics

Why is it important for bioethics to understand that health, illness, and disease are socially shaped, culturally constructed, and historically situated? Basically, those ethnomedical beliefs and values inform people's health-related behavior. More specifically, culture shapes the ways in which people make decisions in the context of morally charged healthcare situations. Culture also shapes the kinds of ethical situations that can arise in a particular healthcare or healing setting and the frameworks for understanding and models for responding to those ethical dilemmas. Anthropology's cross-cultural or comparative perspective, combined with ethnographic methodological approaches, helps people (1) recognize that moral norms vary cross-culturally and (2) challenge tacitly held cultural assumptions in biomedicine and bioethics about what counts as human, self and other, normal and abnormal, life and death, right and wrong, and other key moral concepts (Marshall and Koenig, 1996, 2001; Haimes).

Anthropological investigation into contemporary debates about bioethics raises new questions, provides insights into the ways in which people experience ethical issues, and broadens the scope of inquiry. Anthropological research on genetics, for example, shows that women's decisions to undergo prenatal genetic testing are informed by cultural definitions of risk, perceived acceptable forms of disability, and social dynamics between women and genetics counselors (Browner et al.; Rapp). These factors may come as a surprise to bioethicists, who may expect attitudes toward abortion to take a primary role in women's prenatal decisions. With regard to examining the genetic basis of medical conditions such as Alzheimer's disease and sickle-cell anemia among African Americans, anthropologists have been at the forefront in pointing out the problems with using the term *race*. For instance, using that term risks perpetuating essentialism about clinical phenomena. They also have identified how notions of heredity hinge on cultural ideas of kinship and the implications of genetics research for defining claims to group identity (Koenig and Silverberg; Brodwin, 2002; Gordon; Wailoo, 1997).

The ability to explicitly recognize the cultural basis of bioethical constructs, such as the concept of autonomy, can help bioethics scholars rethink the premises of moral arguments. Furthermore, by recognizing that medical systems maintain their own logic, bioethicists and biomedical practitioners are more likely to attempt to understand patients rather than label them as irrational or incompetent. Patients' perceived levels of competency—from both legal and ethical perspectives—can affect their involvement in medical decision making.

As an example one might consider the case in which a Mien mother from Laos brings her daughter to a pediatrician for her four-month immunizations (Crigger). The pediatrician observes a number of burns on the child's stomach and considers whether to call the Department of Child and Family Services, thinking that the mother has abused her child. The burns actually were the result of a healing ritual designed to ameliorate the child's symptoms that were identified as meaningful to Mien culture. Understanding that the burns are a result of a therapeutic regimen can help the pediatrician realize that the mother was not abusive or neglectful; instead, she was attentive to improving the health of her child (Brown and Jameton). In contrast, one might consider the physician's attempt to pierce skin with a needle as unnecessarily harmful even though it is intended to improve health. Different cultures have different conceptions of what therapeutic interventions constitute acceptable harms or risks and benefits. This case illuminates how culturally shaped ethical notions of risk and benefit are. With a cultural perspective in mind bioethicists can reconstruct arguments regarding risk-benefit ratios. Biomedical healthcare practitioners who recognize these cultural dynamics can better provide not just culturally competent care but also high-quality care.

Conclusion

A community's medical beliefs do not correspond to a homogeneous set of meanings. Both in complex societies and in *traditional* and *tribal* societies individuals are drawn by sickness into multiple and often contradictory systems of meanings and action. The appearance of unity and homogeneity within a specific community is not accidental, however. Usually it is an expression of power, of the capacity of one segment of the community—its medical experts, political leaders, moral authorities, and others—to define and control which of the alternative sets of medical meanings will be carried over into public discourse. In this sense power is the

ability to convince people that the socially dominant meanings of sickness are also the authentic meanings (Young, 1982).

ALLAN YOUNG (1995)
REVISED BY ELISA J. GORDON

SEE ALSO: *Anthropology and Bioethics; Bioethics, African-American Perspectives; Body; Eugenics: Historical Aspects; Feminism; Insanity and the Insanity Defense; Lifestyles and Public Health; Medicine, Anthropology of; Medicine, Philosophy of; Medicine, Sociology of; Mental Illness; Race and Racism; Sexual Identity; Women, Historical and Cross-Cultural Perspectives;* and other *Health and Disease* subentries

BIBLIOGRAPHY

Boddy, Janice P. 1989. *Wombs and Alien Spirits: Women, Men, and the Zar Cult in Northern Sudan.* Madison: University of Wisconsin Press.

Brodwin, Paul. 2002. "Genetics, Identity, and the Anthropology of Essentialism." *Anthropological Quarterly* 75: 323–330.

Brodwin, Paul, ed. 2000. *Biotechnology and Culture: Bodies, Anxieties, Ethics.* Bloomington: Indiana University Press.

Brown, Kate, and Jameton, Andrew. 1998. "Commentary." In *Cases in Bioethics: Selections from the Hastings Center Report,* 3rd edition, ed. Bette-Jane Crigger. New York: St. Martin's Press.

Browner, Carole H.; Preloran, H. M.; and Cox, S. J. 1999. "Ethnicity, Bioethics, and Prenatal Diagnosis: The Amniocentesis Decisions of Mexican-Origin Women and Their Partners." *American Journal of Public Health* 89(1): 1658–1666.

Crigger, Bette-Jane, ed. 1998. *Cases in Bioethics: Selections from the Hastings Center Report,* 3rd edition. New York: St. Martin's Press.

Csordas, Thomas J., ed. 1994. *Embodiment and Experience: The Existential Ground of Culture and Self.* Cambridge, Eng., and New York: Cambridge University Press.

Evans-Pritchard, E. E. 1937. *Witchcraft, Oracles, and Magic among the Azande.* Oxford: Clarendon Press.

Gaines, Atwood, ed. 1992. *Ethnopsychiatry: The Cultural Construction of Professional and Folk Psychiatries.* Albany: State University of New York Press.

Good, Byron. 1994. *Medicine, Rationality, and Experience: An Anthropological Perspective.* Cambridge, Eng., and New York: Cambridge University Press.

Good, Byron, and Kleinman, Arthur, eds. 1985. *Culture and Depression: Studies in the Anthropology and Cross-Cultural Psychiatry of Affect and Disorder.* Berkeley: University of California Press.

Gordon, Elisa J. 2002. "What 'Race' Cannot Tell Us about Access to Kidney Transplantation." *Cambridge Quarterly for Healthcare Ethics* 11: 134–141.

Hahn, Robert A., and Gaines, Atwood D., eds. 1985. *Physicians of Western Medicine: Anthropological Approaches to Theory and Practice.* Dordrecht, Netherlands: D. Reidel.

Haimes, Erica. 2002. "What Can the Social Sciences Contribute to the Study of Ethics? Theoretical, Empirical and Substantive Considerations." *Bioethics* 16: 89–113.

Kleinman, Arthur. 1980. *Patients and Healers in the Context of Culture: An Exploration of the Borderland Between Anthropology, Medicine, and Psychiatry.* Berkeley: University of California Press.

Kleinman, Arthur. 1988. *Rethinking Psychiatry: From Cultural Category to Personal Experience.* New York: Free Press.

Koenig, Barbara A., and Silverberg, H. L. 1999. "Understanding Probabilistic Risk in Predisposition Genetic Testing for Alzheimer Disease." *Genetic Testing* 3: 55–63.

Latour, Bruno, and Woolgar, Steve. 1986. *Laboratory Life: The Construction of Scientific Facts.* Princeton, NJ: Princeton University Press.

Leslie, Charles M. 1976. "Introduction." In *Asian Medical Systems: A Comparative Study,* ed. Charles M. Leslie. Berkeley: University of California Press.

Leslie, Charles M., and Young, Allan, eds. 1992. *Paths to Asian Medical Knowledge.* Berkeley: University of California Press.

Lewis, Gilbert. 1975. *Knowledge of Illness in a Sepik River Society: A Study of the Gnau, New Guinea.* London: Athlone.

Lindenbaum, Shirley, and Lock, Margaret, eds. 1993. *Knowledge, Power and Practice: The Anthropology of Medicine and Everyday Life.* Berkeley: University of California Press.

Lock, Margaret M. 1993. *Encounters with Aging: Mythologies of Menopause in Japan and North America.* Berkeley: University of California Press.

Lock, Margaret M. 2002. *Twice Dead: Organ Transplants and the Reinvention of Death.* Berkeley: University of California Press.

Lock, Margaret M., and Gordon, Deborah R., eds. 1988. *Biomedicine Examined.* Dordrecht, Netherlands: Kluwer.

Lock, Margaret M.; Young, Allan; and Cambrosio, Alberto, eds. 2000. *Living and Working with the New Medical Technologies: Intersections of Inquiry.* New York: Cambridge University Press.

Marshall, Patricia A., and Koenig, B. 1996. "Bioethics and Anthropology: Perspectives on Culture, Medicine, and Morality." In *Medical Anthropology: Contemporary Theory and Method,* rev. edition, ed. C. F. Sargent and T. F. Johnson. Westport, CT: Praeger.

Marshall, Patricia A., and Koenig, Barbara. 2001. "Ethnographic Methods." In *Methods in Medical Ethics,* ed. Jeremy Sugarman and Daniel Sulmasy. Washington, D.C.: Georgetown University Press.

Nichter, Mark. 1989. *Anthropology and International Health: South Asian Case Studies.* Dordrecht, Netherlands: Kluwer.

Rapp, Rayna. 1999. *Testing Women, Testing the Fetus: The Social Impact of Amniocentesis in America.* New York: Routledge.

Wailoo, Keith. 1982. "The Anthropologies of Illness and Sickness." *Annual Review of Anthropology* 11: 257–285.

Wailoo, Keith. 1983. "The Relevance of Traditional Medical Cultures to Modern Primary Health Care." *Social Science and Medicine* 17(16): 1205–1211.

Wailoo, Keith. 1997. *Drawing Blood: Technology and Disease Identity in Twentieth-Century America.* Baltimore: Johns Hopkins University Press.

Young, Allan. 1982. "The Anthropologies of Illness and Sickness." *Annual Review of Anthropology,* 1982: 257–285.

Young, Allan. 1983. "The Relevance of Traditional Medical Cultures to Modern Primary Health Care." *Social Science and Medicine* 17(16): 1205–1211.

IV. PHILOSOPHICAL PERSPECTIVES

Concepts of health and disease—as well as of sickness, wellness, deformity, disability, dysfunction, and disfigurement—direct social energies. They inform medicine and healthcare policy regarding what is wholesome, what is to be avoided, and what is to be treated—all else being equal. Concepts of health and disease either directly or indirectly describe, evaluate, and explain reality and help to assign social roles. Decisions about the meaning and scope of concepts of health and disease profoundly influence the character of healthcare. For example, if alcoholism, homosexuality, menopause, or aging are considered diseases, then medical treatment, resources, and research will be focused on treating them. These concepts therefore become the focus of public-policy debates, and they may conceal value judgments that should be treated more explicitly as bioethical issues.

Diseases and sicknesses are usually distinguished from sins, crimes, and social problems in that they are not directly under the control of the will and are explainable, predictable, and (usually) treatable by an appeal to somatic or psychological laws, generalizations, and associations. Pains that are directly under one's own control or that of others (e.g., the pain from standing on one's own foot), difficulties of a moral sort (e.g., being blameworthy), problems of a spiritual sort (e.g., refusing to repent for one's transgressions), or legal disabilities (e.g., being a convicted felon) are thus contrasted with states of disease or illness. This contrast discloses a boundary between disparate human practices (e.g., blaming the immoral, convicting felons, exorcising demons, treating diseases), and the criteria used to distinguish between any of these practices will vary from culture to culture and shift within the history of a particular culture. In addition, the line between medical and other problems is, in part, a function of the competencies of those making the judgment. Diseases and illnesses are what medicine treats.

Illnesses and diseases are generally identified because they involve a failure of function, a pain that is considered abnormal (compare the pain of teething with that of migraine [King]), a deformity, or the threat of premature death. Insofar as judgments regarding proper function, normal pain, correct human form, and normal span of life can be made without reference to culture-dependent values, concepts of disease will not depend on social norms of proper human function. The same can be said with regard to concepts of health. Though much is said regarding healthcare, health, and wellness, one may question whether such notions can be understood only in positive terms. The positive concepts of health must be understood in relation to the absence of particular dysfunctions, pains, or deformities, and there may be numerous concepts of human well-being and exemplary function (Boorse,1975). It is also difficult to provide a positive account of health and well-being that will not include concepts of economic, political, and social health. For example, the World Health Organization's 1958 definition of health as a "state of complete physical, mental, and social well-being" (WHO, p. 459) has been criticized for being too broad and ill defined to guide the formation of health policy (Callahan). The philosophical literature, aside from addressing these difficulties with concepts of health, has focused mainly on concepts of disease and illness.

Philosophical concerns regarding concepts of health and disease can be organized under six questions:

1. Are disease entities to be discovered or are they and their classifications instrumental constructs that are created to achieve certain ends?

2. How do explanatory models shape the boundaries between health and disease and determine the meaning of disease?

3. What values shape concepts of health and disease, and to what extent are these culturally determined?

4. Is the definition of mental disease and health different from that of somatic (or physical) disease and health?

5. Do concepts of animal disease function in the same way as concepts of human disease?

6. How can concepts of health and disease be used for overt political and social ends?

The *ens morbi*

The history of medicine is replete with talk of clinical findings constituting an *ens morbi* (disease entity). Disease entities have been conceived of as metaphysical entities, clinical entities, pathological entities, etiological entities, and genetic entities. These ways of considering diseases generated a significant dispute in the nineteenth century between those who held that disease entities (and the classifications within which they are understood) identify realities in the world and those who held that disease classifications are at best distinctions imposed on reality to achieve certain goals (e.g., of diagnosis, therapy, and prognosis). The first were termed *ontologists,* while those who took a more conventionalist, instrumentalist, or nominalist position were termed *physiologists.* This distinction appears to have been articulated in 1828 by François-Joseph-Victor Broussais (1772–1838), who denounced ontological accounts of disease (1821). Carl Wunderlich (1815–1877), Ernst von Romberg (1865–1933), Alasdair MacIntyre, Samuel Gorovitz, and others have, in various ways, taken positions in sympathy with Broussais.

Ontological theories have held that disease terms or classifications name things in the world. Though Broussais had directed his criticisms against clinical classifications, disease ontologists can be taken to include any who perceived diseases as entities, including metaphysical views advanced by individuals such as Paracelsus (1493–1541), who held that diseases are specific entities that arise outside the body.

Disease entities have also been understood as clinical realities, or as recurring constellations of findings. Thomas Sydenham (1624–1689), in classifying disease entities, construed them as enduring types and patterns of symptoms: "Nature in the production of disease is uniform and consistent; so much so, that for the same disease in different persons the symptoms are for the most part the same; and the selfsame phenomena that you would observe in the sickness of a Socrates you would observe in the sickness of a simpleton" (p. 15). It is within such a view of disease that one can speak of a person having a typical case of typhoid. Such language expresses the view that there is a central identity for a disease that is its essence, or *type.* One can therefore classify diseases by type, as well as speak of instances of a disease as approximating a *typical* case. Within this understanding, one can also talk of typical cases as rare: "One rarely sees a typical case of secondary syphilis." Patients embody clinical realities where *typical* means the full and complete expression of a disease, or an ideal type, but not necessarily its usual expression. It was against this genre of account that Broussais spoke.

Etiological accounts, like metaphysical views, focused on the cause of the disease as the disease entity, but regarded disease entities as empirical, and usually infectious, agents. Rudolf Virchow (1821–1902) characterized this view as "ontological in an outspoken manner" (p. 192). Virchow considered this understanding of disease entities to rest on a confusion between a disease and its cause. "The parasite," he wrote, "was therefore not the disease itself but only its cause" (p. 192). The confusion of the disease with its cause led to a "hopeless, never-ending confusion, in which the ideas of being (*ens morbi*) and causation (*causa morbi*) have been arbitrarily thrown together, [and] began when microorganisms were finally discovered" (p. 192). The mature Virchow embraced a view of disease entities grounded in pathological findings, and he held that a disease entity is "an altered body-part, or, expressed in first principles, an altered cell or aggregate of cells, whether tissue or organ" (p. 192). Further, "this conception is expressly ontological. That is its merit, not its deficiency. There is in actuality an *ens morbi,* just as there is an *ens vitae* (life force); in both instances a cell or cell-complex has the claim to be thus designated" (p. 207).

Genetic accounts can also interpret the disease entity as an empirical reality, to be found in genetic abnormalities (Anderson; Fowler, et al). The promise of somatic-cell gene therapy raises the question of a disease entity once again. That is, does the disease exist in the genetic structure, or is the structure the cause of the disease?

Current uses of the term *disease* in standard nomenclatures and nosologies (classifications) have a predominantly nonontological character. A conventionalist view allows one to choose, for example, whether one wishes to treat tuberculosis as an infectious, genetic, or environmental disease (recognizing that all three sorts of factors contribute to the development of tuberculosis), based on which variables are most easily manipulated. One may decide that it would be best to treat tuberculosis as an infectious disease because little is known about the inheritance of resistance against tuberculosis, or because any eugenic programs to eliminate tuberculosis would be very slow in taking effect. It may also be seen as an environmental disease that is brought about by socioeconomic conditions such as housing, food, and other such factors. It is meaningless to ask whether such a definition of disease is true or false, only whether it is useful (Wulff).

Diseases as Clinical Findings and Explanatory Accounts

Many people take the term *illness* to identify a subjective experience of failed function, pain, distress, or unwellness. *Disease,* in contrast, is then an explanatory concept, or part of an explanatory account (Boorse, 1975). Or one might identify illnesses as constellations of signs and symptoms and diseases as illnesses joined to disease models or explanations, where the content of the illness is augmented by the phenomena found on the basis of a disease model. But to recognize a state of unwellness as a state of disease is already to have begun to explain it and to recast the meaning of the findings within an interpretive context. A constellation of phenomena is held to be recurrent, and if such a constellation of phenomena is encountered again in the future, it can

be identified. A specific set of symptoms, for example, can be identified as a case of chronic fatigue. Diagnoses of syndromes, of recurrent patterns of signs and symptoms, allow predictions to be made (prognoses) as well as the management of outcomes (therapy). Such predictions and attempts at therapy can succeed even in the absence of causal explanations.

During much of its history, medicine has been concerned with classifying patterns of signs and symptoms so that they can be recognized in the future with greater ease. Thomas Sydenham's classic *Observationes medicae* (1676) suggested classifying diseases in definite species, following the methods of botanists in classifying plants. His work was followed by Carolus Linnaeus's Genera morborum in auditorum usum (1759), François Boissier de Sauvages de la Croix's Nosologia methodica sistens morborum classes juxta Sydenhami mentem et botanicorum ordinem (1763), and William Cullen's Synopsis nosologiae methodicae (1769). These classifications functioned without causal explanations, though these were also given. Such medical descriptions and explanations at a clinical, phenomenological level are still employed whenever a new illness is identified for which a causal explanation is not yet forthcoming. For example, acquired immunodeficiency syndrome (AIDS) was first identified as a clinical, phenomenological entity.

Medicine also explains health and disease by relating what is observed via general laws of physiology, anatomy, psychology, genetics, and so forth to other phenomena. The result is a two-tier account of diseases. The first tier is that of the observed constellations of phenomena, such as a clinical description of yellow fever. The second tier is that of a model advanced within the laboratory medical sciences to explain the observed clinical phenomena, such as an explanation of the clinical findings in yellow fever in terms of the effects of a group B arbovirus (a group of viruses transmitted by mosquitoes and ticks) that causes the death of essential cells in the liver.

The laws of pathophysiology (the physiology of disordered function) and pathopsychology (the psychology of mental disease) relate new phenomena to the original clinical constellations of signs and symptoms. Some of these phenomena are then recognized as the causes of the illness. The concept of disease thus comes to identify disease models that support the search for unnoticed causal factors and expressions of disease. For example, Giovanni Battista Morgagni (1682–1771) in his *De Sedibus et causis morborum per anatomen indagatis* (1761) correlated clinical observations with postmortem findings, and Philippe Pinel (1745–1826) incorporated anatomical considerations into his *Nosographie philosophique* (1798), producing nosologies that embraced not only clinical observations, but anatomical considerations as well. This change in focus was strengthened when Marie-François-Xavier Bichat (1771–1802) argued that constellations of symptoms and signs could be explained in terms of underlying pathological processes. According to Bichat, medical advances are best achieved through autopsies (Foucault). This shift to the study of pathological findings as a way to explain clinical observations was then supplemented by accounts drawn from microbiology, endocrinology, biochemistry, genetics, and other fields, producing contemporary explanations of illnesses.

In the process of moving from accounts of illness that were predominantly clinical observations to accounts based on observable illnesses of the anatomy, the meanings of diseases were altered. Individuals who once were thought to die of acute indigestion were now understood to die of a myocardial infarction. The meanings of the phenomena observed (e.g., clinical signs and symptoms) were reinterpreted in terms of disease models. As a result of this recasting, medical complaints often came to be considered legitimate only to the extent that they had a demonstrable, underlying pathophysiological or pathoanatomical lesion.

Health and Diseases: Discoveries or Cultural Inventions?

If certain physiological and psychological functions can be identified as natural or essential to humans, then their absence can be used to define disease states. Leon Kass and Christopher Boorse have argued that one can specify those functions that are integral to being human, and thus secure accounts of disease that are not relative to a particular culture or set of values. Such understandings of health and disease could then be used to sort out essential from nonessential (if not proper from improper) applications of medicine. However, such naturalistic views may depend on particular understandings of what is *natural*. Others appeal to an evolutionary account of what should count as species-typical levels of species-typical functions appropriate for age and gender (Boorse 1976).

In contrast, Joseph Margolis, H. Tristram Engelhardt, and others have argued that definitions of disease and health depend on sociological, culturally determined value judgments, and that these definitions can be understood only in terms of particular cultures and their ideologies (Margolis). A value-free account of disease cannot be given, some have argued, because diseases are defined not by their causes, but by their effects (Resnek)—and their effects gain significance within a cultural context. K.W.M. Fulford has also indicated deeply hidden but still crucial evaluative elements in medicine. He has done this through a linguistic-analytic examination of how disease language appears to be value-free, while still entailing values, with the result that controversies in medical health are engendered where relevant values are sufficiently diverse. Fulford also argues that part-function analysis, which focuses on the proper function of each part of the body, fails with psychotic mental disorders where the rationality of the person as a whole is disturbed. Others have explored the nature of disease through the use of action theory and by placing concerns about disease and illness within the larger holistic context of health (Nordenfeldt, 1995, 2001). Still others ground disease language in a notion of malady dependent on the universal features of human rationality, thus eliminating culture as a factor (Clouser).

The view that the concepts of health and disease are culturally determined has been supported by feminist writings on healthcare. Many authors have pointed out that the practice of medicine has had an androcentric (masculine) focus, that women's issues have largely been ignored, and that experiences reported by women that could not be documented have been treated as invalid (Rosser; Oakley).

Partisans of the view that social and cultural ideas influence concepts of health and disease stress that a definition of disease tied to evolution makes disease concepts dependent on particular past environments and past adaptations. Successful adaptation must always be specified in terms of a particular environment, including a particular cultural context. A culture-dependent account of concepts of health and disease need not deny that there will be great similarities as to what will count as diseases across cultures, for certain symptoms and conditions will probably be understood as diseases in most cultures. Supporters of a value-infected, culture-dependent account of disease have argued that those who would attempt a purely evolutionary account of disease have not reconstructed the practice of medicine, but rather some practice of characterizing individuals as members of particular biological species (Engelhardt, 1975). The practice of medicine, in this view, depends on culturally constructed understandings of health and disease.

How one understands health and disease will in turn influence how one conceptualizes medical practice. Henrik Wulff has argued that an exclusively biological or empirical model of illness contributes to paternalistic medical practice, for if concepts of health and disease can be fully understood in biological terms, then there may be no need to assign the patient an active role in the decision-making process. If, however, determinations of health and disease are not just empirical concepts, but are also related to cultures and values, the patient will have a more active role in determining the burden of the disease and the extent of treatment.

The conceptualization of medicine will certainly be influenced by developments in genetic research, which hold the promise not only to correct diseases in patients, but to prevent them in future generations of patients (Anderson; Zimmerman). Thus, as the capacities of genetic medicine increase, preventive medicine will expand. Somatic and germ-line therapies will also be affected as choices are made about which genetic variances should be treated as disease abnormalities (e.g., homosexuality, alcoholism, shortness of stature).

Physical, Mental, and Social Diseases

It has been argued that only somatic diseases are legitimately diseases, while *mental diseases* are problems with living (Szasz). Following similar lines of argument, individuals have contended that enterprises such as psychotherapy are tantamount to applied ethics (Breggin), or that the cure of somatic disease constitutes the prime goal of medicine (Kass).

In response, some argue that such stark dichotomies or dualisms fail to offer satisfactory accounts of reality. If mental life is dependent on brain function, then all mental diseases can, in some sense, be tied to physical pathology or abnormal anatomy. For example, depression can be presumed to be dependent on a neurophysiological substrate, and thus, in principle, is open to pharmacological treatment. If one views diseases as explanatory models for the organization of signs and symptoms, then it does not matter whether the signs and symptoms identify physiological states ("I have a rash") or psychological states ("I feel depressed"). Nor does it matter whether models employed to correlate these phenomena are pathophysiological or psychological. Most accounts of disease will, in fact, mingle physical and psychological symptoms. As a consequence, one may come to view distinctions among somatic, psychological, and social models of disease in terms of pragmatic needs—of accenting the usefulness of particular modes of therapeutic intervention. One may even advance sociological models of disease, construing diseases primarily in terms of social variables and giving secondary place to the pathophysiological.

Distinctions between medical and nonmedical models of therapy, unlike somatic, psychological, and sociological accounts of disease, are often meant to contrast the autonomy of clients in nonmedical therapeutic models with the dependence of patients on healthcare practitioners in medical models. Talcott Parsons characterized the "sick role" as: (1) excusing ill individuals from some or all of their usual responsibilities; (2) holding them not responsible for being ill (though they may be responsible for becoming sick); (3) holding that they should attempt to become well (a therapeutic imperative) and seek out experts to treat their illness. Medical models tend to support paternalistic interventions by healthcare practitioners and to relieve patients of responsibility for directing their own care. Nonmedical models, in contrast, tend to accent the patient's responsibility.

Somatic models of disease may be employed within both medical and nonmedical models of therapy. For example, hypertension may be treated with antihypertensive agents or by enjoining the afflicted individuals to find ways to change their lifestyles with regard to stress, eating patterns, and so on. The same is true of psychological models of disease. Depression can be treated chemotherapeutically or by enjoining individuals to make changes in their ways of living.

As predisposing factors toward particular diseases become better known and easier to control or avoid, individuals are held increasingly responsible for becoming ill, even though they will remain nonresponsible for being ill. A person is not held to be responsible for having bronchogenic carcinoma in the same way that one is responsible for being a willful malingerer. In other words, one cannot be told to stop having cancer, but one can be held responsible for having developed cancer through one's smoking habits. As the impact of lifestyle on the development of diseases becomes clearer, the responsibility of individuals for their health may increase the possible scope of nonmedical models of therapy.

Animals and Disease

If concepts of human illness, disease, and health are, in part, social constrictions, there will be differences between the ways in which diseases are identified for humans and the ways they are identified for other animals. Illnesses and diseases in animals will be judged through the social or cultural criteria of human beings. Pets or domestic animals may be regarded as having disease or being healthy depending on how they are viewed through human purposes and constructs. The diseases or illnesses of those animals that are not pets, however, along with those of plants, may be understood less in terms of human social or cultural criteria and more in terms of generalized knowledge about the species. In the case of animals in the wild, there may not be concern for individual suffering, disability, or deformity, but rather with the general health of the species. Identifying the role human values play in the concepts of animal disease and illness expands the discussion of the ethical treatment of nonhuman animals in bioethics.

The Social Force of Diagnosis

Concepts of disease have been used to impose political judgments. For example, in the United States prior to the

Civil War it was proposed that the flight of a slave to the North and the absence of a wholesome inclination to do effective plantation work were diseases for which explanatory accounts and treatments could be provided (Cartwright). Masturbation was once viewed as a serious disease for which castration, excision of the clitoris, and other invasive therapies were employed. Individuals were even determined to have died of masturbation, and postmortem findings "substantiated" this cause (Engelhardt, 1974). In the case of the diseases of slaves, the motivation may have been to protect slaves from punishment. In the case of masturbation, the influence of cultural values on the psychology of discovery was not appreciated.

Historical perspective can increase our awareness that medical practitioners and researchers have tended to "discover" what already was assumed. More recent political uses of disease concepts (e.g., in psychiatry) have been closely connected with repressive goals and political agendas of certain governments. Social employment of disease definitions is often meant to be benevolent, however, such as advocating a view of alcoholism and drug addiction as diseases so as to recruit the forces of medicine to aid in their control. Moreover, such conditions may be termed diseases in order to relieve alcoholics and drug addicts of the social opprobria that attend what is often viewed as immoral behavior.

Summary

Concepts of health and disease shape descriptions of medical reality, convey explanations, advance value judgments, and structure social reality. They influence not only the scope of medicine, but healthcare policy as well. Because they may involve not only moral values but values associated with physical and mental excellence, they raise questions pertinent to both bioethics and the philosophy of medicine. These special concerns regarding medical explanation may sufficiently define a distinctive problem area so as to establish the philosophy of medicine as a field in its own right, despite arguments to the contrary. In any event, the concepts of health and disease, as well as their application, will continue to be the subject of debate in societies that are morally and culturally pluralistic.

H. TRISTRAM ENGELHARDT, JR.
KEVIN WM. WILDES (1995)
REVISED BY AUTHORS

SEE ALSO: *Anthropology and Bioethics; Bioethics, African-American Perspectives; Eugenics: Historical Aspects; Feminism; Lifestyles and Public Health; Medicine, Anthropology of; Medicine, Philosophy of; Medicine, Sociology of; Mental Illness; Women, Historical and Cross-Cultural Perspectives;* and other *Health and Disease* subentries

BIBLIOGRAPHY

Anderson, W. French. 1989. "Human Gene Therapy: Why Draw a Line?" *Journal of Medicine and Philosophy* 14(6): 681–693.

Boorse, Christopher. 1975. "On the Distinction Between Disease and Illness." *Philosophy and Public Affairs* 5(1): 49–68.

Boorse, Christopher. 1976. "Wright on Functions." *Philosophical Review* 85(1): 70–86.

Boorse, Christopher. 1997. "A Rebuttal on Health." In *What is Disease?* ed. James Humber and Robert Almeder. Totowa, NJ: Humana Press.

Breggin, Peter Roger. 1971. "Psychotherapy and Applied Ethics." *Psychiatry* 34(1): 59–74.

Broussais, François-Joseph-Victor. 1821. *Examen des doctrines médicales et des systèmes de nosologie,* 2 vols. Paris: Mequignon-Marvis.

Callahan, Daniel. 1990. *What Kind of Life: The Limits of Medical Progress.* New York: Simon & Schuster.

Cartwright, Samuel A. 1851. "Report on the Diseases and Physical Peculiarities of the Negro Race." *New Orleans Medical and Surgical Review* 7: 691–715.

Clouser, K. Danner; Culver, Charles M.; and Gert, Bernard. 1997. "Malady." In *What is Disease?* ed. James Humber and Robert Almeder. Totowa, NJ: Humana Press.

Engelhardt, H. Tristram, Jr. 1974. "The Disease of Masturbation: Values and the Concept of Disease." *Bulletin of the History of Medicine* 48(2): 225–248.

Engelhardt, H. Tristram, Jr. 1975. "The Concepts of Health and Disease." In *Evaluation and Explanation in the Biomedical Sciences,* ed. H. Tristram Engelhardt Jr., and Stuart F. Spicker. Dordrecht, Netherlands: Reidel.

Engelhardt, H. Tristram, Jr. 1996. *The Foundations of Bioethics.* New York: Oxford University Press.

Foucault, Michel. 1973. *The Birth of the Clinic: An Archeology of Medical Perception.* New York: Pantheon Books.

Fowler, Gregory; Juengst, Eric T.; and Zimmerman, Burke K. 1989. "Germ-Line Gene Therapy and the Clinical Ethos of Medical Genetics." *Theoretical Medicine* 10(2): 151–165.

Fulford, K. W. M. 2001. "What is (Mental) Disease?" *Journal of Medical Ethics* 27(2): 80–85.

Kass, Leon R. 1975. "Regarding the End of Medicine and the Pursuit of Health." *Public Interest* 40: 11–42.

King, Lester. 1981. "What Is Disease." In *Concepts of Health and Disease: Interdisciplinary Perspectives,* ed. Arthur L. Caplan, H. Tristram Engelhardt Jr., and James McCartney. Reading, MA: Addison-Wesley.

Margolis, Joseph. 1976. "The Concept of Disease." *Journal of Medicine and Philosophy* 1(3): 238–255.

Nordenfelt, Lennart. 1995. *On the Nature of Health,* 2nd edition. Dordrecht, Netherlands: Kluwer Academic Publishers.

Nordenfelt, Lennart. 2001. *Health, Science, and Ordinary Language.* Atlanta, GA: Rodopi.

Oakley, Ann. 1993. *Essays on Women, Medicine, and Health.* Edinburgh: Edinburgh University Press.

Paracelsus. 1941. *Four Treatises of Theophrastus von Hohenheim, Called Paracelsus,* ed. C. Lillian Temkin, George Rosen, G. Zilboorg, and Henry E. Sigerist. Baltimore: Leidecker.

Parsons, Talcott. 1971. *The System of Modern Societies.* Englewood Cliffs, NJ: Prentice Hall.

Rosser, Sue V. 1989. "Re-Visioning Clinical Research: Gender and the Ethics of Experimental Design." *Hypatia* 4(2): 125–139.

Sydenham, Thomas. 1848. *The Works of Thomas Sydenham,* vol. 1: *Medical Observations Concerning the History and Cure of Acute Diseases,* tr. Dr. Greenhill. London: Sydenham Society.

Szasz, Thomas. 1974. *The Myth of Mental Illness: Foundations of a Theory of Personal Conduct,* rev. edition. New York: Harper & Row.

Virchow, Rudolf Ludwig Karl. 1958. *Disease, Life, and Man: Selected Essays,* tr. Lelland J. Rather. Stanford, CA: Stanford University Press.

Wartofsky, Marx W. 1975. "Organs, Organisms, and Disease: Human Ontology and Medical Practice." In *Evaluation and Explanation in the Biomedical Sciences,* ed. H. Tristram Engelhardt Jr., and Stuart F. Spicker. Dordrecht, Netherlands: Reidel.

World Health Organization (WHO). 1958. "Constitution." In *The First Ten Years of the World Health Organization.* Geneva: Author.

Wulff, Henrik R. 1981. *Rational Diagnosis and Treatment: An Introduction to Clinical Decision-Making,* 2nd edition. Oxford: Blackwell Scientific Publications.

Zimmerman, Burke K. 1991. "Human Germ-Line Therapy: The Case for Its Development and Use." *Journal of Medicine and Philosophy* 16(6): 593–612.

V. THE EXPERIENCE OF HEALTH AND ILLNESS

Some would argue that given the wide range of historical, cultural, and individual differences concerning health and illness, little could be said on the topic that would have universal validity. Others would point toward certain invariant features of the human body, psyche, or society that could ground cross-cultural commonalities. Presented here is a description of health and illness as experienced within a contemporary Western context. While this description may not be universally applicable, it nonetheless provides a starting point for elucidating similarities and differences among cultures and individuals.

The Experience of Health

In setting out to portray the experience of health, one is struck by how little people are used to focusing on it. This tendency to overlook health—to take it for granted—is also reflected in the paucity of descriptive literature on the subject. In many ways this is precisely the point. To be healthy is to be freed from some of the limitations and problems that promote self-reflection. A healthy person need not pause before scheduling a dinner for later in the week or grabbing a shovel to clear the driveway of snow. The state of health that allows for such engagements remains the tacit background of what Maurice Merleau-Ponty, drawing on the work of Edmund Husserl, calls the bodily "I can": I can get out of bed, move across the room, brush my teeth, and so forth, without a need to explicitly define or acknowledge these abilities—or the wellness that make them possible.

Sometimes people are provoked to reflect on their good health: they revel in their renewed strength after a bout of flu, for example. Health is thus illuminated by contrasting experiences. Certain practices, such as yoga, tai chi, and exercise programs, can systematically teach one to cultivate and appreciate the healthy state, heightening self-awareness.

However, Western culture has tended to neglect or demean bodily experience in favor of a detached rationality or cultivation of the soul (Leder, 1990). People learn to overlook or overcome the body until it seizes their attention, as it does at times of pain and illness. Even preventative *health education* tends to focus on external guidelines concerning exercise, diet, and the like, but do little to cultivate an inner awareness of the body's own voice. Perhaps many illness states could be avoided if people were better listeners to the subtler messages of the body that signal a departure from good health. Yet to be healthy is ever a temptation to overlook, or look beyond, the body. The word *health* comes from the same root as the word *whole*. The healthy body operates as a harmonious whole, allowing one to feel at home in the world (Svenaeus) without the need for undue self-reflection.

Disease and Illness

Illness makes one aware of the precariousness of the world. To capture the profound dislocations caused by illness, it is useful first to distinguish between *illness* and *disease* (Cassell, 1985; Engelhardt, 1982). Modern medicine has been largely concerned with understanding and treating specific diseases. Yet to diagnose an individual as having a disease means looking beyond that particular individual: one notes a cluster of signs and symptoms that have repeatedly presented in a range of cases. The disease label also frequently (and ideally) invokes an explanatory etiology, a prognostic picture, and a set of treatment options, all drawing upon the theories and knowledge base of medical science. Since the eighteenth century, disease classifications have progressively moved from a basis in the patient's reported symptoms to one grounded on the pathological lesions and processes exposed after death or, by medical technologies, in the living (Engelhardt, 1986; Foucault). Hence, *dyspepsia* has become *peptic ulcer disease*. This shift has greatly advanced the explanatory and therapeutic powers of modern medicine, but it has also diminished the attention paid to the patient's experience.

In contrast to the medical characterization of disease, the term *illness* refers to the *experience* of sickness. To fall ill is to undergo a series of transformations that distinguish this state from health. In a sense, any illness is inescapably individual. Even if one shares the same disease with another, the challenges, limitations, and suffering involved can vary considerably from person to person. Yet just as the physician-researcher can uncover the repeated patterns typical of a disease, one can describe certain features that commonly accompany the illness experience (Toombs, 2001).

ILLNESS AND THE EXPERIENCE OF THE BODY.
If health is a kind of wholeness—an integration along a number of dimensions—illness involves a set of experienced *dis-integrations*. This is first seen in relation to the body. Ordinarily, the body operates as a seamless whole (Merleau-Ponty, 1962): in response to one's perceptions one moves through and acts upon the surrounding world, with the internal organs supplying the needed life energy. In illness, however, the body can split into problematic parts and functions. An aching stomach or a pulled muscle suddenly stands out from the rest of the body, demanding attention. As one's organic harmony is disrupted, so too is one's integration with the world. The ill body is no longer at home in its world, but is awkward and limited, and even simple physical acts become difficult.

This dis-integration of the body within itself and from its world also brings about a felt split between the body and the self. Ordinarily, the body is an inseparable part of one's identity, grounding one's interactions with the environment. When one falls ill, however, this body becomes something alien (Leder, 1990; Zaner, 1981), causing pain, limiting movement, or humiliating the ill person with an unpleasant look or odor. One's own flesh seems capable of thwarting and opposing one in a way health had not fully revealed.

This experience presents a severe challenge to one's usual sense of selfhood and autonomy. The ill person may neither understand nor control what is happening within the body, though one's life may depend upon the outcome. One's knowledge of the body becomes mediated through others: the physician who diagnostically probes it, or the surgeon who opens it up, scrutinizing organs the patient has never seen.

ILLNESS AND THE EXPERIENCE OF SPACE AND TIME.
These modes of embodied dis-integration typical of illness also suffuse experiences of space and time. When a person is healthy, space unfolds as a field of possible movement, of activity, of desires to be fulfilled (Straus, 1963), whether it be a flight of steps one knows one can climb or an open street one can cross. With many forms of illness this spatial field is disrupted. One may remain confined in a bed or unable to climb a flight of stairs due to arthritis or a neuromuscular disease.

As space is thus altered by illness, so too is time. Ordinarily, human beings dwell largely in the future (Heidegger), with present activities geared toward the future accomplishment of desired goals—on the way to the paint store, one is envisioning the fully painted room. But when one is sick the way toward the future is blocked, and a claustrophobic world of concern closes in on the sufferer. Even a world traveler or delightful raconteur can transform into an intolerable bore who obsesses about illness minutiae.

There are avenues of escape for the ill person. One can "lose oneself" in a good book or television. One can dwell in nostalgia for a pain-free past or dream of a future restored to health. But these wanderings never fully lose their character as modes of escape from the confinements of illness.

ILLNESS AND THE EXPERIENCE OF OTHERS.
This dis-integration of our spatiotemporal world is often matched by a felt disunity with others. When healthy, one is a part of the mainstream, involved with work, family, and socializing. Yet as simple a sensation as pain can suddenly open a profound distance (Scarry). Though just inches away and sympathetic, another person cannot experience one's pain. It may not even be possible to communicate one's pain, for this most private of experiences is notoriously resistant to expression.

Illness can cut one off from others not only through pain, but through disabling effects. One lingers in bed while everyone else heads off to the duties of a busy life. The energy to work and socialize may be lost. "I don't want you to see me like this" is a frequent refrain of the person reduced by illness to sallow skin or loose bowels, and the healthy may often wish to avoid the world of the sick, which only serves as a reminder of one's own vulnerability.

Loneliness can thus contribute greatly to the suffering of the ill. There is a sense of exile—from one's body, from one's activities and goals, and from one's fellows. In the face of this exile, social connection often takes on heightened importance for the sick person. The compassion (etymologically, "to suffer with") that grounds another's willingness to listen to, touch, and care for the sick person can do much to alleviate suffering (Kane).

ILLNESS AND THE EXPERIENCE OF THE COSMOS. The term *cosmos* refers to the world discerned as an ordered and harmonious whole. This is precisely what illness can bring into question. Imagine discovering in the midst of an ordinary day a growth that is subsequently diagnosed as malignant. Questions scream forth: "Why has this happened?" "Why now?" "Why to me?" The possibility arises that these questions have no good answers. Ordinary structures of meaning are shattered.

This felt meaninglessness can prove all but intolerable. Any meaning may be preferable, even a negative one such as: "I have been bad and this illness is my punishment" (Kopelman). The ill often search for their offending infractions, be it smoking, eating fatty foods, having a "cancer-prone personality," or transgressions against God. This association of sickness and sin preserves the coherence of a just universe, as well as the sense of one's own power within it. However, this reading of illness brings its own sense of painful exile. Sickness remains a scarlet letter, branding the ill person's moral failings. The healthy, eager to strengthen their own illusions of security and superiority, may be willing to collude with this judgment.

Illness, then, is not simply a biological event; it is also an existential transformation. One may be stripped of one's trust in the body, reliance on the future, taken-for-granted abilities, professional and social roles, and even one's place in the cosmos.

Of course, this need not always be the case. The experience of illness varies widely, and much depends on the nature of the attacking disease, the vagaries of individual psychology, and the social milieu. Some of this diversity is captured in the growing literature on medical phenomenology and so-called pathographies—accounts of illness written by or about the sufferers (Brody; Hawkins). One can ultimately imagine textbooks of illness, as there are now for diseases, that would describe experiences typically or possibly associated with severe psoriasis, heart attacks, neurological diseases (Sacks), and other conditions.

ACUTE ILLNESSES AND INFLICTED TRAUMAS. With acute but transitory illnesses, such as the flu, discomfort and disability can shrink one's world and distance it from that shared by others, but the horizon of health remains visible. One is buoyed by the assurance that this illness is temporary,

that after this brief visit to a foreign land one will surely return home. The sense of suffering and cosmic dislocation are thus held in check.

Then there are illnesses and traumas of acute onset but more catastrophic consequences. One may have a car accident, for example, or suffer a serious heart attack that threatens one's life even after recovery. The sudden anomalous nature of such events leaves its own psychic scars. The world and one's body seem less safe, more a house of horrors in which dangers can leap forth from anywhere. This sense may be especially acute when trauma is inflicted by another, as through a gunshot wound or sexual assault (Brison). The embodied self is revealed as profoundly vulnerable to disruption, penetration, or violation by others.

In the face of acute catastrophe, William F. May suggests that a person may experience something of an existential obliteration. He describes a patient suffering from severe burns covering two-thirds of his body, who calls out: "Don't you see, I am a dead man" (May, p. 16). However, this "death" can be followed by rebirth. This is not simply a reclamation of one's previous self, but the forging of a new self, with its own strengths and virtues (Brison).

This can be especially difficult, however for those victimized by others, as in cases of child molestation or spousal battering. Here, the confinements imposed by illness take on new dimensions. The victim is entrapped not only within physical suffering but by a double imprisonment, both external and internal. There are external barriers to breaking free of the violence—in the case of molestation, the power adults exert over children; in the case of a battered wife contemplating escape, the difficulty in attaining employment, financial independence, shelter, and child care. There are internal barriers as well. The victim often feels guilty, tainted, or shamed by his or her participation, and may thus become secretive and complicitous. Feelings of powerlessness and low self-esteem set in: "This will never change. There's nothing I can do. I'm not worth it anyway." Finally, as awful as this abusive world is, it is familiar, and one may cling to it for security amid the fear. Many break free, but social and psychological forces can also pull victims back, making escape an arduous struggle.

CHRONIC ILLNESS AND DISBILITY. Many illnesses are neither transitory nor based on acute events: Instead, they are chronic, lifelong, and involve relatively stable or progressive patterns of disability (Toombs et al., 1995). Forms of arthritis, bronchitis-emphysema, kidney disease, diabetes, Alzheimer's disease, colitis, and autoimmune diseases, for example, fall into this category. While onset may come early in life, the elderly often suffer from such degenerative conditions. Due to the aging of the overall population, along with advances in the prevention and cure of acute disease, chronic illness is increasingly the staple of medical practices and hospital care.

Chronic illness can bring with it all of the dis-integrations described above. Unlike acute and treatable illness, there may be no horizon of health that allows one to look beyond present suffering. The day-in, day-out persistence of pain and disability, without hope of relief, can bring about a kind of existential fatigue that leads to despair. With severe arthritis, for example, even tying one's shoe can become difficult. But the chronic nature of such conditions can also give one time to work through its meanings, and to build strategies for physical and psychological coping. One needs to realistically accept limitations, while also claiming the possibilities that remain for fulfillment.

The burgeoning field of *disability studies* has supported sustained reflection on the phenomenology of specific conditions, such as paralysis (Robillard) or blindness (Hull), and the way these are socially constructed (Michalko). There is a danger to assimilating such conditions, sometimes present from birth, to an illness model that emphasizes suffering and limitation. The disabled individual has often developed alternative abilities that are powerfully life enhancing. It is therefore important to develop attitudes and social policies that respect the diversity of human embodiment.

Disability resulting from chronic progressive illnesses can pose a particular challenge to the individual. S. Kay Toombs, in her book *The Body in Multiple Sclerosis* (1992), discusses her condition in this light. The disease is typified by sudden exacerbations and remissions (e.g., of visual disturbance or bowel and bladder incontinence), but with a gradual buildup of neurological deficits over time. There is thus a continual need to redefine the self in the face of new incapacities. Adjusting to muscle weakness, one becomes accustomed to using a walker until, as the disease advances, one becomes wheelchair-bound. The dignity associated with the upright posture is thus lost, together with passage to regions formerly accessible. The ill person faces the Sisyphean task of repeated readjustment without promise of rest. Yet even under such trying conditions, individuals find modes of strength, support, courage, and consolation to meet the existential challenge.

Medical Treatment and Healing

Taken seriously, the experience of illness leads to the question of what impact the medical profession has upon the sufferer (Toombs, 1992b). When illness results from an easily curable disease, medical treatment surely plays a powerful role in restoring the individual to wholeness. Such

a remedy is not always possible or immediate, however, nor are the experiential impacts of healthcare always benign.

While the concept of *iatrogenic disease* (disease caused by medical intervention) is well known, there is also the possibility of *iatrogenic illness*. Many of the experiential dis-integrations associated with illness can also be brought about or exacerbated by the process of medical treatment. When illness fragments the body into problematic parts and functions, and renders it alien to the self, the process is often intensified in the doctor's office. The physician has the patient disrobe, probes and palpates different organs, investigating the body as if it were a malfunctioning machine, and the patient learns to internalize an objectifying gaze on the body.

Similarly, treatment can exacerbate the disruption of space, time, and social relations. Hospitalization provides a vivid example. One's clothes, a mark of personal identity, are replaced by a hospital gown embarrassingly open at the back. One is dislocated from the routines of everyday life, leaving friends, family, home, and community for a world of strange rules and protocols, frightening technologies, and authorities who loom and disappear. Just when one's world most needs shoring up, it is further fragmented.

Medical language also effects subtle but pervasive displacements. Struggling to make existential sense of what is happening and why, the patient may find little help in diagnostic labels. In Tolstoy's story "The Death of Ivan Ilych," Ivan grapples with the profound issue of his life and death, but for the doctor, "the real question was to decide between a floating kidney, chronic catarrh, or appendicitis" (Tolstoy, p. 121). This exclusive focus on disease leaves the illness unaddressed. Loneliness is intensified when one most needs communion; the search for meaning is truncated by a heap of scientific words.

Some of these deficiencies so characteristic of contemporary medicine emerge from its basis in a mechanistic worldview. The seventeenth-century philosopher René Descartes, who helped lay the groundwork of modern science and medicine, took a dualist position. The human being, he argued, is a conjunction of two very different parts—the mind, imbued with rationality and free will, and the body, a mechanism governed by the same physical laws as the rest of nature. In this view, bodily disease can be understood according to the model of machine breakdown. Doctors become scientists or technicians who fix or replace broken parts. This Cartesian paradigm has generated the search for precision drugs and surgical procedures, the emphasis on scientific (rather than humanistic) training for the physician, and the hospital conceived as a temple to technology. Much of the efficacy of modern medicine rests on its dualist and mechanist foundations. But this focus on the body-as-machine has also led to a neglect of the ill person struggling with profound existential dislocations (Leder, 1992).

Nonetheless, many sensitive clinicians do seek to be healers of illness. To "heal" is to begin reweaving into wholeness the tapestry of life shredded by illness. Even when disease is not curable, the practitioner can try to relieve pain and preserve physical function, explain what is happening within the patient's body, and encourage the patient to be an active participant in treatment. Thus, the ill person regains a measure of knowledge and control.

Cut off from others by the privacy of pain and the loss of function, the sick person may reach out to the provider with the longing of a shipwrecked castaway who spies a sail on the horizon. When the patient is permitted to tell his or her story—to voice fears, ask questions, and hear genuine responses—a social reconnection is forged. The practitioner furthers this process by informing and mobilizing the patient's support system. The participation of family and friends is welcomed, and isolating modes of treatment such as hospitalization can, when possible, be avoided.

Just as the body seeks to heal itself, so individuals seek an interpretive healing by trying to make sense of what has occurred (Kleinman) and telling stories about it (Frank, 1995). Anne Hawkins has studied written accounts of illness and charted out the mythic motifs the sick often use. People suffering from disease may see themselves in an heroic struggle against a dangerous foe, or as journeying to the underworld to retrieve a great prize. These myths can sometimes turn disabling, however. For example, the battle metaphor provides little guidance or solace when the disease finally emerges as the victor. Susan Sontag, in *Illness as Metaphor* (1990) focuses on such dangers of understanding disease metaphorically, suggesting that the practitioner may need to challenge a patient's unhelpful fantasy. But these mythic interpretations can also play a healing role, helping the ill person to render events coherent, to rise to the occasion, and to work creatively with the challenges faced (Hawkins). The practitioner who resists the temptation to rely on reductionist "medicalese" or on metaphors foreign to the needs of the patient can support the patient's own healing narrative.

Ultimately, healing is not just a reconstruction of a prior life, but the building of something new. Through illness people often develop a deeper compassion for others, a greater intimacy with loved ones, an attentiveness to the joys of ordinary living, or a reordering of lifestyle and priorities. It is not unusual to hear a patient say "This cancer [or heart attack, etc.] is the best thing that could have happened to me." For such people, illness is not the diametrical opposite of health. Rather, it is the first stage on a healing journey, summoning the person to needed changes, whether physical, emotional, social, or spiritual.

The suggestion that illness can be a grace is not a license to grow callous to the suffering involved, however. Few seriously ill people wish to be told, "Cheer up, this disease is great for you." But the patient and practitioner alike can remain open to the healing gifts that illness may bring, albeit wrapped in a dark package.

Bioethical Implications

The illness experience has implications not only for clinical practice but for the field of bioethics. Bioethical reflections need not be *top-down* starting from overarching theories and principles that then are applied to cases. They can be *bottom-up* commencing with the concrete situation of the ill and drawing out the needs and moral claims that follow. Indeed, some suggest that bioethics is undergoing a paradigm shift, with a new openness toward methodologies that pay close attention to the experiences of illness and caregiving (DuBose et al.; Welie). Several consequences might ensue for the field.

First, taking lived experience more seriously may shed new light on the traditional issues of bioethics. For example, *truth-telling* and *informed consent* are often supported by reference to a Kantian framework of "respect for persons." Within this framework, emphasis is placed on preserving the individual's autonomy. However, when moving from this abstraction to the concrete situation of the ill, new features come into view. It is not simply the *autonomous individual* of ethical theory who arrives at the doctor's office in pain. By this time the person's sense of lived autonomy may already be compromised by uncertainty and confusion, emotional turmoil, a threatened future, and a body run amok. In this light, informed consent becomes not simply a way to preserve autonomy prior to treatment; it also becomes a part of the treatment itself, restoring autonomy through enhancing the patient's knowledge, control, and trust in others.

Of course, much depends on how the *truth* is conveyed. Medical jargon that sets forth *the facts of the case* can actually disempower the ill person. As with Ivan Ilych's doctor, the physician's terms may obliterate the patient's narrative. Moreover, the theater in which this conversation is enacted is the physician's domain. He or she is in a position of power, with privileged knowledge, authority, and professional status (Zaner, 1988). To really understand informed consent these inequalities of power that define the doctor-patient encounter must be understood. In such ways, paying close attention to the experience of health and illness could reshape the current approach to traditional issues of bioethics—including those of organ transplantation, abortion, the termination of life-support, and many others (Toombs, 2001).

At the same time, an experience-based bioethics might call attention to other issues that have hitherto been neglected. Bioethical discourse has typically focused on particular quandaries brought about by new technologies and conflicting moral intuitions. When should one "pull the plug"? Who has the right to refuse treatment? When can confidentiality be breached? While such issues are real, they often leave unquestioned the general context of medical practice, as if only special dilemmas call for bioethical thought. But the experience of illness and treatment is intrinsically a moral theater. The ill person is confronted with the dis-integration of his or her world and must grapple to restore "the good" or forge a new vision of it. The individuals and institutions involved in healthcare participate in this drama in myriad ways—the language used, the texture of personal relations, the fees exacted, and the structuring of space and time all have ethical significance.

One promising topic for an experience-based bioethics is thus the *moral ecology* of healthcare institutions. One example is George Agich's 1993 study of long-term care, which details how the lived experience of autonomy is enhanced or diminished by environmental patterns. Are schedules set for the convenience of a nursing home bureaucracy, or are the client's needs kept in mind? Are there spatial cues to orient the elderly resident, or does the layout of the home contribute to confusion, powerlessness, and isolation? Is infantilizing baby talk the everyday language, or is there an atmosphere that enhances dignity? Such issues are not as dramatic as those that make bioethics headlines, but they are at least as significant to the lives of many. One can imagine the day when institutional ethics committees attend to such issues of moral ecology, not simply the exceptional-quandary cases.

An experience-based bioethics would also look at the burden placed upon the individual practitioner by the special situation of the ill. This is not just a matter of "What action do I take?" (the focus of deontological and utilitarian ethics), but of "What kind of person should I, the caregiver, be?" (the focus of virtue ethics). The isolation and incapacity of the ill underscore the importance of needed virtues in the practitioner, such as compassion and trustworthiness (Pellegrino and Thomasma).

An experience-based bioethics also demonstrates that it is not simply the practitioner who is a moral actor, but also the ill person (Zaner, 1993). Though defined as *patient*, he or she is also an agent wrestling with a profound existential challenge (May) as described in illness narratives (Broyard;

Price). In the face of the dis-integrations described above, the sick person cannot evade responsibility, literally the ability to respond to circumstances. Depending upon the qualities of this response, the individual can either forge a good life even in the face of suffering or yield in to bitterness and despair. Special virtues are called for in meeting the challenge of illness, including courage, patience, hope, humility, and proper assertiveness. Sickness is an arena that calls people to test and reforge who they really are and who they wish to be. For too long the ill person as agent has been absent from bioethical reflection, and from much of clinical practice. Close attention to the illness experience can help remedy this situation.

DREW LEDER (1995)
REVISED BY AUTHOR

SEE ALSO: *African Religions; AIDS; Alcoholism; Anthropology and Bioethics; Bioethics, African-American Perspectives; Care; Compassionate Love; Epidemics; Family and Family Medicine; Genetics and Racial Minorities; Grief and Bereavement; Healthcare Systems; Human Dignity; Informed Consent; Life, Quality of; Mental Illness; Narrative; Patients' Responsibilities;* and other *Health and Disease* subentries

BIBLIOGRAPHY

Agich, George J. 1993. *Autonomy and Long-Term Care.* New York: Oxford University Press.

Baron, Richard J. 1985. "An Introduction to Medical Phenomenology: I Can't Hear You While I'm Listening." *Annals of Internal Medicine* 103(4): 606–611.

Berg, Jan Hendrik van den. 1966. *The Psychology of the Sickbed.* Pittsburgh: Duquesne University Press.

Brison, Susan J. 1993. "Surviving Sexual Violence: A Philosophical Perspective." *Journal of Social Philosophy* 24(1): 5–22.

Brody, Howard. 1987. *Stories of Sickness.* New Haven, CT: Yale University Press.

Broyard, Anatole. 1992. *Intoxicated by My Illness and Other Writings on Life and Death.* New York: Fawcett Columbine.

Cassell, Eric J. 1985. *The Healer's Art.* Cambridge, MA: MIT Press.

Cassell, Eric J. 1991. *The Nature of Suffering and the Goals of Medicine.* New York: Oxford University Press.

DuBose, Edwin R.; Hamel, Ronald P.; and O'Connell, Laurence J., eds. 1994. *A Matter of Principles? Ferment in U.S. Bioethics.* Valley Forge, PA: Trinity Press International.

Engelhardt, H. Tristram, Jr. 1982. "Illnesses, Diseases, and Sicknesses." In *The Humanity of the Ill: Phenomenological Perspectives,* ed. Victor Kestenbaum. Knoxville: University of Tennessee Press.

Engelhardt, H. Tristram, Jr. 1986. *The Foundations of Bioethics.* New York: Oxford University Press.

Foucault, Michel. 1973. *The Birth of the Clinic,* tr. Alan M. Sheridan Smith. New York: Vintage.

Frank, Arthur. 1991. *At the Will of the Body: Reflections on Illness.* Boston: Houghton Mifflin.

Frank, Arthur. 1995. *The Wounded Storyteller: Body, Illness, and Ethics.* Chicago: University of Chicago Press.

Hawkins, Anne Hunsaker. 1993. *Reconstructing Illness: Studies in Pathography.* West Lafayette, IN: Purdue University Press.

Heidegger, Martin. 1962. *Being and Time,* tr. John Macquarrie and Edward Robinson. San Francisco: Harper San Francisco.

Hull, John M. 1990. *Touching the Rock: An Experience of Blindness.* New York: Pantheon Books.

Kane, Jeff. 2001. *The Healing Companion: Simple and Effective Ways Your Presence Can Help People Heal.* San Francisco: Harper San Francisco.

Kleinman, Arthur. 1988. *The Illness Narratives: Suffering, Healing and the Human Condition.* New York: Basic Books.

Kopelman, Loretta M. 1988. "The Punishment Concept of Disease." In *AIDS: Ethics and Public Policy,* ed. Christine Pierce and Donald Van DeVeer. Belmont, CA: Wadsworth.

Leder, Drew. 1990. *The Absent Body.* Chicago: University of Chicago Press.

Leder, Drew. 1992. "A Tale of Two Bodies: The Cartesian Corpse and the Lived Body." In *The Body in Medical Thought and Practice,* ed. Drew Leder. Dordrecht, Netherlands: Kluwer.

May, William F. 1991. *The Patient's Ordeal.* Bloomington: Indiana University Press.

Merleau-Ponty, Maurice. 1962. *Phenomenology of Perception,* tr. Colin Smith. London: Routledge.

Michalko, Rod. 2002. *The Difference that Disability Makes.* Philadelphia: Temple University Press.

Pellegrino, Edmund D., and Thomasma, David C. 1993. *The Virtues in Medical Practice.* New York: Oxford University Press.

Price, Reynolds. 1994. *A Whole New Life.* New York: Atheneum.

Robillard, Albert B. 1999. *Meaning of a Disability: The Lived Experience of Paralysis.* Philadelphia: Temple University Press.

Sacks, Oliver W. 1985. *The Man Who Mistook His Wife for a Hat, and Other Clinical Tales.* New York: Summit.

Scarry, Elaine. 1985. *The Body in Pain: The Making and Unmaking of the World.* New York: Oxford University Press.

Sontag, Susan. 1990. *Illness as Metaphor; and, AIDS and Its Metaphors.* New York: Anchor.

Straus, Erwin W. M. 1963. *The Primary World of Senses: A Vindication of Sensory Experience,* tr. Jacob Needleman. New York: Free Press.

Straus, Erwin W. M. 1966. *Phenomenological Psychology: The Selected Papers of Erwin M. Straus,* tr. in part by Erling Eng. New York: Basic Books.

Svenaeus, Fredrik. 2000. *The Hermeneutics of Medicine and the Phenomenology of Health: Steps Towards a Philosophy of Medical Practice.* Dordrecht, Netherlands: Kluwer.

Tolstoy, Leo. 1960. *The Death of Ivan Ilych, and Other Stories.* New York: New American Library.

Toombs, S. Kay. 1992a. "The Body in Multiple Sclerosis: A Patient's Perspective." In *The Body in Medical Thought and Practice,* ed. Drew Leder. Dordrecht, Netherlands: Kluwer.

Toombs, S. Kay. 1992b. *The Meaning of Illness: A Phenomenological Account of the Different Perspectives of Physician and Patient.* Dordrecht, Netherlands: Kluwer.

Toombs, S. Kay, ed. 2001. *Handbook of Phenomenology and Medicine.* Dordrecht, Netherlands: Kluwer.

Toombs, S. Kay; Barnard, David; and Carson, Ronald A., eds. 1995. *Chronic Illness: From Experience to Policy.* Bloomington: Indiana University Press.

Welie, Jos V. M. 1998. *In the Face of Suffering: The Philosophical-Anthropological Foundations of Clinical Ethics.* Omaha, NE: Creighton University Press.

Zaner, Richard M. 1981. *The Context of Self: A Phenomenological Inquiry Using Medicine as a Clue.* Athens: Ohio University Press.

Zaner, Richard M. 1988. *Ethics and the Clinical Encounter.* Englewood Cliffs, NJ: Prentice Hall.

Zaner, Richard M. 1993. *Troubled Voices: Stories of Ethics and Illness.* Cleveland: The Pilgrim Press.

HEALTHCARE INSTITUTIONS

• • •

Healthcare institutions are often overlooked in discussions of healthcare policy, biomedical ethics, and the allocation of resources. Institutions, however, are major players within the ethical and policy arena of healthcare and should be considered when one examines the forces at work in any specific issue in healthcare.

A healthcare institution usually has been thought of as a hospital, a nursing home, a rehabilitation facility, or another such single-site entity. Such an institution consists of the human beings who work in many different capacities within it, the leaders who direct and manage it, and its governing body—usually a board of directors or board of trustees that is responsible for hiring (and firing) the chief executive officer (CEO) or president of the institution and for setting policy and direction in partnership with the employed leaders. Many institutions now, however, are much larger than a single facility. For example, there are integrated hospital healthcare networks that include everything from physician group practices to long-term-care facilities. There are also networks that provide a single level of care, such as nursing home chains and hospital chains. As the competitive environment of healthcare continues to drive efforts to reduce costs and capture market share, institutions made up of multiple components will become increasingly more common. Nonetheless, whether institutions are single units or made up of multiple units, they have important characteristics in common that must be considered.

Institutional Missions

One of the most important functions of leadership and governance in an institution is to establish and articulate that institution's mission. This is usually written in a mission statement. An academic health center may have a mission that includes research, education, and patient care as equally strong components. A community hospital may point to excellent patient care and improvement of community health as its mission. A for-profit hospital or hospital chain may articulate excellent patient care and optimal return to shareholders as its mission. As one can imagine, this latter bipartite mission can lead to troubling conflicts of interest, which have been examined by ethicists in some detail (Gray).

The mission of an institution may also be articulated in the framework of its membership in a larger institution such as a church or religious network. Thus, some Catholic hospitals provide care to a large number of American patients (who are not necessarily Catholic), and their mission specifically derives from values espoused by the Catholic Church. Similarly, many other hospitals have emerged from religious systems because of the latter's commitment to helping the vulnerable and caring for the sick and suffering. Institutional missions may sometimes conflict with bedside ethical decisions, such as the decision to forgo life-sustaining therapy or to have an elective abortion. In these settings it is important for patients and providers alike to be clear about the underlying moral environment of the institution and the degree to which it may or may not be flexible on certain issues. Patients who feel strongly that they do not want care with those articulated standards should then have access to other institutions. Besides the question of abortion, the issue of forgoing life-sustaining treatment has been one of the most prominent in this kind of conflict. For example, the member of the patient's family who makes a decision about discontinuing nutrition and hydration in a comatose or unresponsive patient with far advanced dementing illness may find that the institution housing that patient does not allow nutrition and hydration to be withdrawn. If the underlying reason is fear of malpractice or liability concerns, it is sometimes possible for the institution to figure out a way to work together with and respect the wishes of the patient and family. If, however, the underlying reason is a moral or

religious belief consistent with the underlying values of the governance of this institution, then it is less likely that a compromise can occur (Miles, Sinder, and Siegler).

Value Systems

To generalize about these many and varied institutions—both secular and religious, for-profit and not-for-profit—is not a simple matter, but it is useful to explore certain issues relating to the value systems that undergird their several missions and roles in society. Many of the older institutions were launched on the bedrock principle of simply caring for the sick and suffering, and many in the public still, quite unrealistically, think of all healthcare institutions in this way. Because the United States as a nation has not yet realized the right of equal access to healthcare for all its citizens and embraced the concept of healthcare as a social good, there is no consistent underlying covenant between the society and these institutions. A social covenant would lead to some kind of centralized planning for healthcare needs, and institutional missions would flow from this. Instead, the United States relies on marketplace values combined with a variable and often unreliable "safety net" of public institutions. It has proven to be very difficult for any of these institutions to live up to their traditional charitable-based institutional values and at the same time survive the economic and social realities of U.S. culture. The one shared ethical principle that all would espouse is the commitment to competence and excellence, values that have permeated Western medicine through its physicians since the time of the Greek physician Hippocrates (c. 460–c. 377 B.C.E.). This principle is not purely altruistic, however, because a minimum of quality is required for accreditation, and because evidence of excellent quality gives some institutions a market edge in attracting paying patients.

The public institutions created by a county, city, or state for the purpose of delivering health services to a specific population have an unambiguous mission and foundational institutional ethic: to carry out the function for which they were created and for which they continue to receive operating funds from the public sector. The objective of these institutions is to provide care in an appropriate and highly competent fashion to the specified population, usually those who are poor and without access to other sources of care. Whereas, on paper, the goals and objectives of these institutions never change, the public's commitment wavers from year to year, with the obvious result that there is considerable variation in the level of financial support the public is willing to provide; serious underfunding for many public hospitals thus significantly compromises the quality of care in many places. So there remains the paradox, despite an unambiguously consistent mission statement: Compromised public commitment to provide services for the poor has translated to a serious loss of quality in some of these institutions. The profit motive seldom creates an untoward tension among workers at these institutions; the limits imposed by funding sources may, however, lead to the curtailing or closing of certain expensive services, perhaps to the detriment of the patients.

The private, not-for-profit institutions that were established for the purpose of serving the community may share a public-service vision with the public hospitals. Private, not-for-profit hospitals also, however, experience extreme pressures that run counter to their community-service mission. In the United States, since the early 1980s, these institutions have often thrived financially by maximizing income from insurance and philanthropy, both of which have supported the enormous growth of specialty medicine and heroic high-technology care. Governed by boards of directors made up of citizens of the community, these institutions can be expected to have an awareness of community needs. On the other hand, the charity care these hospitals may provide generally must be paid for in one of two ways: (1) by using available reserve funds, or (2) by shifting costs, overcharging those who can pay more, in order to make up for the losses in primary care, chronic care, and general care for the poor or uninsured.

The CEOs of the larger of these hospitals, especially those at the more prominent academic and tertiary-care institutions, are treated and paid as though they were corporate executives. This trend toward providing top-level management for these institutions came from the growing awareness beginning in the early 1970s that these institutions were administratively out of control or at the very least generally ill-prepared to fulfill their potential in a volatile marketplace. Few would argue that the majority of these institutions have become heavily bottom-line oriented. Balancing cross-subsidization among the various payers with issues of access for the poor is a fine art. Many of these hospitals, though losing money on every Medicaid and uninsured patient, manage to produce an overall surplus. They do this by increasing the volume of high-paying expensive procedures on insured patients. This goes far afield from a care mission of investing in prevention to foster healthier populations. Positive bottom lines are often then used to implement programs aimed at increasing "market share" for the hospital, rather than increasing services for the most needy.

Some not-for-profit institutions have extraordinarily idealistic community-service orientations, expressed through their written missions and goals. These orientations have sometimes become so consumed by the direction provided by bottom-line oriented, high-priced management teams that a variety of less-desirable and short-sighted practices have been implemented to produce a positive bottom line. These include the following:

(1) salary incentives to unit managers based primarily upon the financial performance of their cost centers;

(2) high-tech and manpower investment strategies determined primarily by their potential for high earnings;

(3) transfer policies that favor keeping patients whose care will add to the bottom line ("cream-skimming");

(4) policies to reduce existing teaching programs because of uncompensated expenses and negative impacts upon marketing strategies designed to reach more desirable clienteles; and

(5) different patterns of care based on whether or not patients possess ample insurance coverage or other financial resources.

Whether or not one finds these practices appropriate or inappropriate, whether they are more or less typical of not-for-profit as compared with for-profit institutions, the main lesson from these examples is that the pressures and forces inherent in the competitive market-oriented environment that has become dominant since the early 1980s have served to overtake the charitable values and philosophies that were central to the creation of many of these institutions. There is a tendency for healthcare institutions to believe that they are involved in a competitive fight for survival, and they all, in various ways, try to combine that pressure as best they can with the imperative to serve the sick.

Even institutions sponsored by religious organizations charge paying patients more than cost in order to cover the costs of nonpaying patients. Financial stability is the key to survival and thus to carrying out an altruistic mission. It is therefore more realistic to stop envisioning Saint Francis of Assisi when thinking about not-for-profit hospitals and begin thinking instead of "Saint Robin of Hood," robbing the rich to care for the poor.

Most observers see this behavior less as human frailty than as a system failure, the result of an environment that is filled with perverse incentives. In their detailed analysis of the ethics of for-profit as compared to not-for-profit healthcare institutions published in 1986, Dan W. Brock and Allen Buchanan concluded that there are no rationally compelling grounds upon which to find ethical fault with the profit motive in healthcare under the ground rules by which U.S. society now operates. Improvements can come only when the ground rules and societal expectations are altered; it is not enough simply to hope that institutions will take the lead in changing their behavior, in the face of existing incentives to the contrary.

Governance

The role of governance is very important in the character of institutions. In many healthcare institutions, including those in the not-for-profit sector, the board of trustees may be made up largely of prominent businesspeople with a great deal of experience in running large and successful businesses, as well as otherwise wealthy and influential members of the local social circle who may themselves be important philanthropic supporters of the hospital and able to draw others into making major donations. Thus, it is often a minority of individuals on the board who have direct experience with healthcare, such as physicians or nurses, or whose major concerns are with education or research. Therefore it is not surprising that as healthcare has become a trillion-dollar business in the United States, even not-for-profit hospitals and health systems have looked at the bottom line as a marker of how well they are doing. Even though there are no shareholders to pay, an excess of revenue over expenses allows a nonprofit institution to initiate new programs and, in many cases, to salt away substantial reserves that both provide interest income and allow for a cushion in case of adversity.

Because so much money is involved and because of the business orientation of much of hospital governance, it is not surprising that the investments in new programs or the capital investments that are made when excess funds are available are not always, or even primarily, directed toward care of the poor and underserved but are often directed toward ensuring a continuing stream of revenue for the hospital. This usually means investing in additional high-technology medical care that will be marketed to insured patients. For this reason it is not hard to see why the Internal Revenue Service in recent years has begun to ask whether the not-for-profit hospital sector really ought to remain tax exempt. In order to maintain their tax exemption, these institutions must demonstrate that they are community-service organizations and that the educational research missions remain important to them, if not central.

Pressures for Change

In their comprehensive 1986 treatise, Brock and Buchanan made an important distinction between for-profit chains, generally owned by investors and listed on a stock exchange,

and individual for-profit institutions, usually owned by an individual or small group of individuals (frequently physicians from the community). These organizational differences create different incentives and different institutional behavioral responses. In this entry it is the latter subset of for-profit institutions that are of interest, but this in no way ameliorates the validity of these conclusions. The thrust toward identifying healthcare as a commodity distributed according to business rules has, since the early 1980s, been the overwhelming ethical reality for private and not-for-profit private institutions. All of these factors have fueled the debate about the appropriateness of maintaining the tax-free status of not-for-profit hospitals (Gray). If the societal pendulum swings back toward the treatment of healthcare as a right, alterations in institutional behavior may occur that, nevertheless, need not drive the individual for-profit institution out of business.

It is probable that the implementation of national and regional policy decisions about healthcare (such as the trend toward capitation, community rating of insurance, universal access to care, and regional databases capable of rendering comparative institutional quality-of-care estimates) will have more to do with affecting the behavior of these independent institutions than anything else. The most far-reaching impact may result from the pressure on these institutions to join effective consortia or networks of healthcare providers; they may well need to become part of an organized delivery system in order to survive. Thus, by around the year 2005, the number of independent institutions may be severely reduced. Certainly, one already sees a trend in the direction of independents moving into organized systems, not only in the hospital industry but also in the traditionally "Mom and Pop" nursing home arena.

A wide variety of individually governed institutions play a wide variety of roles in the inchoate patchwork quilt of healthcare delivery in the United States. As the forces for systemic reform build, it seems clear that they will have a predominant influence on alterations in the behavior of these various entities. Until such changes occur, one can conclude that this independent sector will in general deliver the best healthcare it can under the vagaries of access, quality, and cost that are in general dictated by the perverse organizational and fiscal incentives created by U.S. society. As a result of a wise reform movement, one can hope for an improved, more equitable, and more uniform performance from this sector of the healthcare distribution system.

Future Trends

In an article in the December 5, 2001, *New York Times,* Milton Freudenheim reported that most of America's largest insurers of healthcare are moving toward insurance design that increases segmentation of the private insurance market, with the sickest having to bear more of the costs while the well will be able to get coverage more inexpensively. This gives further impetus to the movement of employers to defined contribution for health insurance and the growth of high-deductible plans, leaving workers to decide for themselves how much to add from their own sources to acquire coverage. While framed as "choice," this leads to higher costs for patients, especially for the chronically ill or genetically at risk.

All this leads Victor Fuchs (2002) to join others in predicting that there will be a reemergence of interest in social insurance and a national insurance program, essentially because of the inequity and unfairness of what the employment-based system will have become.

At this point, it is safe to assume that healthcare institutions in the United States are caught in a continuing confluence of marketplace forces churning against strong ethical and social currents. Until this ambiguous situation is resolved, it is hard to predict the future for these institutions, but it is clearly more and more difficult for institutions such as hospitals and healthcare systems to be moral leaders.

ROGER J. BULGER
CHRISTINE K. CASSEL (1995)
REVISED BY AUTHORS

SEE ALSO: *Healthcare Resources, Allocation Of; Healthcare Systems; Hospital, Modern History of the; Long-Term Care; Mergers and Acquisitions; Privacy in Healthcare*

BIBLIOGRAPHY

Brock, Dan W., and Buchanan, Allen. 1986. "Ethical Issues in For-Profit Health Care." In *For-Profit Enterprise in Health Care,* ed. Bradford H. Gray. Washington, D.C.: National Academy Press.

Brock, Dan W., and Buchanan, Allen. 1987. "The Profit Motive in Medicine." *Journal of Medicine and Philosophy* 12(1): 1–35.

Bulger, Roger J.; Osterweis, Marian; and Rubin, Elaine R. 1999. *Mission Management: A New Synthesis.* Washington, D.C.: Association of Academic Health Centers.

Devers, Kelly; Brewster, Linda R.; and Casalino, Lawrence P. 2003. "Changes in Hospital Competitive Strategy: A New Medical Arms Race?" *Health Services Research* 38(1): 447–469.

Freudenheim, Milton. 2001. "A New Health Plan May Raise Expenses for Sickest Workers." *New York Times,* December 5. p. A1.

Fuchs, Victor. 2002. "What's Ahead for Health Insurance in the United States." *New England Journal of Medicine* 346(23): 1822–1824.

Gray, Bradford H. 1991. *The Profit Motive and Patient Care: The Changing Accountability of Doctors and Hospitals.* Cambridge, MA: Harvard University Press.

Lesser, Cara S.; Ginsburg, Paul B.; and Devers, Kelly. 2003. "The End of an Era: What Became of the Managed Care Revolution in 2001?" *Health Services Research* 38(1): 337–355.

Miles, Steven H.; Sinder, Peter A.; and Siegler, Mark. 1989. "Conflict between Patients' Wishes to Forgo Treatment and the Policies of Health Care Facilities." *New England Journal of Medicine* 321(1): 48–50.

Rubin, Elaine R., and Lindeman, Lisa M. 2003. *Perspectives 2003.* Washington, D.C.: Association of Academic Health Centers.

Rubin, Elaine R., and Lindeman, Lisa M., eds. 2002. *The Nexus of Research and Business.* Washington, D.C.: Association of Academic Health Centers.

Task Force on Academic Health Centers. 2003. *Envisioning the Future of Academic Health Centers.* New York: Commonwealth Fund.

White, Kerr L., and Connelly, Julian E., eds. 1992. *The Medical Schools' Mission and the Population's Health.* New York: Springer-Verlag.

HEALTHCARE PROFESSIONALS, LEGAL REGULATION OF

• • •

Licensure is "the process by which an agency of government grants permission to persons meeting predetermined qualifications to engage in a given occupation"; certification is "the process by which a nongovernmental agency or association grants recognition to an individual who has met certain predetermined qualifications specified by that agency or institution" (Welch, p. 179). The purpose of licensure, regulation, and discipline is to protect the public at large; the assumption that grounds these practices is that governmental and nongovernmental institutions are competent to judge how such protection should be accomplished.

Background

Public efforts to regulate the health professions, especially by imposing restrictions on those who shall be allowed to practice them, go back to the Babylonian emperor Hammurabi (d. 1750 B.C.E.). Rules for medical practice existed in ancient Greece and tenth-century Baghdad. By the Middle Ages in Europe, it was customary for civil powers to demand a university education, examination, and experience as conditions for permission to practice medicine. In this period the first professional societies were founded, modeled on the merchant guilds (Gross). University and guild combined to link education to licensing—government permission to practice.

The first licensing statutes were passed in the American colonies in the seventeenth century, although not until the eighteenth century did the statutes seek to restrict practice. According to Eliot Freidson (1970), medicine did not emerge as a consulting, as opposed to a teaching, practice until the late nineteenth and early twentieth centuries. Throughout the two millennia since the time of the Greek physician Hippocrates (c. 460–c. 377 B.C.E.), the medical elite created by education and licensed by the state was supplemented by a vast number of unlicensed healers, mostly women (generally barred from medicine), who treated the common folk.

The trend to state regulation, endorsement, and protection of the health professions suffered a brief hiatus in the nineteenth century in the United States, when there arose a deliberate experiment in egalitarian deregulation following from a democratic belief that the common folk were as good as the educated elite in most matters. The experiment was abandoned later in the century, as Texas passed a medical practice act in 1873 and California followed suit two years later; by 1905, thirty-nine states licensed physicians (CSG). Nurses formed a national professional association in 1896; by 1926 forty states required licenses of nurses.

The trend is not, however, universal. Professional recruitment, standard setting, and discipline can be carried out by professional groups and associations without the protection of the state. Typically, groups of serious practitioners band together, agree to set standards, and develop informal review procedures for adherence to standards—for members only. Professional ethics and oaths, including professional standards of education and compensation, can be enforced by the professional association alone, and in some cases (various psychological and holistic health professions, for example) the process goes no further. In several healing professions, there is no regulation beyond that of the voluntary association; the only penalty for professional wrongdoing, if it is discovered, is loss of membership in that association.

Regulation tends to be reserved for those health professions that are widely perceived to have powers the abuse of which can lead to public injury. At one time, only the profession of medicine was included in that category; now it has extended through dentistry, nursing, pharmacy, and others (close to fifty, on one count; CSG/CLEAR), on a state-by-state basis (naturopathy, for instance, is regulated in some states but not in others). Licensure varies in kind as well as in range: As of 1973, nine states still had *permissive* licensing for nurses—an unlicensed nurse could practice without hindrance as long as she did not claim to be licensed. *Scope-of-practice statutes* ordinarily accompany licensure, defining the procedures for which the practitioner is licensed.

The Limited Competence of the State

Well established as the custom is, there is a certain awkwardness of fit between professional standards and state enforcement. The request by the health professions for state protection of their monopoly is certainly plausible. While the state can play little part in instructing or defining the work of the professions, it certainly has always had as part of its police power the protection of the public from outright dangers to health, including health frauds—quacks, charlatans, and sincere professionals whose education was simply inadequate to their tasks (*Dent v. State of West Virginia*, 1889). But a profession is defined in large part by its esoteric knowledge: Only professionals can set professional standards, determine when they have been violated, and, by extension, determine the sanction that would be appropriate as a punishment.

The result is that the public ends up enforcing rules that only a private association can set, presumably for its own benefit as much as for the public good. Nor is it clear that licensing in general, especially in the context of rigid scope-of-practice statutes, is in the public interest. The costs of licensing will normally be passed along to the consumer in the form of higher costs, and the license requirement restricts entry into the profession to those who can afford the initial outlay. The scope-of-practice acts make sure that auxiliary professions, with less expensive preparation and lower fees, cannot perform certain procedures that they may in fact be perfectly competent to perform (CSG/CLEAR). Built into the arrangement, if it is to be tolerable, is a strong presumption of altruism on the part of the professional and trust on the part of the public. Let either fail, and the system is in danger.

Professional Exclusion: The Flexner Report

In 1906 Abraham Flexner, an educator, obtained a grant from the Carnegie Foundation for the Advancement of Teaching to review the quality of medical schools. When his report was published in 1910, it revealed wide discrepancies among the 155 schools studied and produced a strong impetus to regulate medical education at the state and federal levels. Having no independent standards of their own, nor any idea of how to develop them, the states appealed to the American Medical Association's (AMA) Council on Medical Education, which set new standards for accreditation of the medical schools. Physicians also staffed the state licensing boards. The consequence of this major public intervention in the healthcare professions was that by the mid-1920s the AMA had a virtual monopoly, guarding the gate to the medical profession at several levels: admission to medical school, choice of specialty, and obtaining a license to practice.

Such a state-sponsored monopoly is clearly subject to abuse, but it was widely imitated as succeeding levels of health professions sought and obtained state endorsement and protection. By tradition, the major regulatory role in the United States is played by the states, and the licensing laws are typically administered by state agencies and boards dominated by professionals.

Disciplinary Procedures

Disciplinary procedures responding to charges of fraud, incompetence, or malpractice occur at several levels. A certain amount of discipline is carried out by the professional association and is entirely a private matter among the professionals. At the state level, the procedure for disciplining delinquent practitioners varies, but generally it requires that some aggrieved party—a dissatisfied patient, a cost-conscious insurance company, or the plaintiff's lawyer in a malpractice case—register a complaint with the disciplinary board of the state. The agency in charge of these matters will investigate the case, assemble evidence, schedule a hearing, make a finding, and recommend appropriate action. Possible actions include dismissing the complaint, requiring some hours of community service, and removing a license. Increasingly, part of the decision is a refresher course in medical ethics.

The state medical boards are empowered to revoke a physician's license. Short of actual revocation of license, all actions taken against a professional are recorded and circulated through the National Practitioner Data Bank, where misconduct and malpractice findings are logged. The data bank is available to regulators in all fifty states. There are exceptions, but most health professions and practitioners are in the data bank.

Consumers' Protest

The federal government was active in the regulation of health matters for most of the twentieth century. The Pure Food and Drug Act, under which all drugs are approved for sale in the United States, was passed in 1906; since then the federal government has taken an active role in protecting occupational health and public accountability. Early in the 1970s, corresponding to the general wave of public skepticism regarding professional and corporate claims of authority and trustworthiness, a citizen/consumer rebellion turned on the health professions. Seminal works by Eliot Freidson and others spearheaded a literature of public protest against professional privilege and urged vigorous and vigilant oversight of the health professions, medicine in particular.

The protest tended to portray state legislatures as weak, ignorant, or pawns of the powerful professions and urged a drastic widening of the federal oversight function. Such expansion was made possible by the passage of Medicare legislation (1965), followed by Medicaid and other programs that cast the federal government in the role of major funder of healthcare. In a 1976 report titled *A Proposal for Credentialing Health Manpower,* the U.S. Public Health Service recommended that a national certification commission be established "to develop, evaluate and oversee national standards" for agencies that certify healthcare personnel. The National Commission for Health Certifying Agencies was formed on that recommendation, charged with developing universal standards for credentialing healthcare personnel. This effort was supported through the 1980s by the U.S. Department of Health and Human Services, through the Health Resources and Services Administration (CSG/CLEAR).

The origins of consumerism are generally attributed to Ralph Nader, whose investigations of the safety of the American automobile alerted a generation to the possibility that the goods and services available from the trusted providers of the American marketplace might not be as good as advertised. A Nader offshoot, Public Citizen's Health Research Group, maintains that the disciplinary and regulatory powers and laws currently available to the American public are completely inadequate to the task. These groups have changed the broad direction of legislative action. In the era of consumerism, the people's authority exercised at the state or federal level now protects the consuming public from the professional provider instead of aligning itself with the professional against fraudulent competition.

In a return to the democratic assumptions of the nineteenth century, the mantle of legal and moral credibility as protector of the public has passed from the profession to the elected legislature: In the areas of technical expertise and professional wisdom, as well as in the areas of economic self-interest, the American voters are now assumed to be the best guardians of their own interests. Patients' autonomy vis-à-vis their physicians has been generalized to public autonomy vis-à-vis the profession as a whole.

Typical of consumerist initiatives in healthcare is congressional action requiring nationwide licensing of nurses' aides. The bill was demanded by, among others, AARP, an interest group of older Americans with a strong stake in the conduct of nursing homes and chronic-care facilities. The passage of the legislation at the federal level (incorporated into the Omnibus Budget Reconciliation Act [OBRA] of 1987) made the law immune to the objections of state organizations of such facilities. Now the states must implement this law.

Also typical are the regulations proceeding from the work of the National Commission for the Protection of Human Subjects of Biomedical and Behavioral Research, established by Congress in the 1970s in response to claims that patients were being abused by their physicians in pursuit of scientific research (and that aborted fetuses were being used for research). The commission's work resulted in an immense number of federal regulations to protect the rights of human subjects of clinical research, including the formation of institutional review boards in any institution where such research is carried on, charged with reviewing all research that receives any federal money (in effect, all research in the institution).

A third example of such initiatives is the Patient Self-Determination Act, passed as part of the Omnibus Budget Reconciliation Act of 1990, which requires that healthcare providers inform adult inpatients of their rights to refuse treatment; to submit to the provider a document, generally known as a *living will,* specifying their desires regarding treatment or nontreatment should they become terminally ill and unable to give consent to treatment on their own; and to appoint any adult to speak for them to ensure that the living will's instructions are carried out, should they become unable to speak for themselves.

The contrast between profession-oriented and consumer-oriented approaches can be seen in the norms governing confidentiality of investigations of professionals charged with incompetence or negligence. If government is to protect the profession, then the identity of credentialed professionals who are under investigation for wrongdoing must be kept secret until it is determined that they are unsalvageable in the profession, so as to maintain their good name and practice. Consumer advocate groups, on the contrary, demand that the names of accused professionals be made public as soon as the investigation begins, so that the public can take steps to protect themselves.

Rejoinders to consumerism in healthcare have come from diverse sources. One very influential reply, from the perspective of the medical profession, is Charles L. Bosk's 1979 account of a surgical training program, *Forgive and Remember.* In the training of surgical residents, as chronicled by Bosk, supervision was strict, the patients' interests were paramount, and discipline was swift, although generally informal, and highly effective. Bosk found in place an unwritten but well-understood set of rules, rapidly internalized by all surgical residents as a condition of success as surgeons and regularly enforced at all levels. The suggestion that emerged, although not explicitly, was that bureaucratic regulations could not possibly be as effective as this method of professional socialization in producing successful surgeons—at least at the level of the elite practitioners. On the other side, libertarian theorists have attacked regulation of all kinds, formal or informal, arguing that any regulation puts an artificial and uneconomic barrier in the free market. The libertarians achieved major gains in the last decade of the twentieth century.

Alternatives to licensing can easily be imagined. In 1984 Stanley J. Gross outlined a system of state registration of unlicensed practitioners whose competence is determined by the consuming public on the basis of full disclosure of background and skills. Given full disclosure and the absence of coercion, on the principle of freedom of contract, any two persons of mature years should be free to make between themselves any contract for goods and services. The point is primarily theoretical but of very wide application: If accepted, this doctrine would abolish a few dozen federal agencies and all state licensing and disciplinary functions. Concretely, this doctrine has been invoked as primary in cases in which patients request drugs not approved for distribution or sale, such as laetrile and other unproven cancer remedies or experimental AIDS drugs, or marijuana for medicinal purposes.

The Unwanted Participant: Business and the Professions

In the last decade of the twentieth century and the first few years of the twenty-first, the whole philosophy of licensing and regulation of the healthcare professions has undergone a sea change. By 1990, there was a strongly felt undercurrent that healthcare was taking up too much of the national budget (13 percent, higher than any other developed nation) and that it was badly distributed. Often the poor in this rich country had only minimal access to healthcare: They could not afford private fees, they received no health benefits through their employment, and they fell somehow through the cracks of the government-sponsored programs, Medicare (federally funded, for the elderly and disabled) and Medicaid (state funded, for the poor.) In 1992 Bill Clinton was elected U.S. president, and aided by his wife, Hillary

Rodham Clinton, he set out to create a single-payer system, a national health insurance plan, to provide universal access to decent healthcare. Overwhelmed by special interests (especially the private insurance companies, who wanted to run the system themselves), the Clinton plan failed in 1994.

In the aftermath of this failure, major insurance companies took over payment arrangements for the practice of healthcare, under a confusingly diverse pattern of plans. Some insurance company plans simply employ physicians, or contract with physicians' group practices, to provide services for all their subscribers. In such plans, a patient has to consult either physicians employed by the company or those in the groups under contract to the insurance company whose policy the patient purchased (or more likely, whose policy the patient's employer purchased). Other plans offer a choice from a select list of physicians and specialties. Most require preapproval for at least some medications and treatments, and some require preapproval for visits to the emergency room. No two plans cover quite the same list of consultations, treatments, medications and devices, under quite the same terms. The insurance companies arrange the terms, as they have had every right and duty to do, to serve the financial interests of their shareholders. Such arrangements include deliberate policies of delaying reimbursement payments to physicians and medical groups, because all funds retained can be invested for interest; refusal of authorization for payment for medical procedures or hospital days for those cases in which it seems that the patient would have no choice but to avail himself or herself of the service and pay anyway, out of pocket; and *selective deselection* of physicians who cost the plan more than the average over the course of the year because of referrals to specialists or the ordering of tests.

Deselection means that the plan subscribers can no longer receive reimbursement for consulting that physician. In effect, a deselected physician can no longer have those subscribers as patients. If the physician's income heavily depends on that group of patients, she may effectively find herself unemployed; if she belongs to a medical group that depends on a contract with that company, she may find herself rapidly separated from that group in order to preserve the contract. In both cases, because most practices depend heavily on insurance contracts and no group can afford an "outlier" who will attract negative attention to the group, the physician may be separated from all chance of making a living in the practice of medicine. Under the circumstances, it is not surprising that physicians feel that they have little choice but to stay well within the unspoken insurance guidelines, even if that means effectively turning away or deceiving certain patients.

The insurance contracts place healthcare professionals in a clear conflict of interest, a conflict that can affect the lives and health of their patients. (A conflict of interest, for a professional, involves any arrangement in which the personal interest of the professional [physician] is adverse to the interest of the client [patient].) Because all parties to the contract are competent adults, there is nothing the law can do to prevent such contracts from being signed. (Incidentally, according to the code that governs the ethical practice of law, which has legal force, any lawyer who put himself in such a position vis-à-vis a client could be disbarred.) The accrediting body for most U.S. hospitals, the Joint Commission for the Accreditation of Healthcare Organizations (JCAHO), has a special section on "Organizational Ethics" in the 2001 edition of its *Comprehensive Accreditation Manual for Hospitals.* The requirement of the main standard (RI.4) is simply the following: "The hospital operates according to a code of ethical behavior." Of particular interest in the context of bioethics is Standard RI.4.4: "The hospital's code of ethical business and professional behavior protects the integrity of clinical decision making, regardless of how the hospital compensates or shares financial risk with its leaders, managers, clinical staff, and licensed independent practitioners." Translated, this means that whatever impossible conflicts of interest physicians may have signed themselves into, it is the hospital's job to make sure that patient care is not affected. It is not clear how this standard might be met.

Bringing Miscreants to Justice

Notorious problems attend the disciplining of professionals for negligent, fraudulent, or otherwise unacceptable conduct. It is not the wealth or social status of the offenders that obstructs justice; there is no difficulty with trying these people for common crimes. But conflicting expectations arise around professional discipline—that the profession will discipline itself; that the hospitals will take responsibility for the competence of the professionals on their staffs; that state agencies will police the health marketplace and arrest wrongdoers; that the federal and state governments will use their power to withhold Medicare and Medicaid reimbursement to drive crooks and incompetents from the profession; that somehow insurance companies will act for and not against the interests of the patient; and that because the contract between professional and patient is a private one, private litigation is the best protector of rights.

The end product of these conflicting expectations is a nightmare of overlapping jurisdictions. There are, for example, clear cases of the *impaired physician,* usually a physician involved in substance abuse, where there is a clear trail of substance consumption (e.g., bills from the liquor store, prescriptions not justified by patient need) and substandard practice. These are handled at the state level, with reasonable penalties and conditions of rehabilitation. For the remainder of allegations of inadequate care, no one is clearly in a position to initiate action. But once a health professional has been accused of misconduct, every agency—federal, state, or professional—involved at all with the profession typically attempts to get into the case. Routine involvement in all cases is the only way the agencies can ensure public perception of their importance and continued public support. Private lawyers preparing malpractice or negligence suits often alert public agencies to the possibility of professional (usually medical) incompetence because public citation will strengthen their case. When all the agencies take off after a physician at once—threatening loss of hospital privileges and/or the right to prescribe drugs, fines for incorrect billing of Medicare or Medicaid and insurance companies, and devastating publicity for the whole affair—the result can be personally and professionally catastrophic, and quite unjust. On the other hand, complaints continue that physicians work essentially without supervision, that it is very difficult for patients to criticize or check their work, and that bad physicians are practicing, able to evade all scrutiny.

Not all problems are technical or supervision problems. There are conflicting principles at the root of some problems. One of the most common is the conflict between patient autonomy and the protection of patient welfare. If adults regularly choose treatments or interventions that serve very little medical purpose (e.g., liposuction, cosmetic surgery or implants, experimental drugs), who shall be held responsible for the undesirable outcomes? To what extent shall the medical profession be forbidden, by law, to provide such services?

Another typical conflict is that between the salvaging of a professional career and patient protection. A health professional's training is long, difficult, and expensive, and society cannot afford to lose the investment that it represents. There is good reason, then, to try to rehabilitate health professionals who have mismanaged their practices. The problem lies in deciding which lapses are remediable and which are not. There is always a danger that the professional who has offended once will do so again, no matter how tight the supervision. The problem is compounded by the need, given the nature of the professional–client relationship in healthcare, to keep the professional's problems absolutely confidential. Typically, if the physician or other practitioner is *impaired*—psychologically incapacitated, found not guilty of a crime by reason of insanity, alcoholic, drug abusing, or

otherwise unable to practice until a course of therapy has been completed—the records will be kept confidential while the person undergoes therapy. Should the physician leave therapy or breach other agreements (by testing positive for controlled substances, for instance), the matter becomes one of *misconduct* rather than *impairment* and is no longer confidential.

Another typical case of conflict, becoming more common, is between the patient and the insurance company, with the health professional caught in the middle. If the physician says that a treatment, test, or referral is needed, and the insurance company disagrees, whose side is the physician on? Since Hippocrates, the physician has been expected to advocate for the patient; under the new market dispensation, such advocacy may threaten a professional career.

The Future

In the future, licensing, regulation, and disciplinary action will no doubt respond to greater consumer insistence on quality and cost control, thus limiting professional autonomy still further. Meanwhile, new communication modalities will make possible much greater communication with all healthcare professionals as well as with the public. Three major trends can be discerned.

First, higher and more public standards for certification can be expected. Nonprofessional members have already been added to licensing boards in most states (CSG/CLEAR). It is likely that legal statutes will be enacted requiring that health professionals be recertified at some point or at regular intervals in their careers. The public is acutely aware that the scientific foundations of healthcare are rapidly changing, and that professional education has a half-life of less than ten years—five, in the case of certain medical specialties. Mandatory continuing-education requirements are already part of the licensing laws for medicine and nursing; it is not a large step from there to provisions for occasional retesting. Some observers foresee that "good moral character" requirements—already part of the licensing statutes in most states but undefined—will be made more precise and will be more vigorously enforced (CSG/CLEAR).

Second, the effort to control costs will be continued, whatever the fate of current insurance arrangements. There is still a widely held perception that health costs are too high and out of control. Major initiatives to limit them have been less than fully effective and have roused ire among health professionals and the general public alike. Yet to this moment there are no laws specifically excluding commercial arrangements from the healthcare marketplace, even those that entail the exclusion of sick people from private health insurance. The Health Insurance Portability and Accountability Act of 1996 (HIPPAA) at least ensures that a person who becomes ill when insured, and then must change insurance plans, can enroll in the new one. In the past, the illness would constitute a *pre-existing condition,* a sufficient disqualification for enrollment in a new plan. But we have still no way to care for those suffering from serious chronic conditions prior to any insurance coverage.

Third, the entire process of licensing, regulating, and disciplining health professionals will become much more transparent. Both professionals and consumers have demanded this. As an encouraging start, many states have created web sites containing information on how to apply for licensure, listing job openings, and publishing all state laws regarding licensure.

The United States entered the twentieth century with the assumption that only one consent was needed for medical treatment: that of the physician or other health professional. In the last decades of that century it became clear that three consents are needed: the professional's, the patient's, and the payer's—the government agency or the private insurance company. That third consent may become much more problematic. Patients are also taxpayers and ratepayers. There is an increasing mandate to limit the amount of the national wealth that goes into healthcare, and there is no telling how far this new stringency will go in reshaping the health professions.

LISA H. NEWTON (1995)
REVISED BY AUTHOR

SEE ALSO: *Impaired Professionals; Just Wages and Salaries; Labor Unions in Healthcare; Malpractice, Medical; Mistakes, Medical; Nursing, Profession of; Research, Unethical; Nursing as a Profession; Nursing Ethics*

BIBLIOGRAPHY

Bosk, Charles L. 1979. *Forgive and Remember: Managing Medical Failure.* Chicago: University of Chicago Press.

Bosk, Charles L. 1985. "Social Controls and Physicians: The Oscillation of Cynicism and Idealism in Sociological Theory." In *Social Controls and the Medical Profession,* ed. Judith P. Swazey and Stephen R. Scher. Boston: Oelgeschlager, Gunn & Hain.

Boston Women's Health Collective. 1985. *New Our Bodies, Ourselves.* New York: Simon and Schuster.

Collins, Randall. 1979. *The Credential Society: An Historical Sociology of Education and Stratification.* New York: Academic Press.

Committee for the Study of Credentialing in Nursing. 1979. *The Study of Credentialing in Nursing: A New Approach,* vol. 2. Kansas City, MO: American Nurses Association.

Council of State Governments (CSG). 1952. *Occupational Licensing Legislation in the States.* Chicago: Author.

Council of State Governments and National Clearinghouse on Licensure, Enforcement, and Regulation (CSG/CLEAR). 1987. *State Regulation of the Health Occupations and Professions, 1986–1987.* Lexington, KY: Authors.

Dent v. State of West Virginia. 129 U.S. 114 (1889).

Flexner, Abraham. 1910. *Medical Education in the United States and Canada.* New York: Carnegie Foundation for the Advancement of Teaching.

Freidson, Eliot. 1970. *Profession of Medicine: A Study of the Sociology of Applied Knowledge.* New York: Dodd, Mead.

Friedman, Milton, and Friedman, Rose. 1980. *Free to Choose: A Personal Statement.* New York: Harcourt Brace Jovanovich.

Grad, Frank P., and Marti, Noelia. 1979. *Physicians' Licensure and Discipline: The Legal and Professional Regulation of Medical Practice.* Dobbs Ferry, NY: Oceana Publications.

Gross, Stanley J. 1984. *Of Foxes and Hen Houses: Licensing and the Health Professions.* Westport, CT: Quorum Books.

Joint Commission for the Accreditation of Healthcare Organizations. 2001. *Comprehensive Accreditation Manual for Hospitals Refreshed Core,* January 2001 edition. Oakbrook Terrace, IL: Author.

Larson, Magali S. 1977. *The Rise of Professionalism: A Sociological Analysis.* Berkeley: University of California Press.

Mogul, Kathleen M. 1985. "Doctor's Dilemmas: Complexities in the Causes of Physicians; Mental Disorders and Some Treatment Implications." In *Social Controls and the Medical Profession,* ed. Judith P. Swazey and Stephen R. Scher. Boston: Oelgeschlager, Gunn & Hain.

U.S. Public Health Service (USPHS). Health Manpower Coordinating Committee. Subcommittee on Health Manpower. 1976. *A Proposal for Credentialing Health Manpower.* Washington, D.C.: Government Printing Office.

Welch, Claude E. 1976. "Professional Licensure and Hospital Delineation of Clinical Privileges: Relationship to Quality Assurance." In *Quality Assurance in Health Care,* ed. Richard H. Egdahl and Paul Gurtman. Germantown, MD: Aspen Systems.

INTERNET RESOURCES

Business.com. "State Licensing Boards for Physicians." Available from <http://www.business.com/directory/healthcare/practice_areas/physicians/>.

Rhode Island. Department of Health. "Health Professions Regulation." Available from <http://www.healthri.org/hsr/professions/professions_reg.htm>.

Texas. Department of Health. "Health Professions Resource Center." Available from <http://www.tdh.state.tx.us/dpa/Coverpg.htm>.

HEALTHCARE RESOURCES, ALLOCATION OF

• • •

I. Macroallocation

II. Microallocation

I. MACROALLOCATION

The allocation of healthcare resources involves distributing health-related materials and services among various uses and people. The concept of allocation can imply that a designated individual or group is responsible for each level of decision making within a system that is designed to distribute fixed amounts of resources. Nevertheless, the degree to which such a system exists and such explicit allocation decisions occur varies widely. In the United States, for example, allocation of resources to and within healthcare has long been more the product of millions of individual clinical decisions and various market forces than the result of an overall social policy. Even in the United States, however, arenas exist where more explicit allocation occurs, such as the U.S. Veterans Health Administration with its Veterans Equitable Resource Allocation System (U.S. Veterans).

Healthcare allocations are commonly classified in terms of two levels of decision making: microallocation and macroallocation. Microallocation focuses on decisions regarding particular persons. It often involves "patient selection": determining which patients among those who need a particular scarce resource, such as a heart transplant, should receive treatment. Sometimes, however, microallocation entails deciding for an individual patient which of several potentially beneficial treatments to provide, particularly when only a limited time is available for treatment.

Macroallocation, on the other hand, entails decisions that determine the amount of resources available for particular kinds of healthcare services. Macroallocation decisions include how particular health-related institutions such as hospitals or government agencies such as the U.S. National Institutes of Health budget their spending (sometimes referred to as mesoallocation). Macroallocation also encompasses the decisions a nation makes concerning what resources to devote to particular institutions or, more broadly, to high-technology curative medicine as opposed to, for example, research or primary and preventive care. The extent to which health is fostered through medical care as opposed to nonmedical interventions such as environmental regulation is also a matter of macroallocation, as is the amount of money, time, and energy a society allocates to the pursuit of health rather than to education, defense, and other activities.

The term *rationing* is a much less clearly defined term that appears in discussions of macroallocation and microallocation alike. Because the debate over rationing raises issues at the foundation of healthcare allocation, it is the focus of the opening section below. The remainder of this entry discusses substantive standards for judging macroallocation, under three headings: the individual's right to healthcare, the community's responsibility for healthcare, and the importance of efficiency in healthcare.

Rationing

Rationing involves leaving some people, at least temporarily and against their wishes, without particular forms of healthcare that might benefit them. Some use the label "rationing" only if a person is barred from treatment by an explicit policy or decision. Those operating from this definition often oppose rationing because they believe there are sufficient resources, if managed and distributed correctly, to address at least the most important health needs of all. Others view the unavailability of care as rationing, whether or not explicit policies or decisions are involved. While part of this group also holds that there are sufficient resources to avoid rationing for the most part, the majority see implicit or explicit rationing as unavoidable and tend to favor developing explicit, ethical criteria (Ubel; Blank; Wikler).

A fundamental ambiguity, then, attends the word rationing. Moreover, the word's association with a short-term policy for handling a temporary crisis, such as a shortage of goods in wartime, makes it a misleading word to designate society's long-term task of healthcare provision. So the less ambiguous terminology of macroallocation and microallocation is probably more helpful in most discussions. Nevertheless, the debate over the term rationing has identified two important issues that should be examined before embarking on a more detailed consideration of macroallocation: (1) Does implicit allocation of desired and potentially beneficial healthcare actually occur? (2) Will some form of allocation be necessary in the future?

There is little dispute that implicit allocation of beneficial care does take place. For example, waiting lists for certain types of healthcare have been commonplace in Canada and Europe. There the structure of the system (referral and reimbursement policies, acquisition and location of technologies), rather than the explicit exclusion of people or services from coverage, has limited overall national spending on healthcare (Grogan). In less developed countries, some resources are typically located only in major urban centers and have been unavailable to most of the population (Attfield).

Even in the United States, where per capita spending on healthcare exceeds that of any other country, many have not been able to obtain certain forms of beneficial healthcare. In recent decades, tens of millions annually have gone without any health insurance, and at least as many more have been underinsured—predicaments that have resulted in reduced access to healthcare and in poorer health (U.S. Congress). Employer decisions to limit employee health-benefits packages, as well as governmental decisions to omit services from the Medicaid and Medicare programs, have excluded certain people from potentially beneficial healthcare. So have decisions by health facilities not to operate in the most accessible locations or at the most convenient times, and insurance company decisions to exclude from coverage people with preexisting conditions or other high-risk factors.

Greater controversy surrounds the second question, whether healthcare resources can be allocated so that no one has to go without potentially beneficial healthcare (Kilner, 1990). The possibility of avoiding rationing in this sense of the term hinges on achieving sufficient cost containment. Proposed strategies include reducing expenditures on items less vital to society (e.g., potato chips and advertising); eliminating medical procedures with little health benefit; placing greater emphasis on preventive care that preempts the need for more expensive acute care; reforming tort law to reduce the need to practice defensive medicine; simplifying administration; imposing global budgets on the entire healthcare system; and limiting the large gap between the incomes of physicians and other full-time workers. Various forms of "managed care" arrangements pursue several of these strategies simultaneously by restricting patients to approved providers (e.g., in preferred provider organizations or health maintenance organizations) who agree to limit their charges or forgo fee-for-service entirely in exchange for a salary or per-enrollee payment.

Some commentators contend that significant cost savings could be obtained through each of these strategies. Others disagree, arguing that the scope and cost of potential healthcare benefits are so vast that any savings will prove insufficient to fund needed benefits for everyone. Time will tell how effective various cost containment strategies can be in reducing the need for limiting the access to healthcare. After initial cost savings, however, managed care in the United States apparently has been unable to check the growth of healthcare costs (Ginzberg). Meanwhile, ethical

questions have arisen concerning the extent to which physicians can truly pursue patient well-being if they must also serve as "gatekeepers" to conserve society's resources (Willems; S. Daniels). At the same time, the experience of other countries such as the Netherlands, with healthcare systems more nationally coordinated than that of the United States, suggests the pragmatic limits of cost containment (The Netherlands, Government Committee on Choices). Such challenges underscore the importance of making allocation decisions explicit if allocation is not to be shaped by unknown factors and unethical considerations.

Major Macroallocation Standards

Numerous people have proposed ways to prioritize the potential uses of limited resources. These proposals tend to be rooted in one or more of three major ethical concerns: the individual's claim to healthcare, the community's responsibility for healthcare, and the importance of efficiency in healthcare. Within these three concerns, different understandings of justice are at work, and different weights are attached to competing ethical considerations such as liberty, care, and utility.

THE INDIVIDUAL'S CLAIM TO HEALTHCARE. Those who are primarily concerned about the healthcare that is due to each individual often invoke the notion of a right to healthcare. When the World Health Organization in its 1946 constitution affirmed the "enjoyment of the highest attainable standard of health" to be one of the fundamental rights of every human being, the statement both reflected and fostered a growing debate over health-related human rights.

The concept of a human right promotes the idea that each person is entitled to have something or to be free from something. It commonly reflects the basic conviction that each human being has special and great significance. While this conviction is not necessarily religious in nature, it receives special emphasis in theological traditions such as Christianity, Judaism, and Islam (Kilner, 1992; Zoloth; Rahman).

Negative and positive rights are frequently distinguished, as are moral and legal rights. Negative (or liberty) rights guarantee freedom from certain types of interference with the pursuit of one's interests. Positive (or material) rights guarantee access to important services and goods. Accordingly, a right to protection from anything that is seriously harmful to one's health is a negative right; a right to receive certain forms of healthcare is a positive right. Whereas moral rights involve claims about what one ought to have on ethical grounds, legal rights involve claims about what one is actually entitled to by law. Whether everyone has an ethically justifiable right to healthcare is debated in the United States, yet Medicare legislation confers a legal right to healthcare on the country's elderly people.

Differing views. In light of such distinctions and the conflicting conceptions of justice and freedom that underlie them, it is not surprising that people have fundamentally different views about the meaning and legitimacy of a "right to healthcare." Some hold that there is a right to health. The point of the right is to make sure that people actually have health itself, not just access to resources. Others insist on a right to healthcare. Because of the fundamental importance of health, people should have guaranteed access to resources that foster it. Still others reject both positions. While all of these claims represent worthwhile aspirations, they argue, such claims are not rights because no one has the obligation to satisfy them. Probing this last argument first provides useful entry into the debate.

The most prominent basis for rejecting a right to healthcare is a libertarian view of justice that emphasizes negative rights over positive rights (Engelhardt). According to this view, people ought to be free to pursue their own life plans, including their economic livelihood. Government should prevent others from interfering with that pursuit. A right to healthcare that forces healthcare professionals to provide care—or that forces certain people to give up part of what they have earned to pay for other people's care—directly contradicts what justice requires. That some people lack healthcare (or the ability to pay for it) is simply unfortunate rather than unfair. No rights are violated in a market-based system where people are free to buy and sell as their resources permit.

Critics of this position argue that it is self-defeating and mistaken. It is self-defeating because in its zeal to protect people's freedom to use their resources for healthcare and other desired goods, it effectively ensures that those with insufficient resources will not have the freedom to obtain healthcare (Brennan). It is mistaken in three assumptions. First, some note the implausibility of assuming that the present distribution of general resources is fair. In their view, the vastly unequal distribution of the means by which people pay for healthcare is attributable to forces that have affected the fairness of the market over time.

Others doubt a second assumption, namely, that a free-market approach is appropriate for healthcare. Consumers in this case are frequently sick patients with limited knowledge about healthcare. For a free market to function well, consumers would have to be able to understand the costs and benefits of all the available medical options and be willing and able to trade health or even life for money. A free-market approach, then, unfairly discriminates against those who are uneducated as well as those who are poor because of social circumstances or genetic endowments beyond their control.

A third debatable assumption, most frequently questioned by those who operate from a theological perspective, is the understanding of liberty as autonomy. The term *autonomy,* derived from the Greek words *auto* (self) and *nomos* (law), tends to emphasize people's separateness from others. According to a more relational understanding, freedom entails "freedom *for*"—the ability (and obligation) to help others—as much as it involves "freedom *from*" the interference of others.

Some of those who reject a libertarian approach instead affirm the right to health. They insist that health, like life itself, is something so fundamental to human existence that it must be fostered as much as possible. Precisely what the right to health entails, though, is not always clear. It may involve only the negative right that would protect one's freedom from actions that undermine health. This formulation of the right is compatible with the libertarian outlook already discussed. Alternatively, the right to health may entail that people have an entitlement to be healthy and that others have failed in their moral obligations toward individuals who are not healthy.

Those who find this outlook objectionable worry about the prospect of making one person's health another person's responsibility. Such a view tends to undermine people's responsibility for their own health. Opponents also note that it is not possible to maintain someone else's health indefinitely—given that everyone dies eventually—so it seems mistaken to suggest that anyone has an obligation to do so.

A right to healthcare. To avoid these problems some people advocate the right to healthcare. The right to healthcare is a positive right that holds that all people are entitled to receive some measure of healthcare. Whereas some others argue that people are entitled only to an amount of monetary resources that they can spend on whatever they deem important (Brody), supporters of the right to healthcare insist that people must be assured healthcare in particular. Rights, they maintain, do not involve the sort of discretionary items on which people place differing priorities. Rather, they concern goods that all people require in order to pursue their various life courses.

Sometimes the right to healthcare is formulated in comparative terms. According to this view, everyone should have access to whatever healthcare is necessary to provide for a level of access—or even of health itself—equal to that of others (Veatch). Many have resisted this egalitarian outlook because it tends to focus more on the value of equality than on the healthcare people receive. People with chronic illnesses or congenital disabilities may never achieve a level of health equal to that of others and so could claim an infinite amount of healthcare resources by invoking an egalitarian right to healthcare. Alternatively, this right could justify leaving all at a relatively low level of access or health, as long as everyone was treated alike. If, on the other hand, this egalitarian approach requires that everyone be able to receive every treatment that may provide any benefit, then it seems hopelessly unsuited to a world of limited resources.

To correct these deficiencies, various people have proposed identifying the right to healthcare with some sort of achievable standard of healthcare that could be guaranteed to all. They often suggest that because healthcare is provided in response to need, some standard of need should determine the level of healthcare to which all people have a right.

Others would similarly root the individual's claim to healthcare in a person's need for that care, but would appeal to various understandings of justice rather than to the notion of rights. For example, a contractarian approach, which appeals to what all people would agree to in hypothetically fair positions, usually advocates people's access to basic goods that anyone must have in order to carry out a personal life plan. Healthcare is one such good, and whatever amount is essential to enable people to function at a normal level is mandated by justice (N. Daniels; compare Toenjes, who sees the contract as one between physicians and society). Religious traditions that posit a divinely created world also tend to espouse a needs-based understanding of justice. They may, however, view *normal* more in terms of how people were created to be than how they typically are (Mackler).

A utilitarian conception of justice might also undergird a right to healthcare, but the support is tenuous. Because classical (or act) utilitarianism advocates acts that will produce the greatest good for the greatest number of people, it is often criticized for lacking any concept of justice to protect individuals from oppressive majorities. On the other hand, rule utilitarianism, which supports standards that produce the greatest good for the greatest number if followed consistently, might well support a standard of justice.

Standard of need. In light of the important place a standard of need commonly has in formulations of the right to healthcare and in conceptions of justice, it is essential to consider what this standard entails. Defining the standard and delineating its implications are not easy, because even marginal benefits can be considered *needs* (President's Commission). One definitional approach is to think of meeting needs in terms of restoring normal functioning. Another ties the meeting of needs to providing *significant* health benefit. Establishing significance might involve a careful assessment of the quality and length of life that various forms of healthcare would likely provide in various situations, together with some individual or societal evaluation of those benefits.

A broad range of considerations is relevant to the delineation of healthcare needs. In particular, needs less dramatic than the need for acute medical care must receive sufficient attention. Some non-healthcare goods can make an important claim on whatever portion of its resources a society devotes to the pursuit of health. Food, education, and shelter, for example, all contribute directly to health (Tuckson). So do programs that encourage healthy lifestyles. Habits of eating, drinking, sleeping, and drug use can all have a dramatic impact on health, although positive habits resulting in greater longevity may not reduce total healthcare expenditures over the course of an individual's lifetime (L. Russell).

Preventive medicine, supportive care, and medical research must similarly receive sufficient attention along with curative medicine. While preventive medicine is not necessarily less expensive or more effective than curative medicine, it can be both (Hope). Prenatal care for a mother as opposed to neonatal intensive care for her low-birthweight infant is a case in point. Analyses of need must give due attention to the importance of supportive care such as longterm care for elderly persons or effective pain relief for dying patients. Finally, fascination with current curative capabilities can all too easily siphon resources away from medical research. Without sufficient attention to research, there will be fewer new medical resources in the future, to the longterm detriment of society's health.

In the face of such a broad array of healthcare needs, many people believe that not everything that is needed can be provided for all. Accordingly, they conclude that justice or the right to healthcare must mandate only that each individual receive some reasonable level of healthcare—so-called essential care or a *decent minimum* (Eddy). Determining this exact level presents the same challenges as determining need, with the added task of tailoring the determination to the level of overall resources available at the time.

Moreover, people in different locations differ dramatically in their perceptions of need and essential care. Those in European countries, for example, avoid the notion of a decent minimum altogether. Nevertheless, each country's effort to provide comprehensive care is unique in terms of the particular forms of care that receive emphasis (Grogan).

Canada has typically acknowledged differences by allowing each of its provinces to determine which health-related services will be included in the package of guaranteed benefits.

The United States, lacking the nationally coordinated financing system of Canada, has traditionally left its states to develop their own priorities and healthcare systems (Moon and Holahan). For instance, Oregon has explicitly ranked all health-related services in terms of their funding priority. Hawaii has required all employers to provide health insurance to all employees working over twenty hours per week (Hawaii acted in 1974 before federal legislation barred this approach). Minnesota has linked improving healthcare access with an array of measures to control costs.

The differences among these and other state initiatives underscore what an international comparison also illustrates: that varying perceptions of need call forth different healthcare priorities and systems. Cross-cultural sensitivity will be essential if efforts to meet health-related needs are to cross national and international boundaries successfully (Attfield).

Employing need as a basis for allocation, then, presents various challenges. Challenges can be reasons for rejecting an idea. But challenges may be no more than obstacles to overcome so that a good idea may be implemented effectively.

THE COMMUNITY'S RESPONSIBILITY FOR HEALTHCARE. The substantial disagreement over the idea of the individual's claim to healthcare has made many people doubt its usefulness as a basis for allocating healthcare resources. Some have rejected the idea on more principled grounds as well. One prominent concern has been the impact that a preoccupation with the rights of the individual can have on the well-being of the community as a whole (Churchill). A case in point is the United States, a highly individualistic culture in which the use of the language of rights has been particularly prominent. The demand of U.S. taxpayers, patients, health professionals, and healthcare financers for the rights to pursue and satisfy their own various interests may have inhibited the development of an integrated, comprehensive healthcare system.

Those who would not jettison completely the notion of rights may argue—on theological or other grounds—that while people have rights, they have no "right to rights" (Kilner, 1992). According to this view, rights themselves (in the sense of freedoms and goods all people ought to have) are not the problem. The problem is people's preoccupation with their own (right to) rights—a preoccupation that undermines the commitment to pursuing the rights of all. In this sense, group rights are as problematic as individual

rights, because attention to the claims of one's own group tends to encourage the same kind of self-focus and neglect of others as the pursuit of individual rights.

Therefore, some favor deemphasizing the notion of the individual's claim to healthcare—as well as rights language in general—or even replacing the notion with a more explicit conception of the community's responsibility for healthcare. Sensitivity to the needs of individuals and particular groups is not absent in this approach, but the driving concern is the community's obligation to ensure the well-being of the whole community.

In European societies such as Germany and the Netherlands, for example, discussions of healthcare have often invoked social solidarity as a fundamental goal to be pursued through resource allocation (Netherlands, Government Committee on Choices). In the United States, an increasing emphasis on community responsibility has been reflected in the ethics literature (Dyck; Tauber) and in the appearance of such interdisciplinary journals as *The Responsive Community.* Appeals to the common good have also become more frequent, especially in religious circles (Catholic Health Association). Increasingly, people are concluding that ethical macroallocation of healthcare resources in the United States will probably require a different way of thinking about the relationship between the individual and society.

Accordingly, the U.S. President's Commission for the Study of Ethical Problems in Medicine and Biomedical and Behavioral Research, in its 1983 report titled *Securing Access to Health Care,* explicitly rejected the rights-oriented language in the 1952 report of the U.S. President's Commission on the Health Needs of the Nation, titled *Building America's Health.* Instead the 1980s commission affirmed the community's ethical obligation to provide all with equitable access to an "adequate level" of healthcare. In *Securing Access,* the commission argued that a community must ensure that all of its members can obtain such care because healthcare is so important in relieving suffering, preventing premature death, restoring functioning, increasing opportunity, providing information, and strengthening relationships of caring. This approach affirms that ungenerous or uncaring healthcare allocations are clearly as wrong as those that are unjust.

Caring in this context entails looking beyond what theoretical formulations of justice require. It means giving special consideration to those who have been marginalized in the allocation of healthcare resources. Identified in certain religious and liberationist contexts as "the preferential option for the poor," this sensitivity toward disadvantaged persons is characteristic of much feminist analysis as well (Caes; Holmes and Purdy). It embraces the notion of the "common good," but not in the utilitarian or majority-rule sense of the term. It insists that there is no true common good if all do not have the good in common.

Emotional as well as rational, engaged as well as theoretical, a caring commitment to those who are least well-off may or may not justify a different healthcare allocation than that which a rights- or justice-based approach to healthcare allocation would advocate. Its proponents, however, maintain that such a commitment almost certainly will make a difference in the ways in which allocation is implemented. For example, it may be widely acknowledged that justice requires directing more healthcare resources toward African Americans and other disadvantaged groups in the United States (LaVeist). Reallocation, however, is not likely to take place as long as people do not see others' health as their responsibility in any way.

Basing allocation on the community's responsibility for healthcare, then, differs from basing it on the individual's claim to healthcare. But attributing responsibility to the community does not absolve the individual from responsibility. Because individuals are part of the community and share in its well-being, they must share the burden of paying for the cost of the community's healthcare in an equitable manner. Moreover, they have some responsibility for their own health. The implications of this responsibility are controversial. In particular, does an apparently irresponsible person forfeit the community's care?

Both justice and respect for people's liberty may entail that those who voluntarily cause their own health problems should take responsibility for them, particularly when there are insufficient resources to meet the healthcare needs of all. Holding people responsible in this way might have the added benefit of reducing illness and injury resulting from risky behaviors, thereby lowering related healthcare costs as well.

It is extremely difficult in most cases to prove, however, that people caused their illnesses and did so voluntarily. Often there are many causes of an illness, few of which are within a person's control. Even if a person's behavior, such as smoking or overeating, does cause an illness, the voluntary nature of the behavior is difficult to demonstrate conclusively. The person may have engaged in the behavior without understanding that it could cause the resulting illness. Regardless of foreknowledge, other factors—advertising, peer pressure, cultural values, dietary deficiencies, psychological instabilities, or genetic predispositions—may have significantly impaired the ill person's ability to act freely.

Even if a society becomes sufficiently adept at identifying those who have voluntarily caused their own health problems, three further ethical considerations are relevant.

First, fairness may require that an allocation policy based on personal responsibility not apply only to those engaging in the least socially desirable behaviors. In other words, the policy should apply not only to smokers and intravenous-drug abusers but also to those who overwork or overeat, if responsibility can be established in all four types of cases.

Second, the idea that a society would have a responsibility to truly care for its members may call for the provision of more healthcare than strict justice alone requires, even for those who voluntarily engage in risky behavior. The healthcare professions have a long-standing tradition of offering care without making such offers contingent on the extent to which ill people caused their own need. Finally, if caring with fairness requires some form of accountability for risky behaviors, requiring payment of a tax to engage in those behaviors, say on cigarettes and alcohol, would be more humane than denying needed healthcare.

THE IMPORTANCE OF EFFICIENCY IN HEALTHCARE. Efficiency is also a central and disputed issue in ethical resource allocation. How best to eliminate health-related expenditures that are not truly beneficial in order to maximize funding for beneficial healthcare is only part of the efficiency problem. Even greater controversy surrounds proposed mechanisms for determining which forms of beneficial care are most worth their cost.

Two mechanisms for comparing costs and benefits have received particular attention as promising ways to pursue efficiency in healthcare: cost–benefit analysis and cost-effectiveness analysis. While both mechanisms typically involve assessing the costs of various forms of healthcare in monetary units, cost–benefit analysis also uses monetary units exclusively to assess the benefits of care, whereas cost-effectiveness analysis does not.

Cost-benefit analysis. Cost-benefit analysis is well-suited in principle to a broad range of resource allocation decisions both within and outside of healthcare. It employs identical units, such as dollars, to measure all costs and benefits. Accordingly, it can subtract total costs from total benefits to determine if an expenditure is wasteful (i.e., its costs outweigh its benefits). When applied to different health-related and other uses for the same funds, cost-benefit analysis can also determine which use will provide the greatest net benefit. This approach has proven particularly attractive to economists and policy analysts who must prioritize diverse uses of limited funds (Emery and Schneiderman; Oliver, Healey, and Donaldson).

Because cost-benefit analysis is the more familiar efficiency mechanism of the two, and because it alone has the potential to compare all possible uses of available funds, it appears at first glance to be the superior mechanism for allocating healthcare resources. But cost-benefit analysis has a number of pragmatic and substantive weaknesses in its most common forms (B. Russell). Some of these difficulties are inherent in the overall way the mechanism operates. Identifying the numerous ways that people are affected by particular allocation decisions is difficult enough, but reducing the entire range of healthcare outcomes (including continued life itself) to monetary value is virtually impossible. More substantively, while cost-benefit analysis helps to identify the allocation of resources that yields the greatest balance of benefit over cost for a society as a whole, it may fail to consider how fairly the benefits and burdens of that allocation are distributed throughout society. Programs targeting affluent suburbs, for example, can tend to have better cost-benefit ratios than programs in poor inner-city areas because of the bad health fostered by poor social and economic conditions. Ethics, though, must attend to more than economics.

Other difficulties concern the methods cost-benefit analysis uses to convert lives saved and other benefits of healthcare into monetary units. One approach is the *past decisions* approach, which compares how much money a society spent on selected programs to save lives in the past with how many lives were saved as a result of those programs. The unique funding and implementation context of each such program, however, renders generalizations risky.

Two more popular conversion methods involve future earnings (human capital) and willingness to pay. The future-earnings approach determines the monetary value of a health benefit by calculating how much more money patients will earn in the future if they receive treatment than if they do not. Fairness again is a major problem, for this approach implies that the life of a person making twice the income of another person is twice as valuable (i.e., important to save) as that of the other person. Because women and minorities tend to receive less pay than white males for comparable work, this approach devalues the lives of women and minorities. In fact, whatever employment-related discrimination already exists in a society becomes compounded when healthcare allocation reflects salary level.

A willingness-to-pay approach, on the other hand, calculates the value of a health benefit on the basis of the amount of money people would pay to receive a specified increase in the likelihood of receiving that benefit over a particular length of time. This approach, like the previous one, tends to compound certain forms of discrimination. Because wealthy people are generally able to pay more for a program to reduce the risk of illness and death than are poor people, a willingness-to-pay approach systematically reproduces existing injustices in the distribution of wealth.

All forms of cost-benefit analysis, then, are vulnerable to the charges that they are inadequate measures of the value of lives and that they neglect some important ethical considerations in resource allocation. Accordingly, a better mechanism for maximizing the benefit of limited healthcare resources has been sought.

Cost-effectiveness analysis. Cost-effectiveness analysis has generally been the favored alternative because it avoids a major difficulty that troubles cost-benefit analysis: the need to convert health outcomes, including continued life itself, to a monetary equivalent. Cost-effectiveness analysis typically calculates the cost of alternative health initiatives in monetary terms. But it can adopt a nonmonetary unit for comparing the health benefits of these initiatives, such as degree of mobility restored or years of life saved. If, for example, two treatments for hip problems claim to improve mobility, cost-effectiveness analysis can determine which one restores more mobility for the same cost or identical mobility for less cost. It can also determine which use of earmarked funds will produce the greatest health benefits. While this approach cannot determine if costs outweigh benefits or compare all benefits inside and outside of the healthcare field, it can identify the cost per standardized unit of benefit for alternative health-related interventions.

Broad societal healthcare allocations, however, necessitate a more generic measure of health benefit than mobility. Because increased quality and length of life are the two primary goals of healthcare, the standard of *quality-adjusted life years* (QALYs) seems to many to provide a suitable measure (McCulloch; Nord). To determine the number of QALYs that a health-related intervention will produce, the number of years people will likely live after the intervention is multiplied by a percentage reflecting the quality of life to be experienced during those years—0 percent (0.00) signifying death, and 100 percent (1.00) signifying perfect health with no disability.

While QALY-based cost-effectiveness analysis represents an improvement over cost-benefit analysis for the purpose of comparing health-related allocations, it, too, has proven controversial (Harris; Menzel; Stolk, Brouwer, and Busschbach). For example, certain analysts, while affirming the approach in principle, note that studies to date have not yet gathered all of the necessary data on healthcare outcomes, costs, and quality-of-life preferences. More data is needed before cost-effectiveness can be consistently employed as a basis for making comprehensive healthcare allocations.

The state of Oregon, for instance, originally intended to use a form of cost-effectiveness analysis during the early 1990s when it redesigned its approach to allocating public healthcare funds. Through a telephone survey, the state asked people to rank various functional limitations and other symptoms on a quality-of-life scale. The goal was to ascertain a quality-of-life score and cost figure for every health-related intervention so that these interventions could be prioritized for budgetary purposes. Reliable cost data proved so difficult to acquire, though, that the quality-of-life information was employed essentially only to identify which interventions produced the most benefit, irrespective of costs (Garland). Moreover, some rankings had to be altered in the end. The state discovered that interventions producing relatively little health benefit—if inexpensive enough—could rank higher than much more beneficial (even lifesaving) interventions.

Another methodological debate over cost-effectiveness analysis concerns who should assess quality of life (Fleck). The QALY approach determines the quality-of-life percentages for particular outcomes by interviewing large numbers of healthy people concerning the value they place on various qualities of life. Some insist that healthy people are the right ones to make these judgments because resource allocation is like purchasing health insurance. People will appropriately weigh alternative benefit packages before they contract a particular disease, but after contracting it they place disproportionate weight on covering that disease. Others cite studies documenting that healthy people frequently underestimate the quality of life of people who are ill or disabled. One inference drawn is that only those who have experienced such conditions can adequately assess the degree to which they render living more difficult (Lawton, Moss, and Glicksman; Kaplan).

The most heated disputes over the QALY approach, however, involve problems of fairness similar to those attributed to cost-benefit analysis. Although QALY-based cost-effectiveness analysis does not intentionally discriminate against certain groups, it tends to disadvantage patients who are older or disabled—in fact, anyone whose future length or quality of life is comparatively limited. Because QALY calculations are based on precisely these two variables, the treatments most beneficial to such persons tend to receive lower QALY scores and so receive low funding priority. For many who believe in the sanctity of human life, this discrimination is typical of the devaluing of certain types of people that generally results when anticipated quality of life is employed as a basis for ranking patients rather than as a desirable outcome to be sought for each individual patient.

As it turned out, the U.S. government refused the state of Oregon's initial application, which sought legal permission to allocate the state's limited Medicaid funds by ranking health-related interventions based on public quality-of-life judgments. The government's controversial rationale was that the approach discriminated against persons with disabilities. Oregon successfully revised its proposal by eliminating reliance on quality-of-life data. While cost-effectiveness analysis, then, attends well to efficiency, like other efficiency mechanisms it can easily be insensitive to other ethical concerns such as degree of need and fairness (Menzel et al.; Rosenthal and Newhouse).

Conclusion

The individual's claims, the community's responsibilities, and efficiency's importance all represent widely held ethical sensitivities to which resource allocation must attend. The ongoing challenge is to determine how to affirm the best elements of each, where they are not mutually contradictory, in a way that also minimizes their ethically objectionable features.

JOHN F. KILNER (1995)
REVISED BY AUTHOR

SEE ALSO: *Aging and the Aged; Autonomy; Beneficence; Contractarianism and Bioethics; Economic Concepts in Healthcare; Ethics; Human Rights; Justice; Long-Term Care; Managed Care; Medicaid; Medicare; Natural Law; Profession and Professional Ethics; Utilitarianism and Bioethics;* and other *Healthcare Resources, Allocation of* subentries

BIBLIOGRAPHY

Attfield, Robin. 1990. "The Global Distribution of Health Care Resources." *Journal of Medical Ethics* 16(3): 153–156.

Blank, Robert H. 1988. *Rationing Medicine.* New York: Columbia University Press.

Brennan, Troyen A. 2002. "Luxury Primary Care: Market Innovation or Threat to Access?" *New England Journal of Medicine* 346(15): 1165–1168.

Brody, Baruch A. 1991. "Why the Right to Health Care Is Not a Useful Concept for Policy Debates." In *Rights to Health Care,* ed. Thomas Bole III and William B. Bondeson. Dordrecht, Netherlands: Kluwer.

Caes, David, ed. 1992. *Caring for the Least of These: Serving Christ among the Poor.* Scottdale, PA: Herald.

Catholic Health Association. 1991. *With Justice for All? The Ethics of Healthcare Rationing.* St. Louis, MO: Author.

Churchill, Larry R. 1987. *Rationing Health Care in America: Perceptions and Principles of Justice.* Notre Dame, IN: University of Notre Dame Press.

Daniels, Norman. 1985. *Just Health Care: Studies in Philosophy and Health Policy.* Cambridge, Eng.: Cambridge University Press.

Daniels, Scott E. 1998. "Managed Care's Financial Incentives." In *The Changing Face of Health Care: A Christian Appraisal of*

Managed Care, Resource Allocation, and Patient–Caregiver Relationships, ed. John F. Kilner, Robert D. Orr, and Judy A. Shelly. Grand Rapids, MI: W. B. Eerdmans.

Dolan, Paul, and Olsen, Jan Abel. 2003. *Distributing Health Care: Economic and Ethical Issues.* New York: Oxford University Press.

Dyck, Arthur J. 1994. *Rethinking Rights and Responsibilities: The Moral Bonds of Community.* Cleveland, OH: Pilgrim Press.

Eddy, David M. 1991. "What Care Is 'Essential'? What Services Are 'Basic'?" *Journal of the American Medical Association* 265(6): 782–788.

Emery, Danielle D., and Schneiderman, Lawrence J. 1989. "Cost Effectiveness Analysis in Health Care." *Hastings Center Report* 19(4): 8–13.

Engelhardt, H. Tristram, Jr. 1991. *Bioethics and Secular Humanism.* London: SCM Press.

Fisher, Anthony, and Gormally, Luke. 2002. *Healthcare Allocation: An Ethical Framework.* London: Linacre Center.

Fleck, Leonard M. 1992. "Just Health Care Rationing: A Democratic Decisionmaking Approach." *University of Pennsylvania Law Review* 140(5): 1597–1636.

Garland, Michael J. 1992. "Justice, Politics, and Community: Expanding Access and Rationing Health Services in Oregon." *Law, Medicine, and Health Care* 20(1–2): 67–81.

Ginzberg, Eli. 1999. "The Uncertain Future of Managed Care." *New England Journal of Medicine* 340(2): 144–146.

Grogan, Colleen M. 1992. "Deciding on Access and Levels of Care: A Comparison of Canada, Britain, Germany, and the United States." *Journal of Health Politics, Policy, and Law* 17(2): 213–232.

Harris, John. 1987. "QALYfying the Value of Life." *Journal of Medical Ethics* 13(3): 117–123.

Holmes, Helen Bequaert, and Purdy, Laura M., eds. 1992. *Feminist Perspectives in Medical Ethics.* Bloomington: Indiana University Press.

Hope, Tony. 2001. "Rationing and Life-Saving Treatments: Should Identifiable Patients Have Higher Priority?" *Journal of Medical Ethics* 27(3): 179–185.

Kaplan, Robert M. 1993. *The Hippocratic Predicament: Affordability, Access, and Accountability in American Medicine.* San Diego, CA: Academic Press.

Kilner, John F. 1990. *Who Lives? Who Dies? Ethical Criteria in Patient Selection.* New Haven, CT: Yale University Press.

Kilner, John F. 1992. *Life on the Line: Ethics, Aging, Ending Patients' Lives, and Allocating Vital Resources.* Grand Rapids, MI: W. B. Eerdmans.

LaVeist, Thomas A. 1993. "Segregation, Poverty, and Empowerment: Health Consequences for African Americans." *Milbank Quarterly* 71(1): 41–64.

Lawton, M. Powell; Moss, Miriam; and Glicksman, Allen. 1990. "The Quality of the Last Year of Life of Older Persons." *Milbank Quarterly* 68(1): 1–28.

Mackler, Aaron L. 1991. "Judaism, Justice, and Access to Health Care." *Kennedy Institute of Ethics Journal* 1(2): 143–161.

McCulloch, Douglas. 2002. *Valuing Health in Practice: Priorities, QALYs, and Choice.* Burlington, VT: Ashgate.

Menzel, Paul T. 1990. *Strong Medicine: The Ethical Rationing of Health Care.* New York: Oxford University Press.

Menzel, Paul T.; Gold, Marthe R.; Nord, Erik, et al. 1999. "Toward a Broader View of Values in Cost-Effectiveness Analysis of Health." *Hastings Center Report* 29(3): 7–15.

Moon, Marilyn, and Holahan, John. 1992. "Can States Take the Lead in Health Care Reform?" *Journal of the American Medical Association* 268(12): 1588–1594.

Netherlands Government Committee on Choices in Health Care. 1992. *Choices in Health Care.* Rijswijk, Netherlands: Ministry of Welfare, Health, and Cultural Affairs.

Nord, Erik. 1999. *Cost–Value Analysis in Health Care: Making Sense Out of QALYs.* New York: Cambridge University Press.

Oliver, Adam; Healey, Andrew; and Donaldson, Cam. 2002. "Choosing the Method to Match the Perspective: Economic Assessment and Its Implications for Health-Services Efficiency." *Lancet* 359(9319): 1171–1174.

Rahman, Fazlur. 1987. *Health and Medicine in the Islamic Tradition: Change and Identity.* New York: Crossroad.

Rosenthal, Meredith, and Newhouse, Joseph. 2002. "Managed Care and Efficient Rationing." *Journal of Health Care Finance* 28(4): 1–10.

Russell, Barbara J. 2002. "Health Care Rationing: Critical Features, Ordinary Language, and Meaning." *Journal of Law, Medicine, and Ethics* 30(1): 82–87.

Russell, Louise. 1986. *Is Prevention Better than Care?* Washington, D.C.: Brookings Institution.

Stolk, Elly A.; Brouwer, Werner B. F.; and Busschback, Jan J. V. 2002. "Rationalising Rationing: Economic and Other Considerations in the Debate about Funding of Viagra." *Health Policy* 59(1): 53–63.

Tauber, Alfred I. 2002. "Medicine, Public Health, and the Ethics of Rationing." *Perspectives in Biology and Medicine* 45(1): 16–30.

Toenjes, Richard. 2002. "Toward Understanding the Ethics of Business in the Business of Medical Care." *HEC Forum* 14(2): 119–131.

Tuckson, Reed. 1992. "A Question of Survival: An Interview with Tuckson Reed." *Second Opinion* 17(4): 48–63.

Ubel, Peter A. 1999. *Pricing Life: Why It's Time for Health Care Rationing.* Cambridge, MA: MIT Press.

U.S. Congress. Office of Technology Assessment. 1992. *Does Health Insurance Make a Difference?* Washington, D.C.: U. S. Government Printing Office.

U.S. President's Commission for the Study of Ethical Problems in Medicine and Biomedical and Behavioral Research. 1983. *Securing Access to Health Care: A Report on the Ethical Implications of Differences in the Availability of Health Services,* Washington, D.C.: U. S. Government Printing Office.

U.S. President's Commission on the Health Needs of the Nation. 1952. *Building America's Health.* Washington, D.C.: U. S. Government Printing Office.

U.S. Veterans Health Administration. 2002. "Veterans Equitable Resource Allocation System," 6th edition. Washington, D.C.: U.S. Department of Veterans Affairs.

Veatch, Robert M. 1986. *The Foundations of Justice: Why the Retarded and the Rest of Us Have Claims to Equality.* New York: Oxford University Press.

Wikler, Daniel. 1992. "Ethics and Rationing: 'Whether,' 'How,' or 'How Much'?" *Journal of the American Geriatrics Society* 40(4): 398–403.

Willems, Dick L. 2001. "Balancing Rationalities: Gatekeeping in Health Care." *Journal of Medical Ethics* 27(1): 25–29.

Zoloth, Laurie. 1999. *Health Care and the Ethics of Encounter: A Jewish Discussion of Social Justice.* Chapel Hill: University of North Carolina Press.

II. MICROALLOCATION

When the need or demand for healthcare resources exceeds the available supply, resources must be distributed on some basis. The more explicit the criteria, the more likely it will be that the term *rationing* will be applied, although the meaning of the term varies considerably in the bioethical, healthcare, economic, and public-policy literature. Rationing often refers to general limitations placed on the availability of certain types of healthcare, but it may also encompass specific treatment decisions for particular patients. Distribution of healthcare at a broad institutional or societal level is referred to as *macroallocation.* Macroallocation includes the way a hospital budgets its spending, as well as the amount of resources a nation devotes to primary and preventive care compared with high-technology curative medicine and nonmedical activities such as education and defense.

Microallocation, on the other hand, focuses on treatment decisions regarding particular persons. It may entail deciding which of several potentially beneficial treatments to provide an individual patient, particularly when only a limited time is available for treatment. Caregivers most commonly employ various medical criteria in order to make such decisions. These decisions, however, take place in institutional and societal contexts of limited resources. Accordingly, the relative merits of devoting particular resources to one patient rather than to others may exert at least an unconscious influence on treatment decisions, and nonmedical considerations may become involved. Patients' values and beliefs often play a role here as well.

Other microallocation decisions, sometimes referred to as *patient selection decisions,* more explicitly involve choices among patients. In the less developed countries of the world, large numbers of people continue to die for lack of vaccines to prevent disease, antibiotics to cure infections, oral rehydration therapy to replenish fluids lost through severe diarrhea, and healthcare personnel to administer such interventions (UNICEF, 1993, 2003). Microallocation decisions constantly determine who will receive the limited care that is available. Some countries not only continue to wrestle with these low-technology scarcities but also face the high-technology microallocation dilemmas commonly encountered in the more developed countries, where expensive medical technologies have proliferated.

Organ transplantation and hospital intensive care are two primary examples of such technologies. The expense of heart, liver, and other types of organ transplantation keep some patients from even considering such operations. Of those seeking transplantation, more than 6,000 patients in the United States alone die each year while waiting for a suitable organ to be donated (Organ Procurement and Transplant Network [OPTN]). Microallocation of hospital intensive care, meanwhile, must occur whenever more patients could benefit medically from access to it than the available space can accommodate—a persistent occurrence even in the more developed countries (Truog; Lantos, Mokalla, and Meadow).

Scarcities of vital healthcare resources are not likely to disappear in the future. The degree of scarcity in the less developed countries will likely decrease through worldwide cooperative efforts. Nevertheless, social, political, and economic constraints will continue to hamper such efforts. Even in the more developed countries, the need for microallocation will persist (and probably grow) for at least three reasons. First, many emerging technologies such as artificial organs and imaging techniques are so expensive that the cost of making them available to all who could benefit from them is prohibitive. Second, the scarcity of some treatments (e.g., organ transplantation) is not simply a matter of funding but reflects the limited supply of the critical resource itself (e.g., the donated organ). Third, technological development will continue to yield new resources that only a limited number of patients can obtain until the capacity to produce those resources expands sufficiently. The history of healthcare is filled with examples of such scarcity, including the early years of the polio vaccine, the antibiotic streptomycin, the hormone insulin to treat diabetes, the iron lung to enable patients with polio to breathe, and the dialysis machine to filter people's blood when their kidneys fail (Mehlman).

Those responsible for microallocation decisions have adopted a wide range of criteria for determining which patients receive available resources. Sometimes a *triage* model has been used, drawing on the experience of prioritizing the treatment of casualties on the battlefield or patients in the emergency room (Rhodes, Miller, and Schwartz; Bell). At other times these criteria have only been implicit, as was common during the early years of kidney dialysis in the

United States, prior to universal funding by the federal government in 1972. Many dialysis centers employed an ad hoc approach, in which particular patients were selected from eligible pools without any set of guidelines developed in advance. The resulting decisions were widely criticized as arbitrary. Of greater concern is the tendency of ad hoc decision making to reflect the biases and preferences of the decision makers (Fox and Swazey).

Ad hoc decision making continues to take place when individual caregivers, ethics committees, or healthcare institutions make microallocation decisions without first developing an explicit set of allocation criteria to guide them. Nevertheless, significant attention in practice and theory has been devoted to formulating a more ethically acceptable decision-making approach. Overall approaches are discussed in the closing section of this entry.

Allocation Criteria

Before examining such approaches, this entry addresses the justifications and weaknesses of the major allocation criteria from which implemented or proposed approaches have been constructed. As one nationwide questionnaire study of microallocation criteria favored by selected medical directors has documented (Kilner, 1990—hereafter, "U.S. Study"), these criteria can be clustered into four major types: social, sociomedical, medical, and personal criteria.

SOCIAL CRITERIA. The characteristic feature of social criteria is that they seek to promote some particular or general social good as a result of the allocation decisions made. There are five such criteria: social value, progress of science, favored group, resources required, and vital responsibilities.

Social value. Of the social criteria, the most basic is a social value criterion. Given some place in microallocation decisions by 56 percent of the U.S. Study participants, this criterion gives preference to patients judged to be of greatest value to society, according to whatever standards of value the decision makers decide to employ. While the criterion may be explicitly invoked, it can also operate covertly to influence treatment decisions. One result in the United States has been that socially privileged groups such as whites and males have received scarce treatments disproportionately often (AMA, 1990, 1991; Institute of Medicine).

The primary attraction of employing a social value criterion is that it helps to maximize the amount of benefit derived from healthcare resources. Because society has invested its resources in a patient's treatment—or at least in developing the possibility of that treatment—it is understandably interested in a good return on its investment.

Absent this criterion, there might well be an undesirable loss of some of society's most gifted people. A social value criterion usually employs a utilitarian calculus, according to which the patients judged most likely to be most valuable to society in the future are favored. Past contributions to society may also enter the calculus on the basis of just reward or gratitude for a patient's past.

In any form, this criterion is highly controversial. Conscientiously ranking people according to social value is a virtually impossible task. Agreeing on a ranking of all possible social contributions—based on an accurate understanding of future as well as present needs—is extremely problematic even in a setting much more homogeneous than the United States. Assessing how particular individuals rank on this scale requires a virtually unobtainable level of knowledge about people's lives. The omniscience and wisdom required has led critics to label the use of this criterion "playing God." The criterion is also criticized for unfairly discriminating against individuals or groups who cannot contribute as much to society as others. Their relative inability may be due to unchangeable genetic factors or uncontrollable social circumstances (e.g., past discrimination that has undermined either their ability or society's appreciation of their contributions). Moreover, the toll on the caregiver–patient relationship can be severe. Patients can no longer be sure that confidential information about embarrassing symptoms or lifestyle habits, which caregivers often must know in order to treat patients effectively, will not be used to deny them treatment in deference to another more socially promising patient.

Progress of science. Closely related to a social value criterion is a progress of science criterion, which received roughly the same support in the U.S. Study (58% of the participants). It gives priority to patients whose treatment will yield the most scientifically useful information. For example, during the years when kidney dialysis was still scarce in the United States, a hypothesis surfaced that dialysis might alleviate the mental disorder schizophrenia as well as replace kidney function. Under such circumstances, a progress of science criterion favors treating patients who have both medical needs. Because the same number of people will be treated with or without the criterion, it is arguably best to learn as much as possible, through careful patient selection, about the full beneficial potential of a scarce resource.

On the other hand, many of the shortcomings of a social value criterion also apply to a progress of science criterion. For example, the pragmatic difficulties of identifying precisely which patients or groups of patients, if treated, will yield the most important scientific information loom large. So does the coercion inherent in the experimentation (with possible added tests or procedures) the criterion entails. Those eligible for priority treatment must either consent or risk a lower priority of being treated—which could mean substantial suffering or even death. Ultimately the criterion may not really be necessary, because patients with scientifically interesting conditions are usually selected through the application of other criteria. Such patients can volunteer for any special tests or procedures, and data on those patients can be pooled in a central location.

Favored group. According to a favored-group criterion, people of a certain type (e.g., children or military veterans) or who live within certain geographic boundaries receive priority. Much of healthcare operates on this basis, both for the sake of convenience and in order to enhance the quality of care for particular groups. Such justifications become problematic, however, when resources are limited and people who are denied care at a particular facility on the basis of this criterion cannot always obtain it in a different location. Accordingly, only 27 percent of the participants in the U.S. Study supported it.

On the other hand, some rationales for this criterion are more strictly medical and may apply to any patient. For example, when either patients receiving treatment and follow-up care or perishable resources such as transplantable organs must travel long distances, medical outcomes may suffer considerably. If medical considerations are central, though, then at issue is really some form of medical criterion, not one's group identity per se. Moreover, it is arguably better to try to remedy barriers to treatment—for example, by relocating people nearer to a treatment facility—than to employ barriers as grounds for denying treatment.

In certain cases, a very different favored-group justification is at work. A group, even an entire state or country, should arguably have the freedom to produce special resources available only to its own members, as long as the resources available to others are not thereby limited. In practice, though, such is rarely the case. Consider organ transplantation. Because the supply of organs itself is limited, giving some people special access means less access for others. Moreover, neither a particular U.S. state nor the country as a whole can claim all the credit for developing every aspect of the technology required. Accordingly, some have proposed eliminating geographic boundaries or at least implementing regional or national quota systems that would establish priorities without completely excluding any group (Task Force).

Resources required. A resources-required criterion received somewhat more support (66% of the participants in the U.S. Study) than the preceding social criteria. It prioritizes treating those who need less of a given resource before patients who need more of it, though it is usually restricted to situations in which its application will likely increase the number of lives saved. Saving lives is a central task of healthcare and a praiseworthy goal from most philosophical and religious perspectives. The requirement of a greater lifesaving potential most clearly distinguishes the criterion from a more general social value criterion. Usually only patients requiring substantially fewer resources than other patients are favored by the criterion. For instance, patients needing temporary rather than long-term use of a scarce drug receive priority, as do patients needing a single-organ rather than multiple-organ transplant. The criterion is not designed to bias patient selection automatically against patients who have previously been treated for the same problem, such as those whose failing organ transplants must be replaced.

A resources-required criterion can be criticized as too attentive, or not attentive enough, to maximizing good results from treatment. It is too attentive if the life-threatening needs of each patient requiring a particular treatment should receive equal weight regardless of the overall number of lives saved. It is not attentive enough if many characteristics of people should be considered other than whether or not they will survive. From this latter perspective, saving the life of one outstanding person could be preferable to saving two who are not.

Vital responsibilities. According to 69 percent of the participants in the U.S. Study, a vital responsibilities criterion has a legitimate role in microallocation decisions. Intended for exceptional situations only, this criterion accords special priority to patients on whom others depend. The broadest form of the criterion favors any patient who has *family dependents.* Generally, though, there must be some sort of unusual social need that requires special treatment for particular people. In a disaster situation, for example, treating those with medical expertise first may make it possible for them in turn to save additional lives. As in the case of a resources-required criterion, the strictest form of the vital responsibilities criterion requires more than producing general social value: Additional lives must be saved every time the criterion is applied.

Without this lifesaving requirement, the criterion is merely a specific type of social value criterion and therefore open to all of the critiques to which that criterion is vulnerable. Invoking the criterion to favor patients with family dependents is particularly problematic because not everyone has equal access to having children. In some cultures, moreover, sustaining the life of one who has not yet maintained the family name by having children is more important than treating one who already has children. On the other hand, if the pursuit of general social value in microallocation decisions is ethically legitimate, then allowing a vital responsibilities criterion to apply only when additional lives are saved by it is unduly restrictive.

SOCIOMEDICAL CRITERIA. Three other microallocation criteria—age, psychological ability, and supportive environment—are similar to the social criteria, in that they generally seek to promote some social good. They are distinctive, however, in that their stated justifications are often medical in nature, and they are therefore known as sociomedical criteria.

Age. Old age has long been employed as a reason for limiting medical treatment on the basis that elderly people do not sufficiently benefit from it because of their weakened physical condition. At issue may be the likelihood of benefit, the length of benefit, or the quality of benefit. So it is not surprising that 88 percent of the participants in the U.S. Study supported an age criterion to some degree.

In response to book-length justifications of an age criterion that addresses far more than aspects of medical benefit (e.g., Callahan; Daniels), a wide body of literature has emerged (e.g., Homer and Holstein; Walters; Thomasma; Hansen and Callahan). Some supporters of the criterion favor younger candidates for treatment over older candidates in order to give all an equal opportunity to live. A healthcare system, first of all, should keep people from dying "early." Others argue that whereas all people may have an equal claim upon available healthcare resources, that claim diminishes once people have achieved their so-called natural lifespan (perhaps seventy-five or eighty years). Furthermore, were people themselves given the choice, they might prefer to concentrate life-sustaining resources in their earlier years if that would make possible better long-term and supportive care in their elderly years.

Those who reject an age criterion find all such justifications unconvincing. Medical justifications arguably support medical criteria rather than a criterion based on age per se. Equal regard for persons appropriately focuses on persons as a whole—persons who should receive needed healthcare whenever that need occurs—rather than on persons as accumulations of life years, the number of which is to be maximized in the name of equal opportunity. Limiting equal access to people who have not yet lived their natural lifespan, meanwhile, relies on the debatable notion that there is a fixed natural lifespan. Moreover, it imposes on older people the judgment that, relatively speaking, their lives are not worth living, even if they disagree. (At least such is the case if age per se, rather than quality or length of life, is at issue.) Finally, if given a choice, people might well prefer criteria other than age for allocating limited resources. They

would likely recognize that in people's actual experience, they would not be denying certain forms of healthcare to their own older selves, but rather the rest of the community would be denying needed life-sustaining care to a certain group of its members. This denial is more discriminatory than it may at first appear, because the group denied is not only old but also largely female (Jecker).

In the end, all rationales for limiting healthcare for elderly persons are often suspected of being fueled, at least unconsciously, by a utilitarian preference for the achievement and economic productivity more characteristic of younger persons. Not only is the unbounded pursuit of social value itself controversial, but the economic productivity orientation of that pursuit also reflects the questionable bias of Western culture toward productivity even at the expense of personal relationships (Kilner, 1992).

Psychological ability. In the U.S. Study, 97 percent of the participants acknowledged that psychological ability plays at least some legitimate role in allocation decisions. The ability of patients to cope emotionally and intellectually with treatment is commonly assumed to be essential to effective healthcare. Without this ability, patients are unable to follow medical instructions and may even reject treatment or life itself after considerable resources have been expended. Such patients are the most difficult to treat and tend to be the least valuable to society.

These justifications also constitute arguments against the criterion. Rationales that are medical in nature actually support medical criteria rather than a psychological ability criterion per se. When psychological ability per se is invoked, the convenience of the staff or the presumed social value of the patient is problematically allowed to override the patient's claim to equal access. Moreover, caregivers' judgments about the coping abilities and cooperativeness of patients are much more subjective than the physical assessments they conduct and are therefore vulnerable to personal bias. Like everyone else, caregivers find that they can work best with those most like themselves, and many observers question the appropriateness of ranking human lives based on how well-matched patients are to caregivers.

Supportive environment. A supportive environment criterion is one that favors those patients who will have the most supportive living environment during and following treatment. Considered potentially valid by 61 percent of the participants in the U.S. Study, this criterion favors patients with the best access to personal and professional caregivers as well as facilities and other material resources relevant to effective treatment. Without sufficient postoperative care, for example, not only may scarce resources be wasted, but a treatment such as a heart transplant may result in a worse death than if the patient had received no treatment at all. Alternatively, the absence of a supportive environment may indicate that the patient warrants low priority on social value grounds.

A supportive environment criterion per se, however, is unnecessary if the concerns it addresses are already accounted for by medical benefit or social value criteria. Even as a form of another criterion, supportive environment is a problematic consideration, because the connection between people's environment and their medical outcomes or social value is far from precise. Helpful supports are not always necessary for a satisfactory medical outcome, and personal bias easily intrudes when assessing lifestyles or home situations quite different from one's own. In fact, this criterion by its very nature can be unjust when it denies treatment to patients (e.g., children with an inadequate home environment) on the basis of the irresponsibility of others (e.g., parents) or society at large. Arguably, the special needs of such situations call for extra care, not less.

MEDICAL CRITERIA. The third cluster of criteria are explicitly medical in nature, having to do with health-related outcomes of treatment. There are five of these criteria: medical benefit, imminent death, likelihood of benefit, length of benefit, and quality of benefit.

Medical benefit. The most basic of the medical criteria is a medical benefit criterion, acknowledged as a legitimate allocation criterion by 95 percent of the participants in the U.S. Study. Unlike many other medical criteria that compare and rank candidates for treatment, this criterion includes for further consideration everyone with a reasonable likelihood of receiving from treatment significant medical benefit in terms of length and quality. This criterion casts a wide net: any degree of likelihood, length, and quality that can reasonably be considered minimally significant is sufficient. Treatments not offering such benefit are commonly excluded as futile, though futility itself is a concept that requires careful definition (Jecker and Schneiderman).

The requirement that patients benefit medically from scarce medical resources is rooted in ethical standards of efficiency and justice. Without this requirement, precious resources would be wasted on patients who would receive no benefit from them. Moreover, according to many theological and philosophical traditions, need constitutes the major exception to the egalitarian presumption generally built into concepts of justice. The notion of need includes the ideas that some disease or injury condition is present (or will be, where the need for preventive care is in view), and that a person's life is thereby undesirably altered. A need for a lifesaving resource, for example, implies that a person's life is in jeopardy without it; no preferable alternatives remain.

The major difficulty with this criterion is the way in which standards of need can be manipulated. A classic illustration is the provision of kidney dialysis in Great Britain (Aaron and Schwartz). Resources allocated for dialysis by the government-run healthcare system have been insufficient to treat all who could benefit medically from dialysis, according to normal standards of need. Yet many have claimed that all who need treatment receive it. Matching of available resources and need has been achieved by tightening standards of need in sections of the country where resources are particularly scarce. Also, general practitioners do not even refer certain patients to kidney specialists for dialysis when practitioners know that sufficient resources are not available.

Imminent death. The second medical criterion, imminent death, takes the standard of need a step further. Sometimes called an *urgency* criterion, it accords special priority to patients who will die soon without treatment (support for it was not measured by the U.S. study). While the term *imminent* is not precise—generally ranging from a few days to a few weeks—it has been found workable by many in clinical and legal contexts alike (Kilner, 1990).

Not only does this criterion recognize situations of special need, it also results in more lives saved. (A necessary stipulation, though, is that it be applied together with the medical benefit criterion, so that priority will not be accorded to patients for whom treatment is futile.) Because patients whose death is not imminent can survive for a period of time while imminently dying patients receive priority care, a new treatment may become available in the interim, enabling patients in both categories to live. Alternatively (and more likely), additional resources may be made available at any point as the life-threatening situation becomes better known. In fact, the scarcity itself may be only intermittent, as is often the case with intensive care space.

An imminent death criterion, though, is more problematic in practice than it may appear to be in theory. In many situations it is impossible to determine with precision whether or not a patient's death is imminent. In others, caregivers can overstate the urgency of their patients' conditions in order to give them priority access to lifesaving resources. While doing so may be unfair, it may represent an understandable attempt to avoid another problem with the criterion. By making patients wait until they have deteriorated almost to the point of death before they receive priority access to treatment, the criterion ensures that resources will be devoted to the sickest patients. Worse medical outcomes for those treated and greater suffering for those who might wait are bound to result. Moreover, additional resources may never become available for those not prioritized by the criterion.

Likelihood of benefit. Each of the three remaining medical criteria addresses a particular aspect of medical effectiveness. The first of these, likelihood of benefit, was affirmed by 96 percent of the participants in the U.S. Study. This criterion assumes that more than a minimal likelihood of medical benefit is a necessary prerequisite for receiving scarce medical resources. Those with the greatest likelihood should be favored to ensure the most productive use of available resources. While this justification resembles the rationale underlying a social value criterion, the benefits in view here are limited to medical benefits experienced by the persons receiving the scarce resources. Moreover, more lives may ultimately be saved if this criterion is applied, although such will not be the case in every situation in which the criterion is applied.

Several obstacles attend this criterion. Precisely quantifying the probabilities of every patient's benefiting from a particular treatment so that all can be comparatively ranked is quite difficult. Furthermore, while a productive use of resources may be applauded, the cost of achieving it is arguably too great. Many patients have significant (albeit lesser) likelihoods of benefiting from treatment; yet the criterion leaves them with no realistic prospect of receiving lifesaving care if enough patients with better prospects are waiting for the same treatment. Patients can no longer trust caregivers with essential information that suggests their cases may be complicated, because caregivers must steer resources to the patient with the best prospects rather than simply attending to the needs of each patient. Ultimately, this criterion tends to discriminate against whichever groups in society have the poorest health in general and thus the lowest likelihood of having optimal outcomes from any treatment. Poor persons, disabled persons, and members of racial minorities are particularly vulnerable on this score.

Length of benefit. With a length of benefit criterion, all patients are ranked according to the length of time, rather than the likelihood, that they will benefit medically from treatment. As in the case of other comparative medical criteria, the underlying concern is to achieve as much medical benefit as possible from the available limited resources. Specifically in this case, the criterion helps to maximize the success of treatment by maximizing the length of time patients live following treatment. Of the participants in the U.S. Study, 96 percent indicated that a length of benefit criterion should have some place in microallocation decisions.

Several of the difficulties with this criterion parallel those of a likelihood of benefit criterion. Accurately predicting the length of time patients will survive following treatment is extremely hard. The criterion also tends to discriminate against the same groups of people disadvantaged by a likelihood of benefit criterion, because these typically less-healthy groups on average do not live as long as others following various types of treatments. This discriminatory effect extends to elderly patients as well, because they tend to have fewer years of life remaining regardless of the treatment in view. The significance of this concern, however, is as debatable as the age criterion itself. The most fundamental problem with a length of benefit criterion may be its presumption that length of life rather than persons per se is the appropriate focus of allocation decisions. Each person's life is uniquely important to that person. Those who argue that all people have a right to life (including life-sustaining resources) add that rights do not diminish the sicker one gets.

Quality of benefit. The final medical criterion, quality of benefit, shares the wide support expressed for other medical criteria, including acknowledgment by 97 percent of the U.S. Study participants. Like the two previous criteria, it ranks patients on a scale, in this case a scale of quality of life following treatment. This criterion rejects the common preoccupation with merely keeping patients alive and insists that healthcare is also responsible for producing lives with as high a quality as possible. Good quality of life is important to patients because it contributes substantially to their happiness as well as to their autonomy (their ability to make uncoerced decisions concerning their own lives). From a social standpoint, higher quality lives have a tendency to be more socially productive lives.

Quantifying all qualitative considerations in order to compare patients on the same scale, however, may be impossible. Even if it were possible, predicting the quality of life that will follow treatment sufficiently precisely to distinguish most patients remains problematic. So does achieving agreement as to what factors characterize a good quality of life and how these factors should be ranked. While such measures as QALYs (quality-adjusted life years) have been developed to assist macroallocation decision making, they have not proven as helpful in distinguishing individual patients at the microallocation level. Another difficulty arises when some people (usually caregivers) must assess the quality of others' lives. People judge others' quality of life on the basis of objective, observable quality of life indicators. Unfortunately, evidence has long suggested that such objective indicators do not correlate well with patients' subjective experience of their own lives (U.S. Congress). In fact, what is unacceptable to the well may be quite acceptable to the sick.

When some people impose their standards of quality on others, moreover, biases against such groups as disabled, poor, and elderly persons can easily intrude.

PERSONAL CRITERIA. The final four criteria may be designated as *personal* because their justifications are rooted in personal values such as liberty and the worth of the individual. These four are: willingness, responsibility, ability to pay, and impartial selection.

Willingness. Supported to some degree by 89 percent of the participants in the U.S. Study, a willingness criterion ensures that only patients who genuinely want treatment receive it. This criterion respects patients' rights to bodily integrity, as well as their autonomy, or freedom, to make vital decisions that primarily concern their own lives. People have unique life plans and values, and only they can accurately assess the balance between the benefits and burdens of their own treatment. For many, a right to the free exercise of religion is at stake. When resources are allocated to willing recipients, the recipients themselves are happier and the resources are less likely to be ineffective or rejected midcourse. Even if people choose to forgo treatment because other qualified patients need the same treatment, the choice can be applauded as an act of giving rather than simply branded as a typical suicide.

Nevertheless, a willingness criterion can also be problematic. For it to be employed ethically, patients must have complete information concerning the healthcare treatment in question, including the costs and benefits of receiving it; they must understand this information; they must be free from the (sometimes subtle) coercion of family, professional, or other caregivers who might want them to accept or reject treatment; and they must have the mental capacity, despite their current health predicament, to make and communicate decisions that reflect their values. A willingness criterion can also easily become a cover for patients' selfish behavior—for example, suicidal rejection of life-sustaining treatment with no regard for others who in some way depend on them.

Responsibility. Responsibility is actually a willingness criterion of a different sort. It steers resources away from people who willingly engage in unhealthy lifestyles or risky activities that result in the need for treatments (support for it was not measured by the U.S. study). Most commonly invoked as a macroallocation criterion, this criterion has provoked significant debate. Proving responsibility in specific cases is particularly controversial (Wikler).

Ability to pay. As a criterion for microallocation of healthcare resources, ability to pay received support from 43 percent of the participants in the U.S. Study. People with insufficient funds or other necessary resources are explicitly excluded by this criterion from access to certain forms of healthcare. The criterion functions in many indirect ways as well. The uninsured, in fact, use health services only about half as much as the insured and are more likely to die from treatable conditions as a result (Evans; Institute of Medicine). The inability of some patients to pay for the support services that necessarily accompany certain treatments—such as travel expenses and postoperative care—has also in effect excluded some patients from treatment. When transplantable organs have been the scarce resource, those with the ability to mobilize the media or key politicians have occasionally gained special access to the necessary organs. The ethical considerations here are essentially those attending a market approach to macroallocation.

Impartial selection. When all other ethically justifiable criteria have been applied, and there remain more eligible candidates for resources than there are resources to provide, caregivers sometimes invoke an impartial selection criterion. Affirmed by 31 percent of the participants in the U.S. Study, this criterion mandates a random selection from among eligible candidates. Its rationale is that each person who has an equal moral claim on a scarce resource should have an equal opportunity to receive it. The apparent arbitrariness of the selection helps to keep the tragedy of the situation clearly in view. It focuses more attention on the need for additional resources to be made available at the macroallocation level, if possible. There is no comforting illusion that the "best" candidates are being treated.

Some forms of impartial selection, though, may be better than others. One option is a first-come, first-served approach. Because the time that each person is stricken with a medical condition and seeks treatment is more or less random, this approach functions as a sort of natural lottery. Its appeal stems from the familiarity of waiting lines inside and outside the realms of healthcare and from the way that this approach does not seem as starkly random as an explicit lottery. True randomness, however, is the whole point of an impartial selection criterion. First-come, first-served is inferior to a genuine lottery on this score. Patients with the greater power, mobility, information, and confidence associated with the relatively wealthy have better access to healthcare generally and to referral networks in particular. Accordingly, they tend to get on the waiting lists for scarce resources sooner than those who are less wealthy and empowered.

Some weaknesses of an impartial selection criterion, though, are not unique to a particular form of the criterion but are inherent in the criterion itself. For instance, many of the social benefits that other criteria generate are lost when an impartial selection criterion is applied. Socially destructive persons such as dangerous criminals are sometimes selected instead of people who have made great positive contributions to society. Rather than respecting human dignity, impartial selection may demean it by not considering the unique features of each person. Admittedly, people cannot make infallible decisions. In the eyes of some, however, human judgments are arguably better than blind chance.

Allocation Approaches

Allocation criteria, the building blocks of microallocation, must be prioritized and arranged into some sort of basic approach if microallocation decisions are to be ethically consistent. This approach can then serve as a framework for designing specific allocation procedures tailored to particular resources and settings. Approaches tend to be justified ethically by appeals to norms such as productivity, equality, and freedom, but relatively little grounding is typically provided for these norms in the context of allocation discussions. Such norms have long had broad intuitive appeal in Western culture. Nevertheless, increasing ethical pluralism together with the tensions among the norms themselves underscore the need for a larger frame of reference (religious, rationalistic, or otherwise) within which such norms can be justified (Palazzani).

The many approaches to microallocation that have been advocated sort ethically into two groups. One group of approaches is oriented primarily toward making the most productive use of resources; the other, toward ensuring that suitable candidates have equal access to treatment through some form of impartial, or random, selection. Impartial selection may play a minor role in productivity-oriented approaches, but usually only to break ties. Furthermore, all approaches generally affirm or assume some sort of willingness criterion because of the importance of respecting people's freedom.

PRODUCTIVITY. Three forms of productivity-oriented approach can be distinguished. One form focuses exclusively on medical considerations (e.g., Leenen). Employing only medical criteria, along with sociomedical criteria whenever they are essential to good medical outcomes, this approach seeks to allocate resources to those most likely to benefit medically. Medical criteria, particularly when rooted in the notion of meeting needs, can be defended on the basis of ethical concerns other than productivity: for example, a principle of justice. But when all (or virtually all) decision making depends on comparative medical judgments among patients, a more utilitarian concern to maximize productivity is typically at work. The strengths and weaknesses of such approaches will vary depending on which of the three comparative medical criteria (likelihood, length, and quality of benefit) are employed.

A second, related form of productivity-oriented approach attempts to enhance the productivity of an exclusively medical orientation by allowing special exceptions on the basis of value to society. The concern may be to ensure treatment for particularly valuable individuals (e.g., Langford) or to exclude particularly unworthy candidates (e.g., Bayles). In the former case, the relevant rationales are those supporting social value and/or vital responsibilities criteria; in the latter, rationales undergirding a responsibility criterion also apply.

The third form of productivity-oriented approach takes this concern about social value one step further. It makes social considerations primary, combining whatever criteria are necessary to yield the most productive use of scarce resources. The ethical justifications and weaknesses of this form of approach are fundamentally those of the social value criterion itself—most obviously when such approaches affirm social value per se as the overarching consideration (e.g., Basson). When social criteria such as social value and progress of science are combined with comparative medical criteria and/or sociomedical criteria (e.g., Rescher), the additional justifications and weaknesses of those criteria come into play secondarily.

IMPARTIALITY. The major alternative to productivity-oriented approaches seeks to give suitable candidates equal access to treatment through some form of impartial selection. The pool of suitable candidates typically includes all who meet the medical benefit criterion. Priority groups within this pool are identified on the basis of nonutilitarian criteria: vital responsibilities alone (e.g., Childress), vital responsibilities plus resources required (e.g., Winslow), or both of these criteria plus imminent death (e.g., Kilner, 1990). (A priority may also be given to any group of people whose likelihood of benefit is substantially higher than that of all others, though the productivity-oriented nature of this priority creates ethical tension within an impartiality-oriented approach.) Finally, candidates are ordered within each priority group through impartial (usually random) selection.

In contrast to the explicit or implicit utilitarian bent of productivity-oriented approaches, in which benefit to society is the primary goal, the justification of this last type of approach is more egalitarian in nature. Within certain limitations designed to save as many lives as possible, all potential recipients of scarce resources are ensured an equal opportunity to receive them. This commitment to life and equality may simply be intuitive or reflect popular sentiment. Alternatively, respect for life and equality may be grounded in a philosophical or religious understanding of ethics. One philosophical example would be social contract theory, in which such respect may be seen as something to which all people would agree, if they had to decide upon ethical standards to govern society under certain ideal conditions (Winslow; Rawls). A religious example would be the biblical accounts of God's exemplary commitment to even the poorest, which is foundational to Christianity and Judaism (Mitchell; Ramsey; Zoloth; Mackler).

PARTICULAR SETTINGS. Implementing any approach requires tailoring it to particular settings. For instance, medical assessments are handled differently when allocating intensive care (Zoloth-Dorfman and Carney; Lantos, Mokalla, and Meadow) as opposed to transplantable organs (Caplan; Schmidt) or kidney dialysis (Cummings; Rutecki and Kilner). In the intensive care setting, a tool often used has been the APACHE (Acute Physiology and Chronic Health Evaluation) System. Through laboratory tests and bodily measurements, the APACHE System is able to predict patient death rates and length of intensive care stay when patients are first admitted to intensive care (Knaus et al. 1993; "Medical Algorithms Project"). A different quantitative system has been developed for assessing both medical and nonmedical considerations in organ transplantation. The United Network for Organ Sharing (UNOS) has developed a national point system to prioritize patients needing transplants. In the case of kidney transplants, for instance, candidates whose blood type is compatible with that of the donated organ are ranked according to point totals. These totals represent the sum of points given for medical considerations such as antigen matching and for nonmedical considerations such as time on the waiting list (OPTN). Methods of quantifying social value rankings in particular geographic settings have also been developed (Charny, Lewis, and Farrow).

Numerical systems are helpful in facilitating consistent comparisons among potential recipients of healthcare. Nevertheless, the need for judgment in microallocation is unavoidable (AMA, 1993). Caregivers must help identify medically appropriate courses of action, assess the likely outcomes of those courses, and assist potential recipients in their decision making. Potential recipients must evaluate the benefits and burdens of all available courses of action in light of their own sets of values and beliefs. Interdisciplinary committees and healthcare teams in public-policy and institutional settings must not only craft ethically sound allocation criteria into workable allocation approaches; they must also determine what shape such approaches take in specific

settings and discern how they apply to particular people. Microallocation, like healthcare itself, remains an art as well as a science.

JOHN F. KILNER (1995)
REVISED BY AUTHOR

SEE ALSO: *Dialysis, Kidney; Long-Term Care; Managed Care; Medicaid; Medicare; Organ Transplants;* and other *Healthcare Resources, Allocation of* subentries

BIBLIOGRAPHY

Aaron, Henry J., and Schwartz, William B. 1984. *The Painful Prescription: Rationing Hospital Care.* Washington, D.C.: Brookings Institution.

American Medical Association (AMA). Council on Ethical and Judicial Affairs. 1990. "Black–White Disparities in Health Care." *Journal of the American Medical Association* 263(17): 2344–2346.

American Medical Association (AMA). Council on Ethical and Judicial Affairs. 1991. "Gender Disparities in Clinical Decision Making." *Journal of the American Medical Association* 266(4): 559–562.

American Medical Association (AMA). Council on Ethical and Judicial Affairs. 1993. "Ethical Considerations in the Allocation of Organs and Other Scarce Medical Resources among Patients" Report 49. Chicago: Author.

Basson, Marc D. 1979. "Choosing among Candidates for Scarce Medical Resources." *Journal of Medicine and Philosophy* 4(2): 313–333.

Bayles, Michael D. 1990. "Allocation of Scarce Medical Resources." *Public Affairs Quarterly* 4(1): 1–16.

Bell, Nora K. 1981. "Triage in Medical Practices: An Unacceptable Model?" *Social Science and Medicine* 15F(4): 151–156.

Callahan, Daniel. 1987. *Setting Limits: Medical Goals in an Aging Society.* New York: Simon and Schuster.

Caplan, Arthur L. 1992. *If I Were a Rich Man Could I Buy a Pancreas? And Other Essays on the Ethics of Health Care.* Bloomington: Indiana University Press.

Charny, M. C.; Lewis, P. A.; and Farrow, S. C. 1989. "Choosing Who Shall Not Be Treated in the NHS." *Social Science and Medicine* 28(12): 1331–1338.

Childress, James F. 1981. *Priorities in Biomedical Ethics.* Philadelphia: Westminster Press.

Cummings, Nancy B. 1993. "Ethical Considerations in End-Stage Renal Disease." In *Diseases of the Kidney,* 5th edition, ed. Robert W. Schrier and Carl W. Gottschalk. Boston: Little, Brown.

Daniels, Norman. 1988. *Am I My Parents' Keeper?* New York: Oxford University Press.

Evans, Roger W. 1989. "Money Matters: Should Ability to Pay Ever Be a Consideration in Gaining Access to Transplantation?" *Transplantation Proceedings* 21(3): 3419–3423.

Fox, Renée C., and Swazey, Judith P. 1978. *The Courage to Fail,* 2nd edition. Chicago: University of Chicago Press.

Hansen, Mark, and Callahan, Daniel, eds. 1999. *The Goals of Medicine.* Washington, D.C.: Georgetown University Press.

Homer, Paul, and Holstein, Martha, eds. 1990. *A Good Old Age? The Paradox of Setting Limits.* New York: Simon and Schuster.

Institute of Medicine. 2002. *Unequal Treatment: Confronting Racial and Ethnic Disparities in Health Care.* Washington, D.C.: National Academy Press.

Jecker, Nancy S. 1991. "Age-Based Rationing and Women." *Journal of the American Medical Association* 266(21): 3012–3015.

Jecker, Nancy S., and Schneiderman, Lawrence J. 1992. "Futility and Rationing." *American Journal of Medicine* 92(2): 189–196.

Kilner, John F. 1990. *Who Lives? Who Dies? Ethical Criteria in Patient Selection.* New Haven, CT: Yale University Press.

Kilner, John F. 1992. *Life on the Line: Ethics, Aging, Ending Patients' Lives, and Allocating Vital Resources.* Grand Rapids, MI: W. B. Eerdmans.

Knaus, William A.; Wagner, Douglas P.; Zimmerman, Jack E.; et al. 1993. "Variations in Mortality and Length of Stay in Intensive Care Units." *Annals of Internal Medicine* 118(10): 753–761.

Langford, Michael J. 1992. "Who Should Get the Kidney Machine?" *Journal of Medical Ethics* 18(1): 12–17.

Lantos, John D.; Mokalla, Mani; and Meadow, William. 1997. "Resource Allocation in Neonatal and Medical ICUs: Epidemiology and Rationing at the Extremes of Life." *American Journal of Respiratory and Critical Care Medicine* 156(1): 185–189.

Leenen, H. J. J. 1988. "Selection of Patients: An Insoluble Dilemma." *Medicine and Law* 7(3): 233–245.

Mackler, Aaron L. 1991. "Judaism, Justice, and Access to Health Care." *Kennedy Institute of Ethics Journal* 1(2): 143–161.

Mehlman, Maxwell J. 1985. "Rationing Expensive Lifesaving Medical Treatments." *Wisconsin Law Review* 1985(2): 239–303.

Palazzani, Laura. 1994. "Personalism and Bioethics." *Ethics and Medicine* 10(1): 7–11.

Ramsey, Paul. 1970. *The Patient as Person: Explorations in Medical Ethics.* New Haven, CT: Yale University Press.

Rawls, John. 1971. *A Theory of Justice.* Cambridge, MA: Harvard University Press.

Rescher, Nicholas. 1969. "The Allocation of Exotic Medical Lifesaving Therapy." *Ethics* 79(3): 173–186.

Rhodes, Rosamind; Miller, Charles; and Schwartz, Myron. 1992. "Transplant Recipient Selection: Peacetime versus Wartime Triage." *Cambridge Quarterly of Healthcare Ethics* 1(4): 327–331.

Rutecki, Gregory W., and Kilner, John F. 1999. "Dialysis as a Resource Allocation Paradigm." *Seminars in Dialysis* 12(1): 38–43.

Schmidt, Volker H. 1998. "Selection of Recipients for Donor Organs in Transplant Medicine." *Journal of Medicine and Philosophy* 23(1): 50–74.

Thomasma, David C. 1999. "Stewardship of the Aged: Meeting the Ethical Challenge of Ageism." *Cambridge Quarterly of Healthcare Ethics* 8(2): 148–159.

Truog, Robert D. 1992. "Triage in the ICU." *Hastings Center Report* 22(3): 13–17.

United Nations Children's Fund (UNICEF). 1993. *Annual Report.* New York: Author.

United Nations Children's Fund (UNICEF). 2003. *The State of the World's Children, 2003.* New York: Author.

U.S. Congress. Office of Technology Assessment. 1987. *Life-Sustaining Technologies and the Elderly.* Washington, D.C.: U. S. Government Printing Office.

U.S. Task Force on Organ Transplantation. 1986. *Organ Transplantation: Issues and Recommendations.* Rockville, MD: U.S. Department of Health and Human Services, Office of Organ Transplantation.

Walters, James W., ed. 1996. *Choosing Who's to Live: Ethics and Aging.* Urbana: University of Illinois Press.

Wikler, Daniel. 1987. "Who Should Be Blamed for Being Sick?" *Health Education Quarterly* 14(1): 11–25.

Winslow, Gerald R. 1982. *Triage and Justice.* Berkeley: University of California Press.

Winslow, Gerald R., and James W. Walters, eds. 1993. *Facing Limits: Ethics and Health Care for the Elderly.* Boulder, CO: Westview Press.

Zoloth, Laurie. 1999. *Health Care and the Ethics of Encounter: A Jewish Discussion of Social Justice.* Chapel Hill: University of North Carolina Press.

Zoloth-Dorfman, Laurie, and Carney, Bridget. 1991. "The AIDS Patient and the Last ICU Bed: Scarcity, Medical Futility, and Ethics." *Quality Review Bulletin* 17(6): 175–181.

INTERNET RESOURCES

"The Medical Algorithms Project," Chapter 30: "Critical Care." Quanta Healthcare Solutions. 2003. Available from <http://www.medal.org/ch30.html>.

Organ Procurement and Transplantation Network (OPTN). 2003. "Organ Distribution." Available from <http://www.optn.org/policiesAndBylaws/policies.asp>.

Organ Procurement and Transplantation Network (OPTN). 2003. "Removal Reasons by Year." Available from <http://www.optn.org/data/annualReport.asp>.

HEALTHCARE SYSTEMS

• • •

A healthcare system can be defined as the method by which healthcare is financed, organized, and delivered to a population. It includes issues of access (for whom and to which services), expenditures, and resources (healthcare workers and facilities). The goal of a healthcare system is to enhance the health of the population in the most effective manner possible in light of a society's available resources and competing needs. By the beginning of the twenty-first century access to healthcare had come to be regarded by most countries and the United Nations as a special good that is necessary either as a matter of or pursuant to basic human rights. An examination of healthcare systems therefore includes consideration of the ways in which a particular system addresses commonly held values.

The extent and form of a specific system are influenced by a variety of factors, including the unique culture and history of a population or country. What is considered healthcare can vary markedly in accordance with a country's level of development, culture, and social values. Some populations put emphasis on the prevention of disease, whereas others emphasize only the care for or cure of particular illnesses. Definitions of health and disease and of *appropriate* healthcare providers also are subject to cultural variability.

A second major influence derives from the priorities given to various ethical values: "There is no way to adjudicate disputes among the Holy Trinity of cost, quality and access unless a court of values is available to dispense its wisdom" (Reinhard, pg. 1). Those values include respect for the autonomy of both patients and providers, the maximization of benefit, and the promotion of justice or fairness, understood as equality or liberty.

Balancing those values has posed a dilemma in the United States. Public opinion polls have revealed that most Americans see access to healthcare as a fundamental right. However, Americans' equally strong belief in individual autonomy and responsibility, the use of the market as a means for distributing goods and services, and fears about government interference create conflict and have led to a fragmented healthcare system.

A third influence on the structure of a healthcare system is the level of economic resources available. There is a strong positive correlation between economic resources as measured by the per capita gross domestic product (GDP) and both healthcare expenditures and the proportion of a nation's GDP that is spent on healthcare (Gerdtham and Jonsson). This indicates that although healthcare generally is valued, countries and individuals may consider food, shelter, and in some instances spending for the military more important. However, although the economic resources available to a country have a great effect on that country's overall expenditures on healthcare, there is nearly as much variation in the forms of the healthcare systems in countries that are economically poor as there is in wealthy countries.

Public versus Private Control

All governments have some degree of involvement in healthcare because essentially all countries have a centrally funded agency that is concerned with public health issues. The proportion of healthcare expenditures spent on public health tends to be higher in low-income countries, although the level of effort varies greatly from country to country. Government involvement usually includes surveillance of communicable diseases and interventions to prevent or curtail epidemics. Some countries have more extensive government involvement through direct delivery of services (e.g., immunizations, well-child care, screening for developmental disabilities, and treatment of communicable diseases) and programs of health promotion. Public health efforts in the United States are fragmented but have begun to receive more attention as the costs of personal, disease-oriented healthcare and concerns about bioterrorism have increased.

Beyond public health measures, healthcare systems vary dramatically with regard to the degree of public versus private control (Anderson et al.). In fact, the extent of government control is probably the most distinguishing characteristic among systems. In most member countries of the Organization for Economic Cooperation and Development (OECD) the healthcare system is dominated by the public sector. The OECD countries with a high percentage of revenues from the public sector in 2000 included Luxembourg (93%), the Czech Republic (91%), and the Slovak Republic (90%) (OECD). In a few countries the majority of revenues come from the private sector. In the United States the private sector accounts for about 56 percent of healthcare expenditures. The only other OECD countries that receive a majority of funds (more than 50%) from the private sector are South Korea (56%) and Mexico (54%).

The public side of healthcare systems in industrialized countries can be placed into two categories: countries with comprehensive programs and strong government control of virtually all aspects (financing, delivery, quality monitoring) of the system, such as Great Britain, the Scandinavian countries, and the countries of the former Soviet Union, and countries in which the government's role is limited to financing or guaranteeing enrollment for all citizens in a health insurance plan, such as Germany, Belgium, France, and Canada. Both types of systems are characterized by public financing or mandates that guarantee universal coverage, payment that is negotiated between the public sector and providers, and policies regarding facilities and healthcare workers that are modulated predominantly by the public sector.

In countries in which the private sector is the dominant payer for healthcare universal coverage is less common, payment varies from provider to provider and insurance company to insurance company, and policies regarding healthcare workers are negotiated in the marketplace. In the United States, for example, patient and professional autonomy are dominant (Reinhard). Most individuals or employers are free to choose from among multiple insurers and providers, and most provider groups have the freedom to choose whom to serve, how much to charge, and what credentials are required to join the group.

Especially notable has been the strong distrust of government interventions except when they are deemed necessary to guarantee access to a group that is seen as *entitled* because of a special service it has rendered (retirees, veterans) or special need (disability, poverty). However, even in the United States there have been a number of occasions (as in 1910, 1935, 1948, 1965, 1972, and 1994) when a reasonably strong attempt was made to provide a substantial increase in government involvement in the healthcare system. Except in 1965 those attempts failed because of a combination of factors, including provider opposition, lack of public consensus, fears of increased government involvement, and relatively comprehensive healthcare benefits that most working Americans receive from employment-based private insurance.

Financing

The means of financing healthcare, perhaps more than any other aspect of a healthcare system, mirror the values and priorities of a society. As was noted above, unlike the case in the majority of the OECD countries, healthcare financing in the United States is mostly private. There is also little public financing of healthcare in most low-income countries. Because of the high cost of many interventions and the unequal distribution of healthcare costs among individuals, lack of a broad-based system of public financing creates a system in which healthcare is rationed on the basis of the ability to pay.

Beginning with Germany in 1883, most industrialized nations have implemented a government-coordinated or government-controlled system of financing for personal healthcare services. This varies from the systems in countries such as Great Britain and the former Soviet Union, in which

virtually all healthcare is financed through general tax revenues collected by the national government, to systems, such as Canada's, that are financed from both state and national revenues, to those of Germany, France, Belgium, and the Netherlands, in which financing is mandated by the national government through required participation in a community- or employment-based insurance funds.

In the third type of system most funds are obtained through required contributions based on wages. All countries with strong central control have at least a small market of privately financed healthcare that is used predominantly by the rich and the politically connected. For example, in Germany and the Netherlands the most affluent people are not required to purchase health insurance, and most choose to purchase private health insurance, which gives them better access to medical services. Some countries with mixed systems (e.g., Japan and Australia) have a small market for private health insurance that complements the public-sector benefits.

The proportion of public financing of healthcare in the United States has been increasing steadily, rising from about 23.3 percent in 1960 to nearly 44.3 percent in 2000 (OECD). In spite of these increases, there is no universal government-guaranteed or compulsory health insurance. Employer-based or individually purchased private insurance is the most common way people obtain health insurance coverage. A variety of publicly financed programs (e.g., Medicare and Medicaid) provide insurance to persons over age sixty-five and some poor people. They are financed by a spectrum of public financing mechanisms, including federal and local government revenues, the use of income and employment-based taxes, and in some states the revenues from a lottery.

Financing for active-duty military personnel, veterans, and Native Americans mirrors the centrally controlled healthcare systems of Great Britain and the former Soviet Union. Revenues come from the federal income tax, and services are provided by public-sector employees. The Medicare program is financed primarily from a wage tax, whereas Medicaid (for certain categories of disabled and low-income persons) is financed from a combination of state and federal general tax revenues. Financing for some care for the poor who are not eligible for Medicaid comes from general tax revenues at the state or local level that are paid to city and county public hospitals and state mental hospitals.

The dominance of a private system of financing in the United States is a reflection of not only that nation's values but also of a number of historical events. The Blue Cross program began in Texas when Baylor Hospital enrolled schoolteachers in an insurance system during the Great Depression as a method to guarantee that hospitalized patients could pay their health bills. Private health insurance grew slowly during the 1930s.

The real spread of private health insurance occurred during World War II, when wages but not fringe benefits were frozen as a wartime price-control measure. As more firms began to offer health insurance as a benefit, private insurance companies saw the potential for expanding their markets and encouraging those enrolled in health-insurance plans to buy their other insurance products. Another impetus to the market was the decision by the federal government to exempt healthcare benefits from federal income tax. The large number of insurance plans in the United States, each with its own marketing, benefit packages, premiums, deductibles or copayments, billing, and payment requirements, together with the thousands of private physicians, clinics, and hospitals, has created an immense administrative bureaucracy with aggregate administrative spending of $89.7 billion in 2001 (Center for Medicare and Medicaid Services; Levit et al.).

Access and Delivery

A second major characteristic of a healthcare system is access, which has multiple definitions, including the following:

1. The ability to obtain needed care
2. The potential and actual entry of a given population into the health system
3. The timely use of personal health services to achieve the best possible outcome
4. The timely use of needed, affordable, convenient, acceptable, and effective personal health services

Different countries approach the issue of access in various ways and define the term differently. Health systems with strong central control, such as those in Great Britain, the Scandinavian countries, and the countries of the former Soviet Union, emphasize equal access to care for all their citizens. Those countries have a single-payment system, with most healthcare providers working as salaried government employees and a single government-defined set of benefits. There tends to be strong emphasis on primary care by general practitioners and relatively tight control of the number and distribution of providers and facilities that provide highly technical services. In some countries this degree of government control results in substantial waiting times for some services and limited access to advanced technologies. Thus, whereas this approach produces an apparently high level of equal opportunity to obtain needed

health services, it may deny some individuals access to lifesaving technologies and restrict both provider and patient choices. This depends on the level of spending a country is willing to commit to healthcare.

Countries with less centralized systems vary more in regard to the level of access. In some countries access to healthcare for the poor is restricted by the ability to pay. Moreover, providers' freedom to choose their patients can restrict access to medical services among insured low-income individuals. For example, many providers in the United States refuse to serve Medicaid recipients because of the low payment rates. In countries with less centralized health systems working individuals employed in low-paying jobs often face financial barriers (high out-of-pocket expenses for copayments, deductibles, or premiums) to receive needed care (Lee and Tollen). Similarly, the limited control of healthcare workers and facility location tends to result in geographic maldistribution of providers and healthcare facilities.

The degree of access varies widely in the United States. Financial barriers to access are substantial for more than 41 million Americans without health insurance coverage and about the fifth of insured individuals who have inadequate insurance (Mills; Hadley and Holahan; Kaiser Commission on Medicaid and the Uninsured). Studies have shown that those who are poor and have no health insurance have a markedly lower use of almost all forms of healthcare despite their tendency to have a lower baseline health status. This lack is especially great in terms of primary care and preventive services (Bayer and Fiscella). Although the uninsured have some access to high-technology care, especially in urban areas, through use of the emergency rooms and outpatient clinics of public hospitals, research has shown that they have poorer outcomes of hospitalization (controlling for severity) and a markedly lower use of high technology compared with those who have insurance. There is also growing evidence that limited access to primary care results in not only poorer health outcomes but also higher overall costs through delayed treatment, reduced patient adherence to therapeutic regimens, and increased emergency room and hospital admissions.

Payment

The level and means by which providers of healthcare are paid has a substantial effect on access, costs, and the quality of care. In countries that rely on a private healthcare delivery system (the United States, Canada, France, and Belgium) the predominant mode of payment for physicians who provide ambulatory care is fee-for-service. In most instances physicians bargain with insurers or the government over a fee schedule. In some countries there is a provision that physicians can charge patients more than the allowed fees in certain circumstances. There is concern that the financial incentives inherent in a fee-for-service system result in over utilization of services, especially those reimbursed at higher levels relative to other services. However, the autonomy of providers is preserved, and there is an incentive for increased productivity. Additionally, there is no conflict between the financial interests of providers and their duty to provide all services that are of benefit to patients. Cost- or charge-based reimbursement for institutions (hospitals, nursing homes, etc.) has similar risks and benefits.

Some insurers in the United States and the Netherlands use capitation (a set payment per person per year) or a set payment per case to pay providers. Capitation payments provide an incentive for healthcare workers and facilities to limit the volume of provided services and allow providers to determine precisely which services to provide. At the same time, case-based payment and capitation create a conflict between the financial incentive of the provider and the interest of the individual patient in receiving all services that are of possible benefit. This can be a problem for people with multiple chronic conditions, who are often the most expensive to treat.

In many countries, hospitals are paid on prospectively negotiated global budgets and hospital-based providers, including physicians, are paid on a salaried basis. These methods of payment have little apparent effect on the provision of services to individuals. However, the level of payment may have a profound effect on which technology is acquired and on whether providers expend the time and effort required to provide a given service in general.

Expenditures and Cost Controls

Since 1960 in virtually every country expenditures for personal healthcare services have been rising in absolute terms and in relation to GDP (Anderson et al.). Health expenditures have been increasing at a rate nearly double that of other major sectors of some national economies. In some countries concerns are being raised that spending on medical care is occurring at the expense of other socially desirable goods and services. This is especially true in the United States, where despite the highest per capita and GDP-adjusted healthcare spending in the world, healthcare is still not accessible to all, and there is growing concern about other social problems such as deteriorating schools, homelessness, poverty, and crime.

One reason for controlling health spending is that there is strong evidence that more healthcare spending does not necessarily buy better health (Newhouse). Even more compelling is the growing evidence that a substantial number of medical-care services may provide only small marginal benefits. Although small benefits and high cost are the norm in industrialized countries, many developing and economically disadvantaged countries cannot provide their populations with even basic public health measures such as immunization and sanitation.

In many industrialized countries cost controls have created the potentially unpopular phenomenon of waiting lists. Some countries, notably the United Kingdom and the Scandinavian countries, have implemented a policy of increasing health spending to eliminate waiting lists.

The response of different healthcare systems to the growing problem of cost has in general reflected the basic organization and values of each country. In countries with strong central control there has been increasing pressure to create fixed budgets and establish tight control over the acquisition of advanced technologies (supply-side control). Access to basic health services for everyone has been maintained at the expense of not providing expensive services that are potentially lifesaving for a few individuals.

By contrast, in the United States there are relatively fewer advocates for global budgeting. Efforts to reduce costs have focused primarily on enhanced competition (demand-side control). These cost-control mechanisms appear to have produced some one-time reductions in healthcare spending but have had a very modest effect on the rate of growth of expenditures.

Because of the seemingly inexorable rise in costs in the United States, employers have been shifting more of the cost of healthcare to employees by increasing employee-paid premiums, eliminating coverage for dependents, increasing copayments and deductibles, or eliminating coverage altogether. The response of private insurance companies to growing cost concerns has been to refuse to insure high-risk employees (medical underwriting) or to tie premiums directly to the previous year's expenditures by a particular group (experience rating). Employers became more aggressive in eliminating benefits such as health insurance for retirees when the labor market became looser and profits decreased. All these factors, along with a rise in the number of part-time workers and employment in small, nonunion service industries that lack medical benefits, have been primary determinants in the increase in the number of working-age individuals in the United States who are without health insurance.

Resources

The most visible aspects of any healthcare system are the facilities and personnel involved in the delivery of healthcare. Centralized systems have attempted to provide greater equality in the distribution of facilities and healthcare workers by focusing on the needs of a community rather than on the autonomy of providers and patients. In some centralized systems the national government may determine how many and which types of physicians, nurses, and other healthcare workers are produced; the location of hospitals and the technology they may purchase; and the location of hospital-based and outpatient-care providers. Care is strongly regionalized, with easily accessible primary care for most common healthcare problems, some specialty care available in regional hospitals, and subspecialty and tertiary care confined to a few large teaching centers.

In contrast to most other countries, the healthcare system in the United States provides little central control. There has been almost complete autonomy for providers, starting with a system of health-professional education with a substantial number of private schools and little or no restriction on specialty choice, practice, or hospital location or on the availability of technology. Because of the prestige and generous payments for new technology nearly all hospitals provide a full array of high-technology services. This complements a strong trend toward subspecialization among health professionals. In the case of physicians the percentage of generalists versus specialists declined from nearly 50 percent in 1961 to the current 28 percent; if OB/GYN and emergency medicine physicians are included in the generalist category, the figures are 32 percent primary care physicians and 68 percent specialists (Bureau of Health Professionals; Council on Graduate Medical Education). The abundance of specialists, especially those who are trained to perform high-technology procedures, is thought to exacerbate the over utilization of some healthcare services. Conversely, the decline in the number of generalists is believed to be a contributing factor in the poor access to healthcare experienced by persons in rural areas and those with low incomes in urban areas.

Choices for the Future

All countries are continuing to search for better cost-containment and cost-effectiveness mechanisms, including the difficult task of placing limits on the healthcare technologies that provide small marginal benefits to a few individuals at a great cost to the community.

Tension will grow between the values of individual autonomy (reflected in the assumption by patients that the *right* to healthcare includes all interventions that are of possible benefit and the assumption by providers that they have the *right* to set prices and choose where and whom to serve) and concern for the good of the community and other societal needs. Attempts to achieve equality in the systems of financing, payment, cost control, and delivery will have to take into account increasing competition for limited resources and the perceived infringement on personal freedom. Balancing these competing claims will be especially difficult in the United States with its multiple systems and distrust of government involvement in human services.

A renewal of a sense of community and a careful balancing of values will be necessary in achieving a reasonable solution. Although the future is unclear, the United States probably will reconsider policies for rational allocation between healthcare and other sectors of the economy, government regulation to require universal and equitable access to defined *basic* insurance policies, mandated employer-based insurance with a publicly financed safety net, payment based on capitation with some adjustment for the severity of illness in a specific group of patients, and incentives (including scholarships and loan forgiveness) for providers who choose to provide primary care in shortage areas.

L. GREGORY PAWLSON
JACQUELINE J. GLOVER (1995)
REVISED BY VARDUHI PETROSYAN
GERARD F. ANDERSON

SEE ALSO: *Advertising; Health Insurance; Health Policy in International Perspective; Health Policy in the United States; Healthcare Institutions; Healthcare Resources, Allocation of; Hospital, Contemporary Ethical Problems of*

BIBLIOGRAPHY

Anderson, Gerard; Reinhardt, Uwe; Hussey, Peter; and Petrosyan, Varduhi. 2003. "It's the Prices, Stupid: Why the United States Is So Different from Other Countries." *Health Affairs* 22(3): 89–105.

Bayer, William H., and Fiscella, Kevin. 1999. "Patients and Community Together: A Family Medicine Community-Oriented Primary Care Project in an Urban Private Practice." *Archives of Family Medicine* 8: 546–549.

Blank, R. H. 1988. *Rationing Medicine.* New York: Columbia University Press.

Council on Graduate Medical Education.1994. *Recommendations to Improve Access to Health Care through Physician Workforce Reform,* fourth report. Washington, D.C.: U.S. Department of Health and Human Services.

Gerdtham, Ulf-G., and Jonsson, Bengt. 2000. "International Comparisons of Health Expenditure." In *Handbook of Health Economics,* ed. A. J. Culyer and J. P. Newhouse. New York: Elsevier Science.

Kaiser Commission on Medicaid and the Uninsured. 2002a. *The Uninsured: A Primer: Key Facts about Americans without Insurance.* Washington, D.C.: Kaiser Family Foundation.

Kaiser Commission on Medicaid and the Uninsured. 2002b. *Underinsured in America: Is Health Coverage Adequate?* Washington, D.C.: Kaiser Family Foundation.

Levit, Katharine; Smith, Cynthia; Cowan, Cathy; et al. 2003. "Trends in U.S. Health Care Spending, 2001." *Health Affairs* 22(1): 154–164.

Montenegro-Torres, Fernando; Engelhardt, Timothy; Thamer, Mae; and Anderson, Gerard. 2001. "Are Fortune 100 Companies Responsive to Chronically Ill Workers?" *Health Affairs* 20(4): 209–219.

Newhouse, Joseph. 1992. "Medical Care Costs: How Much Welfare Loss?" Journal of Economic Perspectives 6(3): 3–21.

Organization for Economic Cooperation and Development (OECD). 2002. *OECD Health Data, 2002.* Paris: Organization for Economic Cooperation and Development.

Reinhard, Priester. 1992. "A Values Framework for Health System Reform." *Health Affairs* 11(1): 84–107.

Roemer, Milton Irwin. 1991. *National Health Systems of the World.* New York: Oxford University Press.

Shi, Leiyu. 1998. *Delivering Health Care in America: A Systems Approach.* Gaithersburg, MD: Aspen Publishers.

INTERNET RESOURCES

Bureau of Health Professionals: National Center for Health Workforce Information and Analysis. 2003. *Health Workforce Factbook.* Health Resources and Services Administration. Available from <http://bhpr.hrsa.gov/healthworkforce/factbook.htm>.

Center for Medicare and Medicaid Services. Office of The Actuary, National Health Statistics Group. 2003. Available from <http://cms.hhs.gov/statistics/nhe/definitions-sources-methods/>.

Hadley, Jack, and Holahan, John. 2003. "How Much Medical Care Do the Uninsured Use, and Who Pays for It?" *Health Affairs—Web Exclusive.* Available from <http://www.healthaffairs.org/WebExclusives>.

Lee, Jason, and Tollen, Laura. 2002. "How Low Can You Go? The Impact of Reduced Benefits and Increased Cost Sharing." *Health Affairs—Web Exclusive.* Available from <http://www.healthaffairs.org/WebExclusives>.

Mills, Robert J. 2002. *Current Population Report: Health Insurance Coverage 2001. P60–220.* Washington, D.C.: U.S. Department of Commerce, Economics and Statistics Administration, Census Bureau. Available from <http://www.census.gov/prod/2002pubs/p60–220.pdf>.

HEALTH INSURANCE

• • •

The social and economic vulnerability of wage laborers gave rise to nineteenth-century reforms that are the forerunners of modern health insurance. When the flow of resources to a household depends on wage labor, sickness for any prolonged period threatens the family's ability to secure food and shelter. The practice of organizing workers to contribute a portion of their wages to health (or sickness) insurance funds was a response to this vulnerability, and set a social pattern in industrialized nations that has continued for more than a century. The two principal ethical concepts associated with health insurance are social solidarity and social justice.

Health Insurance and Social Solidarity

As was evident in the European sickness funds, the insurance compact expresses an underlying solidarity among insurance pool subscribers. Persons facing a common vulnerability organize into a group whose shared resources, built up from relatively small individual contributions, will assist members who suffer financial loss as a result of illness or injury. Since the anticipated harm is a matter of probability, the group that pools its resources must be large enough and composed of persons with sufficiently variable risk levels so that, in a given period of time covered by the contributions (or premiums), only a minority of those at risk will actually experience illness or injury. The majority will contribute without needing to draw on the pooled resources. Those who do not encounter harm stand in a relationship of fiscal solidarity with those who do. The smaller the group, the more vulnerable it is to being overwhelmed by a small number of very large claims. If the group includes a large number of persons with high probability of need (the elderly, for example), a high level of member contributions will be required to guarantee adequate resources to cover every claim.

In addition to the purely fiscal relationship among contributors, reigning social and political ideas affect the conscious feelings of solidarity they experience as members of an insured group. Compulsory sickness insurance for workers, providing for both lost wages and the cost of medical care, was first organized at a national level in 1883 in Germany by the conservative chancellor Otto von Bismarck as a defensive maneuver against the rising influence of the German Social Democratic Party. As Paul Starr noted in his 1982 work, Bismarck believed workers were less likely to demand more radical reforms if certain harsh realities of the industrial revolution could be tempered with benevolence flowing from the monarchy.

In the closing decades of the nineteenth century, several other European nations took similar actions to protect workers' vulnerability, but the United States showed little interest in the idea until the Progressive reformers began to press the issue in the early years of the twentieth century (Hirshfield). They promoted compulsory health insurance as a form of enlightened self-interest on the part of the middle class: The survival of individual freedoms essential to capitalism required taming the tendency of free enterprise to pursue profit without concern for the precarious circumstance of wage laborers. Robert N. Bellah, et al. (1985) noted that the vocabulary of individualism typical of the culture of private consumption has shaped public discourse about health insurance in the United States, and the concept of social solidarity is only faintly evident in the debate that has evolved since the early twentieth century (Churchill).

In some societies, social consciousness about health insurance sees it as a component of the nation's system of social insurance—that is, a public guarantee that certain basic human needs will be met at some minimum level for all members of the community. This has typically been the meaning of health insurance in Western Europe. Conversely, health insurance may be seen as a marketable service properly residing in the private sector, which has been the dominant, though not unanimous, social understanding in the United States (Greenlick, 1988).

The Progressives' compulsory insurance campaign had failed prior to 1920, and by the late 1930s, the idea of voluntary health insurance for workers as a fringe benefit of employment had taken over as the prevailing rationale for social change. The appeal of voluntary insurance, supported by tax subsidies for employers and workers, was fully compatible with the Progressives' individual freedoms argument. Indeed, the voluntary approach seemed capable of solving the solidarity problem, as the percentage of the whole population with voluntary hospital insurance shot up from less than 10 percent in 1940 to 57 percent in 1950 and to nearly 90 percent by the early 1970s (Anderson). With health insurance spreading widely through the working community, yet systematically leaving those not in the workforce outside the fold, the idea of national health insurance based on explicit appeals to solidarity and social justice emerged periodically but each time failed to pass into law (Hirshfield; Starr).

Health Insurance, Social Justice, and Rights

The concept of justice is the second major ethical theme associated with health insurance. Concerns about justice and health insurance derive from the question whether it is fair for some, but not all, citizens to have insured access to healthcare. Originally, health insurance was viewed as required by social justice not for everyone, but only for those made vulnerable by the conditions of wage labor. Compulsory insurance schemes were designed to help capitalism by making the working class more secure. The U.S. middle class broadly committed itself to the voluntary purchase of health insurance when, as a means of winning better fringe benefits through collective bargaining (intensified under wage and price controls during World War II), getting health insurance as a benefit became a normative expectation of workers.

Once the idea of health insurance takes hold in a society and is widely believed to give access to a fundamental benefit of social existence, it comes to be seen as the way members of the society purchase their healthcare, not merely the way they protect themselves from potential financial loss. Having insurance and getting needed healthcare become closely linked in the logic of justice. (For an account of how social expectations give rise to the perception of entitlement and societal obligation, see the work of Michael Walzer.)

The idea of a right to healthcare as a requirement of social justice is intimately connected to the practice of collectively financed healthcare. The notion that healthcare might count among positive human rights derives from the widespread belief that healthcare successfully meets fundamental human needs, such as security, relief from suffering, prevention of premature death, and maintenance of functional capacity. (For a philosophical argument about the grounds and limits of universal entitlement, see Norman Daniels's work and Charles J. Dougherty's publication.) Creating legal protections for that right becomes a problem of political will.

The injection of rights language into political arguments about health insurance is itself evidence of the evolution of the concept and expansion of its original limited goal of protecting wage laborers from the effects of major illness. In the absence of a constitutional or statutory declaration of a right to healthcare, opinion leaders use human rights language to motivate members of society and to provoke legislative action aimed at helping persons whose needs are being ignored. While specific contractual rights to healthcare exist between insured persons and their insurance carriers, that is not what advocates of a right to healthcare have in mind. When reformers argue for a right to healthcare, they mean that basic relationships of solidarity and interdependence among all members of society create a societal obligation to ensure access to healthcare for all. (For a discussion of issues raised by rights discourse in relation to health insurance and access to healthcare, see the U.S. President's Commission Report, and the 1994 work edited by Audrey Chapman.)

During the second half of the twentieth century, aggregate expenditures for healthcare rose at such a dramatic rate that by the 1980s, cost control in healthcare became a central issue for reformers. However, the question of setting limits makes debate about a right to healthcare politically difficult. Unlike rights to liberty or the pursuit of happiness, which entail noninterference by others, a right to healthcare entails paying someone to provide costly services. By 1990, the need to speak of a limited right was clear to many leaders, although negative reaction to the idea of rationing healthcare led many to deny its necessity, and how to define limits was hotly debated (Strosberg). In 1989, the state of Oregon intensified the debate when it organized a unique social experiment to guarantee coverage to uninsured persons while setting limits on what would be covered based on a prioritized list of healthcare services (Garland, 1992, 1994, 2001).

Organization and Financing of Health Insurance

The fundamental concept of any form of insurance is risk sharing: A large number of people who face a common threat of harm (auto accident, fire damage, costs of treatment for illness or injury) share their risks by paying premiums to an insurer who promises to finance payments to those who in the future actually suffer misfortune. All members of the risk-sharing group get a sense of security in return for their contributions even if they do not receive specific insurance payments (as a result of being personally harmed).

Ethical issues in risk sharing through health insurance are shaped by the insurer's decisions about how to organize and finance the common fund that members of a group rely on for protection against potential financial loss. For example, insurers may organize risk-sharing pools among individual subscribers, various age groups, business firms, or labor organizations. Financing might be done through a single, community-wide premium or through variable premiums tied to past utilization, health-risk or ethnic group or age or gender. The European approach was to develop social insurance mechanisms, or sick funds, initiated by the public sector. In the United States, the free market casualty insurance model was adapted in a unique form to fulfill the social

insurance function. The resulting hybrid fails to satisfy either free market norms or social insurance ideals.

The major development in U.S. health insurance in the 1930s and 1940s was led not by government or business but by nonprofit corporations such as Blue Cross (hospital insurance service corporations), Blue Shield (physician insurance service corporations), and a variety of consumer and producer cooperatives that provided coverage for hospital and medical services. The corporate missions and characteristics of these organizations gave U.S. health insurance a strong social insurance tendency without fully incorporating the European approach.

Because they believed that the nonprofit organizations' approach to health insurance violated the basic tenets of casualty insurance, commercial insurers initially showed no interest in this market (Iglehart). Casualty insurance assumes that a hazard insured against is measurable and not something the insured person wants (such as checkups or preventive services), or can control (such as pregnancy).

From the beginning in the United States strict casualty insurance principles were ignored. While health insurance protects subscribers from the financial impact of relatively rare high-cost medical services, plans commonly also cover many low-cost services used every year by most members of the insured group. The typical health insurance plan provided to employees of large corporations includes coverage for some ambulatory care costs (office visits, X-rays, and laboratory services) and the major portion of emergency room and hospital charges. About 80 percent of the population will use some ambulatory care services, while only 10 percent of the population will need hospital care in any given year.

By the time the commercial insurers overcame their suspicion of the field, the nonprofit insurers had already brought much social insurance philosophy into the market. Consequently, while the health insurance language includes many standard insurance terms ("adverse selection," "moral hazard," "product lines," "lives covered by plans"), leading the casual observer to conclude that the field is a traditional casualty insurance market, it is, in reality, a form of social insurance peculiar to the United States. However, the competitive practices of commercial insurers have led to widespread use of experience rating, which undermines the social insurance spirit by making health insurance more expensive for those in greatest need. Health insurance plans use three basic methods to protect subscribers: indemnity benefits, service benefits, or direct provision of service. Indemnity insurance, typical of commercial insurers, reimburses a patient for a portion of incurred medical expenditures. Service benefits, typical of nonprofit insurers, pay physicians and hospitals directly on behalf of subscribers. Health maintenance organizations, by contrast, actually organize and deliver services directly to their members at clinics and hospitals that the plans usually own and operate, paying for professional services by salary or contract, not on a fee-for-service basis.

In a widespread effort to control medical care costs in the 1990s, managed care systems, especially those who were not associated with organized delivery systems, used various discounting and risk-sharing reimbursement mechanisms to pay medical service providers. By 2000, providers and patients had grown increasingly unhappy with the restrictions imposed by managed care strategies and the organizations could claim little success in controlling medical costs (Levit, Smith, and Cowen). New strategies relied on shifting costs to patients and members of insurance plans (Draper, Hurley, and Lesser; Christianson, Parente, and Taylor; Trude, Christianson, and Lesser). Six major tendencies characterize the way U.S. health insurance adapted casualty insurance concepts to serve a social insurance function: leadership by nonprofit corporations; a gradual shift from financing based on equal shares (community-rated premiums) to financing based on unequal shares (experience-rated premiums); consumer preference for comprehensive benefits; use of service and indemnity methods of benefit definition; carriers' preference for group rather than individual marketing of plans; and persistent ambivalence in the general public about the role of government in health insurance.

NONPROFIT STATUS OF HEALTH INSURANCE PIONEERS.
Because the pioneers in U.S. health insurance were nonprofit, charitable organizations, they were developed to provide a social function beyond creating a profit for shareholders or syndicate owners. However, the social objective was not always to benefit consumers. Blue Cross was first organized to provide for the financial survival of the American voluntary, nonprofit hospital system during the period of the Great Depression. Although organized medicine initially opposed the new insurance schemes as unwanted intrusions into the privacy of the patient-physician relationship, Blue Shield was eventually formed as a preventive measure to keep mechanisms for paying physicians under the direct control of organized medicine. Provider cooperative prepaid group practices, such as Kaiser Permanente, were formed because some reform-minded physicians believed that prepaid group practice was a more satisfying and socially responsible way to practice medicine.

These nonprofit institutions were chartered in the public domain and were guided by boards of directors who were reminded that they represented society at large, rather than a group of stockholders. The corporate cultures that emerged under this influence generally produced organizational behavior different from that found in commercial insurance companies (Greenlick, 1988). The nonprofit corporations possessed a sense of mission to the community, a sense nurtured by their close ties to community hospitals and physicians' organizations. In the 1970s, pressured by their large corporate customers to contain costs, the nonprofit insurers began to behave like their competitors, the commercial insurance companies, and moved from community rating of premiums to experience-rating practices. Consequently, premiums increased for high-risk groups, making it difficult for the most needy to maintain health insurance coverage.

COMMUNITY-RATED VERSUS EXPERIENCE-RATED PREMIUMS. In an institutionalization of the concept of solidarity, the pioneer U.S. health insurance organizations originally used community-rating principles to fund their programs. In pure community rating, the premium is set by estimating the required budget for the covered population for the next year and dividing the total budget by the number of people expected to be covered. The result is the premium charged to each member of the population for the coming year. Thus, all employers in an insurer's service area would be charged the same per capita premium for their employees.

By contrast, in an experience-rated system, the approach favored by commercial carriers, the most recent available claims experience is analyzed to define a risk profile for specific groups. These risk profiles are applied to the next year's expected total budget to calculate group-specific premiums. Experience rating increases the premiums for groups that include high-use subscribers and reduces premiums for groups that include infrequent users. Consequently, people with serious and chronic health problems, who most need the risk-sharing of health insurance, are forced to pay higher and higher premiums, until they can no longer afford the cost of coverage (Greenlick, 1989).

As experience rating became more common, people with preexisting health conditions were frequently excluded from insurance coverage. This led many states during the 1980s to create special high-risk pools for "uninsurables." The practice also made health insurance too expensive for thousands of firms with small numbers of workers, especially those where even one worker had recently experienced a high-cost illness episode. The shift toward experience rating by nonprofit insurers has led to a disturbing incongruity between a social policy that favors free market practices in U.S. health insurance and a prevailing public expectation that private health insurance should fulfill a social insurance function.

COMPREHENSIVE BENEFIT PACKAGES. Because pioneer health insurance organizations had among their objectives supporting the providers of care, they designed insurance plans based on comprehensive benefits that would cover not only infrequently needed high-cost services but also many low-cost services that might be used regularly by most subscribers. The idea of comprehensive benefits was very popular with the employees whose employers were paying most, or all, of the premiums for health insurance. This popularity was supported by the post-World War II belief that economic growth could permanently keep pace with new demands. During the 1960s and 1970s, most Blue Cross Blue Shield and prepaid group practice plans covered, with little deductible or coinsurance cost to the insured, most of the costs of physician, laboratory, X-ray, emergency room, and hospital medical and surgical services. During the 1970s, insurers increasingly added coverage for prescription drugs. To keep pace, commercial insurance companies increased the breadth and depth of their coverage, particularly for low-risk groups.

The preference for comprehensive benefits contributed to the explosive rate of growth in the health services industry during the postwar era. In 1940 healthcare accounted for 4.1 percent of the gross national product (GNP). It had expanded to 7.2 percent by 1970, reaching 10.7 percent in 1985 (Eastaugh). By the late 1970s, a chronic sense of crisis afflicted business and government administrators of health insurance budgets. Cost-containment strategies that used deductibles and coinsurance to reduce the use of health services by insured persons achieved only modest success. However, these typical casualty insurance mechanisms conflicted with the social insurance function of health insurance and were hotly debated among health insurance reformers in the early 1990s.

SERVICE BENEFITS VERSUS INDEMNITY BENEFITS. A distinguishing characteristic of the Blue Cross/Blue Shield programs and the prepaid group practices is that they sell their customers a promise to provide medical care services (service benefits) rather than a promise to reimburse incurred expenses (indemnity benefits). Service benefit organizations concern themselves with issues of delivery of care more than indemnity insurers, who cover only a specified portion of medical care expenses.

Preferred provider organizations (PPOs) and multiple forms of health maintenance organizations (HMOs) emerged from the cost-controlling strategies of the 1970s and 1980s. These service-delivery reforms sought cost savings through peer group review of practice patterns, favoring those that produced effective care while reducing frequency and length of hospitalizations, using fewer repeat visits, and increasing the use of outpatient care in place of costly hospital services. U.S. insurers took a hand in designing and administering these delivery system reforms, giving them a significant role in healthcare that went far beyond merely paying the bills.

GROUP ENROLLMENT VERSUS INDIVIDUAL MARKETING. Like the European social insurance movement, the development of health insurance in the United States was based on enrollment through employment groups. As more Americans left rural occupations and moved to the cities during and after the Great Depression of the 1930s, they found work in large industrial companies that increasingly offered comprehensive health insurance coverage as a fringe benefit of employment. The health insurance industry focused on enrolling members through work groups. As long as employment in these industries grew, so did the proportion of U.S. citizens covered by health insurance. Labor market forces seemed to be producing social insurance goals without the need of centralized decisions.

Employment-based group enrollment ultimately comes up short from the social insurance perspective, however, since many persons with significant healthcare needs are not in the work force and will not have access to health insurance. This way of distributing health insurance leaves workers doubly vulnerable to fluctuations in the labor market: Low-wage jobs frequently do not include health insurance benefits, and business cycles or industry competition may cause work force reductions leading to loss of health insurance for employees and their dependents (homemakers and children).

Inequities in the labor market carry over to health insurance when employment is the basis for its distribution (Jecker). Women's groups argue that healthcare services important to women, such as mammography, have tended not to be covered. Women who work are less likely than men who work to have employer or union contributions to their insurance. Women are also more likely to work part-time and receive no fringe benefits. Women are less likely to belong to a labor union and they change jobs more frequently than men, making them more vulnerable to preexisting condition exclusions from insurance. Women predominate in low-paying jobs where insurance is usually not offered as a benefit. Many of these distribution inequities also affect minorities, leading some reformers to argue for uncoupling health insurance from employment.

After vigorous growth between 1940 and 1960, the employment-based system had generated health insurance coverage for nearly 70 percent of the population under sixty-five, while only slightly more than 40 percent of the elderly were covered, leading to the establishment of Medicare and Medicaid in 1965 (Anderson). These two programs brought health insurance protection to virtually all of the elderly, and to a significant proportion of those living in poverty, as well. They did not, however, provide coverage for everyone, so that the United States entered the 1990s with more than thirty million citizens having no health insurance. This fueled a vigorous revival of interest in a national health insurance program capable of guaranteeing coverage for every citizen.

During the 1980s, self-insurance emerged as a cost-control strategy among large corporations. These firms stopped buying health insurance for their workers and set themselves up as the at-risk entity for healthcare costs incurred by their employees. The practice put these corporations beyond the reach of state insurance regulations because of a 1974 federal law, the Employee Retirement Income Security Act (ERISA). The intent of ERISA was to protect pension trust funds in companies with employees in several states from inconsistent and burdensome state regulations. The effect on health insurance, while not a primary goal of ERISA, so complicated health-insurance reform that, by the late 1980s, it became a critical element in all proposals that relied on employee benefits as the primary vehicle for distributing health insurance to citizens.

At the beginning of the twenty-first century, the concept of *defined contribution* to employee benefit packages (rather than defined benefits) became popular among free market reformers (Christianson et al.). This concept responded to employers' desire to be less involved in insurance purchasing and shift decision making to their employees. The strategy combined a set amount of employer contribution with a responsibility on employees to purchase their own health insurance. Employees could use a portion of the defined contribution for direct purchase of services. In the final analysis, employees in such a plan would be individually responsible to cover the costs of their care with a combination of out-of-pocket spending, insurance protection, and limited access to the defined contribution pool created by the employer. This approach can be understood as an effort to deemphasize the social insurance model by insisting on increased consumer responsibility for non-catastrophic healthcare needs.

The Government Role in U.S. Health Insurance

The U.S. government has had a role in health insurance since the eighteenth century, when it accepted the responsibility to provide medical care for the U.S. Merchant Marine. During the growth period of private health insurance in the United States prior to Medicare and Medicaid (1940–1965), the federal government let the private market work, limiting

itself to indirect involvement through tax incentives for employers and employees who favored the purchase of health insurance as a fringe benefit. State and local governments were expected to provide care to the indigent and to the mentally ill. As a large employer, the federal government became a major purchaser of health insurance for its employees.

Finally, the federal government is a major supplier of social insurance for medical care for Native Americans, active-duty military personnel and their dependents, and veterans. The total public expenditure for medical care services in 2000 was $590 billion, 45 percent of the $1.3 trillion total national expenditure for health services and supplies during the year.

Government involvement in U.S. health insurance differs distinctly from paths followed by most other industrial nations. In Europe, several nations have made the direct delivery of healthcare a national government responsibility (e.g., the United Kingdom and the Scandinavian countries); others have taken up the role of coordination in mixed public-private systems (e.g., Germany, the Netherlands, Switzerland); others have assumed the role of providing health insurance to the citizenry, allowing hospitals and physicians to operate in a fee-for-service environment (France).

In the late 1960s, Canada adopted an approach similar to France's: Each province has a monopoly on health insurance for basic services, while the federal government plays a coordinating role. Canadian Medicare rests on five essential principles: universal entitlement, accessibility of services, comprehensive benefits, portability of benefits across provincial boundaries, and public administration of the system within each province.

Questions about the proper role of government in health insurance continue to be central issues in debates among U.S. health insurance reformers. Proposals put forward in the first decade of the twenty-first century will succeed or fail on the basis of their ability to make the case that they have found an acceptable balance point on the public-private continuum where private markets (insurance carriers, providers, suppliers) come together under public policy constraints to produce an acknowledged common good.

Conclusion

As the twenty-first century dawned, the evolution of health insurance in the United States and elsewhere had reached a point where significant new public policy decisions were increasingly demanded by the consumer groups, business, politicians, and health professionals (see Rashi Fein's work).

In all industrial nations, the rates of growth in total expenditures for healthcare were creating economic strains and social concern (see the report of the Government Committee on Choices in Healthcare). Particularly in the United States—with the highest percentage of its GNP devoted to healthcare—business, government, and consumer groups insisted on effective control of total healthcare expenditures. Some argued that the solution had to come from submitting healthcare to a competitive market. Others preferred government regulation through global budgets, delivery system reforms, and limitations on services that qualify for collective financing. Most reformers insisted that health insurance had to stop fueling uncontrolled growth in healthcare spending.

Expenditure control has major consequences for the social insurance aspect of health insurance schemes. Many European nations and Canada have sought to control total expenditures without sacrificing the healthcare component of their social insurance commitments. In the United States, many providers, social reformers, and the general public have demanded explicit commitment to the social insurance dimension of health insurance: a universal system that would guarantee a decent minimum of healthcare to every citizen. Reformers were particularly concerned to have the nation address the equity issue. During a thirty-two-month period in 1990–1992, one-fourth of the entire population outside of institutions were without health insurance for at least one month; more than one-third of the African-American population and nearly one-half of the Hispanic population found themselves excluded from coverage (Pear).

Growing public awareness of the size of the uninsured population and the vulnerability of the middle class to loss of job-related health insurance have led to growing dissatisfaction with the system and sparked a renewed interest in health insurance reform. Dozens of proposals emerged in the late 1980s and 1990s driven by several key questions. Should America continue its multiple payer, public-private system, or embark on a new path with a streamlined single-payer system? Should the single payer be the federal government or each state? If there were to be multiple payers, who would conduct the negotiations needed to coordinate their practices so that universal coverage would be achieved and maintained?

The multiple-payer approach continues the path of adapting casualty insurance and free-market forces to serve the social insurance function. In the mid-1990s, President Bill Clinton proposed a market-structuring, multiple-payer solution (White House Domestic Policy Council; Zelman), and was immediately criticized by sponsors of competing market proposals for interfering too much with market forces and not trusting them to achieve efficient allocations (Enthoven and Singer). Single-payer advocates, arguing that Clinton was fundamentally mistaken and that the private health insurance market was simply the wrong vehicle for achieving universal coverage and cost control, invoked the social insurance model, abandoning market pluralism in favor of uncomplicated universality and administrative efficiency achievable through centralized financing.

Finally, the Clinton proposal failed politically. Backing away from universal coverage, the Clinton Administration launched a special program to increase children's access to coverage in 1997 (Title XXI of the Social Security Act, the State Children's Health Insurance Program). By 1999, all fifty states had approved programs that either created a special program for children, an expansion of Medicaid, or some combination of the two. Despite success in reaching children, the percentage of Americans without health insurance has grown, costs have not come under control, and the critics of the status quo remain unable to attract sufficient political consensus to bring about universal coverage.

Health insurance in the United States continues to evolve. The tension between the casualty insurance practices and social insurance ideals frustrate reformers in both camps. The enduring challenge is to formulate policies that can control total expenditures while allocating resources fairly and promoting the common good.

MICHAEL J. GARLAND
MERWYN R. GREENLICK (1995)
REVISED BY AUTHORS

SEE ALSO: *Conflict of Interest; Corporate Compliance; Economic Concepts in Healthcare; Genetic Discrimination; Healthcare Institutions; Managed Care; Medicaid; Pharmaceutical Industry; Profit and Commercialism; Race and Racism; Sexism*

BIBLIOGRAPHY

Anderson, Odin W. 1985. *Health Services in the United States: A Growth Enterprise Since 1875.* Ann Arbor, MI: Health Administration Press.

Bellah, Robert N.; Madsen, Richard; Sullivan, William M.; et al. 1985. *Habits of the Heart: Individualism and Commitment in American Life.* New York: Harper and Row.

"Caring for the Uninsured and the Underinsured (Special Issue)." 1991. *Journal of the American Medical Association* 265(19).

Chapman, Audrey, ed. 1994. *Health Care Reform: A Human Rights Approach.* Washington, D.C.: Georgetown University Press.

Christianson, Jon; Parente, Stephen T.; and Taylor, Ruth. 2002. "Defined-Contribution Health Insurance Products: Development and Prospects." *Health Affairs* 21(1): 49–64.

Churchill, Larry R. 1994. *Self-Interest and Universal Health Care.* Cambridge, MA: Harvard University Press.

Daniels, Norman. 1985. *Just Health Care.* Cambridge: Cambridge University Press.

Dougherty, Charles J. 1988. *American Health Care: Realities, Rights, and Reforms.* Oxford: Oxford University Press.

Draper, Debra; Hurley, Robert E.; Lesser, Cara S.; et al. 2002. "The Changing Face of Managed Care." *Health Affairs* 21(1): 11–23.

Eastaugh, Steven R. 1987. *Financing Health Care: Economic Efficiency and Equity.* Dover, MA: Auburn House.

Enthoven, Alain C., and Singer, Sara J. 1994. "A Single-Payer System in Jackson Hole Clothing." *Health Affairs* 13(1): 81–95.

Fein, Rashi. 1989. *Medical Care, Medical Costs: The Search for a Health Insurance Policy.* Cambridge, MA: Harvard University Press.

Garland, Michael J. 1992. "Justice, Politics and Community: Expanding Access and Rationing Health Services in Oregon." *Law, Medicine and Healthcare* 20(1–2): 67–81.

Garland, Michael J. 1994. "Oregon's Contribution to Defining Adequate Healthcare." In *Healthcare Reform: A Human Rights Approach,* ed. Audrey Chapman. Washington, D.C.: Georgetown University Press.

Garland, Michael J. 2001. "The Oregon Health Plan Ten Years Later." In *Changing Health Care Systems from Ethical, Economic, and Cross Cultural Perspectives,* ed. Erich Loewy and Roberta Springer Loewy. New York: Kluwer Academic/Plenum Publishers

Government Committee on Choices in Healthcare. 1992. *Choices in Health Care: A Report.* Zoestermeyer, Netherlands: Author.

Greenlick, Merwyn R. 1988. "Profit and Nonprofit Organizations in Health Care: A Sociological Perspective." In *In Sickness and in Health: The Mission of Voluntary Health Care Institutions,* ed. J. David Seay and Bruce C. Vladeck. New York: McGraw-Hill.

Greenlick, Merwyn R. 1989. "Healthcare for Adults." In *Handbook of Medical Sociology,* 4th Edition, ed. Howard E. Freeman and Sol Levine. Englewood Cliffs, NJ: Prentice-Hall.

Health Insurance Association of America. 1990. *Source Book of Health Insurance Data,* 30th edition. Washington, D.C.: Author.

Hetherington, Robert W.; Hopkins, Carl E.; and Roemer, Milton I. 1975. *Health Insurance Plans: Promise and Performance.* New York: Wiley.

Hirshfield, Daniel S. 1970. *The Lost Reform: The Campaign for Compulsory Health Insurance in the United States from 1932 to 1943.* Cambridge, MA: Harvard University Press.

Iglehart, John K. 1992. "The American Healthcare System: Private Insurance." *New England Journal of Medicine* 326(5): 1715–1720.

Jecker, Nancy S. 1993. "Can an Employer-Based Health Insurance System Be Just?" *Journal of Health Politics, Policy and Law* 18(3, pt. 2): 657–673.

Levit, Katharine; Smith, Cynthia; Cowen, Cathy; et al. 2002. "Inflation Spurs Health Spending in 2000." *Health Affairs* 21(1): 172–181.

Pear, Robert. 1994. "Gaps in Coverage for Healthcare." *New York Times* (March 29): D23.

Starr, Paul. 1982. *The Social Transformation of American Medicine.* New York: Basic Books.

Strosberg, Martin, et al., eds. 1992. *Rationing America's Medical Care: The Oregon Plan and Beyond.* Washington, D.C.: Brookings Institution.

Taylor, Malcolm G. 1990. *Insuring National Healthcare: The Canadian Experience.* Chapel Hill: University of North Carolina Press.

Trude, Sally; Christianson, Jon B.; Lesser, Cara S.; et al. 2002. "Employer-Sponsored Health Insurance: Pressing Problems, Incremental Changes." *Health Affairs* 21(1): 66–75.

U.S. President's Commission for the Study of Ethical Problems in Medicine and Biomedical and Behavioral Research. 1983. *Securing Access to Health Care: A Report on the Ethical Implications of Differences in the Availability of Health Services.* Washington, D.C.: Author.

Walzer, Michael. 1983. *Spheres of Justice: A Defense of Pluralism and Equality.* New York: Basic Books.

White House Domestic Policy Council. 1993. *Health Security: The President's Report to the American People.* Washington, D.C.: Author.

Zelman, Walter A. 1994. "The Rationale Behind the Clinton Health Reform Plan." *Health Affairs* 13(1): 9–29.

INTERNET RESOURCE

Title XXI of the Social Security Act, the State Children's Health Insurance Program. 1997. Available from <http://cms.hhs.gov/schip>.

HEALTH POLICY IN INTERNATIONAL PERSPECTIVE

• • •

Health polices of international agencies and individual countries reflect choices involving diverse ethical issues, including rights and responsibilities of individuals versus society, choices over who benefits and who pays for healthcare services, trade-offs between saving identifiable lives and statistical lives, and choices involving interpersonal and intergenerational equity. This entry begins by examining the role of international agencies in providing public health services, ethical issues raised by testing and use of new drugs, and government involvement in purchasing and providing healthcare. It then outlines four generic models for healthcare financing and delivery that many countries have adapted to their unique circumstances. These four healthcare financing and delivery models reflect different choices about an individual's right to basic healthcare services, and views about whether an individual's ability to pay should influence access to certain services.

Public Health and Preventive Services

International agencies play a critical role in health policy, first by setting public health and health-status goals, and then by monitoring an individual country's progress toward these goals. For example, over the past twenty years the World Health Organization (WHO) has established goals and specific targets for the *Health-for-All* initiative. Two fundamental objectives of this initiative are: (1) making health central to human development and (2) building sustainable health systems (Antezana, et al.). In order to monitor these objectives, Health-for-All in the 21st Century has identified global health targets that each country should meet, such as eliminating certain infectious diseases through childhood immunization and improving access to water, sanitation, food and shelter (Visschedijk and Simeant). In 2000 the WHO began ranking and assessing health systems's performance in 191 countries based on five composite indicators. The WHO hopes to make this assessment a regular activity, which will help policy-makers to monitor their performance in comparison to other countries (WHO, 2000a).

In most countries, public health agencies have the primary responsibility for creating programs that will achieve specific health objectives. International agencies like the World Bank and the United Nations and some affluent countries have programs to assist developing countries. The U.S. Agency for International Development (USAID), for example, operates programs that help developing countries to establish and operate a variety of public health activities.

While there is generally a consensus that government agencies should finance and provide public health and disease-prevention services, policy differences and financial commitments affect the success of specific programs. For example, the childhood immunization rates for six major infectious diseases (diphtheria, pertussis, tetanus, measles, poliomyelitis, and tuberculosis) vary greatly from country to country. In 2000 the immunization rates for diphtheria, pertussis, measles, and poliomyelitis ranged from 55 percent of infants in Africa to over 90 percent of infants in Europe (WHO, 2001). In most countries the WHO's target rate of 90 percent coverage for the year 2000 was not achieved (WHO, 2001).

Another public health activity, the testing and approval of drugs, highlights conflicting ethical values. Beneficence, in terms of concern for public welfare, is reflected when nations employ comprehensive but time-consuming approval processes in order to ensure a safe and efficacious drug supply. The U.S. Food and Drug Administration, for example, has adopted strict regulatory standards that prevent the domestic adoption of new drugs and devices until their safety and efficacy are established beyond reasonable doubt (Sheinin and Williams). In contrast, a respect for autonomy, in terms of individual access to healthcare, is obstructed when the length of the drug approval process delays access to potentially lifesaving treatments—particularly for patients who have exhausted current treatment options and are willing to take experimental drugs.

Since the early 1990s, people with acquired immunodeficiency syndrome (AIDS) have been the most vocal proponents of allowing individuals unrestricted access to unproven medical treatments. Advocates of placing greater weight on beneficence, on the other hand, point to the approval of thalidomide by the United Kingdom in the 1960s, while it was still in testing stages in other countries. The drug was never approved in other countries and was pulled from the British market after it became apparent that severe congenital deformations resulted from maternal use of the drug (Burger).

The principle of justice can be jeopardized when drug trials are carried out in developing countries by investigators and sponsored by agencies from developed countries (Beyrer and Kass; Council for International Organization of Medical Sciences [CIOMS]). Some developing nations have used drugs not approved in industrialized countries. Lower costs of unapproved drugs make them a relatively affordable medical treatment option for poorer nations. In some cases, individuals in low-income nations benefit from access to various drugs, while in other cases individuals are harmed by access to unsafe or inefficacious therapies. For example, HIV/AIDS accounts for about 20 percent of all deaths in Africa, which creates urgent need for new drugs and effective vaccines for HIV infection (Creese, et al.). This urgency is being used to lower the ethical standards of international research and result in ethically controversial actions (e.g., not providing drugs after the conclusion of the clinical trial or make the drugs available at unaffordable prices) (Greco,

Stolberg, Okie). In order to assist the efficient purchase of safe and efficacious drugs by developing nations, the WHO and other international agencies have established *essential drug lists* that identify drugs satisfying the healthcare needs of the majority of the population, and are revised every two years (WHO, 2000b).

Medical Services

Particular attention should be paid to ethical choices in the financing and delivery of medical services, since these services account for a large portion of most countries's total healthcare spending (Organization for the Economic Cooperation and Development [OECD]). The provision of medical-care services requires policymakers to debate myriad ethical values and conflicts, and each country's medical-care system reflects its choices about underlying ethical matters.

Unlike public health activities, which are considered to benefit all members of society, medical-care services are generally considered as private goods, since it is the individual who benefits directly from them. Some countries consider access to medical care a merit good—a good that, although private, benefits society as well. Health insurance is a major determinant of access to care. In most industrialized countries health insurance coverage is universal. In the United States, however, 14 percent of Americans did not have health insurance in 2000 (Mills).

Similar value choices are exemplified by the benefits package that countries's health systems offer. Some countries's health systems cover only hospital and physician care, while others include such items as long-term care, drugs, dental care, home health services, and eyeglasses (Healy). In addition, many European countries incorporate housekeeping, spa vacations and social services into their provision of healthcare services. Cultural norms also affect countries's health systems. Japan, for example, did not establish a formal system of long-term care until recently, in part because of the tradition that the eldest son and his wife have had responsibility for the son's parents (Campbell and Ikegami).

Countries's decisions about government involvement in provider issues can highlight conflicts between the individual liberty of providers and patients's access to care. Some countries, such as Israel, have adopted policies that restrict providers's ability to practice in areas that exceed a certain physician-population ratio and have developed policies that encourage them to operate in underserved locations (Anderson and Antebi). Other policies may limit the total income that can be generated by health professionals, either through

restrictions on the salaries that physicians can earn or by limiting the volume of services the physicians may provide (White). In addition, some countries, such as the United Kingdom, permit providers to operate publicly (through a national health service) and have a private practice (Healy). Other countries, like most of the provinces in Canada, require a provider to work completely in the publicly financed plan or completely in the privately financed sector (Flood and Archibald).

Countries use three basic mechanisms, in addition to out-of-pocket payments, to finance medical-care services. One option is to use general tax revenues. With this method, citizens pay for medical services based on the structure of the overall tax system. This option is considered by economists to be the most progressive. For economists, progressive means that the income tax rate increases as the taxpayer's income rises. A second basic method to generate funds for medical-care services is through a payroll tax earmarked for the health system. This is referred to as a proportional or flat tax since the tax rate does not vary with income. The third basic method to finance medical-care services is through health-insurance premiums. This method is considered to be regressive by economists because the rate falls as income rises.

A related financing and access issue is that of the cost sharing by individuals. Cost sharing, such as coinsurance, copayments, and deductibles, is introduced when health insurance systems want to give patients a financial incentive not to use certain health services—especially services they believe to be only marginally beneficial. However, the patients' ability to make appropriate choices is debatable especially when they are poor (Fuchs). Poor patients's demand for care depends more on whether they have money at the time than on their own judgment of the seriousness of the condition (White). Some countries, such as the United Kingdom, Canada, and Germany, operate with no or nominal deductibles and coinsurance (Glaser, U.S. General Accounting Office 1991a, 1991b). Other countries have substantial cost-sharing requirements. For example, 10 to 20 percent coinsurance requirements are typical in the United States and France, and 20 to 30 percent coinsurance requirements are typical in Japan and Korea (U.S. General Accounting Office 1991b, Anderson).

Four Healthcare Financing and Delivery Models

As individual countries design their own healthcare financing and delivery systems, they make a number of policy decisions that are based upon ethical considerations. These decisions involve choices regarding who is covered, the method of financing the medical-care delivery system, and whether the delivery system is public or private. These healthcare financing and delivery systems are categorized below into four models and specific countries are identified that exemplify each type of model. It is important to recognize, however, that no country fits any model precisely, and that healthcare systems are dynamic. The four generic models are national health service, national health insurance, social insurance, and private voluntary health insurance.

NATIONAL HEALTH SERVICE. National health service systems usually collect revenues from general taxation, mandate the use of public facilities, and have limited cost sharing. As a result, countries with national health service generally offer the greatest equality in access to care and employ the most progressive financing methods. However, some critics have expressed concern that national health services may be relatively inefficient and unresponsive to individuals's healthcare service preferences (Enthoven).

The United Kingdom's National Health Service (NHS) is the archetypal example of this model. Since its creation in 1948, the guiding principal of the NHS has been equity— equal access to healthcare services for all inhabitants. The NHS offers a comprehensive array of government-provided services, a national benefits package, and is financed by general tax revenues. During the early 1990's, the concerns about inefficiencies and customer service led to introducing some market incentives and development of a system of competition within the NHS (Enthoven). However, subsequent reforms initiated by the Labor government largely abolished the quasi-market and emphasized the idea of collaboration with a return to strong elements of command and control (Le Grand).

NATIONAL HEALTH-INSURANCE PROGRAM. National health-insurance systems usually generate revenues from general taxation, have private providers and facilities, allow the government to set payment rates for healthcare providers, and may have limited cost sharing. The major difference between national health insurance and national health service is the ownership of the facilities.

The Canadian health system is an example of a national health-insurance system. Revenues are generated from general taxation, the government sets payment rates for the providers who participate in the system, and there is no cost sharing. Healthcare professionals must choose between participating in the national health-insurance system and opting out of the system entirely to work in the privately financed sector (Flood and Archibald).

SOCIAL INSURANCE. In social insurance systems, revenues are generated from payroll taxes, the private sector provides health insurance, private facilities are common, and the government sometimes sets payment rates for providers. Although insurance is compulsory, and thus accessible to all, the scope of healthcare benefits may vary by plan.

Social insurance, the first type of health insurance to be developed, was introduced in Germany by Otto van Bismarck [1815–1898] in 1883. Germany has continued to use the social insurance system, and several European nations and other countries like Japan and Korea have modified the basic social insurance model to meet their own needs (Glaser, Powell and Anesaki, Anderson).

PRIVATE VOLUNTARY HEALTH INSURANCE. In the private voluntary health insurance system revenues are generated by a variety of sources including premiums, payroll taxes, and general taxation, private facilities are the norm, the government may or may not set provider payment rates, and coinsurance is common (Maxwell, Storeygard and Moon). This system is likely to have the greatest disparity in access to healthcare services, since access is based upon ability to pay. In addition, it is common for a proportion of the population to be uninsured. In theory, this system should be more efficient than government-run health systems, because free-market competition should result in greater efficiency (Enthoven and Kronick). However, it is believed by many that free-market principles, such as a free flow of product information and price sensitivity among consumers, do not fully apply to the healthcare sector, and consequently competition and greater efficiency do not always occur (Rice et al.). The United States and many low and middle-income countries use a system of voluntary private health insurance.

Summary

Health financing and delivery systems are influenced by divergent views on a number of ethical issues. Countries must resolve ethical dilemmas such as (1) whether access to basic healthcare services is one of the fundamental rights of every human being, and (2) how scarce resources should be allocated between the old and the young, between medical and preventive care, and between healthcare and other social needs, as they develop their healthcare systems.

GERARD F. ANDERSON
STEPHANIE L. MAXWELL (1995)
REVISED BY GERARD F. ANDERSON
VARDUHI PETROSYAN
STEPHANIE L. MAXWELL

SEE ALSO: *Access to Healthcare; Aging and the Aged: Healthcare and Research Issues; AIDS; Beneficence; Children; Economic Concepts in Healthcare; Freedom and Coercion; Future Generations, Reproductive Technologies and Obligations to; Healthcare Resources, Allocation of; Human Rights; International Health; Justice; Labor Unions in Healthcare; Managed Care; Medicaid; Medicare; Patients' Rights; Pharmaceutical Industry; Public Health; Research Policy*

BIBLIOGRAPHY

Anderson, Gerard F. 1989. "Universal Health Care Coverage in Korea." *Health Affairs* 8(2): 24–34.

Anderson, Gerard F., and Antebi, Shlomi. 1991. "A Surplus of Physicians in Israel: Any Lessons for the United States and Other Industrialized Countries?" *Health Policy* 17(1): 77–86.

Antezana, Fernando S.; Chollat-Traquet, Claire M.; and Yach, Derek. 1998. "Health for All in the 21st Century." *World Health Statistics Quarterly* 51(1): 3–6.

Beyrer, Christopher, and Kass, Nancy. 2002. "Human Rights, Politics, and Reviews of Research Ethics." *Lancet* 360(9328): 246–251.

Burger, Edward J. 1976. *Protecting the Nation's Health: The Problems of Regulation.* Lexington, MA: Lexington Books.

Campbell, John C., and Ikegami, Naoki. 2000. "Long-Term Care Insurance Comes to Japan." *Health Affairs* 19(3): 26–39.

Council for International Organization of Medical Sciences (CIOMS) in collaboration with the World Health Organization. 2002. *International Ethical Guidelines for Biomedical Research Involving Human Subjects.* Geneva, Switzerland: Author.

Creese, Andrew; Floyd, Katherine; Alban, Anita; et al. 2002. "Cost-Effectiveness of HIV/AIDS Interventions in Africa: A Systematic Review of the Evidence." *Lancet* 359: 1635–1642.

Enthoven, Alain C. 2000. "In Pursuit of an Improving National Health Service." *Health Affairs* 19(3): 102–119.

Enthoven, Allen, and Kronick, Richard. 1989. "A Consumer-Choice Health Plan for the 1990s: Universal Health Insurance in a System Designed to Promote Quality and Economy." *New England Journal of Medicine* 320(1): 29–37 and 320(2): 94–101.

European Observatory on Health Care Systems (EOHCS). 2002. "Health Care Systems in Eight Countries: Trends and Challenges," commissioned by the Health Trend Review, HM Treasury. London: Author.

Flood, Colleen M., and Archibald, Tom. 2001. "The Illegality of Private Health Care in Canada." *Canadian Medical Association Journal* 164(6): 825–830.

Fuchs, Victor R. 2002. "What's Ahead for Health Insurance in the United States?" *New England Journal of Medicine* 346(23): 1822–1824.

Glaser, William A. 1991. *Health Insurance in Practice: International Variations in Financing, Benefits, and Problems.* San Francisco: Jossey-Bass.

Greco, Dirceu B. 1999. "Clinical Trials in 'Developing Countries': The Fallacy of Urgency or Ethics vs. Economics." *Bulletin of Medical Ethics* 150: 33–34.

Healy, Judith. 2002. *Treasure Report. Health Care Systems in Eight Countries: Trends and Challenges.* London: The European Observatory on Health Care Systems and London School of Economics & Political Science Hub.

Le Grand, Julian. 2002. "Further Tales From the British National Health Service." *Health Affairs* 21(3): 116–128.

Maxwell, Stephanie; Storeygard, Mathew; and Moon, Marilyn. 2002. *Modernizing Medicare Cost-Sharing: Policy Options and Impacts on Beneficiary and Program Expenditures.* New York: The Commonwealth Fund.

Mills, Robert J. 2001. *Current Population Report: Health Insurance Coverage 2000.* Washington, D.C.: U.S. Department of Commerce, Economics and Statistics Administration, Census Bureau.

Okie, Susan. 1997. "A Look at Ethics and AIDS." *Washington Post,* September 28.

Organization for the Economic Cooperation and Development (OECD). 2002. *OECD Health Data 2002.* Paris: Author.

Powell, Margaret, and Anesaki, Marahira. 1990. *Health Care in Japan.* London: Routledge.

Rice, Thomas; Brown, Richard; and Wyn, Roberta. 1993. "Holes in the Jackson Hole Approach to Health Care Reform." *Journal of the American Medical Association* 270(11): 1357–1362.

Sheinin, Eric, and Williams, Roger. 2002. "Chemistry, Manufacturing, and Controls Information in NDAs and ANDAs, Supplements, Annual Reports, and Other Regulatory Filings." *Pharmaceutical Research* 19(3): 217–226.

Stolberg, Sheryl G. 1997. "U.S. AIDS Research in Poor Nations Raises Outcry on Ethics." *New York Times,* September 18.

U.S. General Accounting Office. 1991a. *Canadian Health Insurance: Lessons for the United States,* GAO/HRD–91–90. Washington, D.C.: Author.

U.S. General Accounting Office. 1991b. *Health Care Spending and Control: The Experience of France, Germany, and Japan,* GAO/HRD–92–9. Washington, D.C.: Author.

Visschedijk, Jan, and Simeant, Silvere. 1998. "Targets for Health for All in the 21st Century." *World Health Statistics Quarterly* 51(1): 56–67.

White, Joseph. 1999. "Targets and Systems of Health Care Cost Control." *Journal of Health Politics, Policy and Law* 24(4): 653–696.

World Health Organization. 2000a. *The World Health Report 2000: Health Systems: Improving Performance.* Geneva: Author.

World Health Organization. 2000b. *Technical Report Series 895: The Use of Essential Drugs, Ninth Report of the WHO Expert Committee.* Technical Report Series 895. Geneva: World Health Organization.

World Health Organization. 2001. *WHO Vaccine-Preventable Diseases: Monitoring System: 2001 Global Summary.* Geneva: World Health Organization. Department of Vaccine and Biologicals.

HEALTH POLICY IN THE UNITED STATES

• • •

Issues of health and healthcare are rather similar across countries, and there are many commonalities in the ways that governments deal with them through health policies. All industrialized nations, for instance, have public health programs and license and regulate healthcare providers to some extent. But there are many differences among their health policies as well—policies that both address and raise issues of justice. Much of the variation in approaches can be traced to the histories, ideologies, and institutions of respective political systems. The relatively unique character of the American political tradition is an essential context for understanding the distinctive aspects of health policies in the United States and their bioethical implications.

Impact of Liberal Ideology

Compared with other industrialized nations, the political ethos of the United States emphasizes the importance of the individual rather than the collectivity (see Gøsta Esping-Andersen). U.S. political ideas, institutions, and behavior uniquely reflect a virtually unanimous acceptance of the tenets of seventeenth-century English political philosopher John Locke, whose liberal philosophy was in harmony with the laissez-faire economics subsequently propounded by Adam Smith in *The Wealth of Nations* (2000 [1776]). As Locke propounded in *Of Civil Government, Two Treatises* (1924 [1690]), the individual should be much more important than the collective, and one of the few important functions of a limited state is to ensure that the wealth that individuals accumulate through the free market is protected. The framers of the U.S. constitution, strongly influenced by the atomistic individualism of Locke's philosophy and his views on the sanctity of private property, took pains to limit the power of government. The constitutional rights they established for American citizens are largely protections for the individual and his property from governmental actions.

This ongoing ideological tradition helps to explain an important distinctive feature of the American political system's approach to health policy. Although U.S. governments intervene a great deal in the health arena, on some matters they are more inclined to rely on the individual and the free market than most other industrialized nations.

Unequal distribution of access to healthcare is a prime example of the effects of this approach. Most industrialized nations, for instance, use the power of government to assure health insurance coverage for virtually 100 percent of their citizens. The rate of government-assured health insurance in the United States, however, is only 33 percent, by far the lowest among industrialized nations (Anderson and Poullier), because the expectation is that most financing of personal healthcare is the responsibility of individuals and their employers (some exceptions are discussed below). Consequently, in 2000, 14 percent of Americans, nearly forty million persons, had no health insurance (U.S. Census Bureau). Lack of insurance, of course, limits access to care, and has been documented by researchers such as David W. Baker, Joseph J. Sudano, Jeffrey M. Albert, et al., (2001) as increasing the risk of poor health.

Impact of Power Fragmentation

Even as the framers of the Constitution were enamored of Locke's political philosophy, they and many other early Americans were heavily influenced by French philosopher Baron de Montesquieu's *The Spirit of the Laws* (1949 [1748]), in which he urged that the powers of governments should be separated in order to thwart the development of tyrannical states. Accordingly, the framers divided the very limited powers of the national government they established into executive, legislative, and judicial branches—each with the power to check the actions of the others. This structure, of course, made it difficult for government to act and thereby interfere with individuals and their property.

The separation of powers exacerbated what was already a characteristic of the American political system, the endemic fragmentation of power in a federal form of government. Not only did the state governments retain most of their power in the federal system but, reflecting the influence of Montesquieu, the powers in each of them were also separated. The fragmentation of governmental power in the United States is astounding: Altogether, there are some 80,000 governments—including counties, municipalities, special district governments, and independent school districts, as well as the state and national governments—and the powers of each of these are usually separated, and even further fragmented. Therefore, generally speaking, government intervention of a sweeping nature is difficult in the American political system. Health policies and other policies tend to be incremental rather than systemic or comprehensive.

One consequence in the health arena, for example, is that various American presidents since the 1920s have failed in their efforts to secure national health insurance, including President Bill Clinton who declared it the prime legislative goal of his first term (1992–1996). One of them may well have succeeded if he had been the head of a disciplined ruling party in a parliamentary system of government, with no separation of powers. Another consequence is that many important health policies are carried out in disparate and uneven fashions throughout the nation because they are primarily the responsibility of state and local governments. These responsibilities include: public health; regulation of hospitals, nursing homes, home health agencies, hospices, and other healthcare provider organizations; licensing of healthcare professionals; and regulation of private health insurance plans. Still another and related consequence is that it is difficult to establish national standards for healthcare.

Government Health Insurance and Direct Care

Despite a political culture that emphasizes individualism and the free market, about three-fifths of all U.S. spending on personal healthcare is financed, directly or indirectly, by governments (Woolhandler and Himmelstein). About 25 percent of this amount is used to support the employer-sponsored system of private health insurance through tax subsidies and public employee benefits. About 20 percent of it is spent on direct government provision of healthcare to veterans and members of the armed forces (and their dependents), and to Native Americans (under treaty obligations). Almost all of the remaining 55 percent is spent on Medicare and Medicaid, two government health insurance programs for selected groups of Americans that have been politically legitimized as especially deserving of collective help. A central rationale for the establishment of these two programs has been "market failure"—the fact that employer-sponsored private insurance does not tend to reach these particular groups.

Medicare, enacted by Congress in 1965, provides national health insurance for about forty million persons. One group covered by the program is all persons aged sixty-five and older who are eligible for Social Security benefits (or Railroad Retirement Benefits)—over 99 percent of Americans in this age range—about thirty-five million people at the turn of the twenty-first century. The political threshold for legitimating older people as a special deserving group worthy of collective assistance had already been crossed during the Great Depression when the Social Security Act of 1935 created government-funded old-age retirement benefits at the age of sixty-five. The rationale for establishing Medicare was that older persons, retired from employment,

had no way to obtain group health insurance. Comparatively few had employer-sponsored retiree health insurance. Moreover, most older people could not afford the comparatively steep premiums charged for individual insurance policies, and many could not obtain them because of pre-existing medical conditions.

Medicare coverage was extended in 1973 to another select group, younger individuals who become eligible after they have received Disability Insurance (DI) benefits from the federal government for at least two years; about five million such persons were covered at the turn of the century. These are persons who, due to a medically certified physical or mental impairment (but not other circumstances), are unable to engage in any kind of *substantial employment* (earning $500 monthly or more) for at least a year. They have been politically legitimized as deserving of Medicare coverage because without employment they cannot obtain group health insurance or afford it on their own. Until the year 2000, DI recipients who were able to return to substantial employment lost their Medicare coverage after two years. However, in recognition of the fact that many employers of former DI recipients do not provide health insurance, this disincentive to work was attenuated by the Ticket to Work and Work Incentives Improvement Act of 1999. It enables DI recipients who become substantially employed to participate in the Medicare Program for an additional four and one-half years.

The Medicaid program, established by the federal government along with Medicare in 1965, is a jointly-funded cooperative venture between the national and state governments that provides healthcare insurance coverage for some poor Americans. But Medicaid policy does not fully equate poverty with *deservingness.* Federal law only requires states to provide coverage for specific categories of deserving groups among the poor that, in their nature, are unlikely to be able to obtain employer-sponsored insurance through the market. Although the list of these requirement categories is long and detailed, the principal eligible groups are children, adults with dependent children, disabled persons (who are not eligible for federal DI benefits), blind persons, and older people (to cover their long-term care costs and certain other expenses not covered by Medicare). Persons within these categories are eligible for Medicaid if their income and financial assets fall below thresholds determined by each state (within minimum federal guidelines). Poor working age men generally do not qualify for Medicaid; the vast majority of those who are eligible in the "adults with dependent children" category are single women. Altogether, the program covers over forty million persons.

Because state governments have considerable latitude in setting income and asset thresholds for Medicaid eligibility, there are substantial interstate inequalities in program participation by persons within the categorical groups designated in federal legislation. An example is the range of low-income thresholds used by states to determine whether infants are eligible for Medicaid. At the most generous end of the range of low-income thresholds used by states in 1999 was Tennessee's 400 percent of the federally-established poverty line; at the other extreme were eight other states with a threshold of 133 percent (Ku, Ullman, and Almeida).

Federal Regulation

The federal government's Food and Drug Administration has long played a role in protecting consumers through regulation. The agency is responsible for ensuring that medicines, medical devices, blood supplies, and certain experimental medical treatments (e.g., gene therapy) are safe and effective, and that foods and cosmetics are truthfully labeled and not harmful. It is only since the late 1980s, however, that the federal government has entered the broader arena of regulating healthcare providers and health insurers, traditionally the bailiwick of state and local governments. It has done so principally to address bioethical issues.

Some policies have been enacted to compensate for perceived inadequacies in state regulation, such as measures in the Omnibus Budget Reconciliation Act of 1987 established to reform the quality of nursing home care. Others have responded to new developments in thinking about ethical patient care. For instance, in the context of growing concerns about protecting patient autonomy, the federal Patient Self-Determination Act was enacted in 1990. It requires healthcare organizations to immediately inform new patients of their rights to refuse medical and surgical treatment and to execute written legal documents, called *advance directives,* regarding their preferences in this regard.

In 1996 alone, the federal government enacted three regulatory laws intended to protect consumers by addressing ethical issues. The Mental Health Parity Act of 1996 responded to inequities in coverage for mental healthcare by requiring that if a group insurance plan covers mental health, the annual and lifetime benefits available must be equivalent to those available for medical and surgical services. The Newborns' and Mothers' Health Protection Act of 1996 addressed perceived issues in quality of care by mandating minimum inpatient stays for mothers and their newborns following deliveries and caesarean sections. And the Health Insurance Portability and Accountability Act of 1996 made obtaining group health insurance easier for individuals with pre-existing health problems and disabilities or previous illnesses, and for those who lost their coverage because of changing jobs or job termination.

The role of the federal government in addressing ethical issues through regulatory policy is likely to expand continually. Technological and biomedical discoveries and innovations inevitably generate questions of fairness and equity that lend themselves to the possibility of government intervention, such as whether genetic tests should be used as screens to exclude applicants for private insurance, whether or in what circumstances stem cell research should be allowed, or how scarce societal resources (e.g., organs for transplantation) should be distributed.

Major Ongoing Issues

The agenda for government policy action grows larger and larger because new issues do not obliterate ongoing concerns. Perhaps the two broadest and most important ongoing issues from a bioethical perspective are: (1) how government will deal with issues of increased longevity; and (2) whether government will remedy the unequal distribution of access to care by securing insurance for the uninsured.

INCREASED LONGEVITY. One set of issues involving increased longevity is generated by the aging of the baby boom, a cohort of 76 million Americans born between 1946 and 1964. During the early decades of the twenty-first century the ranks of older Americans will swell enormously. By 2030, the population of Americans aged sixty-five and older will double, from about 35 million in 2002 to 70 million, and make up 20 percent of the population. Because of this population aging, and ongoing developments in medical technology, the nation will need to greatly increase its financial commitment to the Medicare program if it is to be sustained.

Various commentators are alarmed by this prospect. Bioethicist Daniel Callahan, for example, has described future healthcare costs of older persons as "one of the great fiscal black holes" (p. 216) and argues that these costs will pose an enormous and unsustainable economic burden for the nation and drain resources that could be used for other worthy social causes—an issue of so-called intergenerational equity. Thus, he and others maintain that rationing healthcare on the basis of old age is essential from an economic point of view. Moreover, from a philosophical perspective, Callahan regards it as inappropriate for older people to live beyond what he terms a "natural life span." Accordingly, for both economic and philosophical reasons he has urged that the Medicare program should not pay for life-saving care for anyone aged about 80 or older, and he hopes that this practice will extend to the private sector. Others (e.g., Binstock and Post) have sharply critiqued the arguments of Callahan and other proponents of old-age-based rationing on both economic and ethical grounds. It is not clear that such rationing at the age range suggested would save a great deal of money. And among the ethical arguments against it is the specter raised by the notion that a demographically-defined group might be singled out as unworthy of life-saving care, and be the first of many groups to which such a designation might be applied.

Another dimension of longevity that raises important bioethical policy questions is the quest to slow, arrest, or reverse processes of aging. The U.S. National Institutes of Health (NIH) not only support research to understand the basic biological processes of aging, but promote efforts to substantially increase average life expectancy or the human life span. In 1999, for example, two NIH institutes convened a clinical advisory group of more than fifty scientists to set a research agenda for slowing the fundamental processes of aging and extending maximum life span (Masoro). The desirability of such a policy has been questioned from a number of quarters.

Among bioethicists, Leon Kass, appointed in 2001 as chairman of the U.S. President's Council on Bioethics, opposes such efforts. He believes that even if the human life span were increased by only 20 years, we would lose the benefits that finitude confers:

1. interest and engagement in life;
2. seriousness and aspiration;
3. beauty and love; and
4. virtue and moral excellence (Kass).

Even one of the premier biological researchers in the field of aging, Leonard Hayflick (1994), rejects the goals of substantially extending life expectancy and life span because of distributional justice issues that would arise regarding access to longevity technologies and because of various other social and economic consequences. Other biologists, however, particularly those who are engaged in efforts to slow or reverse the processes of aging, acknowledge such concerns but do not feel that they warrant a halt to their quest to achieve increased longevity (e.g., de Grey, Ames, and Anderson; Miller). And bioethicist John Harris argues that it is doubtful that coherent ethical objections can be generated against the achievement of immortality and urges that we "start thinking now about how we can live decently and creatively with the prospect" (p. 59).

INSURING THE UNINSURED. Finally, as noted above, about forty million Americans have no health insurance in the early years of the twenty-first century. Trends in the labor market suggest that the outlook for expansion of health insurance coverage through the private sector is dim for the foreseeable future. Although the percentage of employed

Americans grew to its highest level in many decades during the economic expansion that took place in the 1990s, employer-sponsored healthcare benefits did not grow apace. When the economy began to flag in the early years of this century, the ranks of the uninsured grew. In the absence of a new government health insurance initiative that reaches beyond the present selected, politically legitimated groups, it is unlikely that many of the uninsured will be covered; indeed, their number could grow.

Since 1994, when Congress rejected President Clinton's initiative for national health insurance, no such policy has been on the political agenda. When and how might such an effort be renewed, and how might it have a chance of success?

The proportion of voters who are poor and members of racial and ethnic minority groups will grow sharply over the next several decades, and these groups are disproportionately represented among the uninsured. Perhaps they will be mobilized effectively in a demand for access to the healthcare that their fellow citizens are receiving.

Another possible scenario is that the swiftly changing dynamics of American healthcare will threaten profits in the healthcare industry. Government insurance for an additional forty million persons (and perhaps a larger number in the future) would be a bountiful source of revenue. Unlike the American Medical Association, which vigorously opposed initiatives to secure universal insurance during the twentieth century, the contemporary healthcare industry might appreciate what government can do for it. As Bruce Vladeck observed in 1999, Medicare financing has largely built and sustained the modern medical industrial complex. The political power of the healthcare industry, although fragmented into various interests, is substantial; it might very well carry the day for universal coverage if united by a vision of what further governmental largesse could do for it. If so, despite a political tradition that has been dominated by emphasis on individualism and the free market, the United States will be able to eliminate major inequalities in access to healthcare.

ROBERT H. BINSTOCK

SEE ALSO: *Access to Healthcare; Health Insurance; Health Policy in International Perspective; Managed Care; Medicaid; Medicare*

BIBLIOGRAPHY

Anderson, Gerard F., and Poullier, Jean-Paul. 1999. "Health Spending, Access, and Outcomes: Trends in Industrialized Countries." *Health Affairs* 18(3): 178–192.

Baker, David W.; Sudano, Joseph J.; Albert, Jeffrey M.; et al. 2001. "Lack of Health Insurance and Decline in Overall Health in Late Middle Age." *New England Journal of Medicine* 345: 1106–1112.

Binstock, Robert H., and Post, Stephen G., eds. 1991. *Too Old for Health Care?: Controversies in Medicine, Law, Economics, and Ethics.* Baltimore: The Johns Hopkins University Press.

Callahan, Daniel. 1987. *Setting Limits: Medical Goal in an Aging Society.* New York: Simon and Schuster.

de Grey, Aubrey D.N.J.; Ames, Bruce N.; Andersen, Julie K.; et al. 2002. "Time to Talk SENS: Critiquing the Immutability of Human Aging." *Annals of the New York Academy of Science* 959: 452–462.

Esping-Andersen, Gøsta. 1999. *Social Foundations of Postindustrial Economics.* New York: Oxford University Press.

Harris, John. 2000. "Intimations of Immortality." *Science* 288: 59.

Hayflick, Leonard. 1994. *How and Why We Age.* New York: Ballantine Books.

Kass, Leon R. 2001. "L'chaim and Its Limits: Why Not Immortality?" *First Things* 13(May), 17–24.

Ku, Leighton; Ullman, Frank C.; and Almeida, Ruth A. 1999. *What Counts? Determining Medicaid and CHIP Eligibility for Children.* Washington, D.C.: The Urban Institute.

Locke, John. 1924 (1690). *Of Civil Government, Two Treatises.* London: J.M. Dent and Sons, Ltd.

Masoro, Edward J., ed. 2001. "Caloric Restriction's Effects on Aging: Opportunities for Research on Human Implications." *Journals of Gerontology: Biological Sciences and Medical Sciences* 56A(special issue 1).

Miller, Richard A. 2002. "Extending Life: Scientific Prospects and Political Obstacles." *The Milbank Quarterly* 80: 155–174.

Montesquieu, Charles-Louis de Secondat de. 1949 (1748). *The Spirit of the Laws,* tr. Thomas Nugent. New York: Hafner.

Smith, Adam. 2000 (1776). *The Wealth of Nations.* New York: Modern Library.

Vladeck, Bruce C. 1999. "The Political Economy of Medicare: Medicare Reform Requires Political Reform." *Health Affairs* 18(1): 22–36.

Woolhandler, Steffie, and Himmelstein, David U. 2001. "Paying for National Health Insurance and Not Getting It." *Health Affairs* 21(4): 88–98.

INTERNET RESOURCE

U.S. Bureau of the Census. 2002. *Health Insurance Coverage: 2000.* Available from <http://www.census.gov/hhes>.

HEALTH SERVICES MANAGEMENT ETHICS

• • •

Health services management ethics encompass the myriad ethical issues, virtually all of which directly or indirectly affect clinical services, faced by the managers of organizations that deliver health services and the moral context in which these decisions are made. Health services managers plan, organize, control, direct, and staff health services organizations (HSOs) and lead, coordinate, and integrate their activities so that clinical care can be provided. In essence, by managing the HSO, managers provide the workshop and wherewithal that enable clients and patients to receive health services. These preventive, acute, restorative, and supportive services may be provided in and through a variety of organizational settings that include inpatient services, outpatient (clinic) care, and home health services. The most intensive or acute services are provided to hospitalized inpatients; the least acute are provided in the home and in hospice, where the emphasis is comfort care and pain control. The types of health services management ethical issues that arise in the various settings are similar and run a gamut that includes macro-level resource allocation, conflicts of interest, staffing levels, and providing the structure and support for patients and families as they decide whether to withhold or withdraw life-saving treatment.

Health services managers are commonly educated in professional masters degree programs where there is emphasis on the skills of business and the ethics of medicine. In other words, these programs socialize health service managers to understand that they are entering a field in which they manage a social enterprise with business dimensions, rather than a business enterprise with social dimensions. This fact in itself makes the HSO and those working in it unique and unlike any other type of service organization. The persons served by the HSO have a unique relationship with it. This relationship is expressed through a level of trust in the organization and implicitly in its management that is rarely found in the service industry.

Health Services Management as a Profession

Health services management was recognized as a distinct academic discipline in the early 1930s. This makes it a relative late-comer to a field including the long-established professions of medicine and nursing. In seeking professional status, health services managers have established and joined professional associations that, in turn, have developed and adopted codes of ethics. These vary in their level of proscription and prescription and the methods of enforcement, but all have the common thread of doing what is in the patient's best interest—usually as defined by the patient. The codes tend to emphasize beneficence, nonmaleficence, respect for persons (autonomy, truth-telling, fidelity, and confidentiality), and justice. Applying the ethical principles often used in clinical ethical decision making is sometimes strained, nevertheless they provide a useful starting point that is supplemented as needed by other principles.

A few states flirted with licensure of hospital administrators, but this appears to be a dead issue. In response to federal regulation that was stimulated by scandals in nursing homes, however, nursing home administrators are licensed in all states. Future scandals and abuses in the health services field likely will stimulate new government regulatory forays. As with state licensing of health professions such as medicine and nursing, regulation of HSO managers probably will include codification of ethical expectations.

It is noteworthy that managers in the health services field are often held to a higher standard than managers in business and other sectors of the economy. This may result in part from their association with the healing professions of medicine and nursing. It may also be a function of the not-for-profit tradition that is so dominant in the health services field. The higher standard also may arise from the expectation that none of those served by such an organization should have their trust breached—the trust inherent in the intimate, emotional, and vital relationship established in the process of delivering health services.

Personal Ethic

In addition to the guidance provided by the codes of ethics of professional associations, health services managers should develop a personal code of professional moral conduct—a personal ethic. Formal academic instruction in ethics is an expected part of graduate-level health services management education. Students enter health services management education with a moral framework developed from life experience, family environment, religious values, introspection, and self-study. The academic preparation in their professional education sensitizes them to the managerial and clinical ethical issues that they are likely to encounter and provides a framework for analysis and problem-solving ethical issues. Because of the pragmatic and applied nature of their work, health services management ethics tend to be

normative and ask the question "What ought I (we) to do in this situation?"

Even with additional academic preparation, however, health services managers are likely to understate the importance of having a prospectively-developed, coherent, comprehensive, and consistent personal ethic. Their academic preparation is likely to give them a mind set that they can reason through and solve almost any problem that arises. While partially true, such an approach will not aid managers in anticipating ethical issues and prospectively working to prevent them or minimizing their effect when they arise. Lack of a personal ethic is likely to result in a relativistic approach to ethical problem solving, which is generally undesirable and certainly inconsistent with the value frameworks so ubiquitous in HSOs. It is difficult to overstate the importance of a well-developed personal value system.

Organizational Culture and Values

HSOs have mission and vision statements framed within the context of stated organizational values. The values identified reflect the culture of the organization; this implies that the organization's culture has been *discovered*. All organizations have a culture—the shared values that make each HSO unique. Rather than having *discovered* the culture and organized these discoveries into a mission statement, however, it is more typical that senior management developed a statement of values that they hold themselves or that they think should be the HSO's. The resulting organizational values statement may or may not reflect the culture of the HSO. Culture (and values) can be affected over time, but it is a slow, almost glacial process. Managers must beware of the trap of failing to model the organization's stated (desired) values, but asking of staff that which they are unwilling to do themselves. This will do naught but lead to cynical, noninvolved staff. Leading by example is essential.

The organization's values should be key to and provide the context for all HSO activities. These values must be the context in which staff are recruited, screened, and hired. Failure to measure candidates against the framework in which they will work invariably lead to mismatches of context and staff. The result will be higher costs and unnecessary and counterproductive levels of dissatisfaction, or worse. In terms of the HSO's services and how they are provided, its values should be inviolate. This is to say that, despite the demands of users, the organization can maintain its integrity only if it refuses to act in ways inconsistent with its values. It must be true to itself.

Questions arise as to the need for congruence between the organization's values and the personal ethic of staff, especially staff in management positions. Sectarian HSOs are likely to demand that senior leadership be adherents to their faith, a decision within the prerogatives of private organizations. It is more important, however, and often forgotten, that the values (personal ethic) of staff at all levels be congruent with the HSO's. Only by achieving a high level of congruence is the HSO able to live its values by developing a strong, pervasive culture. Managers may assume staff members have a *tabula rasa* or a generally compatible value system, and then must teach the HSO's culture tothem; the HSO's values must be reinforced by the actions of all, especially those in leadership positions. A strong culture, with clearly defined and shared values, will drive from it those whose interests and actions are contrary and this in itself is a worthy goal. High levels of cultural conformity do tend to stifle innovation, but this risk can be overcome in other ways, such as including innovation as an identified, important value in the culture.

Addressing Ethical Issues in the HSO

Health services managers have a multi-faceted role in preventing, identifying, and solving ethical problems. The importance of a personal ethic has been discussed. As a resource allocator, the health services manager is obligated to provide the support needed by the organization and its staff so that they are educated about ethics issues, have learned a methodology for addressing the ethical dimensions of management problems, and have the systems and procedures to support these efforts. Education about the HSO's values is an essential first step toward these goals; celebrating heroes of the culture and providing case examples are very useful. In addition, the manager is the driving force in ascertaining that the policies and procedures of the HSO address all of the areas where it is likely ethical problems will arise. For example, a comprehensive policy about accepting gratuities that is communicated to staff will go far to prevent conflicts of interest.

Ethics committees are required by institutional and programmatic accreditors and, thus, are ubiquitous in HSOs. Most commonly these committees are involved in clinical ethical issues and in this regard are charged with clinical case consultation, developing and reviewing clinical policies, and educating staff. Clinical staff tend to predominate on ethics committees, although social workers, clerics, and managers usually participate. Ethics committees are less likely to be involved in management ethics problems. Managers seem reluctant to allow ethics committee involvement in reviewing ethical implications of macro-resource allocation, for example. Support for ethics committees by management should include a modest budget, some staff assistance, and

the prestige of recognizing their importance to the organization. Ethics committees commonly use ethicists as consultants.

Key Issues in Managerial Ethics

CONFLICTS OF INTEREST. Conflicts of interest arise when someone has two sets of duties or obligations and meeting one set makes it impossible to meet the other. They embody the biblical admonition against serving two masters. Whether a conflict of interest is present is fact-dependent, and accurate determination requires careful scrutiny. The potential for a conflict of interest does not necessarily mean that there is a conflict of interest. It is useful to distinguish differing interests that might lead to conflicts of interest from actual conflicts of interest. Even when differing interests are present it is possible to avoid actual conflicts of interest, but the slope is slippery.

Differing interests are present, for example, when an HSO manager has an ownership interest in a supplier that could service the HSO. If the manager approves purchases from that supplier at higher-than-market prices, a conflict of interest has occurred. However, if the price is lower than available elsewhere the differing interests continue, but no conflict of interest has occurred. In fact, the better pricing is an advantage to the HSO. However, if the manager uses the position of authority to cover up inadequacies in the supplies being provided, the differing interest has produced a conflict of interest.

All HSOs should have a policy defining conflicts of interest. Conflicts of interest can be avoided by disclosing the conflicting interest and recusing oneself from the decision. Using competitive bids also reduces the probability of conflicts of interest. Managers must avoid even the appearance of a conflict of interest. Few revelations are as devastating to one's moral leadership as the suggestion of improper gain from a position of authority. Health services managers, generally, are held to a higher standard than managers in the business sector, and the mere appearance of impropriety is considered more stringently than would be the same activity if performed in another enterprise.

CONSENT. Although it is commonly considered a purely clinical ethics issue, consent is an issue that should concern the HSO manager. If it is to operationalize the patient's autonomy, the HSO must assure itself that the patient has been adequately informed as to the services that are to be rendered under its auspices. The legal requirement is that the physician obtain the patient's consent after explaining benefits, risks, and alternatives to the services that are to be rendered. However, the HSO should have policies and procedures that involve nursing or other appropriate clinical staff in ascertaining that the patient adequately understands what is happening. The manager is obliged to recognize that assuring the adequacy of consent is important; establishing the means by which it can be done and providing the staffing will make it a reality.

RESOURCE ALLOCATION. Resource allocation in HSOs occurs at the macro and micro level. The macro level includes new plant, capital equipment, and services. These decisions have major resource implications for the HSO. In turn, macroallocation decisions have major implications on the microallocation decisions made by clinicians. For example, a decision not to expand the intensive care unit (ICU) (macroallocation) means that decisions about individual patients (microallocation) will be constrained by the number of ICU beds. This, in turn, may mean that patients who might benefit from ICU services may be unable to readily receive them. Macroallocation decisions invariably have clinical implications, whether direct or indirect, and successful managers involve physicians in making these decisions. Nevertheless, resource constraints mean that not all that is clinically desirable is available.

RESOURCE CONSTRAINTS. Concomitant with ethical issues of macroallocation is the problem of resource constraints. Reimbursement from all funding sources is increasingly sparse. Most HSOs are barely achieving a modest surplus; many are running deficits. This change has occurred because of the dramatic funding reductions that began in the 1980s, after the halcyon days of the 1960s and 1970s. It is likely that the problem of inadequate reimbursement will continue unabated as patients demand more from HSOs and third-party payers are increasingly unwilling to pay at adequate levels and in a timely manner.

STAFFING. Severe shortages of several health professions plague HSOs. Registered nurses have received the most attention, although other health professions such as pharmacists and imaging technologists have also attracted too few. In addition, it has been projected that the emphasis on primary care in the 1980s and 1990s will result in too few physicians in some procedure-based specialties in the twenty-first century. HSOs have responded to nursing shortages by reducing the ratio of registered nurses to other types of staff who provide direct care to patients and instituting tuition benefits programs to encourage staff to enter nursing. Although health services managers and HSO trade associations assert that these shortages have not led to a diminution in quality of care, it stands to reason that doing more with less will eventually affect quality negatively, thus raising questions of beneficence and nonmaleficence.

COSTS. As the costs of providing health services continue to climb at double the rate of inflation in the general economy, and as the rate of reimbursement declines, the health services manager is caught in a double squeeze. Higher costs mean that more resources must go into providing basic services, and there is less capital for new equipment, programs, services, and innovation. This further exacerbates the resource allocation issue discussed above.

QUALITY OF CARE. It is estimated by researchers and quality improvement experts that 30 percent of the costs of providing a good or service occurs because of waste, delay, and rework. Such costs in the HSO setting are even more significant because to them must be added the discomfort, pain, morbidity, and mortality that can occur. The HSO manager has an ethical obligation to undertake quality improvement throughout the organization in all of the many clinical and administrative processes.

CLINICAL ETHICS ISSUES. Managers must assure that clinical staff have the support needed to prevent, minimize, and solve clinical ethical issues that arise. In addition, managers must be aware of clinical ethics issues that arise and make changes and improvement in the support available. Managers are expected to participate in ethics committees and institute and participate in ethics grand rounds in the HSO. Only by such hands-on involvement can the manager be aware of failings and issues that arise in the HSO.

The Future

The future promises to be even more challenging to health services managers than the past has been. The types of problems noted above are likely to continue, both in their present forms and in new permutations. New or exacerbated problem areas include terminal illness and futility care, advance directives, serving the underserved, marginal practitioners, multiculturalism (especially the differing meanings of life, death, disease, and treatment held by American subcultures), corporate compliance, employment practices, and whistleblowing. Three of these areas are noteworthy.

FUTILITY CARE. Futility care has been discussed since the early 1990s, but remains inadequately addressed. Acute care hospitals face families (and, less often, patients) who demand that care offering no hope of benefit be continued.

Fear of legal action and bad publicity have prevented hospitals from acting to withhold or withdraw services in such situations.

MULTICULTURALISM. Effectiveness in a multicultural society requires that the HSO's values are clearly communicated to patients, lest the HSO be pulled in many directions with inconsistent demands. Patient interests must be accommodated when possible, but not in contravention of the organization's values.

CORPORATE COMPLIANCE. Corporate compliance is the hot button issue of the new millennium. An organization whose culture and values include honesty, respect, and fair dealing will require little attention to corporate compliance, even though compliance officers are mandated by law. Its values already encourage staff to act honestly. Managers must assure that the organization's culture has no incentives for staff to do otherwise.

Conculsion

Health services managers face a future paradoxically marked by a bleak economic outlook and a challenging, hopeful outlook for providing services. Even as they endeavor to bring high quality health services to all who need them, health services managers will have to do so with fewer resources and under heavier constraints then ever in the profession's history.

KURT DARR

SEE ALSO: *Corporate Compliance; Hospital, Contemporary Ethical Problems of; Medicaid; Medicare; Mental Health Services; Mergers and Acquisitions; Organizational Ethics in Healthcare; Pharmaceutical Industry; Profit and Commercialism*

BIBLIOGRAPHY

Beauchamp, Tom L., and Walters, LeRoy, eds. 1999. *Contemporary Issues in Bioethics,* 5th edition. Belmont, CA: Wadsworth Publishing Company.

Boatright, John R. 2003. *Ethics and the Conduct of Business,* 4th edition. Upper Saddle River, New Jersey: Prentice Hall.

Darr, Kurt. 1997. *Ethics in Health Services Management,* 3rd edition. Baltimore: Health Professions Press.

Hall, Robert T. 2000. *An Introduction to Healthcare Organizational Ethics.* New York: Oxford University Press.

Pellegrino, Edmund D., and Thomasma, David C. 1988. *For the Patient's Good: The Restoration of Beneficence in Health Care.* New York: Oxford University Press.

HINDUISM, BIOETHICS IN

• • •

The following is a revision and update of the first-edition entry "Hinduism" by A. L. Basham. Portions of the first-edition entry appear in the revised version.

Hinduism is a religious system that has grown and developed from the Vedic religion identified with Aryans who invaded the Indian subcontinent over a period of centuries in the second millennium B.C.E. It is rooted in an oral tradition that gave rise to four groups of sacred texts during a period that is difficult to pinpoint more precisely than 1500 to 900 B.C.E. Based on this informal collection of traditions, beliefs, and practices and the corpus of formal written treatises, which together provided a context for development of the medical system known as *Ayurveda,* Hinduism encompasses a range of values and codes of conduct highly relevant to a study of Indian bioethics.

Hinduism as we might recognize it today took shape in the Gupta Period (c. 300–500 C.E.), often regarded as the classical age of Hindu India. This entry will identify and briefly discuss basic concepts, which clarify the setting for analysis of bioethics in Hindu India, before focusing on medical ethics in *Ayurveda.* Just as they do now, social and cultural values defined standards of medical education and practice, ideas about ethical behavior as a determinant of health and disease, the balance of commercial and altruistic motives of clinicians, access to care and humane treatment, and the rights and responsibilities of patients and physicians.

Hindu Worldview

The doctrine of transmigration is a definitive concept for Hinduism. It postulates the existence of an innermost self (*ātman*) for all beings, ranging from the highest god to the meanest insect, that is essentially immutable. By becoming incarnate, this self becomes further involved with matter, which some philosophical systems hold to be fundamentally illusory and others regard as the primordial source of intellect, ego, elements, and the material world. According to the conduct of the embodied being, the soul or self is carried at death to another body, in which it flourishes or suffers according to previous behavior (the law of *karma*). This process is called *samsāra.* From an outsider's perspective, the force of *karma* operates as a tangible manifestation of an ethical system associated with principles of righteous conduct and moral values inherent in the concept of *dharma,* a difficult-to-translate term that embodies cosmic order, sacred law, and religious duty. Within the system, however, the effects of *karma* are typically conceived more as the operation of natural law governing the effects of behavior than a statement of moral and ethical values.

Transmigration links all living beings in a single system. Unlike the Judaeo-Christian and Islamic religious systems, Hinduism makes no sharp distinction between human and animal. *Dharma* as a guide to proper behavior is relative, not the same for different people or different beings. The ideas of *karma* and *samsāra* motivate values of nonviolence (*ahimsā*) and vegetarianism. Nonviolence, which was never so prominent a value in Hinduism as it was in Jainism and Buddhism, has less stringent implications for laypersons than for ascetics, and it does not interfere with righteous warfare, punishment of criminals, or self-defense.

The process of transmigration is considered painful, and the main quest of classical Hinduism has been to find "release" (*mokṣa*) from the cycle of birth and death and thereby enter a state of timeless bliss. For the orthodox schools of Hindu philosophy and systems of Buddhism and Jainism that sprang from them, knowledge provides a means of escaping this repetitive cycle of birth, death, and rebirth. Each of these schools has a somewhat different interpretation of the problem and the solution. Both the *Sāṃkhya* school, identified with yoga practice and once very influential, and the heterodox sect of Jainism, define release as the complete separation of the individual soul from matter. The *Advaita* Vedanta system, which exerts the greatest influence on intellectual Hinduism, interprets it as a full realization of the illusory character of the material world, the speciousness of individual personality, and the recognition of the soul's identity with an underlying impersonal world spirit, often called *Brahman.* Theistic Hinduism of the *ViśIṣtādvaita* school, which has had the greatest influence on popular ideas, interprets release as union with the personal God not through knowledge but through devotion to *Viṣṇu,* who is identified with *Brahman,* the ultimate reality of the universe and out of whom the world repeatedly emerges in the course of cosmic cycles.

Ideally, release is the aim of all striving, but Hinduism recognizes the validity of other aims, which for laypersons are fully legitimate. The ascetic (*sannyāsi*), on the other hand, "who has given up the world," should pursue only release. Ordinary people approach this goal through gradual stages over many lives. For them there are three legitimate aims: *dharma,* adherence to religious and ethical norms in order to ensure a happier rebirth; *artha,* amassing wealth for the benefit of oneself and one's family; and *kāma,* seeking pleasure and the satisfaction of personal desires. These three aims are valued in descending hierarchical order, but each is fully acceptable for different persons at a particular stage of life and for caste-based communities, which may emphasize one of them.

The Hindu pantheon begins with one primeval being, or God, and innumerable supernatural beings, all of whom are endowed with individual volition. Some of these beings adhere to the will of the higher gods, but others oppose the work of creation. Battles between gods and demons, light and darkness, and good and evil were important features of the earliest Hindu literature, and these themes are widely represented in popular beliefs and practices. Complementing more intellectual naturalistic explanations that are also a prominent feature of Hinduism, some look upon the world as a place full of demons, which are normally at war with gods, and which can be potent factors in causing misfortune and disease.

Hindu cosmology refers to four ages (*yuga*) over the period of a great cycle (4,320,000 years). The current cycle, the *Kali yuga,* is the worst, but fortunately the shortest, lasting 432,000 years, about 5,100 of which have elapsed. Looking backward to better times provides a guide in this troubled age. Neither the doctrine of *karma* nor that of cosmic decline, however, implies fatalism. Human effort may influence the process, and it holds potential for gaining release from the personal cycles of birth and rebirth. Hindu texts emphasize the virtue of human effort (*puruṣakāra*), rather than passive acceptance of adversity that may follow from destiny or chance.

Social Norms

The four great classes (*varṇa*), constituting an eternal hierarchical social order, were believed to have emerged at the beginning of time from the body of the Creator as the fundamental basis of society. The *Brahman* (priest), the *Kṣatriya* (warrior and ruler), the *Vaiśya* (merchant), and the *Sūdra* (worker) formed these four classes, each with different roles, responsibility, and status. Maintaining differences that distinguish each of them was a prerequisite of the social order, and any effort to violate the boundaries of social organization and behavior was an affront to nature and the gods, degrading for those at the top and punishable for those at the bottom. Below the four great classes were the untouchables, theoretically outside, but operating at the bottom of the social order. They performed important social functions that others considered polluting, such as removing garbage, cremating corpses, working in leather, and so forth. Contact between them and the other classes was strictly limited.

Although aspects of this class structure persist in Hindu society today, social conditions rarely operated according to textbook norms. More important and more complex in everyday life was the caste (*jāti*), a group of families generally following the same profession and theoretically contained within one of the four classes, though not always recognizably so in practice, especially in South India. Castes were also hierarchically graded and normally endogamous. Local councils of elders exerted great power over their members.

Family

Social research in recent years has emphasized the primacy of the family over the individual in Hindu and other societies outside North America and western Europe. Hindu individuals were more likely to define themselves with reference to the extended family (*kula*) as a corporate unit. Social responsibilities, which constitute underpinnings for the concept of *dharma*, rather than individual rights, were clearly the priority among ethical concerns. Except in some parts of South India, primarily Kerala, the family was patrilinear, patriarchal, and patrilocal, though the authority of the patriarch was limited by traditional law. He did not have the right to dispose of family property arbitrarily, nor did he have complete control over the lives of family members.

The ritual of *śrāddha*, whereby dead ancestors retained a presence, sustained by the living, was a powerful force in shaping the character of Hindu family life. A male descendant to perform the *śrāddha*, a ritual offering of rice balls (*piṇḍa*), was needed not only to sustain the ancestral lineage but also to avoid one's own suffering in the afterlife. In view of heavy child mortality, it was incumbent upon families to produce as many children as possible, in the hope that at least one surviving son would maintain the lineage, attend to the spiritual needs of the ancestors, and contribute to the economic well-being of the family.

A Hindu wife was integrated into her husband's family, and theoretically (though not always in practice) completely subordinate to him. In many communities it was considered indecent to leave a girl unmarried after her first menstruation, and marriage normally required the payment of a heavy dowry. Thus, the birth of a daughter was often looked on as a misfortune. Although female infanticide has been practiced and persists in some parts of India, the practice is completely without foundation in the Hindu scriptures, which look upon abortion and infanticide as grave forms of murder.

Prospective parents employed various techniques to increase their chances of bearing a male, rather than female, child. Diet and activities of a pregnant woman were believed to influence the sex, physical features, and character of the offspring. Treatises of *Ayurveda* advise that intercourse on even days after the onset of menstruation produces sons, and on odd days it produces daughters (Caraka, iv. 8. 5). *Pumsavana* rites to alter the sex of a recently conceived embryo and ensure the birth of a male child are discussed in the texts of *Ayurveda*. They are also discussed in religious treatises of the Veda and other texts that detail proper Hindu codes of conduct (*dharmaśāstra*) (Kane).

In recent years profitable ultrasound clinics have proliferated in India, in some states illegally, to make use of modern technology to identify and abort female fetuses. Responding to a culturally based gender bias and a persisting dowry system that taints perceptions of female children as economic liabilities, this ultrasound technology challenges the viability of *pumsavana* clinics previously established in some *Ayurvedic* hospitals and employing traditional Hindu medical methods for assuring the birth of male children.

Individual Conduct

Within the framework of the three aims of life (*puruṣārtha*) acceptable for the high-caste individual were a series of ritual observances and taboos throughout life. Sacraments beginning before birth and continuing after death marked the progress of life. The Brahman was expected to devote a considerable amount of time each day to prayer and ritual, and members of other castes were encouraged to imitate him.

The aim of many of these sacraments and taboos was to maintain ritual purity. Although conceived with reference to another conceptual framework, many practices also maintained a hygienic standard contributing to health in a tropical climate. Notable examples include insistence on a daily bath, the custom of eating with the right hand and washing the anus and sexual organs with the left, the ban on eating cooked food left overnight, and a strict taboo against contact with human corpses and animal carcasses. The bodily fluids of others, such as saliva and mucus, are considered polluting, and contact with anything contaminated by them, such as used dishes or drinking glasses, was to be avoided.

Social values and a conflicting emphasis in various texts of classical Hinduism portray an ambivalent attitude that both exalts and denies sexuality. *Vedic* texts regard sexuality as a metaphor for a ritual sacrifice. The *Bṛhadāraṇyika Upaniṣad* (vi. 2. 13), among the best known of this speculative genre of Hindu scriptures (*Upaniṣad*), identified woman as a sacrificial fire fueled both by her own and her male partner's genital organs in the act of sexual intercourse.

Semen is an offering to this fire, which may generate a person.

In later texts, however, sex is affirmed as a valid source of gratification, a legitimate pursuit among the three aims of life: righteousness, wealth, and pleasure. Erotic temple art and texts devoted to the details of enhancing sexual gratification, such as the *Kāma Sutra,* document a cultural sanction of pleasure seeking for men. These texts acknowledge female sexuality but consider it primarily from a male perspective—how to attract and please a man. Hindu texts concerned with moral codes of conduct (*Dharmaśāstra*) emphasize chastity and procreation more from the classical period onward than previously (Bhattacharyya).

Even for men, classical Hinduism confines sexual activity to one stage of a man's life. An initiation ceremony (upanayana) that preceded a long period of celibate studentship was a milestone for upper-caste boys. Afterwards, a young man was married, normally to a bride chosen by his parents, and raised a family. According to the ideal, he was expected to give up family cares in late middle age to devote the rest of his life to religion and to strive for liberation. Ascetic values discouraged sexual activity, which not only distracts the individual from a quest for release from the cycle of rebirth but also results in the loss of physical and spiritual power.

In addition to the emphasis on a moral code of religious practices, Hinduism also emphasizes ethical principles of social relations. The principle of nonviolence has often been interpreted in a positive sense, as actively benefiting others. Though subject to the constraints of conflicting values in a comprehensive social order, Hindu texts and practices encourage virtues of honesty, hospitality, and generosity. Explicit codes detailing how guests are to be received, fed, and looked after emphasize hospitality as a social value (see chap. 21 on receiving guests in Kane). The *Taittirīya Upanisad* (i. 11. 2) admonishes students to treat parents, teachers, and guests as gods.

Hindu Medicine

A complex medical system, known as *Ayurveda,* "the science of (living to a ripe old) age," developed in India over the first millennium B.C.E. The theory of health and disease according to *Ayurveda* refers to a humoral physiology based on the balance of three substances (*dosas*): wind (*vāta*), bile (*pitta*), and phlegm (*kapha*). They are recognizable indirectly by their impact on health and illness. The excess of one or another and their locus in the body or among bodily elements (*dhātu*) determines the nature of specific physical and mental diseases, their manifestations, and subtypes.

Although *karma,* demons, and deities may also play a role in producing ill health, it is a relatively minor role in the medical texts and more of a concern in other settings. The role of a physician practicing *Ayurveda* is to restore the harmony of humoral balance with medicines, purification, massage, diet, and directives for appropriate lifestyle. Experience with an exceptionally wide pharmacopoeia and careful observations of the symptomatology, clinical course, and treatment response of various diseases—especially chronic conditions for which Western medicine does not provide a clearly superior alternative—have enabled practitioners of the system to maintain the respect of a large number of South Asians who continue to use it.

Health, Disease, and Morality

Ayurveda, despite its emphasis on the humoral basis of health and disease, also recognized external (*āgantu*) causes that provided a better account than endogenous (*nija*) causes—that is, humoral imbalance—to explain some medical conditions. *Karma* referred to the impact of misdeeds in a previous life. Irreverent, unethical behavior and other violations of codes of conduct (*prajñā-aparadha*) in one's current life were not limited to effects on that individual; they could also affect offspring (Caraka, iv. 8. 21, 30). Serious transgressions of the king might also produce epidemic disease and disasters (*janapadoddvamsana*) in his kingdom (Caraka, iii. 3). Moral conduct, affecting individuals, distinct from epidemics affecting populations, operated through the all-embracing doctrine of karma; in some instances, *karma* explained health or disease if the humoral theory or demonic possession could not, and in other instances, it provided a complementary explanation.

Illnesses might be caused by the sins or shortcomings of a previous existence; longevity was also explained by this idea of *karma.* The doctrine encouraged inner acceptance of disease and gave a ready-made explanation of its cause, but nowhere is a person advised to submit to illness without attempting its cure. *Karma* could explain otherwise mysterious congenital defects. Someone born with a deformed hand, for example, could be said to have incurred this misfortune as a result of an evil deed (for instance, striking a *Brahman*) committed by the same hand in a previous life. This did not necessarily discourage efforts to improve the condition by surgery, since the duration of the punishment through *karma* was not known, and the trouble might be only temporary. Since the evil brought about by *karma* cannot be estimated with certainty, and the bad effects of sins can be offset by the merit gained by good deeds, there was every reason why a sick person should seek all available medical help to achieve health.

Other factors besides *karma* were believed to promote health or disease. Devotion (*bhakti*) to God, who might set aside the law of *karma* for the faithful, promoted longevity and health. Neglect of religious duties and lack of faith, on the other hand, might lead to the withdrawal of divine protection, increasing the risk that demons might exert their influence, leading to disease or madness.

More closely linked with ethics was the general view in the medical treatises that equanimity and kindness are therapeutic in their effects. Excess in every respect is looked on with disfavor by the medical texts. An impressive emphasis on the values of moderation, altruism, and love to promote health and longevity is found in the seventh-century text of the Buddhist physician Vāgbhata, the *Aṣṭāṅgahṛdayasaṃhitā* (1965, i. 2). This work, along with the *Caraka Samhitā* and the *Suśruta Samhitā*, is among the so-called great-three (*bṛhattrayī*) texts of classical *Ayurveda*. After reviewing the benefits of exercise and symptoms resulting from overexercise, it enjoins the physician to support those who are sick, poor, or needy and to treat them with respect.

Mental and spiritual training in concentration and meditation, commonly known as yoga, was also believed to promote health and longevity. Yoga is still widely practiced both as treatment for clinical problems in yoga clinics of some Indian hospitals and more generally to promote health and well-being. Different forms of yoga practice involve physical postures and exercises (*hatha-yoga*), meditation (*rāja-yoga*), or both. These produce not merely health and longevity; they also provide a way for the most advanced adepts to attain liberation from the cycle of rebirth, and hence immortality.

Ethics of Medical Practice

The activities of the physician (*vaidya*) were closely linked with the doctrine of the three aims of Hindu life (Caraka, i. 30. 29; Vāgbhaṭa, i. 2. 29). Viewed as complementary, rather than contradictory, they guide appropriate behavior. By relieving suffering and adding to the sum of human happiness, a physician (assumed in the texts to be a man) fulfills the first aim, carrying out his religious duty; from the generous fees of his wealthy patients he achieves the second aim, riches; while the third aim, pleasure, is achieved by the satisfaction he obtains, first, from a high reputation as a healer and, second, from the knowledge that he has cured many people whom he loves and respects.

The last two aims were not to be disparaged. The few famous physicians described in story and tradition were not selfless servants of humanity but very wealthy men—in that regard resembling successful practitioners of modern times.

There appears to have been no ban to keep a physician from advertising his skill. As the example of Vāgbhata indicates, Hindu and Buddhist medical traditions were closely linked. A Buddhist text, the *Mahāvagga,* provides more biographical detail than the Hindu sources about medical practice in the same society. It refers to the material interests of a renowned doctor in his youth, *Jīvaka,* recently qualified and in search of patients. As he entered an ancient Indian city, to earn money for his onward journey, he walked through the streets inquiring, "Who is ill here? Who wants to be cured?" (Mahāvagga, viii. i. 8–13).

Although Jīvaka's concern for his fees was matched by qualifications and skill, it appears that quackery was also rampant in ancient India; charlatans would come canvassing as soon as they heard that a well-to-do person was sick (Caraka, i. 29. 8–12). Recognizing such problems, Suśruta (i. 10. 3) referred to a system of licensing qualified medical practitioners. Texts on politics and statecraft suggested punishments for doctors whose ineffective treatment resulted in injury or death (*Kauṭilya,* iv. 1; Kane). Caraka also advocated a high moral standard for a proper physician, based on religious duty (*dharma*). At the outset, a physician's training began with a solemn initiation, at which his teacher (*guru*) instructed him that he was to live a frugal and ascetic life, celibate and vegetarian, while undergoing training. He must obey his teacher implicitly "unless instructed to commit a mortal sin." The prescribed instruction continues:

> When you have finished your studies, if you want to have a successful, wealthy, and famous practice, and to go to heaven when you die, you must pray every day, when you get up and go to sleep, for the welfare of all beings, especially cattle and brahmans, and you must strive with all your power to heal the sick. You must not betray your patients, even at the risk of your own life.... You must always be pleasant of speech ... and always strive to improve your knowledge.... Having entered a patient's home, a physician's speech, mind, intellect, and senses should be devoted to nothing other than caring for the patient. Any peculiarities of the household you may learn about should not be disclosed outside. (Caraka, iii. 8. 13. 4–5, 7)

This well-known passage has been compared with the Hippocratic oath. The text also addressed other persisting dilemmas of medical practice. If it becomes clear that a patient in treatment has a fatal condition, the matter of whether or not a doctor should disclose this information was left largely to the doctor's discretion. Caraka advised that if a physician concludes that the condition of the patient is hopeless and if he believes that it might shock the patient or others, he should keep this knowledge to himself.

The same chapter of the Caraka Saṃhitā also contains advice about when a physician should refuse to provide treatment. He should not treat the king's enemies, women unattended by a husband or guardian, or patients for whom a request for treatment comes as they are about to die (Caraka, iii. 8. 13.6). Accepting a terminal case might damage his reputation.

The Hindu medical tradition is based on a relatively stable theory of health and illness, but it advocates a policy of openness to new ideas about treatments. Although the theoretical basis rooted in the doctrine of the three humors has always guided *Ayurveda* and undergone little modification over the course of time, the *vaidya* was advised to be constantly on the lookout for new drugs and treatment methods. Compared chronologically, the texts show a steady increase in the number of items in the pharmacopoeia. Even after his long apprenticeship was over, the physician was counseled to continue to improve his knowledge by studying his patients and inquiring about unusual but potentially useful remedies from hermits, cowherds, and hillmen (Suśruta, i. 36. 10).

Professional gatherings of physicians were regarded as valuable opportunities for the exchange of knowledge that could enhance a clinician's skills. The descriptions of these colloquiums distinguish friendly discussions from hostile debates, and the exchange of information was not necessarily free and open. Many physicians guarded proprietary knowledge not recorded in professional textbooks, knowledge they might reveal to prove a point in the heat of impassioned debate. Entering into professional discussions, the clinician is advised not to boast, embarrass others, or fear discomfort. In the company of knowledgeable colleagues, he is advised to listen attentively and speak freely. The text also advises how to handle hostile discussions with superiors, inferiors, and equals. "The wise never applaud a person engaging in hostile discussion with a superior … but the following methods help in quickly overpowering an inferior disputant…." (Caraka, iii. 8. 15–21; see also the remainder of chap. iii. 8).

The texts encouraged the physician, though he might be wealthy and unfettered by any rules of an ascetic character, to consider himself a sort of secular priest with a special, almost supernatural charisma bestowed on him by the initiation ceremony at the beginning of his studies. The high-caste man who had undergone the normal Hindu initiation (*upanayana*) was "twice-born" (*dvija*), and thus superior to the Śudra or woman, who had only one birth. The *vaidya* was even a step beyond, "thrice-born" (*trija*). As the prescribed words of his teacher show, this exalted status required a high standard of fortitude and conduct. The student was taught that as a physician he should always be "of calm mind, pleasant speech, … the friend of all beings" (Suśruta, i. 10. 3). To some extent professional identity relieved him of the burden of caste taboos. He could enter the homes of people of a lower caste than his, handle their bodies, and even taste their urine when making a diagnosis.

Notwithstanding vegetarian cultural values, treatment employed animal products to compound drugs, and they appear to have been prescribed freely. The taboo that proscribed handling a corpse, however, may have applied to most physicians. Most medical texts do not advocate the actual dissection of a cadaver; *Suśruta Saṃhitā* (iii. 5), however, is an exception. It advises that for a surgeon to study the position of internal organs, a carefully selected dead body should be placed in a cage after removing excrement from the entrails, positioned in a stream with a swift current, and examined after seven days as it begins to decompose. In that way the body might be studied in each anatomical layer, beginning with the skin.

Although concerns about ritual pollution and principles of nonviolence inhibited anatomical study and surgery in *Ayurveda,* in recent years they appear to have had surprisingly little influence on modern medicine in India, known as allopathy, with respect to the burgeoning surgical practice of organ transplantation. Concern about the adverse impact on the transmigration of souls has had a negligible effect on the transmigration of vital organs from one person to another. Bombay has acquired a dubious distinction as a world center for transplants from unrelated live donors, spawned by a profitable private-practice medical industry, an impoverished subpopulation willing to donate organs for a fee, and enterprising brokers whose activities reflect little concern for the ethics of these practices.

Access to Healthcare

The provision of free medical care to the poor was looked on as part of a king's duty to protect his subjects, which was generally interpreted in a positive sense (Caraka, i. 30.29; see also the background essay in vol. 1, pp. 254–264 of P. M. Mehta's translation). From the days of the benevolent Buddhist emperor Aśoka in the third century B.C.E., the better rulers of India responded in some measure to this responsibility. Medical clinics of one kind or another, where professional doctors provided free services to the poor, existed in many cities. These were sometimes supported by the states, but others were often financed by private charity. In South India especially, hospitals and dispensaries were often attached to the great temples. Medical services might have been subsidized by doctors themselves, for they were encouraged to treat the poor, learned Brahmans, and ascetics without charge (Suśruta, i. 2. 8; vi. 11. 12–13). Free medical services in South and Southeast Asia, however, were more extensive in Buddhist Sri Lanka and Cambodia.

Reasoned Suicide and Mental Health

The aim of the idealized ascetic to attain release and end the cycle of rebirth provided an acceptable rationale for suicide in highly selected circumstances. *Sallekhaná* is a Jain practice sanctioned for elderly mendicants involving ritual fasting that ends in death; its aim is for the individual to meet the final moment with utmost tranquillity (Settar). The *Dharmaśāstra* literature, which outlines Hindu codes of conduct, also refers to another form of religious suicide, the "great journey," justified by incurable disease or great misfortune (Kane). Those who undertake this ultimate renunciation in the final stage of life proceed in a northeasterly direction, "subsisting on water and air, until his body sinks to rest" (*The Laws of Manu*, 6. 31). Other means of accomplishing religiously motivated suicides include jumping from a height (*bhrgupāta*), often associated with pilgrimage sites where these suicides were most frequent, such as Śravana Belgola, west of Bangalore in South India, and Prayaga (modern Allahabad) in the North.

Questions about these carefully reasoned suicides, usually sanctioned only for the elderly, were framed in religious rather than medical contexts, unlike current debates about euthanasia and assisted suicide in the West. Nevertheless, issues identified as appropriate justification by those who advocate these practices in both settings are comparable, especially the role of terminal illness and functional disability. Whether one regards these socially sanctioned self-willed deaths as suicide or something else is a debatable matter. Some scholars avoid the stigmatized English term (Settar), although more commonly suicide is used descriptively, regardless of whether it is proscribed.

Although Hindu texts were very much concerned about ethical questions that ultimately lead to sanctioning or condemning suicides, based on their circumstances, the context of the discourse was strikingly different from that of present-day debates about physician-assisted suicides. Suicide in the West typically raises questions about deviance and mental disorder. Concerns for victims are framed in clinical terms with a focus on prevention and cure of psychopathology associated with suicidal impulses. Hindu traditions that consider suicide are concerned with a different set of questions, which focus not on deviance but on cultural values. Religious suicides of ascetics and pilgrims and the self-immolation of a widow on the funeral pyre of her husband (*anumarana*)—an act that has come to be known as *sati*, after the Sanskrit term for the "righteous woman" who undertakes it—were not discussed in medical contexts. Modern criticism of *sati* proceeds from social, economic, and feminist perspectives; it focuses on questions about the deviance and disorder not of the victims but of societies that disvalue women, especially widows.

Suicide was regarded neither as a defining feature nor an important symptom of mental disorder. Mental disorders (*unmāda*), however, were recognized and classified according to threatening, disorganized, and disordered behaviors, and by disturbing emotional states. The classification of some of these mental disorders fit the characteristic humoral framework, but others did not. Like some childhood diseases discussed in the texts (but few other health problems), they were explained by the influence of demons and deities. The texts prescribe a mix of gentle, humane treatment, as well as not-so-gentle efforts to restrain and shock patients into normalcy with threats of harm and false reports of the death of loved ones. Offerings to demons and deities (*bali*) and medicines to correct a humoral imbalance of excessive wind, bile, or phlegm were also prescribed for mental illnesses attributed to these respective causes.

Conclusion

Many issues that remain concerns in modern medical practice were recognized and addressed by Hindu religious texts, codes of conduct, and Sanskrit treatises of *Ayurveda*. The medical texts discussed responsibilities of the physician to society, patients, and colleagues in terms that recognized the professional nature of these interactions, distinctive social values, and political forces. Medical theory, which was primarily humoral, incorporated a moral basis for explaining health and illness of individuals. Some questions that have become major concerns for medical ethics in the West, such as the status of rational suicide, were considered in the context of Hindu traditions other than medicine.

Recent developments in biotechnology have placed controversial questions about bioethics and cultural values near the top of an agenda for equitable social policy in South Asia. The ongoing debate that follows from the impact of new technologies should be informed by an appreciation of the cultural and historical contexts in which these questions emerge.

MITCHELL G. WEISS (1995)

SEE ALSO: *Buddhism, Bioethics in; Confucianism, Bioethics in; Daoism, Bioethics in; Death, Eastern Thought; Ethics, Religion and Morality; Eugenics and Religious Law: Hinduism and Buddhism; Healing; Health and Disease; Jainism, Bioethics in; Sikhism, Bioethics in*

BIBLIOGRAPHY

Basham, Arthur Llewellyn. 1967. *The Wonder That Was India: A Survey of the History and Culture of the Indian Sub-Continent Before the Coming of the Muslims,* 3rd rev. edition. London: Sidgwick and Jackson.

Bhattacharyya, Narendra Nath. 1975. *History of Indian Erotic Literature.* Delhi: Munshiram Manoharlal.

Caraka. *Caraka Samhitā.* 1949. 6 vols, ed. by P. M. Mehta with translations in Hindi, Gujarati, and English by the Shree Gulabkunverba Ayurvedic Society. Jamnagar, India: Gulabkunverba Ayurvedic Society.

Coward, Harold G.; Lipner, Julius J.; and Young, Katherine K. 1989. *Hindu Ethics: Purity, Abortion, and Euthanasia.* Albany: State University of New York Press.

Desai, Prakash N. 1988. "Medical Ethics in India." *Journal of Medicine and Philosophy* 13(3): 231–255.

Dossetor, John B., and Manickavel, V. 1991. "Ethics in Organ Donation: Contrasts in Two Cultures." *Transplantation Proceedings* 23(5): 2,508–2,511.

Filliozat, Jean F. 1949. *La doctrine classique de la médecine indienne: Ses origines et ses parallèles grecs.* Paris: P. Geuthner & Imprimerie nationale, tr. Dev Raj Chanana under the title *The Classical Doctrine of Indian Medicine: Its Origins and Its Greek Parallels.* Delhi: Munshiram Manoharlal, 1964.

George, Sabu; Abel, Rajaratnam; and Miller, Barbara D. 1992. "Female Infanticide in Rural South India." *Economic and Political Weekly* 27(22): 1,153–1,156.

Jeffery, Roger; Jeffery, Patricia; and Lyon, Andrew. 1984. "Female Infanticide and Amniocentesis." *Social Science and Medicine* 19(11): 1,207–1,212.

Jolly, Julius. 1901. *Medicin.* Strasbourg: K. J. Trubner, tr. and ed. Chintaman Ganesh Kashikar under the title *Indian Medicine.* Poona, India: C. G. Kashikar, 1951.

Kane, Pandurang Vaman. 1968–. *A History of Dharmasastra: Ancient and Mediaeval Religious and Civil Law in India,* 2nd rev. edition. Poona, India: Bhandarkar Oriental Research Institute.

Kauṭiliya. 1969. *The Kauṭiliya Arthasastra.* 2nd edition. 2 vols. ed. and tr. by R. P. Kangle. Bombay: University of Bombay. Text and translation.

Lannoy, Richard. 1971. *The Speaking Tree: A Study of Indian Culture and Society.* London: Oxford University Press.

The Laws of Manu. 1988. tr. Georg Buhler. Delhi: Motilal Banarsidass.

Mahāvagga [The Great Division]. 1881–1882. tr. T. W. Rhys Davids and Hermann Oldenberg, ed. Friedrich Max Müller. Oxford: Clarendon Press.

Majumdar, R. C. 1971. "Medicine." In *A Concise History of Science in India,* 213–273, ed. D. M. Bose, S. N. Sen, and B. V. Subbarayappa. New Delhi: Indian National Science Academy.

Menon, I. A., and Haberman, H. F. 1970. "The Medical Students' Oath of Ancient India." *Medical History* 14(3): 295–299.

Monier-Williams, Monier. 1883. *Religious Thought and Life in India: Vedism, Brāhmanism and Hinduism.* London: John Murray.

Reddy, D. V. Subba. 1941. "Medical Relief in Medieval South India: Centres of Medical Aid and Types of Medical Institutions." *Bulletin of the History of Medicine* 9: 385–400.

Reddy, D. V. Subba. 1961. "Medical Ethics in Ancient India." *Journal of the Indian Medical Association* 37(16): 287–288.

Settar, Shadakshari. 1990. *Pursuing Death: Philosophy and Practice of Voluntary Termination of Life.* Dharwad, India: Institute of Indian Art History, Karnatak University.

Sharma, Priya Vrat, ed. 1992. *History of Medicine in India: From Antiquity to 1000 A.D.* New Delhi: Indian National Science Academy.

Suśruta. *Suśruta Samhitā.* 1947. 3 vols, tr. Kaviraj Kunja Lal Bhishagratna. Varanasi, India: Chowkhamba Sanskrit Series.

Vagbhata. 1965. *Aṣṭāngahṛdayasaṃhitā. The First Five Chapters of Its Tibetan Version,* ed. and tr. Claus Vogel. Deutsche Morgenländische Gesellschaft. With original Sanskrit text. Wiesbaden: Franz Steiner.

Weiss, Mitchell G. 1980. "Caraka Saṃhita on the Doctrine of Karma." In *Karma and Rebirth in Classical Indian Traditions,* 90–115, ed. Wendy Doniger O'Flaherty. Berkeley: University of California Press.

Williams-Monier, Monier. 1883. *Religious Thought and Life in India: Vedism, Brāhmanism and Hinduism.* London: J. Murray.

Zysk, Kenneth G. 1991. *Asceticism and Healing in Ancient India: Medicine in the Buddhist Monastery.* New York: Oxford University Press.

HOLOCAUST

• • •

Bioethics is a type of *discourse,* defined as "any collective activity that orders its concerns through language" (Zito). As members of a discourse community, bioethicists use rhetorical strategies to make arguments, define terms, and influence the direction of the discourse as a whole. One of those strategies is to invoke the Holocaust as a way to warn, cajole, criticize, or silence those who have opposing or divergent views. The use of the Holocaust as a rhetorical instrument raises important ethical and strategic questions for bioethics.

The Holocaust

The Holocaust lies like a specter behind modern bioethics. Contemporary bioethical discourse derives much of its moral legitimacy from the legacy of the Holocaust. The unfathomable cruelty of the Holocaust is paradigmatic of the degree to which the unfettered power of the majority over despised minorities can distort human relationships. The eugenic philosophy that undergirded social engineering and extermination campaigns informs all current debate about genetic engineering and population genetics. The genocidal strategy of the Nazis, coupled with the complicity of large segments of the German public, including medical professionals, showed the depths to which human beings could go in the pursuit of misguided philosophies of science and in-group politics. The atrocities committed in the name of medical research revealed individual subject vulnerability in the hands of investigators so starkly that virtually all modern standards for protecting human research subjects originated in the aftermath of the Holocaust.

The events that occurred in Germany under National Socialism have come to represent evil in pure form, without caveat or ambiguity. The Holocaust thus has come to signify the ultimately evil act; the Nazi enterprise, the ultimately evil political and social movement; and Hitler, the ultimately evil leader. By extension, those who were inactive in the face of evil are invoked as the paradigm of complicity and those who did not speak out are emblems of culpable silence. It thus is not surprising that evoking the Holocaust as a rhetorical strategy has enormous symbolic power.

However, such power cannot be wielded without risk. Drawing on symbols of ultimate evil to buttress arguments about the undesirability of lesser evils may be emotionally satisfying, but it is rarely a persuasive rhetorical strategy. If the analogy is seen as inapt, it tends to weaken rather than strengthen the case being made. Still, the temptation to employ the Holocaust is strong, and it has become a central metaphor for a variety of social movements (Stein), special interests (Novick), and political actors (Lin and Gur-Ze'ev) as well as in popular culture (Hungerford, Mintz, Zelizer).

The use of the Holocaust in bioethics has taken on a particular character. Bioethics is a normative discourse, and the Holocaust is a signifier with great normative power. The Holocaust frequently is invoked in bioethical discourse to draw analogies, suggest threats to vulnerable groups, or warn against perceived slippery slopes. After a brief historical summary, some of those strategies will be examined in this entry to explore their impact on bioethical discourse.

Rhetoric and the Holocaust

The term *holocaust* is derived from the Greek *holokauston*, meaning "burnt whole," which was a derivation of the Greek translation of the Hebrew *olah*, a biblical term for a burnt sacrifice. Historically, the term was used to denote great destruction of human life, especially through conflagration. For that reason it was employed often by journalists in

World War II to refer not only to the destruction perpetrated by the Nazis on Jews and others but also to Allied acts such as the bombing firestorms that destroyed much of Hamburg and Dresden. It is ironic that the German press used the term first to refer to the bombing of German cities.

The use of *holocaust* in reference to the destruction of the European Jewish community at the hands of the Nazis gained currency by being the preferred English translation of the Hebrew word *shoah*. The 1948 Israeli Declaration of Independence, for example, makes reference to the *shoah,* which is rendered as "the Nazi holocaust" in official English translations (Novick). However, in the decades after World War II the destruction of European Jewry was rarely part of American public discourse. It was only during the 1960s, particularly with the advent of the trial of the Nazi official Adolf Eichmann, that the term *holocaust* began to be used in common discourse to refer to World War II. At first the term often was used to refer to the death of all the millions of people who were killed by the Nazis. By the late 1960s, however, *the Holocaust* (capitalized and usually preceded with the word *the*) was defined in dictionaries as the genocidal killing of millions of Jews by the Nazis during World War II.

The lowercased term *holocaust,* however, still is used commonly to describe great loss of human life at the hands of others, as occurred in Biafra in the 1960s, Cambodia in the late 1970s, Afghanistan in the 1980s, and Rwanda and Serbia/Bosnia in the 1990s. Over 2,000 books in print include the word *holocaust* in their titles, many of which do not refer to World War II: *The Real Holocaust* depicts the African slave trade, *The Silent Holocaust* describes victims of famine, and two books titled *The Forgotten Holocaust* discuss South American Indians and the rape of Nanking; *Holocaust Island* is a book of poetry about Australia by an aboriginal poet.

Despite the widespread and diverse use of the term, controversy over its proper usage outside the Nazi context remains. The *American Heritage Book of English Usage* reports that 99 percent of its Usage Panel, composed of over 180 experts who determine the correct employment of terms, accept the term *nuclear holocaust.* However, only 60 percent accept its use for the 1 million to 2 million victims of the Khmer Rouge, only 31 percent for the millions of victims of drought in Africa, and a mere 11 percent in reference to the AIDS epidemic.

The use of the term *holocaust* in other contexts is confounded by the fact that the rhetorical power of the word largely has been taken over by its single exemplar; every use of the term, even in lowercase or in other contexts, inevitably becomes a referent. Another complication is that the penetration of the term into the American consciousness has been astonishing. Ninety-seven percent of the public in one poll knew what the Holocaust was, a higher percentage than could identify Pearl Harbor or knew that the United States had dropped an atomic bomb on Japan. The majority in a second poll said that the Holocaust "was the worst tragedy in history" (Novick, p. 232). The casual use of the term outside the Nazi experience can provoke the sensitivities and strong voice of the Jewish community, which was affected singularly by the Nazi campaign of eugenic eradication and for which the Holocaust remains a powerful and personalized event. Such factors complicate the term's use in contexts other than the Nazis' actions in World War II.

The Uniqueness of the Holocaust

The controversy surrounding the use of the Holocaust as a metaphor revolves in part on claims of the Holocaust's *uniqueness.* The targeting of one ethnic group said to be singularly evil; the use of medical and public health justification for the destruction of that group; the relentless and single-minded searching out and destruction of all men, women, and children in that group as an end in itself; the widespread collaboration of the public in each new country conquered; the dedication of enormous economic, military, and social resources to that end; and the systematic technological extermination of the group are said to set the Holocaust apart from all other cases of genocide in human history.

Lucy Dawidowicz (*Hastings Center Report*) has argued that the Nazi experience cannot be used to gain insight or help resolve the conflicts of other eras. If the Holocaust is *unique* and thus is a singular, exceptional, disjunctive moment in the course of human history, it lies outside the flow of normal events and cannot serve as a historical lesson. It therefore cannot be used to understand *normal* evil or even the periodic emergence of extraordinary evil. Conversely, if the Holocaust is just one, however singularly tragic, example of many historical examples of genocide or hatred, what is to keep its particularities intact when it is used constantly as the referent for the killing of the Armenians, African slaves, or embryos? The Nobel Prize winner Elie Wiesel, who is known for his advocacy of the uniqueness of the Holocaust, has tried to resolve the dilemma by arguing that the Holocaust was "a unique Jewish tragedy with universal implications" (quoted in Novick, p. 239). However, it is difficult to maintain that an event is both absolutely unique and universally applicable.

Arguments against the use of the Holocaust as an analogy to other cases of suffering take two major forms. One suggests that the Holocaust had a uniquely Jewish context and that to use the term as a referent cheapens and discounts the Jewish experience of suffering and loss. Edward Alexander in an article titled "Stealing the Holocaust" indicts those who use the Holocaust to call attention to other instances of injustice, arguing that they *use up* something accumulated by Jews through their suffering. A second argument suggests that use of the referent blunts the true horror and extremism of the event. Discussing the related use of the label *Nazi* in a Hastings Center Report Conference on bioethics and the Holocaust, Milton Himmelfarb lamented the "overly hasty invocation of 'Nazism' and the rather free and easy use of Nazism to brand practices with which we disagree.... By universalizing Nazism, one makes it shallow, and one removes the actual reality of Nazism. If everything is Nazi, then nothing is Nazi, and even Nazism wasn't Nazi" (*Hastings Center Report,* p. 7).

Insisting that the Holocaust lies outside history and has no role in creating an understanding of other cases of mass killing is also problematic. The argument for the incomparability of the Holocaust trivializes other crimes and can lead to discussions such as the reported argument about whether the Bosnian slaughter was "truly holocaustal or merely genocidal" (Novick, p. 14). Some analogies are clearly apt. The discussion of the *Rwandan holocaust* in a medical journal, indicating with the lowercase *h* that the term is used as a noun and not explicitly as a reference to the Jewish Holocaust, seems a proper usage (Decosas). The tragic events in Rwanda are well described as a holocaust.

The Holocaust in Bioethical Discourse

In bioethical contexts the Holocaust often is invoked as a form of moral approbation. The development of the Nuremberg Code in the wake of the Holocaust was the clear precursor to the emergence of modern protection measures for human subjects and therefore often is referenced legitimately (Caplan). However, the Holocaust-Nazi analogy also is invoked regularly to condemn a wide range of practices (e.g., abortion, physician-assisted suicide), healthcare strategies (e.g., managed care, age rationing), and even people (e.g., by opponents of the work of philosopher Peter Singer). Sometimes the analogies are so overblown as to be easily dismissed, for example, when the breast implant controversy was referred to at an Institute of Medicine meeting as the "silicone holocaust" (Ault). However, it is instructive to look at a number of cases in which the use of Holocaust metaphor or imagery is employed to make a bioethical argument in a professional or public forum.

ANIMAL RIGHTS. Animal rights activists have called fur farms *Buchenwalds for animals* and have likened animal experimentation to the human medical experiments of the

Nazi doctor Josef Mengele. A best-selling book in the animal rights movement called *Eternal Treblinka* (Patterson) argues that there are many parallels between animal exploitation and the Nazi exploitation of people and points out that the slaughterhouse was the model for the death camps. In 2003 People for the Ethical Treatment of Animals (PETA) mounted a graphic campaign and exhibit called *Holocaust on Your Plate,* which placed 60-square-foot panels displaying gruesome scenes from Nazi death camps side by side with disturbing photographs from factory farms and slaughterhouses. One exhibit shows a starving man in a concentration camp next to a starving cow. The campaign, which highlighted medical research using animals along with other forms of animal exploitation, used the slogan "To animals, all people are Nazis" (Specter). Jewish leaders, as well as many others, objected strongly to the exhibition.

AIDS. AIDS activists often use the slogan "silence equals death" to liken the purported indifference among bystanders in the face of the epidemic to the inaction of those who let the Holocaust occur. It also has become common for activists to refer to AIDS as the "Gay Holocaust" (Bamforth). At the 2000 AIDS summit in South Africa delegates accused drug companies of a "holocaust against the poor" for refusing to provide Africans with inexpensive AIDS drugs (Smith). Used in tandem with the slogan about silence, that phrase is an implicit rebuke of the claimed unwillingness of the drug companies and others to dedicate the resources and attention to its eradication that the activists believe AIDS deserves.

ABORTION AND EMBRYONIC STEM CELLS. In the abortion debate and more recently in the human embryonic stem cell (hES) debate both sides have made use of Holocaust metaphors to defend their positions. The pro-life and anti-hES movements commonly refer to the destruction of embryos as "the American Holocaust" and use symbols and images from the Holocaust as a primary metaphor in their literature (Neustadter). When he was surgeon general of the United States C. Everett Koop warned of a progression "from liberalized abortion … to active euthanasia … to the very beginnings of the political climate that led to Auschwitz, Dachau, and Belsen" (quoted in Novick, p. 241). At a Senate Labor and Health and Human Services Appropriations Subcommittee meeting in April 2003 Senator Sam Brownback of Kansas likened embryo research to Nazi research on Holocaust victims.

Conversely, the pro-choice side often argues that state control of women's bodies is the first step toward state ownership of people and ultimately toward genocide. The Holocaust thus is also used to argue against state involvement in reproductive freedom. Pro-choice advocates point out that abortion was illegal in Nazi Germany and that the state prominently expressed an interest in controlling women's reproduction through antimiscegenation and compulsory sterilization laws.

END-OF-LIFE ISSUES. Public discussions about end-of-life options, from disconnecting life supports to physician-assisted suicide, inevitably raise comparisons to the *euthanasia* campaign in World War II, especially in Germany (Kottow, Spannaus et al.). In a *Hastings Center Report* commentary, the *Village Voice* columnist Nat Hentoff compared Dan Callahan's argument in *Setting Limits* (in which Callahan argued that some categories of people, notably the elderly, should not be entitled to the same access to healthcare as others) to the Nazi policy of *lebensunwertes leben,* "life unworthy of life." Hentoff also stated that the Hastings Center's 1987 Guidelines on the Termination of Life-Sustaining Treatment and the Care of the Dying would have been welcomed by defense attorneys for Nazi doctors. Although the respondents, including Callahan, addressed some of Hentoff's arguments against Callahan's points, the responses focused predominantly on the appropriateness of the Nazi analogy. Ironically, the epithet also was hurled from the other side of the issue as Jack Kevorkian assailed doctors who were not willing to help patients die as Nazis (*New York Times*).

THE HOLOCAUST AS AN IMPEDIMENT TO PROGRESS. Some people argue that the focus on the Holocaust has become an impediment to medical progress. In a keynote speech to molecular biologists in Berlin in 2002 the Nobel laureate James D. Watson, the codiscoverer of the structure of DNA and the first director of the Human Genome Project, told his German audience that the time had come to "put Hitler behind us" and embrace the good that genetic science can do (Koenig).

Rhetorical Strategies

The uses of the Holocaust in bioethical argumentation tend to follow a number of rhetorical strategies. The Holocaust may be used comparatively to suggest that a targeted act or position is morally equivalent: "What is happening here is no different from (or no better than) what was done during the Holocaust." Others use the Holocaust as a referent for a slippery slope argument: "Actions like these, if they continue, will lead to a Holocaust." Some use the term to chastise their colleagues or adversaries: "Your actions are no different from those of the Nazis or those who stood silent in the face of the Nazis." Conversely, the Holocaust can be used to justify an action by arguing that a criticism is misplaced: "After all, this is not like the Holocaust."

Conclusion

The cautions enumerated above are not meant to suggest that there are not appropriate and thoughtful attempts to use the Holocaust in bioethical argumentation. The Holocaust stands as a signal moment in the human encounter with euthanasia, unconscionable medical experimentation, victimization of the marginalized and powerless, relentless bureaucracy, eugenic extremism, and other acts and philosophies that bioethics forgets at its peril. Clearly, the considered use of the Holocaust can illuminate and strengthen a moral position. For example, many antiabortion and anti–embryo research scholars have tried to use the Holocaust as a thoughtful and nonsensational analogy to explore issues of vulnerability and medical justification (Neuhaus).

Bioethics is most effective when it pursues reasoned moral discourse, and the use of hyperbole and rhetorical strategies that depend on shock and insult cheapens the enterprise as a whole. In such cases the Holocaust does not inform bioethical debate but instead erodes it. The lessons of the Holocaust have profound meaning for modern bioethics, and the atrocities committed must stand as a bellwether against moral recidivism. Invoking the Holocaust to score rhetorical points, however, fails as a rhetorical strategy and degrades the genuine lessons that the Holocaust offers to bioethical discourse.

PAUL ROOT WOLPE

SEE ALSO: *Bioterrorism; Eugenics: Historical Aspects; Genetic Discrimination; Harm; Homicide; Life Sustaining Treatment and Euthanasia: Historical Aspects of; Medical Codes and Oaths; Metaphor and Analogy; Minorities as Research Subjects; Moral Status; Race and Racism; Research, Unethical; Warfare: Medicine and War*

BIBLIOGRAPHY

Alexander, Edward. 1980. "Stealing the Holocaust." *Midstream* 26(9): 47–51.

The American Heritage Book of English Usage. 1996. Boston: Houghton Mifflin.

Ault, Alicia. 1998. "U.S. Institute of Medicine Panel Deliberates on Breast-Implant Safety." *Lancet* 352(9125): 380.

Bamforth, Iain. 2001. "Literature, Medicine, and the Culture Wars." *Lancet* 58: 1361–1364.

Caplan, Arthur., ed. 1992. *When Medicine Went Mad: Bioethics and the Holocaust.* Totowa, NJ: Humana Press.

Decosas, Josef. 1999. "Developing Health in Africa." *Lancet* 353: 143–44.

Hastings Center Report, Supplement. 1976. "The Nazi Experience: Origins and Aftermath." August, pp. 3–19.

Hentoff, Nat. 1988. "The Nazi Analogy in Bioethics." *Hastings Center Report,* August/September, pp. 29–30.

Hungerford, Amy. 2003. *The Holocaust of Texts.* Chicago: University of Chicago Press.

Koenig, Robert. 2002. "Watson Urges 'Put Hitler Behind Us.'" *Science* 276(5314): 892.

Kottow, M. H. 1988. "Euthanasia after the Holocaust—Is it Possible? A Report from the Federal Republic of Germany." *Bioethics* 2(1): 58–59.

Linn, Ruth, and Gur-Ze'ev, Ilan. 1996. "Holocaust as Metaphor: Arab and Israeli Use of the Same Symbol." *Metaphor and Symbolic Activity* 11(3): 195–206.

Mintz, A. 2001. *Popular Culture and the Shaping of Holocaust Memory in America.* Seattle: University of Washington Press.

Neuhaus, Richard John. 1990. "The Way They Were, the Way We Are: Bioethics and the Holocaust." *First Things* 1: 31–37.

Neustadter, Roger. 1990. "'Killing Babies': The Use of Image and Metaphor in the Right-to-Life Movement." *Michigan Sociological Review* 4: 76–83.

New York Times. 1991. "Doctor in Suicides Assails U.S. Ethics." November 3, p. 14.

Novick, P. 1999. *The Holocaust in American Life.* Boston: Houghton Mifflin.

Patterson, Charles. 2002. *Eternal Treblinka: Our Treatment of Animals and the Holocaust.* New York: Lantern Books.

Smith, A. D. 2000. "AIDS Summit: Drug Companies 'Inflicting Holocaust on the Poor.'" *The Independent* (London), July 10, p.11.

Spannaus, N. B.; Kronberg, M. H.; and Everett, L., eds. 1988. *How to Stop the Resurgence of Nazi Euthanasia Today.* Washington, D.C.: EIR News Services.

Specter, M. 2003 "The Extremist: The Woman behind the Most Successful Radical Group in America." *New Yorker,* April 14, p. 52.

Stein, A. 1998. "Whose Memories? Whose Victimhood? Contests for the Holocaust Frame in Recent Social Movement Discourse." *Sociological Perspectives* 41(3): 519–540.

Zelizer, Barbie., ed. 2001. *Visual Culture and the Holocaust.* New Brunswick, NJ: Rutgers University Press.

Zito, George. V. 1983. "Toward a Sociology of Heresy." *Sociological Analysis* 44: 123–130.

HOMICIDE

• • •

Homicide has been defined as "the killing of one human being by the act, procurement, or omission of another"

(Black, p. 867). However, federal homicide statistics reflect the police classification of homicide deaths as either murder or nonnegligent manslaughter, with deaths caused by negligence, suicide, or accident excluded. Some deaths that are not included in these federal statistics may ultimately be ruled homicides by a coroner or a court. Reported statistical data derive from various sources, including the FBI's Uniform Crime Reporting (UCR) Program and the FBI's Supplementary Homicide Report (SHR). Homicide figures reported from these databases are estimates, rather than exact numbers, because: (1) the classification is based on police investigation rather than coroner findings or judicial determinations; (2) many homicides are unsolved, resulting in the omission of data related to offender, and sometimes victim, characteristics; and (3) state agencies may fail to report details relating to homicides. These omissions in the available data may result in biased conclusions. For instance, the SHR does not include details related to approximately 8 percent of the homicides reported in the UCR, so conclusions from the SHR may be biased.

Despite these limitations, it is believed that homicide is the least underreported of any serious crime in the United States. Available data underscore the increasing frequency with which homicide occurs in U.S. society. As an example, the nation's murder rate in 1997 was 6.8 per 100,000 persons, compared to a rate of 4.6 per 100,000 in 1950.

Once considered to be an issue for law enforcement only, homicide is now recognized as a major public health problem (Novello, Shosky, and Froehlke). Because of disparities in the risk of homicide across subgroups, homicide must be considered as an issue of ethical, as well as public health, concern.

Epidemiology

Homicide data for the years 1976 to 1999 indicate that, compared to whites, blacks are six times more likely to be homicide victims and eight times more likely to commit homicide. Males represent nearly 75 percent of all homicide victims and almost 90 percent of all offenders. Compared to females, males are three times more likely to be killed and eight times more likely to commit homicide. Younger individuals are also at greater risk; almost one-third of victims and nearly one-half of offenders are under the age of twenty-five (Fox and Zawitz).

Homicide among intimate partners and family members remains a major concern, despite decreases in the rates of such events. In comparison with males, females are more likely to be killed by their intimate partners (defined as current or former spouses and current or former boyfriends and girlfriends, including those of the same sex). Women in the United States are at higher risk of homicide victimization than women in any other high-income society (Hemenway, Shinoda-Tagawa, and Miller). In 1998 the deaths of almost three-quarters of all women murdered were attributable to their intimate partners (Rennison and Welchans). For the period from 1993 through 1999, intimate partners killed 32 percent of all female murder victims ages twenty to twenty-four (Rennison, 2001). Analysis of homicide data for the years 1981 through 1998 indicate that the highest rates of intimate partner homicide during these years were among black and white females in the southern and western states (Paulozzi, Saltzman, Thompson, et al.), and most female victims were killed by an unarmed partner. Additionally, homicide is a major contributor to deaths occurring during pregnancy (Dannenberg, Carter, Lawson, et al.).

Women who kill their intimate partners often do so in response to repeated batterings. These beatings may result in the development of trauma symptoms, such as anxiety and psychic numbing, as well as lowered self-esteem and the development of self-destructive coping responses to the violence. The victimization may also lead to a total loss of the woman's social self. In general, a battered woman does not attack her abuser when harm is imminent but, instead, during a hiatus in the assaults. The incidence of female-perpetrated partner homicide appears to be lower in states that have strong domestic-violence legislation and greater access to supportive services such as shelters, crisis lines, and support groups (Dutton).

Disparities also exist in the disposition of cases involving intimate partner homicide. Of the 156 wives and 256 husbands convicted in 1988 in the United States for murdering their partners, wives received prison sentences that, on average, were twenty years shorter than those received by convicted husbands, even when comparing only those husbands and wives who were not provoked prior to the homicide (Langan and Dawson).

The United States has the highest rate of childhood homicide of any industrialized nation in the world (CDC). In fact, homicide represents the leading cause of infant deaths due to injury in the United States (Overpeck, Brenner, Trumble, et al.). An estimated 37,000 children were killed in the United States between 1976 and 1994, and one-fifth of these murders were committed by a family member (Greenfield). Of all children under the age of five who were murdered from 1976 to 1999, 61 percent were killed by parents or stepparents, and an additional 29 percent were killed by other relatives or by a male acquaintance. Most of the children killed were male and most of the offenders were male (Fox and Zawitz). Children under the age of eighteen accounted for nearly 11 percent of all murder victims in the United States in 1994, and nearly half of these children were between the ages of fifteen and seventeen. Among those killed in this age group, nearly 70 percent were killed with a handgun, while almost 20 percent were killed by another child. In addition, infants born to very young mothers have an increased risk of homicide (Overpeck, Brenner, Trumble, et al.).

The number of homicides involving adult or juvenile gang violence has increased fourfold since 1976 (Fox and Zawitz), and an increasing proportion of these homicides are now associated with firearm use. In Los Angeles County, for example, firearms were used in 94.5 percent of homicides in 1994, compared to 71.4 percent in 1979. Homicides committed with semiautomatic weapons also increased substantially during this period (Hutson, Anglin, and Kyriacou).

As of 2000, firearm use accounted for approximately 70 percent of all murders in the United States (Rennison, 2001). From 1973 to 1999, more than 80 percent of all workplace homicides were committed with a firearm (Duhart). The rate of homicides involving firearms has historically been higher in the southern states than in other regions (USDOJ, Homicide Trends). This regional variation has been attributed to both sociocultural factors and to the ease of access to firearms in the South.

Despite the increase in gun-related homicides, numerous state legislatures eased restrictions on the availability and use of firearms during the closing decades of the twentieth century, allowing citizens to carry concealed weapons even into churches and some government buildings. Public surveys indicate, however, that such increased gun-carrying actually reduces, rather than increases, public perceptions of safety (Hemenway, Azrael, and Miller).

The risk of homicide is also associated with the use of alcohol or illicit substances by the perpetrator and/or the victim immediately prior to the killing (Pernanen). Chronic alcohol use has been found to increase by up to tenfold an individual's risk of being a homicide victim (Rivara, Mueller, Somes, et al.). It is believed that the use of alcohol and illicit substances may adversely affect an individual's ability to process and interpret information correctly, thereby increasing the likelihood of miscommunication, which may lead to violence. Additionally, because alcohol use may impair an individual's judgment, intoxicated persons may be more likely to place themselves in situations that entail a high risk of violence. Chronic alcohol use may also indicate that an individual has an antisocial personality disorder, which is associated with increased rates of violence and victimization (Rivara, Mueller, Somes, et al.).

Prevention

Prevention efforts may focus on one or more of three levels. Primary prevention efforts attempt to prevent the onset of a condition—such as preventing violent behavior. These efforts often utilize a broad-based approach aimed at the general public, including messages urging the use of nonviolent means to resolve disputes and problems. Secondary prevention efforts target populations considered to be at high risk, such as individuals who have already committed some act of violence. Tertiary prevention is analogous to damage control after an event has already occurred, and most frequently consists of arrest and incarceration following the commission of a homicide.

Various primary prevention strategies have been utilized in an attempt to reduce the relatively high rates of homicide in the United States. Numerous jurisdictions have adopted *child access prevention laws,* which hold adults criminally liable for the unsafe storage of firearms in environments where children live or are present (Webster and Starnes). Such laws remain controversial, however, due to the ease with which children can obtain firearms outside of the household (Hardy). Pediatric-based counseling of parents to increase their safety-related behavior has also been recommended, but the effectiveness of this approach is questionable due to physicians' lack of time, their inability to accurately assess actual gun ownership among parents, and their perceived lack of credibility as a source of information (Hardy).

Homicide prevention efforts must also address the use of alcohol and other substances. Primary prevention efforts have included the imposition of increased excise taxes on alcohol, the use of anti-alcohol advertising and promotion, and the development of responsibility training programs for servers of alcohol (Rivara, Muller, Somes, et al.).

Secondary prevention efforts have included the counseling of individuals through court-ordered programs in an effort to intervene before violence becomes a pattern and before the violence escalates to the level of homicide. Healthcare providers are now more likely to ask female patients about domestic violence—in large part due to focused training of providers and recent accreditation requirements and legal mandates imposed on healthcare institutions. It is believed that the early identification of violence in the home, coupled with modifications in legal policy—such as the increased enforcement of laws prohibiting and punishing violence—will decrease the rate of intimate partner homicide. However, efforts also require that healthcare providers assess individuals' risk for becoming violent offenders before violence has begun, and to then refer those at high risk for appropriate intervention. Patient counseling by primary care providers to reduce excessive alcohol use and binge drinking may also help to reduce the rate of homicide by reducing the use of alcohol (Rivara, Muller, Somes, et al.).

Secondary prevention strategies also include the issuance of civil protection orders by courts. These orders prohibit individuals who have committed an act of intimate partner violence from further abusing their victims. In general, victims are more likely to seek such orders if they are financially independent from the perpetrator, if they are no longer living with him or her, and if they have seen family members or friends threatened or abused by the perpetrator (Wolf, Holt, Kernic, et al.).

TOM CHRISTOFFEL (1995)
REVISED BY SANA LOUE

SEEALSO: *Abortion; Abuse, Interpersonal; Bioterrorism; Death; Death Penalty; Embryo and Fetus; Harm; Infanticide; Insanity and Insanity Defense; Medicine, Profession of; Mistakes, Medical; Pain and Suffering; Race and Racism; Right to Die: Policy and Law; Sexism; Smoking; Warfare*

BIBLIOGRAPHY

Black, Henry Campbell. 1951. *Black's Law Dictionary,* 5th edition. St. Paul, MN: West Publishing.

Centers for Disease Control and Prevention (CDC). 1997. "Rates of Homicide, Suicide, and Firearm-Related Deaths among Children—26 Industrialized Countries." *Morbidity and Mortality Weekly Reports, CDC Surveillance Summaries* 46(5): 101–105.

Craddock, Amy; Collins, James J.; and Timrots, Anita. 1994. *Fact Sheet: Drug-Related Crime.* Washington, D.C.: United States Department of Justice, Office of Justice Programs, Bureau of Justice Statistics [NCJ–140286].

Dannenberg, Andrew L.; Carter, Debra M.; Lawson, Hershel W.; et al. 1995. "Homicide and Other Injuries as Causes of Maternal Deaths in New York City, 1987 through 1991." *American Journal of Obstetrics and Gynecology* 172(5): 1557–1564.

Duhart, Detis T. 2001. *Special Report: Violence in the Workplace, 1993–1999.* Washington, D.C.: United States Department of Justice, Office of Justice Programs, Bureau of Justice Statistics [NCJ–190076].

Dutton, Donald G. 1995. *The Domestic Assault of Women: Psychological and Criminal Justice Perspectives.* Vancouver: UBC Press.

Greenfield, Lawrence A. 1996. *Child Victimizers: Violent Offenders and Their Victims.* Washington, D.C.: United States Department of Justice, Office of Justice Programs, Bureau of Justice Statistics [NCJ–158625].

Gundersen, Linda. 2002. "Intimate Partner Violence: The Need for Primary Prevention in the Community." *Annals of Internal Medicine* 136: 637–640.

Hardy, Marjorie S. 2002. "Behavior-Oriented Approaches to Reducing Youth Gun Violence." *Future of Children* 12(Summer/Fall): 101–117.

Hemenway, David; Azrael, Deborah; and Miller, Matthew. 2001. "National Attitudes Concerning Gun Carrying in the United States." *Injury Prevention* 7: 282–285.

Hemenway, David; Shinoda-Tagawa, Tomoko; and Miller, Matthew. 2002. "Firearm Availability and Female Homicide Rates among 25 Populous High-Income Countries." *Journal of the American Medical Women's Association* 57: 100–104.

Hutson, H. Range; Anglin, Deirdre; Kyriacou, Demetrios N.; et al. 1995. "The Epidemic of Gang-Related Homicides in Los Angeles County from 1979 through 1994." *Journal of the American Medical Association* 274: 1031–1036.

Kalin, Jack R., and Brissie, Robert M. 2002. "A Case of Homicide by Injection with Lidocaine." *Journal of Forensic Sciences* 47: 1135–1138.

Langan, Patrick A., and Dawson, John M. 1995. *Spouse Murder Defendants in Large Urban Counties.* Washington, D.C.: United States Department of Justice, Office of Justice Programs, Bureau of Justice Statistics.

Novello, Antonia C.; Shosky, John; and Froehlke, Robert. 1992. "From the Surgeon General, U.S. Public Health Service: A Medical Response to Violence." *Journal of the American Medical Association* 267: 3007.

O'Connor, James F., and Lizotte, Alan. 1979. "The 'Southern Subculture of Violence' Thesis and Patterns of Gun Ownership." *Social Problems* 25: 420–429.

Overpeck, Mary D.; Brenner, Ruth A.; Trumble, Ann C.; et al. 1998. "Risk Factors for Infant Homicide in the United States." *New England Journal of Medicine* 339: 1211–1216.

Paulozzi, L. J.; Saltzman, L. E.; Thompson, E. P.; et al. 2001. "Surveillance for Homicide among Intimate Partners—United States—1981–1988." *Morbidity and Mortality Weekly Report, CDC Surveillance Summaries* 50: 1–15.

Perkins, Craig. 1997. *Special Report: Age Patterns of Victims of Serious Violent Crime.* Washington, D.C.: United States Department of Justice, Office of Justice Programs, Bureau of Justice Statistics [NCJ–162031].

Rennison, Callie Marie. 2001a. *Bureau of Justice Statistics National Crime Victimization Survey: Criminal Victimization 2000: Changes 1999–2000 with Trends 1993–2000.* Washington, D.C.: United States Department of Justice, Office of Justice Programs, Bureau of Justice Statistics.

Rennison, Callie Marie. 2001b. *Special Report: Intimate Partner Violence and Age of Victims, 1993–1999.* Washington, D.C.: United States Department of Justice, Office of Justice Programs, Bureau of Justice Statistics.

Rennison, Callie Marie, and Welchans, Sarah. 2002. *Special Report: Intimate Partner Violence.* Washington, D.C.: United States Department of Justice, Office of Justice Programs, Bureau of Justice Statistics.

Rivara, Frederick P.; Mueller, Beth A.; Somes, Grant; et al. 1997. "Alcohol and Illicit Drug Abuse and the Risk of Violent Death in the Home." *Journal of the American Medical Association* 278: 569–575.

Webster, Daniel W., and Starnes, Marc. 2000. "Re-examining the Association between Child Access Prevention Gun Laws and Unintentional Shooting Deaths of Children." *Pediatrics* 106: 1466–1469.

Wolf, Marsha E.; Holt, Victoria L.; Kernic, Mary A.; et al. 2000. "Who Gets Protection Orders for Intimate Partner Violence?" *American Journal of Preventive Medicine* 19: 286–291.

INTERNET RESOURCE

Fox, James A., and Zawitz, Marianne W. 2002. "Homicide Trends in the U.S." United States Department of Justice, Bureau of Justice Statistics. Available from <http://www.ojp.usdoj.gov/bjs/homicide>.

HOMOSEXUALITY

• • •

I. Clinical and Behavioral Aspects

II. Ethical Issues

III. Religious Perspectives

I. CLINICAL AND BEHAVIORAL ASPECTS

It is believed that 2 to 10 percent of the U.S. population is gay or lesbisan (Gadpaille). However, there is no consensus among clinicians and behavioral scientists about the definition of homosexuality (Mondimore) and there are multiple definitions of the terms *bisexual, gay,* and *lesbian* (Francoeur, Perper, and Scherzer). Researchers, for instance, often fail to distinguish between sexuality (I am gay/lesbian), sexual behavior (I have sex with men/women), and community participation (I am a member of a gay/lesbian community) (Rothblum). These three dimensions, although somewhat overlapping, are not synonymous. Additionally, individuals' self-identity may change over time and in different contexts (Rothblum), as may the meanings ascribed to these terms by society.

Historically, homosexuality has been defined by reference to a person's physical behavior. An individual's orientation was determined by his or her biological sex and by the sex of his or her sexual partners. This view focuses on behavior as determinate and assumes that (1) only two sexual orientations—homosexuality and heterosexuality—exist and (2) an individual acquires his or her sexual orientation when he or she has sex for the first time.

Additional perspectives, however, may be critical to an understanding of sexual orientation. The self-identification view posits that sexual orientation may be discordant with behavior. Accordingly, the fact that an individual self-identifies as a homosexual does not preclude the possibility of that person having sexual relations with an individual of the opposite sex. Similarly, self-identity as a heterosexual allows for the possibility of sexual intimacy with a person of the same sex. The dispositional view of sexual orientation also considers an individual's sexual desires and fantasies and the sexual behaviors in which he or she is disposed to engage in ideal circumstances.

Dimensionality of Sexual Orientation

In the past sexual orientation was understood somewhat simplistically. Sexual orientation was treated as a binary construct: An individual was either heterosexual or homosexual. However, that understanding failed to explain bisexuality. The bipolar view of sexual orientation utilized by Alfred Kinsey conceived of sexual orientation along a continuous scale, with exclusive homosexuality at one end and exclusive heterosexuality at the other. According to this view, bisexuals are individuals who (1) are strongly attracted to people of the same sex and to those of the opposite sex, (2) are moderately attracted to those of the same sex and to those of the opposite sex, or (3) are weakly attracted to those of the same sex and to those of the opposite sex. The bipolar conceptualization of sexual orientation has been criticized for being one-dimensional and characterized as being similar to seeing masculinity and femininity as the opposite ends of a scale.

Most recently clinicians and researchers have employed either a two-dimensional or a four-dimensional scale to determine sexual orientation. The two-dimensional view posits that one dimension represents the degree of an individual's attraction to individuals of the same sex whereas the second dimension represents the degree of that person's attraction to those of the opposite sex. The four-dimensional view, which considers the varying levels of complexity inherent in defining sexual orientation, focuses also on an individual's choice of a sexual object, that is, the sex and sexual orientation of the individual and of those to whom that individual is sexually attracted, such as gay men, gay women, and straight men.

Theories on the Cause of Homosexuality

Same-sex eroticism and sexual behavior often have been viewed as abnormal or maladaptive. For instance, Richard von Krafft-Ebing, a late nineteenth-century neurologist, concluded that homosexuality represents an aberration in sexual behavior that results from the effect of worldly stress on a neuropathic disposition; thus, it constitutes a pathological condition rather than an immoral, criminal act (Mondimore). Havelock Ellis, a late nineteenth-century physician with a strong interest in anthropology, viewed homosexuality, or *sexual inversion,* as an inborn trait that reflects a permanent deviation in sexual development.

In contrast to those views, Kinsey concluded from his research that homosexuality is the product of cultural and socialization processes and therefore should not be considered criminal or the basis for the social ostracism of individuals (cited in Pomeroy). John Money, a sexologist, ultimately determined that homosexuality is a normal variation of sexual expression that results from prenatal influences interacting with environmental influences at critical unspecified periods.

A number of biological models have been developed in an attempt to explain sexual orientation and, specifically, homosexuality. The permissive model asserts that biological factors shape the brain structure on which experiences inscribe sexual orientations, whereas genetic factors constrain the period during which that experience can affect an individual's sexual orientation. The direct model attributes the responsibility for sexual orientation directly to genes, hormones, and other biological factors and their direct influence on the brain structures that underlie sexual orientation. The indirect model posits that biological factors shape an individual's temperament and/or personality, which in turn shapes the development of sexual orientation; genes may predispose a person to homosexuality in certain environments.

Proponents of biological theories of homosexuality have claimed support for their view from various findings. First, precursors of the reproductive organ systems of both sexes are present in the both male and female embryos. Second, various conditions related to sexual differentiation are thought to support the role of biology in determining sexual orientation. For instance, androgen insensitivity syndrome results from an inherited defect in the receptor molecule for testosterone; in persons with this syndrome testosterone has no effect on any of the target tissues. Individuals with this condition appear to be women and most often are attracted to men. Individuals with congenital adrenal hyperplasia experience abnormally high levels of circulating testosterone during embryonic development. As a result, genetic females develop masculinized genitalia. The condition 5-alpha-reductase deficiency results in the absence in genetic males of the enzyme required to develop external genitalia. At puberty females with this condition may experience an enlargement of apparently female organs into a penis-size organ, the secretion of testosterone, and a deepening of the voice.

Experiential theories of homosexuality encompass four major perspectives. One view focuses on the nature of an individual's early sexual experience and posits that through the process of operant conditioning an early pleasurable experience with an individual of the same sex will result in same-sex attraction. This theory has provided the basis for the seduction and first-encounter theories of homosexuality, which assert that individuals are *recruited* into a *homosexual lifestyle.* Other experientialists focus on the importance of family dynamics, theorizing that male homosexuality results from the influences of a strong mother and a distant father. This theory has served as the basis for many of society's stereotypes about the development of homosexuality and the characteristics of homosexuals and their families. Childhood gender roles are also a focus: It is believed that gender-atypical children such as girls who are "tomboys" and boys who are "sissy boys" develop into homosexuals.

Unlike these first three perspectives, experience-based developmental theory recognizes the potential role of biology and posits that biological factors code for childhood personality types and temperaments, which then are molded into gender roles. Once children develop gender roles, those who are different are seen as exotic and other. Lesbians develop from girls who fit masculine gender roles, and heterosexual women develop from girls who fit feminine gender roles. This theory is similar in many respects to the indirect biological model of homosexuality.

These biological models have proved to be controversial for a number of reasons. First, replication studies are lacking. Second, the results have significant implications for society's response to individuals who self-identify or are labeled as homosexuals. Some individuals argue that if homosexuality results from biology and does not signify a *lifestyle choice,* homosexuals cannot be considered morally depraved or criminal and consequently should receive the same legal rights and social recognition as any other identified group. Others fear that the identification of a biological basis for homosexuality ultimately will lead to attempts to correct what is perceived of as a biological *mistake.*

Only relatively recently has psychiatry declassified homosexuality per se as a mental illness by eliminating it as a category of illness in the *Diagnostic and Statistical Manual,* which guides clinicians in the diagnosis of mental disorders. However, the concept of illness has been retained through the incorporation into that text of a category for "sexual disorder not otherwise specified," which applies to individuals who experience "persistent and marked distress about sexual orientation" (American Psychiatric Association, p.

582). This definition does not recognize that the distress may result not from a person's sexual orientation but from the societal response to that orientation. Despite these changes some professionals and laypersons continue to view homosexuality as the result of an abnormal process of development and as reflective of an underlying pathology (Socarides).

The Formation of Gay Identity

Research suggests that individuals develop their sexual identity in stages. However, the specific process by which people develop sexual identity is not well understood and is subject to great variation across individuals.

Troiden (1989), who has written extensively about the process of identity formation among homosexuals, has posited that identity formation proceeds through four phases: sensitization, identity confusion, identity assumption, and commitment. Troiden observed that children may first feel a sense of "differentness." For example, boys may feel less interested in sports than do their male peers. Often this sense of differentness is experienced at an early age. Troiden has labeled these years of sensitization to one's differentness as the "sensitization stage," which generally spans the ages of six through twelve. During these years, children do not think of themselves as sexually different and the term *homosexual* has little, if any, meaning for most of them. In addition to feelings of differentness, children may become sensitized to a set of labels and attitudes inflicted on them by their peers; those labels may include terms such as *faggot, dyke,* and *queer.* An antihomosexual bias may be absorbed by children from their parents and peers, resulting in an internalized homophobia that causes extreme psychic damage during adolescence and adulthood.

It is during adolescence, generally before the age of fifteen, that children may recognize an incongruity between their sexual feelings and those reported by their peers. This stage in the process of identity formation has been labeled *identity confusion* (Cass; Troiden, 1988). The confusion often results from the conflict between an awareness of their sexual feelings toward members of their own sex and the others' assumption that they are like everyone else. A child's confusion may exacerbated by fears that he or she is not *normal* but instead is *abnormal, perverted,* or *sinful.*

As a result the child may experience cognitive dissonance, a psychological state that results when one is confronted by contradictory facts that both appear to be true. This disorienting state often is accompanied by intense fear and anxiety. The conflict may be resolved through an acceptance of one's homosexuality or a complete refusal to acknowledge one's feelings, that is, denial. Adolescents who are in denial may isolate themselves from individuals of the opposite sex or, conversely, engage in a frenzy of heterosexual dating. Denial may be accompanied by alcohol and drug use in an attempt to create distractions from these uncomfortable feelings. Some individuals may experience *identity foreclosure,* in which they use their energy to deny, avoid, or redefine homosexual thoughts and feelings in an attempt to prevent their incorporation into their identity (Cass). It is believed that most homosexuals go through a period of cognitive dissonance.

Once individuals have self-labeled as homosexuals, that is, have reached the stage of *identity assumption or acceptance* (Troiden, 1989), they must decide how to incorporate that information into other aspects of their lives. This decision may be extremely difficult because of the potential for stigmatization and rejection by their families and friends and in the workplace. Individuals may become increasingly aware of the discrepancy between their positive attitudes toward homosexuality and society's disparaging views and discriminatory treatment. In an effort to cope with this stigmatization some individuals may seek to separate themselves completely from the heterosexual world, viewing everything that is gay as "good" and everything that is not gay as "bad." This approach constitutes one variation of identity foreclosure (Cass). Others may proceed to the *commitment* phase, in which they disclose their sexual orientation to others, experience same-sex intimacy, and become involved with the homosexual community (Troiden, 1988).

A number of factors have been found to be helpful to individuals as they struggle with their identity. They include the presence of a gay or lesbian family member who has disclosed his or her own sexual orientation, the presence of a gay or lesbian role model, the support and acknowledgment of heterosexual friends, the presence of gay-positive media messages, the increasing visibility of gay issues, and open discussions in the course of receiving confidential healthcare services (Perrin).

Medical and Social Attitudes toward Homosexuals

Medical professionals have participated in widespread discrimination against individuals who self-identify as gay or lesbian. A study of 278 nursing students found that 38 percent believed that lesbians try to seduce heterosexual women and provide a negative role model for children (11%) (Eliason, Donelan, and Randall). A survey of 100 nursing educators found that 24 percent believed that lesbian behavior is wrong, 23 percent believed that lesbianism is immoral, and 15 percent felt that lesbians are perverted (Randall). Heterosexist and homophobic attitudes also have been noted among social workers (Berkman and Zinberg) and physicians (Douglas, Kalman, and Kalman; Matthews et al.; Oriel et al.; Pauly and Goldstein). These attitudes have been found to affect the quality of the care provided (Schatz and O'Hanlan; Wise and Bowman) and may interfere with the ability of gay and lesbian parents to obtain pediatric care for their children (Perrin and Kulkin).

A number of professional organizations have attempted to dispel prejudice among their members. The American Academy of Pediatrics, for example, stated:

> Teenagers, their parents, and community organizations with which they interact may look to the pediatrician for clarification of the medical and social issues involved when the question or fact of adolescent homosexual practices arises.... The American Academy of Pediatrics recognizes the physician's responsibility to provide healthcare for homosexual adolescents and for those young people struggling with the problems of sexual expression. (pp. 249–250)

Various other changes reflect an increasing acceptance of homosexuals, including the adoption of antidiscrimination provisions by many state and local governments, the availability of healthcare and other benefits to partners of gay and lesbian employees, and the ability of gay and lesbian couples to adopt children (Cain). However, there also has been an escalation in the number of hate crimes reported. National attention most recently was focused on antigay sentiment as a result of the 1998 murder of Matthew Shepard in Wyoming (Loffreda).

Ethical Issues in Psychiatric and Psychological Care

Ethical issues arising in the context of psychiatric and psychological care provided to homosexual patients are similar, for the most part, to issues that arise in the context of providing care to individuals who are heterosexual. Ethical issues related to the "conversion" of homosexuals to heterosexuality arise only for those who continue to believe that homosexuality is abnormal or an illness. There is no evidence that therapy will result in long-term change in the sexual orientation of adults (Coleman). Although parents may place their children in therapy to ensure that they are or will become heterosexual, evidence indicates that such experiences may be psychologically injurious (Isay).

Nevertheless, some psychoanalysts believe that attempts to change an individual's sexual orientation are ethical as long as the individual wants that change (Nicolosi; Socarides).

Significantly, Gerald C. Davidson (pp. 97–98), one of the original pioneers of conversion therapy, ultimately concluded:

> Change of orientation therapy programs should be eliminated. Their availability only confirms professional and societal biases against homosexuality, despite seemingly progressive rhetoric about its normalcy. Forsaking the reorientation option will encourage therapists to examine the life problems of some homosexuals, rather than focusing on the so-called problem of homosexuality.
>
> It is critical that health professionals create an atmosphere in which their patient can openly discuss issues related to sexuality and sexual behavior. As with heterosexual patients, the focus should be on the patient's sexual behavior, not his or her sexual orientation. (quoted in Perrin)

Additional research is needed to address many unresolved issues. Physicians and therapists may be called on to offer their professional opinions in cases involving adoption by gay or lesbian parents. There is no evidence of mental health problems among children raised by lesbian mothers in the absence of a biological father. However, a related but relatively unexplored issue is the extent to which children may be especially vulnerable to societal stressors as a result of the societal bias against homosexuality.

Further research is needed to examine whether the sexual orientation of a clinician should be a factor in the selection of a healthcare provider, whether a provider should disclose his or her sexual orientation during the therapeutic process, and what effect the disclosure of the sexual orientation of a provider may have on the therapeutic process and its outcome.

ELI COLEMAN (1995)
REVISED BY SANA LOUE

SEE ALSO: *Lifestyles and Public Health; Mental Health, Meaning of Mental Health; Mental Illness: Conceptions of Mental Illness; Psychiatry, Abuses of; Sexual Behavior, Control of; Sexual Ethics; Sexual Identity; Sexuality, Legal Approaches to;* and other *Homosexuality* subentries

BIBLIOGRAPHY

American Academy of Pediatrics, Committee on Adolescence. 1983. "Homosexuality and Adolescence." *Pediatrics* 72: 249–250.

American Psychiatric Association. 2000. *Diagnostic and Statistical Manual of Mental Disorders,* 4th edition, text rev. [DSM–IV–TR].

Berkman, C. S., and Zinberg, G. 1997. "Homophobia and Heterosexism in Social Workers." *The Social Worker* 42(4): 319–332.

Cain, Patricia A. 2000. *Rainbow Rights: The Role of Lawyers and Courts in the Lesbian and Gay Civil Rights Movement.* Boulder, CO: Westview Press.

Cass, Vivian C. 1979. "Homosexual Identity Formation: A Theoretical Model." *Journal of Homosexuality* 4: 219–235.

Coleman, Eli. 1978. "Toward a New Model of Treatment of Homosexuality: A Review." *Journal of Homosexuality* 3: 345–359.

Davidson, Gerald C. 1982. "Politics, Ethics, and Therapy for Homosexuality." In *Homosexuality: Social, Psychological and Biological Issues,* ed. William Paul, James D. Weinrich, John C. Gonsiorek, and Mary Hotvedt. Beverly Hills, CA: Sage.

Douglas, Carolyn J.; Kalman, Concetta M.; and Kalman, Thomas P. 1985. "Homophobia among Physicians and Nurses: An Empirical Study." *Hospital and Community Psychiatry* 36: 1309–1311.

Eliason, Michele; Donelan, Carol; and Randall, Clara. 1992. "Lesbian Stereotypes." *Health Care for Women International* 13: 131–144.

Francoeur, Robert T.; Perper, Timothy; and Scherzer, Norman A. 1991. *Descriptive Dictionary and Atlas of Sexology.* New York: Greenwood Press.

Gadpaille, W. 1995. "Homosexuality and Homosexual Activity." In *Comprehensive Textbook of Psychiatry,* 6th edition, vol. 1, ed. Harold I. Kaplan and Benjamin J. Sadock. Baltimore: Williams & Witkins.

Isay, R. A. 1999. "Gender in Homosexual Boys: Some Developmental and Clinical Considerations" *Psychiatry* 62(2): 187–194.

Loffreda, Beth. 2000. *Losing Matt Shephard: Life and Politics in the Aftermath of Anti-Gay Murder.* New York: Oxford University Press.

Mathews, W. Christopher; Booth, Mary W.; Turner, John D.; et al. 1986. "Physicians' Attitudes towards Homosexuality—A Survey of a California Medical Society." *Western Journal of Medicine* 144: 106–110.

Mondimore, Francis Mark. 1996. *A Natural History of Homosexuality.* Baltimore: Johns Hopkins University Press.

Money, John. 1988. *Gay, Straight, and In-Between: The Sexology of Erotic Orientation.* New York: Oxford University Press.

Nicolosi, Joseph. 1993. *Healing Homosexuality: Case Stories of Reparative Therapy.* Northvale, NJ: Jason Aronson.

Oriel, Karen A.; Maldon-Kay, Diane J.; Govaker, David; et al. 1996. "Gay and Lesbian Physicians in Training: Family Practice Program Directors' Attitudes and Students' Perceptions of Bias." *Family Medicine* 28: 720–725.

Pauly, Ira B., and Goldstein, Steven. 1970. "Physicians' Attitudes in Treating Male Homosexuals." *Medical Aspects of Human Sexuality* 4: 26–45.

Perrin, Ellen C. 2002. *Sexual Orientation in Child and Adolescent Health Care.* New York: Kluwer Academic/Plenum.

Perrin, Ellen C., and Kulkin, Heidi. 1996. "Pediatric Care for Children Whose Parents Are Gay or Lesbian." *Pediatrics* 97: 629–635.

Pomeroy, Wardell. 1972. *Dr. Kinsey and the Institute for Sex Research.* New York: Harper & Row.

Randall, Carla E. 1989. "Lesbian Phobia among BSN Educators: A Survey." *Journal of Nursing Education* 28: 302–306.

Rothblum, Esther D. 1994. "'I Only Read about Myself on Bathroom Walls': The Need for Research on the Mental Health of Lesbians and Gay Men." *Journal of Consulting and Clinical Psychology* 62: 213–220.

Schatz, Benjamin, and O'Hanlan, Katherine A. 1994. *Anti-Gay Discrimination in Medicine: Results of a National Survey of Lesbian, Gay, and Bisexual Physicians.* San Francisco: American Association of Physicians for Human Rights.

Socarides, Charles W. 1988. *Preoedipal Origin and Psychoanalytic Therapy of Sexual Perversions.* Madison, CT: International University Press.

Troiden, Richard R. 1988. "Homosexual Identity Development." *Journal of Adolescent Health* 9: 105–113.

Troiden, Richard R. 1989. "The Formation of Homosexual Identities." *Journal of Homosexuality* 17: 43–73.

Wise, Amy J., and Bowman, Sarhon L. 1997. "Comparison of Beginning Counselors' Responses to Lesbian vs. Heterosexual Partner Abuse." *Violence and Victims* 12: 127–135.

II. ETHICAL ISSUES

The practice of medicine involves a body of knowledge, a body of practitioners, and the people who seek healthcare services. Homosexuality is of moral interest to medicine in all these areas. The term *homosexuality* was coined in 1869 by Karoly Maria Benkert to refer to same-sex eroticism, and it has prevailed over other proposed names, such as sodomy, contrary sexual feeling, inversion, and Uranism (Kennedy). To be sure, same-sex eroticism predates contemporary terminology and has a long—if contested—cultural history. The relationship between medicine and homosexuality has reflected both cultural prejudices as well as scientific advances.

History and Prevalence

In ancient Greek and Roman cultures, same-sex interactions were part of the cultural background, notwithstanding critics in those very societies. Educational relations among the Greek aristocracy took the form of mentoring relationships between older men and adolescent males, and schools for women sometimes followed this model (Marrou). It is not surprising that intimate mentoring relationships would sometimes become sexual. Roman civilization also had its share of same-sex eroticism, with some notorious emperors having harems of male lovers at their disposal (Gibbon). The

Emperor Hadrian was so distraught after the death of a beloved youth, Antinous, that he deified him, erected statues of him through the empire, and founded a city in his name (Birley).

In later times, the social and religious circumstances of medieval Europe worked to limit the visibility of homosexuality, but subcultures and literary and artistic expressions of same-sex love were far from unknown even in ecclesiastical communities (Boswell). Homosexuality has expressed itself elsewhere around the globe, as well, including Africa, China, and among Native American cultures.

In ways without precedent in human history, a same-sex culture has emerged in the large contemporary cities of the developed world and, it is a social force in communication, entertainment, business and commerce, and politics. Men and women who acknowledge their homosexuality hold prominent and influential social positions, as do men and women who choose not to disclose their homosexuality. The social visibility of homosexuality has not dispelled all moral and religious condemnation. In less developed parts of the world, homosexuality is sometimes far less visible but not altogether absent.

The extent of homosexuality in a given human society is difficult to estimate, for a number of reasons. Studies of sexual behavior face certain methodological problems, including adequate study samples and reluctance to discuss sex freely. Several ambitious studies have nevertheless tried to estimate the extent of homosexuality among men and women in the United States. In the mid–twentieth century, one Kinsey study of approximately 6,000 men showed that about 4 percent of them behaved exclusively as homosexuals after adolescence, and that 37 percent of men overall had some sexual experience with another man to the point of orgasm at some point during their lives (Kinsey). Another study showed that 1.32 to 2 percent of approximately 6,000 women behaved exclusively as homosexuals after adolescence, and that 13 percent of the women overall had had sexual experience with another woman to the point of orgasm at some point during their lives (Kinsey). At the end of the century, Laumann and colleagues also found that many people engage in homosexuality at some point. They found that 2.8 percent of their 1,749 male subjects and 1.4 percent of their females subjects claimed a homosexual identity (Laumann et al.).

Taken together, these studies show that many adolescents, and adult men and women, have same-sex fantasies and desires and engage in same-sex behavior. That said, there is often a fluidity to human sexuality that does not allow any easy division of humanity into homosexuals and heterosexuals, even if most people come to have entrenched sexual interests in males or females alone. This fluidity sometimes stands in the way of precise definitions of homosexuality, and of scientific accounts of why people behave a certain way.

Scientific Study

For most of human history, the origins of homosexuality did not elicit scientific interest. Neither was homosexuality treated as a pathological state. Instead, homosexuality was evaluated in moral and religious terms, and it was often condemned. In nineteenth-century Europe, however, many researchers and physicians began to study homosexuality in a systematic way and treat it as pathological. Describing homosexuality as a disease or disorder laid the foundations for discovering its causes and for developing treatments. For a variety of reasons, these researchers were often more interested in the origins and treatment of male homosexuality than female homosexuality. This emphasis may have resulted from greater social visibility of male homosexuality and a bias toward the selection of male subjects in medicine.

Many studies worked to show that homosexuality represented a kind of degenerate or defective human biology (Kraft-Ebing). Locating the origins of homosexuality in biology did not, however, always impose a pathological interpretation. For example, the German sex researcher Karl Heinrich Ulrichs (1825–1895) argued that homosexual men and women represented a *third sex,* and he offered an elaborate account of how the biological natures of men and women were blended in this sexual variation (Ulrichs). This view led Ulrichs to argue that homosexual men and women should not be punished by the law or mistreated by medicine for acting according to their biological natures (Hirschfeld).

Biology was only one field of study, of course, and not all theorists held that biology dictated the nature of one's sexual interests. Many psychologists looked to experiences in development for the factors that determined the nature and scope of homosexuality in men and women (Ellis). By contrast, the father of psychoanalysis, Sigmund Freud (1856–1939), drew no sharp distinctions between biology and psychology. He looked rather to an interplay of psychology and biology, believing that some people developed homosexually for psychological reasons, while biology played a more decisive role in the sexual development of others (Freud, 1953). In any case, Freud did not think that homosexuality was inherently pathological, though he did not think it represented full sexual maturity.

In the United States, organized psychiatry in the twentieth century first affirmed, and later repudiated, the view that homosexuality was pathological (Bayer). In 1952 the

American Psychiatric Association (APA) described its categories of disease for the first time, and it labeled homosexuality as a "sociopathic personality disorder" (APA, 1952). A 1968 revision of this classification described homosexuality as a "personality disorder," and in 1973 the APA formally abandoned the view that homosexuality was pathological. Yet another revision, in 1980, led the APA to identify homosexuality as an "ego-dystonic disorder," meaning that it could be treated as a disorder if an individual suffered from it. There is no specific mention of homosexuality in the most recent versions of the APA diagnostic nomenclature, but the APA does recognize "sexual orientation distress," which involves persistent and marked distress about sexual orientation (APA, 1994). However, sexual orientation distress would apply to all unwanted and distressing orientations, not just homosexuality. In 1981 the World Health Organization removed homosexuality from its list of diseases. Despite this sea change in the views of the medical profession generally, some physicians and psychologists still maintain that homosexuality is a serious disorder.

Even after the APA depathologized homosexuality, debates about the relationship of homosexuality to health, disease, and illness continued. Some commentators in bioethics tried to describe health and disease in *naturalist,* or objective, terms that transcended cultural and social variation. These commentators described disease in terms of impediments to the central species functions of survival and reproduction. Heart dysfunction, for example, poses a threat to individual survival no matter the culture in which it occurs. Other commentators were not persuaded that categories of disease and health could be identified apart from moral evaluations about the worth and merit of particular states. For these *normativist* commentators, human moral evaluations always played a role in determining how a given society defined its states of disease and health (Engelhardt). From either the naturalist or normativist perspectives, it is hard to make the case that homosexuality is necessarily pathological.

Arguing from a naturalist perspective, the philosopher Christopher Boorse has maintained that homosexuality can be treated as a disease because of its interference with reproduction—whatever else it is, homosexuality is sterile (Boorse). In fact, however, homosexuality does not rule out having children, and some cultures manage to accommodate the marriage and parenting of people whose sexuality is primarily homosexual.

It is also doubtful that homosexuality is always a threat to species survival. Sociobiologists have hypothesized that homosexuality might even confer survival advantages to groups, since homosexual men and women may play roles in a society that offset any reduced number of children they

might have (Ruse). As to their own survival, homosexual men and women may face individual health risks that others do not, but these risks may be tied to social circumstance rather than to homosexuality itself. For example, even if homosexual men face increased risks of disease and death, those risks are contingent, in the sense that successful treatments and vaccines could significantly dispel the danger.

As for normativist evaluations, it is clear that many men and women embrace their homosexuality without complication, and many cultures have also accommodated those people in one way or another. It is therefore hard to argue that—all other things being equal—homosexuality must lead to disorder and suffering. This is not to deny that some people and some cultures may disapprove of homosexuality, but the variance of response seems to show that it is not homosexuality per se, but how it is valued and treated that sometimes provokes its designation as disease.

For most of human history, medicine did not think of homosexuality in terms of disease. As both naturalist and normativist approaches show, what counts as disease—and what therefore deserves biomedical study and treatment—very much depends on one's theoretical starting points.

More recent commentary has challenged not the roles of health and disease in the study of homosexuality, but the very idea that homosexuality has root causes that science can discover. Indeed, the very fluidity of sexuality—both in individuals and in the sexual roles of various cultures—leads some commentators to maintain that sexual orientations are socially constructed. In this view, there are no homosexuals or heterosexuals in the sense that these are distinct kinds of people (Halperin). It would therefore be a mistake to look for genetic or hormonal causes of sexual orientation, just as it would be a mistake to study the biology of human beings in order to learn why some people are baseball fans and some people are not. Circumstance and society shape baseball fans, not human nature, and some commentators, known as *social constructionists,* hold the same view of sexual orientation.

In contrast, *essentialists* argue that human beings have sexual orientations by reason of their given nature, and that sexual orientation is likely rooted in biology. In other words, people are of *natural kinds* in regard to their sexual nature, and there are homosexuals and heterosexuals in the same way that there are elm trees and maple trees or people with blue eyes and people with brown eyes. From this perspective, sexual orientation amounts to an essential trait, and people express sexuality according to their natural kind (Stein). To essentialists, it is not a mistake to search out the root causes that distinguish people by sexual orientation.

The scientific study of fantasies, desires, and behaviors does not commit social-science researchers to either social constructionism or essentialism. It is possible to study many aspects of sexual psychology and behavior whether sexual orientation is rooted in nature or is simply a reflection of habits and patterns that people acquire in the course of their social development. However, the debate between constructionism and essentialism does have important implications for the causal study of sexual interests. It would be a mistake to look for the root biological causes of sexual interest where they do not exist. There is no well-validated account of how human beings come to have the entrenched sexual interests they have, though it is clear that genetics, anatomy, hormones, and psychological history all play a role. So it is not unscientific to ask why homosexuality comes to the fore in some people, why heterosexuality comes to the fore in others, and why others blend their sexual interests. There may well be genes or neurological features that dispose some people to the sexual interests they have. To be sure, there may be dubious motives behind some researchers' quest to understand the pathways of sexual development, but it is not unscientific to investigate the origins and determinants of sexual orientation.

The origins of sexuality—and homosexuality in particular—have attracted a good deal of scientific interest. Researchers across the life sciences have looked to see whether homosexual men and women have traits in body or mind that others do not have, and to learn whether those traits are causally connected to their sexual interests. Researchers have looked at body shape, the nervous system, hormones, genetics, and so on to discern the influences behind sexual orientation. They have also looked at psychological and behavioral differences, including the ability to whistle, the preference for certain colors, and relationships with family members (LeVay, 1996). There has been no shortage of studies along these lines, and contemporary researchers have continued to add to this domain of research.

In 1991 the neuroanatomist Simon LeVay published a report showing that some brain structures in homosexual men are statistically smaller than the same structures in heterosexual men. But because the size of these structures does not correspond exactly with sexual orientation, this study could not establish any definitive link between neuroanatomy and sexual interests. In 1993 the geneticist Dean Hamer and colleagues published a study showing that homosexual men are more likely than others to have male homosexual relatives, and the pattern of distribution of these male homosexual relatives suggests a genetic inheritance passed through mothers. The study also showed that male homosexual brothers are more likely to share a genetic region in common than nonhomosexual brothers, which also suggests there is a genetic contribution to sexual orientation. Again, however, because this shared genetic region does not

correspond exactly with sexual orientation, these patterns do not prove that there is a "gay gene."

Both the LeVay and Hamer studies are preliminary and suggestive, but they are not definitive. Some commentators have nevertheless interpreted these studies as showing that homosexuality is *natural,* in the sense that there is a describable biology behind it (LeVay, 1993). These commentators think scientific study will protect homosexuality from social condemnation by confirming it as part of human biological nature. Others fear that these studies will revive theories that homosexuality is pathological (Bersani).

Where there is scientific uncertainty, there will be speculation and disagreement. For this reason, many analysts turn to ethics rather than science as a guide to the meaning and significance of homosexuality. Ethical analysis of homosexuality has a far longer history than its scientific study, and it will continue to have a role as the findings of science unfold.

Ethical and Legal Evaluation

Ethical theories try to describe an overarching view of what is good for human beings and to describe ways of distinguishing among states, choices, and behaviors that contribute to—or at least do not detract from—that overarching good. Ethical theories vary in their interpretations of homosexuality.

PREMODERN ETHICAL THEORIES. In ancient Greece, there were disagreements among intellectuals about erotic interactions between males. According to his chroniclers, Socrates (470–399 B.C.E.) experienced attraction toward other males, but he saw it as a means to achieve spiritual wisdom rather than physical gratification. Plato's (427–347 B.C.E.) views modulated over his long lifetime—from prudential accommodation of the spiritual aspects of homosexuality to more or less outright condemnation of this sexuality as being contrary to nature (Dover). His sympathetic references to erotic attraction between adult and adolescent males do not undercut his more fully considered view. Aristotle (384–322 B.C.E.) had less to say about homosexuality, though he also disapproved, describing homosexuality, in his *Nicomachean Ethics,* as a pleasure of those with bad natures.

In Medieval Europe, it was Thomas Aquinas (1225–1274) who—from a Catholic background—offered the next major treatment of homosexuality, calling it the most sinful species of lust. He did so in the context of *natural law*—a law defined in terms of the goals said to be inherent in human life. In his *Summa Theologiae,* he describes homosexuality as a violation of animal nature and of the order of sexual acts generally. The historian John Boswell has criticized this view by arguing that bodies and body parts have multiple purposes, and that the use of human genitals is meaningful only in sexual acts capable of begetting children. It is also the case that that there are analogues to homosexuality in other animals (Bagemihl), though even if there were not, it is unclear why animal behavior should be taken as a guide for human beings capable of reasoned evaluations of their choices.

MODERN ETHICAL THEORIES. The German philosopher Immanuel Kant (1724–1804) had a number of things to say about homosexuality, though he found doing so distasteful. Kant defended the categorical imperative as the central guide to human action. There are various formulations of the categorical imperative. What they share in common is the counsel to abide by rules that one would wish to see function as universal law. To use a negative example of how this would apply, one should not like because one would not wish to live in a world where lying was the universal norm. To use a positive example, one should be charitable because one could possibly want charity from others in the future. Kant argued that homosexuality was wrong because it could not function as a universally accepted practice. Applied to everyone, the sterility of homosexuality would put an end to the birth of children. Kant also found same-sex erotic behavior especially degrading to the parties involved.

By way of response to the Kantian view, it should be noted that it is sometimes difficult to see how precisely, or how broadly or narrowly, a moral maxim should be drawn. For example, it might be possible to frame a maxim of behavior this way: if—and only if—people find themselves sexually attracted to their own sex, then they should act accordingly, but not otherwise. In this way, the future of the human race would be secure and people would not have to act contrary to their actual sexual interests. And, of course, some heterosexual acts are just as disrespectful of sexual partners as homosexual acts—selfish sexual gratification is not the province of one sexual orientation alone.

In striking contrast to Kant, the British utilitarian philosopher Jeremy Bentham (1748–1832) came to almost the opposite conclusion about the morality of homosexuality. In works that were not published in his lifetime, he defended homosexuality for those inclined to it, saying it gives them pleasure and leads to happiness. In keeping with his utilitarian view that actions should be judged in terms of their capacity to contribute to human happiness through pleasure, Bentham thought it undeniable that homosexuality was one way to human pleasure. For some people, therefore, the pursuit of same-sex relations would be a

positive good. Bentham was not especially worried that social accommodation of homosexuality might lead to more homosexuality, for if there is nothing wrong with homosexuality (for those interested in it), then increasing the amount of homosexuality in a society is not wrong either. He was convinced, too, that the forces of heterosexual lust were stronger than any threat to the birth rate that homosexuality might pose. In a strict sense, from this point of view, homosexual orientation and behavior are not of inherent moral interest.

Another utilitarian philosopher, John Stuart Mill (1806–1873), also believed that actions were moral to the extent that they promoted happiness. Given that adults are ordinarily the best judges of what makes them happy, Mill wanted to limit social interference with individual pursuits. He articulated his "liberty principle" in order to define a sphere of behavior that did not warrant social action. To Mill, social interference with the actions of others is justified only to prevent harm to others. Harm to one's own self is not a sufficient reason for interfering with an adult's beliefs and choices. With this conceptual background, it is possible to articulate a formidable boundary against social interference with homosexuality. Unless their behavior harms others—as in rape, for example—men and women should be able to pursue same-sex partners without social interference.

Alan H. Goldman, a commentator on sexual ethics, has argued that there are no moral rules specific to sexuality alone. He argues that the moral rules or precepts that apply across the range of human relations are the rules that should apply to sexuality as well. This means that the same rules that apply in heterosexual relationships should apply in others as well: if sexual fidelity is promised, it should be honored; there should be no deception or mistreatment; and so on. In one sense it is this very attempt to make social relations consistent across sexual orientations that has led to ambitious attempts to reform laws that criminalize homosexuality.

DEVELOPMENTS IN THE LAW. The ethical standards reflected in laws around the world are widely variable. In some nations, sex between males or between females is strictly forbidden and severely punished. In others, homosexuality is illegal as a matter of formal statutes but is not punished in practice. In other countries, homosexuality is not an object of legal interest in itself, only insofar as sexual relations may be involuntary or public. In 1957, in England, the Committee on Homosexual Offenses and Prostitution issued a report, commonly known as the *Wolfenden Report,* that recommended that the United Kingdom decriminalize consensual "sodomy" among adults. In coming to this conclusion, it drew heavily on notions of privacy and protection from social intrusion. In this regard, the report shared parallels with the Napoleonic Code, put in place in 1804. In that code there was no explicit mention of homosexuality, only of criminalization of involuntary and public sexual crimes, regardless of the sex of the parties involved. Lord Patrick Devlin argued against the conclusions of the *Wolfenden Report* by saying that society's moral revulsion toward homosexuality should count as a valid reason for legal restrictions. Devlin argued that a society requires shared moral values and political beliefs and that even acts that occur in private threaten the existence of society, and are not beyond the reach of social suppression. Nevertheless, Britain did decriminalize homosexuality among adults.

In 1986 the U.S. Supreme Court, in *Bowers v. Hardwick,* affirmed the right of states to enact laws prohibiting homosexuality among adults. In the case of *Romer v. Evans* (1996), however, the Court maintained that states could not deprive homosexual men and women of particular rights. As of this writing, the Court has heard a sodomy case which may undercut the conclusions of *Bowers v. Hardwick.*

In general, there is a trend in the United States to decriminalize homosexuality. In many other jurisdictions around the world, the legal battles have shifted away from the simple question of whether sexual relations between men and between women should be criminal or not. Newer legal battles have engaged such topics as protection from discrimination in employment, housing, and public accommodations, and many jurisdictions are debating broader civic rights for same-sex couples. For example, the Netherlands and Belgium have recognized same-sex marriage. In the United States, the state of Vermont recognizes a *civil union* that parallels marriage. Other issues advancing on the legal frontier for homosexual men and women are the right to custody of children and the right to serve openly in the military.

The Uses of Sexual-Orientation Science

Despite social and legal acceptance in many quarters, the place of homosexual men, women, and adolescents is not secure in all societies. Many societies, for example, lack basic protections for homosexual men and women. For this reason, some observers are wary of going forward with sexual-orientation research. Some observers believe that sexual-orientation science is not valuable (Suppe), while others believe it will be harmful to homosexual men and women (Bersani). Such research might be used to "treat" homosexuality in adults, or even to control the sexual orientation of children, sometimes through prenatal interventions. Each of these uses raises moral concerns.

SEXUAL-ORIENTATION THERAPY. As a matter of ethics, sexual-reorientation therapies should be guided by the standards of informed consent that guide clinical treatment in other areas. At the very least, patients should understand and freely consent to treatment, appreciate the risks and benefits of treatment, and be advised about alternatives to treatment. These conditions have not always been met in sexual orientation therapy, especially involuntary treatment imposed by family and the state. As a matter of science, a broad array of techniques has been used with men and women to redirect sexual orientation from homosexuality to heterosexuality. Techniques used toward this end have generally reflected prevailing treatment methods of the time. Drug and hormone treatment, behavioral therapy, surgery, and psychotherapies have all been deployed at one time or another (Murphy, 1992). While some of this therapy has gone forward with professional integrity, there has also been involuntary treatment, gruesome castrations in the Nazi camps, and chemical and electrical aversive therapies that can only be called abusive.

While there are some reports in the scientific literature that describe successful re-orientations (Spitzer), it is unclear that sexual orientation therapies consistently deliver what they promise, especially when applied to randomly selected groups of people. Reports of success in reorientation come most typically from psychoanalysts, behavior therapists, and religious programs. These reports have been criticized for problems related to method, sample size, the lack of long-term assessment, a focus on behavior change (instead of psychic change), and the lack of control groups.

For therapists and their patients who still maintain that homosexuality is pathological, research that led to truly effective therapy would be all to the good. Other therapists do not maintain that homosexuality is pathological, but still believe that some treatments are justified in the name of respecting wishes about unwanted traits (Schwartz and Masters). For these therapists, research into treatments is also highly desirable, but it would remain a matter of debate whether the extinguishing of unwanted traits is a legitimate objective for medicine. Some commentators have argued that sexual-orientation therapy is immoral because it contributes to social prejudice against gay men and lesbians. For these commentators, further investigation into causes and therapies for sexual orientation is objectionable. The psychologist Gerald C. Davison has held that the mere availability of such therapy encourages its use, thereby perpetuating oppressive views about homosexuality. In contrast, the philosopher Frederick Suppe has pointed out that such an argument is persuasive only if the therapy: (1) presupposes that homosexuality is inherently inferior to heterosexuality, and (2) is socially influential in perpetuating injustice. It is not always clear that therapy programs meet these two conditions. It can be said, however, that pursuit of sexual orientation therapy may be an artifact of social injustice rather than an injustice in itself. In other words, people might look to therapy as a remedy for mistreatment in society at large.

THERAPY WITH ADOLESCENTS. Sexual orientation therapy is not confined to adults. In the past, parents have turned to punishment, moral exhortation, religious counsel, reform school, and even electroshock therapy in order to bring their children to heterosexuality. Both ethics and the law converge in the view that the people with the strongest immediate interest in protecting children are their parents. For this reason, parents are ordinarily entrusted to make even profoundly life-affecting decisions about their children. However, if parents' choices interfere with their children's well-being, then those children are entitled to protection. For example, the state can intervene when parents endanger children, deprive them of essential food and medical treatment, interfere with their education, and so on. Should ethics and the law recognize the right of parents to choose the sexual orientation of their children? The answer is "it depends."

To the extent that children do not have an interest in one sexual orientation over another, it would seem that parents should be able to plot the course of their children's lives, provided their actions are not harmful. For example, if parents wanted to ensure that they have only heterosexual boys, they might encourage their young boys to act in ways that they think (rightly or wrongly) will ensure that sexual orientation. They could therefore encourage boys to play vigorous contact sports and socialize with other boys. Unless it is hectoring and abusive, this encouragement does not by itself interfere with the child's well-being.

However, as they mature, children develop some degree of moral right to protection from parents' choices, even if those choices are well-meaning. Both ethics and the law recognize, for example, the rights of maturing adolescents to enroll in clinical trials and to refuse life-sustaining treatment when they are profoundly ill. That is, maturing adolescents are entitled to act in ways that protect their interests, even if their parents profoundly disagree with the choices made. This model can be extended to sexual orientation therapy as well: if maturing adolescents are profoundly unhappy about their emerging sexual interests, they might well accede to their parents' wishes and seek therapy. If, however, adolescents are not unhappy about their emerging sexual identity,

it is unclear, as a matter of morality, why their parents' choice ought to prevail, especially if therapies or treatments carry risks that outweigh the possible gains of success.

PRENATAL INTERVENTIONS. Some commentators worry that research programs aimed at identifying the origins of homosexuality may lead to the elimination of homosexual progeny through prenatal interventions. They worry that markers for sexual orientation might be discovered that could predict a child's eventual sexual orientation. If this were possible, some parents might want to use various interventions to control the sexual interests of their children. This might be done—hypothetically speaking—through gamete selection, embryo biopsy, genetic manipulations, fetal treatments, or even abortion. This discussion is speculative, but it does illuminate key moral issues in parents' choices about their children.

In the United States, women are entitled, as a matter of ethics and law, to the prenatal information that bears on their choice whether to have children or not, as well as information related to fetal well being. They are also entitled to make abortion decisions for reasons of their own. The question under debate is whether this general approach is appropriate for choices about the sexual orientation of children. On one level, it would be idiosyncratic to forbid the use of prenatal diagnostics or even abortion when there are no legal barriers to doing so in regard to other traits of children (LeVay, 1996; Murphy, 1999). Some commentators worry, however, that the use of prenatal interventions could jeopardize the status and well-being of homosexual men and women in general (Stein). If used widely, these interventions could reduce the total number of homosexual men and women in the world, making group self-protection more difficult. By the same token, legal interference with parents' choices about the use of prenatal diagnostics could lead to circumstances in which homosexual children are born into families that do not want them. Parents could also use these techniques as a way of having homosexual children, and some parents no doubt would choose this option.

These considerations weigh against a moral conclusion that society should forbid prenatal interventions in the name of protecting homosexual men and women in general. In order to reach that conclusion it would have to be shown that sexual minorities could only be protected by such intrusive measures, and that these measures are ultimately more important than allowing parents to have children according to their own best judgments. It is to be remembered that this discussion is hypothetical, and there are no known means for ensuring the sexual orientation of a child.

Beyond Diagnosis and Treatment

Since the 1800s, the debate about the pathology of homosexuality has occupied center stage in the relationship between homosexuality and medicine. That focus notwithstanding, the vast majority of homosexual men and women never wanted, sought, or received therapy for their sexual orientation. Each one of these men and women has, however, other healthcare needs. At the very least, males who have sex with males and females who have sex with females have specific risks to their health, and this is especially true for homosexual youth who seem to be at increased risk of suicide (Gibson). Against this background, it is important to ask whether health professionals have the knowledge and communication skills necessary to meet the health needs of this group. Certainly some health professionals and academic commentators have paid attention to the healthcare needs of homosexual people (Solarz). However, medicine's own history in regard to homosexuality can stand in the way of appropriate degrees of study and effective healthcare.

No matter what their sexual interests, patients already face a problematic relationship with healthcare: medicine is distant from them by reason of its complex and intricate knowledge, cultural expectations about the role of the physician, and professional commitments within medicine (Engelhardt, p. 291). People with same-sex interests are perhaps at a further disadvantage because they cannot uniformly expect to encounter healthcare practitioners who are conversant with the specific health risks of homosexual men and women and who are comfortable with the nature of their sexual lives.

Indeed, some practitioners may believe that health risks associated with homosexuality are *deserved* and therefore require less social attention than other problems. In the 1980s, for example, some commentators argued that the AIDS epidemic was a divine punishment for immoral homosexuality. This view is hard to credit for a variety of reasons. In the first place, the view is suspect because the "punishment" is applied inconsistently. Some men who have sex with other men have developed AIDS, but most others—across history and even in the present—have not. Further, why should homosexuality receive this sort of punishment while other moral transgressions go unpunished? How is the punishment proportionate in its effect, and why should consensual behavior be punished so severely?

Rather than tie AIDS to divine punishment, some commentators pointed to social injustice as a root cause of the epidemic. These commentators argue that the sexual behavior of many homosexual men is affected by social prejudice. In other words, some men take sexual risks as *adverse preferences,* something they would not do if they had the same array of options in relationships and social status as others. Because they do not, they make poorer choices. According to these commentators, society has an obligation to make amends to those whose disease can be traced back to social inequality (Mohr).

Are there social factors that stand in the way of the health of homosexual men, women, and adolescents? One factor might be obstacles to the formation of long-term relationships and families that are especially important when it comes to healthcare and caregiving. Some homosexual people have no access to health insurance through their partner's employment, as married partners have, and others have no presumptive right of inheritance or decision making at the bedside of a partner who cannot direct his or her medical choices. The law does allow homosexual men and women to make health decisions for their partners who lose the ability to do so, but this recognition ordinarily requires advance directives such as a power-of-attorney for healthcare. When such arrangements are not put in place, some partners are excluded from decision making. Some healthcare services are not available to homosexual people. Some commentators think infertility clinics should not offer services to people in same-sex relationships, and some clinics do exactly that (Ford). For reasons like these, it is certainly worth asking whether deficits in the health and well-being of homosexual men and women are rooted in social injustice, with injustice minimally defined as the social failure to treat like cases alike.

Patients are not the only people in healthcare relationships, of course, and it is important to note that many gay and lesbian health professionals—physicians, nurses, and others—believe that certain social attitudes work against their full acceptance in the medical community. For example, some residency directors do not wish to have homosexuals in their graduate training programs. These hurdles may not have the same force everywhere and for everyone, but they nevertheless work against the equal standing of gay, lesbian, and bisexual healthcare practitioners (Potter).

The debate about the ethics of homosexuality has extended into discussions about cloned human beings. Some commentators have argued broadly that no one—single people, coupled partners, or married people—ought to use cloning to have children (President's Council on Bioethics). Others open the door to the use of cloning by some infertile couples and would allow same-sex female couples to use cloning technologies if they become safe and effective, since these couples have fewer options available to them. Still other commentators have argued that if cloning technology is safe and effective, there is no obvious reason why all same-sex couples should not have access to it. In cloning, as in other aspects of social and moral life, unwritten ethical rules and social opinion often guide the application of biomedical technologies and the distribution of healthcare benefits. When it comes to homosexuality and healthcare, it is often these unwritten rules of social opinion that are decisive and most in need of analysis.

TIMOTHY F. MURPHY

SEE ALSO: *AIDS; Autonomy; Behavior Modification Therapies; Epidemics; Freedom and Coercion; Human Nature; Natural Law; Human Rights; Law and Morality; Lifestyles and Public Health; Narrative; Public Health; Sexual Ethics;* and other *Homosexuality* subentries

BIBLIOGRAPHY

American Psychiatric Association. 1994. *Diagnostic and Statistical Manual of Mental Disorders,* 4th edition (*DSM-IV*). Washington, D.C.: American Psychiatric Association.

Bagemihl, Bruce. 1999. *Biological Exuberance: Animal Homosexuality and Natural Diversity.* New York: St. Martin's.

Bayer, Ronald. 1987. *Homosexuality and American Psychiatry: The Politics of Diagnosis.* Princeton, NJ: Princeton University Press.

Bentham, Jeremy. 1978 (1785). "Offences against One's Self: Paederasty." *Journal of Homosexuality* 3: 389–405; 4: 91–107.

Bersani, Leo. 1995. *Homos.* Cambridge, MA: Harvard University Press.

Birley, Anthony R. 1997. *Hadrian: The Restless Emperor.* New York: Routledge.

Boorse, Christopher. 1975. "On the Distinction between Diseases and Illness." *Philosophy and Public Affairs* (5): 49–68.

Boswell, John. 1980. *Christianity, Homosexuality, and Social Tolerance.* Chicago: University of Chicago Press.

Bowers v. Hardwick. 478 U.S. 186 (1986).

Committee on Homosexual Offenses and Prostitution. 1963 (1957). *The Wolfenden Report.* New York: Stein and Day.

Davison, Gerald C. 1976. "Homosexuality: The Ethical Challenge." *Journal of Clinical and Consulting Psychology* 44(2): 686–696.

Devlin, Patrick. 1965. *The Enforcement of Morals.* Oxford: Oxford University Press.

Dover, Kenneth J. 1989. *Greek Homosexuality.* Cambridge, MA: Harvard University Press.

Ellis, Havelock. 1936. "Sexual Inversion." In *Studies in the Psychology of Sex,* vol. 2. New York: Random House.

Engelhardt, H. Tristam, Jr. 1996. *The Foundations of Bioethics,* 2nd edition. New York: Oxford University Press.

Ford, Norman. 2002. "Access to Infertility Clinics for Single Women and Lesbians." *Chisholm Health Ethics Bulletin* (6): 1–3.

Freud, Sigmund. 1953. "The Psychogenesis of a Case of Homosexuality in a Woman." In *The Standard Edition of the Complete Psychological Works of Sigmund Freud,* vol. 18, ed. and tr. James Strachey. London: Hogarth Press.

Freud, Sigmund. 1953. "Three Essays on Sexuality." In *The Standard Edition of the Complete Psychological Works of Sigmund Freud,* vol. 7, ed. and tr. James Strachey. London: Hogarth Press.

Gibbon, Edward. 1983 (1776). *The Decline and Fall of the Roman Empire.* vol. 1. London: The Folio Society.

Gibson, P. 1989. *Gay Male and Lesbian Youth Suicide: Report of the Secretary's Task Force on Youth Suicide.* Washington, D.C.: U.S. Department of Health and Human Services.

Goldman, Alan H. 1976–1977. "Plain Sex." *Philosophy and Public Affairs.* (9): 267–287.

Halperin, David. 1990. *One Hundred Years of Homosexuality and Other Essays on Greek Love.* New York: Routledge.

Hamer, Dean H.; Hu, Stella; Magnuson, Victoria; et al. 1993. "A Linkage between DNA Markers on the X Chromosome and Male Sexual Orientation." *Science* (261): 321–327.

Hirschfeld, Magnus. 2000. *The Homosexuality of Men and Women,* tr. M. A. Lombardi-Nash. Buffalo, NY: Prometheus.

Kennedy, Hubert. 1997. "Karl Heinrich Ulrichs, First Theorist of Homosexuality." In *Science and Homosexualities,* ed. Vernon A. Rosario. New York: Routledge.

Kinsey, Alfred C.; Pomerory, Wardell B.; and Martin, Clyde E. 1948. *Sexual Behavior in the Human Male.* Philadelphia: Saunders.

Kinsey, Alfred C.; Pomeroy, Wardell B.; Martin, Clyde E.; et al. 1953. *Sexual Behavior in the Human Female.* Philadelphia: Saunders.

Laumann, Edward O.; Gagnon, John H.; Michael, Robert T.; et al. 1994. *The Social Organization of Sexuality: Sexual Practices in the United States.* Chicago: University of Chicago Press.

LeVay, Simon. 1991. "A Difference in Hypothalamic Structure between Heterosexual and Homosexual Men." *Science* 253: 1034–1037.

LeVay, Simon. 1996. *Queer Science: The Use and Abuse of Research into Homosexuality.* Cambridge. MA: MIT Press.

Marrou, Henri I. 1997. *History of Education in Antiquity.* Madison: University of Wisconsin Press.

Mill, John Stuart. 1978 (1859). *On Liberty,* ed. Elizabeth Rapoport. Indianapolis, IN: Hackett.

Mohr, Richard. 1988. *Gays/Justice: A Study in Ethics, Society, and Law.* New York: Columbia University Press.

Murphy, Timothy F. 1992. "Redirecting Sexual Orientation: Techniques and Justifications." *Journal of Sex Research* 29: 501–523.

Murphy, Timothy F. 1998. *Gay Science: The Ethics of Sexual Orientation Research* New York: Columbia University Press.

Murphy, Timothy F. 1998. "Our Children, Our Selves: The Meaning of Cloning for Gay People." In *Flesh of My Flesh: The*

Ethics of Cloning Humans, ed. Gregory E. Pence. Lanham, MD: Rowman & Littlefield.

Murphy, Timothy F. 1999. "Abortion and the Ethics of Genetic Sexual Orientation Research." *Cambridge Quarterly of Healthcare Ethics* 4: 340–345.

Potter, Jennifer E. 2002. "Do Ask, Do Tell." *Annals of Internal Medicine* 137: 341–343.

President's Council on Bioethics. 2002. *Human Cloning and Human Dignity: An Ethical Inquiry.* Washington, D.C.: Author.

Romer v. Evans. 116 S.Ct. 1620 (1996).

Ruse, Michael. 1988. *Homosexuality: A Philosophical Inquiry.* New York: Basil Blackwell.

Solarz, Andrea L., ed. 1999. *Lesbian Health: Current Assessment and Directions for the Future.* Washington, D.C.: National Academy Press.

Spitzer, Robert L. "Psychiatry and Homosexuality." *Wall Street Journal,* May 23, 2001.

Stein, Edward. 1999. *Mismeasure of Desire: The Science, Theory, and Ethics of Sexual Orientation.* New York: Oxford University Press.

Suppe, Frederick. 1994. "Explaining Homosexuality: Philosophical Issues, and Who Cares Anyway?" In *Gay Ethics: Controversies in Outing, Civil Rights, and Sexual Science,* pp. 223–268. Binghamton, NY: Haworth Press.

Ulrichs, Karl Heinrich. 1994. *The Riddle of "Man-Manly" Love: The Pioneering Work on Male Homosexuality,* tr. Michael A. Lombardi-Nash. Buffalo: Prometheus.

III. RELIGIOUS PERSPECTIVES

Homosexuality is one of the most contentious issues of contemporary times, though important scholarship has indicated that it was not always so. This article will trace Western religious perspectives on homosexuality in Judaism, Roman Catholicism, and Protestantism from Greco-Roman times to the twenty-first century, as well as summarize homosexuality's position in Islam.

Pre-Christian Greece and Rome

In the Greco-Roman ancient world, same-sex relationships were parts of the warp and woof of civilization, though there is no evidence that the word *homosexuality* existed in either Greek or Latin. However, same-sex unions paralleling heterosexual marriage appear to have existed from ancient times through the Middle Ages (Boswell, 1994). Both Jonathan Ned Katz and John Boswell argue that *homosexuality* is a nineteenth-century invention. Anne Zachary reports that "the term, 'homosexuality,' was first coined as recently as 1869 by Benkert."

Scholars have long known that in ancient Greece, adult male citizens engaged in pederasty (sex between men and boys), a practice that was a thoroughly acceptable part of Greek social and cultural anthropology. It was common for adult male citizens (not slaves) to initiate young boys into the rituals of manhood, which included sexual partnering. This same practice was not followed in ancient Rome, though same-sex relationships did exist there.

In the Mediterranean world, social stratification was commonplace and included rigid demarcations between free men and slaves, as well as between adult males and adult free women. Bernadette Brooten has argued that attitudes toward same-sex relationships between women in the ancient world ought to be viewed within the context of attitudes towards women in general (1996). Since gender stratification undergirded the Mediterranean worldview, the ancients commonly regarded women as inferior to males, and they held derivative positions by virtue of their relationships to their husbands and fathers. Such a realization is important in understanding the place of same-sex relations within the Greco-Roman context.

In Greek and Roman anthropology, human nature was bifurcated—either active or passive. Under this view, males were thought to possess an active nature and women a passive nature. In terms of sexuality, the ancients recognized a fluidity that extended to any sexual expression of the male nature. Sexual expression would have taken place between "one active and one passive partner, regardless of gender...." (Brooten, 1996, p. 2). Some scholars point to social condemnation of the penetrated male because he was thought to violate the male *nature* by assuming a role fitted for women. The male penetrator did not appear to be similarly reviled, since he was acting in accord with man's *active nature.*

Within the context of this worldview, sex between two women simply had no place in the social and gender hierarchy of the ancient world. However, the ancients may have been less condemnatory of the partner who was penetrated as she was at least behaving according to nature (*kata physin,* in Greek). Both Roman and Greek sources indicate a knowledge of female homoeroticism: *frictrix/fricatrix* and *tribas/tribades* in Latin, for women who "rubbed" other women, as well as the Greek words, *tribas* and *Lesbia.* Although ancient authors were certainly aware of female homoerotic relationships, it remains unclear whether this was regarded as a matter of particular concern since it was out of the bounds of gender hierarchy on which the ancient world was based.

Was there an anti-homosexual attitude in ancient Greece and Rome? The question is itself reflective of a twenty-first-century bias. It has been established that the term was unknown to the ancients, and scholars such as Brooten (1996) argue that what the ancients condemned was the transgression of rigid gender hierarchies (the active/passive distinction), rather than *homosexuality*. Boswell (1994) argues that same-sex relationships were not condemned, though he did not apply a gender analysis to his research. R. T. France, an Evangelical scholar, holds that "Homosexual partnerships, whether pederastic or between adults, are accepted without comment, and described with appreciation, across a wide range of Greek literature" (France, p. 248).

Some scholars argue that a bias against same-sex relations did exist, though most write chiefly of male-male relations. Ward, for example, argues that such a bias can be found in Plato (*The Timaeus*, and *Laws*), as well as in Philo, a first-century C.E. Hellenistic Jewish philosopher, and in the *Sentences of Pseudo-Phocylides*, contemporary with Philo (Ward). The bias articulated in these sources, according to Roy Bowen Ward, is one of anti-hedonism and pro-procreationism. In this view, homoeroticism in the Greco-Roman world was seen to be *para physin* (against nature) because it is hedonistic behavior that cannot lead to procreation.

Biblical Issues

By far the most contentious terrain in the battle over homosexuality and religion is that of the Bible; this is particularly so for Christians. Genesis 19: 1–11 and Judges 19: 22–30 each contain a reference to a similar story in which God punishes ancient Israel for its behavior. Exactly what *kind* of behavior is the hermeneutical issue for biblical scholars. Theological conservatives tend to interpret Genesis 19 and Judges 19 as stories of God's condemnation for attempted homosexual rape, while more liberal exegetes have taken the position that the violations condemned are violations against the ancient code of hospitality so central in the Biblical world. Feminist biblical scholars have pointed to the misogyny of Judges 19 as an interpretive key.

There are only two places in the Hebrew Scriptures (Old Testament) that contain explicit prohibitions against what is referred to as homosexuality, though the word itself is never mentioned in the Bible. Both are contained in the book of Leviticus, mentioned in the context of the codes of ritual purity by which Israel is to set itself apart from other people. The New Revised Standard Version (NRSV) of the Bible translates as follows: Leviticus 18:22, "You shall not lie with a male as with a woman; it is an abomination"; Leviticus 20: 13, "If a man lies with a male as with a woman, both of them have committed an abomination; they shall be put to death; their blood is upon them."

Scholars debate both the meaning of word choices (what does it mean to "lie with a male as with a woman"? what does *abomination* mean?), and of historical/cultural context. Not surprisingly, Evangelical and conservative Christian exegetes tend to interpret the passages to mean that God condemns acts of same-sex eroticism between men; a few Biblical literalists use Leviticus 20:13 to argue for the death penalty for homosexuals today (see <www.godhatesfags. com>). If the writer of Leviticus does intend to signal God's condemnation of homosexual sex between men, what is the basis for the condemnation? Conservative exegetes argue that the *abomination* (*toevah* in Hebrew) in question is quite simply *sodomy,* or anal intercourse between two men; hence the meaning of to "lie with a male as with a woman." Lynne C. Broughton claims that *toevah* signifies something inherently wrong and contradictory to nature.

More liberal Christian exegetes make two kinds of hermeneutical claims. The first view is that the ritual codes of ancient Israel were written for a particular context and that few of these commands are observed today (Borg). Indeed, few Christians observe other prohibitions found in Leviticus, such as having sex with a menstruating woman (18:19), eating certain foods (19:26), cutting beards (19:27), wearing clothes made from two kinds of fabrics (19:19), or tattooing (19:28). Marcus J. Borg maintains that Christians who set aside these laws must assume the burden of proof for following any one of them, including the proscription on *homosexuality*. Others who view the New Testament as superceding the Old Testament might claim that the New Testament already invalidates much of the Levitical ritual concerns, rendering them less authoritative for Christians.

A second view, characteristic of William L. Countryman and Brooten, holds that the concerns of Leviticus 18–20 are not those of ritual and morality, but rather, as Brooten puts it, "holiness, impurity, defilement, shame and abomination" (1996, p. 288). On this view, the Levitical codes exist to secure the holiness of the people of Israel, a people bound to God. It is important to recognize the centrality of group welfare in ancient Israel—the writer's concern is not for securing individual purity, but the purity and survival of the whole people. This runs counter to the modern sense of individual liberties and rights. When seen from the perspective of group purity, many of the pieces of the Levitical codes that contemporary readers find objectionable (execution for adulterers, execution for perpetrators and victims of pederasty, and so on) can be understood as relevant to group survival and holiness: the offending violation and the violators must be cleansed from the midst of the community.

Similarly, Daniel Helminiak holds that the Levitical proscriptions are not against male homogenital relations (women are never mentioned), but must be seen within the context of ritual purity; the taboo (a translation of *toevah*) that concerns Leviticus is one of uncleanliness or defilement in a religious sense, but not in an ethical or moral sense. The chief concern of the writer is the purity of the people of Israel over and against the Gentiles; all of the purity violations in the holiness codes are cited as *abominations* or *taboo*.

Scholars generally agree that Paul relies on Leviticus in his proscriptions against same-sex expression, particularly in Romans 1:26–27, though also in I Corinthians 6:9 and again in I Timothy 1:10. The latter texts concern lists of behaviors to be avoided by Christians (lying, adultery, idolatry, and so on), and included among the lists we find the Greek word, *arsenokoitai,* which is generally translated as "men lying with men." While this word has been translated "homosexual," it has been variously translated "sodomites" or "male prostitutes," "homosexual perversion," and even as "abusers of themselves with mankind" (Borg, p. 4; Helminiak). Boswell (1980) argues that *arsenokoitai* refers to male prostitution and not homosexuality generally. *Arsenokoitai* also appears in the Septuagint Greek translation of Leviticus 18:22, 20:13. Some scholars hold that it refers to the specific practice of pederasty in ancient Greece and that it is this practice, along with male prostitution, that is condemned by Paul, and not homosexuality per se (Scroggs; Borg, 1994; Ackerman). Others disagree with this interpretation (e.g., Furnish; Wright).

First Corinthians 6:9 also contains the word *malakoi*, which refers to soft or weak persons, though Brooten translates this term as "men who assume a passive sexual role with other men" (1996, p. 260). This translation undergirds her argument that what was reviled by the ancients, including Paul, was the violation of the active/passive distinction on which society was based. Countryman and Boswell (1980) argue that *malakoi* does not refer to homosexuality at all.

Romans 1:26–27 is cited by most Protestant religious denominations, as well as the Roman Catholic Church, as the cornerstone of a variety of positions opposed to homosexual sexual expression. It merits citing here: "For this reason God gave them up to degrading passions. Their women exchanged natural intercourse for unnatural, and in the same way also the men, giving up natural intercourse with women, were consumed with passion for one another. Men committed shameless acts with men and received in their own persons the due penalty for their error" (NSRV). Scholarly debate generally turns on the context of the passage: what is it that Paul is concerned to communicate to his audience? and what is meant by the terms *natural (kata physin)* and *unnatural (para physin)*?

Does *para physin* mean contrary to nature in keeping with the Stoic insight on the right and natural order of things (Hays, contra Boswell), or does it mean, as Boswell suggests, beyond nature, meaning extraordinary or peculiar, but not unnatural (1980)? Boswell's claim is that the term was in some sense morally neutral for Paul, since he used it with respect to salvation of the Gentiles as well as to sex between men. Picking up from Boswell, Helminiak suggests that Paul meant *surprising* behavior, which is to say, "When people acted as was expected … they were acting 'naturally.' When people did something … out of character, they were acting 'unnaturally'" (Helminiak, p. 64). Thus "exchanging natural intercourse for unnatural" would have indicated sex that was surprising and out-of-the-ordinary, but not inherently wrong or disordered in the Stoic sense of "the laws of nature."

Stoic philosophy did make use of the term *para physin* and the Stoic philosophy of the *natural law* was pervasive in the Roman Empire. Robin Scroggs, however, maintains that *para physin* was "a commonplace Greco-Roman attack on pederasty" (p. 115), while Ward sees in it echoes of the emphasis on the importance of procreation typical of the Hellenistic Jewish community (and Stoic thought) of which Paul was a part. In terms of the procreation concern, Helminiak believes it would have been inconsistent for Paul to have made a priority out of this issue since, as we know, the early Christian community expected the imminent return of Jesus; thus marriage and procreation were not their chief concerns.

Among the more persuasive arguments is Brooten's (1996), that *para physin* did mean *contrary to nature,* but that what is referred to as *kata physin* (according to nature) is the non-biological active/passive distinction: any sex act had to have an active and a passive partner. Accordingly, sex between two women would certainly be thought of as shameful, unnatural and impure because *natural* sex meant penetration, characterizing the active dimension of the male. "Impurity applied to gender thus means that people are not maintaining clear gender polarity and complementarity" (Brooten, 1996, p. 235).

Similarly, for a man to have intercourse with a man, instead of a woman, would be a violation of the social order in which the *male nature* was believed to be active and penetrating. Boswell, on the other hand, argues that to exchange natural for unnatural intercourse refers to heterosexuals engaging in homosexual sex, since Paul presumes that such persons are capable of *natural intercourse.* He further maintains that Paul is making a distinction between homosexual persons and homosexual acts, and is really concerned only with the latter (Boswell, 1980). Richard B.

Hays disputes Boswell on this point, arguing that for Paul homoerotic expression does constitute a willful upending of the sexual differences that God intended for creation. Brooten adds that neither scholar takes a gendered analysis of Paul's position and his cultural assumptions into account, and that "Gender ambiguity is also the best framework within which to view Paul's understanding of unnatural relations in Romans I" (Brooten, 1996, p. 252).

Homosexuality and Judaism

Rabbinic Judaism, emphasizing the *halakhic* or legal side of the Talmud, has been largely opposed to same-sex sexual expression between males. Such expression between women is not addressed in the Torah, although it was later condemned by the rabbis (e.g., *Sifra* 98 and *Mishneh Torah Issurei Biah* 21:8). Perhaps silence on same-sex eroticism between women in the biblical period of ancient Judaism reflects the patriarchal nature of culture; one cannot really be certain. However, it is clear that male homoeroticism was condemned as an "abomination" (*toevah*) in Leviticus 18:22 and punishable by death in Leviticus 20:13. The reasons for the condemnation have been debated both in the Talmud and by scholars up to the present.

In contemporary Judaism, Saul Olyan, for example, argues that what the Torah actually prohibits in Leviticus is male anal intercourse and not other instances of male-male coupling (see also Boyarin). For contemporary explanations on the differing treatment of male and female homoeroticism in Jewish law, see the work of Rebecca Alpert and Rachel Biale. One of the debates in contemporary Judaism has been whether or not *halakhah* is open to change on homosexuality in light of new realities, or whether its character is fixed. In one sense, within *halakhic* Judaism it is apparent that homoerotic acts (though not necessarily inclinations) between men are to be regarded as an abomination, and as an aberration from the commonly held norm of heterosexual acts that ensure procreation and the promotion of family life, primary values in Judaism. David M. Feldman, for instance, does not agree that the proscription in Leviticus has anything to do with procreation. He summarizes three possible reasons for the prohibition according to his reading of rabbinic sources: that male homosexuality cannot result in procreation; that such sexual activity will result in men leaving their wives and families; that it constitutes "going astray" (*toeh attah bah,* play on *toevah*) from the Creator's design for creation (Feldman, p. 428).

Following the rabbis, Feldman regards homosexual acts as sinful, but makes the distinction that "If the aberration is the result of 'sickness,' no guilt can attach to it; if it is

advocated as an 'alternative lifestyle,' this then is consciously immoral and soberly sinful"; thus volition plays a key part in the condemnation (Feldman, p. 426). Under this view, *halakhah* and homosexuality are regarded as incompatible, and it is interesting to note that the rabbis apparently regarded male homosexuality and Judaism as an unlikely combination—that Jews could not really *be homosexual.* There is much discussion, from Talmud to Maimonides, on *yihud,* "being alone together." Generally, proscriptions against *yihud* reflect concerns with heterosexual adultery so that the Talmud actually allows two men to be alone together and even to sleep under the same blanket. This might reflect the relative lack of attention paid to homosexuality as a reality in ancient Judaism, in contrast to the gentile communities in Greece and Rome.

Robert Kirschner, opposing Feldman and David J. Bleich, argues that *halakhah* is capable of change on this matter, as it has been on many others (e.g., the debate over *heresh* deaf mute), since the power of interpretation is a cornerstone of rabbinic tradition. Kirschner makes a case for Judaism taking into consideration scientific evidence about sexuality, including theories on the etiology of homosexuality. Contemporary science confirms, for example, what the rabbis did not think to be the case—that sexuality and its expression is variable, fluid and not dichotomous; therefore, homosexuality can be seen "not as a perversion but, rather, in its multiple manifestations, a state of sexual being" (Kirschner, p. 457).

Currently, the four branches of Judaism in the United States (Orthodox, Conservative, Reform, and Reconstructionist) take a variety of positions on homosexuality. Orthodox Judaism is largely settled on these questions and it accepts the Levitical condemnation on male same-sex acts as an abomination. Some more liberal Orthodox Jews maintain a distinction between the act and the person (the sin and the sinner), regarding the homosexual Jew as sinning, but a Jew nonetheless. In recent years, support networks of Orthodox homosexual Jews have emerged, despite the fact that Orthodoxy does not recognize homosexuality as an orientation or state of being. Examples of these networks include: Gay and Lesbian Yeshiva Day School Alumni Association (GLYDSA), Orthogays, and Orthodykes, all of which have a presence on the Internet. In 1999, Rabbi Steven Greenberg became the first Orthodox rabbi to *come out* as a homosexual Jew, a subject of great controversy in Orthodox Judaism (see Grossman). In 2000, the Rabbinical Council of America condemned the position taken by the Reform rabbis to affirm same-sex relationships in Jewish ritual. In 1999, the Council publicly opposed the state of Vermont's ruling legalizing same-sex civil unions, on the grounds that marriage is only between heterosexuals.

In 1991, the Conservative Movement in Judaism (both the Rabbinical Assembly and the United Synagogue of Conservative Judaism) passed a resolution affirming its *halakhic* commitment to heterosexual relationships, while simultaneously opposing civil restrictions on and expressions of hatred against gays and lesbians. The movement officially welcomes gay and lesbian persons at synagogue and encourages education among Jews about homosexuality. Since 1992, the official policy of the Conservative movement's Committee on Jewish Law and Standards has been to prohibit the ordination of gay and lesbian rabbis, as well as to prohibit same-sex marriages or commitment ceremonies. That policy was under discussion at the beginning of the twenty-first century, and is opposed by some rabbis within the movement. Conservative rabbis are permitted to serve gay and lesbian congregations, but they are *halakhicly* prohibited from officiating at commitment ceremonies. For a helpful and balanced overview on homosexuality in Judaism, see *Matters of Life and Death,* by Conservative rabbi Elliot Dorff (1998). The Rabbinical Assembly of Conservative Judaism published an official rabbinical letter on human intimacy in which it stated, with reference to the Levitical codes, that some acts of sexual expression are abominations (cultic, oppressive, or promiscuous sex, whether by homosexuals or heterosexuals), but that monogamous, loving sex is sacred and should be sanctified, whether heterosexual or homosexual (see Dorff, 1996).

For the Reform Movement and for Reconstructionist Judaism, homosexuality is almost a non-issue, in that the Union of American Hebrew Congregations (UAHC) voted in 1973 to accept full membership of a synagogue that had a specific outreach to homosexual Jews. In the 1980s the official seminary of Reform Judaism, Hebrew Union College, voted to accept gay or lesbian rabbinical students; the Reconstructionist Rabbinical College preceded Hebrew Union in doing so. In 1993, UAHC adopted a resolution calling for full legal equality for gay and lesbian monogamous partnerships. In 1997, the UAHC reaffirmed its commitment to welcoming gays and lesbians into full participation in all aspects of Jewish life, and officially resolved (1) to support efforts towards civil gay and lesbian marriages; (2) to urge Reform congregations to honor monogamous gay and lesbian partnerships; (3) to support the Central Conference of American Rabbis (CCAR) in its study of the possibility of religious commitment ceremonies for gay and lesbian unions between Jews. In March 2000, the CCAR became the first major congregation of American clergy to give its clergy permission to perform gay and lesbian commitment ceremonies. Although the UAHC and the CCAR have been very supportive of gay rights issues, there is no official position on the adoption of children by homosexuals.

Homosexuality and Roman Catholicism

Since Roman Catholicism and Christianity were synonymous until the Reformation, Christian attitudes towards homosexuality were, *de facto,* Roman Catholic attitudes, although popular attitudes were not necessarily synonymous with official Catholic teaching, as is true today. Boswell (1994) contends that evidence from liturgical texts and cultural history indicates that Christians once accepted same-sex relationships. Moreover, he argues that a distinctive contribution of early Christianity was an emphasis on the celibate life as spiritually superior to the heterosexual married state; eroticism thus became suspect and marriage was seen as a distraction from the important preparation of the Second Coming, and at best a compromise with the material world. These attitudes held sway in the church for the first thousand years of its existence (Boswell, 1994). Mary Rose d'Angelo shows how pairs of women missionaries in the New Testament can be seen as evidence of commitment both to the mission and to each other. Boswell, too, discusses the influence of "paired saints," such as Perpetua and Felicity, Serge and Bacchus, and even Jesus and John, on ordinary Christians.

Christian thinkers from late antiquity to the high Middle Ages have had an influence on official Catholic teaching on homosexuality. Among these are Augustine of Hippo, John Chrysostom, Clement of Alexandria and Thomas Aquinas. St. Augustine (354–430) contributed heavily to the Catholic view that marriage was for procreation, monogamy, and fidelity, or as Augustine put it, *fides, proles, sacramentum* (Boswell, 1994; Augustine, 2000). So influential was this view that traces of it are found in papal documents up through the twentieth century. Augustine was influenced by his membership in the Manichean movement that viewed the natural world as an inherent evil. Hence one finds in Augustine an insistence on sex within marriage exclusively for the purpose of procreation—husbands were encouraged to make use of prostitutes if they had a need for non-procreative sex (Augustine, 2000). Boswell (1980) maintains that Augustine's view of *nature* is to be understood in the sense of *out of the ordinary,* not the *normal* use of something. Thus Augustine condemned same-sex eroticism since it was certainly not the *normal* use of sex with which he was familiar. *Contra naturum* meant that which did not conform to *ordo,* or order of the world, the divine plan (see Augustine's "De ordine.") In this view, conformity was the issue for Augustine, not *nature* itself. Part of the order of things, as Brooten tells us, is the maintenance of gender boundaries. Augustine was one of the Christian thinkers who, perhaps reflecting the culture around him, insisted on the male nature as superior to the female.

Clement of Alexandria (150–c. 215) argues against homosexuality in the *Paedagogus,* an instruction manual for Christian parents. Clement did espouse the procreation argument for moral intercourse, but his rationale against same-sex eroticism was grounded primarily in the Epistle of Barnabas's view that such acts were *animalistic.* (The comparison to animals figured prominently in theological treatises up through Thomas Aquinas.) This popular first century Epistle (now part of the Catholic Apocrypha) equated the eating of certain animals in Leviticus (notably the hare, the hyena, and the weasel) with sexual sins. Though regarded as erroneous, the Epistle's influence is evident in Clement's writing, which itself was influential in the early church. Clement is one of the few sources who explicitly opposed *woman-woman marriage,* believing it to be unnatural in that it flaunts God's plan for woman as the receptacle of male seed. Drawing on both Plato and St. Paul, Clement held that same-sex relations were *para physin.*

John Chrysostom or John of Antioch (347–407) was another of the early Christian thinkers who was influenced by the Manichees, as well as by the Stoics, a combination of belief systems that "led him into the paradoxical position of condemning sexual pleasure … while at the same time denouncing homosexual acts for not providing pleasure: 'Sins against nature … are more difficult and less rewarding, so much so that they cannot even claim to provide pleasure, since real pleasure is only in accordance with nature.'" (Boswell, 1980, p. 156). Chrysostom, also a product of Mediterranean misogynistic culture, was repulsed by the idea of a male taking on the role of a woman and this transgression was part of his opposition to same-sex eroticism. Both Boswell and Brooten agree on this. Brooten notes that Chrysostom began to use the language of disease with respect to same-sex eroticism, adding this to the language of sin in early Christianity and ancient Judaism (1996).

Thomas Aquinas (c. 1225–1274), the influential Dominican scholar, argued that same-sex acts were to be regarded as sinful because they thwarted the *natural law,* as ordained by God. The thirteenth century is the period in which civil laws against homosexuals arose; anti-homosexual rhetoric became vitriolic and remained so through the twentieth century. In this light, Boswell (1980) regarded Aquinas as reflecting the popular attitudes of his time rather than responding to the substance of church tradition on this issue. It is important to recall that Aristotle, the Stoics, and *natural law* discussions of the first centuries of Christian history heavily influenced Aquinas. His articulation of what constitutes *nature* and *natural law,* particularly in his *Summa theologiae,* has been given decisive weight in Roman Catholic moral theology up through the present day. Aquinas devotes much of the *Summa* to considerations of *natural law*; one succinct definition is as follows: "It is clear that natural law is nothing other than the participation of rational creatures in eternal law" (Aquinas, 1952, Ia.2ae.91.2). Aquinas held that reason is that which distinguishes what is natural to humans from what is natural to animals. Therefore, one might expect Aquinas to argue that homosexual acts are contrary to reason, and in this sense unnatural. But this was not the rationale that he employed.

In the *Summa* there are three places of commentary on same-sex eroticism (Ia.2ae.31.7; Ia.2ae.94.3 ad 2; 2a.2ae.154.11–12), though "only the last has received scholarly attention in the context of Scholastic attitudes towards homosexuality" (Boswell, 1980, p. 323). In 2a.2ae.154.11–12, Aquinas discusses "vices against nature," which for him included heterosexual intercourse without intent to procreate, intercourse with animals, homosexual intercourse, and masturbation. These constitute the most sinful forms of lust, though Aquinas does not here discuss what order of nature is violated by these sins; he does hold that all sins are unnatural because they are "against the order of reason, which must order all things according to their ends" (Aquinas, 1952, 2a.2ae.153.2 Resp.). Why then is homoeroticism particularly unnatural? One might expect Aquinas to ground his opposition in the "spilling of seed" argument that had been popular (nature intended semen to find its end in procreation of children), and indeed he did consider this rationale (Aquinas, 1923). But he disposed of the argument after considering that nature fitted other body parts for uses to which they were not always put and therefore, misusing a part of the body could not be the sin; the sin was rather to impede the propagation of the species, which itself is a good. If homosexual sex precludes procreation, he the might have applied the same argument to celibacy and to virginity, but he did not.

However, Aquinas considered that there were some things that might seem against human nature generally, though peculiar to certain individuals and, therefore, *natural* to those individuals as everything in nature was believed to be ordered by God to some good end. One might have a *defect* of nature, but that defect of nature could be quite *natural;* indeed this was the way in which Aquinas regarded females (as "defective" males) (see Aquinas, 1952, Ia.92.I). As he writes, "In fact, because of the diverse conditions of humans, it happens that some acts are virtuous to some people, as appropriate and suitable to them, while the same acts are immoral for others, as appropriate to them" (Aquinas, 1952, Ia.2ae.94 ad 3). And in a footnote to history, Boswell writes, "It would seem that Saint Thomas would have been constrained to admit that homosexual acts were 'appropriate' to those whom he considered 'naturally' homosexual"

(1980, p. 327). Perhaps reflecting the attitudes of his day, Aquinas did not do so, as he also did not show why homosexual acts were immoral theologically, apart from being unnatural—neither is this point considered in official Catholic teaching on homosexuality.

The Roman Catholic Church has issued five key statements that are meant to instruct the faithful as to its official teaching on homosexuality:

1. in December 1975, homosexuality is considered within the document, "Declaration on Certain Problems of Sexual Ethics" ;
2. in October 1986, the Vatican issued "The Pastoral Care of Homosexual Persons";
3. in July 1992, "Responding to Legislative Proposals on Discrimination Against Homosexuals" was issued;
4. in 1995 the Catechism of the Catholic Church was revised, containing three sections on homosexuality (paragraphs 2357, 2358, 2359);
5. in 1997, the United States Catholic Bishops issued a pastoral letter on homosexuality, "Always Our Children."

With remarkable consistency, the church has always held that homosexual acts are *disordered* and against nature. Thus the church has never sanctioned such acts, though its documents on the matter do indicate a shift from a complete condemnation in the documents from 1975 and 1986 (Congregation for the Doctrine of the Faith, 1982; Congregation for the Doctrine of the Faith, 1986) to a more recent distinction between the act and the actor, or the sin and the sinner in the documents from 1995 and 1997. For an alternative claim by a contemporary Catholic moral theologian, see Margaret Farley, "An Ethic for Same-Sex Relationships."

If the church is now making a distinction between homosexual acts, which it condemns as against the natural law, and homosexual persons, who deserve compassion, it does so because it believes that homosexuality is not chosen (Roman Catholic Church). Earlier, the church had distinguished between curable and incurable homosexuals, yet it counseled the faithful to instill hope "in them of one day overcoming their difficulties and their alienation from society" (Congregation for the Doctrine of the Faith, 1982, para. 8). It would seem that Pope John Paul II is aware of the scientific data about the origins of homosexuality and that his position in the Catechism accounts for some openness to science and social science. In rather non-judgmental language, the *Catechism* observes: "Homosexuality refers to relations between men or between women who experience an exclusive or predominant sexual attraction toward persons of the same sex. It has taken a great variety of forms throughout the centuries and in different cultures. Its psychological genesis remains largely unexplained" (Roman Catholic Church, p. 2357).

All of this notwithstanding, the Roman Catholic Church does not condone homosexuality and recommends celibacy as the only acceptable form of sexual expression for homosexuals. Accordingly, it does not approve of civil unions, such as the state of Vermont's; nor does it condone homosexual marriages or unions in its churches, nor adoption of children by gay and lesbian persons. It should be noted, however, that there is a substantive gay-affirming movement within the Roman Catholic tradition known as Dignity. During the 1970s, 1980s and into the mid-1990s, a Catholic priest, Robert Nugent, and a Catholic nun, Jeanine Gramick, ran New Ways Ministry, a ministry to gay and lesbian Catholics. In 2000, they were ordered by the Vatican to cease teaching publicly or face expulsion from their respective orders.

Homosexuality and Protestantism

Most of the major Protestant denominations in the United States have positions on homosexuality. Since Martin Luther's movement back to the authority of the Bible defined Protestantism, interpretations of scripture tend to play the major role in shaping Protestant denominations. Protestantism in the United States exists on a kind of continuum with conservative Protestant denominations on one end (Southern Baptist Convention, Assemblies of God, independent Evangelical churches), liberal Protestant churches on the other end (Episcopal Church, American Baptist Church, United Church of Christ), and moderate Protestant churches in the middle (Presbyterian Church U. S. A., United Methodist Church, the Evangelical Lutheran Church in America).

In general terms, conservative Protestants tend to regard homosexuality as a perversion of God's intent for creation (heterosexual marriage and children). They regard the institution of the heterosexual family as the bedrock of God's plan and are opposed to anything that thwarts this plan. Homosexuality is a grave sin and homosexuals are regarded as sinners; some conservative Protestants believe that there is an inherent contradiction between being Christian and being homosexual. Such Protestants hold that the Bible condemns homosexuality unequivocally and Christians are called to do likewise and to help homosexuals repent of their sin (see, for example, <www.sbc.net>). *Conversion ministries,* in which ex-homosexuals help homosexual persons convert to heterosexuality through Jesus Christ, are a suggested means of dealing with this aberrant lifestyle (see Exodus International, for example). Conservative Protestants view homosexual *inclinations* as either a depravity of nature or a willful choice to violate God's intent, and thus these denominations retain an ambivalent attitude with regard to developments in science and genetics (Green and Numrich).

Liberal Protestant denominations, on the other hand, tend to regard homosexuality as an alternative expression of the variety and goodness of sexuality given by God. While affirming the inherent dignity of homosexual persons, such churches have taken advocacy positions for full civil rights for gay, lesbian, and transgendered persons, usually including recognizing legal status of domestic partners, and adoption of children. Some of these churches perform holy unions or commitment ceremonies for same-sex members of their churches, and some also ordain "out" homosexual clergy. Liberal Protestants tend to embrace developments in science; in fact many are sanguine about the benefits of science for humankind, particularly genetic science. One finds openness to the possible genetic etiology of homosexuality among liberal Protestants. The United Church of Christ has taken several public stands affirming gay and lesbian persons and "it was also one of the first American churches to affirm and ordain gays and lesbians in ministry" (Green and Numrich, p. 23). The Episcopal Church has called for full participation in the life of the church for gay and lesbian persons, including church leadership, and is studying the possibility of holy unions. Still, many of these churches struggle over the issue of how to regard homosexuality within the confines of their respective traditions.

Moderate Protestant denominations are a hotbed of struggle over homosexuality. The question of whether homosexuality is compatible with Christian teaching (especially the Bible) is intensely debated, and some have speculated that it could produce a schism in the church. Moderate Protestants are clear, however, that homosexuals are children of God and deserve a place in their congregations. Commitment ceremonies for same-sex unions have been intensely debated in recent years in these denominations, as has the ordination of *practicing* homosexual clergy. The Presbyterian Church (U.S.A.) agreed to lift its ban on ordination of gay and lesbian clergy in, though the issue appears far from settled. The Methodist Church has been in conflict over the disciplining of clergy who perform same-sex union ceremonies in its churches, as well as over the sanctioning of clergy who have "come out" as homosexual. The Evangelical Lutheran Church will spend until 2005 studying issues of ordination of homosexual clergy, same-sex blessing ceremonies, and so on.

Currently, "out" homosexual clergy in most denominations are expected to be celibate. Moderate Protestants are not settled on these questions, or on the issue of whether homosexuals may adopt children. However, rooted in an affirmation of Biblical justice, all moderate Protestant denominations reject efforts to curb the civil rights of homosexuals, and advocate non-discrimination of gay and lesbian persons.

There are also movements within a variety of Protestant denominations to affirm the rights and dignity of homosexuals. For example, in the Presbyterian Church there are "More Light churches"; the United Church of Christ has the "Open and Affirming Movement"; the Episcopal Church has a national gay and lesbian affirmation movement called "Integrity."

Homosexuality and Islam

The Western concept of *homosexuality,* as sexual orientation and lifestyle, is unknown in the Islamic world. As Amreen Jamal notes, "the term 'homosexuality' is erroneous when it is used in Islam, unless it is used by Muslims who identify also with the Western description of the queer lifestyle which includes both behavior and orientation" (Jamal, p. 69). It must be stated that just as there are many versions of Christianity and Judaism, so Islam is not monolithic in its expression. For the purposes of this discussion, however, it may be assumed that Islam is in wide agreement in its outlook and teachings on same-sex activity.

The authoritative text for Muslims, *Al-Qur'an* (believed to be the divine revelation from God to the Prophet Muhammad as told to him by Gabriel) is generally thought to be explicit in its condemnation of same-gender sexual activity. Al-Qur'an (Koran) references the same story that some Jewish and Christian scholars reference in the Hebrew Bible, the story of Lot and the destruction of Sodom (Genesis 19), as evidence of God's condemnation of same-gender sex. "In Islamic terminology," Khalid Duran notes, "homosexuals are called *qaum Lut,* Lot's people, or, briefly, *Luti*" (Duran, p. 181). Traditional Islamic scholars tend to interpret this story as evidence of God's disproval of the actions of Lot's people, anal penetration.

Beyond the Lot narrative (mentioned five times in Al-Qur'an), the Qur'an permits sex for pleasure, but indicates that the express purpose of sex is procreation. Marriage and procreation are central values of Islam, and the Prophet Muhammad is reported to have said, "Marriage is half the religion." In light of this, the *shari'a* (traditional Islamic law) finds same-sex activity, particularly between men, to be a punishable offense, though the offense must offend publicly and solid evidence of the offense must be established. In other words, the *shari'a* has little concern for what occurs in private, but what is publicly offensive is punishable. While there is a range of opinion among scholars, traditionalists interpret homosexuality as a crime and not just a sin; since the penalty is not specified in the Qur'an, it is a matter for contemporary authorities to debate, and death has been interpreted as one of punishments. In summary, Islam generally teaches that such sexual acts are against the natural order God intended for humans and are therefore sinful violations, and a deviation of the proper intent for human sexuality, marriage and procreation.

At least one scholar notes that there may be some openness to reform of the Muslim position within the context of its mystical branch, Sufism, and the freedom and justice teachings of Ustadh Mahmud Muhammad Taha (d. 1985) of Sudan. Ustadh Mahmud's teachings involved the development of a new or revised *shari'a* that was not dependent on the social constructs of seventh-century Islam (Duran). For an interesting contemporary study of the possibility of reform interpretations of homosexuality in Islam, see Amreen Jamal, 2001.

SUZANNE HOLLAND

SEE ALSO: *African Religions; Authority in Religious Traditions; Christianity, Bioethics in; Judaism, Bioethics in;* and other *Homosexuality* subentries

BIBLIOGRAPHY

Ackerman, Susan. 2000. "When the Bible Enters the Fray." *Bible Review* October: 6, 50.

Alpert, Rebecca T. 1997. *Like Bread on the Seder Plate: Jewish Lesbians' Transformation of Tradition.* New York: Columbia University Press.

Aquinas, Saint Thomas. 1923. *The Summa contra gentiles of Saint Thomas Aquinas,* tr. English Dominican Fathers from the latest Leonine edition. New York: Benziger.

Aquinas, Saint Thomas. 1952. *The Summa theologica of Saint Thomas Aquinas,* tr. Fathers of the English Dominican Province. Chicago: Encyclopaedia Britannica.

Augustine, Saint, Bishop of Hippo. 1948. *De Ordine,* tr. Ludwig Schopp, Denis J. Kavanagh, Robert P. Russell, and Thomas F. Gilligan. New York: Cima Pub. Co.

Augustine, Saint, Bishop of Hippo. 2001. *De bono coniugali; De sancta uirginitate (Augustine On the Good of Marriage),* ed. and tr. P.G. Walsh. Oxford: Clarendon Press.

Biale, Rachel. 1984. *Women and Jewish Law: An Exploration of Women's Issues in Halakhic Sources* New York: Schocken.

Bleich, David J. 1980. "Halakhah as an Absolute." *Judaism* 29(1).

Borg, Marcus, J. 1994. "Homosexuality and the New Testament." *Bible Review* December: 20, 54.

Boswell, John. 1980. *Christianity, Tolerance, and Homosexuality: Gay People in Western Europe from the Beginning of the Christian Era to the Fourteenth Century.* Chicago: University of Chicago Press.

Boswell, John. 1994. *Same-Sex Unions in Premodern Europe.* New York: Villard Books.

Boyarin, Daniel. 1995. "Are There Any Jews in 'The History of Sexuality'?" *Journal of the History of Sexuality* 5: 333–55.

Brooten, Bernadette. 1985. "Paul's Views on the Nature of Women and Female Homoeroticism." In *Immaculate and Powerful: The Female in Sacred Image and Social Reality,* ed. Clarissa W. Atkinson, Constance H. Buchannan, and Margaret M. Miles. Boston: Beacon.

Brooten, Bernadette. 1996. *Love Between Women: Early Christian Responses to Female Homoeroticism.* Chicago: University of Chicago Press.

Broughton, Lynne C. 1992. "Biblical Texts and Homosexuality: A Response to John Boswell." *Irish Theological Quarterly* 58: 141–153.

Congregation for the Doctrine of the Faith. 1982. "Declaration on Certain Problems of Sexual Ethics." In *Vatican Council, II,* vol. 2.

Congregation for the Doctrine of the Faith. 1986. "The Pastoral Care of Homosexual Persons." *Origins* 16(22): 377, 379–81.

Congregation for the Doctrine of the Faith. 1992. "Responding to Legislative Proposals on Discrimination Against Homosexuals." *Origins* 22(10): 174–77.

Countryman, William L. 1988. *Dirt, Greed, and Sex: Sexual Ethics in the New Testament and Their Implications for Today.* Philadelphia: Fortress Press.

D'Angelo, Mary Rose. 1990. "Women Partners in the New Testament." *Journal of Feminist Studies in Religion.* 6(1): 65–86.

Dorff, Elliot N. 1996. "'This Is My Beloved, This Is My Friend': A Rabbinic Letter on Intimate Relations." Written for and with the Commission on Human Sexuality of the Rabbinical Assembly. New York: Rabbinical Assembly.

Dorff, Elliot N. 1998. *Matters of Life and Death: A Jewish Approach to Modern Medical Ethics.* Philadelphia: Jewish Publication Society.

Duran, Khalid. 1993. "Homosexuality and Islam." In *Homosexuality and World Religions,* ed. Arlene Swidler. Valley Forge, PA: Trinity Press International.

Farley, Margaret A. 1983. "An Ethic for Same-Sex Relations." In *Challenge to Love: Gay and Lesbian Catholics in the Church,* ed. R. Nugent and J. Gramick. New York: Crossroads.

Feldman, David M. 1983. "Homosexuality and Jewish Law." *Judaism* 32 (Fall): 426–29.

France, R. T. "From Romans to the Real World: Biblical Principles and Cultural Change in Relation to Homosexuality and the Ministry of Women." In *Romans and the People of God: Essays in Honor of Gordon D. Fee on the Occasion of His 65th Birthday,* ed. Sven K. Soderlund and N. T. Wright. Grand Rapids: Eerdmans.

Furnish, Victor P. 1979. "Homosexuality." In *The Moral Teaching of Paul.* Nashville, TN: Abingdon Press.

Green, Christian M., and Numrich, Paul D. 2001. *Religious Perspectives on Sexuality: A Resource Guide.* Chicago: The Park Ridge Center.

Grossman, Naomi. 2001. "The Gay Orthodox Underground." *Moment.*

Hays, Richard B. 1986. "Relations Natural and Unnatural: A Response to John Boswell's Exegesis of Romans 1." *Journal of Religious Ethics* 14: 184–215.

Helminiak, Daniel. 1994. *What the Bible Really Says about Homosexuality.* San Francisco: Alamo Square Press.

Jamal, Amreen. 2001. "The Story of Lot and the Qur'an's Perception of the Morality of Same-Sex Sexuality." *Journal of Homosexuality* 41: 1–88.

Katz, Jonathan Ned. 1990. "The Invention of Heterosexuality." *Socialist Review* 20: 1, 7–34.

Kirschner, Robert. 1998. "Halakhah and Homosexuality: A Reappraisal." *Judaism* 37(Fall): 450–58.

Maimonides. *Mishneh Torah, Issurei Biah* 21: 8.

Moberly, Walter. 2000. *Theology* 103(814): 251–258.

National Conference of Catholic Bishops/United States Catholic Conference. 1997. "Always Our Children."

Olyan, Saul. 1994. "'And With a Male You Shall Not Lie the Lying Down of a Woman': On the Meaning and Significance of Leviticus 18:22 and 20:13." *Journal of the History of Sexuality* 5: 179–206.

Roman Catholic Church. 1995. *Catechism of the Catholic Church.* New York: Image/Doubleday.

Scroggs, Robin. 1983. *The New Testament and Homosexuality: Contextual Background for Contemporary Debate.* Philadelphia: Fortress Press.

Sifra 98.

Ward, Roy Bowen. 1997. "Why Unnatural? The Tradition Behind Romans 1:26–27." *Harvard Theological Review* 90(3): 263–84.

Weiss, J. H., ed. 1862. *Sifra.* Vienna: Schlossberg.

Wright, David. F. 1984. "Homosexuals or Prostitutes: The Meaning of *ARSENOKOITAI* (1 Cor. 6:9, 1 Tim. 1:10)." *Vigilae Christianae* 38: 125–153.

Zachary, Anne. 2001. "Uneasy Triangles: A Brief Overview of the History of Homosexuality." *British Journal of Psychotherapy* 17(4): 489–492.

INTERNET RESOURCE

Grossman, Naomi. 2001. "The Gay Orthodox Underground." Beliefnet. Available from <http://www.beliefnet.com/story/96/story_9647.html>.

HOSPICE

SEE *Palliative Care and Hospice*

HOSPITAL, CONTEMPORARY ETHICAL PROBLEMS OF THE

• • •

Hospitals are complicated institutions that bring together technological innovations and social services, salaried and unsalaried personnel, private and public funding, a charitable mission and a business orientation. Hospitals are accountable to patients, physicians, board members, employees, the local community, third-party payers, business partners, and other providers. It is no wonder that hospitals encounter ethical issues and problems.

Ethical concerns confronting hospitals in the United States are discussed in the following categories: identity and mission; special sponsorship; clinical issues; and relationships with healthcare professionals.

Identity and Mission

Perhaps the most fundamental ethical issue has to do with identity and mission. Is a hospital a business like any other, subject to the pressures of the marketplace, and primarily motivated by commercial interests and incentives? Or is it a social institution, primarily responsible for serving the health needs of the community and sometimes suffering financial loss in the process? These questions fall within the purview of the relatively recently established field of organizational ethics in healthcare. Two edited volumes (by Boyle, DuBose, Ellingson, et al.; and Spencer, Mills, Rorty, et al.) elaborate on these questions and show how hospitals experience tensions between their role as community servants and their role as entrepreneurs. These roles can coexist, as for-profit hospitals have tried to show. However, the public has come to expect more from the nonprofits—for example, that they provide care that is not reimbursed, support unprofitable services, and be alert to community healthcare needs.

Hospitals in the United States face more difficult questions of identity and mission than do hospitals in countries where healthcare is typically regarded as an essential service, not subject to the usual marketplace forces. A confluence of factors—including the growth of scientific medicine, the alliance of physicians and hospitals, the phenomenon of specialization, enormous capital investments, commercial ventures, and the payment system—has caused U.S. hospitals to behave much like businesses. Public policy has encouraged this by endorsing antitrust laws that discourage hospitals' collaboration with one another; by inadequate government-reimbursement programs; and by the failure to ensure universal entitlement to healthcare. These factors create financial incentives for hospitals that conflict with their stated mission, namely, to serve all people and to meet the needs of their communities.

Most hospitals remain not-for-profit and therefore tax-exempt. Voluntary hospitals, whose boards of trustees receive no pay because they are understood to serve the community, believe that this community orientation is the most effective way to deliver care. In their rhetoric, they cultivate an image of benevolence and moral worth that obscures their business orientation, seeking government subsidies but eschewing government control. Some business practices adopted by both for-profit and not-for-profit hospitals have tarnished this image of benevolence. These practices include aggressive marketing, advertising, and competition for paying patients; the creation of for-profit ventures, often with physicians, thus creating the potential for conflict of interest; resistance or refusal to care for the indigent; and expensive duplication of services to compete with other hospitals.

Until the latter part of the twentieth century, hospitals could count on the public's trust and support. The special nature of healthcare and the religious affiliation of many hospitals fostered this trust. Contemporary hospitals, however, face increasing skepticism and criticism from patients and the public at large. This dissatisfaction with hospitals' behavior arises from an expectation that hospitals will behave differently from ordinary businesses, that they have a "higher purpose." Distrust also stems from the Institute of Medicine's 2000 report, *To Err is Human,* which documents high rates of medical errors or unanticipated outcomes occurring in hospitals. It is imperative for hospitals to establish policies toward disclosure of such outcomes, since disclosure facilitates patient trust and reduces legal liability. Yet some hospitals are regaining public trust by various innovations that aim to empower patients to participate in their care (Nolon, Dickinson, and Bolton). Thus, one of the most pressing ethical issues facing hospitals is whether to rededicate themselves to a mission based on altruism and community service. The decision may be compounded by new hospital networks, mergers, and acquisitions. Hospitals still have fundamental ethical choices about whom they serve, how they allocate their resources, and what sort of

leadership and vision they bring to providing quality healthcare.

Special Sponsorship

Hospitals under religious sponsorship—Catholic, Jewish, Episcopal, Lutheran, Adventist, Presbyterian, Methodist—have special concerns. They were founded by traditions having particular beliefs and aspirations, yet they provide care in a pluralistic society. They neither employ nor provide care solely for persons of the faith of their founders. Like other hospitals, they are heavily dependent on state and federal payment for services rendered. In some cases, a hospital under religious sponsorship may be the only hospital serving a particular community. Ethical conflicts may arise between hospitals' allegiance to their religious sponsors and their obligation to provide needed services to the community.

This is especially the case in rural settings where, with government funding cuts, hospital closures or consolidations are increasingly common and Catholic health systems acquire nondenominational hospitals in the process. When Catholic hospitals become the primary source of healthcare in a region, rural residents, especially lower-income women, may find it difficult to obtain reproductive health services (Bennett; Bellandi).

Identity and mission are of particular concern here. In the United States, the majority of hospitals are *private,* that is, they are free to follow their own moral mission in religious matters. A hospital may therefore choose, on religious grounds, to offer different services from others in the community; for example, to follow certain dietary practices, or not to perform blood transfusions, abortions, or sterilizations. Hospitals are also heavily affected by the liability insurance crisis which has lead to the elimination of medical services, such as trauma, and to considerations of tort reform (Haugh; Taylor).

Thus far, the policies of hospitals with religious affiliations have not been proscribed by law, and arguably should not be proscribed ethically, unless they create undue hardship for patients. This would occur if patients could not gain reasonable access to needed services in any other way. The definition of what is reasonable will be interpreted variously, of course, depending on whether the perspective adopted is that of the sponsor and its adherents or of those who desire the service. Sponsored hospitals occasionally find themselves with conflicting loyalties, as they strive to be faithful to both their religious tradition and their constituents.

The growth of managed care and alliances among hospitals of different sponsorships creates another set of ethical conflicts for religious hospitals. If they are part of the new system of healthcare delivery, they will be closely associated with those who practice differently from them. This will result in their cooperating with and financially profiting from the very practices they prohibit in their own hospitals. How hospitals work this out requires careful consideration of their various ethical commitments.

Clinical Issues

With advances in medical technology, hospitals have encountered a number of new and perplexing ethical questions, some of the most contentious arising in relation to the use of life-sustaining treatment. When is it appropriate to withhold or withdraw medical treatment from a critically ill patient? Who should make the decision if the patient cannot? What are the rights and obligations of nurses, physicians, family members? What role should the hospital play in disputes among these groups? What policies should the hospital have in place to deal with these questions?

In 1991, the Joint Commission on Accreditation of Healthcare Organizations (findings published 1992) mandated that hospitals have a process for addressing ethical issues in patient care to protect patients' rights. To satisfy this policy, most hospitals created interdisciplinary ethics committees and used ethics consultants to aid physicians, hospital staff, and patients and their families in mediating individual cases as well as to recommend new policies on forgoing treatment that recognized the preeminence of patient choices. Resuscitation, ventilation, tube and intravenous feeding, renal dialysis, and antibiotic therapy continue to be some of the treatments discussed. Regardless of treatment, patients became entitled to full disclosure about the risks, benefits, and alternatives of treatment; and they, or surrogates, now have the ethical and legal right to accept or refuse any treatment. Many, but not all, physicians and hospitals changed their policies and developed new practices to reflect this situation.

The principle of patient autonomy caused additional ethical dilemmas for hospitals. In the early 1990s, some well-publicized cases arose in which patients' surrogates wanted life-sustaining interventions, but physicians and hospitals did not want to provide them. A claim of medical futility was the usual reason for this reluctance, although disputes about whether research had shown the desired treatment, such as cardiopulmonary resuscitation (CPR), to be reasonably effective also arose. Patients and surrogates invoked the principle of autonomy to justify their demands for treatment. These demands were particularly strong if the patient, or the patient's insurer, was willing to pay for the treatment.

Physicians and hospitals thus faced new issues: What are the limits of patients' or surrogates' rights to medical treatment? Are there situations in which physicians are justified in refusing to provide it? Is it ethical for physicians to have in mind scarce hospital resources when treating individual patients? What is the meaning, and what are the ethical implications, of medical futility? What are the economic and/or ethical conflicts of interest for hospitals in these cases?

These questions are inextricably related to the nature of insurance coverage. If insurance companies pay on a per diem or fee-for-service basis, it is to the hospital's advantage that patients have extensive treatment and long hospital stays, particularly if the insurance pays close to the actual cost of caring for the patient. In the late 1980s, many insurers changed the method of payment to capitation. Under this method, hospitals are *at risk* and receive a predetermined reimbursement for each patient, regardless of the actual costs of caring for the patient. Capitation creates very different economic incentives for physicians and hospitals than they have under a fee-for-service system. Thus, money becomes a factor in responding to the ethical question of *who* should decide when treatment should be provided. If the public thinks it is not receiving the medical care it needs because hospitals and/or physicians fear losing money, trust between healthcare providers and those they serve will be further eroded. Hospitals must therefore demonstrate their commitment to community service and educate the public about the importance of cost control. In order for trust to be renewed, the public must understand the connection between limiting expensive treatments for some patients and providing more basic care for others. They will need to agree that such changes are not primarily for the economic benefit of healthcare providers but are for the benefit of society as a whole.

Public trust in hospitals and clinical care is also waning due to greater awareness or experiences of sociodemographic disparities in healthcare (Smedley, Stith, and Nelson). The U.S. Department of Health and Human Services has established as a top priority the elimination of health disparities across racial/ethnic groups, sex, age, and geographic location. Hospitals have the capacity to contribute substantially toward this aim by ensuring the availability of qualified interpreters, employing healthcare professionals of diverse ethnic backgrounds, and providing culturally competent care. When justice can be secured through the provision of healthcare to individuals regardless of their cultural or religious backgrounds, the quality of healthcare will improve (Smedley, et al.; Committee on Quality of Health Care in America).

Relationships with Healthcare Professionals

Hospitals and physicians have always had an uneasy alliance: They need each other but often do not trust each other. For the first half of the twentieth century, hospitals were referred to as the "physicians' workshop." Hospitals provided the beds, equipment, nurses, and other personnel, and physicians provided the patients. Except in teaching institutions, hospitals and physicians had few common goals and mutual responsibilities beyond providing a place to care for patients. Physicians directed all aspects of patient care, and expected hospitals and their personnel to provide whatever the physicians deemed necessary. Until the middle of the twentieth century, hospitals themselves were not legally responsible for the care provided by physicians. At that time, courts began finding hospitals and their employees liable for not intervening to protect the patient when physicians provided inferior care. Since that time, hospitals have instituted mechanisms to monitor and intervene when necessary in physicians' care of patients.

This change was good for patients, but strained the relationship between hospitals and physicians. It created ethical conflicts for hospitals when, for example, physicians who admitted large numbers of patients were questioned or disciplined regarding quality of care. Some of these physicians left the hospitals, taking a large source of revenue with them. Accountability to patients required that hospitals and their organized medical staffs be vigilant about monitoring and intervening in the quality of care practiced by physicians. Economic self-interest, however, tempted hospitals to be more lenient with physicians.

Toward the end of the twentieth century, relationships between hospitals and physicians began to change again. Integrated delivery systems, through which healthcare providers and payers (such as insurance companies) collaborate to deliver care to patients in a particular geographic region, align the economic incentives affecting both physicians and hospitals. Capitation, a fixed fee paid to a group of providers to provide care for a fixed number of patients, resolves some of the ethical problems of the past related to hospital reimbursement. But capitation creates new ethical issues due to economic incentives to provide the least expensive care to patients. This change is good for some patients, but may not be good for others. Hospitals will continue to face ethical dilemmas of conflicting loyalties to patients and physicians.

The introduction of integrated delivery systems changes the relationships between hospitals and physicians in other ways. Some managed care plans require that primary-care physicians be the "gatekeepers," seeing patients first and referring them to specialists only if absolutely necessary.

This, combined with capitation systems, creates incentives for hospitals and primary-care physicians to offer their services as one unit. However, the retreat of managed care has signaled increased access to healthcare providers while increasing healthcare costs (Robinson, 2001). Many hospitals that purchase physicians' medical practices manage the business side of the practices. This is extremely difficult to accomplish with ethical integrity on both sides, because physicians and hospitals have historically operated independently of one another—both psychologically and practically—even though they are in the same building.

A related problem is that, after having courted specialists for years, hospitals now rely on primary-care physicians to direct patients to specialists. Nevertheless, ethical issues of loyalty and integrity are raised, as physicians in specialty practices find themselves in professional and economic jeopardy when their interests no longer match those of their hospital.

In response to the restrictions healthcare organizations impose upon physicians to control costs and medical decision-making, the American Medical Association established a union, Physicians for Responsible Negotiations, in 1999. Subsequently, medical residents separately unionized in 1999, limiting the number of work hours required per week. These unionizations can have a profound impact on hospitals (Yacht; Cohen). Some hospitals and physicians are concerned that unionization will lead to strikes, interfere with education and patient care, and add to hospital finances, as well as undermine the meaning of medical professionalism. Accounts of unionization at some hospitals, however, reveal that such fears do not materialize, given that these labor organizations have banned strikes to prioritize patient care (Yacht).

Hospitals face other problems with the delivery of medical care in relation to physicians and managed care. Managed care plans are increasingly utilizing evidence-based medicine guidelines to enhance efficiency in medical care by eliminating overtreatment and undertreatment (Sackett, Straus, Richardson, et al.). Many physicians fear that such guidelines interfere with personalized patient care, which deters their willingness to implement them. Consequently, hospitals may not be able to reach levels of clinical practice to which they aspire.

Much attention has also turned to the relationship between hospitals and nurses, given the critical shortage of nurses. This shortage results from efforts to contain hospital costs, and it contributes to medical errors and poor patient care. Although technicians and nursing aids have been hired to perform some nursing duties, it remains to be determined how hospitals will recruit a sufficient number to provide appropriate nursing care.

Conclusion

Contemporary hospitals encounter many ethical concerns and problems. All constituents—patients, physicians, employees, board members, volunteers, the community at large, payers, business partners—have a stake in the way these ethical issues are considered and resolved.

CORRINE BAYLEY (1995)
REVISED BY ELISA J. GORDON

SEE ALSO: *Advance Directives and Advance Care Planning; Artificial Nutrition and Hydration; Cancer, Ethical Issues Related to Diagnosis and Treatment; Compassionate Love; Conscience, Rights of; Healthcare Resources, Allocation of; Informed Consent; Malpractice, Medical; Managed Care; Mistakes, Medical; Nursing Ethics; Organ Transplants; Patients' Responsibilities; Patients' Rights; Pharmaceutics, Issues in Prescribing; Professional-Patient Relationship; Research Policy; Right to Die: Policy and Law; Teams, Healthcare; Women as Health Professionals, Contemporary Issues of*

BIBLIOGRAPHY

American Hospital Association. 1992. *Management Advisory: Ethics—Ethical Conduct for Health Care Institutions.* Chicago: American Hospital Association.

Bellandi, Deanna. 1998. "Access Declines: Reproductive Services Fall with Hospital Consolidation." *Modern Healthcare* 28: 26.

Bennett, Trudy. 2002. "Reproductive Health Care in the Rural United States." *Medical Student JAMA* 287: 112.

Boyle, Philip J.; DuBose, Edwin R.; Ellingson, Stephen J.; et. al. 2001. *Organizational Ethics in Health Care: Principles, Cases, and Practical Solutions.* San Francisco: Jossey-Bass.

Bulger, Ruth Ellen, and Reiser, Stanley Joel. 1990. *Integrity in Health Care Institutions: Humane Environments for Teaching, Inquiry and Healing.* Iowa City: University of Iowa Press.

Burke, Marybeth. 1991. "Hospitals Tackle Image Problems at Many Levels." *Hospitals* 65(5): 24–31.

Cohen, Jordan J. 2000. "Sounding Board: White Coats Should Not Have Union Labels." *New England Journal of Medicine* 342(6): 431–434.

Committee on Quality of Health Care in America, Institute of Medicine. 2001. *Crossing the Quality Chasm: A New Health System for the 21st Century.* Washington, D.C.: National Academy Press.

Department of Health and Human Services. 2000. *Healthy People 2010.* Washington, D.C.: Department of Health and Human Services.

Gray, Bradford H. 1991. *The Profit Motive and Patient Care: The Changing Accountability of Doctors and Hospitals.* Cambridge, MA: Harvard University Press.

Gray, Bradford H., ed. 1986. *For-Profit Enterprise in Health Care.* Washington, D.C.: National Academy Press.

Hastings Center. 1987. *Guidelines on the Termination of Life-Sustaining Treatment and the Care of the Dying: A Report.* Briarcliff Manor, NY: Author.

Haugh, Richard. 2002. "Feeling the Pressure?" *Hospital Health Network* 76(3): 42–45, 2.

Institute of Medicine. 2000. *To Err is Human: Building a Safer Health System.* Washington, D.C.: National Academy Press.

Joint Commission on Accreditation of Healthcare Organizations. 1992. *Patients Rights: 1992 Accreditation Manual for Hospitals.* Chicago, IL: The Joint Commission on Accreditation of Healthcare Organizations.

Jonsen, Albert R.; Siegler, Mark; and Winslade, William J. 1986. *Clinical Ethics: A Practical Approach to Ethical Decisions in Clinical Medicine,* 2d edition. New York: Macmillan.

Marty, Martin E., and Vaux, Kenneth L., eds. 1982. *Health/Medicine and the Faith Traditions: An Inquiry into Religion and Medicine.* Philadelphia: Fortress Press.

McCormick, Richard A. 1984. *Health and Medicine in the Catholic Tradition.* New York: Crossroad.

Nolon, Anne K.; Dickinson, Duo; and Boltin, Ben. 1999. "Creating a New Environment of Ambulatory Care: Community Health Centers and the Planetree Philosophy." *Journal of Ambulatory Care Management* 22(1): 18–26.

Quinlan, In Re. 1975. 348 A.2d 801 (N.J. Ch. Div.); 355 A.2d 647 (N.J. 1976).

Robinson, James C. 2001. "The End of Managed Care." *Journal of the American Medical Association* 285(20): 2622–2628.

Rosenberg, Charles E. 1987. *The Care of Strangers: The Rise of America's Hospital System.* New York: Basic Books.

Sackett, David L.; Straus, Sharon E.; Richardson, W. Scott; et al. 2000. *Evidence-Based Medicine: How to Practice and Teach EBM,* 2nd edition. New York: Churchill Livingstone.

Seay, J. David, and Vladeck, Bruce C. 1987. *Mission Matters: A Report on the Future of Voluntary Health Care Institutions.* New York: United Hospital Fund of New York.

Smedley, Brian D.; Stith, Adrienne Y.; and Nelson, Alan R., eds., Committee on Understanding and Eliminating Racial and Ethnic Disparities in Health Care, Board on Health Sciences Policy, Institute of Medicine. 2002. *Unequal Treatment: Confronting Racial and Ethnic Disparities in Health Care.* Washington, D.C.: National Academy Press.

Spencer, Edward M.; Mills, Ann E.; Rorty, Mary V.; and Werhane, Patrick, eds. 2000. *Organization Ethics in Health Care.* New York: Oxford University Press.

Starr, Paul. 198). *The Social Transformation of American Medicine.* New York: Basic Books.

Stevens, Rosemary. 1989. *In Sickness and in Wealth.* New York: Basic Books.

Taylor, Mark. 2002. "Cashing in on a Crisis." *Modern Healthcare* 32(23): 30–32.

U.S. President's Commission for the Study of Ethical Problems in Medicine and Biomedical and Behavioral Research. 1983. *Deciding to Forgo Life-Sustaining Treatment.* Washington, D.C.: Author.

Yacht, Andrew C. 2000. "Sounding Board: Collective Bargaining Is the Right Step." *New England Journal of Medicine* 342(6): 429–431.

HOSPITAL, MEDIEVAL AND RENAISSANCE HISTORY OF THE

• • •

Hospitals have become the primary theaters of modern medical practice. The early history of these institutions dates from about 400 to 1600, and includes these developments: (1) the origins of hospitals; (2) their development in the Byzantine and Islamic worlds; (3) their history in medieval western Europe; and (4) their flowering in Renaissance Italy. For purposes of this discussion, the term *hospital* refers to an institution that focused on caring for patients and, if possible, curing them. *Hospice* describes an institution that offered food and shelter to the poor, travelers, and the homeless sick but did not maintain specific services, such as the attentions of physicians, to treat those who were ill.

Hospital Origins

Several early cultures developed institutions to care for the sick. Ancient Indian sources describe centers that dispensed medicines and engaged specially trained personnel to care for the ill. Classical Greek society produced the *asklepieia*, the temples of the god of medicine, where the sick sought divine and natural cures. The Roman Empire supported *valetudinaria* (infirmaries) providing medical care to legionaries stationed on the barbarous northern frontier. None of these institutions, however, was strong enough to survive the upheavals that destroyed much of ancient civilization in Eurasia between 200 and 600. Modern hospitals trace their origins, and even their name, not to Indian treatment centers, Greek *asklepieia*, or Roman *valetudinaria* but to the hospices and hospitals established by the Christian church during the late Roman Empire.

From its earliest days, Christianity demanded that its adherents aid sick and needy people. Christians believed that on the Last Day, God would judge according to the love one had shown those in need. Had one fed the hungry, sheltered the homeless, visited the sick (Matt. 25:31–46)? By the early second century, bishops such as Polykarp of Smyrna expected Christian clergy to take care of the sick, orphans, and widows.

Local Christian clergy assisted the unfortunate without any formal charitable institutions until the fourth century. Thereafter, in the eastern Greek-speaking provinces of the Roman Empire, the demand for charity became so great, especially in the larger cities, that specialized institutions called *xenodocheia* (hospices) appeared. By the 320s the church in Antioch operated a hospice to feed and shelter the poor of Syria. By the mid-fourth century, the pagan emperor Julian referred to hospices as common Christian institutions.

Before 360, Christian hospices did not focus attention on the sick; but during the 370s Basil, bishop of Caesarea in Asia Minor, opened an institution where physicians and nurses treated patients. Two decades later, Bishop John Chrysostom supervised hospitals in Constantinople where doctors tended the sick. By about 410, the monk Neilos of Ankyra considered the hospital physician a common figure in the Greek Christian world. These early hospitals thus evolved from simpler hospices by expanding their services to include free medical care for needy guests.

Christian bishops built hospices during the fourth century and subsequently created more specialized hospitals for the sick, not only because they wished to follow Christ's command to practice charity but also because they sought support for the new religion among the urban lower classes. During the fourth century the cities of the Eastern provinces experienced an influx of rural poor who migrated to towns in search of food and employment. Classical civic institutions could not feed, house, and care for these new residents. The local bishops used the expanding resources of the Christian church to build hospices and hospitals for these migrants, and thereby won support both from the many poor and from the urban aristocrats. When Emperor Julian (361–363) tried to halt the spread of Christianity, he emphasized that the "Galilaeans" had succeeded in part because of their charitable institutions.

Early hospitals met their expenses from the revenue of lands that local bishops had donated. Subsequently, wealthy aristocrats and the emperors augmented these resources. As Christianity expanded it destroyed some aspects of classical civilization, but others it simply reoriented. For example, Christianity wholeheartedly accepted the classical obligation of aristocrats to benefit local cities, but the Christian church encouraged donors to endow institutions such as hospitals rather than traditional theaters, baths, and ornamental colonnades. By supporting hospitals a Christian aristocrat not only acted charitably but also fulfilled the classical duty toward the city. Moreover, such benefactions cemented local political support. This same combination of Christian morality, classical traditionalism, and political realism motivated emperors in their benefactions (Miller, 1985).

Hospitals of the Byzantine and Muslim Worlds

Hospitals developed most rapidly where they had first appeared, in the eastern half of the Roman Empire. The large cities of the eastern Mediterranean and the stable political conditions of the eastern Roman, or Byzantine, Empire fostered their hospitals' further evolution. By the late sixth century, Christian hospitals such as the Sampson Xenon (hospital) of Constantinople maintained specialized wards for surgery patients and those with eye diseases. Moreover, the premier physicians (*archiatroi*) of the Byzantine capital were assigned monthly shifts to treat patients in the Sampson and in other hospitals of the city. By the twelfth century the hospitals of Constantinople had evolved into relatively sophisticated medical centers. The Pantokrator Xenon maintained five specialized wards, seventeen physicians, thirty-four nurses, eleven servants, and a store of medicines supervised by six pharmacists. The Pantokrator treated outpatients as well as those who were hospitalized. Emperor John II (1118–1143), the founder of the Pantokrator, reminded the hospital's staff that the sick were God's special friends and that caring for patients was more important than maintaining buildings (Volk).

From their beginnings, the Christian hospitals of Byzantine cities were designed for the poor, but as these institutions became increasingly sophisticated medical centers served by the best physicians, some middle-class and a few wealthy patients began to use them. In this regard Byzantine practice differed markedly from the medieval West, where the bourgeoisie and nobility shunned hospitals as institutions solely for the destitute.

Medieval Islamic society maintained hospitals (in Persian, *bimaristani*) that equaled those of Byzantium. The first Islamic hospitals were founded in Baghdad during the reign of the caliph Harun al-Rashid (786–809). According to a governor of the caliph, Islamic hospitals had become common by the 820s; subsequently Muslims considered support of hospitals a mark of true piety.

Like Byzantine hospitals, *bimaristani* had evolved from earlier Christian philanthropic institutions in large cities of the Byzantine Empire. When Emperor Zeno expelled Nestorian Christians from Syria in 489, many sought refuge in Persia, where they established institutions, including hospitals, modeled on those in Byzantine cities such as Antioch. After the Muslims conquered Sassanid Persia in the seventh century, they came in contact with Nestorians. Impressed by Nestorian medical skills, they adopted many Syrian medical traditions—teaching methods, scientific texts, and hospitals—as models for shaping Islamic institutions.

Although Islamic hospitals evolved from Christian institutions, they experienced a unique development. They differed strikingly from their Byzantine counterparts by including separate sections for mental patients. Gradually these psychiatric wards became the most prominent features of *bimaristani*. Neither Byzantine nor medieval Western hospitals had wards for mental patients (Dols).

Medieval Western Europe

Hospitals developed more slowly in the western Roman Empire. Saint Jerome (ca. 331–420) mentioned two small hospitals near Rome about 400. During the early Middle Ages, however, social conditions retarded hospital development in western Europe. Barbarian invasions from the north and Muslim advances in Africa inhibited political, economic, and social life. Few towns of the size and complexity that could support medical centers such as the Byzantine and Muslim hospitals survived. In the domains of Charlemagne (768–814), hospitals did not evolve beyond simple hospices. As late as the thirteenth century, hospitals were rare in Europe. None of the 112 houses for the sick in medieval England provided physicians for their patients, nor did they stock any medicines (Carlin).

In the twelfth century, a new religious order, the Knights of the Hospital of Saint John of Jerusalem (known today as the Knights of Malta) reintroduced into Europe specialized medical care for the sick when they organized their renowned hospital in Jerusalem. Under Byzantine influence, the Knights' rule for this hospital mandated a permanent medical staff of four physicians and four surgeons to treat patients. Moreover, the Knights developed a unique philanthropic ethic by adapting feudal notions to the traditional Christian command to aid those in need. The Knights were to treat the sick in the Jerusalem hospital as vassals served their overlords. As the Knights expanded, they built many smaller hospitals in the towns of Europe where they introduced practices they had established in Jerusalem (Sire).

The Knights' hospital in Jerusalem inspired many similar institutions throughout western Europe. Using its rule as a model, Pope Innocent III established in 1200 the famous Hospital of the Holy Spirit in Rome. In 1217 the church in Paris reorganized its ancient hospice, the Hôtel-Dieu, by drafting a new constitution based on the regulations of the Jerusalem hospital (Miller, 1978).

The Knights of Saint John had such a wide-ranging effect not only because their rule inspired western Europeans to help the needy, especially the sick, but also because Latin Christendom was entering a new phase of urban growth. As country dwellers migrated to the towns in growing numbers, these newcomers were exposed to a wider range of diseases. Hospitals became necessary to treat the rapidly growing number of sick among the urban poor. In fact, the economic and social conditions in the expanding towns of thirteenth-century Europe were remarkably similar to those in the fourth-century Byzantine cities where hospitals had first appeared.

An examination of the rule for the Roman Hospital of the Holy Spirit, however, indicates one important difference between the new institutions of the West and the Jerusalem hospital. The Roman rule mandated many of the Knights' practices, but it omitted any reference to physicians or surgeons. The same is true of the rule for the Hôtel-Dieu of Paris. Only gradually did physicians come to serve in these hospitals. The records of the Hôtel-Dieu do not mention a permanent staff physician until 1328. As late as the eighteenth century a physician visited Saint Bartholomew's Hospital in London only once a week. That trained doctors did not assume a major role in caring for patients in Western medieval hospitals distinguishes them from Byzantine *xenones* and Moslem *bimaristani*, where doctors not only treated the sick but supervised hospital administration.

It is also clear that some of the Western medieval hospitals did not provide care on the same level as did the Eastern medical facilities. The twelfth-century hospital at Saint-Pol in northern France maintained only six nurses (or nursing sisters) for sixty patients. Iconographic evidence indicates that at the Hôtel-Dieu in Paris patients sometimes shared beds. The wards of many medieval hospitals were also poorly heated. Conditions such as these no doubt made it difficult for hospitals to heal the sick and provided some support for the charges of later Enlightenment reformers that all medieval hospitals had in fact been death traps (Miller, 1985).

Renaissance Italy

Inspired by the Jerusalem hospital, the communes of Tuscany began building hospitals during the thirteenth century. Before 1300, for example, the town of Siena built an institution that differed from the Hôtel-Dieu of Paris in that it maintained on its staff a physician, a surgeon, and a pharmacist. In 1288 Folco Portinari, the father of Dante's Beatrice, founded the Hospital of Santa Maria Nuova in Florence; by the fifteenth century, this institution had developed into an elaborate center for medical treatment. A document dated 1500, but reflecting earlier arrangements, reveals that Santa Maria paid six of the best physicians of Florence to visit patients each morning. In addition, three young interns lived permanently at the hospital. In return for room and board and a valuable opportunity to gain experience in medical practice, they served the hospital's 300 patients by monitoring their conditions and making daily reports to the senior physicians.

Santa Maria Nuova was not a death trap, as were some less well-organized hospitals, nor was it a hospice where poor sick people were simply nourished. It provided its patients access to society's best physicians and boasted an excellent rate of cure. Hospital records reveal that about 85 percent of the patients recovered from their ailments (Park; Henderson).

At Santa Maria Nuova, the interns were willing to serve patients for free not only because such service was virtuous but also because it offered them an unparalleled opportunity to observe the course of many diseases. During the sixteenth century, the medical professors of Padua (in Venetian territory) established formal clinical instruction at the Hospital of San Francesco. Many students from northern Europe came to study at Padua because of its excellent empirical training (Bylebyl).

Conclusion

Modern scholars have not been inclined to examine medieval hospitals because of the prevailing view that these were poorly equipped asylums that offered the sick only minimal medical care. Such institutions supposedly had nothing in common with today's hospitals. This view has its origins in Enlightenment skepticism concerning religious institutions. Eighteenth-century intellectuals contrasted the efficacy of science in curing human ills, including disease, with the helplessness of Christian charity, which at best provided only comfort, not true remedies.

However, hospitals in Renaissance Italy, as well as those in medieval Constantinople and Baghdad, demonstrate that philanthropic institutions were not necessarily isolated from scientific medicine. In fact, hospital service in Italy came to form a vital part of medical training, first in Florence and then at the University of Padua. In hospitals such as Santa Maria Nuova, the Christian command to aid the needy interacted with a sense of civic pride and with a concept of professional ethics on the part of physicians to create institutions that were both truly philanthropic and efficient in curing the sick.

TIMOTHY S. MILLER (1995)
BIBLIOGRAPHY REVISED

SEE ALSO: *Care; Christianity, Bioethics in; Islam, Bioethics in; Medical Ethics, History of: Europe; Professional-Patient Relationship: Historical Perspectives; Public Health: History*

BIBLIOGRAPHY

Amundsen, Darrel W. 1986. "The Medieval Catholic Tradition." In *Caring and Curing: Health and Medicine in the Western Religious Traditions,* pp. 65–107, ed. Ronald L. Numbers and Darrel W. Amundsen. New York: Macmillan.

Amundsen, Darrel W. 2000. *Medicine, Society, and Faith in the Ancient and Medieval Worlds.* Baltimore: Johns Hopkins University Press.

Brodman, James. 1998. *Charity and Welfare: Hospitals and the Poor in Medieval Catalonia* (Middle Ages Series). Philadelphia: University of Pennsylvania Press.

Bylebyl, Jerome J. 1982. "Commentary." In *A Celebration of Medical History: The Fiftieth Anniversary of the Johns Hopkins Institute of the History of Medicine and the Welch Medical Library,* pp. 200–211, ed. Lloyd G. Stevenson. Baltimore: Johns Hopkins University Press.

Carlin, Martha. 1989. "Medieval English Hospitals." In *The Hospital in History,* pp. 21–39, ed. Lindsay P. Granshaw and Roy Porter. London: Routledge.

Dols, Michael W. 1987. "The Origins of the Islamic Hospital: Myth and Reality." *Bulletin of the History of Medicine* 61(3): 367–390.

Henderson, John. 1989. "The Hospitals of Late-Medieval and Renaissance Florence: A Preliminary Survey." In *The Hospital in History,* pp. 63–92, ed. Lindsay P. Granshaw and Roy Porter. London: Routledge & Kegan Paul.

Lee, Gerard A. 2002. *Leper Hospitals in Medieval Ireland: With a Short Account of the Military and Hospitaller Order of st Lazarus of Jerusalem.* Dublin, Ireland: Four Courts Press.

Miller, Timothy S. 1978. "The Knights of Saint John and the Hospitals of the Latin West." *Speculum* 53(4): 709–733.

Miller, Timothy S. 1985. *The Birth of the Hospital in the Byzantine Empire.* Baltimore: Johns Hopkins University Press.

Miller, Timothy S. 1997. *The Birth of the Hospital in the Byzantine Empire.* Baltimore: Johns Hopkins University Press.

Park, Katharine. 1985. *Doctors and Medicine in Early Renaissance Florence.* Princeton, NJ: Princeton University Press.

Risse, Guenter B. 1999. *Mending Bodies, Saving Souls: A History of Hospitals.* New York: Oxford University Press.

Schreiber, Georg. 1948. "Byzantinisches und Abendländisches Hospital." In *Gemeinschaften des Mittelalters: Recht und Verfassung, Kult und Frömmigkeit,* pp. 3–80. Münster: Regensberg.

Shatzmiller, Joseph. 1995. *Jews, Medicine, and Medieval Society.* Berkeley: University of California Press.

Sire, H. J. A. 1994. *The Knights of Malta.* New Haven, CT: Yale University Press.

Thompson, John D., and Goldin, Grace. 1975. *The Hospital: A Social and Architectural History.* New Haven, CT: Yale University Press.

Volk, Robert. 1983. *Gesundheitswesen und Wohltätigkeit im Spiegel der byzantinischen Klostertypika.* Munich: Institut für Byzantinistik und Neugriechische Philologie der Universität.

HOSPITAL, MODERN HISTORY OF THE

• • •

Although a few Renaissance institutions supplemented charitable assistance with professional medical care, the hospital's gradual *medicalization* occurred from the seventeenth century onward, within changing social and scientific frameworks. Three distinct periods can be identified within this development: (1) the early shift of the hospital from welfare to medical establishment, 1650–1870; (2) the evolution of a successfully medicalized institution for all social classes, 1870–1945; and (3) the creation of a specialized showcase of scientific medicine, 1945 to the present.

From Welfare to Medicine: 1650-1870

During the early modern period, hospitals in Europe's urban centers were charitable shelters for the poor and working classes, functioning primarily as instruments of religious charity and social control with minimal involvement of the medical profession. Whether the patients were Catholic or Protestant, hospitalization continued to be an opportunity for physical comfort as well as moral rehabilitation. However, in time of epidemics such as plague and syphilis, specialized hospitals were created to ensure the isolation of the sick and thus avoid the spread of contagion. Given the expanding institutionalization of charity, the decline of religious institutions, and new roles in the preservation of public health, hospitals increasingly came under lay control, including municipal governments, fraternal organizations, and private patrons.

After 1650, new geopolitical agendas designed to increase the power and prosperity of the emerging national states pressed hospitals into new roles. Human life was given greater financial value as population policies were aimed at increasing the number of inhabitants as a base for state power, economic development, and military strength. Proponents of emerging European mercantilism viewed labor as the key source of wealth and urged that the nation's workforce be mobilized and kept at an optimum state of productivity. Within such a framework, the desire to promote the health of citizens inspired new programs of public health, hygiene, and medical care.

At the same time, more optimistic visions of health preservation and rehabilitation elaborated by Enlightenment thinkers suggested that sickness, instead of an inevitable, sinful, and often long-term human burden, could be controlled and eliminated. In addition to their traditional moral and physical aims, hospitals were now envisioned as institutions for physical rehabilitation and cure, places of early rather than last resort, especially for military personnel and the labor force. This agenda implied a greater involvement of the healthcare professions with large sectors of the population hitherto without such contacts.

To implement their new health policies, national governments, local authorities, and corporate professional bodies organized efforts to reform the existing medical and surgical professions. Physicians and surgeons were granted new forms of access to hospitals and given new rules to guide their institutional activities. Early models for the medicalization process came from military and naval establishments that provided for the sick and wounded members of Europe's expanding military forces. Later, medical professionals working in civil hospitals also began to argue successfully that their management of patients provided a valuable addition to the rest and food traditionally furnished to inmates in religious shelters. During the late eighteenth and early nineteenth centuries, medical objectives dramatically reshaped hospital routines from admission to the discharge or death of the patient. Acute rather than chronic illnesses were preferred; young rather than old patients were accepted. Rehabilitation and cure were the new goals.

HOSPITALS AS TRAINING INSTITUTIONS. At the same time, surgeons—and later physicians—recognized the great opportunities hospitals offered to improve their clinical skills and thus increase their power and status. By the eighteenth century, shifts in scientific ideology emphasized the importance of empirical studies and the construction of knowledge based on observed facts. Surgeons in France and

Great Britain were especially keen to acquire practical knowledge of anatomy, pathology, and clinical management. After the French Revolution, physicians in that country initiated a new strategy of professional and social advancement under the banner of what was generically called the *medicine of observation*. With significant numbers of sick people assembled in hospital wards, doctors could observe at the bedside the evolution of individual diseases and their diagnoses on a much larger scale than they could in private practice. Postmortem dissections performed on former hospital inmates provided further information on the pathology responsible for the symptoms. Moreover, patient management offered unequaled opportunities to check the usefulness of the traditional medical regimens, especially the effects of older remedies. Efforts to upgrade the preparation and uses of drugs involved clinical trials and statistical analysis. Hospitals became the focal points of comprehensive bedside research programs.

Finally, the expanding medical and surgical presence in European hospitals made such institutions increasingly attractive as places for education and training of rank-and-file practitioners. Hospitals were seen as "great nurseries" that could "breed some of the best physicians and chirurgeons because they may see as much there in one year as in seven any where else" (Bellers, 1714). In certain establishments, the authorities created special teaching wards where professors and attendants, followed by their students, made regular rounds of the patients. Instruction varied greatly, from passive observation to supervised and even independent, hands-on examination and management of the patients by students and apprentices.

REORGANIZATION OF THE HOSPITAL STRUCTURE. How did the hospital as an institution adapt to these new agendas? France possessed several types of organizations, including massive *hôpitaux générales,* or hospices, for the elderly poor, beggars, vagrants, incurables, and prostitutes. There were also small welfare establishments at the parish level for similar cases. In larger urban areas, the traditional *Hôtels-Dieux* now limited admissions to the sick but excluded incurables, the insane, and venereal cases. All original ward layouts were based on medieval principles, providing in a shelter as many beds as possible and still crowding three to four individuals into each bed. Hospital size was fiercely debated, with advocates of medicalization arguing for smaller institutions to prevent cross-infections.

In Great Britain and the young American republic, major population centers possessed a number of *voluntary infirmaries,* or private hospitals, founded and operated by local philanthropists and often financed by a system of yearly subscriptions solicited from local merchants and professionals. Except for accident cases, these establishments admitted only a very restricted number of the sick poor. These persons, recommended for admission by the subscribers, were judged by the community to be willing to work and thus *deserving* of hospital care and rehabilitation. In addition, there were a number of private special hospitals, especially in London after 1800, supported by contributions and patient fees and operating under the direction of medical professionals. By contrast, English "poor law" infirmaries were supported financially by parish taxes and linked to local workhouses, which provided free care to the sick poor deemed able bodied, or vagrant, and thus *undeserving* of other charitable assistance. Later, in the nineteenth century, many of these workhouse infirmaries evolved into municipal hospitals and were placed under the direction of salaried medical superintendents. At the same time, and with financial support from leading local citizens, Great Britain also created a string of small cottage hospitals, providing paid medical care to those who could afford it.

To support expanding medical services and teaching activities, nineteenth-century hospitals required more money and changes in their physical plants and administrative organizations. By the 1870s, hygienic principles had come to dominate the construction and functioning of new establishments, now equipped with single beds for the sick and providing ample ventilation in their pavilion-type wards. Isolation chambers, surgical amphitheaters, emergency rooms, morgues, libraries, and outpatient facilities became indispensable adjuncts. Medical control also shifted power from patients and caregivers to attending physicians, thereby creating conflicts between traditional charitable practices and scientific goals of disease identification and management. Medicalization implied a shift from the primary focus on shelter and food for the needy to the diagnosis and treatment of diseases exhibited by sick patients.

A Hospital for All Social Classes: 1870–1945

Thanks in part to advances in medical knowledge and technology, the medicalization process of Western society was significantly advanced before the end of World War II. By 1900, upper- and middle-class patients in Europe and the United States were seeking and paying for medical care in hospitals. Staffed by competent medical and nursing professionals, and equipped with clinical laboratories and other diagnostic tools, hospitals became the preferred destination of those who were acutely sick and in need of surgical and medical care. The newly created demand for hospital care, spurred by urbanization and industrialization, expanded further to include the needs of birthing and child care.

In the United States, such requirements were eagerly met by the establishment of a vast, decentralized system of voluntary hospitals fiercely competing for community resources, physicians, and their patients. Local private citizens provided the necessary funds and volunteer service required to create general community hospitals. Alongside schools, police stations, and firehouses, U.S. general hospitals became emblems of community life, the pride of Main Street. In Europe, many hospitals became governmental facilities managed by paid professionals.

The new hospital mission was a result of converging ideologies, policies, and needs, some traditional, others new. Religious values and charitable donations still played an important role in the early 1900s, while developing economic tenets based on capitalism suggested that the health of workers in the industrial world was of great importance both to the state and to the private sector. In the United States, new social conditions favored the creation and utilization of more hospitals. Urbanization was accelerating at a rapid pace, bringing an ever-increasing number of adults into crowded city quarters. Among them were waves of new immigrants with multiple healthcare needs and few resources. Industrialization, in turn, created a new panorama of occupational diseases and accidents. Without the means or family networks to get the necessary help, many sick or injured individuals were thus forced to seek medical care in hospitals.

Under the new banner of scientific medicine, hospitals became the institutions of first rather than last resort. Thanks to the increasingly sophisticated diagnostic and therapeutic procedures offered in hospitals after 1900, optimistic Enlightenment notions of physical rehabilitation and cure were becoming a reality. Radiology, electrocardiography, and the clinical laboratory greatly improved the ability of hospital personnel to refine diagnoses. In addition to providing rest and a healthier diet, hospitals focused increasingly on managing acute diseases, especially life-threatening conditions that required intensive and highly technical care. A new generation of chemotherapeutic agents and vaccines improved the odds of success in the battle against certain diseases. Following the adoption of anesthesia and antisepsis, hospitals became the primary centers for surgical operations. Surgeons recognized the advantage of centralizing their new and expensive equipment within the *surgical suites* of a hospital.

THE CHANGING STATUS OF NURSES, PHYSICIANS. For patient care, hospitals relied increasingly on a new generation of nurses, drawn from the middle class and trained in professional education programs based on the model established by Florence Nightingale (1820–1910). Shedding their previous low-status role of cleaning women and servants, these new hospital nurses gradually displaced the dwindling number of religious staff members who had traditionally performed patient services. In time, the Nightingale nurses became valuable assistants to the medical profession in patient management.

By the 1910s, more physicians joined hospital staffs, staking their professional reputations on the achievements of scientific medicine such institutions seemed to make possible. In U.S. voluntary hospitals, medical staff organizations remained flexible, bestowing admission privileges on both local general practitioners and specialists who could deliver paying patients. In Great Britain, however, traditional social and professional barriers between general practitioners, on the one hand, and hospital-appointed physicians and surgeons, on the other, created insurmountable barriers in voluntary establishments. Although referring their patients to hospitals, the former were not allowed to practice within them. As so-called consultants, the latter operated small units and exclusively took care of a specific number of patients.

Since the hospital was rapidly becoming the physician's primary workshop in the 1920s, medical goals, including specialization, education, and research, needed to become top institutional priorities. Twentieth-century hospitals witnessed a dramatic growth of specialized care through the creation of clinical departments, an increase in student doctors, called *house staff*, and the performance of clinical research. Such activities became central to educational and licensing requirements, and conferred prestige and higher professional status on those allowed to work in the most preeminent institutions.

THE CHANGING FOCUS OF HOSPITALS. Once again the hospital as an institution adapted to these new agendas. Some new hospitals were associated or affiliated with medical and nursing schools. Others, especially in the United States, sprouted between 1890 and 1920 in ethnic urban neighborhoods, or strategic suburban locations, their creation influenced by state and local governments, population, philanthropy, or industry. Sectarian Jewish, Catholic, and Protestant institutions, German- and French-speaking clinics, municipal and state hospitals, private establishments sponsored by railroads and universities—all formed a constellation of autonomous units across the U.S. landscape.

In Europe, governments became increasingly involved in sponsoring and managing hospitals. In Great Britain, the Public Health Act of 1875 encouraged municipalities to establish isolation hospitals for persons suffering from infectious diseases. The poor law infirmaries were gradually taken over by local health departments and converted to general hospitals. The National Health Insurance Act of 1911 eliminated the charitable character of the voluntary hospitals and brought their services under the umbrella of regional healthcare schemes.

In the United States, hospital organizations in the 1920s changed to serve the new medical objectives and compete for paying patients, an ever-greater source of needed revenue. The rapid growth of medical technology generated further budgetary pressures, forcing voluntary hospitals to redouble their fundraising efforts and use endowment income for capital expenditures. As they became individual corporations in a competitive healthcare market, demands for greater efficiency prompted hospitals to bolster their administrations and institute stringent financial measures. Institutional care became a commodity, a product to be furnished mostly to those willing to pay for it directly or through health-insurance policies.

By the 1930s, economic conditions stemming from the Depression forced the creation of new funding systems, such as the Blue Cross health-insurance companies, organized by physicians. As competition for philanthropic support and patient revenue accelerated, accountability and public relations dominated the hospitals' administrative agendas. Since each U.S. institution was the proud product of individual community efforts, cooperation among hospital administrations was resisted.

As the hospital became the preferred locus for the application of scientific principles to medicine, new ethical problems appeared. The medicalization of life processes expanded the range of life experiences now addressed as medical problems by health professionals in hospital settings: Birth and death, formerly events that occurred in the home, now took place in the hospital. Since the early nineteenth century, a depersonalized, disease- and organ-centered approach had already replaced earlier holistic notions of sickness. As hospital routines became increasingly technical and standardized, patients came to be seen as merely embodiments of diseases that were the primary objects of inquiry and treatment. This approach affected the nature of the physician-patient relationship, as professionals focused primarily on successful problem solving in diagnosing and arresting human pathology. The physician's moral authority, hitherto based on personal qualities, now became grounded in scientific competence. Clinical experimentation became rampant, sometimes abusive, with few safeguards provided for the patients.

The Hospital as Biomedical Showcase: 1945 to the Present

Following World War II, the hospital rapidly consolidated its position as the embodiment of scientific and technologically sophisticated medicine. An explosion in medical knowledge led to the expansion of diagnostic and therapeutic services at hospitals. This development had far-reaching implications for institutional access, cost, and quality of care as delivered to a broad spectrum of the public under various private and state-sponsored health plans. The hospital's mission continued to reflect converging agendas, including the religious, political, economic, and scientific goals set in preceding decades.

In the United States, the federal government's involvement in sponsoring hospital care gradually expanded as the demand for institutional beds and services multiplied. Beginning with the Hill Burton Act in 1946, the federal authorities supported the existing system of decentralized, private hospitals—first, through the provision of construction subsidies, and later, through reimbursement schemes for services, such as the Medicare and Medicaid programs in 1966. This supportive rather than regulatory role preserved a network of independent and competing municipal, sectarian, and academic hospitals in each community. In marked contrast with events in Europe, the 1950s through the 1970s witnessed an impressive growth in U.S. hospital facilities, including neonatology and intensive-care units, imaging facilities, and transplantation services. Individual hospitals continue to operate as independent business organizations within a burgeoning healthcare *industry*. Periodic institutional accreditation by a joint commission of the American Medical Association and the American Hospital Association ensures compliance with a number of performance standards.

To work in hospitals of their choice, all practicing physicians in the United States must secure admission *privileges* in such institutions. Most hospital care is indeed rendered by private practitioners who briefly visit the hospital to check on the status of their patients. This system allows the establishment of larger and more mobile medical staffs whose authority remains diffuse. To exert some measure of control, medical staffs usually create a number of committees to deal with the issues of credentials, admissions, education, and quality control. (Hospital ethics committees grapple with a host of issues, from informed consent and patient autonomy to advance directives and the definition of death.) The resulting administrative complexity and instability require a great deal of consensus building, achieved through frequent meetings and written communications. This record keeping effort is especially important among the attending physicians and more permanent hospital personnel to achieve a necessary degree of internal standardization of medical and administrative procedures.

Hospitals in Europe, even those owned by municipalities or private bodies, continue to be closely supervised by central governments. All hospital planning, construction, management, and recruitment of medical personnel remains subject to state control. In Great Britain, the government has assumed responsibilities for ensuring free access to hospital care as a social right. The implementation of the National Health Service Act of 1946 brought about the outright nationalization of all hospitals and placed them under the authority of regional boards appointed by the government and responsible to the Ministry of Health. In many European communities, the larger municipal and voluntary hospitals erected more than a century earlier remain in full operation. Greater administrative uniformity has allowed for smaller staff requirements. Given these hospitals' outdated physical plants, limited technology, and often a lingering stigma from their charitable past, well-to-do patients still prefer smaller, privately owned hospitals or clinics, many of which are still owned or managed by religious orders.

European hospitals operate with closed, full-time medical staffs hierarchically organized within smaller, autonomous divisions, each of which operates its own clinical, diagnostic, and rehabilitative services. While such internal arrangements reduce administrative overhead and foster more stable relationships among patients, physicians, and nurses, the schism between hospital and private practice remains. In Great Britain, this decentralized staffing framework follows the traditional, voluntary models of allocating a specific block of beds to each hospital physician or consultant, who is assisted by a stratified junior medical staff in training for specialist status.

Financial Difficulties of Hospitals

Although outpatient facilities are quickly becoming an integral component of professional education, hospital-based training continues to be the backbone of all medical education programs. Given the range of diagnostic and therapeutic options available, hospital practice remains at the center of biomedicine, providing the specialized clinical experience and technical proficiency required for today's professional status. With medical specialization and subspecialization on the rise, U.S. hospitals have expanded dramatically and have extended their residency training programs. As a result, physicians in training exercise greater management responsibility and are better remunerated than ever before.

Due to restrictive reimbursement schemes instituted by government and the private insurance industry, and the escalating costs of technologically assisted medical care, together with a gradual fragmentation of the medical marketplace, many U.S. hospitals find themselves increasingly under siege, victims, in part, of their previous success. Excessively bureaucratized and inefficient, their physical facilities overexpanded, hospitals are struggling to maintain their patient volumes as costs continue to increase. Unable to survive in a highly competitive environment, some institutions have already merged while others are closing wards or their doors altogether, thus forcing a major restructuring of the entire medical-care delivery system. Many hospitals are being reorganized into for-profit corporations, extending their services into networks of clinics and practitioners, and offering health insurance and service plans.

Conclusion

Ultimately, the evolution of the hospital in recent centuries poses the central question of whether care is still the primary function of this institution. While subjected to competing agendas—including religious beliefs, social control, secular philanthropy, scientific curiosity, communal pride, and economic autonomy—the hospital's original purpose was to shelter and comfort all sufferers in need. To a great extent, hospitals now restrict admission to seriously ill patients who require the most sophisticated diagnostic and therapeutic measures. The tilt toward acute episodes of physical illness, complex technological interventions, and the increasing costs of confinement have made hospital stays episodic and brief. Bureaucratization, financial constraints, and the pervasive presence of instrumentation only accentuate the essential impersonality of institutional care. The trade-offs are clear. Three centuries of medicalization transformed the hospital from a caring shelter for the poor into a disease-oriented machine for the sick who can afford to be cured.

GÜNTER B. RISSE (1995)
BIBLIOGRAPHY REVISED

SEE ALSO: *Aging and the Aged, Societal Aging; Care; DNR; Ethics: Institutional Ethics Committees; Informed Consent; Long-Term Care; Medicaid; Medical Education; Medicare; Mergers and Acquisitions; Patients' Rights; Research Ethics Committees*

BIBLIOGRAPHY

Abel-Smith, Brian. 1964. *The Hospitals in England and Wales, 1800–1948: A Study in Social Administration.* Cambridge, MA: Harvard University Press.

Ackerknecht, Erwin H. 1967. *Medicine at the Paris Hospital 1794–1848.* Baltimore: Johns Hopkins University Press.

Bellers, John. 1714. *Essay Towards the Improvement of Physick.* London: J. Sowle.

Dowling, Harry F. 1982. *City Hospitals: The Undercare of the Underprivileged.* Cambridge, MA: Harvard University Press.

Foucault, Michel. 1973. *The Birth of the Clinic: An Archeology of Medical Perception,* tr. Alan M. Sheridan Smith. New York: Pantheon.

Freidson, Eliot, ed. 1963. *The Hospital in Modern Society.* New York: Free Press.

Hollingsworth, J. Rogers, and Hollingsworth, Ellen J. 1987. *Controversy About American Hospitals: Funding, Ownership and Performance.* Washington, D.C.: American Enterprise Institute for Public Policy Research.

Honigsbaum, Frank. 1979. *The Division in British Medicine: A History of the Separation of General Practice from Hospital Care, 1911–1968.* London: Kogan Page.

Long, Diana E., and Golden, Janet L., eds. 1989. *The American General Hospital: Communities and Social Contexts.* Ithaca, NY: Cornell University Press.

Nelson, Sioban. 2001. *Say Little, Do Much: Nurses, Nuns, and Hospitals in the Nineteenth Century.* Philadelphia: University of Pennsylvania Press.

Prochaska, F. K. 1992. *Philanthropy and Hospitals of London: The King's Fund, 1897–1990.* Oxford: Clarendon Press.

Risse, Günter B. 1986. *Hospital Life in Enlightenment Scotland: Care and Teaching at the Royal Infirmary of Edinburgh.* New York: Cambridge University Press.

Rivett, Geoffrey. 1986. *The Development of the London Hospital System, 1823–1982.* London: King Edward's Hospital Fund.

Roemer, Milton I. 1962. "General Hospitals in Europe." In *Modern Concepts of Hospital Administration,* ed. Joseph K. Owen. Philadelphia: W. B. Saunders.

Rosen, George. 1974. "The Hospital: Historical Sociology of a Community Institution." In *From Medical Police to Social Medicine: Essays on the History of Health Care,* ed. George Rosen. New York: Science History Publications.

Rosenberg, Charles E. 1987. *The Care of Strangers: The Rise of America's Hospital System.* New York: Basic Books.

Stevens, Rosemary. 1989. *In Sickness and in Wealth: American Hospitals in the Twentieth Century.* New York: Basic Books.

Vogel, Morris J. 1980. *The Invention of the Modern Hospital, Boston, 1870–1930.* Chicago: University of Chicago Press.

Woodward, John H. 1974. *To Do the Sick No Harm: A Study of the British Voluntary Hospital System to 1875.* London: Routledge & Kegan Paul.

Yaggy, Duncan, and Hodgson, Patricia, eds. 1985. *Physicians and Hospitals: The Great Partnership at the Crossroads: Based on the Ninth Private Sector Conference, 1984.* Durham, NC: Duke University Press.

HUMAN DIGNITY

. . .

Few terms or ideas are more central to bioethics or less clearly defined than human dignity. Although the core idea of human dignity has to do with the worth of human beings, the precise meaning of the term is controversial. Respect for human dignity is an ethical mandate to which both sides of many bioethical debates appeal. For example, the state of Oregon legalized physician-assisted suicide by passing the Death with Dignity Act, but opponents claimed that legalizing that practice would undermine the dignity of elderly, disabled, and dying patients. Similarly, in response to claims that respect for the dignity of those patients demands the pursuit of cures through the production of embryos by means of cloning for embryonic stem cell research, others claim that producing human beings in embryonic form and destroying them for the benefit of others is an affront to human dignity.

Views of Dignity

This term also is surfacing more frequently in important bioethical and other public documents. It has played a role in the constitutions of a politically diverse array of countries, including Afghanistan, Brazil, Canada, Costa Rica, the former Federal Republic of Germany, Greece, Guatemala, Ireland, Italy, Nicaragua, Peru, Portugal, South Korea, Spain, Sweden, and Turkey. In some of those countries, such as Germany, the role of human dignity is substantial. Affirming that "the dignity of the human being is inviolable," the German constitution recognizes various human rights that the law must respect. Even in countries where the term has not been influential in constitutional language, it has come to play an important role. For example, the U.S. Supreme Court has employed the term in its deliberations over the meaning of the First, Fourth, Fifth, Sixth, Eighth, and Fourteenth Amendments to the Constitution.

International documents that are relevant to issues in bioethics also have affirmed the critical importance of human dignity. The United Nations, whose charter celebrates the "inherent dignity" of "all members of the human family," issued a Universal Declaration of Human Rights in 1948 whose preamble contains the same language. Article 1 specifically affirms that "all human beings" are born "equal in dignity." Two other documents—the International Covenant on Economic, Social and Cultural Rights and the International Covenant on Civil and Political Rights—were joined to that document in 1966 to constitute the so-called International Bill of Rights. All three documents ground the various rights of all human beings in their human dignity. In line with this outlook, the Council of Europe's 1996 Convention on Human Rights and Biomedicine was designed explicitly to "protect the dignity" of "all human beings."

These documents reflect the primary sense in which human dignity is invoked today: as an attribute of all human beings that establishes their great significance or worth. The word *dignity* comes from the Latin words *dignitas* ("worth") and *dignus* ("worthy"), suggesting that dignity points to a standard by which people should be viewed and treated. Although the standard usually has an egalitarian bent today, in ancient Greece and Rome the standard more commonly was attached to inegalitarian traits such as physical prowess and intellectual wisdom, as exemplified in figures such as Hercules and Socrates. People differed in dignity according to the degree to which they manifested the relevant traits, and the honor due them varied accordingly. This sense of dignity persists today when one speaks of dignitaries who warrant special honor or behavior that is dignified or undignified. Dignity in this sense can increase or decrease, can be gained or lost (Spiegelberg).

Dignity can refer to something that is variable in other ways as well. There is a difference between having dignity, on the one hand, and having an awareness of dignity or being treated with dignity, on the other hand. Someone may not be aware of having dignity though possessing it nevertheless; someone may not treat people in a particular group as having dignity though they may possess it. Such variability, however, should not be confused with the contemporary concept of dignity that is beyond the perceptions or actions of particular individuals and is rooted in what all human beings have in common. This is the concept that typically is operative when human dignity is invoked as the basis for the ways in which human beings should be viewed or treated.

Respect for human dignity is connected to a virtue as well as an ethical standard. A virtue-oriented approach to human dignity may take different forms. For example, exhibiting human dignity (usually referred to simply as dignity) can be a virtue in a way that is reminiscent of the notion of dignified behavior discussed above. To say that certain people exhibit dignity or are dignified can be a way of commending their courageous attitudes or actions in the face of adversity. However, the virtue of human dignity may refer to a person's capacity to recognize and live in accordance with a particular standard of human dignity. This form of the virtue serves as a reminder of how important it is that respect for human dignity be lived out in practice rather than existing only as an abstract concept. Exercising such a virtue still requires specifying what human dignity is.

People most commonly view human dignity in one of two basic ways. Some see it as grounded in particular characteristics of human beings; others view it as attached to being human per se. Both understandings are examined below, and then this entry surveys some of the bioethical implications of those views. First, it is necessary to clarify the significance and meaning of the concept by noting arenas in which it has been denied.

Challenges to Human Dignity

In the twentieth century perhaps the most widely decried denial of human dignity took place under the fascist regime in Germany; this accounts for the emphasis on dignity in the German constitution and the international and European documents discussed above. Millions of people were forced to be subjects of experimentation against their will or were tortured or killed for other reasons. As a result, the importance of human freedom and bodily integrity became much clearer and the danger of compromising them in the interests of the larger society became widely evident.

A tension necessarily exists between the idea of human dignity and ethical outlooks, such as utilitarianism, that, at least in their more popular and influential forms, affirm human dignity only to the degree that doing so is recognized to be sufficiently beneficial. Although the good of society is important, it potentially can justify doing anything to certain individuals, no matter how destructive, unless some standard of human dignity prevents that from happening. From a utilitarian perspective, what ultimately matters is the benefit itself (e.g., pleasure or preference satisfaction), not the individuals who benefit.

Others who are not well disposed to the notion of human dignity reject its high regard for freedom of choice or bodily integrity. Those who are most skeptical about freedom of choice include some in the social and biological sciences. Psychiatrists and psychologists who follow Sigmund Freud, for example, argue that freedom of choice is an illusion: Choices are driven largely by unconscious and irrational forces. Behaviorists who follow B. F. Skinner see such freedom as illusory because in their view behavior is driven more by environmental stimuli than by freely willed choices. Some biologists are skeptical about attributing any

special dignity to humans because they are less impressed by any apparent differences between the abilities of people and animals to make free choices than they are by biological similarities between humans and animals. Those similarities go beyond the ability to experience pleasure and pain to encompass certain genetic, physiological, and other mental similarities.

Those who are skeptical about the high regard for bodily integrity in the notion of human dignity include so-called postmodernists and posthumanists. Postmodernists reject the "modernist" notion of a universally binding objective truth that has a wide range of implications for the ways in which people should be treated. Many postmodernists would characterize as oppressive the idea that certain applications of technology to the human body are inherently unethical (i.e., violations of human dignity). Posthumanists, in contrast, doubt the value of the human body. Bodily form is seen as an accident of history that eventually will be replaced through developments in cybernetics and artificial intelligence. According to this view, because human beings have no lasting significance, human dignity is an illusion.

Characteristics That Give Humans Dignity

In the face of such challenges there has persisted a widely shared commitment to human dignity: the conviction that human beings have a special worth that warrants respect and protection. The big question is: For what reason? Many people have addressed this question, and their responses are basically of two types. The first type of response maintains that human beings have dignity because of one or more characteristics that are typically human. This view can be traced back at least to Marcus Aurelius and earlier Stoic philosophers who held that human beings have a basic equality that is rooted in their common ability to reason. It can be spotted occasionally in later periods—for example in Renaissance thinkers such as Pico della Mirandola and Enlightenment philosophers such as John Locke.

A full-blown account of human dignity rooted in reason took on its most complete form in the work of Immanuel Kant, especially in his *Groundwork of the Metaphysics of Morals,* where he argues that "morality, and humanity so far as it is capable of morality, is the only thing which has dignity" (p. 102). In other words, human beings do not have dignity simply because they are human but because and to the extent to which they are capable of morality. Because for Kant "morality lies in the relation of actions to the autonomy of the will" (p. 107), he concludes that "autonomy is therefore the ground of the dignity of human nature" (p. 103). Simply put, human beings have dignity because autonomous reason rather than impulses or the pursuit of personal or social benefit governs their actions.

According to Kant's principle of autonomy, a human being "is subject only to laws which are made by himself and yet are universal" (p. 100). Both parts of this principle are essential. Moral decisions must be self-made rather than imposed by others, even by God, but they also must be decisions that could be made consistently and acted on by everyone rather than products of an individual's personal view of reality, as in postmodern autonomy. In Kant's words, "all merely relative" ends are excluded: "The principle of autonomy is 'Never to choose except in such a way that in the same volition the maxims of your choice are also present as universal law'" (p. 108). Because they have autonomy, human beings have dignity, as opposed to price: "Everything has either a price or a dignity. If it has a price, something else can be put in its place as an equivalent; if it is exalted above all price and so admits of no equivalent, then it has a dignity" (p. 102). Accordingly, human dignity requires that a human being be treated "never merely as a means" but "always also as an end" (p. 105).

Deryck Beyleveld and Roger Brownsword, among others, have tried to go beyond Kant and develop a reason-based approach to human dignity together with its implications for bioethics. They affirm Kant's attempt to root human dignity in people's reason and capacity to be moral agents, but they prefer to follow Alan Gewirth in adopting an understanding of agency that is focused more on choice. For Beyleveld and Brownsword "the essence of the dignity of agents resides in their capacity to choose, to set their own ends" (p. 5). Consequently, they prefer to see human dignity more as empowerment than as constraint. Whereas Kant's emphasis on people as "ends in themselves" fosters significant attention to limits on the ways in which people may be treated, even by themselves, these authors see the protection of each individual's right to choose as the primary mandate flowing from the rooting of human dignity in reason.

Despite the preoccupation with individual rights in many discussions of human dignity, especially in the West, the focus on the individual as opposed to the community is not inherent in the concept. A communitarian approach can champion human dignity in various ways. For example, it can establish respect for autonomy and choice as the hallmark of what should characterize a society. However, it also can promote a vision of how people should and should not be treated that limits individual choices.

Regardless of its individualistic or communitarian bent, any attempt to root human dignity in human characteristics

such as reason and autonomy faces at least two important hurdles. First, it is possible for a living human being to lack such characteristics yet still be recognized as a human being. Are there human beings who lack human dignity? If having human dignity requires possessing the ability currently to exercise moral capacity or autonomy, for example, those who have mental disabilities, are comatose, are children, or are still in the womb do not have human dignity even if they are recognized as human beings (Gaylin). Often these are the individuals who are most in need of the protection that a concept of human dignity is designed to give.

Proponents of autonomy-based approaches have tried to give at least partial status and protection to those human beings in various ways. For example, Gewirth ties the level of a being's moral status to the degree to which that being has the necessary characteristic or characteristics. However, if human dignity is something one either has or does not have, as is affirmed typically, and if autonomy is the characteristic on which human dignity is based, then anyone without true autonomy does not have human dignity. Beyleveld and Brownsword agree but think it possible to grant those persons moral status on the basis and to the degree to which they may be moral agents who have autonomy. However, in cases in which there is a significant possibility that beings with autonomy are present, many people would consider it better to recognize and respect their human dignity rather than giving partial respect even to the simplest life forms under the assumption that they may be autonomous beings.

The second hurdle for this approach to human dignity is the plausibility of holding that what matters about human beings can be reduced to specific characteristics. Kant, for example, has been criticized for reducing what ultimately matters about human beings to the mind—to the rational—for that demeans bodily existence, which is essential in matters of bioethics (Kass). In fact, the focus on characteristics is vulnerable to the very criticism that it uses against its alternatives: It reduces human beings to what people in general or a particular community values about them and so in principle invalidates ascribing human dignity to them. The view that a particular characteristic such as moral capacity or autonomy is a sufficient basis for granting human beings an exalted status called human dignity may seem intuitively plausible to many, but it does not seem so to others. Accordingly, this approach is "based upon an anthropological 'creed'—not necessarily a religious creed" (Hailer and Ritschl, p. 99).

Dignity Rooted in Being Human

Because basing human dignity on particular human characteristics has difficulties, it may be preferable to root that dignity in being human per se. One way to do that is to focus on a basis from which all characteristics may be said to flow, such as the human genetic code. The 1997 Universal Declaration on the Human Genome and Human Rights of the United Nations Educational, Scientific, and Cultural Organization, for example, affirms that all human beings are equal in dignity because of the underlying unity provided by the human genome. Although this commonality may suggest a basic equality in all human beings, it does not address the significance of all human beings.

If their significance cannot be rooted in who people are, that is, in the specific characteristics discussed above, perhaps it can be found in something or someone beyond themselves. One candidate would be the sort of universal force acknowledged in Buddhism (Inoue). Because that force is in all living things, though, whatever dignity it imparts is not particularly human. However, if there is a God who establishes a special relationship with human beings that confers special worth on them, all people may be said to have a dignity that is distinctively human.

No such account of human dignity has had greater influence than the one portrayed in the authoritative writings of several major religious traditions, in which human beings are described as the "image of God." In addition to its role within religious traditions such as Judaism (Cohn), Christianity (Moltmann), and Islam (Bielefeldt et al.), this account has had a substantial impact on public formulations of the concept of human dignity (Bayertz). For illustrative purposes, this entry will consider this notion as it appears in the Christian Bible, since much of the Bible's relevant content is shared by other religious traditions.

The Bible uses two basic terms for *image*: the Hebrew *tselem*/Greek *eikon* (generally translated as *image*) and the Hebrew *demut*/Greek *homoiosis* (generally translated as *likeness*). Although there have been attempts to distinguish the two terms, it generally is recognized that they are used almost synonymously throughout the Bible. Usually one or the other appears, but occasionally, as in the account of the original creation of humanity in Genesis, both are employed. The sense conveyed is that of an image that is truly representative of God (Bray). In this view human dignity is not tied to a claim that human beings are divine or inherently worthy apart from God, and it is not because of human autonomy independent of God that people assume the authority to declare their own worth. Instead, human dignity is grounded in humanity's unique connection with God, by God's own initiative. This connection has three aspects: creation, alienation, and renewal. The first two have special significance for human dignity as an ethical standard, and the third for human dignity as a virtue.

In terms of creation, Genesis 1 (with a reaffirmation in Genesis 9) indicates that the image of God attaches to that which is human as opposed to that which is animal or plant. As a human child was considered the *tselem* of a parent (Genesis 5) and a *tselem* in the ancient Near East could refer to a statue reminding people of a king's presence (Westermann), human beings were created to have a special, personal relationship with God that includes their being God's representative in the world. Accordingly, the Bible speaks of human beings not only as being created in the image of God but also as being the image of God. This is striking because images of God are strictly forbidden in the Bible (e.g., Deuteronomy 4). However, the consistent message is that people are not to fashion images to make God the way they want God to be any more than they are to be God themselves. They are to manifest God to the world in accordance with the way God has made them and continues to direct them to be.

There have been attempts to attach more specific content to being the image of God. Some have seen its essence as involving humanity's (like God's) ability to reason, relate to others, or rule the world. However, others have maintained that those interpretations are read into the biblical text rather than read from it. For instance, Genesis does identify creation in God's image as unique to human beings, as opposed to other living things, and does instruct people about their responsibility to exercise stewardship over the rest of creation. However, the second instruction, some note, is not part of the description of what creation in God's image is; it is a separate matter that exemplifies what can be expected of one who is created in God's image. Similarly, they add, it is not surprising to find rational and relational abilities in those created in God's image, but they are never identified as what constitute that image (Cheshire). Angels, for instance, appear to have similar abilities but never are identified as being created in God's image. The picture presented in the biblical writings is that human beings themselves, not particular attributes or functions, are through God's creation the image of God.

The Bible goes on to record, however, that human beings were not and never have been content simply to be who God made them to be. In deciding to do things their own way, to give in to the temptation to "be like God" on their terms rather than God's (Genesis 3), they have experienced alienation not only from God but also from their own best selves, other people, and the rest of creation. Their capacities to reason, relate, and rule well have been damaged severely (Psalm 14, expanded in Romans 1, 8), and people now seek to create images to worship (including themselves) because they have lost sight of the fact that they are images of

God created to reflect and direct worship toward God rather than to be worshiped themselves.

Even in this alienation human beings remain the images of God, for God will not allow all connection with their Creator to be broken. The ethical standard of respect for human dignity gains its force precisely from this ongoing connection, for those who are dealing with human beings are dealing in a significant sense with God. Killing an innocent human being is equivalent to destroying an image of God without warrant from God and for that reason is unacceptable (Genesis 9), as is the attempt to tear down a human image of God verbally through cursing (James 3). Human dignity as constraint thus joins human dignity as empowerment once alienation has occurred and protection of human beings has become necessary.

The ethical standard of respect for human dignity rooted in the biblical accounts of creation and alienation, as was noted above, is affirmed in various religious traditions, as is the virtue of recognizing the dignity of human beings in words and actions, along with the difficulty of doing that once one is alienated from God. What the remainder of the biblical story adds is a particularly Christian account of how that marred image of God can be renewed, and with it the ability to live out the virtue of human dignity. For alienation to be replaced by reconciliation—for renewal to occur—according to this account, people literally must undergo a new creation (2 Corinthians 5). They must recognize the hopelessness of their alienation, give up all attempts to improve their situation through their own (futile) efforts, and invite God to re-create them in the image of God revealed in Jesus Christ. Although the creation is new, the image on which it is based is not, for Christ is identified not only as the image of God but also as God who created humanity in God's image in the first place (Colossians 1).

The new creation is portrayed as both ontological and logical. It is ontological in that it is an event in time that involves a change in being; it is logical in that it involves a process that flows logically from that event. People become in practice who they already are in being. This is said to be God's doing—people "are transformed" into the image/likeness of Christ (2 Corinthians 3)—but it also requires them to "be who they are" and "put on the new self, created to be like God" (Ephesians 4).

When people are renewed "in the image of their Creator," the result is described in terms of not only renewed individuals but also a renewed community: "Here there is no Greek or Jew, circumcised or uncircumcised, barbarian, Scythian, slave or free" (Colossians 3). Differences no longer divide; they disappear or in some cases can even enhance

community, in which the human dignity of all is recognized. Those who are renewed images of God warrant no better treatment than does any other human being in this view because all human beings have human dignity by virtue of their original creation in God's image. However, those who are renewed images are characterized as increasingly more capable of exercising the virtue of human dignity than they would be otherwise.

God makes covenants with human beings, became a human being in Jesus Christ, retains that humanity eternally, died in humanity's place to pay the penalty for human rebellion against God, and will appear personally to bring humanity into an unending celebration of life with God, at which point people finally will understand all that being in the likeness of God entails (1 John 3). All these historical developments fill out the biblical account of human dignity but also rest on the basis that human beings are images of God, which some identify as the *essence* of what it means to be human (Berkouwer).

Rooting human dignity in being human, like basing it on specific human characteristics, faces at least two important hurdles. First, although it avoids the problematic idea that there could be human beings without human dignity, it begs the question of who is a human being. Does anyone with a human genome qualify, and if so, how much of the human genetic code must be missing or nonfunctional before status as a human being is lost? Are certain capacities instead or in addition what constitute a human being, and if so, must the exercise of those capacities be actual or may it be potential?

The second hurdle for this approach also has to do with its plausibility. Those who reject the existence of God or the notion of the image of God necessarily reject this approach. Some go further and find the idea of according a special dignity to the human race per se to be a form of "speciesism" that is ethically akin to racism or sexism (Singer). Just as that critique is not necessarily a religious one, attempted refutations do not necessarily depend on religious argument (Chappell). In any case, as was noted above, every approach to human dignity rests on some form of an *anthropological creed* whose plausibility must be assessed.

Specific Implications for Bioethics

As has been suggested here, people most commonly invoke human dignity in situations in which the worth of human beings is brought into question when they are used, forced, or injured. Human beings should not be used because their dignity requires that they be treated as having intrinsic, not merely instrumental, worth. They should not usually be forced because their dignity mandates that their wishes be respected. They should not normally be injured because their dignity entails that their well-being be preserved.

In some bioethical issues these dignity-related concerns argue persuasively against other considerations and typically claim to trump them. For example, in evaluating a form of human experimentation people commonly insist on obtaining the informed consent of participants lest the participants' dignity be violated when something is done to them against their wishes. No amount of benefit to society warrants such a violation. In matters of resource allocation some people invoke human dignity to argue that the allocation producing the greatest overall social benefit is not the right one if the burden that certain individuals must bear to bring it about is too heavy. Not only may some people be injured, the very process by which anything can be done to them if it results in greater benefit to society is demeaning. Human dignity also is invoked to protest the injury involved in human cloning for reproductive purposes as long as animal studies show that attempts to clone humans almost certainly would result in the birth of children who eventually would develop serious deformities.

In other bioethical debates human dignity is not so unambiguously on one side of the issue. The reason for this is that more than one anthropological creed is influential, leading to competing conceptions of human dignity. Sometimes the clash involves a conflict between those concerned about injuring people and those concerned about forcing people. In the debate over abortion, for instance, people who consider the freedom to choose as central to human dignity often see no conflict. In regard to the mother and the fetus there is only one human being with the ability to choose, and so her decision prevails. Opponents of abortion with a different view of anthropology may hold that two human beings are present. Accordingly, they see the situation as a conflict between two affronts to dignity in which a greater violation would be done by fatally injuring the unborn child than would be done by forcing the mother to carry the child to term. The debate over embryonic stem cell research can be construed similarly, with supporters championing the dignity (choice) of researchers and the potential beneficiaries of the research and opponents decrying the greater violation that would occur if embryonic human beings were destroyed.

Other bioethical debates are even more complicated in that two elements of human dignity—preventing people from being injured and preventing people from being used—are in conflict with a third element: preventing people from being forced. For this reason the groups of people on each side of these debates are not the same groups as those in the debates mentioned above. For example, in the debate over germline intervention to enhance future generations of human beings those who see the only threat to human dignity as the limitation of people's choices tend to favor giving parents and society freedom to pursue such avenues. Others, more concerned to protect people against injury even if their choices are limited in the process, identify a threat to human dignity in subjecting young human beings to such procedures when the potential negative effects of genetic alterations for enhancement purposes are not well understood. That opposition is strengthened for many by seeing not just the potential injury involved but also the fact that the people doing the enhancement unacceptably use other human beings by altering them to exhibit traits that parents or society may like but that the ones who are altered may not. Similar issues arise in the debate over the genetic determination of human beings through cloning; the indignity involved is made worse for some if the cloning is done with the intentional injury, that is, death, of the cloned embryo in view.

In end-of-life debates a similar complex of considerations involving human dignity commonly arises. On one side are those who insist that human dignity requires that people have all choices open to them at the end of their lives, including physician-assisted suicide. On the other side are those concerned that the dignity of patients will be demeaned by overt or subtle pressures to give up their lives or by the necessity for them to justify their continued existence in the face of familial and societal burdens. As some see it, patients who are mentally disabled may even be injured directly by inadequate treatment or acts of euthanasia.

Conclusion

Human dignity plays a significant role in many bioethical debates. Because human dignity can be invoked on both sides of various issues, there is a pressing need for those who use that term to clarify what they mean by it. At some point they also need to defend the plausibility of the *anthropological creed* that underlies their view.

JOHN F. KILNER

SEE ALSO: *Aging and the Aged; Autonomy; Care; Compassionate Love; Competence; Confidentiality; Dementia; Death: Cultural Perspectives; Disability; Emotions; Environmental Ethics; Life, Quality of; Life Sustaining Treatment and Euthanasia; Moral Status; Palliative Care and Hospice;*

Reproductive Technologies; Research Policy; Transhumanism and Posthumanism

BIBLIOGRAPHY

Baker-Fletcher, Garth. 1993. *Somebodyness: Martin Luther King and the Theory of Dignity.* Minneapolis: Fortress.

Bayertz, Kurt. 1996. "Human Dignity: Philosophical Origin and Scientific Erosion of an Idea." In *Sanctity of Life and Human Dignity,* ed. Kurt Bayertz. Dordrecht, Netherlands: Kluwer.

Bednar, Miloslav, ed. 1999. *Human Dignity: Values and Justice.* Washington, D.C.: Council for Research in Values and Philosophy.

Berkouwer, G. C. 1975. *Man: The Image of God.* Grand Rapids, MI: Eerdmans.

Beyleveld, Deryck, and Brownsword, Roger. 2001. *Human Dignity in Bioethics and Biolaw.* New York: Oxford University Press.

Bielefeldt, Heiner; Brugger, Winfred; and Dicke, Klaus, eds. 1992. *Würde und Recht des Menschen.* Würzburg, Germany: Königshausen & Nevmann.

Bloch, Ernst. 1986. *Natural Law and Human Dignity,* tr. Dennis J. Schmidt. Cambridge, MA: MIT Press.

Bray, Gerald. 1991. "The Significance of God's Image in Man." *Tyndaly Bulletin* 42: 200–201.

Chappell, Tim. 1997. "In Defense of Speciesism." In *Human Lives: Critical Essays on Cosequentialist Bioethics,* ed. David S. Odenberg and Jacqueline A. Laing. London: Macmillan.

Cheshire, William P. 2000. "Toward a Common Language of Human Dignity." *Ethics and Medicine* 18(2): 7–10.

Chochinov, Harvey M. 2002. "Dignity-Conserving Care—A New Model for Palliative Care." *Journal of the American Medical Association* 287: 2253–2260.

Cohn, Haim H. 1983. "On the Meaning of Human Dignity." *Israel Yearbook on Human Rights* 13: 226–251.

Collste, Goran. 2002. *Is Human Life Special? Religious and Philosophical Perspectives on the Principle of Human Dignity.* Bern and New York: Peter Lang.

Du Toit, D. A. 1994. "Anthropology and Bioethics." *Ethics and Medicine* 10(2): 35–42.

Egonsson, Dan. 1998. *Dimensions of Dignity: The Moral Importance of Being Human.* Dordrecht, Netherlands: Kluwer.

Gaylin, Willard. 1984. "In Defense of the Dignity of Being Human." *Hastings Center Report* 14: 18–22.

Gewirth, Alan. 1978. *Reason and Morality.* Chicago: University of Chicago Press.

Gotesky, R., and Laszle, E., eds. 1970. *Human Dignity: This Century and the Next.* New York: Gordon and Breach.

Hailer, Martin, and Ritschl, Dietrich. 1996. "The General Notion of Human Dignity and the Specific Arguments in Medical Ethics." In *Sanctity of Life and Human Dignity,* ed. Kurt Bayertz. Dordrecht, Netherlands: Kluwer.

Hansson, Mats G. 1991. *Human Dignity and Animal Well-Being: A Kantian Contribution to Biomedical Ethics.* Stockholm: Almqvist & Wiksell.

Hill, Thomas E. 1992. *Dignity and Practical Reason in Kant's Moral Theory.* Ithaca, NY: Cornell University Press.

Inoue, T. 1988. "Dignity of Life." In *Human Dignity and Medicine, Proceedings of the Fukui Bioethics Seminar, Japan,* ed. Jean Bernard, Kinichiro Kajikawa, and Norio Fujiki. Amsterdam: Elsevier.

Kant, Immanuel. 1964 (1785). *Groundwork of the Metaphysics of Morals,* tr. H. J. Paton. New York: Harper and Row.

Kass, Leon R. 2002. *Life, Liberty and the Pursuit of Dignity: The Challenge for Bioethics.* San Francisco: Encounter Books.

Kavanaugh, John. 2001. *Who Counts as Persons?* Washington, D.C.: Georgetown University Press.

Kilner, John F.; Miller, Arlene B.; and Pellegrino, Edmund D., eds. 1996. *Dignity and Dying.* Grand Rapids, MI: Eerdmans.

Knoppers, Bartha M. 1991. *Human Dignity and Genetic Heritage.* Ottawa: Law Reform Commission of Canada.

Kolnai, Aurel. 1976. "Dignity." *Philosophy* 51: 251–271.

Meyer, Michael J. 1989. "Dignity, Rights and Self-Control." *Ethics* 99: 520–534.

Meyer, Michel J., and Parent, William A., eds. 1992. *The Constitution of Rights: Human Dignity and American Values.* Ithaca, NY: Cornell University Press.

Moltmann, Jurgen. 1984. *On Human Dignity: Political Theology and Ethics.* Philadelphia: Fortress.

Moser, Leslie E. 1973. *The Struggle for Human Dignity.* Los Angeles: Nash Publishing.

Peters, Ted. 2001. "Embryonic Stem Cells and the Theology of Dignity." In *The Human Embryonic Stem Cell Debate: Science, Ethics, and Public Policy,* ed. Suzanne Holland, Karen Lebacqz, and Laurie Zoloth. Cambridge, MA: MIT Press.

Pritchard, Michael S. 1972. "Human Dignity and Justice." *Ethics* 82: 106–113.

Pullman, Daryl. 2001. "Universalism, Particularism and the Ethics of Dignity." *Christian Bioethics* 7(3): 333–358.

Schachter, Oscar. 1983. "Human Dignity as a Normative Concept." *American Journal of International Law* 77: 848–854.

Singer, Peter. 1993. "Animals and the Value of Life." In *Matters of Life and Death,* 3rd edition, ed. Tom Regan. New York: McGraw-Hill.

Skinner, B. F. 1971. *Beyond Freedom and Dignity.* New York: Knopf.

Smith, Michael A. 1995. *Human Dignity and the Common Good in the Aristotelian-Thomistic Tradition.* Lewiston, NY: Mellen University Press.

Spiegelberg, Herbert. 1970. "Human Dignity: A Challenge to Contemporary Philosophy." In *Human Dignity: This Century and the Next,* ed. Rubin Gotesky and Ervin Laszlo. New York: Gordon and Breach.

Westermann, Claus 1984. *Genesis 1–11,* tr. John J. Scullion. Minneapolis: Augsburg.

INTERNET RESOURCE

Center for Bioethics and Human Dignity. 2003. Available from <http://www.cbhd.org>.

HUMAN EVOLUTION AND ETHICS

• • •

The idea of evolution—that all organisms living and dead come by a naturalistic process of development from one or just a few forms—dates to the eighteenth century, but it was not until 1859 that Charles Darwin (in his *Origin of Species*) proposed the causal mechanism that today is generally thought the main force behind evolutionary change. Noting the potential population explosion existing among animals and plants, Darwin argued that there will be an inevitable struggle for existence and that this in turn leads to a natural selection of the ones with certain advantageous features. *Adaptations* like the eye and the hand are, therefore, the key mark of living beings.

The earliest of evolutionists all saw humans as being part of the process—usually the end point of a progressivist march upwards, from the primitive to the complex. Darwin initially said little about *Homo sapiens,* not because he did not want to include them in the evolutionary picture, but because he wanted first to establish the main outlines of the general case. In 1871 he did turn explicitly to humankind, and in the *Descent of Man* he argued that humans are completely and utterly part of the natural, living world. Drawing on a secondary mechanism, sexual selection, Darwin argued that the differences between men and women and between races are adaptive, although generally less for the immediate needs of survival and reproduction and more for the competition for mates between humans themselves.

Hominid History

It was around the time of the publication of the *Origin of the Species* that the first evidence of fossil humans were uncovered, remains of so-called Neanderthal Man, although it was not until the end of the nineteenth century that bones of the first unambiguous link between humans and their ancestors were discovered (Java Man, by the Dutch doctor Eugene Dubois). Since then a great deal of evidence has been unearthed about humans and their ancestors—the *hominids.* Most famously there is Lucy, *Australopithecus afarensis,* a being that lived in Africa about 4 million years ago, that walked upright and yet had an ape-size brain.

Modern thinking—based both on fossils and on molecular evidence—is that humans and the great apes (especially gorillas and chimpanzees) broke apart about 6 million years ago (Lewin). Most likely humans are more closely related to chimps than they are to gorillas. There was an upward growth of brain to the present size (about 1200 cubic centimeters), although there was a fair amount of diversification rather than one single line leading just to humans. Apparently all modern humans came from Africa about 150,000 years ago and are probably not related directly to the Neanderthals (who, incidentally, had slightly larger brains than present day humans). Sophisticated powers of speech are probably fairly recent (some argue that that was the key advantage of *Homo sapiens* over the Neanderthals), and full-blown culture and agriculture is very recent—only 10,000 years or more old.

Social Adaptations

As Darwin noted in the *Descent of Man,* apart from speech, one of the most distinctive aspects of humankind is that they are ethical beings. Humankind has a sense of right and wrong, and thus is led to act morally or ethically. Humans do things for others because they think them right rather than simply because they appeal to the self-interest of the doer. In fact sometimes people do things that are very much not in their own self-interest, like attempting to save a drowning child from a rapid river. If one takes a hard-line Darwinian position, arguing that adaptations are produced by selection to aid their possessors—I have eyes and hands because they help me—then the existence of the ethical sense is somewhat of a puzzle (Wright). Why do something for others when it puts the doer at risk? In the family situation, where the mother for instance aids her child, this is readily understandable. If the child does not survive then the mother does not reproduce. But what about the cases in which there is no relationship? One does not jump into the river only to save one's own children.

It has been stressed by students of animal behavior, especially by students of the behavior of higher organisms like the great apes, that there is no necessity to the appearance of an ethical sense and consequent behavior (Goodall,

1986). Ethical sense will not come into existence as a matter of course, even if the brain grows in size and power. There has to be a reason, and this reason most obviously is that this is an adaptation for social beings. There are great advantages to being social. Two or three can often do that which is impossible for one animal on its own—especially when the animals are foraging or hunting, practices that provide the high-protein supplies needed by organisms with high-maintenance adaptations like brains. At the same time, there are costs to being social, like the potential for spread of disease. Hence social animals tend to have (and need) special adaptations to exploit their sociality and to prevent the costs. Often, for instance, social animals have much better degrees of immunity against disease than do solitary animals.

Social animals—and humans are beyond all others, social animals—need abilities to help each other and at the same time to reduce intragroup strife. (It is for this reason that researchers often find that a better model for humans than close relatives like the orangutans—who are asocial—are less close relatives like the wolves—who are very social.) On the negative side, as one might say, humans are notable for not having very good physical methods of attack—their teeth, for instance, are puny besides those of chimpanzees. If one turns on a fellow human, the attacker is not very likely to rip the victim apart physically. Another important negative aspect of humans is the way in which the females do not come into heat or advertise their ovulation. There has been much discussion about the reason for this—sociobiologist Sarah Hrdy argues that a major reason for this behavior is that it keeps males guessing and hence in doubt about paternity, if they do not stay around and help with the family. Another reason obviously is that it keeps the group quieter and more stable—imagine trying to run complex social lives if women were often in heat.

On the positive side, a sense of morality is surely (in the opinion of Darwinian biologists) an adaptation for sociality. Organisms that take seriously their obligations to others are more stable and work together better than those that do not. Expectedly one finds what might at least be called proto-morality—with senior group members enforcing behavior—in other social animals, especially (as emphasized by ethologist Frans de Waal) the chimpanzees.

What sort of morality might one expect an evolutionary process to produce? Will it decide, for instance, between utilitarians and Kantians? Probably not, for it will be too coarse grained for that—giving just basic directions that will then be fleshed out by culture. Significant is that both utilitarians (like Peter Singer) and Kantians (like John Rawls) have welcomed an evolutionary approach. Rawls particularly points out that it solves the big lacuna in any social contract approach to morality, namely how did the contract get put in place in the first place. It was not a group of old men around a fire but the genes. "The theory of evolution would suggest it is the outcome of natural selection; the capacity for a sense of justice and the moral feelings is an adaptation of mankind to its place in nature. As ethologists maintain, the behavior patterns of a species, and the psychological mechanisms of their acquisition, are just as much its characteristics as are the distinctive features of its bodily strictures; and these patterns of behavior have an evolution exactly as organs and bones do. It seems clear that for members of a species which lives in stable social groups, the ability to comply with fair cooperative arrangements and to develop the sentiments necessary to support them is highly advantageous, especially when individuals have a long life and are dependent on one another. These conditions guarantee innumerable occasions when mutual justice consistently adhered to is beneficial to all parties." (Rawls, p. 502–503).

Altruism

The technical biological term for organisms giving to others, at cost to themselves, is *altruism* (Wilson, 1975). It is important to note that this is a metaphor—it does not necessarily mean the altruism to which one refers when speaking of a good person, as in: Mother Teresa showed great altruism towards the poor of India. Ants helping others in the nest would be called altruistic, even though (as against the literal sense) there is clearly no implication that the ants consciously set out to do the right thing. Human altruism, or goodness as one might say, is therefore a sub-class of the general biological notion of altruism.

But why have humans developed so elaborate a method of interacting as a moral sense? Why, unlike the ants, are humans simply not hard-wired? There is a simple reason. Being hard-wired has virtues—there is no need for learning. The cost however is high. One cannot regroup and do something else if the situation changes. An ant will behave instinctively even though (because of changed circumstances) it may be doing itself or its nest a harm. Generally this does not matter, because ants are produced cheaply—a queen can afford the loss of a few thousand. Humans on the other hand are beings that require a great deal of care and only a few can be produced. (Technically humans are K-selected as opposed to ants that are r-selected.)

Humans need the ability to respond to change, especially to change brought on by fellow species members. A moral sense allows humans to do this. They can assess different or changing situations and act in the best interests of themselves and their brood. As philosopher Daniel Dennett has pointed out, this fact diffuses the oft-brought charge that any evolutionary approach to ethics must fail because it presupposed that humans have no real choices, they are *genetically determined.* It is true that humans are part of the causal chain, but they have a dimension of freedom not possessed by the ants. (In a sense humans are like the rockets that can adjust to moving targets, whereas ants are like cheap rockets that cannot change direction once fired.)

Selfish Genes

How does selection bring on altruism (using this now in the biological sense)? There is much debate. After Darwin most biologists assumed that selection could work for the group and that morality would emerge automatically—a species member that helped another was thereby helping the species. Famous was the notion of *mutual aid,* promoted by the Russian-born anarchist, Prince Petr Kropotkin. In the 1960s there was a sea change in opinion (going back in fact to the insights of Darwin himself). It was pointed out that group selection (selection for the benefit of the group over the individual) was too open to cheating. A selfish individual could take advantage of others (Williams). Hence came what Richard Dawkins has labeled the *selfish gene* view of the evolutionary process—in some sense, all adaptations (including social and behavioral adaptations) must be related back to self-interest. If they do not help the individual first and foremost, they will be wiped out.

The selfish-gene way of thinking was applied very fruitfully to the problem of altruism. William Hamilton (1964a, 1964b) introduced the idea of *kin selection,* arguing that altruistic behavior could be a very good strategy if one is helping others who share the same copies of genes as oneself—one is thereby reproducing by proxy as it were. Most dramatically Hamilton solved the question of why sterile workers (always female) in the hymenoptera (ants, bees, and wasps) devote their lives to their nest mates. In the hymenoptera only females have two parents, hence females are more closely related to sisters than to offspring and so it pays to raise fertile sisters rather than fertile daughters. More generally Hamilton showed that in any animal, if the conditions are right, then altruism will come into being.

Robert Trivers introduced a more general mechanism, that can function between non related organisms (even organisms of different species). *Reciprocal altruism,* so-called, suggests that if one gets a benefit by helping others, especially if others will thereby be more likely to help in response,

then altruistic adaptations should come into play. Essentially, as Darwin himself realized, this is a case of: "If you scratch my back, then I will scratch your back." In complex, thinking animals like humans, one could expect this to be a powerful mechanism. There will be times—when one is young, old, or sick—when even the most powerful will appreciate aid. In conjunction with this will be memory, so that humans are able to enforce reciprocation, and learn quickly to exclude those who do not play the game. Those who receive and do not give will soon be excluded.

More generally the ideas and techniques of game theory have been applied profitably to questions of sociability generally and morality particularly (Maynard Smith 1982). Sophisticated models can now be built showing how and when particularly moral traits might be expected to emerge (Skyrms). At the same time, experimentation can show whether or not specific hypotheses are well-taken. There have, for instance, been serious studies on questions about when commitments are kept and when broken. Also on how people respond to fairness or the lack thereof.

Group Selection

Criticisms of this whole selfish-gene approach tend to be of two kinds. On the one hand, there are more philosophical objections. Mary Midgely objects that the whole point about morality is that it is not selfish, nor is it simply enlightened self-interest. Morality means giving without hope or expectation of reward. But this objection is to misunderstand both the theory and the metaphor. Selfish genes do not necessarily cash out as selfish people. In fact humans might operate more efficiently (in their biological interests) if what they do is done precisely because they do not think it self-centered. One must make a distinction between what Dawkins (1982) labels the *replicators* (the genes) and the *vehicles* (the whole organism). To speak of selfish genes is to say that selection makes characteristics that rebound ultimately on the actor. Genes themselves are neither selfish nor unselfish. They just are. Individuals (vehicles) might be selfish at times and (genuinely) altruistic at times. It just depends on the situation.

On the other hand, there are objections of a more biological nature. Every biologist recognizes that sometimes a group selective force might overcome the individual selective force. For instance in a constantly fragmenting and reuniting population (that is with many sub-populations forming and disappearing) and with strong pressure towards altruistic behavior, group attributes might emerge before they can be eliminated by individual forces—these attributes might persist by being merged into the whole group. It has been suggested that the maintenance of sexuality might result from such a group force (Maynard Smith, 1978). (Others however, including Hamilton, think that sexuality can be explained at the individual level [Hamilton et al.].)

In particular, with the human case, some think that a group selective force might be the key factor in altruism (human, literal altruism, that is). Biologist David Sloan Wilson and philosopher Elliott Sober argue this way. Illustrating their position with a short story by Stephen Crane, in which a group are caught in a life boat and can survive if and only if they all work together, Wilson and Sober conclude that only a group analysis will explain the successful outcome. Because of our ability to think and plan, humans can and do overcome the forces of individual selection and are shaped by group forces. "Behaving as part of a coordinated group is sometimes a life-or-death matter in which the slightest error—or the slightest reluctance to participate—can result in disaster for all. Situations of this sort—in which the members of a group are bound together by the prospect of a common fate—have been encountered throughout human evolution, with the important fitness consequences, so it is reasonable to expect that we are psychologically adapted to cope with them" (Sober and Wilson, p. 335–336). In 2002 Wilson extended his analysis to look at issues to do with the evolution of religion and its moral codes. He argues that something like the Calvinism of sixteenth century Geneva can be explained in terms of a kind of group selection, where adaptations appear for the benefit of the whole against the individual.

This is still very contentious. English sociobiologist John Maynard Smith argues that nothing here makes even probable the group selection hypothesis. He argues that even humans are unable to overcome the strong tug of the selfish gene. In the lifeboat case, there is no need to suppose other than that each individual saw that it was in his own interests to cooperate. As Ben Franklin said on signing the Declaration of Independence: "Gentlemen, we must all hang together or assuredly we shall all hang separately."

Conclusion

In conclusion therefore the best assessment is that evolutionary biology has brought many new insights to our thinking about human nature, including human moral nature. It would nevertheless be overly optimistic to think that we are even close to ending all debate or offering all the materials needed to solve all outstanding problems.

MICHAEL RUSE

BIBLIOGRAPHY

Darwin, Charles. 1859. *On the Origin of Species.* London: John Murray.

Darwin, Charles. 1871. *The Descent of Man.* London: John Murray.

Dawkins, Richard. 1976. *The Selfish Gene.* Oxford: Oxford University Press.

Dawkins, Richard. 1982. *The Extended Phenotype: The Gene as the Unit of Selection.* Oxford: W.H. Freeman.

De Waal, Frans. 1982. *Chimpanzee Politics: Power and Sex Among Apes.* London: Cape.

Dennett, Daniel C. 1984. *Elbow Room.* Cambridge, MA: M.I.T. Press.

Goodall, Jane. 1986. *The Chimpanzees of Gombe: Patterns of Behavior.* Cambridge, MA: Belknap.

Hamilton, William D. 1964a. "The Genetical Evolution of Social Behaviour I." *Journal of Theoretical Biology* 7: 1–16.

Hamilton, William D. 1964b. "The Genetical Evolution of Social Behaviour II." *Journal of Theoretical Biology* 7: 17–32.

Hamilton, William D.; Axelrod, R.; and Tanese, R. 1990. "Sexual Reproduction as an Adaptation to Resist Parasites." *Proceedings of the National Academy of Science, USA* 87(9): 3566–3573.

Hrdy, S. B. 1981. *The Woman that Never Evolved.* Cambridge, MA: Harvard University Press.

Kropotkin, Petr. 1902 (reprint 1955). *Mutual Aid.* Boston: Extending Horizons Books.

Lewin, R. 1993. *The Origin of Modern Humans.* New York: Scientific American Library.

Maynard Smith, John. 1978. *The Evolution of Sex.* Cambridge, Eng.: Cambridge University Press.

Maynard Smith, John. 1982. *Evolution and the Theory of Games.* Cambridge, Eng.: Cambridge University Press.

Midgley, M. 1979. "Gene-Juggling." *Philosophy* 54: 439–458.

Rawls, John. 1971. *A Theory of Justice.* Cambridge, MA: Harvard University Press.

Singer, Peter. 1981. *The Expanding Circle: Ethics and Sociobiology.* New York: Farrar, Straus, and Giroux.

Skyrms, B. 1996. *Evolution of the Social Contract.* Cambridge, Eng.: Cambridge University Press.

Sober, Elliot, and Wilson, David Sloan. 1997. *Unto Others: The Evolution of Altruism.* Cambridge, MA: Harvard University Press.

Trivers, Robert L. 1971. "The Evolution of Reciprocal Altruism." *Quarterly Review of Biology* 46: 35–57.

Williams, G. C. 1966. *Adaptation and Natural Selection.* Princeton, NJ: Princeton University Press.

Wilson, David Sloan. 2002. *Darwin's Cathedral: Evolution, Religion, and the Nature of Society.* Chicago: University of Chicago Press.

Wilson, E. O. 1975. *Sociobiology: The New Synthesis.* Cambridge, MA: Harvard University Press.

Wright, R. 1994. *The Moral Animal: Evolutionary Psychology and Everyday Life.* New York: Pantheon.

HUMAN GENE TRANSFER RESEARCH

• • •

Human gene transfer research (HGTR) involves the deliberate transfer of genetic material (naturally-occurring, genetically-modified, or synthetic DNA or RNA) into human subjects. Clinical success has come more slowly than was first predicted, but HGTR remains a fundamentally novel approach to medical practice. It may one day enable clinicians to cure genetic disorders at their source, as well as provide oncologists with tools designed to disable or cure specific cancers. Nonetheless, HGTR differs from other clinical modalities in a number of ways. It involves creating genetically novel organisms that are potentially both transmissible and pathogenic, and there is a risk that this could modify the human genome. Human gene transfer techniques may also be extended beyond therapy into other, more controversial, areas (Verma). Consequently, while HGTR continues to capture the public's imagination, it has received an unparalleled level of public oversight. However, only when HGTR finally achieves success will ethical concerns become real issues.

Basic Terminology and Methods

Two distinctions shape the analysis and practice of human gene transfer: between therapy and enhancement, and between somatic and germline cells. The first refers to the transfer's intended outcome. Researchers may seek to prevent or cure disease (therapy), or they may want to alter an individual's characteristics or capabilities (enhancement). The second refers to whether researchers, in order to achieve these ends, seek to alter nonreproductive (somatic) cells or reproductive (germline) cells. Somatic alteration would affect only the individual subject, while germline alteration would change genes passed on to an individual's offspring. As of 2003, federal regulatory bodies will only entertain somatic-cell gene transfer protocols conducted for preventing diseases or developing treatments (U.S. NIH).

Genetic material can be transferred to human subjects in different ways, but most methods share certain similarities. Many protocols can be classified as either *ex vivo* or *in vivo*. *Ex vivo* protocols obtain tissue cells from the subject, genetically modify them in the lab, and return them to the subject's body. *In vivo* protocols employ different techniques to introduce genetic material into a subject's body, hoping that it will reach the appropriate tissues. Most protocols to date have used disabled viruses as the *vector* for transferring genetic material, though other vectors are also under development. Information on how frequently different methods are used can be obtained from the "Human Gene Transfer Protocol List" compiled by the National Institutes of Health (NIH) Office of Biotechnology Activities (OBA).

Clinical Successes and Setbacks

Certain milestones and setbacks mark the progress of HGTR from 1989 through 2003. Within this period, over 545 human gene transfer protocols, involving over 4,000 patients, were registered with the OBA. The field was launched on May 22, 1989, when Steven A. Rosenberg, Michael Blaese, and W. French Anderson injected genetically modified white blood cells into a male subject with advanced skin cancer. This protocol was not designed to intervene in his disease, but rather to track where the "marked" cells went in his body. The first protocol that sought a therapeutic outcome began on September 14, 1990, when W. French Anderson and colleagues transferred genetically modified white blood cells to Ashanti DeSilva, a four-year-old girl with severe combined immune deficiency (SCID). Ashanti's immune system was strengthened, but her underlying condition was not cured. Throughout the 1990s no other protocol was able to report clinical efficacy.

The first unambiguous clinical successes were reported in the spring of 2000. In April 2000 the French researchers Marina Cavazzano-Calvo and Alain Fischer reported that two baby boys (a number later raised to nine) with a version of SCID had normal immune systems ten months after receiving cells that were genetically modified to replace a missing gene. In March 2000 Katherine A. High and Mark A. Kay reported that subjects with hemophilia B experienced an increase in factor IX protein activity for at least six months after the gene transfer.

Yet this long awaited clinical progress has been tempered by setbacks. In December 2002 a subject in the hemophilia-B study developed signs of liver injury, halting the trial. The same trial was briefly halted in December 2001 when the gene-carrying virus was found in subjects' semen, raising the specter of inadvertent germline gene transfer.

And in January 2003 the second of the nine boys treated in France developed a leukemia-like illness.

More troubling for the field was the death of Jesse Gelsinger. On September 17, 1999, Gelsinger, an 18-year-old subject, died from a gene transfer experiment being conducted at the University of Pennsylvania's Institute for Human Gene Therapy. Gelsinger was affected by ornithine transcarbamylase (OTC) deficiency. Patients with OTC deficiency lack an enzyme needed for processing nitrogen with the result that toxic levels of ammonia accumulate in their bloodstreams, leading to severe mental impairment and even death. But Gelsinger's symptoms were manageable so that, unlike subjects in other gene transfer trials, he approximated a healthy volunteer. The viral vector used in this protocol was an adenovirus—a virus that usually causes the common cold. Although used in many protocols prior to Gelsinger's death, in his case the vector triggered a deadly immune response. An inquiry into his death resulted in severe sanctions against the University of Pennsylvania and the researchers involved, and it revealed major problems with HGTR oversight and conduct nationwide.

Public Oversight of Human Gene Transfer Research

HGTR is overseen in the United States by two agencies within the Department of Health and Human Services: the NIH and the Food and Drug Administration (FDA). While FDA review is "public" insofar as it involves federal oversight, NIH review through the Recombinant DNA Advisory Committee (RAC) is truly a forum open to the public. This aspect is unique to HGTR and reflects its historical development.

EARLY CONCERNS ABOUT "GENETIC ENGINEERING."
Serious debate about human gene transfer began in the 1960s, when scientists, theologians, and philosophers raised many concerns about *genetic engineering,* or *genetic manipulation.* Theoretical concerns evolved into real possibilities in 1972 when scientists discovered how to combine genetic material from different organisms. Recognizing that biologically novel organisms created through these techniques could, if inadvertently released, imperil the environment, individuals, or society, the scientific community called for a voluntary moratorium on this research—referred to as *recombinant DNA research* or *rDNA*—until safety issues could be assessed (Berg et al., 1974). The 1974 moratorium was lifted after leading scientists met in Asilomar, California, and issued strict guidelines for the safe conduct of rDNA in 1975 (Berg et al., 1975).

The self-imposed scientific moratorium on rDNA research unnerved the public, who were already disenchanted by a decade of research scandals. In response to these scientific and public concerns, the NIH established the RAC, on October 7, 1974. The RAC embodied a novel approach to federal oversight of a novel biotechnology. Because concerns about rDNA were societal as well as scientific, the RAC was staffed by both scientists and nonscientists, and its meetings were open to the public. In 1976 the RAC issued its first set of guidelines. These guidelines focused on laboratory safety and containment, required federally funded institutions conducting rDNA research to establish an Institutional Biosafety Committee (IBC), and required all rDNA research to be reviewed first by the local IBC and then by the RAC.

HGTR OVERSIGHT.
The RAC's early work focused on laboratory research that created recombinant organisms, and on work with animals and plants. As safety concerns raised by specific novel techniques were allayed, the RAC regularly shifted oversight responsibility to the IBCs.

By 1983 the RAC's attention had turned to HGTR. This shift was catalyzed by a number of events that captured public attention, including two unauthorized and scientifically ill-founded human gene transfer experiments (the 1970 case of Dr. Stanfield Rogers and the 1980 case of Dr. Martin Cline) as well as the controversial decision in *Diamond v. Chakrabarty,* allowing the patenting of genetically engineered organisms (for further information on these cases, see Walters and Palmer). One of the most important outcomes of these events was the 1982 publication of *Splicing Life,* a report on human gene transfer issued by the President's Commission for the Study of Ethical Problems in Medicine and Biomedical and Behavioral Research. The commission argued that only transfer into somatic tissues to prevent or treat disease could be justified.

The President's Commission also recommended that the RAC broaden its responsibilities to include HGTR—and to attend to ethical and social implications as well as safety concerns. In 1983 the RAC created the Working Group on Human Gene Therapy (later renamed the Human Gene Therapy Subcommittee) to develop guidelines for human rDNA research and to review protocols (Walters, 1991). By 1985, this working group had produced "Points to Consider," the first version of the guidelines that would eventually govern HGTR.

CLINICAL TRIALS AND CHALLENGES TO PUBLIC OVERSIGHT.
In April 1988 the RAC received its first actual human gene transfer protocol, and federal oversight of HGTR began. The field grew cautiously at first, and then

exponentially, moving quickly from work with single-gene disorders to cancer research (Ross et al.).

By 1995 the NIH was spending $200 million per year (2% of its budget) on HGTR. Harold Varmus, the director of NIH, commissioned two reports on the state of the field. The first, coauthored by Stuart H. Orkin and Arno G. Motulsky, criticized researchers for exaggerating prospects for therapeutic success. They argued that more basic research was needed before moving to and investing in clinical trials. The second assessed the work of the RAC and concluded that the committee continued to serve important functions (Verma).

From the outset, RAC oversight of HGTR was contested. As early as 1990, RAC review was assailed for delaying vital medical research (U.S. NIH-RAC; Culliton). Biotech companies objected to the public nature of RAC review, while researchers felt that RAC review unnecessarily duplicated FDA review, which holds statutory authority for such approval. Human gene transfer protocols, unlike other areas of research, must be reviewed both by the RAC and by the FDA, either simultaneously or sequentially. At the FDA, responsibility for human gene transfer lies with the Center for Biologics Evaluation and Research (CBER), and review focuses on the safety and efficacy of rDNA products, the safety of the manufacturing process, and the control of the final product (Coutts). To protect proprietary interests, CBER review is closed, and it cannot, by charter, address the ethical or social implications of research. The FDA has developed its own "Points to Consider" document to advise investigators (U.S. FDA, 1998).

In 1996, with the urging of biotech lobbyists, researchers, and politically powerful patient activists, Varmus proposed to abolish the RAC, and only overwhelming public support for the RAC averted its demise. Although not abolished, the RAC was downsized and could no longer recommend approval or disapproval of specific protocols. From 1996 through 2000, the RAC reviewed approximately 10 percent of the HGTR proposals submitted to the NIH (those proposing novel methodologies) and convened occasional Gene Therapy Policy Conferences.

THE AFTERMATH OF THE GELSINGER CASE. The Gelsinger case revealed major problems with the oversight of HGTR. A primary finding concerned the reporting of adverse events (bad reactions or deaths during a human gene transfer experiment). According to the NIH Guidelines, all adverse events must be reported in a timely fashion to the RAC, but Gelsinger's investigators failed to report three adverse events to the FDA in a timely manner. Moreover, only 37 of 970 adverse events that occurred between 1993 and 1999 in trials using the adenovirus vector (approximately 25% of the HGT protocols underway at that time) were properly reported to the NIH (Walters, 2000)—these adverse events were reported to the FDA, but not relayed to the RAC.

The inquiry also uncovered problems in the informed-consent process. The informed-consent document given to subjects in Gelsinger's protocol differed from the one approved by the RAC and FDA, and it did not mention adverse events in animal studies. Public reporting about HGTR had led the Gelsingers to believe that patients had been cured by "gene therapy," and they reported that the investigators had led them to believe subjects in their particular protocol had experienced clinical benefit. Finally, adverse events experienced by other subjects in the protocol were not communicated to the Gelsingers, as required by federal guidelines (Stolberg). Ironically, the RAC's attention to informed consent was one reason given by Varmus for abolishing it (Marshall).

The Gelsinger case led to Congressional inquiries, multiple hearings, and soul-searching at the NIH and FDA. The RAC provided a unique and crucial forum for gathering, analyzing, and publicizing information relevant to this crisis. This resulted in two notable outcomes: (1) the FDA formally agreed to inform the NIH of all adverse events reports it received, and (2) the Advisory Committee to the Director of the NIH recommended that the RAC receive novel protocols at an earlier stage in their development—namely, prior to submission to the IRB and FDA.

Ethical Issues in Human Gene Transfer Research

Early ethical and social concerns surrounding HGTR were outlined in 1985 in the NIH's "Points to Consider." Since then, broader public and commercial contexts of HGTR have raised additional concerns, especially involving subject recruitment and economic conflicts of interest. These issues become increasingly important as HGTR moves toward new applications and methods.

THE ETHICAL COMMITMENTS OF THE "POINTS TO CONSIDER." The "Points to Consider in the Design and Submission of Protocols for the Transfer of Recombinant DNA Molecules into One or More Human Subjects" consists of over 100 specific questions that HGTR investigators must address for RAC approval (U.S. NIH, Appendix M). The RAC Working Group on Human Gene Therapy tested the document and developed its process of protocol review by working through a prototype HGTR protocol submitted in April 1987 by a team led by W. French Anderson (Walters and Palmer).

The ethical commitments of the "Points to Consider" reflect its historical context. The document reflects both the RAC's involvement with debates surrounding rDNA and a decade of national deliberations on the use of human subjects in biomedical research (Juengst). Its ethical framework hinges on six moral concerns. The first three derive from specific concerns about rDNA technology:

1. the need for special biosafety precautions;
2. the need for public participation in genetic research policy; and
3. potential broad and long-range research consequences (Juengst).

The final three concerns reflect the *Belmont Report*'s three central principles (beneficence, respect for the person, and justice) and the federal guidelines for the protection of human subjects issued in 1981:

4. clinical benefit to subjects;
5. free and informed consent by subjects; and
6. fair subject selection (Walters and Palmer; Juengst).

The RAC deliberations based on the "Points to Consider" tended to focus primarily on issues of safety and informed consent. Biosafety concerns focused on whether genetically modified viral vectors might be *shed*, or infect others who come into contact with research subjects. There was concern that viral vectors might revert to *wild-type* strains and become *replication competent*—that is, capable of replicating and infecting subjects or others in unanticipated ways. Further, might transferred genetic material integrate into the wrong place in the subject's genome, thus causing cancer (a hypothesized cause for the illnesses seen in the French SCID boys)? Might it inadvertently integrate into the subjects' germline tissues and be transmitted to their descendants? Scientific and clinical questions further attended to the risks particular protocols might present to subjects themselves. Nonscientific members (patient advocates, ethicists, attorneys) consistently raised concerns about informed consent and subject recruitment.

THE CHALLENGE OF RECRUITMENT. There are also important concerns about subject recruitment. HGTR initially targeted only life-threatening, incurable conditions for which no other effective therapy existed. Theoretical benefits to these subjects were believed to outweigh any possible risks. Initially, disease candidates included only single-gene disorders. By 2002, however, the pool of disease candidates had expanded to include cancers (64% of all protocols), HIV, peripheral artery disease, rheumatoid arthritis, and erectile dysfunction (U.S. NIH-OBA).

Subjects with life-threatening, incurable conditions are often in desperate straits, and it is not clear that consent can be truly voluntary in such situations? Too often, subjects misunderstand experimental protocols as their last or only *hope*, or as *therapy*, when in fact most human gene transfer trials are designed only to test safety, not efficacy. Subjects are aided in this misunderstanding by informed-consent documents that describe experimental interventions as *treatment*, or that mention a possible *benefit*. This, coupled with the misleading label of *gene therapy*, has led the field to be redescribed more accurately as "human gene transfer research" (Churchill et al.)

Misunderstanding gene transfer as therapy has led to questions about fair access to protocols. Before the first protocol was launched, concerns were raised about how to decide which members of even a limited subject pool would have access to the *potential benefits* of the research. Such thinking climaxed in 1993 when, in response to political pressure, Bernadine Healy, then the director of the NIH, allowed researchers to enroll a subject in an unapproved human gene transfer protocol as a last-chance therapy on the basis of "compassionate use." This would not be the last time the RAC faced political pressure to alter protocol approval (Lysaught).

COMMERCIAL INTERESTS AND "ORPHAN DISEASES." Another important issue is that of rare diseases and commercial interests. Early advocates of HGTR emphasized that this novel methodology promised, at long last, to provide cures for some 4,000 single-gene disorders. Ashanti DeSilva was afflicted with just such a disorder. But investigators quickly began applying human gene transfer techniques to clearly non-Mendelian disorders (e.g., cancer). As of 2002 only 10 percent of human gene transfer protocols approved by the RAC involved monogenic disorders. Most monogenic disorders are quite rare, with a small market for eventual therapies, and those involved in HGTR have been accused of abandoning persons with genetic disorders in order to cash in on big market payoffs (Meyers; Anderson).

The Orkin-Motulsky panel raised concerns about economic incentives surrounding human gene transfer in 1995. Due to these incentives, they noted, virtually every NIH institute had created a gene transfer program, whether equipped to do so or not, and they cautioned that the rush to find the gold in HGTR might lead investigators to ignore the pursuit of other, easier-to-achieve, conventional treatments.

Commercial interests, and the potential for conflicts of interest, also emerged in the Gelsinger case and led to a renewed examination of the relationship between academic research and industry. In Gelsinger's case, the University of

Pennsylvania's Institute for Human Gene Therapy received one-fifth of its $25 million annual budget from a company founded by the Institute's director, James M. Wilson. In return, the company had exclusive commercial rights to Wilson's discoveries. None of the subjects in the study had been informed of this relationship or this arrangement. In 2000 the American Society of Gene Therapy established a policy that its researchers should be free of significant financial involvement with companies that sponsor their studies.

FRONTIER ISSUES. Although HGTR has yet to achieve unambiguous clinical success, "frontier issues" such as prenatal gene transfer, nonrecombinant methods of DNA transfer, and the likelihood of enhancement merit mention.

Prenatal gene transfer might offer certain advantages, as early intervention might prevent the devastating effects of some conditions. The prenatal environment may provide better conditions for gene transfer and facilitate sustained gene expression. It could also offer parents at risk for conceiving a child with a genetic disorder an actual therapeutic alternative to selective abortion or preimplantation genetic diagnosis. However, *in utero* research entails unknown risks to the fetus and mother and raises the real possibility of germline modification (Fletcher and Richter). In January 1999 the RAC concluded (based on a Gene Therapy Policy Conference) that allowing prenatal gene transfer research would be premature. However, the RAC indicated its willingness to entertain *in utero* gene transfer protocols if current scientific questions were to be addressed (U.S. NIH-RAC).

Jesse Gelsinger's death and setbacks in the French SCID and hemophilia trials raised anew concerns about the risks of viral vectors. Researchers are therefore pursuing alternative methods of DNA transfer, including approaches that do not involve DNA recombination. Microinjection, where DNA or RNA is directly injected into a cell's nucleus using a glass pipette, is currently used for germline modification in animal research. A similar approach involves the injection of *naked DNA* (DNA not contained within a vector) directly into tissues. Another protocol uses high pressure to push short DNA sequences into graft tissue. Others suggest attaching DNA to other macromolecules, such as liposomes. These complexes can navigate cell membranes without the risks posed by viral vectors. And yet others are developing methods of inserting not just genes but entire *artificial chromosomes*. While these approaches may reduce certain safety concerns, they may also introduce others. For example, transmission of artificial chromosomes to offspring via germline integration raises questions about the creation of individuals with more than the standard complement of forty-six chromosomes. How does this challenge our understanding of what it means to be human? Moreover, given our limited knowledge of chromosomal interaction and gene mutation, the long-term consequences of such modifications cannot be known.

Finally, researchers clearly have an interest in pursuing gene transfer for enhancement purposes. The same techniques used for legitimate medical therapies could be used for decidedly non-therapeutic purposes by athletes for example, looking for a competitive advantage. Somatic-cell interventions might be able to strengthen muscles and bones or boost oxygen efficiency, while germline enhancements could provide a way for parents to engineer children with superior athletic skill. Researchers further anticipate developing techniques that will enable inserted genes to be "turned off" by an additional intervention if necessary. While such developments might prove therapeutically useful, they could also allow a mechanism for avoiding detection of genetic modifications. What responsibilities do researchers and physicians have with regard to such practices? Although clearly decades away at best, the World Anti-Doping Agency is taking this possibility quite seriously. With the advent of stem cell and cloning techniques, the prospect of gene transfer being used for enhancement purposes becomes increasingly probable. Certainly such applications of gene transfer technology raise serious questions about the just allocation of resources in a world where over 2 million people each year die from a lack of adequate sanitation and clean water and 44 million people in the U.S. remain without adequate health insurance.

Conclusion

The possibilities of prenatal or germline gene transfer and genetic enhancement suggest that the need for public oversight of HGTR is far from over. Initial safety and societal concerns surrounding rDNA research and HGTR have not materialized, in part because the research has received careful scrutiny and oversight in a public forum that has earned respect through hard work and responsiveness to changes in its social and scientific contexts. Unlike other biotech developments, HGTR is not perceived as being driven solely by the momentum of the market, with technology racing ahead of society's moral compass. Nor has it become intractably polarized. Public oversight has provided both a forum for discussing ethically controversial applications of human gene transfer and a mechanism for exercising prudence and caution.

Public oversight of HGTR also provides a unique venue for addressing concerns that are not unique to HGTR, but are applicable to the practice of scientific research in general. These include concerns about the commercial influence on scientific research, the practice of informed consent, and about vulnerable patients. But because it proceeds in public view, HGTR may serendipitously lead to significant improvements in the conduct of human-subjects research in the United States and throughout the world.

M. THERESE LYSAUGHT

SEE ALSO: *Genetic Engineering, Human; Genetics and Human Self-Understanding; Public Policy and Bioethics*

BIBLIOGRAPHY

Anderson, W. French. 1994. "Yes, Abbey, You Are Right." *Human Gene Therapy* 5(October): 1199–1200.

Berg, Paul R., et al. 1974. "Potential Biohazards of Recombinant DNA Molecules." *Science* 185(July): 303.

Berg, Paul R.; Baltimore, David S.; Brenner, Sidney; et al. 1975. "Summary Statement of the Asilomar Conference on Recombinant DNA Molecules." *Proceedings of the National Academy of Sciences U.S.A.* 72(6): 1981–1984.

Churchill, Larry R.; Collins, Myra L.; King, Nancy M. P.; et al. 1998. "Genetic Research as Therapy: Implications of 'Gene Therapy' for Informed Consent." *Journal of Law, Medicine, and Ethics* 26(1): 38–47.

Coutts, Mary Carrington. 1994. "Scope Note 24: Human Gene Therapy." *Kennedy Institute of Ethics Journal* 4: 63–83.

Culliton, Barbara J. 1990. "Conflict at the RAC." *Science* 248(4952): 159.

Fletcher, John C., and Richter, Gerd. 1996. "Human Fetal Gene Therapy: Moral and Ethical Questions." *Human Gene Therapy* 7(13): 1605–1614.

Juengst, Eric. 1990. "The NIH 'Points to Consider' and the Limits of Human Gene Therapy." *Human Gene Therapy* 1(4): 425–433.

Lysaught, M. Therese. 1998. "Reconstruing Genetic Research as Research." *Journal of Law, Medicine, and Ethics* 26(1): 48–54.

Marshall, Eliot. 1996. "Varmus Proposes to Scrap the RAC" *Science* 272(5264): 94.

Meyers, Abbey S. 1994. "Gene Therapy and Genetic Diseases: Revisiting the Promise." *Human Gene Therapy* 5: 1201–1202.

Ross, Gail; Erickson, Robert; Knorr, Debra; et al. 1996. "Gene Therapy in the United States: A Five-Year Status Report." *Human Gene Therapy* 7(14): 1781–1790.

Stolberg, Sheryl Gay. 2000. "Youth's Death Shaking Up Field of Gene Experiments on Humans." *New York Times,* 27 January.

Thompson, Larry. 1994. *Correcting the Code: Inventing the Genetic Cure for the Human Body.* New York: Simon & Schuster.

U.S. National Institutes of Health, Recombinant DNA Advisory Committee. 1990. "Minutes of Meeting, February 5, 1990." *Human Gene Therapy* 1(4): 363–369.

Walters, Leroy. 1991. "Human Gene Therapy: Ethics and Public Policy." *Human Gene Therapy* 2(2): 115–117.

Walters, Leroy. 2000. "The Oversight of Human Gene Transfer Research." *Kennedy Institute of Ethics Journal* 10(2): 171–174.

Walters, Leroy, and Palmer, Julie Gage. 1997. *The Ethics of Human Gene Therapy.* New York: Oxford University Press.

INTERNET RESOURCES

American Society of Gene Therapy. 2000. "Policy of The American Society of Gene Therapy on Financial Conflict of Interest in Clinical Research (Adopted April 5, 2000)." Available from <http://www.asgt.org>.

Orkin, Stuart H., and Motulsky, Arno G. 1995. "Report and Recommendations of the Panel to Assess the NIH Investment in Research on Gene Therapy, December 7, 1995." NIH Office of Biotechnology Activities. Available from <http://www4.od.nih.gov/oba>.

U.S. Food and Drug Administration, Center for Biologics Evaluation and Research. 1998. "Guidance for Industry: Guidance for Human Somatic Cell Therapy and Gene Therapy." Available from <http://www.fda.gov/cber>.

U.S. Food and Drug Administration, Center for Biologics Evaluation and Research. 2000. "Human Gene Therapy and The Role of the Food and Drug Administration, September 2000." Available from <http://www.fda.gov/cber>.

U.S. National Institutes of Health. 2002. "Guidelines for Research Involving Recombinant DNA Molecules (NIH Guidelines, April 2002)." NIH Office of Biotechnology Activities. Available from <http://www4.od.nih.gov/oba>.

U.S. National Institutes of Health, Office of Biotechnology Activities. 2002. "Human Gene Transfer Protocol List." Available from <http://www4.od.nih.gov/oba>.

Verma, Inder 1995. "Report of the Ad Hoc Review Committee: The Recombinant DNA Advisory Committee, September 8, 1995." NIH Office of Biotechnology Activities. Available from <http://www4.od.nih.gov/oba>.

HUMAN NATURE

• • •

Theories of human nature offer systematic and comprehensive accounts of human beings' most significant distinguishing characteristics. Such accounts are central in people's perennial attempts to organize their understandings of the cosmos; to figure out their relation to God, to nature, and to each other; and to uncover the possibilities, meanings, and purposes of human life.

Western Understanding of Human Nature

Modern Western theories of human nature, which will be the focus of this essay, typically differ from their classical and medieval predecessors in appealing to the findings of a variety of life and social sciences, including anthropology, medicine, physiology, psychology, economics, sociology, and even ethology. Nevertheless, although these sciences undeniably help us to understand specific aspects of human life, even contemporary theories of human nature are never simply summaries of the results of empirical research—despite their frequent claims to scientific authority.

One reason that theories of human nature are not simply generalizations from the conclusions of scientific study is that they enter into empirical investigations not only as conclusions but also as presuppositions, structuring the conceptual frameworks within which research programs are conducted. Contemporary psychological investigation, for instance, proceeds with a variety of models of the human mind, including the Freudian, the behaviorist, the existentialist or humanist, and the computer models. Empirical research cannot fully evaluate the adequacy of its own framework relative to others; determining the adequacy of an entire framework requires reference to considerations beyond empirical data, including how the framework coheres with other respected theories and even its moral and political implications.

A related reason that theories of human nature go beyond ordinary scientific claims is that typically they aspire to provide a comprehensive conceptual framework that will render coherent the contributions of all those disciplines and discourses that investigate various aspects of human life. These often represent human beings in ways that, at least on the surface, appear quite incompatible with each other; for instance, lawyers assume that people ordinarily are responsible for their actions, while psychologists may suggest that people's behavior is determined ultimately by factors outside their control. Theories of human nature endeavor to resolve these incompatibilities in a variety of ways, ranging from reinterpreting the meaning of a discourse, such as the religious, to setting limits on the domain within which its claims are accepted; occasionally, a theory of human nature may even proclaim the invalidity of a whole realm of discourse, such as the parapsychological. Rather than simply summarizing the conclusions of the various life and social sciences, therefore, theories of human nature typically perform a regulatory function, authorizing some methodological approaches while delegitimating others.

Yet another respect in which theories of human nature differ from scientific theories, at least as science is ordinarily understood, is in the prominence of their normative or evaluative component. Even if one contends that all knowledge is to some degree value-laden, the evaluative element is far more evident in theories of human nature than it is, for instance, in modern theories of the physical universe. All theories of human nature provide a general account of human capacities and human needs, human potentialities and human well-being, and thus contain at least an implicit, and often an explicit, diagnosis of human malaise and a prescription for human flourishing.

Like all theoretical constructions, theories of human nature are developed in specific historical circumstances and are designed to address specific conceptual puzzles or practical concerns; consequently, they shift their emphasis according to the scientific, moral, and political preoccupations of the time. Despite variations in focus and emphasis, however, the Western project of understanding human nature historically has centered on two questions. The first of these addresses the human aspect of *human nature*: How can human be distinguished from nonhuman nature? The second addresses the natural aspect: How can what is natural for humans be distinguished from what is unnatural, abnormal, or artificial? The concerns inherent in these two questions constitute continuing themes that link the variety of Western inquiries into the nature of human beings.

Reflection on these themes reveals that the Western project of providing a systematic theory of human nature has been predicated historically on certain assumptions. They include the following: (1) that it is possible to discover specific qualities or features that characterize human beings universally and transhistorically; (2) that these characteristics decisively distinguish humans from all other beings, notably nonhuman animals; and (3) that, from the discovery of these characteristics, it is possible to derive specific prescriptions about the proper conduct of human life. In other words, the Western project of understanding human nature generally has been motivated by a desire to derive from it universal and unchanging values.

These assumptions went unquestioned and often unarticulated throughout most of Western history. Once they are made explicit, however, it is easy to see that they are all contestable; and we shall see how, in the nineteenth and twentieth centuries, each of them was contested. For instance, Karl Marx (1818–1883) and John Dewey (1859–1952) challenged the first assumption; Charles Darwin (1809–1882) and the twentieth-century sociobiologists challenged the second; and the theorists of positivism and neopositivism challenged the third.

Since the 1970s not only these assumptions but the whole project of developing a comprehensive theory of human nature has been subjected to more fundamental critiques, launched by poststructuralist or postmodern French writers such as Michel Foucault (1926–1984), Jacques Derrida (1930–), and Jean-François Lyotard (1924–). While these authors differ on many points, they are united in rejecting the possibility of any overarching philosophical framework capable of unifying and legitimating the specific disciplines. Such totalizing frameworks or discourses, they claim, reflect unrealizable aspirations to discover universal and absolute truths in morals, politics, or science. These authors deny that any genuinely universal truths can be found, and assert that claims to them typically are propounded by groups who wish to use them for promoting their own political agendas. Truth, they argue, is relative to specific discursive practices that are historically contingent and self-justifying. Consequently, there is no need for, as well as no possibility of, a *master* discourse designed to be the ground or foundation of these more specific discourses.

As described so far, the dominant tendency in Western thought has been to conceptualize human nature as both *universal* and *transhistorical.* Its conceptualizations typically take the form "All human beings throughout history have characteristics x, y, z," implying that x, y, and z are necessary, as well as universal, characteristics of human nature. However, the Western tradition also includes conceptions of human nature that are not universalistic although they are transhistorical. These *relational* theories take the form "Group x is inferior to group y with respect to characteristics x, y, z"; typically, relational theories are used to justify the dominance of one group over another. Finally, some Western conceptions of human nature are *historical* rather than transhistorical, used within theories that claim that as human cultures change, so do certain important human characteristics. Some theories contain elements both universal and relational—for example, the theories of Aristotle and the sociobiologists—or both transhistorical and historical—for example, the theories of Karl Marx and John Dewey.

Three Classic Western Approaches

ARISTOTLE. The origins of Western philosophy, in the sense of systematic and rational inquiries into the nature of reality, knowledge, and value, are often traced to the reflections of ancient Greek thinkers in the fifth and fourth centuries B.C.E. Plato (ca. 428–347) and Aristotle (384–322), two of the three philosophical giants of this period (the third being Socrates, ca. 470–399), developed systematic theories of human nature. Aristotle's view has been particularly influential on the Western tradition because it was incorporated into the Scholastic philosophy that dominated Europe

in the Middle Ages and early Renaissance, and continues to shape the thinking of the Roman Catholic Church.

Aristotle conceptualized human beings as complexes of soul and body. The soul was the distinctively human element—the essence or form or intelligible principle of the body—but it existed only in conjunction with a living human body. Aristotle's conceptualization of the soul as inseparable from its body contrasted with Plato's view that human beings were souls united only temporarily with bodies, but Aristotle also acknowledged the possibility of the actively knowing and thinking part of the soul, the mind or intellect, being "set free from its present conditions … immortal and eternal." When this happened, however, Aristotle asserted that the mind remembered nothing of its former embodied activity and, because all connection with a specific human body was thus lost, he did not regard the human soul as personally or individually immortal.

Aristotle's view of human nature, like Plato's, was *teleological,* which is to say that he regarded human beings, like other things in the world, as having a "function" or activity peculiar to them. He further assumed, again like Plato, that the good life, or *eudaimonia,* consisted in the successful or efficient performance of that function. For Aristotle, the distinctive function of human beings was reasoning, or "an active life of that which possesses reason," and so he inferred that the good life was one in which the rational part of the soul governed the appetitive or desiring part, thus avoiding excess and living in accordance with virtue.

For Aristotle, human beings were, by nature, political animals who needed to live in a community: "He who is unable to live in society, or who has no need of it because he is sufficient to himself, must be either a beast or a god." Within human communities, however, not everyone was capable of citizenship: The nature of some was to rule and of others to be ruled. Among those whose nature was to be ruled were children, barbarians, and Greek women; thus, while Aristotle posited a universal standard for human nature, he simultaneously asserted that some groups of humans were less than fully human. The theme of dominance and subordination runs not only through Aristotle's account of the relations between human beings but even through his account of the nature of individual humans. He compared the controlling relation between form and matter with the relation between male and female, and he asserted that the proper relation between mind and body was like that of master to slave.

AQUINAS. The dominant philosophical figure of the Middle Ages was Thomas Aquinas (1226–1274), later Saint Thomas, who synthesized Greek thought and church doctrine into a Christian philosophy. He conceptualized human nature in terms that were basically Aristotelian, with some (often Platonic) modifications made in order to adapt Aristotelian views to church doctrine.

Aquinas believed, like Aristotle, that there was a distinctive and essential human nature that could be understood teleologically; he also shared the Aristotelian belief that the good life or *eudaimonia* was action in accordance with this function. A proper understanding of the ends or purposes of human life was therefore essential to morality and should be achieved by discovering the precepts of *natural law*. Natural law, as Aquinas conceptualized it, was universal and unchanging. It described supposedly universal human tendencies, such as preserving life, but presented them not simply as empirical facts about human nature but also as manifestations of God's design for humanity. For Aquinas, therefore, natural law simultaneously described how things were and prescribed how they should be. It was discoverable by reason, which, because it gave insight into God's purposes, provided guidance on how humans should live.

Like Aristotle, Aquinas saw humans as combinations of soul and body, with the soul as the form of the body. To allow for the possibility of personal or individual immortality, however, Aquinas diverged from Aristotle, declaring that the soul was a "substantial" form, capable of existing separately from matter. Not only was personal immortality conceptually possible, according to Aquinas; it was humans' destiny. God would not have implanted the universal—and therefore natural—human desire to live forever unless this desire had an object.

While Aquinas shared the Aristotelian view that human nature had an end or purpose, he believed, in accordance with church doctrine, that this end was supernatural rather than natural: It was to spend eternity united with God in heaven, where alone perfect happiness might be enjoyed. Human life as we know it was no more than a preparation for life after death, and this world was simply a testing ground for the next. So long as humans inhabited this world, however, they should strive to live in accordance with natural law, which provided a test for the moral validity of the laws of the state.

DESCARTES. The thought of René Descartes (1596– 1650) is generally considered to mark the beginning of modern philosophy. Refusing to accept the authority of tradition, Descartes developed "rules for the direction of the understanding" and a "method for rightly conducting reason" designed to enable each individual to establish certain truth in science and philosophy. He wrote in the vernacular (French) as well as in Latin, in order to reach lay as well as clerical readers.

Descartes's conception of human nature was even more *dualistic* than that of Aristotle and Aquinas. Living human beings, for Descartes, were composed of two entirely different kinds of entities: souls, which were active, intellectual substances, immaterial and immortal; and bodies, which were unthinking, passive mechanisms, spatially extended and temporally finite. Individual humans were to be identified not with their bodies but with their souls, which were able to survive the death of the body. While Descartes's model allowed for the soul's separation from the body after death, it rendered problematic the relation of the soul to the body during life, since it was unclear how material and immaterial substances could have a causal influence on each other. Descartes never succeeded in providing a satisfactory explanation of mind-body interaction.

As a scientist, Descartes wanted his theory of human nature to be compatible with both the new developments in physical science and the doctrines of the Roman Catholic Church. He attempted to reconcile these two worldviews by postulating two spheres of reality, each governed by entirely different laws or principles. The laws of God governed spiritual or mental reality; the laws of science governed physical reality, understood by Descartes in mechanical terms. Although Descartes never developed a systematic moral philosophy, his assertion that all "men" were potentially equal in their capacity to reason laid the foundation for later egalitarian moves in ethics and politics. Simultaneously, his conceptualization of animals as mere stimulus-response mechanisms, lacking consciousness because they lacked souls, justified the exclusion of animals from moral consideration. Cartesian biologists, in defense of vivisection, have compared the howls of cut-up dogs to the squeaks of unlubricated machines.

SHARED FEATURES OF DOMINANT PRE-DARWINIAN CONCEPTIONS OF HUMAN NATURE. There are at least six common features of pre-Darwinian conceptions of human nature:

1. Human nature is the same transhistorically.
2. It is distinguished primarily by possession of a soul.
3. Human souls are characterized by their capacity to reason. This capacity exists, perhaps in varying degrees, as a potential innate in all humans, sharply distinguishing them from all other beings, including animals.
4. Humans' possession of a rational soul gives them special moral worth.
5. Lacking such a soul, animals lack comparable moral worth or value. Those biological features that are similar in humans and animals comprise humans'

"lower" nature, which humans should strive to rise above.

6. Developing our potential to reason is a key to the good life for humans. Reasoning not only tells us how to live well but actualizes our distinctively human potential. Thus, the concept of human nature is clearly normative: Our task is to realize our humanness by fulfilling our potential for rationality; those who are incapable of fulfilling this potential are less than human.

The Materialist Tradition and the Darwinian Pivot

The features listed above as characterizing pre-Darwinian conceptions of human nature represent the dominant Western tradition prior to the nineteenth century. Running counter to this *rationalist* and dualist tradition, however, Western thought also includes a less prominent *materialist* or naturalist tradition.

Anaximander (ca. 500 B.C.E.), an early pre-Socratic philosopher, developed a speculative theory of evolution in which human beings were descended from lower forms of animal life. Democritus (460–370 B.C.E.), a contemporary of Socrates, developed a speculative atomic theory in which even the human soul was composed of atoms. The English philosopher Thomas Hobbes (1588–1679) assimilated individual behavior and politics to the laws of mechanics, regarding desire as motion toward an object, and human beings as motivated entirely by self-interest. The French philosopher Julien de La Mettrie (1709–1751) accepted Descartes's assertion that animals were like machines but insisted that so, too, were human beings. The German philosopher Baron Paul Henri d'Holbach (1723–1789) argued that thinking could be reduced to the functioning of the brain and explicitly denied the existence of a soul. Another of the French philosophes, Claude-Adrien Helvétius (1715–1771), argued that all mental faculties were ultimately reducible to physical sensation and that all humans were motivated by the desire to achieve physical pleasure and reduce pain. This latter idea was developed into an elaborate ethical calculus by the nineteenth-century British utilitarians, Jeremy Bentham (1748–1832), James Mill (1773–1836), and the latter's more famous son, John Stuart Mill (1806–1873). Collectively, these philosophers suggested an alternative understanding of human nature—one that focused more on the body than on the soul, on the emotions and desires more than on reason, and on the similarities rather than the differences between humans and animals. It remained for Charles Darwin to give this materialist tradition a scientific basis by providing a naturalistic analysis of the relations between humans and animals.

In his landmark work, *On the Origin of Species* (1859), Darwin argued that the distinctive features of human nature were not divinely created in an instant but had evolved over many millennia through a process he called "natural selection". Although the word *selection* suggested conscious purpose, Darwin's use of it was metaphorical, since nature *selects* only in the sense that certain new traits or mutations that appear accidentally are sufficiently adaptive to the environmental conditions within which the organism lives for the new organism to survive. The view that human beings had evolved through accidental mutations implied that there was no preordained nature, no ultimate meaning or cosmic purpose for human life to fulfill. In an attempt to escape this conclusion and reconcile science with Christianity, some later theorists postulated a direction and a goal in evolution, characterizing more recently evolved species as *higher* or otherwise superior; but such teleological and evaluative interpretations were ultimately alien to the basically antiteleological spirit of the concept of natural selection.

When Darwin first proposed his theory of evolution, the wife of the canon of Worcester Cathedral was said to have remarked, "Descended from the apes! My dear, we will hope it is not true. But if it is, let us pray that it may not become generally known." Indeed, the church denounced Darwin, recognizing that his theories challenged not only the beliefs in divine creation and a radical discontinuity between humans and animals but also the idea of an immortal soul with special moral worth. Darwin argued that morality had developed from the social instincts of animals; and he construed the uniquely human capacity for rationality, which Aristotle had seen as the telos of human existence, as the outcome of natural selection operating on accidental mutations.

Biological Determinism: A Critique

Once Darwin had demonstrated an evolutionary continuity between humans and other animals, questions arose about the causal role of human biology in relation to other aspects of human life. For many scientists, the project became the *reductionist* one of showing how the various psychological and social characteristics of human beings were causally determined by human biology.

Many *biological determinist* theories have negative social implications because they present human characteristics like aggression and dominance as biologically determined and therefore inescapable. For instance, Sigmund Freud (1856–1939), the founder of psychoanalysis, insisted that all human motivation could be reduced to two basic drives— the sexual drive, or libido; and the aggressive drive, an ineradicable instinct to hurt, torture, or kill other human beings (Freud). The German ethologist Konrad Lorenz (1903–1989) also posited an aggressive instinct in humans similar to that he found in his study of various animal species in their natural habitats. In each species, the instinct had evolved to serve one or more life-preserving functions, such as territorial dispersion, selection of the strongest for reproduction, defense of the young, and the establishment of a hierarchy that could provide the group with social cohesion. In species armed with sharp teeth, claws, or beaks, the aggressive instinct was generally coupled with an inhibitory mechanism preventing fighting animals from killing each other; Lorenz argued that there had been no need for such an inhibitory mechanism to evolve in humans because they were not naturally armed. With the development of weaponry, however, the absence of such a mechanism was often lethal, and the advent of nuclear weapons made it a threat to the survival of the species (Lorenz).

More recent studies of animal behavior have generated a new form of biological determinism called *sociobiology*. Two precursors of sociobiology, anthropologists Lionel Tiger (1937–) and Robin Fox (1913–1971), proposed the concept of a "biogram," a code or program genetically "wired" into the brain that produced certain forms of social behavior, including patterns of dominance and submission—hierarchy among males and dominance of males over females. Both of these were assumed to be the evolutionary heritage of the hunting life of early hominids (Tiger and Fox). The same general line of thinking was employed by entomologist Edward O. Wilson (1929–), who first coined the term *sociobiology*. Wilson insisted that "genes hold culture on a leash" and play a significant role in determining such human social behavior as altruism toward kin, communal aggression, nationalism, racism, homosexuality, and the dominance of males over females. Wilson has conceded that these biologically based tendencies might be counteracted through extreme social measures, but he argues that humans would pay a high price for doing so (1977).

While Wilson's assertion of a universal genetic tendency toward ethnocentric and racist attitudes was not an attempt to justify racism, there is a long Western tradition of using evolutionary theory to denigrate certain racial or ethnic groups. In the nineteenth century, some scientists in this tradition asserted that Caucasians and Orientals had crossed the *Homo sapiens* threshold before "Negroes," or that *Homo sapiens* had begun in Asia and migrated to Africa, where the original stock had degenerated. Others sought to prove racial, ethnic, and class inequalities in intelligence through the use of IQ (intelligence quotient) theory. Frances Galton (1822–1911), a cousin of Darwin who coined the term *eugenics,* attempted to show that the upper classes had superior intellectual capacities and that blacks were "two

grades" below whites. Many of the early IQ theorists in the United States made similar claims about various immigrant groups.

After World War II, when the Nazis had shown the possible social consequences of eugenic ideas, such theories fell into disrepute. They were revived in 1969 when educational psychologist Arthur Jensen (1923–) published an article in the *Harvard Educational Review* arguing as follows: Intelligence testing has demonstrated that whites score on average about fifteen IQ points above blacks; IQ is 80 percent *heritable*; therefore, the mean difference between the scores proves a hereditary difference in innate intelligence between the two groups (Jensen). Shortly after Jensen's article appeared, Harvard psychologist Richard Herrnstein (1930–) made a similar argument concerning the difference in IQ scores between *upper-class* and *lower-class* people. He concluded that humans should give up any aspirations to democratic equality and accept the idea of a natural meritocracy (Herrnstein).

Biological determinist theories were highly controversial in the late 1960s and 1970s, but in the 1980s and 1990s they became increasingly fashionable—claiming, for instance, genetic factors in alcoholism; locating homosexuality in the structure of the brain; and asserting that men with XYY chromosomes have a tendency toward criminal violence. However, biological determinist theories of human nature are problematic in a number of respects.

Empirically, the evidence for such theories is at best inconclusive. Even within the psychoanalytic tradition, some theorists have argued against Freud that aggressive desires may be explained as derivative manifestations rather than primary instincts, resulting from situations that frustrate other, nonaggressive desires. Ethologists and sociobiologists typically move incautiously from observations of certain animal species or conjectures about early hominids to claims about modern human beings. Sometimes, like Lorenz, they focus on the behavior of fish, birds, and other animals considerably removed from humans—while they ignore studies indicating that many higher mammals, especially primates, display almost no hierarchical organization or intraspecies aggression, being instead peaceful and cooperative. Finally, regardless of how nonhuman species behave, similarities in behavior between humans and nonhuman animals do not establish that the human behavior in question is biologically determined; it may still be a learned response.

Claims for the universality of human aggression, hierarchy, and male dominance also are not confirmed by anthropological evidence. Many hunter-gatherer societies are reported to be remarkably lacking in aggressive behavior, and some enjoy an exceptionally high degree of social equality. Assertions of women's *natural* dependence on men are undermined by evidence that gathering, a task often performed predominantly by women, is a more reliable food source than hunting in many hunter-gatherer societies. The sexual division of labor varies widely cross-culturally, and even where certain constants are observed, such as a tendency for women rather than men to care for young children, this may be a social adaptation to prevailing conditions rather than a biological predetermination.

Claims about the genetic basis of racial and ethnic differences in IQ are equally suspect. The idea of different evolutionary paths for different races is contradicted by the paleontological evidence; indeed, the concept of race itself is now widely discredited, with anthropologists preferring instead to talk about the statistical frequency of certain characteristics within a geographical population. Further, the idea that IQ tests measure innate intelligence is undermined by the recognition that all tests are culturally biased, since they all require prior learning, and that learning experience can significantly raise IQ. Finally, the very concept of *heritability* is a technical one, designating a ratio of the contribution of heredity to environment within a given population; it cannot be used, therefore, to compare one population against another.

Biological determinist theories of human nature are not just empirically unconfirmed; they also fail to acknowledge what is most distinctive of our species. The human genetic constitution determines highly developed learning and cognitive capacities that allow humans to respond flexibly rather than instinctively to environmental problems, as well as to develop a range of distinctively human cultural characteristics. The implications of this were noted by one of the world's foremost geneticists, Theodosius Dobzhansky (1900–1975), who wrote, "In a sense, human genes have surrendered their primacy in human evolution to an entirely new, nonbiological or superorganic agent, culture. However, it should not be forgotten that human culture is not possible without human genes" (p. 113). In short, what has developed in the human evolutionary process is a primate with a genetic structure capable of a new kind of evolution, cultural evolution.

Biological determinist theories of human nature contrast sharply in content with their pre-Darwinian counterparts, but they are often inspired by the same motivation of discovering universal and unchanging social values. Typically, they describe as *natural* aspects of behavior thought to be biologically determined; though few would assert that natural behavior is always to be encouraged or even permitted, characterizing some behavioral tendencies as natural provides a certain legitimation for them. Because they are understood as resulting from natural selection, such tendencies are regarded as having been necessary at least at some time for human survival; in consequence, they cannot be entirely deplored, and they may even be romanticized as clues to a more *natural* way of life. Thus, biological determinist approaches to understanding and evaluating human nature may be seen as secular analogues of Aquinas's theory of natural law.

It may be the social function of biological determinist theories of human nature, rather than their scientific credentials, that accounts for their continuing popularity. Put simply, these theories tend to rationalize existing manifestations of aggression and inequality: Biological determinist analyses of violence, war, and crime tend to deflect attention from the social and economic causes of these phenomena, just as theories about the biological determinants of male and female behavior distract us from the ways in which men and women are socialized for their respective roles. The implication often drawn from biological determinist theories is that significant social movement in the direction of peaceful cooperation and equality is impossible because it is alleged to go against *human nature*. Clearly, those in power benefit from such an assumption and are likely to encourage the development of such theories.

Behaviorism: Another Form of Post-Darwinian Reductionism

The Western materialist or naturalist tradition has not always moved in a biological determinist direction. It also includes thinkers who claim that environmental or cultural factors are the primary determinants of the human mind or behavior. The philosopher John Locke (1632–1704) saw the human mind as a kind of blank tablet to be written upon by sensory impressions, while Enlightenment figures like Helvétius assumed that education could shape human beings into almost any form.

In the first part of the twentieth century, environmentalist ideas became popular in the United States through a psychological movement known as behaviorism. John B. Watson (1878–1958), who first systematically developed the theory, insisted that in order for psychology to become a rigorous experimental science, it must give up its introspective orientation. It should no longer take its task to be analyzing private mental states, such as feelings, desires, and thoughts, but instead should study the relation between publicly observable behavior and the environment. For Watson, the two basic forms of this relation were the *unconditioned* and the *conditioned reflex*. The former was the basic human physiological endowment, consisting of automatic responses to environmental stimuli, such as salivating in the presence of food and contracting pupils in the presence of light. Watson based his analysis of the conditioned reflex on the work of the Russian experimental psychologist Ivan Petrovich Pavlov (1849–1936), who had demonstrated that a hungry dog, repeatedly presented with both food and the ringing of a bell, would eventually salivate at only the bell-ringing. The sound of the bell had become a *substitute stimulus,* and the salivation was now a *conditioned response.* For Watson, all human behavior could be reduced to these two kinds of reflexes.

Watson's version of behaviorism was superseded by that of B. F. Skinner (1904–1990), who argued that reflex action could account for only a small part of human behavior. For Skinner, human behavior was primarily shaped by what he called *operant conditioning,* which *reinforced* certain spontaneous movements of the organism. For example, when a pigeon raised its head above a certain height and food was released into its cage, the result was a higher frequency of that behavior. Unlike the stimulus in Watson's model, the "reinforcer" (the food) was introduced *after* the "response" (the raising of the head to the desired height) occurred. For Skinner, most human behavior other than automatic reflex action, even human language, could be explained as the result of *positive* or *negative reinforcement,* which, by adding something to the situation (food, sex, money, praise, etc.)—or by removing something from it—increased the frequency of some behavior. While not denying that feelings and thoughts existed, Skinner refused to characterize them as residing in a special mental domain, consciousness, and claimed that they had no causal effect on human behavior (Skinner, 1953).

Both Watson and Skinner believed that human beings could be conditioned to develop almost any pattern of behavioral responses. Watson boldly declared that he could take almost any infant "at random and train him to become … doctor, lawyer, artist, merchant-chief, and, yes, even a beggar man and thief." Skinner insisted that operant conditioning "shapes behavior as a sculptor shapes a lump of clay." One evident consequence of the behaviorist program was that human freedom was an illusion. For Skinner, in particular, such concepts as freedom, moral responsibility, and human dignity were the conceits of a prescientific age (Skinner, 1973).

Behaviorism, just as much as biological determinism, is heir to the evolutionary paradigm because human behavior is still explained in terms of genetic dispositions regarded as having survival value. For behaviorism, however, these predispositions are not instincts or drives. Instead, specific unconditioned reflexes have evolved in the human species because they have survival value, while the human organism's susceptibility to conditioning helps it survive by allowing it to adapt to environmental changes more rapidly than its genetic structure could.

There are a number of difficulties with the behaviorist conception of human nature. First are the primary data of consciousness, such as desires, feelings, reflection, and decision making; it is hard to believe that these do not have at least some causal influence on human activity. Second, the fact that pigeons, rats, and human beings can sometimes be controlled by operant conditioning does not mean that all human behavior can be understood in this way. Linguist Noam Chomsky (1928–), for example, has argued against Skinner that linguistic competence requires creativity that goes beyond responses to prior conditioning because we are constantly constructing sentences that we have never before encountered. Finally, there is no room in the behaviorist model for human agency: The environment acts, human beings merely react. In this, behaviorism may be seen as ideologically reflecting a world in which people are continually managed and manipulated by technocratic and bureaucratic elites.

Social and Historical Conceptions of Human Nature

Social and historical conceptions of human nature offer an alternative to seeing human beings either as primarily determined by their biological drives or as passive clay to be molded by their physical and social environment. These approaches, while not ignoring human biology or the role of social conditioning, emphasize the importance of human social activity within specific historical contexts. The work of the revolutionary social theorist Karl Marx, together with his collaborator Friedrich Engels (1820–1895), and of the U.S. pragmatist philosopher John Dewey, provides two examples of this approach.

Marx and Engels's view of human nature (Schmitt) was embedded in their more general theory of human history, *historical materialism.* Human history, they contended, began with humans' attempt to satisfy their basic biological needs through producing their means of subsistence, so that human beings were, first and foremost, producers. Human production differed from that of nonhuman animals in that it was deliberate rather than instinctive, involving imagination, planning, and tool use. It was also inherently social, not only in requiring the coordination of human effort but also in utilizing skills and knowledge transmitted from one individual, group, or generation to another. In societies producing a surplus beyond that needed for immediate survival, human production typically involved a division of labor going beyond a division into separate tasks, to a division between intellectual and physical work and between work considered appropriate for men and for women. Most important for Marx and Engels was the class division of labor between those groups who owned the means of production and those who had to work for them, a division generating the class struggles regarded by Marx and Engels as the motor force in history.

Different economic systems, or what Marx and Engels called modes of production, established forms of social life through which human beings individuated and understood themselves. Peasants and artisans, ladies and gentlemen, merchants and professionals, corporate capitalists and industrial workers would tend to think and act differently from each other. Changes in the mode of production would generate new forms of social life, new ways of understanding the world, and new ways of thinking and acting—in effect, new kinds of *individuals*. Thus, human nature itself would change. Since human beings were active in the class struggle that caused these social and economic changes, however, it could also be said that human beings actively changed their own natures over the course of history.

For John Dewey, as for Marx and Engels, human beings were neither governed by instincts nor passive recipients of environmental forces; rather, they were social agents who changed their own natures in the process of changing their societal conditions. However, in contrast to Marx and Engels, Dewey regarded the motor force of social change not as class struggle but as the product of reflective intelligence.

Dewey acknowledged that human beings had instincts—or impulses, as he preferred to call them in order to discourage associations of inflexibility. Impulses, in his view, were extremely flexible in that they could take on a variety of meanings, depending on the social context. Thus, the impulse of fear might become cowardice, caution, reverence, or respect; while the impulse of anger might become rage, sullenness, annoyance, or indignation. Impulses took on these meanings as habits, predispositions to certain kinds of thinking and acting, ultimately embodied in social customs and institutions. The content of these habits constituted our historical nature. However, when the habits proved inadequate to new social problems, humans could employ their reflective intelligence to redirect their impulses into new habits. For example, as war became increasingly problematic or as certain economic institutions become increasingly outmoded, human impulses could be rechanneled, creating new institutions embodying new habits.

To make sense of the claim that human nature changes, we need to remember the distinction between transhistorical and historical conceptions of human nature. For both Dewey and Marx, it is precisely because a certain transhistorical human nature exists—socially productive and reflectively intelligent—that the content of human nature can be changed historically. To put this point in a more contemporary idiom: Our distinctively human capacity to transform social institutions transforms social roles and, in so doing, transforms historically specific character structures.

Giving more weight to the social and historical aspects of human nature offers a new model of the relation between genetic determination and social conditioning, on the one hand, and social behavior, on the other. What is determined by our genes is our capacity to learn, reflect, and work for change. Humans can, thus, be agents of their own history. Biology determines certain potentialities, but it is only through concrete historical activities that humans develop certain specific cultural and psychological characteristics. Genes dictate the ability to develop general modes of response, such as learning languages, engaging in productive labor, and developing forms of social relatedness; but they do not dictate that humans learn English, produce nuclear weapons, or become selfish and competitive as opposed to altruistic and cooperative. Thus, historical and social conceptions of human nature do not deny biology but refuse to privilege it as the primary cause of human action. Similarly, they do not deny conditioning but equally refuse to privilege it in explaining human action. Certain social conditions undoubtedly encourage the development of certain habits, but these are not merely behavioral responses; instead, they are social patterns of meaning that connect thought to action. Furthermore, human beings do not merely react to social conditions but individuate themselves within them and can reflect intelligently on them. Thus, both individually and collectively humans can decide to change their habits and work to transform the social conditions from which they arose.

A Social and Historical Conception of the Human Body

Although many theorists are willing to acknowledge that people's character or personality or behavior is socially shaped, at least to some degree, the biological constitution, the body, is often viewed as a presocial given, the universal and unchanging foundation on which elaborate cultural edifices are erected. According to this way of thinking, the body constitutes the most natural aspect of human nature. Itself a product of natural selection, the body sets the *natural*, that is, biologically determined, limits of social variability.

While it may be true that there is less systematic cross-cultural and transhistorical variation in people's bodies than there is in their personalities and social institutions, it is too simple to regard the human body as a presocial given. Although the human body may sometimes be experienced as a given, in fact, like the mind or the personality, bodies are socially and historically shaped on several levels.

It is not difficult to recognize some of the ways in which human bodies are influenced by their social context. Different kinds of work and living conditions develop or distort the body in various ways. For instance, scarcity of food results in stunted growth, so that body size and development vary systematically not only between cultures but often also between social classes. While many of these bodily marks are unintended side effects of social practices, others are deliberately induced. Social norms are consciously inscribed on the body in a variety of ways, ranging from foot-binding and circumcision to diet clinics and cosmetic surgery. The varying social meanings assigned to bodily characteristics and functions influence a person's experience of his or her body, which, depending on the social context, may become a source of pride, joy, pain, or embarrassment.

Social influences on the human body operate not only on the level of observable physical structure, the phenotype; in the past, they have also influenced the genotype, our genetic inheritance, and they continue to do so. While human prehistory is highly speculative, it seems likely that some genetically heritable characteristics have been selected not only *naturally,* as adaptive to such nonsocial circumstances as climate and food availability; but also socially, as adaptive to certain forms of social organization or perhaps even as the results of conscious social preferences. For instance, the average size difference between human males and females may have been a consequence as much as a cause of male dominance: If the dominant males fed first and most, only smaller-framed women could survive on the leftover food. Even today, the human gene pool continues to be influenced by social factors. For instance, exposure to environmental pollutants sometimes leads to genetic mutations, and modern medicine now makes it possible for people to survive and reproduce with genetic conditions that otherwise would have led to their early deaths. Finally, genetic engineering is rapidly becoming a real possibility.

The recognition that even the genetic constitution is influenced by social factors has far-reaching consequences for understanding human nature. The point is not simply that most versions of biological determinism are false because they fail to give sufficient weight to the social determinants of human characteristics. It is, rather, that the usefulness of the whole nature-culture distinction as an analytical framework for understanding human beings comes into question. Just as we cannot identify any cultural or social phenomena uninfluenced in some way by human biology, neither can we identify any human biological or *natural* features that are independent of social influence. The biological and the social are so intertwined in the human past and present that it becomes impossible in principle to distinguish the natural from the social or cultural components in the constitution of human beings. As far as human beings are concerned, the relation between nature and culture is mutually constitutive: To oppose one to the other is incomprehensible. Everything that we are and do is revealed as simultaneously cultural and natural.

Ethical Implications for the Life Sciences: A Cautionary Tale

What are the bioethical implications of these various conceptions of human nature? First, a cautionary note. Practical ethics reflects on a host of considerations in practical contexts and cannot simply deduce specific moral conclusions from general ethical principles, let alone from some general conception of human nature. Thus, the relation between the various conceptions of human nature and any specific bioethical position is unlikely to be one of logical entailment. This does not mean, however, that concepts of human nature have no relevance to bioethical issues. They may serve as starting points for bioethical analysis, raise suspicions about certain bioethical claims, or even rule out certain bioethical positions. In general, certain conceptions of human nature may be said to cohere, or provide a better *fit,* with certain bioethical stances than with others.

The dominant pre-Darwinian conceptions of human nature view physical nature, including the human body, as the realm of the material, the immanent, and the profane, and identify God with the spiritual, the transcendent, and the sacred. It is only because human beings are endowed with a soul that they are regarded as capable of partaking in the sacred, and their mission is to transcend their bodies and realize their spiritual nature. Insofar as they are part of God's creation, nonhuman animals are sometimes assigned a degree of moral worth, but the view that they lack souls typically rationalizes the claim that nonhuman animals are merely resources to serve human purposes. Saint Francis of Assisi notwithstanding, the dominant view of the Judeo-Christian tradition is that God created nonhuman animals and, indeed, all of nonhuman nature, primarily for the use of human beings. This sharp bifurcation between human and nonhuman nature not only permits but even legitimates the human subjugation and exploitation of all nonhuman nature, and may therefore contribute to the contemporary ecological crisis.

Within this ontology, the human body occupies a unique and somewhat ambiguous moral status. Although material, and therefore a source of temptation, the body is nevertheless sacrosanct because it is indispensable to human life. God is thought to have a divine plan for humanity, and any attempt to subvert this plan by tinkering with the human body is regarded as at least prima facie wrong. When applied to humans as opposed to nonhuman animals, therefore, reproductive technology, genetic engineering, and euthanasia are viewed with suspicion, if not censure; and *brain death* may not be considered sufficient reason to switch off a life-support system, depending on when the soul is believed to leave the body. If, for example, the soul is thought to remain in the body until the last breath of life, then euthanasia can never be justified: Even the suffering and dying body must be revered as the house of the soul. Finally, because humans are morally distinguished by the possession of a soul, abortion is condemned at whatever point the fetus is believed to acquire a soul. It is interesting to note that the Catholic Church has not always held that fetal ensoulment occurs at the moment of conception: Saint Thomas Aquinas, for instance, argued as an Aristotelian that the fetus did not have a soul until it assumed human form, which he thought occurred after three months' gestation for the male fetus and six months' for the female.

In contrast with the pre-Darwinian dichotomies between human and nature, spiritual and material, sacred and profane, post-Darwinian conceptions of human nature posit an evolutionary continuity between human and nonhuman animals. This continuity is sometimes used as a basis for moral challenges to the human exploitation and domination of animals, especially animals that are close to human beings in evolutionary terms. It is precisely those nonhuman animals most like humans, however, that are most useful for many purposes, such as medical experiments and organ transplants; in consequence, some philosophers have sought to undercut moral challenges to the human exploitation of nonhuman animals by arguing that beings *lower* on the evolutionary scale may be sacrificed for the good of *higher* species. Opposing this position is a growing minority in the bioethics community that argues that such a position is an example of unwarranted human chauvinism or *speciesism*, a term invoked to suggest parallels with racism and sexism.

Although post-Darwinian assumptions of an evolutionary continuity between humans and nonanimals may be used to challenge the view that animals are simply a resource for human use, they have also been used to justify radical interventions in human life processes. If it is legitimate to experiment on nonhuman animals, for instance, it may be equally legitimate to experiment on human beings. If *Homo sapiens* is the accidental outcome of natural selection, if there is no inherent purpose for which we are created, then there is no a priori reason to assume that further modifications in

human biological processes should not be made via reproductive technologies or even genetic engineering. Since the human nervous system is a defining component of human life, the fetus at an early stage of brain development is likely to have a different moral status than it does once the brain has developed. Certainly, the post-Darwinian conception of human nature would generally assume that *brain dead* means dead.

These conclusions reflect the absence of the concept of a soul in post-Darwinian views of human nature, since it was the soul that, in earlier conceptions, provided the philosophical grounding for human dignity. Unless an adequate substitute for the concept of the soul can be found, post-Darwinian conceptions of human nature may permit the drastic manipulation of human beings. Behavior regarded as undesirable may be treated either as a biological abnormality or as a failure of social conditioning. Biological determinists may regard alcoholism, addictive gambling, violent criminal behavior, schizophrenia, depression, and even homosexuality as candidates for treatment with a variety of biological techniques: psychosurgery, shock therapy, hormonal therapy, psychopharmacological interventions, and perhaps, in the future, even genetic manipulation. Behaviorists, of course, emphasize the use of various conditioning techniques to modify human behavior, raising the prospect of a *Clockwork Orange* world. Skinner, in fact, wrote a utopian novel, *Walden Two* (1948), in which behavioral managers conditioned people from birth to make choices in accord with the goals and institutions of that society. Both biological and behavioral interventions often work toward the same goal—direct control of human behavior.

But who will control the controllers, and how far will such control be allowed to extend? There are already biological determinists who advocate the use of genetic manipulation to raise IQ or to alter certain *undesirable* tendencies in the human species, perhaps to create a Superman. Others would clone the embryo and store it for future use, perhaps in case of some failure of the original stock. Brave New World may be just around the corner unless we can reclaim the concept of human dignity. Social and historical conceptions of human nature offer a secular basis for doing so.

Although people who accept a social and historical conception of human nature may still utilize some concept of naturalness in describing various human activities, such as conceiving or giving birth, they recognize that what is taken to be natural or unnatural changes historically and culturally, so that ethical decisions cannot be grounded in some unchangeable concept of human nature. However, this does not prevent us from ethically evaluating various attempts to manipulate and control human nature. Indeed, those who accept social and historical conceptions of human nature are likely to urge caution in the use of biological interventions and conditioning techniques for the purposes of altering human behavior. They will be suspicious of all treatment and research modalities that fail to respect human agency, reflective intelligence, and decision-making capabilities, since it is precisely these transhistorical capacities that make possible the continuous transformation of our historical natures. In short, social and historical conceptions of human nature will tend to reaffirm the concept of human dignity. In the sphere of medicine, for instance, they are likely to insist on the dignity of medical subjects and emphasize informed consent and coparticipation in physician-patient relationships.

The recognition that human beings individuate themselves within and through social processes may also have implications for the abortion controversy; at the very least, it suggests that women and fetuses cannot have the same moral status. Moreover, social and historical conceptions of human nature emphasize that consideration of bioethical problems must be sensitive to concrete social and political contexts; in a society with an expressed commitment to human equality, for example, questions like procreative technology or contract parenting must be evaluated with special reference to their implications for people of different classes, genders, abilities, races, and ethnicities. Finally, social and historical conceptions regard human beings as transhistorically creative, productive, social, and capable of reforming their habits through reflective intelligence; and people who accept these conceptions are likely to valorize those capacities and seek to develop social institutions—including healthcare, psychiatric, and research institutions—through which they would be enhanced.

The open-ended nature of these last implications serves as a reminder that ethical conclusions are not strictly entailed by any general conception of human nature, especially by social and historical conceptions. In addressing particular bioethical problems, therefore, the values implicit in these conceptions must be supplemented by explicitly ethical criteria, such as historically specific understandings of justice, freedom, and human well-being.

ALISON M. JAGGAR
KARSTEN J. STRUHL (1995)
BIBLIOGRAPHY REVISED

SEE ALSO: *Behaviorism; Enhancement Uses of Medical Technology; Eugenics; Freedom and Free Will; Genetics and Human Behavior; Genetics and Human Self-Understanding; Human Dignity; Natural Law; Nanotechnology; Transhumanism and Posthumanism*

BIBLIOGRAPHY

Antony, Louise M. 2000. "Natures and Norms" *Ethics* 111(1): 8–36.

Aquinas, Thomas. 1962 (1272). *Summa Theologiae.* Turin: Marietti.

Aristotle. 1947. "Metaphysics." In *Introduction to Aristotle,* pp. 243–296, tr. W. D. Ross, ed. Richard P. McKeon. New York: Modern Library. Includes Books 1 and 12.

Aristotle. 1947. "Poetics." In *Introduction to Aristotle,* pp. 553–617, tr. W. D. Ross, ed. Richard P. McKeon. New York: Modern Library. Includes Books 1 and 3.

Arnhart, Larry. 1998. *Darwinian Natural Right: The Biological Ethics of Human Nature* Albany: State University of New York Press.

Athanasopoulos, C. 2000. "Good and Evil in Human Nature: Some Preliminary Ontological Considerations." *Philosophical Inquiry* 22(3): 103–115.

Block, Ned J., and Dworkin, Gerald, eds. 1976. *The I.Q. Controversy: Critical Readings.* New York: Pantheon.

Blum, Jeffrey M. 1978. *Pseudoscience and Mental Ability: The Origins and Fallacies of The IQ Controversy.* New York: Monthly Review Press.

Chomsky, Noam. 1959. "Review of B. F. Skinner, Verbal Behavior." *Language* 35: 26–58.

Darwin, Charles. 1936 (1859; 1871). *On the Origin of Species by Means of Natural Selection; or, The Preservation of Favoured Races in the Struggle For Life; and The Descent of Man and Selection in Relation to Sex.* New York: Modern Library.

Descartes, René. 1931 (1637–1650). "Rules for the Direction of the Mind," "Discourse on the Method of Rightly Conducting the Reason," and "Meditations on First Philosophy." In vol. 1 of *Philosophical Works of Descartes,* tr. Elizabeth S. Haldane and George R. T. Ross. Cambridge, Eng.: Cambridge University Press.

Dewey, John. 1957. *Human Nature and Conduct: An Introduction to Social Psychology.* New York: Modern Library.

Dewey, John. 1963. *Freedom and Culture.* New York: Capricorn.

Dobzhansky, Theodosius G. 1966. *Heredity and the Nature of Man.* New York: New American Library.

Ehrlich, Paul R. 2000. *Human Natures: Genes, Culture and the Human Prospect.* Washington, D.C.: Island Press.

Freud, Sigmund. 1962 (1930). *Civilization and Its Discontents,* tr. James Strachey. New York: W. W. Norton.

Gilkey, Langdon. 1995. "Biology and Theology on Human Nature" in *Biology, Ethics, and the Origins of Life,* ed. Holmes Rolston III. Boston: Jones and Bartlett.

Herrnstein, Richard J. 1973. *I.Q. in the Meritocracy.* Boston: Little, Brown.

Jensen, Arthur R. 1969. "How Much Can We Boost IQ and Scholastic Achievement?" *Harvard Educational Review* 39(1): 1–123.

Lee, Richard Borshoy. 1979. *The !Kung San: Men, Women, and Work in a Foraging Society.* New York: Cambridge University Press.

Lewontin, Richard C.; Rose, Steven P. R.; and Kamin, Leon J. 1984. *Not in Our Genes: Biology, Ideology, and Human Nature.* New York: Pantheon.

Lorenz, Konrad. 1974. *On Aggression,* tr. Marjorie Kerr Wilson. New York: Harcourt Brace Jovanovich.

Midgley, Mary. 1995. *Beast and Man: The Roots of Human Nature* New York: Routledge.

Montagu, Ashley. 1978. *The Nature of Human Aggression.* New York: Oxford University Press.

Montagu, Ashley, ed. 1970. *The Concept of Race.* London: Collier.

Passmore, John A. 1970. *The Perfectibility of Man.* London: Duckworth.

Post, Stephen G.; Underwood, Lynn G.; Schloss, Jeffery P.; Hurlbut, William B., eds. 2002. *Altruism and Altruistic Love: Science, Philosophy and Religion in Dialogue.* New York: Oxford University Press.

Radcliffe-Richards, Janet. 2000. *Human Nature after Darwin: A Philosophical Introduction.* New York: Routledge.

Rasmussen, Douglas B. 1999. "Human Flourishing and the Appeal to Human Nature." *Social Philosophy and Policy* 16(1): 1–43.

Reiter, Rayna R., ed. 1975. *Toward an Anthropology of Women.* New York: Monthly Review Press.

Schmitt, Richard. 1987. *Introduction to Marx and Engels: A Critical Reconstruction.* Boulder, CO: Westview.

Skinner, B. F. 1948. *Walden Two.* New York: Macmillan.

Skinner, B. F. 1953. *Science and Human Behavior.* New York: Macmillan.

Skinner, B. F. 1972. *Beyond Freedom and Dignity.* New York: Bantam.

Tiger, Lionel, and Fox, Robin. 1974. *The Imperial Animal.* New York: Dell.

Tucker, Robert C., ed. 1972. *The Marx-Engels Reader.* New York: W. W. Norton.

Watson, John B. 1925. *Behaviorism.* New York: W. W. Norton.

Wilson, Edward O. 1977. *Sociobiology: A New Synthesis.* Cambridge, MA: Harvard University Press.

Wilson, Edward O. 1979. *On Human Nature.* New York: Bantam.

HUMAN RIGHTS

• • •

Human rights constitute a set of norms governing the treatment of individuals and groups by states and nonstate actors on the basis of ethical principles incorporated into national and international legal systems. Because the subject matter of the norms in question relate to the treatment of human beings, human rights overlap to a considerable degree with ethics, but they nevertheless should not be confused with ethics. Similarly, because human rights include the right to health and refer to essential social determinants of health and well-being of people, they overlap with many principles and norms of bioethics. Human rights and bioethics differ, however, in scope, sources, legal nature, and the mechanisms of monitoring and applying the norms.

The *scope* of bioethics is the ethical issues arising from healthcare and biomedical sciences, whereas that of human rights embraces the claims individuals and groups can legitimately make against states and nonstate actors to respect their dignity, integrity, autonomy, and freedom of action as defined in an officially endorsed set of standards or norms. Bioethics regulates clinical encounters with patients on the basis of principles; human rights, by contrast, are the special rules agreed upon in a given society to achieve justice and well-being.

The *source* of human rights is the norm-creating process of national and international legal systems, whereas that of bioethics is the deliberations and published opinions of leading thinkers, constituted review boards, and professional associations on the health-related ethical issues they address. Bioethics and human rights share an ethical concern for just behavior, built on empathy or altruism. The proximate formal source of human rights is typically an international human rights treaty or declaration while that of bioethics is a professional code or review board guidelines. The proximate source occasionally is identical, as when an instrument of international law directly addresses an issue of bioethics and human rights, for example, in the United Nations Educational, Scientific and Cultural Organization's (UNESCO) Universal Declaration on the Human Genome and Human Rights or the Council of Europe's Convention for the Protection of Human Rights and Dignity of the Human Being with Regard to the Application of Biology and Medicine, both of which were adopted in 1997.

The *legal nature* of human rights norms ranges from merely aspirational claims to justiciable and enforceable legally binding obligations. An important distinction is made between *rights* and *human rights.* In ethics a right refers to any entitlement, the moral validity or legitimacy of which depends on the mode of moral reasoning the ethicist is using. In law, a right is any legally protected interest. In human rights discourse, a human right is a higher-order right authoritatively defined using the expression *human rights* with the expectation that such a right carries a peremptory character and thus prevails over other (ordinary) rights. Another distinction is between the natural law and positive law foundations of human rights. The former refers to rights deriving from the natural order or divine origin, which are inalienable, immutable, and absolute, whereas in positive law rights are recognized through a political and legal process that results in a declaration, law, treaty, or other normative instrument. These may vary over time and be subject to derogations or limitations designed to optimize respect for human rights rather than impose an absolute standard. Human rights emerge from claims of people suffering injustice and thus are based on moral sentiment, culturally determined by contextualized moral and religious belief systems. They become part of the social order when an authoritative body proclaims them, and they attain a higher degree of universality based on the participation of virtually every nation in the norm-creating process, a process that is law-based but that reflects compromise and historical shifts. The International Bill of Human Rights (consisting of the Universal Declaration of Human Rights [UDHR] of 1948 and the International Covenant on Civil and Political Rights and the International Covenant on Economic, Social and Cultural Rights, both of 1966), along with the other human rights treaties of the United Nations (UN) and of regional organizations, constitute the primary sources and reference points for what properly belongs in the category of human rights.

The *methods of monitoring compliance* with human rights include moral judgments made with reference to recognized human rights, quasi-judicial procedures of investigation and fact-finding leading to official pronouncements of political bodies, and enforceable judicial decisions. The parallel methods of bioethics focus more on codes of bioethics and official pronouncements of professional bodies that may result in altering research design or the behavior or liability of health professionals in their relations with patients or in policies affecting the health of populations.

The overlap of human rights and bioethical discourse and the differences between the two become clearer as one clarifies the following: the emergence of human rights in political and legal discourse, the content of the right to health as defined in human rights instruments, the other human rights as they relate to health and well-being, and the role and means of promotion and protection of human rights.

Emergence of Human Rights

The early formulation of the norms that are characterized today as human rights is inseparable from historical and philosophical manifestations of human striving for justice. Ultimately, human rights certainly derive from basic human instincts of survival of the species and behavior of empathy and altruism that evolutionary biology is only beginning to understand. Since human evolution is driven by reproductive selfishness, one could wonder why the human species would develop any ethical system, like that of human rights, according to which individuals manifest feeling for the suffering of others (empathy) and—even more surprising— act in self-sacrificing ways for the benefit of others without achieving any noticeable reproductive advantage. And yet, as Paul Ehrlich notes in *Human Natures*, "empathy and altruism often exist where the chances for any return for the altruist are nil" (p. 312). Natural selection does not provide the answer to moral behavior as "there aren't enough genes to code the various required behaviors" but rather "cultural evolution is the source of ethics" (p. 317) and therefore of human rights.

Religion and law have an ambiguous role in this historical process. The history of religions is replete with advances in the moral principles of behavior—many of which directly influenced the drafting of human rights texts—but also in crimes committed in the name of a Supreme Being. Similarly, the emergence of the rule of law has been critical both to advancing justice and human rights against the arbitrary usurpation of power in most societies and to preserving the impunity of oppressors.

Scholars trace the current configuration of international human rights norms and procedures to the revolutions of freedom and equality that transformed governments across Europe and North America in the eighteenth century and that liberated subjugated people from slavery and colonial domination in the nineteenth and twentieth centuries. Enlightenment philosophers derived the centrality of the individual from their theories of the state of nature. Social contractarians, especially the eighteenth-century French philosopher Jean-Jacques Rousseau, predicated the authority of the state on its capacity to achieve the optimum enjoyment of natural rights, that is, of rights inherent in each individual irrespective of birth or status. Rousseau wrote in *A Discourse on the Origin of Inequality* (1755) that "it is plainly contrary to the law of nature … that the privileged few should gorge themselves with superfluities, while the starving multitude are in want of the bare necessities of life" (p. 117). Equally important was the concept of the universalized individual ("the rights of Man"), reflected in the political thinking of Immanuel Kant, John Locke, Thomas Paine, and the authors of the French and American declarations. Much of this natural law tradition is secularized in contemporary human rights.

World War II was the defining event for the internationalization of human rights, with the latter anticipated by Roosevelt's "Four Freedoms" speech (1941), confirmed by the inclusion of human rights in the UN Charter (1945), and applied at the trial of Nazi doctors, leading to the

Nuremberg Code (1946). In the war's immediate aftermath, bedrock human rights texts were adopted: the Genocide Convention and the UDHR in 1948 and the Geneva Conventions in 1949, followed in 1966 by the two international covenants. Nongovernmental organizations (NGOs) played a role in all these developments and in subsequent drafting of treaties, as well as in the creation of investigative and accountability procedures at the intergovernmental level and at the national level. These processes were instrumental in bringing down South African apartheid, transforming East-Central Europe, and restoring democracy in Latin America. Human rights NGOs are now active on all continents.

The Normative Content of Human Rights: The Right to Health

The current catalogue of human rights consists of some fifty normative propositions. They are enumerated in the international bill of human rights, extended by a score of specialized UN treaties, a half-dozen regional human rights treaties, and hundreds of international normative instruments in the fields of labor, refugees, armed conflict, and criminal law.

The meaning, scope, and practical significance of the right to health are particularly relevant for bioethics. The right to health as understood in international human rights law is defined in article 25 of the 1948 Universal Declaration of Human Rights ("Everyone has the right to a standard of living adequate for the health of himself and of his family, including food, clothing, housing and medical care and necessary social services.") and in article 12 of the 1966 International Covenant on Economic, Social and Cultural Rights (ICESCR) ("the right of everyone to the enjoyment of the highest attainable standard of physical and mental health"). Variations on these definitions are found in most of the core UN and regional human rights treaties. In 2000 the Committee on Economic, Social and Cultural Rights (CESCR), which was created to monitor the ICESCR, analyzed the normative content of the right to health in terms of availability, accessibility, appropriateness, and quality of care and specified the duties of the state to respect, protect, and provide this right. The committee also listed fourteen human rights as "integral components of the right to health." These related rights define to a large extent the determinants of health.

The right to health does not mean the right to be healthy, because being healthy is determined only in part by healthcare; it is also determined by genetic predisposition and social factors. The field of social epidemiology has excelled at establishing correlations between discrimination based on race, class, or gender, denial of education and of decent working conditions, as well as other factors that contribute directly to increased rates of mortality and morbidity. These social determinants may also be defined in human rights terms as deprivation of these health-related rights, which are among the most salient social factors that contribute to healthy lives. The summary below seeks to underscore the function of human rights as determinants of health by highlighting their normative content and their relation to health.

Health-Related Human Rights

Health is profoundly related to human rights both because human right violations have health impacts—such as those on torture survivors—and because human rights concern the dignity, integrity, autonomy of action, and conditions of social functioning of people. Some examples will be provided in each of these areas.

Foremost among the human rights relating to physical and mental integrity is the right not to be arbitrarily deprived of life, which does not rule out death resulting from lawful acts of warfare or capital punishment, although international humanitarian law limits the former, and newer protocols and regional conventions, supported by UN resolutions and social movements, define the latter as a violation of human rights. Special treaties and procedures exist for prevention and repression of torture, disappearance, summary and extrajudicial execution, crimes against humanity, genocide, slavery, racial discrimination, and various forms of terrorism. Most of these are also dealt with in international humanitarian law, which was established to protect victims of armed conflict (injured and shipwrecked combatants, prisoners of war, and civilian populations notably under occupation) and codified in the four Geneva Conventions of 1949 and the Additional Protocols of 1977.

The right to "a standard of living adequate for the health and well-being" of oneself and one's family was defined in the UDHR as including "food, clothing, housing and medical care and necessary social services" as well as "the right to security in the event of unemployment, sickness, disability, widowhood, old age or other lack of livelihood in circumstances beyond [one's] control." Subsequently, the rights to health, work, safe and healthy working conditions (occupational health), adequate food and protection from malnutrition and famine, adequate housing, and social security (that is, a regime covering long-term disability, old age, unemployment, and other conditions) have been further elaborated by the International Labour Organisation, the UN Commission on Human Rights, and the work of special rapporteurs and treaty bodies.

Dignity tends to be mentioned as both the basis for all human rights and a right per se. The great civil liberties—freedom of oral and written expression, freedom of conscience, opinion, religion, or belief—as well as freedom from arbitrary detention or arrest, rights to a fair hearing and an effective remedy for violations of human rights, and protection of privacy in domicile and correspondence, all support the autonomy of individuals to act without interference from the state or others. A separate but related human right is that of informed consent to medical experimentation, which was included in post-1945 enumerations of rights because of the extensive abuse of that right during World War II.

Equality and nondiscrimination are human rights that are at the same time principles for the application of all other human rights, because they require that all persons be treated equally in the enjoyment of their human rights and that measures be taken to remove discriminatory practices on prohibited grounds. Freedom of movement means the right to reside where one pleases and to leave any country, including one's own, and to return to one's country. The right to seek and enjoy asylum from persecution is also a human right, which has been developed and expanded by international refugee law, the practice of the UN High Commissioner for Refugees, and recent codes relating to internally displaced persons. This right, like many others, is not absolute; limitations may be imposed, for example, in time of epidemic, as long as certain safeguards, defined in human rights law, are observed.

Social well-being depends in large measure on group identity, education, family, culture, political and cultural participation, gender and reproductive rights, scientific activity, the environment, and development, all of which are the subject of specific human rights. The basic human rights texts affirm a limited number of group rights, notably the rights of *peoples* to self-determination, that is in the terms of the ICCPR and the ICESCR, to "determine their political status and freely pursue their economic, social and cultural development" and to permanent sovereignty over natural resources. They also enumerate the rights of persons belonging to minorities to practice their religion, enjoy their culture, and use their language. Indigenous peoples have defined rights that take into account their culture and special relation to the land.

The right to education is defined in the ICESCR and by the CESCR, as well as specialized instruments of UNESCO. Other rights of the child have been codified in the 1989 Convention on the Rights of the Child. Political rights include the right to run for office and to vote in genuine and periodic elections. Cultural rights refer primarily to the right to participate in the cultural life of the community; the

protection of writers, artists, and performers; and the preservation of cultural heritage.

Health issues loom large in human rights standard-setting and policy determination regarding gender and sexual and reproductive rights. The basic human rights texts have been supplemented by a specialized Convention on the Elimination of All Forms of Discrimination against Women (CEDAW) of 1979. Considerable advances in mainstreaming women's rights as human rights were made at international conferences, a 1993 Declaration on Violence against Women, the work of a special rapporteur on this problem, and statements and programs on traditional practices harmful to health, such as female genital mutilation. Reproductive rights include the right of "men and women … to decide freely and responsibly on the number and spacing of their children" (CEDAW, article 16) and "to be informed and to have access to safe, effective, affordable and acceptable methods of family planning of their choice" (ICPD 1994). Various internationally approved programs and plans of action have set out in considerable detail the specific ways in which this right can be realized.

Bioethical concerns overlap with human rights with respect to the right to enjoy the benefits of scientific progress and rights in scientific research. The former refers to the positive and equitable use of scientific advances, while the latter protect freedom to conduct research and disseminate results and the requirement of informed consent of human subjects.

Occasionally, scholars refer to solidarity or third-generation rights to certain global values such as peace, a healthy environment, development, communication, and humanitarian intervention or assistance. Two rights in this category have become more systematically developed and enshrined in authoritative texts: the rights to a healthy environment and to development. The former has been recognized in many national constitutions and in the regional human rights texts. The latter has been recognized in numerous UN resolutions and specifically in a 1986 declaration, as well as in the African Charter on Human and Peoples' Rights. The 1986 Declaration on the Right to Development defines the right to development as "an inalienable human right by virtue of which every human person and all peoples are entitled to participate in, contribute to, and enjoy economic, social, cultural and political development, in which all human rights and fundamental freedoms can be fully realized."

Finally, article 28 of the UDHR proclaims the right of everyone to "a social and international order in which the rights and freedoms set forth in this Declaration can be fully realized." This right is perhaps the broadest but also the most significant in making human rights the ordering criterion for national societies and international relations. The required social order suggests a democratic constitutional regime in which human rights of all categories are recognized in law and effectively observed in practice. It also suggests that international relations provide support for global efforts to further human rights and to establish means of accountability for persons and groups to obtain redress from countries that fail to fulfill their human rights obligations.

The Enforcement and Implementation of Human Rights

The term *enforcement* refers to coerced compliance, whereas *implementation* refers to supervision, monitoring, and the general effort to hold duty-holders accountable. Implementation is further subdivided into promotion—preventive measures to ensure respect for human rights in the future—and protection—responses to violations that have occurred in the past. The means and methods of implementation may be summarized in three forms of promotion and five forms of protection.

Promotion of human rights is achieved through developing awareness, standard-setting and interpretation, and creating national institutions. Awareness of human rights is a precondition to acting on them and is advanced though dissemination of knowledge and human rights education at all levels, for which the UN proclaimed a decade of action for the period from 1995 to 2004. Standard-setting means the drafting of human rights texts, for which the UN Commission on Human Rights, established in 1946, plays a central role, along with other UN and regional organizations. These norms are interpreted by various international courts and treaty-monitoring bodies. The third preventive or promotional means of implementation is national institution-building, which includes improvements in the judiciary and law enforcement institutions and the creation of specialized bodies such as national commissions for human rights and offices of an ombudsman.

The *protection* of human rights involves a complex web of national and international mechanisms to monitor, judge, denounce, and coerce states, as well as to provide relief to victims. Monitoring compliance with international standards is carried out through the reporting and complaints procedures of the UN treaty bodies and regional human rights commissions and courts. Special procedures of working groups and special rapporteurs study countries or issues, taking on cases of alleged violations, reporting back on their findings, and requesting redress from governments. Among the *thematic* rapporteurs, one is specifically mandated to study the right to health, and others deal with a variety of health-related issues. The second means of protection is adjudication of cases by fully empowered human rights courts, the main ones being the European Court of Human Rights of the Council of Europe, the American Court of Human Rights of the Organization of American States (OAS), and the African Union's African Court of Human and Peoples' Rights, which was not yet functioning in mid-2003.

Political supervision refers to resolutions judging the policies and practices of states adopted by the Commission on Human Rights, the UN General Assembly, the Committee of Ministers of the Council of Europe, the Assembly of OAS, and other political bodies that denounce governments for violations of human rights and demand that they redress the situation or provide compensation to the victims.

The use of coercion is available only to the UN Security Council, which can use its powers under Chapter VII of the UN Charter to impose sanctions, cut off communications, create ad hoc criminal tribunals, and authorize the use of force by member states or the deployment of UN troops to put an end to a threat to international peace and security, which it has on occasion interpreted to include human rights violations (e.g., Haiti, Somalia, Bosnia, Iraq). This forceful means of protecting human rights is complex and dangerous and can have harmful health consequences, as has been the case with sanctions imposed on Haiti and Iraq. If used properly it can be a modern and legitimate form of the nineteenth-century doctrine of humanitarian intervention, according to which states use armed force to halt atrocities committed in another state while respecting the principles of necessity, proportionality, disinterestedness, and collegiality. The North Atlantic Treaty Organization (NATO) sought to employ such a doctrine in Kosovo in 1999 but without the necessary authorization from the Security Council engaged in what most scholars consider a legitimate but illegal use of force. Each case of action (e.g., no-fly zones over Iraq imposed in 1991) or inaction (e.g., Rwanda in 1994) regarding the use of armed force for human rights purposes has complex ethical and legal difficulties.

The final means of responding to human rights violations is through humanitarian relief or assistance. Provision of food, blankets, tents, medical and sanitary assistance, and other forms of aid saves lives and improves the health of persons forcibly displaced often as a result of large-scale human rights violations. Refugees and internally displaced persons come under the protection of the UN High Commissioner for Refugees (UNHCR), which deploys massive amounts of aid, along with the International Committee of the Red Cross, UNICEF, World Food Program (WFP), United Nations Development Programme (UNDP), the

UN Office for the Coordination of Humanitarian Affairs, and other agencies, as well as major NGOs such as Oxfam International, CARE, and the International Rescue Committee.

Conclusion

Every country in the world has accepted that human rights are universal, but all are challenged, in one way or another, to achieve progress with respect to those rights they neglect, however proud they may be of achievements with respect to other rights. Thus Cuba may be rightfully proud of its record on rights to health and education but is challenged to do more for political and civil rights; the United States may pride itself on the degree to which freedom of expression or civil rights are guaranteed but is challenged to take seriously economic, social, and cultural rights, including universal access to healthcare. The normative content of the corpus of human rights standards is probably the most complete catalogue of the determinants of physical, mental, and social well-being. The methods of implementation or intervention to ensure compliance are not directly linked to medical and health practice or to health policy, as is the case with bioethics. They nevertheless constitute a potentially rich framework for the improvement of health policy and practice, which is the objective of the emerging subfield of health and human rights.

STEPHEN P. MARKS

SEE ALSO: *Death Penalty; Ethics: Normative Ethical Theories; Genetic Discrimination; Harm; Human Nature; Justice; Law and Bioethics; Law and Morality; Natural Law; Pain and Suffering; Reproductive Technologies; Warfare; Women, Historical and Cultural Perspectives*

BIBLIOGRAPHY

British Medical Association. 2001. *The Medical Profession and Human Rights: Handbook for a Changing Agenda.* London and New York: Zed Books.

Brody, Eugene B. 1993. *Biomedical Technology and Human Rights.* Brookfield, VT: Dartmouth Publishing Company, and Paris: UNESCO.

Claude, Richard Pierre. 2002. *Science in the Service of Human Rights.* Philadelphia: University of Pennsylvania Press.

Committee on Economic, Social and Cultural Rights (CESCR). 2000. *General Comment 14: The Right to the Highest Attainable Standard of Health,* UN doc. E/C.12/2000/4, 4 July 2000.

Dworkin, Ronald. 1977. *Taking Rights Seriously,* Cambridge, MA: Harvard University Press.

Ehrlich, Paul R. 2000. *Human Natures: Genes, Culture and the Human Prospect.* Washington, D.C.: Island Press.

Falk, Richard A. 2000. *Human Rights Horizons: The Pursuit of Justice in a Globalizing World.* New York: Routledge.

Forsythe, David P. 2000. *Human Rights in International Relations.* New York: Cambridge University Press.

François-Xavier Bagnoud Center for Health and Human Rights. *Health and Human Rights. An International Journal,* published semi-annually by Harvard University.

Gruskin, Sofia, and Tarantola, Daniel. 2001. "Health and Human Rights." In *Oxford Textbook on Public Health,* ed. R Detels and R. Beaglehold. New York: Oxford University Press.

Hannum, Hurst, ed. 1999. *Guide to International Human Rights Practice,* 3rd edition. New York: Transnational Publishers.

Korey, William. 1998. *NGOs and the Universal Declaration of Human Rights: "A Curious Grapevine."* New York: St. Martin's Press.

Lauren, Paul Gordon. 1998. *The Evolution of International Human Rights: Visions Seen.* Philadelphia: University of Pennsylvania Press.

Lauterpacht, Hersch. 1973 (1950). *International Law and Human Rights,* with an introduction by Isidore Silver. New York: Garland.

Lenoir, Noëlle. 1999. "Universal Declaration on the Human Genome and Human Rights: The First Legal and Ethical Framework at the Global Level." *Columbia Human Rights Law Review* 30(Summer): 537–587.

Lenoir, Noélle, and Mathieu, Bertrand. 1998. *Les normes internationales de la bioéthique.* Paris: Presses Universitaires de France.

Mann, Jonathan M.; Gruskin, Sofia; Grodin, Michael A., et al., eds. 1999. *Health and Human Right.* New York: Routledge.

Morsink, Johannes. 1984. "The Philosophy of the Universal Declaration." *Human Rights Quarterly* 6(3): 309–334.

Rousseau, Jean-Jacques. 1762. *A Discourse on the Origin of Inequality,* tr. G.D.H. Cole, rev. and augmented by J. H. Brumfitt and John C. Hall, updated by P.D. Jimack (1973). London: Orion Publishing Group and Rutland, VT: Charles E. Tuttle Co. Inc.

Steiner, Henry J., and Alston, Philip. 2000. *International Human Rights in Context: Law, Politics, Morals,* 2nd edition. Oxford: Oxford University Press.

Sumner, L. W. 1987. *The Moral Foundation of Rights.* Oxford: Clarenden Press.

Symonides, Janusz. 1998. *Human Rights: New Dimensions and Challenges.* Burlington, VT: Ashgate Publishing Company, and Paris: UNESCO.

Symonides, Janusz. 2000. *Human Rights: Concepts and Standards.* Burlington, VT: Ashgate Publishing Company, and Paris: UNESCO.

United Nations. 1986. "Declaration on the Right to Development." General Assembly Resolution 41/128 of 4 December 1986.

United Nations 1993. *World Conference on Human Rights. The Vienna Declaration and Programme of Action,* UN Doc. A/CONF.157/24, 25 June 1993.

United Nations. 1994. *Report of the International Conference on Population and Development,* UN Doc A/CONF.171/13, Oct. 18, 1994.

United Nations Development Programme. 2000. *Human Development Report 2000: Human Rights and Human Development.* New York: Oxford University Press.

United Nations Educational, Scientific and Cultural Organization (UNESCO). 1997. *Universal Declaration on the Human Genome and Human Rights: Twenty-Nine Records of the General Conference 41–46.* Paris: Author.

Weston, Burns H., and Marks, Stephen P., eds. 1999. *The Future of International Human Rights.* New York: Transnational Publishers.

INTERNET RESOURCES

Human Rights Internet. 2003. "Human Rights Databank." Available from <http://www.hri.ca/databank/>.

Office of the High Commissioner for Human Rights. 2003. Available from <http://www.unhchr.ch>.

University of Minnesota. 2003. "Human Rights Library." Available from <http://www1.umn.edu/humanrts/>.